MILLS & STERNBERG'S

# Diagnostic Surgical Pathology *Review*

THIRD EDITION

MILLS & STERNBERG'S

# Diagnostic Surgical Pathology *Review*

THIRD EDITION


**TERI A. LONGACRE, MD**

*Richard L. Kempson Endowed Professor of Surgical Pathology*
*Department of Pathology*
*Stanford University School of Medicine*
*Director of Gastrointestinal & Hepatobiliary Pathology*
*Director of Gynecologic Pathology*
*Stanford Medicine*
*Stanford, California*

**ERNA FORGÓ, MD**

*Assistant Professor of Pathology*
*Department of Pathology*
*Robert J. Tomsich Department of Pathology & Laboratory Medicine, Diagnostics Institute*
*Cleveland Clinic*
*Cleveland, Ohio*

**CINDY WANG, MD**

*Clinical Assistant Professor*
*Department of Pathology*
*Stanford University School of Medicine*
*Stanford Medicine*
*Stanford, California*



Wolters Kluwer

Philadelphia • Baltimore • New York • London
Buenos Aires • Hong Kong • Sydney • Tokyo

*Acquisitions Editor:* Nicole Dernoski
*Development Editor:* Ariel S. Winter
*Editorial Coordinator:* Janet Jayne
*Production Project Manager:* Matthew West
*Manufacturing Coordinator:* Lisa Bowling
*Marketing Manager:* Kirsten Watrud
*Manager, Graphic Arts & Design:* Stephen Druding
*Prepress Vendor:* S4Carlisle Publishing Services

Third Edition



9 8 7 6 5 4 3 2 1

Printed in Mexico

---

**Library of Congress Cataloging-in-Publication Data**

ISBN-13: 978-1-975220-28-0

Cataloging in Publication data available on request from publisher.

---



shop.lww.com

QUADM1124

# PREFACE

The third edition of *Mills & Sternberg's Diagnostic Surgical Pathology Review* has been greatly expanded to include more than 1,000 multiple-choice questions in board format, about two-thirds of which are accompanied by pictures, which are this time reproduced in color from the seventh edition of *Mills & Sternberg's Diagnostic Surgical Pathology*, the sourcebook. The answers and explanations to the questions are reported at the end of each chapter in this edition. We hope that these editorial improvements will make the review a more effective tool for board and recertification examinations.

# ACKNOWLEDGMENTS

We appreciate the productive collaboration with Ariel S. Winter, Senior Development Editor, and Janet Jayne, Editorial Coordinator, who provided considerate and conscientious assistance during manuscript preparation and book production.

# CONTENTS

SECTION VIII

## Alimentary Canal and Associated Organs



SECTION IX

## Urinary Tract and Male Genital System



SECTION X

## Female Reproductive System and Peritoneum

# 1 Nonneoplastic Diseases of the Skin

1. The biopsy shown in Figure 1 is from a 32-year-old female with purple, pruritic, polygonal papules on the flexor surfaces of her extremities. The best diagnosis is

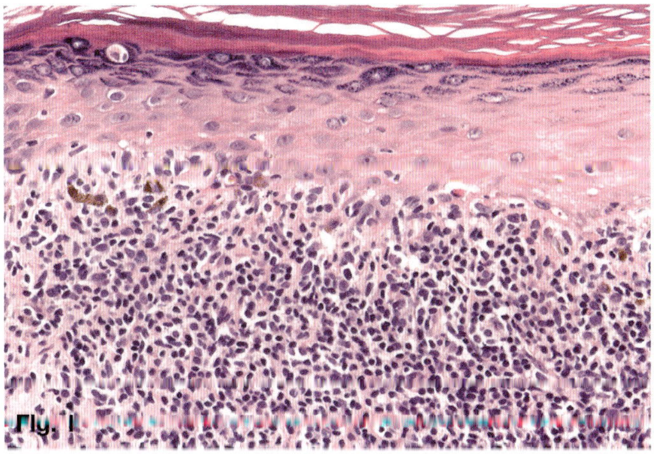

Fig. 1

A. acute graft versus host disease.
B. lichen nitidus.
C. lichen planus.
D. lichen simplex.
E. lichenoid drug eruption.

2. Which histologic feature distinguishes lichenoid drug eruption from lichen planus?

A. Colloid (civatte) bodies
B. Lichenoid interface
C. Mixed dermal inflammatory infiltrate
D. Superficial dermal inflammatory infiltrate
E. Vacuolar interface dermatitis

3. What is the most likely clinical presentation for the biopsy shown in Figure 1?

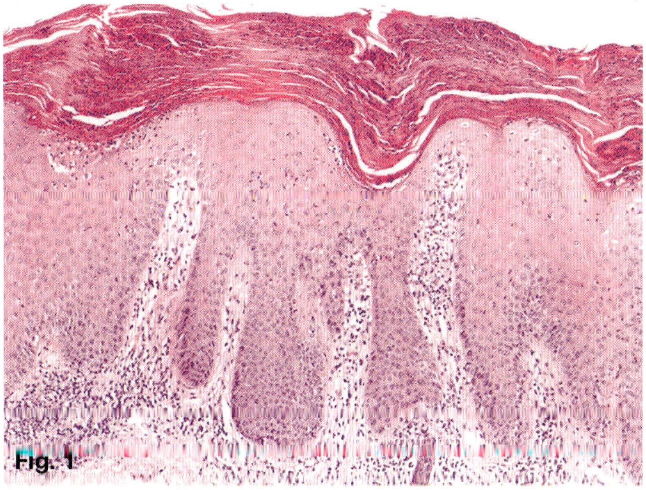

Fig. 1

A. Erythematous plaques covered by silvery scale on extensor surfaces
B. Malar erythema in a butterfly distribution
C. Painful subcutaneous nodule on the anterior surface of the leg
D. Pruritic plaques with accentuation and thickening of skin markings
E. Pruritic purple papules on the flexor surfaces of arms and legs

All figures in this chapter are from Longacre TA, Greenson JK, Hornick JL, Reuter VE, eds. *Mills and Sternberg's Diagnostic Surgical Pathology.* 7th ed. Wolters Kluwer; 2022 except for those noted at the end of this book.

4. What is the most likely clinical presentation for the biopsy shown in Figure 1?

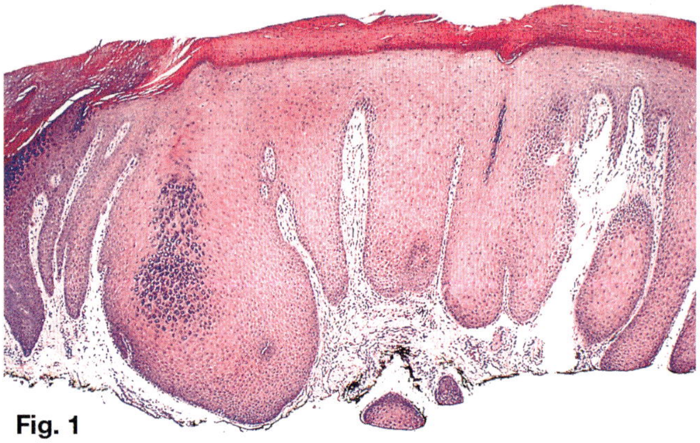

Fig. 1

A. Erythematous plaques covered by silvery scale on extensor surfaces
B. Malar erythema in a butterfly distribution
C. Painful subcutaneous nodule on the anterior surface of the leg
D. Pruritic plaques with accentuation and thickening of skin markings
E. Pruritic purple papules on the flexor surfaces of arms and legs

5. What is the most likely clinical presentation for the biopsy shown in Figure 1?

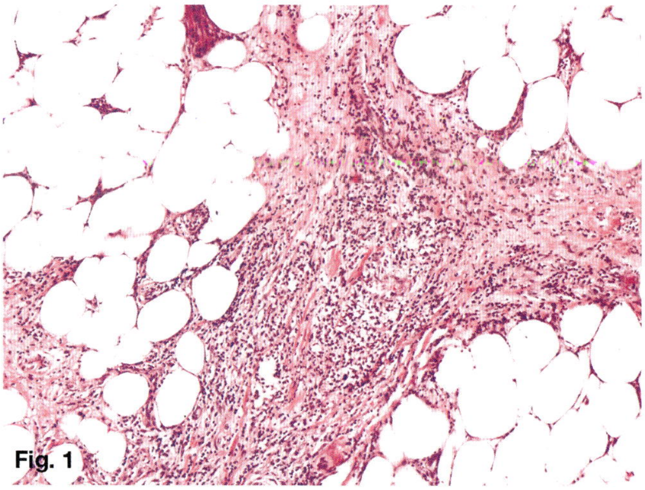

Fig. 1

A. Erythematous plaques covered by silvery scale on extensor surfaces
B. Painful subcutaneous nodule on the anterior surface of the leg
C. Pruritic plaques with accentuation and thickening of skin markings
D. Pruritic purple papules on the flexor surfaces of arms and legs
E. Sharply circumscribed erythematous plaques that may be thick or thin

6. What is the most likely clinical presentation for the biopsy shown in Figure 1?

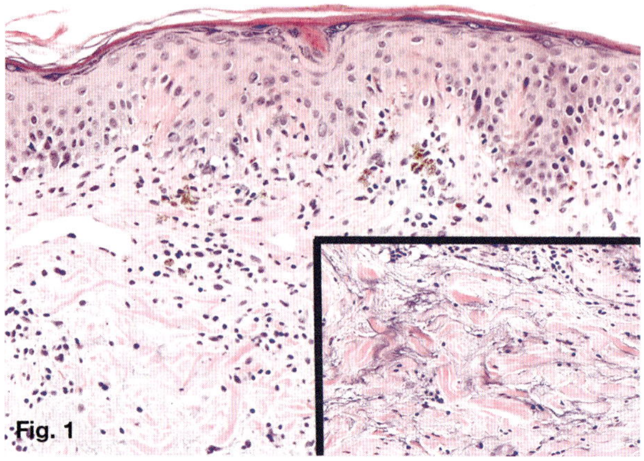

Fig. 1

A. Erythematous plaques covered by silvery scale on extensor surfaces
B. Painful subcutaneous nodule on the anterior surface of the leg
C. Pruritic plaques with accentuation and thickening of skin markings
D. Pruritic purple papules on the flexor surfaces of arms and legs
E. Sharply circumscribed erythematous plaques that may be thick or thin

7. Which of the following is the most common condition associated with erythema nodosum?

A. Bacterial infections
B. Drugs
C. Inflammatory bowel disease
D. Sarcoidosis
E. Tuberculosis

8. A 55-year-old man presents with fever and abrupt eruption of erythematous papules and plaques over his face, neck, and upper extremities. Some of these lesions have evolved into pustules. A biopsy reveals diffuse neutrophilic infiltration of the upper dermis underlying a pustule, as shown in Figure 1. The best diagnosis is

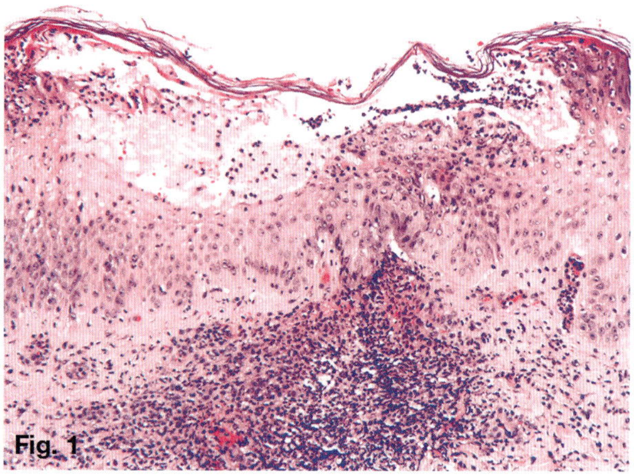

Fig. 1

A. acute febrile neutrophilic dermatosis (Sweet syndrome).
B. fixed drug reaction.
C. Henoch-Schönlein syndrome.
D. pityriasis lichenoides et varioliformis acuta.
E. Stevens-Johnson syndrome.

9. What is the best diagnosis for the biopsy of a large, yellow atrophic plaque on the shin of a 48-year-old female, shown in Figure 1?

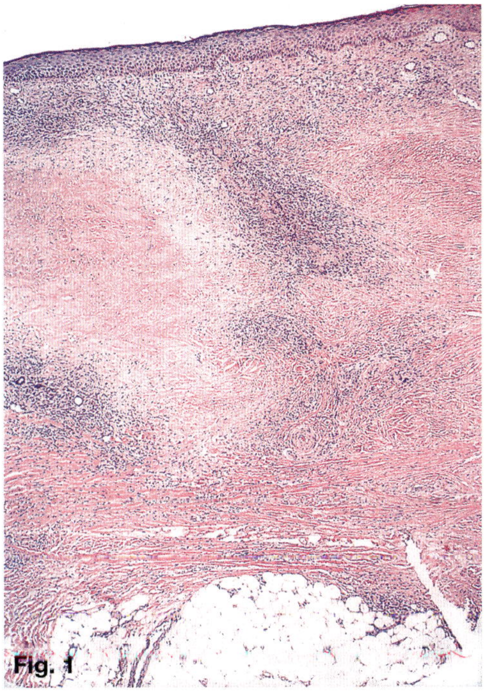

Fig. 1

A. Foreign body granuloma
B. Granuloma annulare
C. Necrobiosis lipoidica
D. Necrobiotic xanthogranuloma
E. Rheumatoid nodule

10. A 32-year-old female develops large tense bullae on the flexor surfaces, trunk, and intertriginous regions. Biopsy of one of the lesions, shown in Figure 1, demonstrates a subepithelial bulla most consistent with

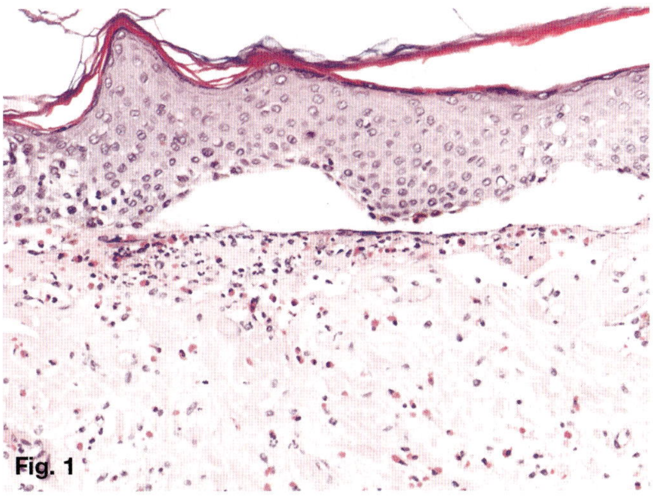

Fig. 1

A. bullous pemphigoid.
B. herpesvirus infection.
C. keratosis follicularis.
D. pemphigus vulgaris.
E. toxic epidermal necrosis.

11. A 50-year-old female develops erythematous papules and plaques in an annular configuration on the extremities. The biopsy of one of the lesions, shown in Figure 1, is best diagnosed as

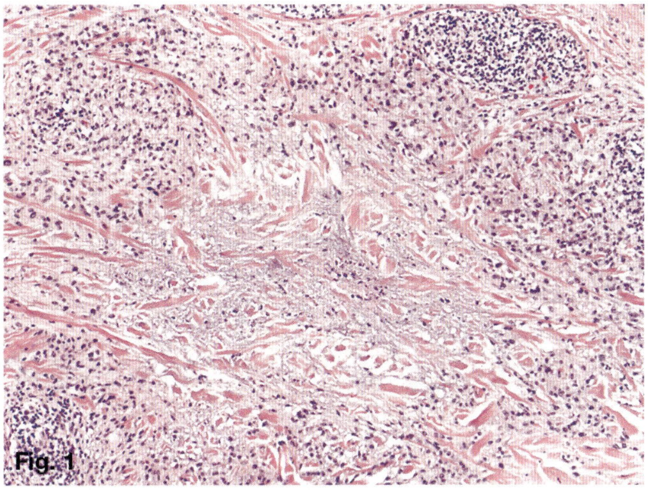

Fig. 1

A. foreign body granuloma.
B. granuloma annulare.
C. necrobiosis lipoidica.
D. necrobiotic xanthogranuloma.
E. rheumatoid nodule.

12. A 24-year-old male undergoes an allogeneic bone marrow transplantation for acute myelogenous leukemia. At day 45, he develops diarrhea and a macular rash on the trunk and extremities. Biopsy of one of the cutaneous lesions, shown in Figure 1, is best attributed to

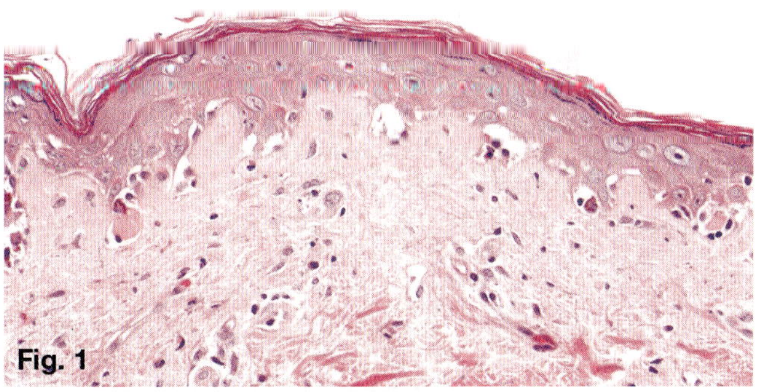

Fig. 1

A. acute graft versus host disease.
B. bone marrow ablative therapy.
C. chronic graft versus host disease.
D. cytotoxic chemotherapy.
E. radiation therapy.

13. A 25-year-old man has multiple subcutaneous masses around the scapular region and elbows. Excision of the mass is performed. Which of the following is the most likely diagnosis?

A. Calcinosis cutis
B. Calciphylaxis
C. Cutaneous amyloidosis
D. Cutaneous gout
E. Osteoma cutis

14. A 24-year-old man presents with a recent onset of blisters on his face and dorsal surfaces of his hands. On physical examination, hypertrichosis is noted on temporal and malar areas. There is no family history of similar skin disorders. One of the blisters is biopsied (shown in Figure 1). The best diagnosis is

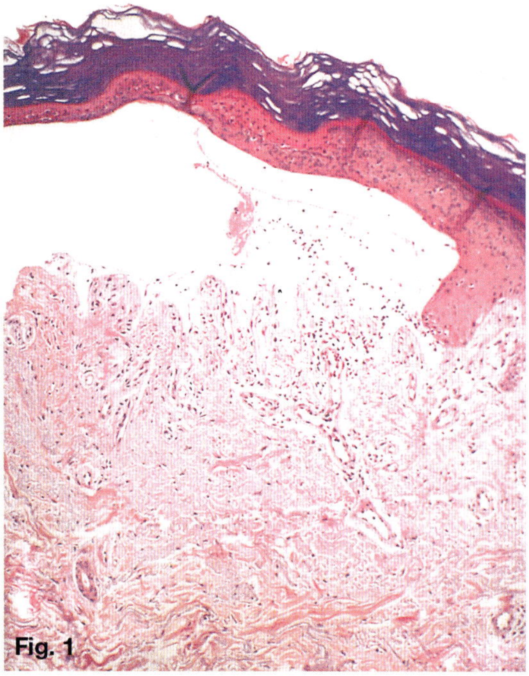

Fig. 1

A. bullous pemphigoid.
B. dermatitis herpetiformis.
C. epidermolysis bullosa.
D. keratosis follicularis.
E. porphyria cutanea tarda.

15. A 45-year-old man suffers from a skin disease characterized by chronic eruption of brown hyperkeratotic lesions on the neck and trunk. Several family members on his father's side suffered from a similar disorder. A biopsy of one of the trunk lesions, shown in Figure 1, is performed. Which of the following is the most likely diagnosis?

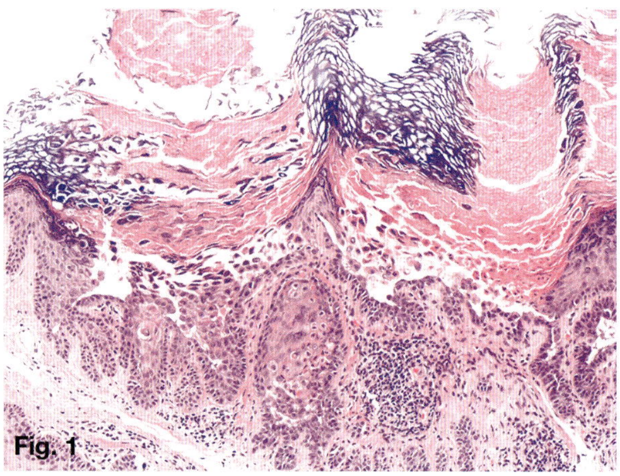

Fig. 1

A. Benign familial pemphigus
B. Epidermolysis bullosa
C. Keratosis follicularis
D. Pemphigus vulgaris
E. Transient acantholytic dermatosis

16. A 22-year-old female presents with mild fever, fatigue, and target lesions on the palms and soles of the feet characterized by papules with central bullae and peripheral erythema. A biopsy, shown in Figure 1, is performed. Which is the most likely diagnosis?

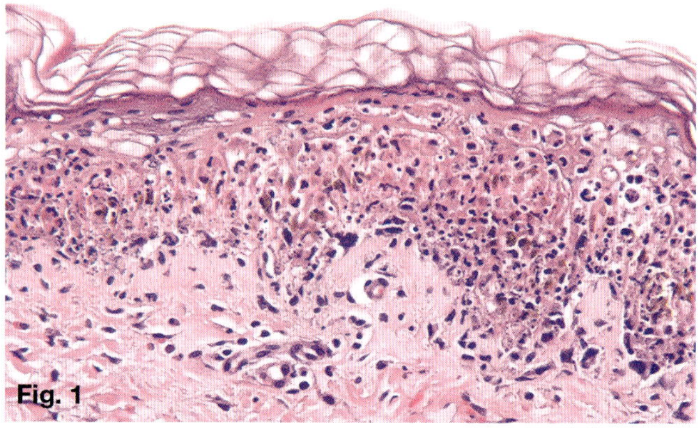

Fig. 1

A. Bullous impetigo
B. Erythema multiforme
C. Fixed drug eruption
D. Guttate psoriasis
E. Toxic epidermal necrosis

17. A 32-year-old female develops numerous small, flaccid bullae on the scalp, trunk, and oral mucosa. A biopsy from one of the trunk lesions, shown in Figure 1, is performed. What is the most likely diagnosis?

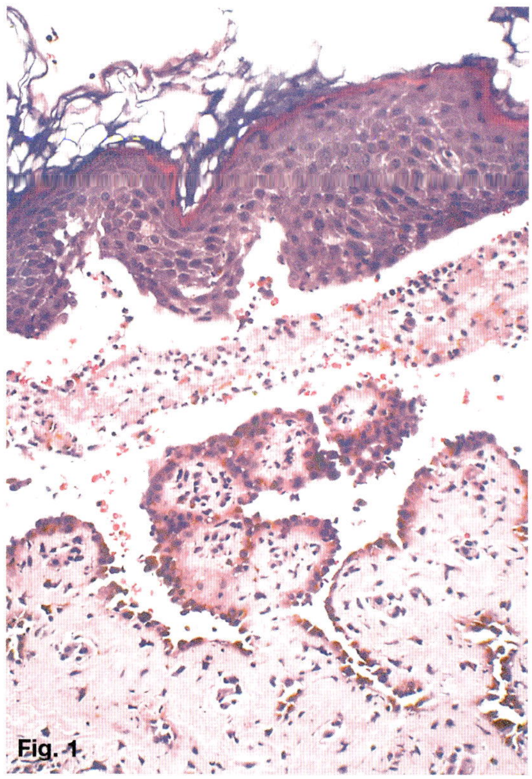

Fig. 1

A. Bullous pemphigoid
B. Dermatitis herpetiformis
C. Epidermolysis bullosa
D. Erythema multiforme
E. Pemphigus vulgaris

18. A 24-year-old female presents to the emergency department with a widespread eruption of macules, papules, and flaccid bullae involving at least 50% of her skin and mucosal surfaces. She reports taking sulfonamides for a urinary tract infection. A biopsy, shown in Figure 1, is performed. Which of the following is the most likely diagnosis?

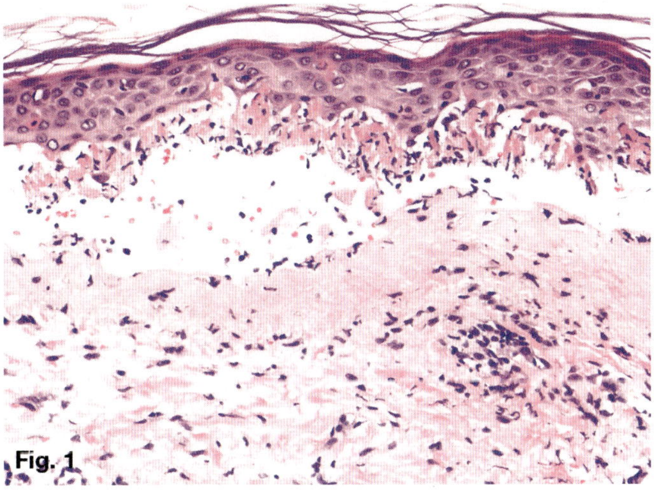

Fig. 1

A. Acute generalized exanthematous pustulosis
B. Lichenoid drug reaction
C. Staphylococcal scalded skin syndrome
D. Stevens-Johnson syndrome
E. Toxic epidermal necrolysis

19. A 22-year-old male develops raised, sharply defined plaques with silvery gray scales over his scalp, elbows, extensor knees, and umbilicus. The features seen in this biopsy, shown in Figure 1, are most diagnostic of which entity?

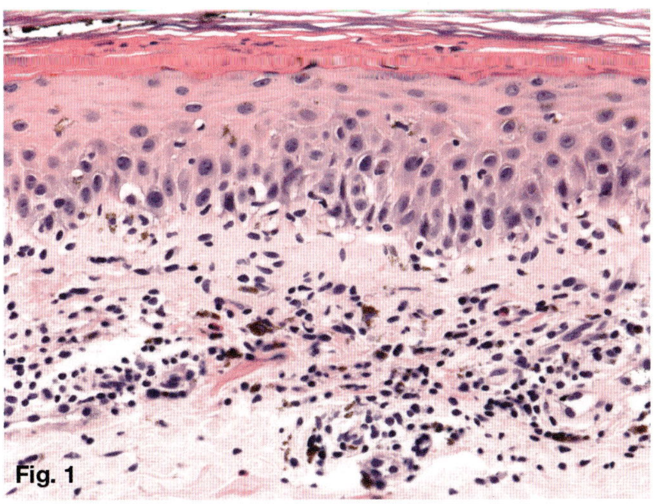

Fig. 1

A. Atopic dermatitis
B. Dermatophytosis
C. Nummular eczema
D. Pityriasis rosea
E. Psoriasis vulgaris

20. The biopsy shown in Figure 1 is from an immunocompromised 70-year-old male with itchy erythematous papules and papulovesicles on the flexor wrist. What is this organism?

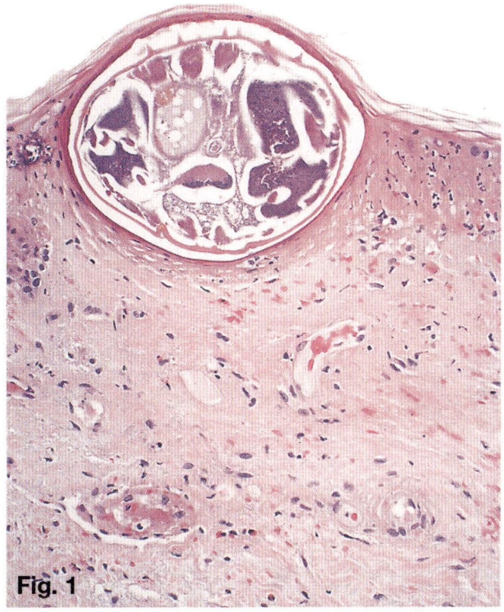

Fig. 1

A. *Ancylostoma braziliense*
B. *Ancylostoma caninum*
C. *Pediculus humanis*
D. *Sarcoptes scabiei*
E. *Tunga penetrans*

21. The biopsy shown in Figure 1 is from a 54-year-old female with pruritic, hypopigmented papules and plaques on her vulva. The best diagnosis is

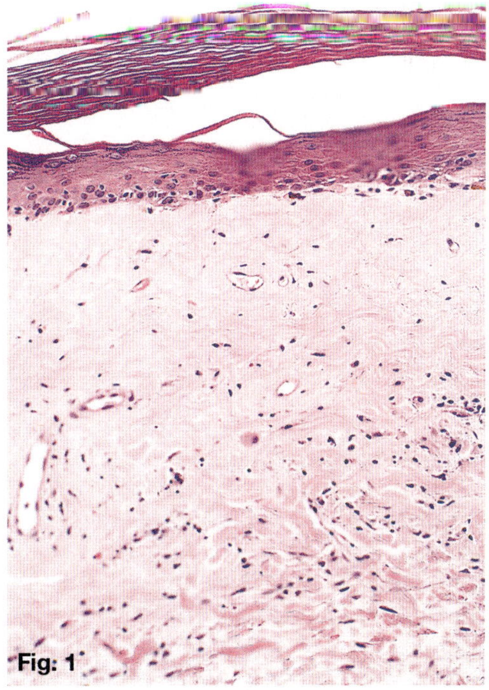

Fig. 1

A. cutaneous amyloid.
B. lentigo simplex.
C. lichen sclerosus.
D. scleroderma.
E. solar lentigo.

# ANSWERS AND EXPLANATIONS

**1. Correct choice: C.**

Lichen planus is an inflammatory, usually self-limiting dermatosis characterized by "pruritic, purple, polygonal papules" symmetrically distributed on the flexor surfaces of elbows and wrists. Oral lesions are often present and consist of white reticulated mucosal changes. Histologically, it is characterized by a band-like lymphocytic infiltrate obscuring the dermal-epidermal junction, hyperkeratosis, hypergranulosis, irregular acanthosis, and colloid bodies. The latter (also called civatte bodies) are apoptotic bodies usually seen close to the basement membrane.

**2. Correct choice: C.**

Lichenoid drug eruption may resemble lichen planus on biopsy, but it is often associated with epidermal parakeratosis and the presence of a mixed dermal inflammatory infiltrate including eosinophils and plasma cells. A clinical history of exposure to various drugs and chemicals, including gold salts, thiazide diuretics, antimalarial drugs, and penicillamine, as well as β-blockers is often present.

**3. Correct choice: A.**

Psoriasiform dermatitis is a common skin disease characterized by raised, sharply demarcated, erythematous plaques covered by silvery scale. The plaques occur on the extensor surfaces, scalp, umbilicus, and sacral region. Key histologic features of psoriasiform dermatitis are epidermal parakeratosis, hypogranulosis, and regular psoriasiform acanthosis with suprapapillary plate thinning and sparse perivascular lymphocytic inflammation. The elongated and narrowed rete ridges have a "comb-like" appearance.

**4. Correct choice: E.**

Lichen simplex chronicus is a chronic itchy skin disorder characterized by well-demarcated, erythematous patches, and plaques of thickened leathery skin. Also known as neurodermatitis, it is caused by chronic rubbing and scratching, which leads to lichenification in predisposed individuals. Raised, pruritic nodules are referred to as prurigo nodularis. The histologic changes can be described as "irregular psoriasiform acanthosis," with marked hyperkeratosis (both orthokeratosis and parakeratosis), prominent granular layer, irregular elongation of rete ridges, fibrotic dermis, and thickening of nerve twigs. Spongiosis is absent or minimal.

**5. Correct choice: B.**

Erythema nodosum is characterized by tender, red bumps, usually found symmetrically on the shins. Up to 55% of cases have no clear identifiable cause. Erythema nodosum is associated with many diseases, including infection and drug reaction. The septal panniculitis is characterized by acute and chronic inflammatory cell infiltration with limited involvement of adjacent fat lobules. Over time, the septal inflammation transitions to histiocytes, including multinucleated giant cells. Granulomas arranged around a central cleft are known as Miescher radial granulomas. In later stages, there is minimal inflammation with septal thickening and fibrosis.

**6. Correct choice: E.**

Discoid lupus is a type of cutaneous lupus erythematosus characterized by round erythematous plaques, usually on the face or scalp. The plaques may be thick or thin. Histologic features include epidermal hypertrophy or atrophy, attenuation (flattening) of rete ridges, hyperkeratosis, and follicular keratotic plugging. Vacuolar degeneration with keratinocyte apoptosis is present in the basilar layer. A mild lymphocytic lichenoid infiltrate with admixed melanophages is seen in the papillary dermis in most hypertrophic cases. Increased interstitial dermal mucin in the reticular dermis may also be present.

**7. Correct choice: A.**

Erythema nodosum is a form of panniculitis with predominant septal involvement. Bacterial infections (usually streptococcal) are the most frequent predisposing conditions. Sarcoidosis, fungal infections, tuberculosis, inflammatory bowel disease, leukemia, pregnancy, and estrogen use are also associated with erythema nodosum.

**8. Correct choice: A.**

Acute febrile neutrophilic dermatosis (Sweet syndrome) is characterized by abrupt eruption of erythematous papules, plaques, and pustules, along with fever and leukocytosis. Although no apparent causes are identified in most cases, some are associated with respiratory infections, hematologic malignancies, or drug reactions. Fixed drug reaction is a vacuolar form of interface dermatitis distinguished by dyskeratotic keratinocytes. Stevens-Johnson syndrome and toxic epidermal necrosis consist of vacuolar interface dermatitis leading to epidermal necrolysis and bulla formation. Pityriasis lichenoides et varioliformis acuta is also a vacuolar interface dermatitis whose skin lesions resemble smallpox (variola). Henoch-Schönlein syndrome presents with palpable purpura due to leukocytoclastic vasculitis.

**9. Correct choice: C.**

Necrobiosis lipoidica presents as atrophic, yellow depressed plaques, often symmetrical, on the lower extremities in the pretibial area. It is associated with diabetes, hypo and hyperthyroidism, inflammatory bowel disease, and vasculitis. Histologic features include palisading, necrobiotic granuloma consisting of a large confluent area of necrobiosis centered in the superficial dermis and subcutaneous fat surrounded by epithelioid histiocytes, giant cells, and sometimes a well-formed granuloma. A linear infiltrate of histiocytes, plasma cells, and lymphocytes is present between collagen bundles. Granuloma annulare presents as painless pale red annular plaques, often grouped in a circinate fashion, most commonly on the dorsal surfaces of hands and feet. Rheumatoid nodules develop on the extensor surfaces of patients with rheumatoid arthritis. Necrobiotic xanthogranuloma occurs on the head and neck of patients with monoclonal IgG (immunoglobulin G) paraproteinemia.

**10. Correct choice: A.**

Bullous pemphigoid is characterized by large tense bullae developing on the flexor surfaces, trunk, and intertriginous areas. The bullae result from the separation of the epidermis from the dermis, associated with an eosinophil-rich inflammatory infiltrate. Bullous pemphigoid, cicatricial pemphigoid, and herpes gestationis are all caused by autoantibodies to basement membrane zone proteins, with linear deposits of IgG (immunoglobulin G) and C3 along the basement membrane in direct immunofluorescence examination. Keratosis follicularis is associated with prominent suprabasal acantholysis, as well as dyskeratotic keratinocytes. In pemphigus vulgaris, there is suprabasal acantholysis-associated blistering and an attached row of distinctive appearing basal keratinocytes. Herpesvirus bullae contain keratinocytes with the typical nuclear inclusions. Extensive keratinocyte necrosis is found in toxic epidermal necrosis.

**11. Correct choice: B.**

Granuloma annulare is a benign skin condition characterized by small, raised bumps that form a ring with a normal or sunken center. The cause of granuloma annulare is unknown and it is found in patients of all ages. The condition tends to be seen in otherwise healthy people. It is characterized by palisaded or interstitial granulomatous inflammation with mucin. Granulomas characterized by central areas of degraded collagen surrounded by lymphocytes and histiocytes, occasionally palisaded, are present in the dermis. Occasional multinucleate giant cells may also be present.

**12. Correct choice: A.**

Graft versus host disease (GVHD) refers to multiorgan syndrome of tissue inflammation or fibrosis that primarily affects the skin. Early stages of GVHD (weeks following transplantation) are characterized by the microscopic picture described in this case. Later stages (months/years) are associated with diffuse dermal fibrosis without significant inflammation, mimicking scleroderma. In the initial stage, the degree of chronic inflammation correlates with prognosis. Histologically, acute GVHD presents with vacuolar interface dermatitis with necrotic keratinocytes surrounded by lymphocytes and chronic GVHD shows either lichenoid or sclerodermoid changes. Late radiation dermatitis shows bizarre, stellate-shaped fibroblasts in the dermis with mild inflammatory changes.

**13. Correct choice: A.**

Calcinosis cutis is a condition in which calcium salts are deposited in the skin and subcutaneous tissue. It is classified into four main types: dystrophic (previously damaged skin), metastatic (secondary to hypercalcemia in chronic renal failure or hyperparathyroidism), idiopathic (tumoral calcinosis and calcinosis of the scrotum), and iatrogenic. Tumoral calcinosis consists of masses of calcium that deposit in the dermis/subcutis around major joints or areas of persistent trauma, surrounded by a giant cell reaction; half are familial. In calcinosis cutis, calcium appears as deeply basophilic or purple, amorphous material on H&E (hematoxylin and eosin) stains. In osteoma cutis, the deposits are eosinophilic with visible osteocytes sitting within small lacunae. Cutaneous amyloidosis is characterized by the deposition of pale, pink amorphous material within the papillary dermis, resulting in a number of scattered and confluent globular deposits, often with a "cracked" appearance. In gouty tophi, the crystal deposits form washed-out pale areas surrounded by a dense inflammatory cell infiltrate containing multinucleated giant cells. Needle-like spaces can be seen in a radial array. Calciphylaxis is a severe condition in which calcium accumulates in the intima and media of small and large subcutaneous vessels, followed by thrombosis and ischemic necrosis of the skin. It occurs in patients with renal failure or altered calcium/phosphate metabolism.

**14. Correct choice: E.**

Porphyria cutanea tarda (PCT) is due to reduction in uroporphyrinogen decarboxylase enzyme (UROD), a key enzyme in heme synthesis. Most cases occur sporadically but 20% are transmitted as an inherited mutation. The subepidermal bullae of PCT are not associated with significant inflammation; the dermal papillae project into the bulla in a "festooned" pattern. The bulla in bullous pemphigoid bullae is associated with an eosinophil-rich inflammatory infiltrate. The bulla in epidermolysis bullosa is also subepidermal and not associated with inflammation but tends to appear at sites of trauma. Keratosis follicularis (Darier disease) exhibits suprabasal acantholysis with dyskeratosis and hyperkeratosis (grains and corps ronds). Dermatitis herpetiformis is characterized by papillary dermal neutrophilic microabscesses followed by the formation of subepidermal bulla with a mild neutrophilic dermal inflammatory infiltrate. Granular deposits of IgA (immunoglobulin A) are present in the papillary dermis of the perilesional skin on direct immunofluorescence examination.

**15. Correct choice: C.**

Keratosis follicularis (Darier disease) is a hereditary, autosomal dominant disorder characterized by a lifelong eruption of crusted, vesicular lesions on the neck and trunk. The lesions consist of suprabasal acantholytic vesicles that contain large dyskeratotic cells called grains in the stratum corneum and corps ronds in the granular layer. The dermal papillae are lined by a single layer of keratinocytes. The condition is caused by a mutation of an intracellular calcium pump gene (ATP2A2). Pemphigus vulgaris is characterized by suprabasal epidermal acantholysis, clefting, and blister formation. The blister cavity may contain inflammatory cells including eosinophils and rounded acantholytic cells with intensely eosinophilic cytoplasm and a perinuclear halo. The floor of the blister may be lined with intact keratinocytes, the so-called "tombstone pattern." Benign familial pemphigus (Hailey-Hailey disease) is similar to pemphigus vulgaris but is autosomal dominant. Epidermolysis bullosa is a group of heritable skin fragility disorders and is characterized by blistering, erosions, and chronic ulcers in the skin and mucous membranes. In some forms, the blistering phenotype is associated with extensive mutilating scarring and blister overlying a papillary dermal scar. Transient acantholytic dermatosis (Grover disease) is similar to Darier disease but related to heat and sweating.

**16. Correct choice: B.**

Erythema multiforme is an acute inflammatory disease characterized by concomitant development of macules, papules, and bullae. The classic target lesion is a papule with a central bulla surrounded by erythema. Frequently involved is the skin of palms and soles as well as mucosae. Up to 90% of cases are secondary to herpes simplex infection. Bullous impetigo is associated with staphylococcal infection. It is characterized by confluent pustules and honey-colored crusts. On biopsy, there is a subcorneal epidermal bulla with acantholysis and a neutrophilic infiltrate. Gram-positive cocci may be present. Fixed drug eruption is characterized by recurrent red-brown patches in the same location after repeated administration of certain drugs. Typical locations are the face and genitalia. The characteristic findings on biopsy are focal vacuolar epidermal alteration with scattered dyskeratotic keratinocytes and perivascular lymphocytic inflammatory infiltrate. Toxic epidermal necrosis (TEN) and Steven Johnson syndrome (SJS) are severe, potentially life-threatening mucocutaneous diseases that are now considered to be distinct from erythema multiforme. In general, SJS is defined as involvement of less than 10% of the body surface area while TEN involves greater than 30%. Both exhibit more widespread erythematous macules, papules, large flaccid bullae, and desquamation. They are often associated with medications, such as sulfonamides, and are distinguished from erythema multiforme by the clinical presentation. Guttate psoriasis appears as small, round papules that are raised and sometimes scaly. They appear over the trunk and extremities. It may start after an infection such as strep throat.

**17. Correct choice: E.**

Pemphigus vulgaris is due to autoantibodies against epidermal desmosomal proteins such as desmoglein 3 that mediate the immune mechanism leading to the destruction of the intercellular junction. The mechanism of bulla development in pemphigus vulgaris is acantholysis (disruption of intercellular attachment), leading to intraepidermal bullae. Pemphigus vulgaris thus results in suprabasal bullae, in which the epidermal cells remaining attached to the basement membrane come to resemble a "row of tombstones." Depending on the level of intraepidermal cleavage, pemphigus can be superficial (foliaceus) or deep (vulgaris and vegetans).

**18. Correct choice: E.**

Toxic epidermal necrosis (TEN) and Steven Johnson syndrome (SJS) are severe, potentially life-threatening mucocutaneous diseases that are now considered to be distinct from erythema multiforme. In general, SJS is defined as involvement of less than 10% of the body surface area while TEN involves greater than 30%. Both exhibit more widespread erythematous macules, papules, and large flaccid bullae with desquamation. They are often associated with medications, such as sulfonamides. Lichenoid drug reaction is an adverse drug reaction characterized by symmetric, erythematous, violaceous papules reminiscent but rarely fully characteristic of lichen planus. Checkpoint inhibitors are the most frequently reported drugs, followed by tyrosine kinase inhibitors and anti-TNF (tumor necrosis factor)-α-monoclonal antibodies. Staphylococcal scalded skin syndrome is a serious skin infection in children. The infection causes peeling skin over large parts of the body. It looks like the skin has been scalded or burned by hot liquid. It's more common in the summer and fall. Acute generalized exanthematous pustulosis is a rare, acute eruption characterized by the development of numerous nonfollicular sterile pustules on a background of edematous erythema. Fever and peripheral blood leukocytosis are usually present. Over 90% of cases are provoked by medications, most often β-lactam antibiotics (eg, penicillins and cephalosporins).

**19. Correct choice: E.**

Key features of psoriasis vulgaris include confluent parakeratosis, regular acanthosis with suprapapillary thinning, and the absence of a granular layer. Perivascular lymphocytic infiltration and focal hemorrhages are present in the upper dermis. The elongated and narrowed rete ridges have a "comblike" appearance. Additional findings include collections of neutrophils in the parakeratotic stratum corneum (Munro microabscesses) or at the surface of the stratum malpighii and stratum corneum (spongiform pustules of Kogoj). Atopic dermatitis (eczema) is a condition that causes dry, itchy, and inflamed skin. It is common in young children but can occur at any age. Atopic dermatitis is long lasting (chronic) and tends to flare sometimes. Pityriasis rosea is another relatively common skin condition that causes a temporary rash of raised red scaly patches on the body. It can affect anyone, but it's more common in older children and young adults. Affected patients develop a large, scaly patch with slightly raised margins that appear first on the trunk in most cases or more rarely on the extremities (herald patch). Nummular eczema (also known as *nummular dermatitis*) appears as itchy, coin-shaped spots on the hands, forearms, and legs. Early lesions show moderate spongiosis with mild acanthosis and exocytosis of inflammatory cells. Dermatophytosis (tinea) also called "ringworm" is a common contagious disease caused by fungi. Lesions appear as scaly, red annular plaques. Biopsy shows a spongiotic dermatitis. A useful clue is the presence of neutrophils in the epidermis or stratum corneum, often within or adjacent to a follicular orifice. Hyphae may be seen on H&E but are also highlighted by periodic acid-Schiff with diastase stain.

**20. Correct choice: D.**

Scabies is an infestation of the skin by the human itch mite (Sarcoptes scabiei var. hominis). The microscopic scabies mite burrows into the upper layer of the skin where it lives and lays its eggs. The most common symptoms of scabies are intense itching (often worse at night) and a pimple-like skin rash. This rash causes little bumps that often form a line. The bumps can look like hives, tiny bites, knots under the skin, or pimples. Some people develop scaly patches that look like eczema. Scabies may be misdiagnosed as eczema, dermatitis prurigo nodularis, or lupus erythematosus. Multiple level sections may need to be performed to identify the mite.

**21. Correct choice: C.**

Lichen sclerosus may affect males and females from infancy to late adulthood, but onset in perimenopausal age is most frequent. It affects the labia majora, labia minora, perianal region, and trunk. When confined to the vulva, it is designated as kraurosis vulvae, whereas the penile form is known as balanitis xerotica obliterans. Grossly, white papules coalesce to form plaques, which in time evolve into a smooth, ivory-colored surface. Pruritus is frequent. Key histologic features include hyperkeratosis with follicular plugging, atrophy of the stratum malpighii, hydropic degeneration of the basal layer, edema and collagen degeneration in the upper dermis, and chronic inflammatory infiltrate in the mid-dermis.

# 2 Nonmelanocytic Cutaneous Tumors

1. The deep dermal biopsy shown in Figure 1 from the thigh in a 34-year-old male is best diagnosed as

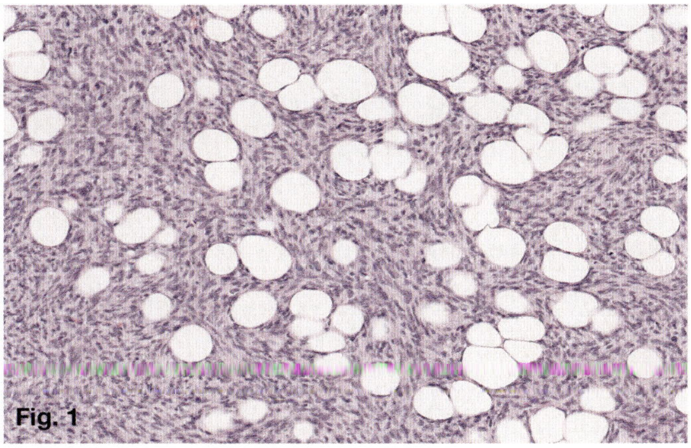

Fig. 1

A. cellular dermatofibroma.
B. dermatofibrosarcoma protuberans.
C. leiomyosarcoma.
D. solitary fibrous tumor.
E. spindle cell melanoma.

2. What immunohistochemical stain can help to confirm the diagnosis of the thigh lesion shown in Figure 1?

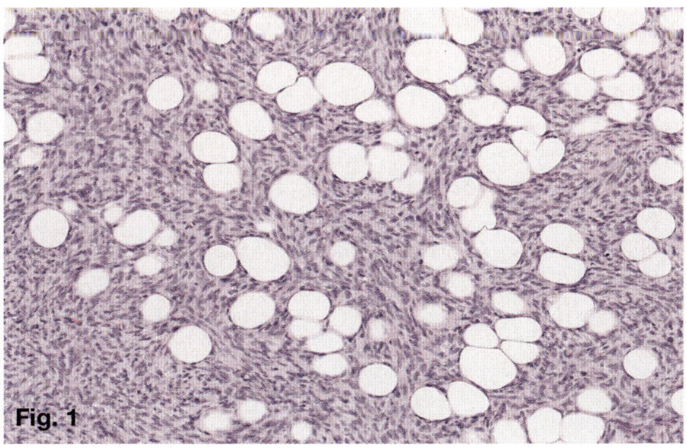

Fig. 1

A. CD34
B. Desmin
C. Factor XIIIa
D. S100
E. STAT6

3. What is the best diagnosis for the biopsy shown in Figure 1 of a firm nodule on the anterior shin of a 32-year-old male?

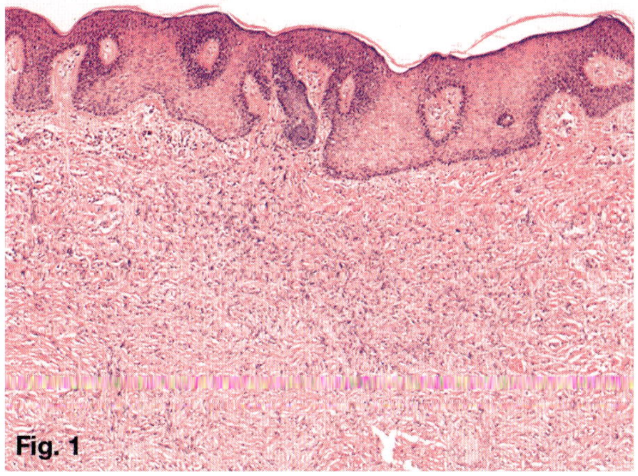

Fig. 1

A. Dermal scar
B. Dermatofibroma
C. Kaposi sarcoma
D. Leiomyoma
E. Neurofibroma

4. The biopsy shown in Figure 1 of a violaceous nodule on the temple of a 70-year-old male showed dotlike paranuclear staining with cytokeratin. What is the best diagnosis?

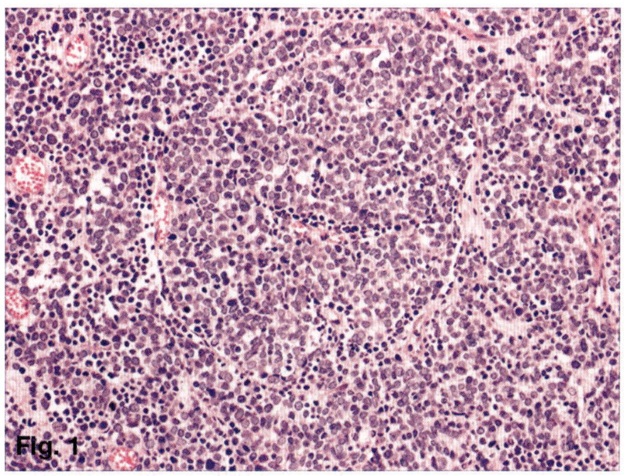

Fig. 1

A. Basal cell carcinoma
B. Leukemia cutis
C. Lymphoma
D. Malignant melanoma
E. Merkle cell carcinoma

All figures in this chapter are from Longacre TA, Greenson JK, Hornick JL, Reuter VE, eds. *Mills and Sternberg's Diagnostic Surgical Pathology.* 7th ed. Wolters Kluwer; 2022 except for those noted at the end of this book.

5. Which gene fusion is associated with dermatofibrosarcoma protuberans?

   A. *COL1A1-PDFGB*
   B. *COL6A3-CSF1*
   C. *ETV6-NTRK3*
   D. *TGFBR3-MGEA5*
   E. *WWTR1-CAMTA1*

6. An 18-year-old female developed multiple small pale pink bumps forming small clusters over her malar region. A biopsy, shown in Figure 1, is performed. What is the best diagnosis?

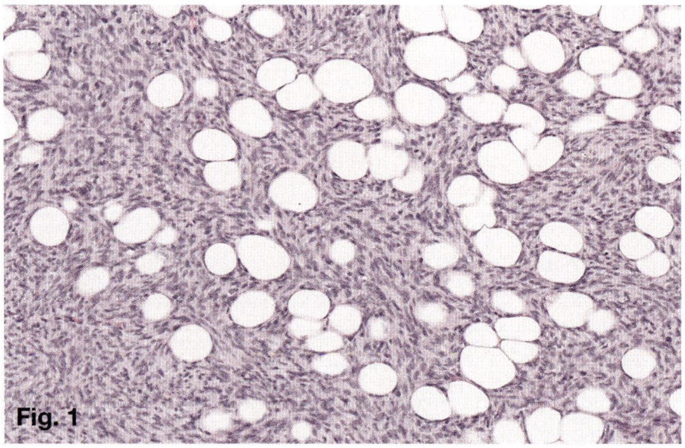

Fig. 1

   A. Desmoplastic trichoepithelioma
   B. Hidrocystoma
   C. Microcystic adnexal tumor
   D. Morpheaform basal cell carcinoma
   E. Syringoma

7. The biopsy shown in Figure 1 is from a subungual mass on the left thumb of a 22-year-old male. What is the best diagnosis?

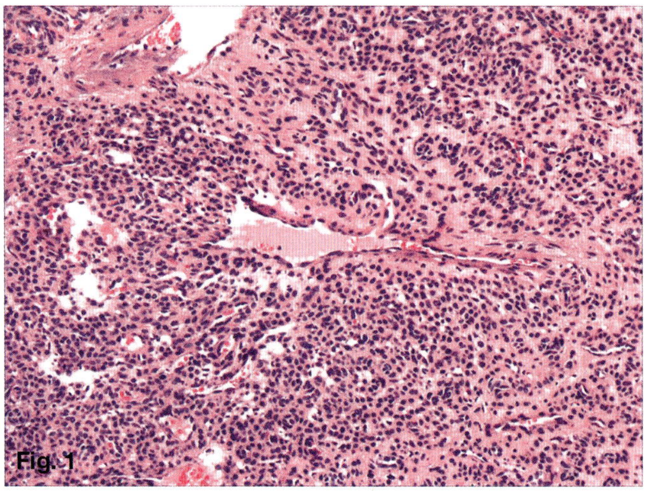

Fig. 1

   A. Angioleiomyoma
   B. Glomus tumor
   C. Myopericytoma
   D. Nodular hidradenoma
   E. Paraganglioma

8. A 12-year-old girl presents with a hard nodule on her forearm. A biopsy, shown in Figure 1, is performed. What is the best diagnosis?

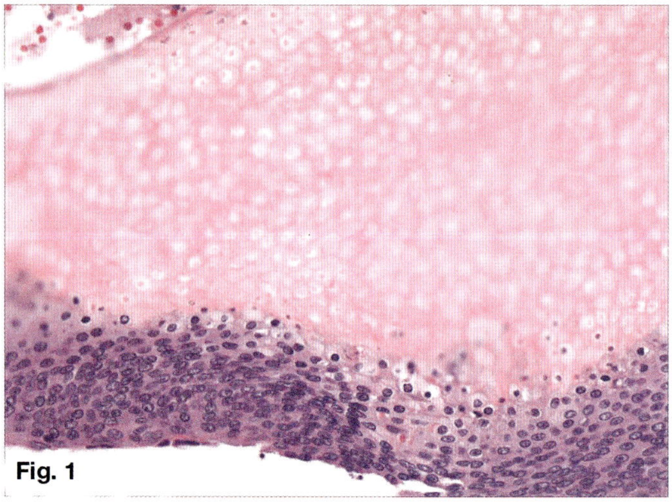

Fig. 1

   A. Basal cell carcinoma
   B. Eccrine poroma
   C. Pilomatrixoma
   D. Trichoblastoma
   E. Trichoepithelioma

9. A 6-year-old boy presents with a hard nodule on his forearm. A biopsy, shown in Figure 1, is performed. Which immunohistochemical stain is helpful in diagnosis?

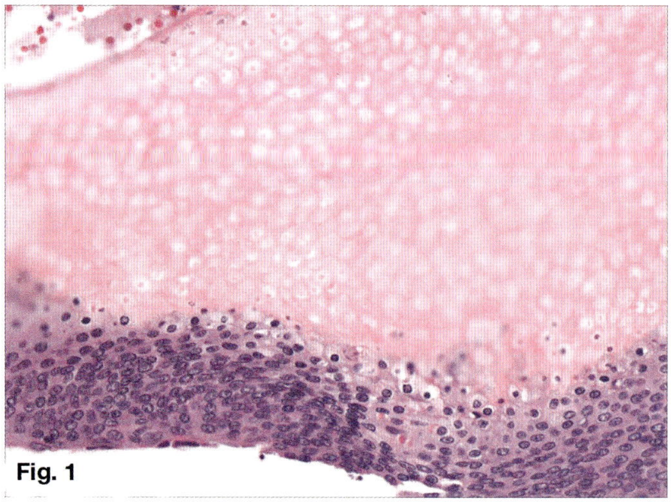

Fig. 1

   A. β-Catenin
   B. CK5/6
   C. Ki-67
   D. p40
   E. S100

10. Which gene fusion is associated with cutaneous glomus tumors?

   A. *COL1A1-PDFGB*
   B. *COL6A3-CSF1*
   C. *ETV6-NTRK3*
   D. *MIR143-NOTCH*
   E. *TGFBR3-MGEA5*

11. The biopsy of a solitary, well-circumscribed, pink nodule on this 44-year-old female's left palm, shown in Figure 1, is best diagnosed as

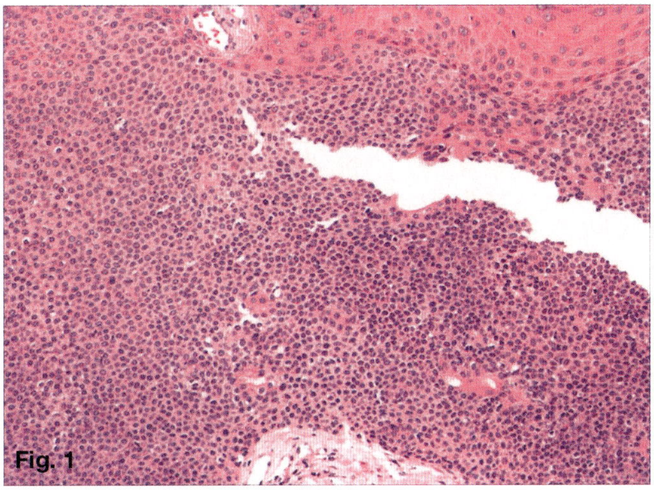
Fig. 1

A. basal cell carcinoma.
B. eccrine poroma.
C. hidradenoma.
D. seborrheic keratosis.
E. trichilemmoma.

12. The biopsy of a rapidly growing erythematous, polypoid mass on the index finger of a 32-year-old female, shown in Figure 1, is best diagnosed as

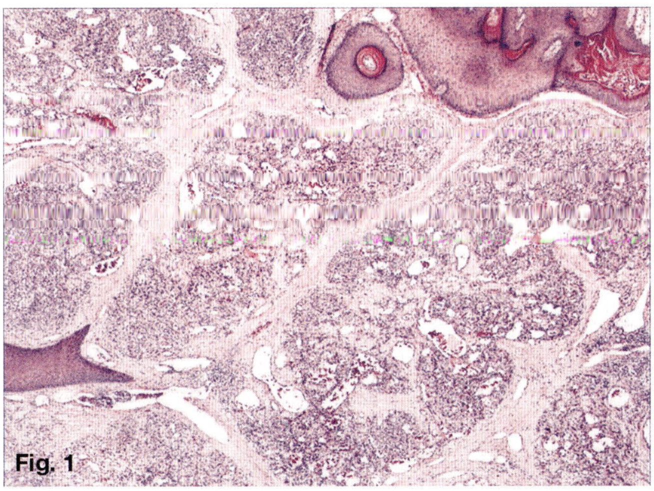
Fig. 1

A. bacillary angiomatosis.
B. glomangioma.
C. glomeruloid hemangioma.
D. glomus tumor.
E. lobular capillary hemangioma.

13. A 52-year-old male developed a slowly growing, brown plaque with a stuck-on appearance on her back. The biopsy of the lesion, shown in Figure 1, most likely represents

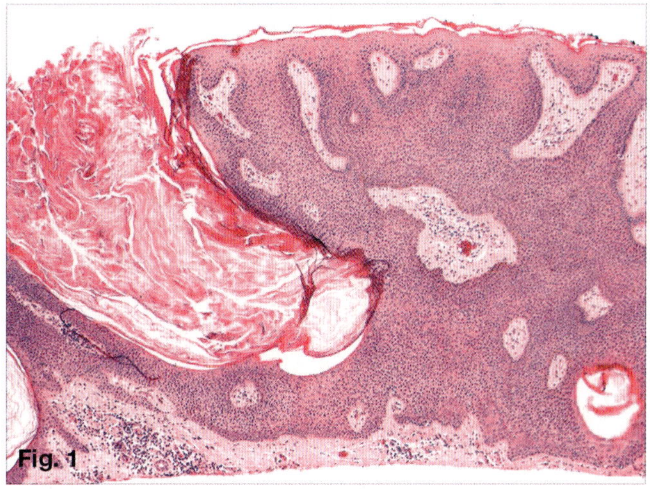
Fig. 1

A. acrochordon.
B. epidermal nevus.
C. inverted follicular keratosis.
D. seborrheic keratosis.
E. verruca vulgaris.

14. A rapid appearance of pruritic seborrheic keratoses on the trunk should prompt which clinical response?

A. Biopsy to exclude cutaneous lymphoma
B. Evaluation for possible colon adenocarcinoma
C. Full body skin examination for atypical nevi
D. Immediate treatment with cryotherapy
E. Skin scraping for underlying infection

15. A 13-year-old girl presents with a slowly growing yellowish polypoid lesion on the posterior scalp. A biopsy, shown in Figure 1, is performed. What is the best diagnosis?

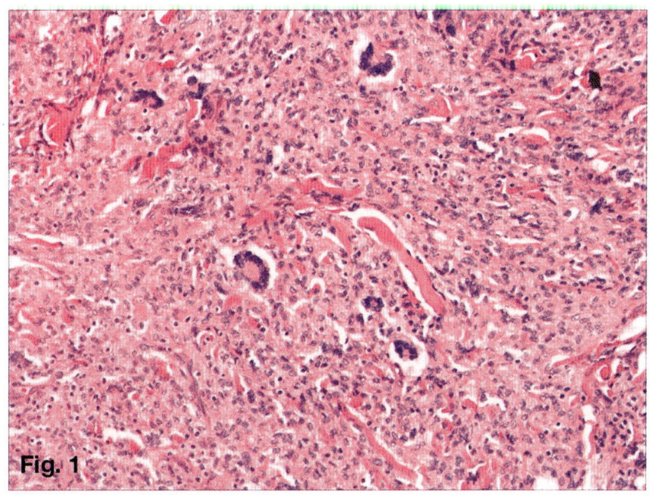
Fig. 1

A. Dermatofibroma
B. Juvenile xanthogranuloma
C. Langerhans histiocytosis
D. Reticulohistiocytoma
E. Tuberous xanthoma

16. A 2-year-old boy presents with generalized lymphadenopathy, hepatosplenomegaly, and a papule on his eyelid. The eyelid lesion is biopsied (shown in Figure 1). What is the most likely diagnosis?

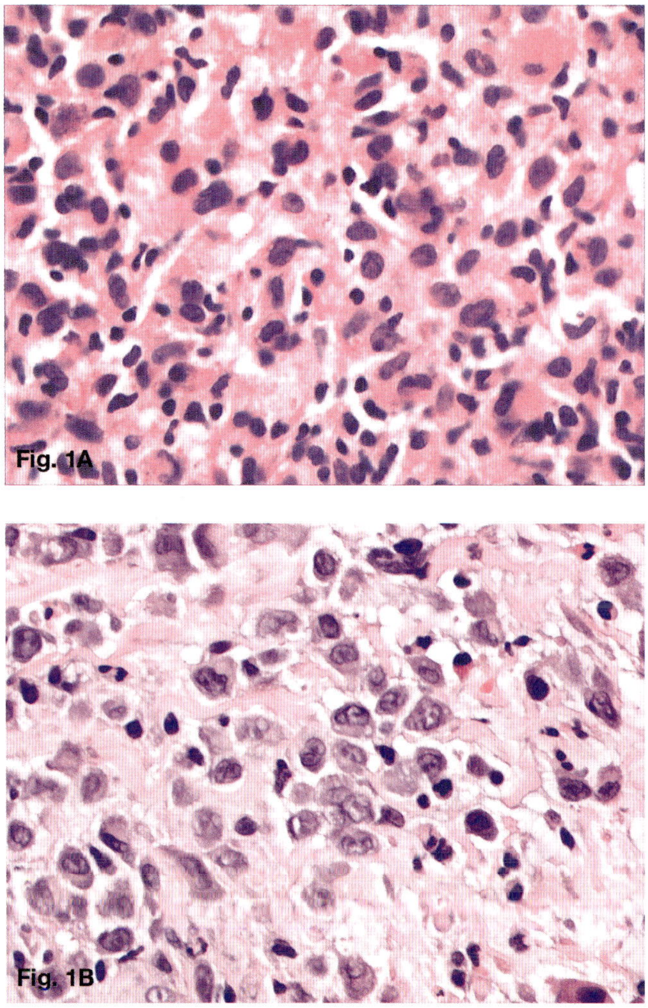


A. Erdheim-Chester disease
B. Juvenile xanthogranuloma
C. Kimura disease
D. Langerhans cell histiocytosis
E. Rosai-Dorfman disease

17. A 34-year-old man presents with diarrhea and multiple pale tan skin nodules. A biopsy, shown in Figure 1, is performed. What is the best diagnosis?

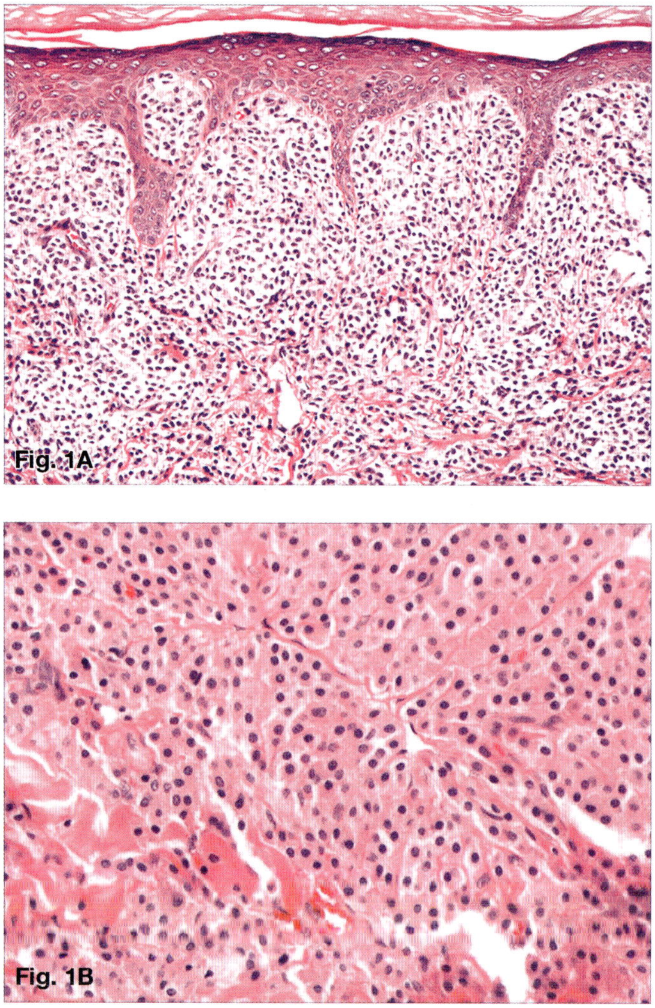


A. Cutaneous mastocytosis
B. Langerhans cell histiocytosis
C. Leukemia cutis
D. Melanocytic nevus
E. Mycosis fungoides

18. A 52-year-old female develops multiple eczematoid or psoriasiform patches and plaques over her buttock, trunk, and proximal limbs (the so-called "bathing trunk" distribution). One of the plaques is biopsied (shown in Figure 1). What is the best diagnosis?

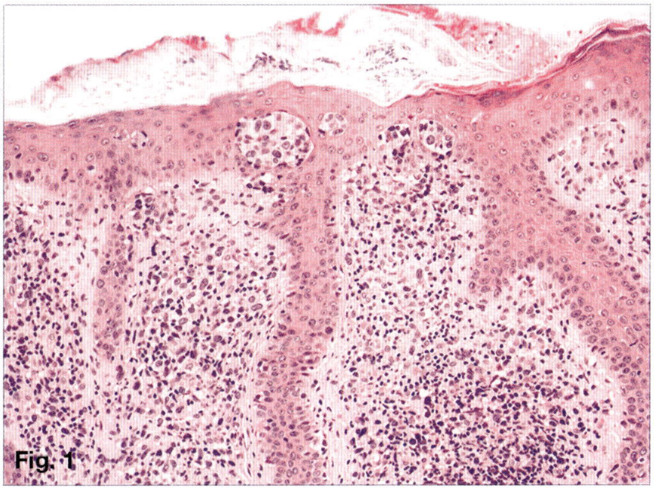

Fig. 1

A. Atopic dermatitis (eczema)
B. Lichenoid dermatitis
C. Lymphomatoid papulosis
D. Mycosis fungoides
E. Vitiligo

19. A 17-year-old female presents with a solitary, superficial, slow-growing mass measuring 1.2 cm on the thumb. The mass is biopsied (shown in Figure 1). What is the best diagnosis?

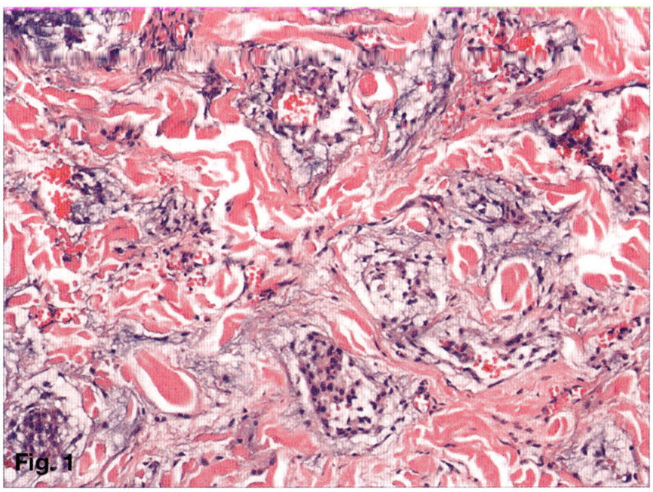

Fig. 1

A. Dermatofibroma
B. Melanocytic nevus
C. Nerve sheath myxoma
D. Neurothekeoma
E. Schwannoma

20. What is the best diagnosis for the excisional biopsy of a rapidly growing verrucous lesion on the forearm of a 66-year-old man, shown in Figure 1?

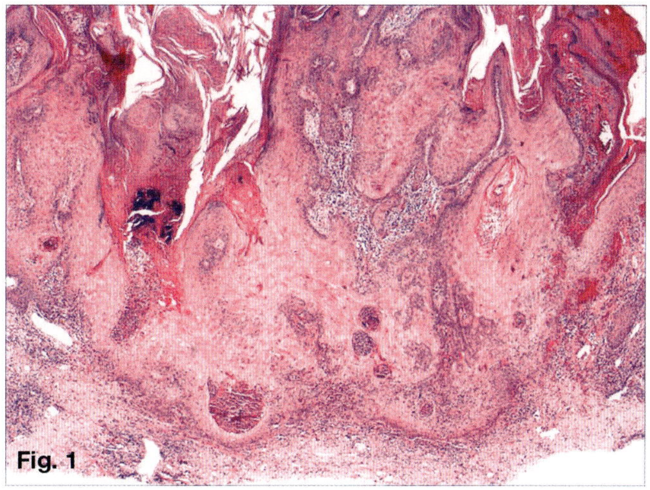

Fig. 1

A. Keratoacanthoma
B. Squamous cell carcinoma
C. Verruca vulgaris
D. Verrucous carcinoma
E. Verrucous psoriasis

21. Telangiectasia macularis eruptiva perstans is a variant of

A. angiocentric lymphoma.
B. cutaneous angiosarcoma.
C. cutaneous mastocytosis.
D. mycosis fungoides.
E. Sézary syndrome.

# ANSWERS AND EXPLANATIONS

**1. Correct choice: B.**

Dermatofibrosarcoma protuberans is a dermal-based low-grade sarcoma characterized by spindle cells with a storiform to whorled pattern. The cytoplasm is generally abundant and eosinophilic; nuclei are monomorphic and ovoid to elongated with variable mitotic activity. Tumors infiltrate and expand fibrous septa; interdigitation among lobules of fat yields a honeycomb pattern. Adnexal structures are typically spared. The stroma may be collagenous, myxoid, or microcystic. A subset of cases undergoes fibrosarcomatous transformation. The differential diagnosis includes dermatofibroma (usually, the deep cellular type), which exhibits peripheral collagen entrapment, but no interdigitation of fat lobules. Solitary fibrous tumors may contain adipose tissue but are based in the deeper soft tissue. They exhibit a patternless distribution, prominent branching vasculature, and keloid-like collagen bundles. Spindle cell melanoma (S100) can be excluded with immunohistochemical stains. Leiomyosarcoma exhibits a more fascicular growth pattern and expresses desmin and/or caldesmon.

**2. Correct choice: A.**

Dermatofibrosarcoma protuberans is positive for CD34, while dermatofibroma is positive for factor XIIIa. Occasionally, CD34 may be present at the periphery of a dermatofibroma, but the central zone is spared. Note that CD34 expression may be diminished in fibrosarcomatous transformation of dermatofibrosarcoma protuberans. Solitary fibrous tumor is also positive for CD34 but also expresses STAT6. S100 and HMB45 (human melanoma black 45) can be useful in establishing a diagnosis of melanoma. Leiomyosarcoma expresses desmin and/or caldesmon, as well as other smooth muscle markers.

**3. Correct choice: B.**

Dermatofibroma (also known as fibrous histiocytoma) encompasses a spectrum of benign dermal-based lesions with fibroblastic and histiocytic differentiation. It is typically painless and varies in size from 5 mm to 2 cm. It consists of a nodular proliferation of fibroblasts and histiocytes. Collagen trapping at the periphery is commonly seen. Although it is relatively circumscribed, it may have irregular and unencapsulated borders. It is characterized by a storiform, pinwheel, or curlicue pattern. Patterns range from diffuse to reticular to hemangioma-like to keloid-like. Early lesions are more cellular, while later lesions are more sclerotic. Dermatofibroma may extend into superficial fat but does not exhibit interdigitation of the fat lobules. Neurofibromas are characterized by lightly wavy spindle cells with loose appearance, poor circumscription, and expression of S100. Leiomyomas are composed of fascicles of spindle cells with cigar-shaped, blunt-ended nuclei; they express smooth muscle markers, such as desmin, caldesmon, and smooth muscle actin. Dermal scars show loss of dermal papilla and adnexal structures and dense collagen fibers run parallel to the dermal-epidermal junction.

**4. Correct choice: E.**

Merkel cell carcinoma is a highly aggressive neuroendocrine carcinoma. It typically presents on the head or neck of older individuals but may present initially as a metastasis. Most Merkel cell carcinomas are associated with a polyomavirus (Merkel cell polyomavirus), which is integrated into the genome of the tumor. The tumor is characterized by aggregates of small, round cells within the dermis. Typically, there is sparse cytoplasm, and the nuclei are round or oval with finely granular chromatin and inconspicuous nucleoli. Mitoses are brisk. Immunohistochemical stains show dotlike paranuclear staining for cytokeratin and cytokeratin 20, as well as positive staining for neuroendocrine markers. PAX-5 (paired box protein-5) and TdT (terminal deoxynucleotidyl transferase) are positive in a subset of cases. Metastatic neuroendocrine carcinoma from elsewhere should be excluded with cytokeratin 20. Lymphoma and leukemia can be excluded with CD45 and CD43, respectively. Melanoma (S100, HMB45 [human melanoma black 45]) and basal cell carcinoma (Ber-EP4) can also be excluded by immunohistochemical stains.

**5. Correct choice: A.**

The translocation involving t(17;22)(q22;q13.1) in dermatofibrosarcoma protuberans creates a fusion transcript involving the *COL1A1-PDFGB* genes. Cases without *PDFGB* fusions can show translocations in the *PDFGD* gene. *COL6A3-CSF1* is seen in tenosynovial giant cell tumors. *WWTR1-CAMTA1* is seen in epithelioid hemangioendothelioma. *ETV6-NTRK3* is seen in infantile fibrosarcoma, while myxoinflammatory fibroblastic sarcoma is associated with *TGFBR3-MGEA5* fusion transcript.

**6. Correct choice: E.**

Syringomas are benign sweat duct (eccrine) tumors. They are most often found in clusters on the lower eyelids, but they may also arise elsewhere on the face, in the armpits, umbilicus, upper chest, and vulva. They start to appear in adolescence and are more common in women than men. There is sometimes another affected member of the family. They are typically skin-colored or yellowish firm rounded bumps, 1 to 3 mm in diameter. Histologically, a syringoma forms a circumscribed dermal lesion with comma-shaped ductules resembling tadpoles and lined by basaloid cells set in a sclerotic stroma. There is no cytologic atypia and mitoses are rare. Hidrocystoma is a benign apocrine tumor often occurring as a cystic lesion on the head and neck (often the cheek). When it occurs on the eyelid it is known as Moll gland cyst. It is usually solitary, but multiple lesions have been documented. Histologically, the cyst is lined by a double layer of epithelial cells: an outer layer of flattened vacuolated myoepithelial cells and an inner layer of tall columnar cells with eosinophilic cytoplasm and basally located, round or oval vesicular nuclei. Decapitation secretion is characteristic but may not be present in distended cysts. Morpheaform basal cell carcinoma is histologically similar to a syringoma with strand-like growth pattern but exhibits more sclerotic stroma with deeply infiltrative, basaloid cells. Microcystic adnexal carcinoma is poorly circumscribed and deeply infiltrative, often with perineural invasion. Desmoplastic trichoepithelioma is typically a single lesion with keratinous cysts next to strands of basaloid cells. Unlike syringoma, neither of the latter two tumors occurs on the vulva.

**7. Correct choice: B.**

Glomus tumors present as painful, blue-red blanchable papules or nodules in the deep dermis or subcutaneous fat, most commonly on the fingers and toes and under the nail plate. They are well circumscribed and composed of glomus cells, vasculature, and smooth muscle cells. They are subclassified as solid glomus tumor—predominantly glomus cells, poor vasculature, and rare smooth muscle cells (75%); glomangioma—prominent vascular component (20%); and glomangiomyoma—prominent vascular and smooth muscle components (5%). Rare variants have microscopically infiltrative and diffuse growth and are known as glomangiomatosis.

Glomus cells have a round shape with indistinct borders with a rounded, sharply punched-out nucleus in amphophilic to eosinophilic cytoplasm. Collars of uniform glomus cells forming nests, sheets, and trabeculae surround branching capillary-sized vessels lined by endothelial cells in a hyalinized or myxoid stroma. Mitoses are rare. The cells stain positive for smooth muscle actin, muscle-specific actin, and calponin. Myopericytoma and other pericytic tumors are derived from perivascular cells and may lie on a spectrum with glomus tumors; they can have histologic and immunohistochemical overlap in areas with more prominent spindled differentiation. Angioleiomyoma may also be painful but is characterized by bundles of smooth muscle cells that lack a prominent round cell component. Desmin is typically positive in angioleiomyoma but not in glomus tumors. Nodular hidradenoma exhibits variable epithelial or sebaceous differentiation, and is positive for cytokeratin (glomus tumors are negative for cytokeratin) but negative for smooth muscle actin. Paraganglioma features a prominent Zellballen growth pattern; it is positive for synaptophysin and chromogranin with S100-positive sustentacular cells.

**8. Correct choice: C.**

Pilomatrixoma is a benign skin adnexal tumor originating from hair matrix and cortex. It is the most common adnexal neoplasm in children; however, a wide age range has been described.

Females are affected slightly more than males. It is usually solitary, but multiple lesions can occur. The head and neck are the most common sites of involvement, followed by upper and lower extremities and then trunk. Pilomatrixoma is associated with mutations in *CTNNB1* gene located in the exon 3 region encoding β-catenin. Although pilomatrixoma is usually not hereditary, familial forms have been seen. Pilomatrixoma presents as a slow-growing, flesh-colored, dermal-based, asymptomatic nodule measuring 0.5 to 3 cm. It is typically very hard, due to calcification. Microscopically, it is a lobulated and circumscribed dermal-based neoplasm composed of islands of basaloid cells exhibiting abrupt keratinization, without intervening granular layer (trichilemmal keratinization). Ghost/shadow cells may predominate. The basaloid cells show mitotic activity; however, abnormal mitoses are absent. Basal cell carcinoma arises in sun-exposed skin and is most often seen in older individuals. However, it may occur in children in association with basal cell nevus syndrome, xeroderma pigmentosum, and organoid nevus. It is characterized by nests of basaloid cells that palisade at the periphery, stromal retraction and mucin, and high mitotic activity. Most show connection to epidermis. Anucleate shadow cells are not a feature of basal cell carcinoma. Trichoepithelioma is also dermal based but has focal epidermal connection, and features branching nests of basaloid cells and small keratinous cysts. Aggregations of fibroblasts are present as abortive attempts to form papillary mesenchyme (papillary mesenchymal bodies). Trichoblastoma is a circumscribed, dermal basaloid tumor without surface connection; it is characterized by the formation of primitive hair bulbs. Neither have anucleate shadow cells. Eccrine poroma is a well-circumscribed tumor that replaces the epidermis and extends into the dermis in broad anastomosing bands. Poroma cells are monomorphic, small, and cuboidal with basophilic round nuclei, inconspicuous nucleoli, and compact eosinophilic cytoplasm

**9. Correct choice: A.**

β-Catenin is the defining molecular alteration in pilomatrixoma, and nuclear staining of basaloid cells is diagnostic. CK5/6 and p40 expression is also seen in some basal cell carcinomas. p53 aberrant expression is associated with malignant pilomatrixoma but does not assist in the identification of this lesion. Ki-67 will show increased staining in basaloid cells and other inflammatory cells (if present in the adjacent stroma). Identification of abrupt keratinization and ghost cells is based on H&E (hematoxylin and eosin) section.

**10. Correct choice: D.**

The *MIR143-NOTCH* gene fusion is common in benign glomus tumors. The *COL1A1-PDFGB* gene fusion is seen in dermatofibrosarcoma protuberans. *COL6A3-CSF1* is seen in tenosynovial giant cell tumors. *ETV6-NTRK3* is seen in infantile fibrosarcoma, while myxoinflammatory fibroblastic sarcoma is associated with the *TGFBR3-MGEA5* fusion transcript.

**11. Correct choice: B.**

Eccrine poroma is a benign glandular adnexal tumor that usually originates from cells of the outer layer of the acrosyringium and terminal eccrine duct. It commonly occurs on the palms and soles or sides of the feet of adults. Typically, it is a single, slow-growing, asymptomatic, well-circumscribed, smooth, skin-colored papule or nodule. Histologically, it is composed of well-circumscribed broad anastomosing bands of poroma cells with sharp demarcation from adjacent keratinocytes. Poroma cells are monomorphic, small, and cuboidal with basophilic round nuclei, inconspicuous nucleoli, and eosinophilic cytoplasm. Basal cell carcinoma forms nodules, nests, or infiltrative cords with proliferation of small basaloid cells and peripheral palisading, stromal retraction artifact, and mucinous stroma. Irritated seborrheic keratosis shows follicular differentiation with keratinizing pseudohorn cysts. Hidradenoma features nests and nodules of epithelial cells lacking epidermal connection, has both solid and cystic components, and has clear cell features. Trichilemmoma is a squamoproliferative lesion in continuity with the epidermis; it shows hyperkeratosis and stromal clefting, with pale eosinophilic or clear cells and a peripheral palisade of cuboidal or columnar cells.

**12. Correct choice: E.**

Lobular capillary hemangioma is a very common cutaneous neoplasm characterized by a rapidly growing polypoid red mass surrounded by a thickened epidermis, often on the finger or lips.

Recurrences, regional satellite lesions, and dissemination have been reported, but it is essentially a benign lesion that may even regress spontaneously. Microscopically, it is a lobular vascular proliferation with inflammation and edema resembling granulation tissue (similar to pyogenic granuloma). The epidermis overlying the lesion is thin with variable ulceration. Acanthosis and hyperkeratosis are present along the sides of the lesion, sometimes forming a collarette.

There is a central branching capillary vessel that forms vascular lobules, with no (or rare) red blood cells, surrounded by endothelial cells. Bacillary angiomatosis is a reactive vascular proliferation due to infection by *Bartonella henselae* or *Bartonella quintana*. It most commonly affects individuals who are immunocompromised (especially those with HIV) and presents as widely distributed red, smooth papules and nodules. It also exhibits a lobular proliferation of capillaries with ectatic vessels lined by prominent endothelial cells, but neutrophils, lymphocytes, and histiocytes are frequently present and purplish gray bacterial colonies may be seen. Glomangioma also has a prominent vascular component and glomus cells that have a round shape with indistinct borders with a rounded, sharply punched-out nucleus in amphophilic to eosinophilic cytoplasm. Glomus tumors present as painful, blue-red blanchable papules or nodules in the deep dermis or subcutaneous fat, most commonly on the fingers and toes and under the nail plate. They are well circumscribed and composed of glomus cells, vasculature, and smooth muscle cells. Both glomangioma and glomus tumors express smooth muscle actin. Glomeruloid hemangioma typically arises in children, with equal gender distribution; it is composed of small capillary-sized blood vessels with a larger feeding vessel commonly present.

**13. Correct choice: D.**

Seborrheic keratosis is a common benign keratinocyte proliferation of middle-aged and older adults.

It appears as a waxy, brown slow-growing papule. Histologically, it features a proliferation of basaloid keratinocytes without atypia, often with acanthosis and hyperkeratosis and horn pseudocysts. An acrochordon is more polypoid and is composed of normal skin lacking adnexal structures. An epidermal nevus is a verrucous lesion typically occurring at birth or early childhood; it may mimic a seborrheic keratosis on biopsy due to the presence of papillomatosis and acanthosis. Inverted follicular keratosis is a benign, endophytic follicular tumor with the characteristic presence of squamous eddies. Verruca vulgaris is an exophytic lesion with inward-curving papillomatosis, coarse hypergranulosis, and koilocytes; it is associated with human papillomavirus.

**14. Correct choice: B.**

Rapid development of multiple seborrheic keratoses, the Leser-Trélat sign, is a paraneoplastic syndrome associated with underlying malignancy, most often colon adenocarcinoma, and should prompt a clinical workup to evaluate. The Leser-Trélat sign is not associated with an increased risk for atypical nevi or lymphoma. Nor is it associated with underlying infection. Seborrheic keratoses can be treated with cryotherapy, but they are benign and treatment is not necessary.

**15. Correct choice: B.**

Juvenile xanthogranuloma is a sporadic, benign disorder that results from the proliferation of factor XIIIa-positive dendritic cells. Typically, a disorder of early childhood, it may also be seen in adults. Histologically it is characterized by the presence of histiocytes, foam cells, and Touton giant cells. Lymphocytes, plasma cells, eosinophils, and some neutrophils can be observed. Early lesions usually have monomorphous histiocytes with abundant eosinophilic cytoplasm, while older lesions contain histiocytes with more lipids in their cytoplasm, imparting a foamy appearance. Dermatofibroma with lipidization may contain Touton giant cells, but they are more irregular in contour, hemosiderin granules may be present, and there is collagen trapping at the periphery. Also, dermatofibroma tends to occur in an older age group. Langerhans histiocytosis does not typically contain Touton giant cells. Langerhans histiocytosis stains for CD1a, langerin, and S100 (S100 may be seen in up to one-third of juvenile xanthogranulomas). Reticulohistiocytoma has sharper-defined nuclear membranes, more prominent nucleoli, and "ground-glass" cytoplasm. Touton giant cells are few or absent. Tuberous xanthoma occurs in areas of pressure and is associated with hypercholesterolemia and high LDL (low-density lipoprotein). It is characterized by dermal aggregates of foam cells, without Touton giant cells.

**16. Correct choice: D.**

Langerhans cell histiocytosis is a clonal proliferation of cells that morphologically and immunophenotypically resemble Langerhans cells. It is more common in childhood (1-3 years old) and may involve multiple sites (the most common site is bone). The lesional cells show prominent nuclear grooves with admixed eosinophils and are positive for CD1a, langerin, and S100. Most cases harbor *BRAF* V600E mutations and other RAS/MAPK (Rat Sarcoma/mitogen-activated protein kinase) pathway-activating mutations. Unifocal disease is generally associated with a good prognosis, whereas multisystem and multifocal disease is associated with a poor prognosis. Erdheim-Chester disease is a multiorgan disease but is rare in children. The histiocytes in Erdheim-Chester disease are negative for CD1a and langerin. Juvenile xanthogranuloma is positive for factor XIIIa, a marker of interstitial dendrocytes but negative for S100, CD1a, and langerin. Kimura disease, also a multiorgan disease, predominantly affects young Asian males and lacks a significant population of Langerhans cells. The histiocytes in Rosai-Dorfman disease exhibit emperipolesis; they are positive for S100 but not for CD1a or langerin.

**17. Correct choice: E.**

Cutaneous mastocytosis occurs most commonly in young children but may also occur in adults. Skin lesions can vary from solitary nodules to widespread maculopapules and plaques, as well as diffuse erythroderma with thickened skin. Adult-onset cutaneous mastocytosis is often associated with systemic disease (in this case, diarrhea is due to gastrointestinal tract involvement). On biopsy, mast cells infiltrate the dermis, sparing the epidermis. These mast cells are often spherical or spindled in shape with round to oval nuclei, clumped chromatin, inconspicuous nucleoli, and plentiful cytoplasm filled with tiny granules. Eosinophils are often present. The mast cells are highlighted by CD117, tryptase, and in systemic disease, CD25. The lesional cells in Langerhans cell histiocytosis show prominent nuclear grooves and are positive for CD1a, langerin, and S100. Leukemia cutis is characterized by a dense infiltrate of atypical cells that track along dermal collagen; they are separated from the epidermis by a grenz zone. Melanocytic nevi typically involve epidermis and dermis and express S100 and HMB45 (human melanoma black 45). Mycosis fungoides shows a band-like papillary dermal atypical lymphoid infiltrate with background fibroplasia, lymphocytes tagging the junction and migrating to the epidermis as single cells and Pautrier microabscesses.

**18. Correct choice: D.**

Mycosis fungoides is the most common form of cutaneous T-cell lymphoma. The classic presentation is multiple eczematoid or psoriasiform patches and plaques over the buttock, trunk, and proximal limbs (the so-called "bathing trunk" distribution). Histologically, it is characterized by infiltrates of lymphocytes and an indolent clinical course, usually slowly progressing from patches to thicker plaques and eventually to tumors. Biopsies from developed patches and plaques show band-like papillary dermal lymphoid infiltrates with background fibroplasia, lymphocytes tagging the junction and migrating to the epidermis as single cells and Pautrier microabscesses. The lymphoid cells exhibit cytologic atypia. Immunohistochemistry is generally more useful to exclude other lymphomas than to confirm a diagnosis of mycosis fungoides.

T-cell gene rearrangement studies demonstrate a clonal population of T cells in the majority of cases. Mycosis fungoides can mimic spongiotic or psoriasiform dermatitis, wax and wane, and elude a definitive diagnosis for years. Atopic dermatitis (eczema) exhibits lymphocytic exocytosis that is proportionate to the degree of spongiosis; however, since intraepidermal edema with eosinophils also can be present in mycosis fungoides, paired clonality studies may be helpful in establishing a diagnosis. Lichenoid dermatitis often has colloid (civatte) bodies. Some forms of lymphomatoid papulosis exhibit epidermotropism and a band-like distribution of small to medium atypical lymphocytes with cerebriform nuclei, without $CD30^+$ expression, mimicking the patch stage of mycosis fungoides. Distinction is based on clinical findings (lymphomatoid papulosis often undergoes spontaneous regression) but may require paired clonality studies.

Early inflammatory phases of vitiligo can mimic mycosis fungoides. This is particularly problematic in cases of hypopigmented mycosis fungoides and often requires paired clonality studies.

**19. Correct choice: D.**

Neurothekeoma is a solitary, superficial, slow-growing mass involving the dermis or subcutis, typically on the head, upper extremities, or shoulder girdle. It is seen slightly more frequently in women. The mean age is 17 years but ranges from 2 to 85 years. Histologically, it appears as a circumscribed mass with whorled or focally fascicular patterns of spindled and epithelioid cells with abundant cytoplasm-forming lobules separated by sclerotic collagen. Individual lesions may be cellular, myxoid, or mixed. Occasional multinucleated giant cells may be present. Nuclear atypia may also be present. Mitotic activity is variable. Neurothekeomas express NKI (nuclear Ki-67)/C3 and PGP9.5 (protein gene product 9.5), but not S100. Dermatofibroma exhibits collagen trapping at the periphery; the epithelioid histiocytes do not typically form solid aggregates or lobules. Melanocytic nevi, nerve sheath myxoma, and schwannoma each express S100.

**20. Correct choice: A.**

Keratoacanthoma is a rapidly growing, well-differentiated, cutaneous squamous cell carcinoma that often spontaneously regresses. Regression is attributed to immune-mediated destruction of the squamous cells. It occurs in older adults with a male-to-female ratio of 3:1. Classic presentation is a dome-shaped tumor with a central keratinous plug on sun-exposed areas, most commonly on the head and neck, followed by extremities. Histologically, it is a well-differentiated squamous tumor with a central keratin-filled crater surrounded by an epidermal lip.

The tumor is composed of bland squamous cells with abundant eosinophilic or glassy cytoplasm and enlarged hyperchromatic to vesicular nuclei. Mitotic activity and cellular atypia are usually seen at the periphery of the tumor. Intraepidermal neutrophilic microabscesses and keratin horn pearls are seen within the tumor. Conventional squamous cell carcinoma shows greater cellular atypia and mitotic activity. Intraepidermal neutrophilic microabscesses and tissue eosinophilia are less common, but they may be difficult to distinguish in superficial biopsies. Verrucous carcinoma also has bland cytologic features but exhibits prominent endophytic and exophytic growth and lacks central crateriform architecture. It may also be difficult to distinguish in superficial biopsies. Verrucous psoriasis is characterized by regular psoriasiform epidermal hyperplasia with acanthosis, hyperkeratosis, and either spongiform neutrophilic or Munro microabscesses. In addition, verrucous psoriasis shows papillomatosis with bowing of the peripheral rete ridges toward the center of the lesion (buttressing). Verruca vulgaris shows hyperkeratosis, papillomatosis, and hypergranulosis; it lacks central crateriform architecture. Columns of parakeratosis typically project from dermal papillae. Vacuolated superficial keratinocytes with pyknotic raisin-like nuclei (koilocytes) may be present.

**21. Correct choice: C.**

Telangiectasia macularis eruptiva persistans is a variant of cutaneous mastocytoma. Patients, typically adults, present with widespread telangiectatic lesions. The features may be subtle, with increased mast cells around dilated superficial capillaries, basal cell hyperpigmentation of the overlying epidermis, and superficial lymphohistiocytic infiltrate. Special stains for mast cells, for example, CD117 and mast cell tryptase, may be required to establish a diagnosis.

# 3 Melanocytic Lesions

1. What is the best diagnosis for the biopsy from a pigmented lesion on the arm of a 12-year-old boy, shown in Figure 1?

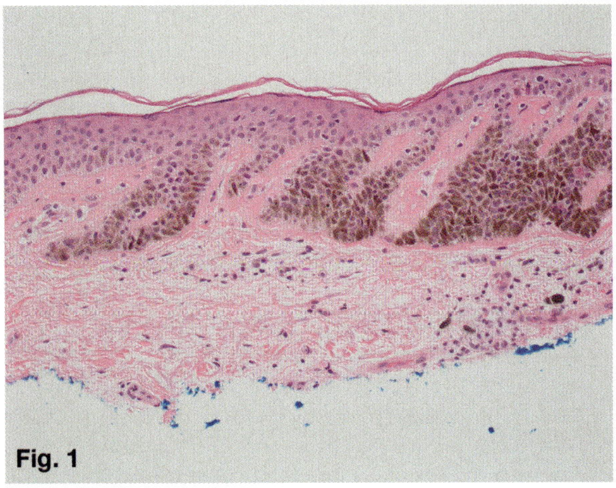

Fig. 1

A. Acquired melanocytic nevus
B. Lentigo simplex
C. Pigmented seborrheic keratosis
D. Pigmented spindle cell nevus
E. Solar lentigo

2. What is the best diagnosis for the biopsy of a pigmented lesion on the thigh in a 23-year-old woman, shown in Figure 1?

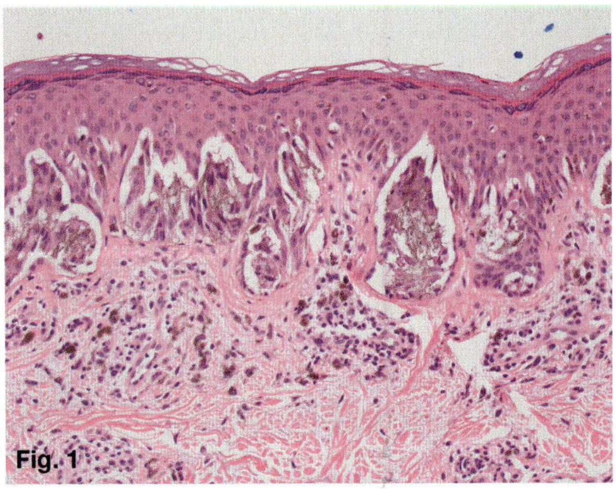

Fig. 1

A. Desmoplastic Spitz nevus
B. Lentigo malignant melanoma
C. Pigmented dysplastic nevus
D. Pigmented spindle cell nevus
E. Superficial spreading melanoma

3. What is the best diagnosis for the biopsy of a dark blue to black dome-shaped lesion on the dorsum of the right hand in a 32-year-old White female, shown in Figure 1?

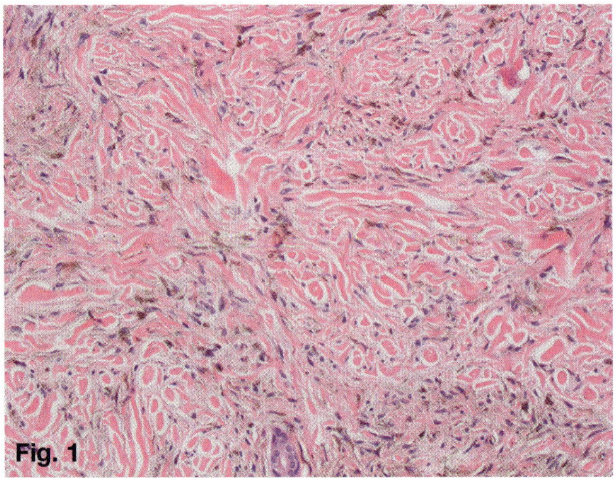

Fig. 1

A. Cellular blue nevus
B. Common blue nevus
C. Congenital melanocytic nevus
D. Nevus of Ota
E. Pigmented epithelioid melanocytoma

4. What is the best diagnosis for the slowly growing blue-black plaque on the scalp of a 25-year-old female, shown in Figure 1?

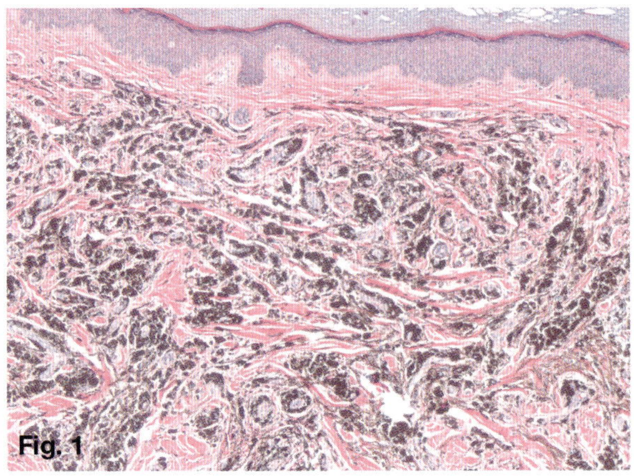

Fig. 1

A. Cellular blue nevus
B. Common blue nevus
C. Congenital melanocytic nevus
D. Nevus of Ota
E. Pigmented epithelioid melanocytoma

All figures in this chapter are from Longacre TA, Greenson JK, Hornick JL, Reuter VE, eds. *Mills and Sternberg's Diagnostic Surgical Pathology.* 7th ed. Wolters Kluwer; 2022 except for those noted at the end of this book.

5. A 76-year-old female former marathon runner with light skin presents with a pigmented lesion on her right cheek. Physical examination reveals a 1.5 × 1.0 cm tan to brown macule with irregular borders. A biopsy, shown in Figure 1, is performed. What is the diagnosis?

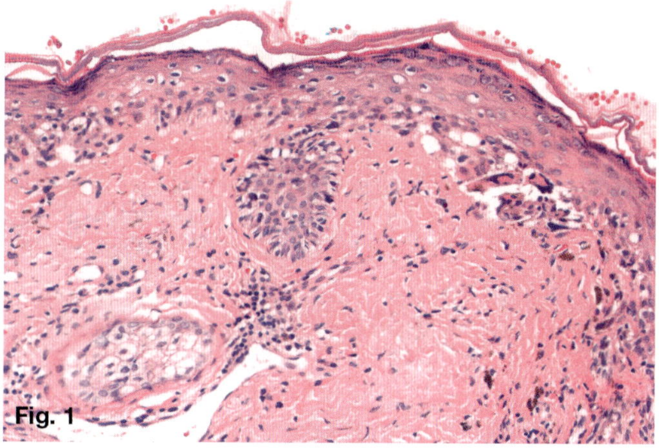

Fig. 1

A. Actinic keratosis
B. Dysplastic nevus
C. Lentigo maligna melanoma
D. Solar lentigo
E. Superficial spreading melanoma

6. A 23-year-old female with a family history of melanoma presents with innumerable pigmented skin lesions. One of the lesions is biopsied (shown in Figure 1). Which is the most likely diagnosis?

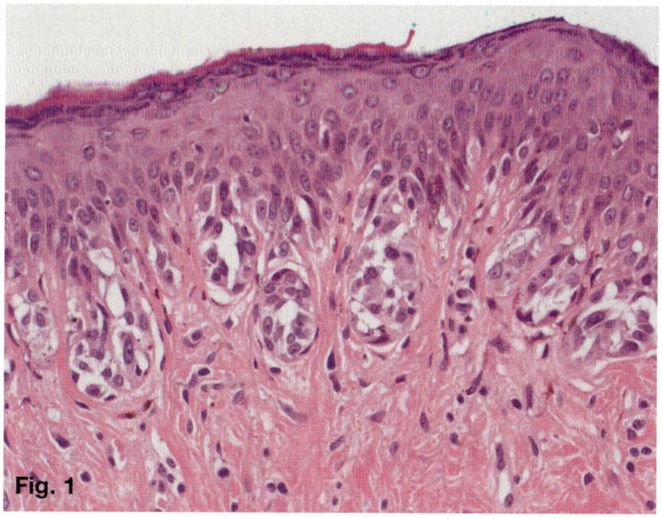

Fig. 1

A. Acquired melanocytic nevus
B. Congenital melanocytic nevus
C. Dysplastic nevus
D. Lentigo simplex
E. Spitz nevus

7. What is the appropriate method of measuring the thickness of a melanoma based on the Breslow system?

A. From the dermal-epidermal junction to the deepest point of invasion
B. From the highest level of melanoma to the deepest point of invasion
C. From the top of the dermal papillae to the deepest point of invasion
D. From the top of the granular layer to the deepest point of invasion
E. From the top of the squamous layer to the deepest point of invasion

8. Which of the following is the most frequent form of melanoma in light-skinned persons?

A. Acral lentiginous melanoma
B. Desmoplastic melanoma
C. Lentigo maligna melanoma
D. Nodular melanoma
E. Superficial spreading melanoma

9. What is the most frequent form of malignant melanoma in individuals of African and Asian descent?

A. Acral lentiginous melanoma
B. Desmoplastic melanoma
C. Lentigo maligna melanoma
D. Melanoma arising in a blue nevus
E. Nodular melanoma

10. What is the most likely diagnosis for the biopsy of a densely pigmented macule on the palm of a 42-year-old Asian female, shown in Figure 1?

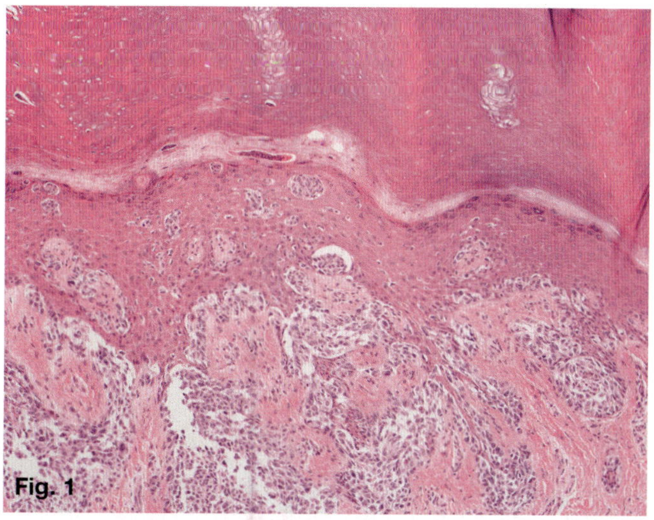

Fig. 1

A. Acral lentiginous melanoma
B. Desmoplastic melanoma
C. Lentigo maligna melanoma
D. Nodular melanoma
E. Spitz melanoma

11. What is the most likely diagnosis for this pigmented skin lesion shown in Figure 1 that has been present since birth?

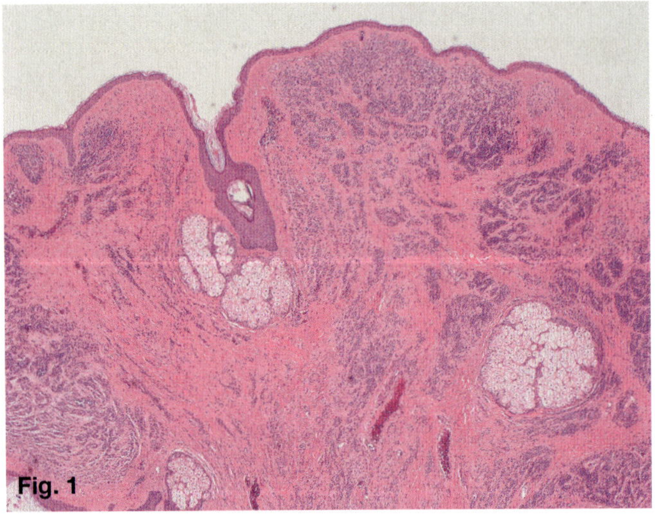

Fig. 1

A. Acquired melanocytic nevus
B. Acral melanocytic nevus
C. Congenital melanocytic nevus
D. Deep penetrating nevus
E. Spitz nevus

12. Which of the following melanocytic nevi is most commonly misdiagnosed as malignant melanoma?

A. Common blue nevus
B. Congenital nevus
C. Deep penetrating nevus
D. Halo nevus
E. Recurrent melanocytic nevus

13. Which of the following histologic features is most useful in establishing a diagnosis of a benign melanocytic proliferation?

A. Absence of neurotization
B. Nuclear atypia
C. Pagetoid spread
D. "Shoulder" of junctional melanocytic hyperplasia
E. Symmetric growth pattern

14. Which senescent change in this dermal nevus is depicted in Figure 1?

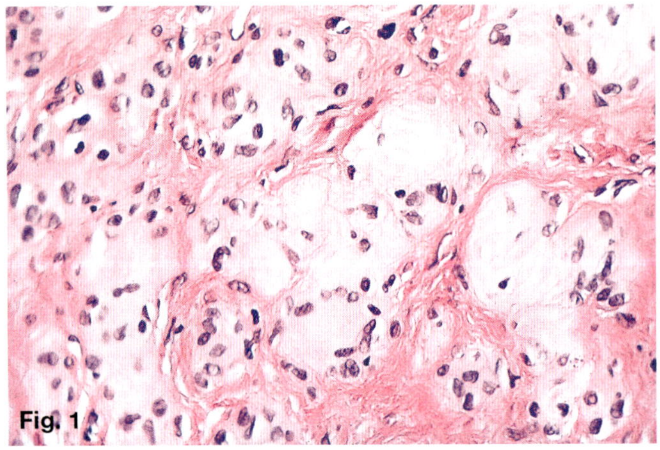

Fig. 1

A. Balloon cell change
B. Inflammatory regression
C. Lipomatous degeneration
D. Neurotization
E. Osseous metaplasia

15. At which of the following specific locations can melanocytic nevi show atypical cytologic and architectural features that can be mistaken as evidence of malignancy?

A. Acral skin, ear, milk line, scalp
B. Acral skin, face, milk line, scalp
C. Extensor surfaces, face, scalp
D. Extensor surfaces, milk line, scalp
E. Flexor surfaces, face, scalp

# ANSWERS AND EXPLANATIONS

**1. Correct choice: B.**

Lentigo simplex is a benign pigmented lesion characterized by accumulation of melanin pigment in basilar keratinocytes and melanocytic hyperplasia. There is no nesting of melanocytes, as is seen in acquired melanocytic nevi. Lentigines acquired during childhood appear as small, dark brown macules. Although they can arise anywhere, there is a predilection for acral sites. Acquired melanocytic nevus is a benign proliferation of melanocytes, which is classified by its location in the epidermis, the dermis, or both: junctional nevi, compound nevi, and intradermal nevi. It is the most common melanocytic tumor in humans. It arises at 6 months of age and reaches peak incidence during the third decade of life. Acquired melanocytic nevus may exhibit a particularly rapid rate of development at puberty and may decrease in quantity with increasing age. It is more common in people of Caucasian descent and the incidence is increased in association with sun exposure and sun burns. Acral and conjunctival nevi are more common in African, African American, and Asian populations. Most acquired melanocytic nevi are derived from activating mutations in *BRAF*. Approximately one third of melanomas are derived from these benign melanocytic nevi. Macular-pigmented seborrheic keratosis is a thicker lesion and features horn cysts/pseudocysts. Pigmented spindle cell nevus occurs on the trunk and proximal extremities of younger adults (median age 25). It is generally less than 1 cm, solitary, deeply pigmented, and well circumscribed. It clinically resembles melanoma, but on biopsy, it is a symmetric lesion with cytologic maturation. Nests and fascicles of spindled melanocytes are present along the dermal-epidermal junction and within dermal papillae. It may be junctional or compound. If compound, it extends no deeper than the reticular dermis. Solar lentigo is a benign melanocytic proliferation due to sun exposure. It occurs on sun-exposed skin of the older adults (the so-called age spots). It appears as a macular area of hyperpigmentation, often greater than 1 cm. An "ink spot lentigo" variant is smaller, darkly pigmented, and stellate in configuration. On biopsy, it exhibits elongation of rete ridges and increased pigmentation at the tips of the retes; pigmentation may be irregular. Solar elastosis, telangiectasia, and variable chronic inflammatory infiltrate in the dermis are also often present.

**2. Correct choice: D.**

Pigmented spindle cell nevus (pigmented spindle cell nevus of Reed) is a heavily pigmented nevus, often with recent onset. It has been considered a variant of Spitz nevus. It occurs on the trunk and proximal extremities of younger adults (median age 25). It is generally less than 1 cm, solitary, deeply pigmented, and well circumscribed. It clinically resembles melanoma, but on biopsy, it is a symmetric lesion with cytologic maturation. Nests and fascicles of spindled melanocytes are present along the dermal-epidermal junction and within dermal papillae. It may be junctional or compound. If compound, it extends no deeper than the reticular dermis. Desmoplastic Spitz nevus also occurs in young adults on the proximal extremities (as well as other sites) but clinically resembles a dermatofibroma or scar. It is characterized on biopsy by a densely collagenized dermis with interspersed spindle and epithelioid cells. Maturation at the base is not common, and so this lesion can be mistaken for a desmoplastic melanoma. Lentigo maligna melanoma typically grows on the cheeks (or otherwise sun-exposed areas) of older individuals with light skin. The designation of lentigo maligna derives from the characteristic lentiginous distribution of atypical melanocytes along the dermal-epidermal junction, either singly or in small nests. Pigmented dysplastic nevus has irregular borders and a variegated appearance. Microscopically, it looks like a common compound nevus but with the following atypical features: (a) lentiginous spread along the dermal-epidermal junction well beyond the lateral margins of the dermal component (shoulder effect); (b) cellular atypia ranging from mild to severe; (c) hyperplasia and fusion of rete ridges by melanocytes; (d) drape-like fibrosis of dermal papillae, known as lamellar fibroplasia; and (e) dermal lymphocytic infiltration. Superficial spreading melanoma is the most common clinicopathologic form of melanoma in White persons. It may develop anywhere in the body and appears as a variably colored flat lesion with irregular notched borders. The most characteristic feature of this form is the pagetoid spread of atypical melanocytes within the epidermis, with nest formation and presence of melanin up to the stratum corneum (pigmented parakeratosis).

**3. Correct choice: B.**

Common blue nevus is composed of cells reminiscent of neural crest–derived dendritic melanocytic precursors (neural, or type C, nevomelanocytes). The lesion occupies the reticular dermis and may extend into the subcutis. Nevus of Ota is an uncommon acquired hamartoma of dermal melanocytes. There is a clear uninvolved zone between the nevus and the overlying epidermis. Melanin is abundant, but most of it is within melanophages (histiocytes), which may obscure the accompanying dermal melanocytic component. If the pigment is mistaken as hemosiderin, a blue nevus may be erroneously diagnosed as fibrous histiocytoma. Cellular blue nevus is most common on the buttocks and consists of a dumbbell-shaped dermal aggregate of interweaving fascicles of spindled cells with and without melanin. Congenital melanocytic nevi are relatively infrequent, found in 1% of newborns. They are generally large and irregular. Histologically, nevus cells extend deep into the dermis up to the subcutis, around pilosebaceous units and arrector pili muscles. Pigmented epithelioid melanocytoma is a low-grade melanoma composed of a deep dermal population of heavily pigmented epithelioid and spindle melanocytes. Sentinel lymph node involvement is frequent (44%), but growth is indolent and the prognosis is good.

**4. Correct choice: E.**

Pigmented epithelioid melanocytoma is a slow-growing low-grade melanocytic tumor with heavily pigmented epithelioid, spindled, and dendritic melanocytes. It does not appear to be related to sun exposure. Although the median age of presentation is 20 to 27 years, it can be seen in infants and children. It affects all racial/ethnic groups. Some cases are associated with the Carney complex. Sentinel lymph node involvement is seen in 30% to 50% of cases, but distant metastases are rare. Death due to rare systemic metastases has not been reported.

**5. Correct choice: C.**

Lentigo maligna melanoma typically grows on the cheeks (or otherwise sun-exposed areas) of adult individuals with light skin. The designation of lentigo maligna derives from the characteristic lentiginous distribution of atypical melanocytes along the dermoepidermal junction, either singly or in small nests. The overlying epidermis is atrophic. Lentigo maligna is an actinic-induced melanocytic lesion, which could be viewed as the melanocytic counterpart of actinic keratosis. The most common driver mutations are *NF1*, *NRAS*, and *KIT*, but *BRAF*V600K mutations may also occur. Solar lentigo is a benign melanocytic proliferation due to sun exposure. It occurs on sun-exposed skin of the older adults (the so-called age spots). Superficial spreading melanoma is the most common clinicopathologic form of melanoma in White persons. It may develop anywhere in the body and appears as a variably colored flat lesion with irregular notched borders. The most characteristic feature of this form is the pagetoid spread of atypical melanocytes within the epidermis, with nest formation and the presence of melanin up to the stratum corneum (pigmented parakeratosis). Development of vertical growth is manifested by the appearance of a nodule within the lesion. The *BRAF*V600K mutation is the most common driver mutation in superficial spreading melanoma, which is also seen in most benign nevi.

**6. Correct choice: C.**

Dysplastic nevus is a precursor of melanoma and exhibits specific atypical features. Clinically, it is often larger than 5 mm, with irregular borders and variegated appearance. Microscopically, it looks like a common compound nevus but with the following atypical features: (a) lentiginous spread along the dermal-epidermal junction well beyond the lateral margins of the dermal component (shoulder effect); (b) cellular atypia ranging from mild to severe; (c) hyperplasia and fusion of rete ridges by melanocytes; (d) drape-like fibrosis of dermal papillae, known as lamellar fibroplasia; and (e) dermal lymphocytic infiltration. Patients with dysplastic nevus syndrome, an autosomal dominant hereditary disorder, have multiple dysplastic nevi and two family members diagnosed with melanoma.

**7. Correct choice: D.**

The Breslow system is based on the measurement of melanoma thickness from the top of the granular layer to the deepest level of invasion of the tumor. It assumes that the overlying epidermis is intact. This microstage system correlates with prognosis and the likelihood of lymph node metastases. Three categories have been identified:

1. Low risk: thickness less than 0.76 mm
2. Intermediate risk: thickness greater than 0.76 but less than 1.5 mm
3. High risk: thickness greater than 1.5 mm

**8. Correct choice: E.**

Superficial spreading melanoma is the most common clinicopathologic form of melanoma in White persons. It may develop anywhere in the body and appears as a variably colored flat lesion with irregular notched borders. The most characteristic feature of this form is the pagetoid spread of atypical melanocytes within the epidermis, with nest formation and the presence of melanin up to the stratum corneum (pigmented parakeratosis).

**9. Correct choice: A.**

Acral lentiginous melanoma develops most commonly in the glabrous (non-hair-bearing) aspects of the palms, soles, and subungual areas but also along mucocutaneous junctions and the anal region. It is more common in people with increased pigmentation because they are not as susceptible to the chronic sun damage subtypes of melanoma.

**10. Correct choice: A.**

Microscopically, acral lentiginous melanoma is similar to lentigo maligna, but the overlying epidermis is hyperplastic instead of atrophic as in lentigo maligna. Acral lentiginous melanoma has a more aggressive behavior compared to lentigo maligna and superficial spreading melanoma.

**11. Correct choice: C.**

Congenital melanocytic nevi are relatively infrequent, found in 1% of newborns. They are generally larger and more irregular than acquired nevi. The giant forms, covering large areas of the body ("bathing trunk nevi"), have a 5% to 10% risk of malignant transformation. Histologically, nevus cells extend deep into the dermis up to the subcutis, around pilosebaceous units and arrector pili muscles. Otherwise, the cellular morphology of congenital nevi is similar to that of acquired nevi. Acral melanocytic nevi are junctional nevi that occur on the hands and feet; they display prominent lentiginous proliferation mimicking acral lentiginous melanoma. Deep penetrating nevus may arise de novo as a blue papulonodular lesion or, more often, within a preexisting nevus. Histologically, this nevus is wedge shaped, with the base at the epidermis and the apex deep into the dermis, sometimes extending into subcutaneous fat. Spitz nevus is a benign melanocytic lesion that can mimic melanoma because of the presence of marked cytologic atypia, mitotic activity, and occasional pagetoid spread. Misdiagnosis as a melanoma is a common cause of malpractice claims. Melanin is usually scanty or absent. The following architectural features are important in differentiating it from melanoma: symmetric growth, triangular shape, fascicles oriented perpendicular to the epidermal surface, and downward maturation of nevus cells. A prominent vascular network may suggest a diagnosis of hemangioma. Head and neck are the most common sites. It is usually first diagnosed in children and adolescents. Variants of Spitz nevus include pigmented spindle cell nevus, desmoplastic Spitz nevus, angiomatoid Spitz nevus, atypical Spitz tumors, and Spitz melanoma.

**12. Correct choice: C.**

Deep penetrating nevus may arise de novo as a blue papulonodular lesion or, more often, within a preexisting nevus. In the latter case, the development of a bluish discoloration may generate suspicion of malignant degeneration. Histologically, this nevus is wedge shaped, with the base at the epidermis and the apex deep into the dermis, sometimes extending into subcutaneous fat. There is maturation and no mitotic activity, but deep infiltration may be mistaken as evidence of melanoma. Melanoma lacks expression of dipeptidyl peptidase IV, which is retained in deep penetrating nevus. Halo nevus is a "regressing nevus" in which a circular rim of depigmentation is due to the destruction of nevomelanocytes by a florid lymphocytic reaction. Recurrent nevi are those that reappear on the site of a previously removed nevus by shaved biopsy. They look worrisome because of the uneven melanin distribution due to scarring.

**13. Correct choice: E.**

Of the features listed in the answer options, symmetry of growth is the most characteristic of benign melanocytic proliferations: The dermal component of the melanocytic expansion is roughly equal, in lateral diameter, to the epidermal component. This can be appreciated on low-power examination. In contrast, with the exception of Spitz nevus, nuclear atypia is usually absent in benign lesions. Neurotization (also called schwannian differentiation) is a common manifestation of senescence in such lesions. Pagetoid spread is seen not only in melanomas but also in Spitz nevi and common acquired nevi in the acral regions. A "shoulder" of melanocytic hyperplasia located at the margins of a melanocytic lesion is more often associated with malignancy.

**14. Correct choice: D.**

Neurotization (also called schwannian differentiation) is a common manifestation of senescence in melanocytic nevi. The formation of these "neural structures" in the loose connective tissue may simulate a neurofibroma. Balloon cell change is a degenerative change due to apoptosis, resulting in the vacuolization of melanosomes and a block in melanin synthesis. Nevus cells have clear or vacuolated cytoplasm. Melanin can be absent or abundant. This change is found in less than 2% of melanocytic proliferations, mostly benign. Inflammatory regression is associated with a pronounced host cell response, typically due to trauma. A prominent inflammatory response is also seen in "halo" nevi, wherein the inflammatory cells destroy melanocytes, resulting in an enlarging peripheral rim of hypopigmentation around a commonly acquired nevus. Lipomatous degeneration is characterized by infiltration of dermal nevi by fat cells, while osseous metaplasia features bone.

**15. Correct choice: A.**

Melanocytic nevi arising in the scalp, around the ear, and along the milk line (from axilla to groin) and genital region (particularly the vulva) are known to exhibit unusual cytologic and architectural features, which may be mistaken for signs of anaplasia. However, maturation and absence of mitotic activity in the dermal component are still appreciable in such lesions. The etiology of these changes is unknown.

# 4 Muscle Biopsy in Neuromuscular Diseases

1. Mitochondrial abnormalities are recognized by

   A. lobulated fibers.
   B. moth-eaten fibers.
   C. ragged red fibers.
   D. ring fibers.
   E. target fibers.

2. A 2-year-old male presents with a history of progressive awkwardness and frequent falls. A clinical diagnosis of Duchenne muscular dystrophy can be confirmed by which of the following?

   A. Biochemical studies of mitochondrial metabolism
   B. Genetic analysis for detection of trinucleotide repeats
   C. Immunohistochemistry for dysferlin
   D. Immunohistochemistry for dystrophin on muscle biopsy
   E. Measurement of blood creatine kinase

3. This oxidative preparation (nicotinamide adenine dinucleotide) on the muscle biopsy shown in Figure 1 demonstrates

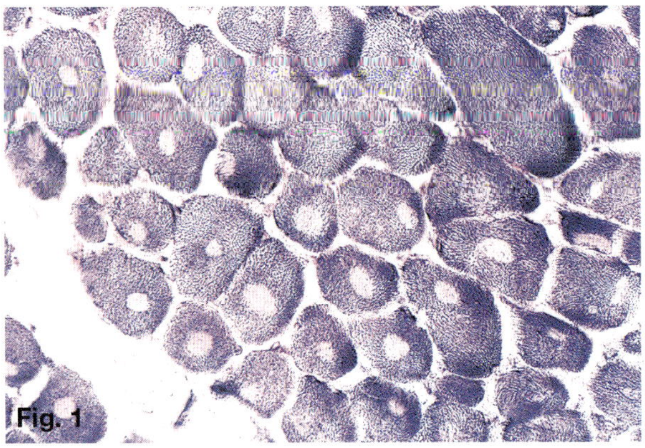

Fig. 1

   A. cores.
   B. lobulated fibers.
   C. moth-eaten fibers.
   D. target fibers.
   E. vacuolar change.

4. Which of the following is most likely to be seen in a muscle biopsy in the setting of neurogenic atrophy?

   A. Chronic inflammatory infiltration of the endomysium
   B. Group atrophy and fiber type grouping
   C. Hyaline fibers and endomysial fatty infiltration
   D. Internalization of nuclei and myofiber splitting
   E. Ragged red fibers on modified Gomori trichrome

5. The muscle biopsy, shown in Figure 1, from an 18-year-old male with progressive muscular weakness most likely represents

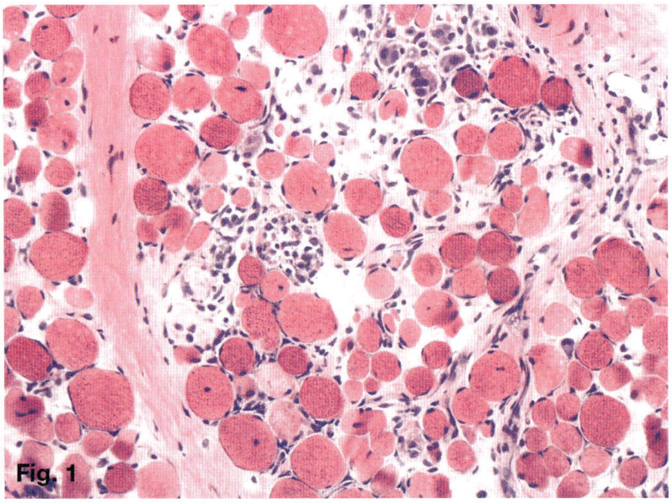

Fig. 1

   A. autoimmune necrotizing myopathy.
   B. inclusion body myositis.
   C. mitochondrial myopathy.
   D. muscular dystrophy.
   E. polymyositis.

6. Which of the following lipid storage diseases is responsive to riboflavin?

   A. Carnitine palmitoyltransferase I deficiency
   B. Multiple acyl-coenzyme A dehydrogenase deficiency
   C. Neural lipid storage disease
   D. Primary carnitine deficiency

7. What is the enzyme defect in glycogen storage disease type 2 (Pompe disease)?

   A. Acid maltase
   B. Glycogen branching
   C. Glycogen debranching
   D. Myophosphorylase
   E. Phosphofructokinase Tarui

All figures in this chapter are from Longacre TA, Greenson JK, Hornick JL, Reuter VE, eds. *Mills and Sternberg's Diagnostic Surgical Pathology.* 7th ed. Wolters Kluwer; 2022 except for those noted at the end of this book.

# ANSWERS AND EXPLANATIONS

**1. Correct choice: C.**

Ragged red fibers constitute the morphologic expression of mitochondrial diseases. Classic ragged red fibers are identified on Gomori trichrome. Intensely red sarcolemmal protrusions from the cell surface impart an irregular, ragged appearance of involved fibers. Target fibers are considered pathognomonic for denervation with reinnervation, typically of type 1 fibers. Lobulated fibers are nonspecific but when found in significant numbers may be associated with trabecular myopathy. Moth-eaten fibers are nonspecific but appear to be associated with reversible injury. Ring fibers may be seen in a variety of diseases, but they are most consistently observed in limb-girdle dystrophies and when present in large numbers, myotonic dystrophy 1.

**2. Correct choice: D.**

Duchenne muscular dystrophy (DMD) is caused by mutations of the X-linked gene encoding dystrophin. Lack of expression of this protein results in DMD, whereas partial expression of dystrophin leads to Becker muscular dystrophy (BMD). H&E (hematoxylin and eosin) changes in muscle biopsies from patients with DMD are characteristic, but the diagnosis is established by immunohistochemistry (or immunoblot) for dystrophin. In DMD, there is complete absence of the normal sarcolemmal immunoreactivity, whereas in BMD, immunoreactivity is patchy and discontinuous. Ragged red fibers would suggest a mitochondrial disorder. Expansion of trinucleotide CGT repeats in the MyD (myeloid differentiation) gene is the cause of myotonic dystrophy, characterized by myotonia (inability to relax muscle), ptosis, and weakness in facial and acral muscles. Lack of dysferlin is found in a limb-girdle dystrophy known as dystrophinopathy. Elevation of blood creatine kinase is a nonspecific effect of any kind of myopathy associated with myofiber necrosis.

**3. Correct choice: A.**

Cores (sharply demarcated areas of reduced enzyme oxidative activity), when numerous and present in type 1 muscle fibers, are associated with central core myopathy. Moth-eaten (or mottled) fibers are characterized by central, patchy areas of poor staining, while lobulated fibers are characterized by several muscle fibers that are divided into lobules by septa occupied by mitochondria. Both are nonspecific. Target fibers are characterized by an inert, unstained central zone surrounded by a rim of increased enzyme activity.

**4. Correct choice: B.**

In neurogenic atrophy (resulting from axonal damage or motor neuron loss), atrophic fibers are angulated and usually clustered in groups (group atrophy). If reinnervation takes place, the same neuron will reinnervate neighboring myofibers, imparting the same fiber phenotype (either type I or type II) to a large group of myofibers: hence fiber type grouping. Chronic inflammation is associated with inflammatory myopathies such as polymyositis. The endomysial compartment is not expanded by fibrosis or fatty infiltration. Internalization of nuclei and fiber splitting are characteristic of primary muscle diseases (myopathic changes). Ragged red fibers are due to the accumulation of abnormal mitochondria.

**5. Correct choice: D.**

The classic histologic features of muscular dystrophy are myonecrosis and regeneration with variable lymphocytic inflammation, internally placed nuclei, muscle fiber atrophy or hypertrophy, and endomysial fibrosis. Polymyositis and autoimmune necrotizing myopathy/myositis are autoimmune disorders in which lymphocytes have become sensitized to muscle antigens. This cell-mediated response leads to necrosis of muscle fibers and subsequent regeneration. Muscle fiber atrophy may occur in long-standing disease and simulate a dystrophic appearance. Inclusion body myositis is the most common sporadic muscle disease over the age of 55. Because initial biopsies may simulate several disease processes, it may be misdiagnosed as a nonspecific inflammatory myopathy. The presence of many, small angular and grouped muscle fibers, fiber hypertrophy, and fiber splitting are typical features. Mitochondrial myopathies often have an onset in infancy or young adulthood but are typically multiorgan diseases.

**6. Correct choice: B.**

Multiple acyl-coenzyme A dehydrogenase deficiency (MADD) is a rare autosomal recessive disorder caused by deficiency of electron transfer flavoprotein. Late-onset form of MADD typically presents with slowly progressive proximal weakness, myalgia, lethargy, vomiting, hypoglycemia, and metabolic acidosis. Almost all patients with late-onset MADD are responsive to riboflavin.

**7. Correct choice: A.**

Glycogen storage diseases are inherited metabolic disorders of glycogen metabolism due to a lack of specific enzymes that control the synthesis, regulation, and degradation of glycogen. There are at least 15 types, most of which are autosomal recessive. Glycogen storage diseases are classified numerically in the order of recognition and identification of the enzyme defect causing the disorder. Von Gierke disease was the first glycogen storage disease to be recognized and is called type 1 glycogen storage disease. The most common presenting symptoms are hypoglycemia and exercise intolerance. Pompe disease (also known as glycogen storage disease 2) is a rare genetic disorder that causes progressive weakness in the heart and skeletal muscles; it is due to a deficiency in acid maltase enzyme. Anderson disease is due to a defect in glycogen-branching enzyme, while a defect in glycogen debranching enzyme is seen in Cor/Forbes. McArdle disease is associated with myophosphorylase deficiency. A defect in the phosphofructokinase enzyme is seen in Tarui disease.

# 5 Soft Tissues

1. Which of the following soft tissue tumors is strongly immunoreactive for STAT6?

    A. Atypical fibroxanthoma
    B. Desmoplastic melanoma
    C. Solitary fibrous tumor
    D. Spindle cell carcinoma
    E. Synovial sarcoma

2. A 2-cm nodule is excised from the right forearm of a 32-year-old man, who says that it grew rapidly over 2 weeks. It is diffusely positive for smooth muscle actin (see Figure 1). Which of the following is the most likely diagnosis?

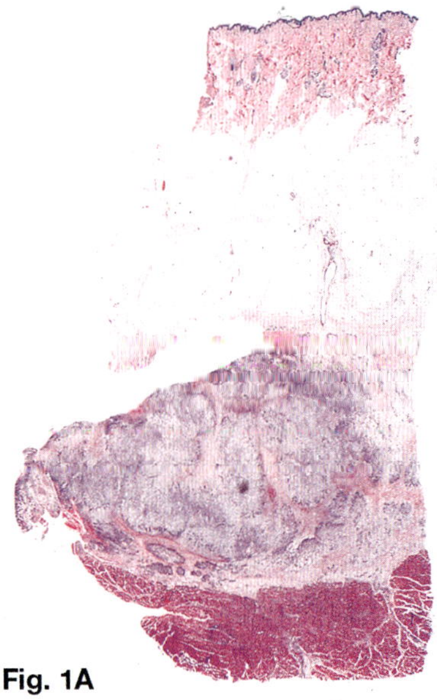

Fig. 1A

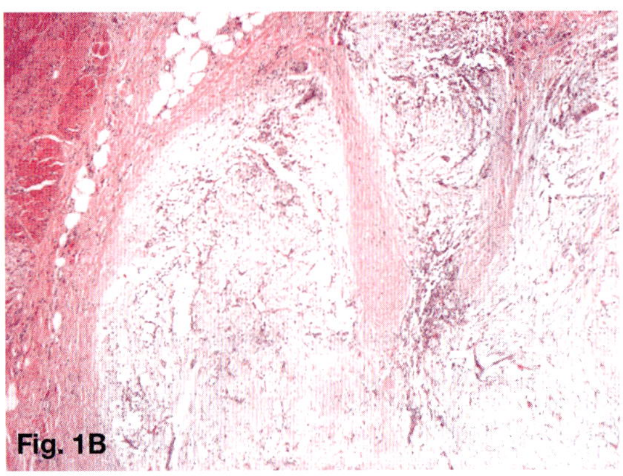

Fig. 1B

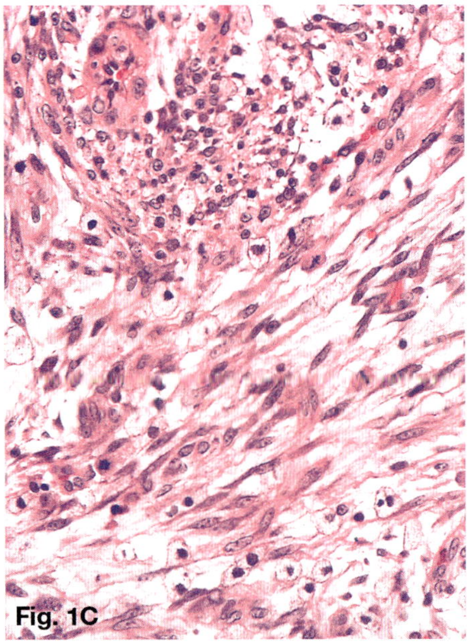

Fig. 1C

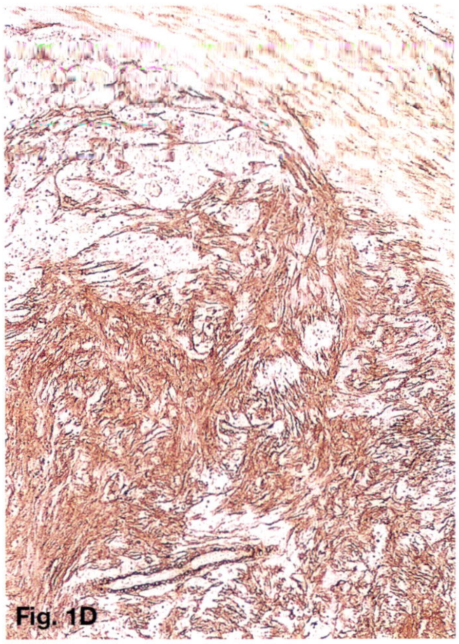

Fig. 1D

    A. Desmoid-type fibromatosis
    B. Fibrous histiocytoma
    C. Lipoblastoma
    D. Myxoid liposarcoma
    E. Nodular fasciitis

All figures in this chapter are from Longacre TA, Greenson JK, Hornick JL, Reuter VE, eds. *Mills and Sternberg's Diagnostic Surgical Pathology*. 7th ed. Wolters Kluwer; 2022 except for those noted at the end of this book.

3. The biopsy shown in Figure 1 is from the back of the neck of a 64-year-old man. What is the best diagnosis?

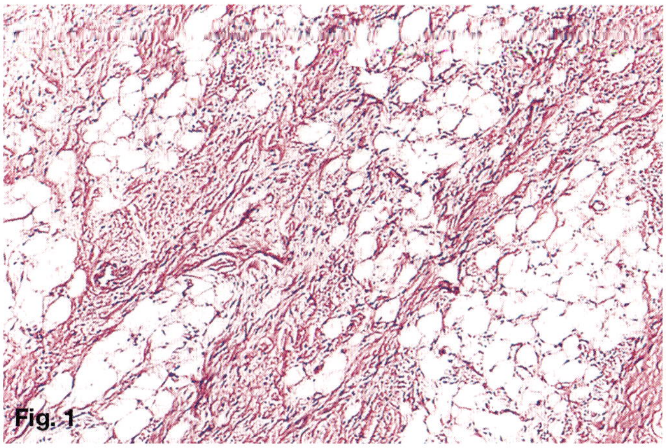

Fig. 1

A. Angiolipoma
B. Chondrolipoma
C. Intramuscular myxoma
D. Pleomorphic lipoma
E. Spindle cell lipoma

4. A 40-year-old woman undergoes excision of a slowly growing, poorly circumscribed mass in the thigh (see Figure 1). What is the best diagnosis?

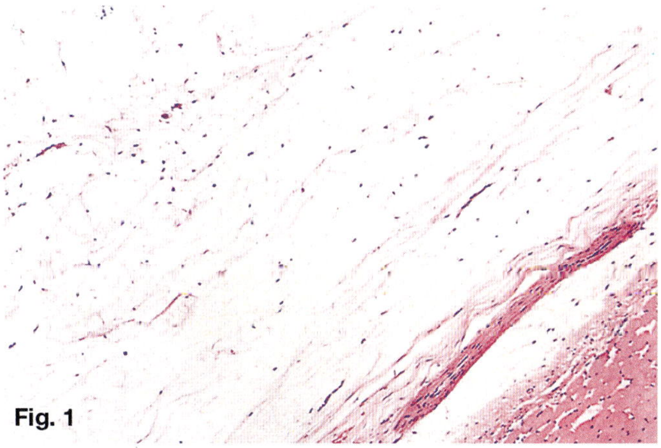

Fig. 1

A. Intramuscular lipoma
B. Intramuscular myxoma
C. Myxofibrosarcoma
D. Myxoid chondrosarcoma
E. Myxoid liposarcoma

5. The fetal form of rhabdomyoma may develop in the vulvovaginal region of middle-aged women. Which of the following is the most common location in children?

A. Extremities
B. Head and neck
C. Mediastinum
D. Perineal region
E. Retroperitoneum

6. A poorly circumscribed nodular mass (see Figure 1) is removed from the right subscapular region of a 55-year-old man. What is the most likely diagnosis?

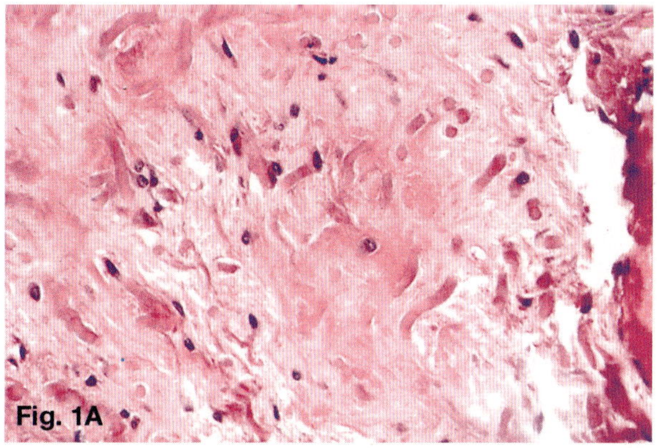

Fig. 1A

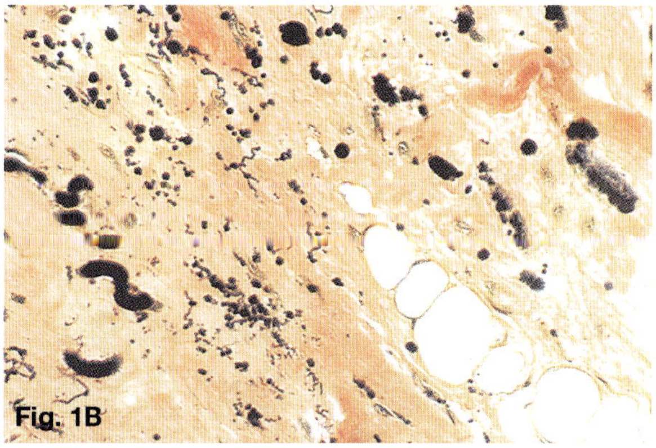

Fig. 1B

A. Elastofibroma
B. Fibroma of the tendon sheath
C. Fibromatosis
D. Keloid scar
E. Nodular fasciitis

7. Which of the following types of fibrosarcomas arises in the hands and feet and is associated with the characteristic histologic picture shown in Figure 1?

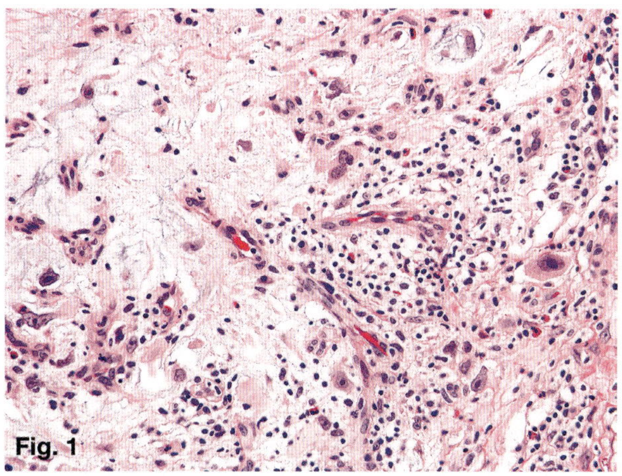

Fig. 1

A. Low-grade fibromyxoid sarcoma
B. Myxofibrosarcoma
C. Myxoinflammatory fibroblastic sarcoma
D. Sclerosing epithelioid fibrosarcoma
E. Superficial angiomyxoma

8. A 34-year-old male undergoes excision of a slow-growing, 9-cm, painless soft tissue mass in the thigh, shown in Figure 1. What is the best diagnosis?

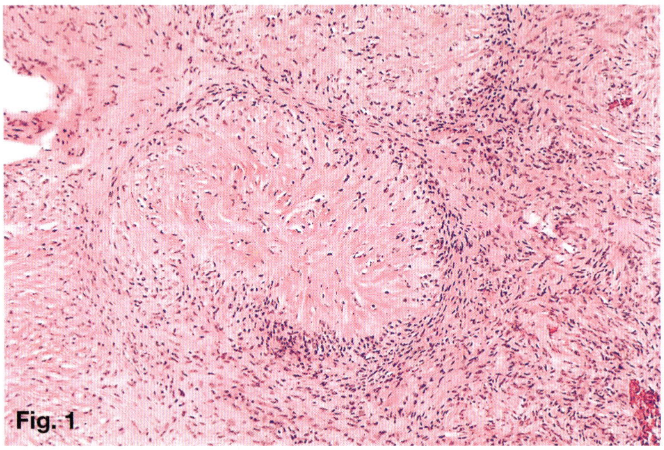

Fig. 1

A. Desmoid-type fibromatosis
B. Desmoplastic fibroblastoma
C. Giant cell fibroblastoma
D. Low-grade fibromyxoid sarcoma
E. Sclerosing epithelioid fibrosarcoma

9. A 28-year-old man presents with four painful 1- to 2-cm nodules in the skin, subcutaneous tissue, and skeletal muscle of the right lower leg. One of the nodules is excised, as shown in Figure 1. The tumor is immunoreactive for AE1/AE3, ERG (erythroblast transformation specific-related gene), and CD31 and negative for EMA (epithelial membrane antigen) and CD34. This clinical and pathologic presentation is diagnostic of

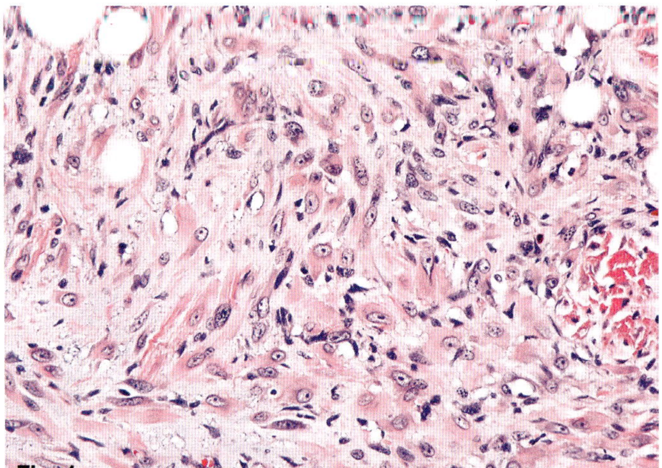

Fig. 1

A. epithelioid hemangioendothelioma.
B. epithelioid sarcoma.
C. kaposiform hemangioendothelioma.
D. pseudomyogenic hemangioendothelioma.
E. retiform hemangioendothelioma.

10. On histologic examination, a soft tissue tumor reveals a spindle cell population in a background of vascular channels displaying a staghorn appearance, as seen in Figure 1. The neoplastic cells and the vascular endothelial lining are immunoreactive for CD34 and STAT6 (depicted here). Cytokeratin and EMA (epithelial membrane antigen) are negative. Which of the following is the most likely diagnosis?

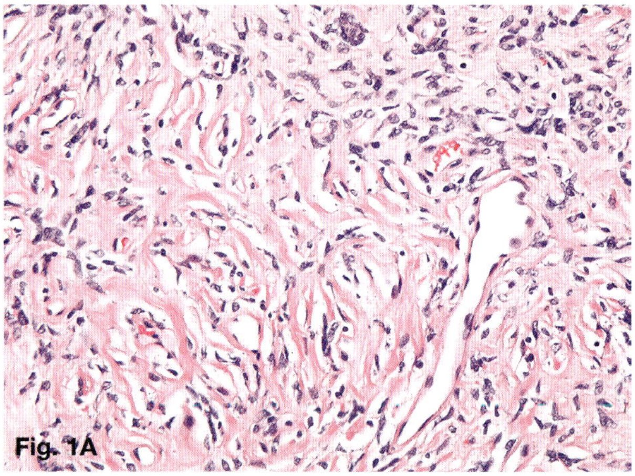

Fig. 1A

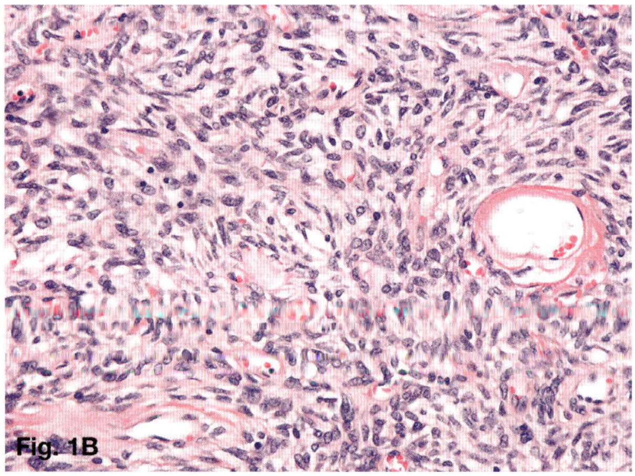

Fig. 1B

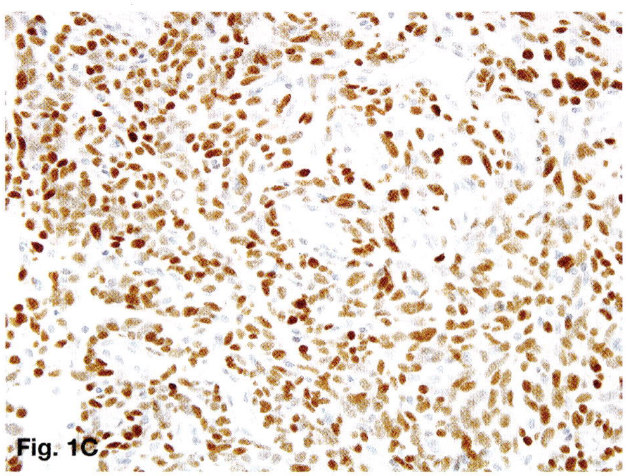

Fig. 1C

A. Dermatofibrosarcoma protuberans
B. Fibrosarcoma
C. Peripheral nerve sheath tumor
D. Solitary fibrous tumor
E. Synovial sarcoma

11. This biopsy of a soft tissue mass from the thigh of a 25-year-old woman, shown in Figure 1, is associated with an unbalanced translocation der(17)t(X,17), resulting in the *ASPSCR1-TFE3* fusion gene. What is the most likely diagnosis?

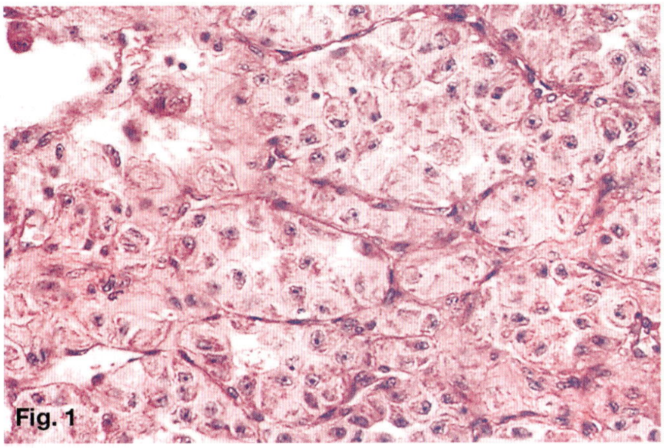

Fig. 1

A. Alveolar rhabdomyosarcoma
B. Alveolar soft part sarcoma
C. Epithelioid sarcoma
D. Granular cell tumor
E. Malignant melanoma

12. Biopsy of the enlarged, painless inguinal lymph node, shown in Figure 1, in a 34-year-old female is best diagnosed as

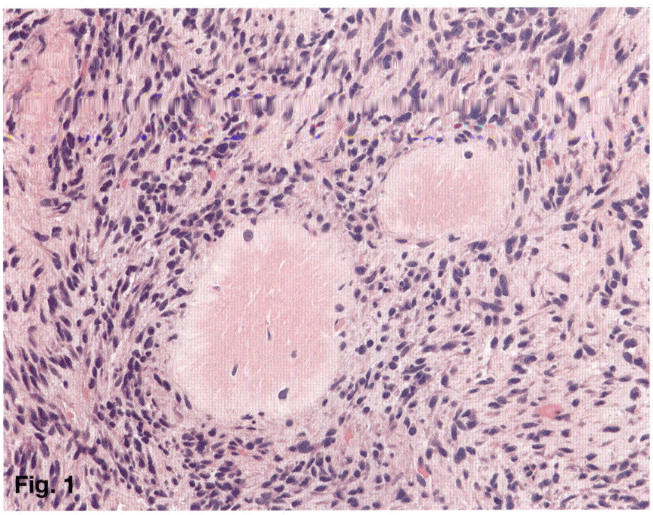

Fig. 1

A. benign metastasizing leiomyoma.
B. dendritic cell sarcoma.
C. intranodal schwannoma.
D. metastatic leiomyosarcoma.
E. palisaded myofibroblastoma.

13. Low-grade fibromyxoid sarcoma is associated with which of the following gene fusions?

A. *BCOR-CCNB3*
B. *FUS-CREB3L2*
C. *FUS-DDIT3*
D. *NAB2-STAT6*
E. *YAP1-TFE3*

14. Which immunohistochemical marker is most useful in establishing a diagnosis of low-grade fibromyxoid sarcoma?

A. BCOR
B. MUC4
C. PLAG1
D. RB1
E. ROS1

15. A 45-year-old male presents with a deep thigh mass with recent enlargement and pain. The mass is biopsied, shown in Figure 1. Which of the following is the most likely diagnosis?

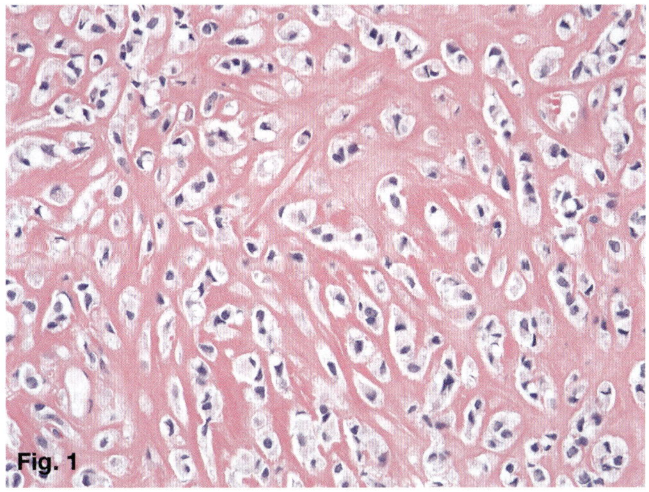

Fig. 1

A. Metastatic signet-ring carcinoma
B. Ossifying fibromyxoid tumor
C. Parosteal osteosarcoma
D. Sclerosing epithelioid fibrosarcoma
E. Sclerosing rhabdomyosarcoma

16. What is the best diagnosis for the inguinal mass, shown in Figure 1, in a 55-year-old man?

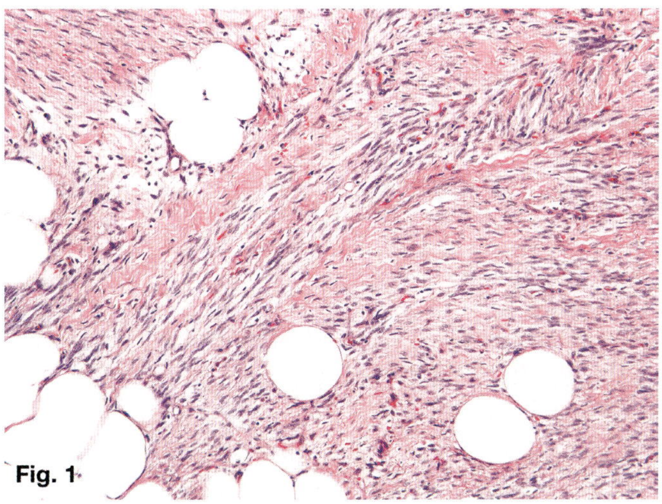

Fig. 1

A. Desmoid-type fibromatosis
B. Myofibroblastoma
C. Nodular fasciitis
D. Solitary fibrous tumor
E. Spindle cell lipoma

17. What is the best diagnosis for the subcutis soft tissue mass, shown in Figure 1, in a 54-year-old man?

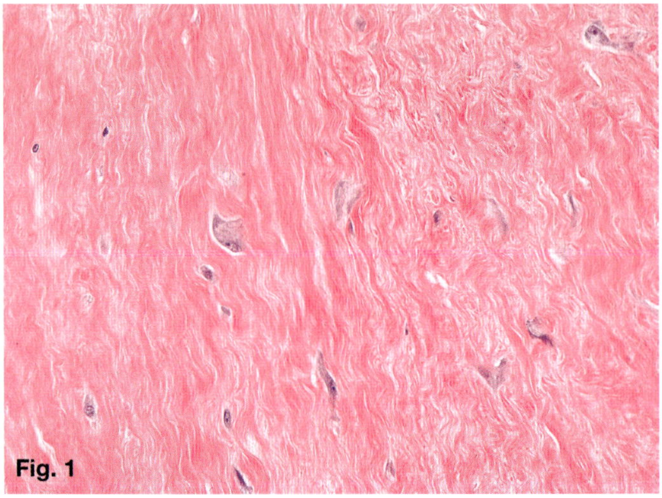
Fig. 1

A. Desmoid-type fibromatosis
B. Desmoplastic fibroblastoma
C. Fibroma of tendon sheath
D. Gardner fibroma
E. Hypertrophic scar (keloid)

18. What is the best diagnosis for the soft tissue mass, shown in Figure 1, excised from a 2-year-old boy?

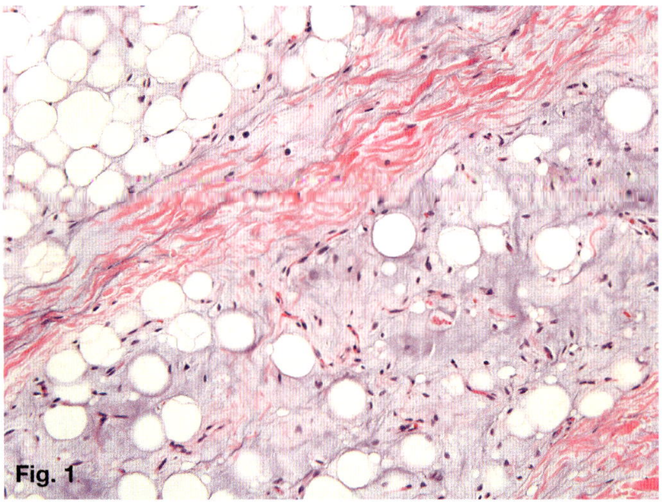
Fig. 1

A. Chondroid lipoma
B. Hibernoma
C. Lipoblastoma
D. Lipoma
E. Spindle cell lipoma

19. What is the best diagnosis for the painless, slow-growing mass, shown in Figure 1, in the subcutaneous tissue of the lower thigh region in a 70-year-old man?

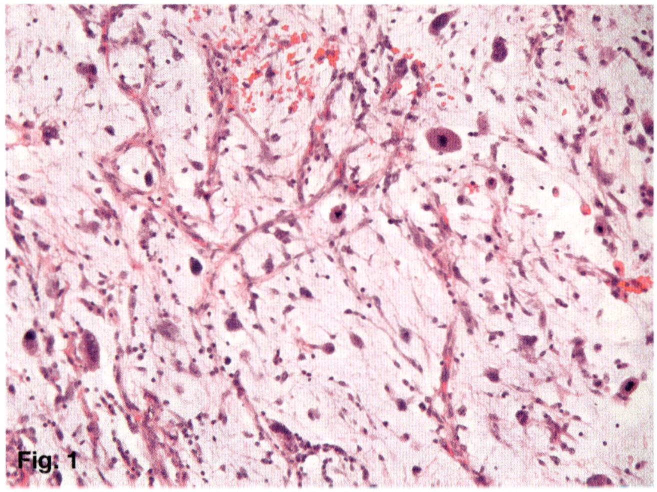
Fig. 1

A. Myxofibrosarcoma
B. Myxoid liposarcoma
C. Myxoid pleomorphic liposarcoma
D. Myxoinflammatory fibroblastic sarcoma
E. Undifferentiated pleomorphic sarcoma

20. The locally recurring, rarely metastasizing subcutaneous tumor, shown in Figure 1, arising in the antecubital fossa of a 12-year-old boy is associated with which of the following fusion genes?

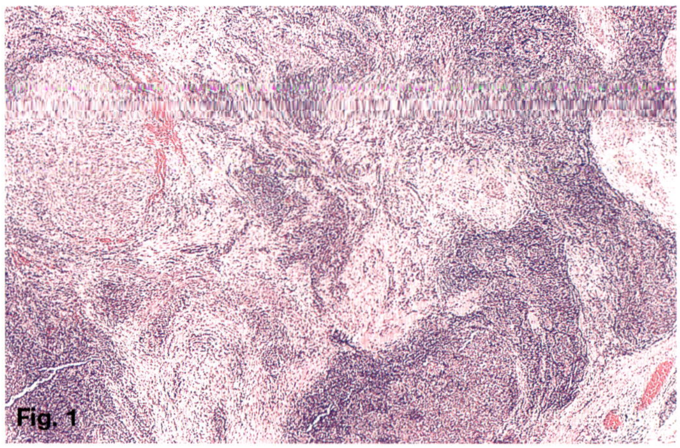
Fig. 1

A. *BCOR-CCNB3*
B. *EWSR1-CREB1*
C. *FUS-CREB3L2*
D. *FUS-DDIT3*
E. *NAB2-STAT6*

21. What is the best diagnosis for the mediastinal mass, shown in Figure 1, in a 28-year-old female?

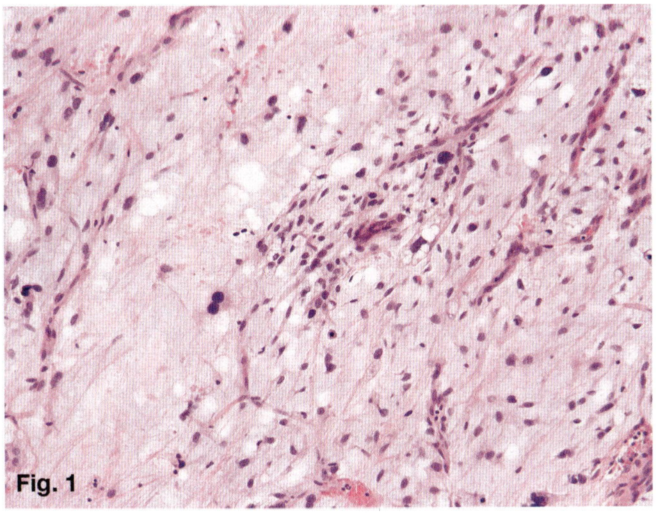

Fig. 1

A. Atypical pleomorphic lipomatous tumor
B. Myxoid liposarcoma
C. Myxoid pleomorphic liposarcoma
D. Myxoinflammatory fibroblastic sarcoma
E. Nodular fasciitis

22. What is the best diagnosis for the thigh mass, shown in Figure 1, in a 55-year-old man?

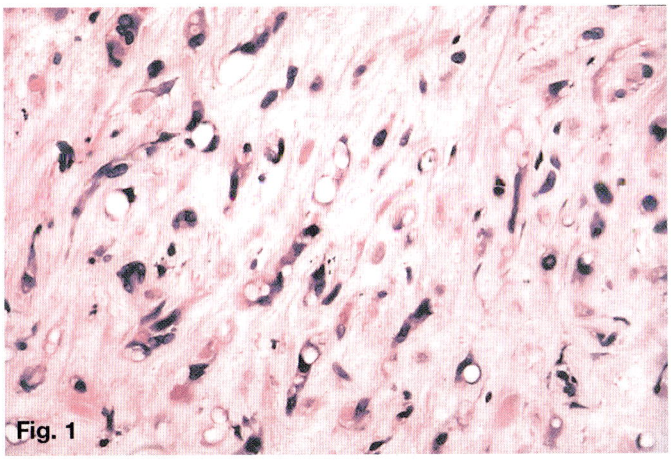

Fig. 1

A. Epithelioid angiosarcoma
B. Epithelioid hemangioendothelioma
C. Metastatic signet-ring carcinoma
D. Metastatic signet-ring melanoma
E. Pseudomyogenic hemangioendothelioma

23. What is the best diagnosis for the solitary soft tissue mass, shown in Figure 1, in the arm of a 24-year-old female?

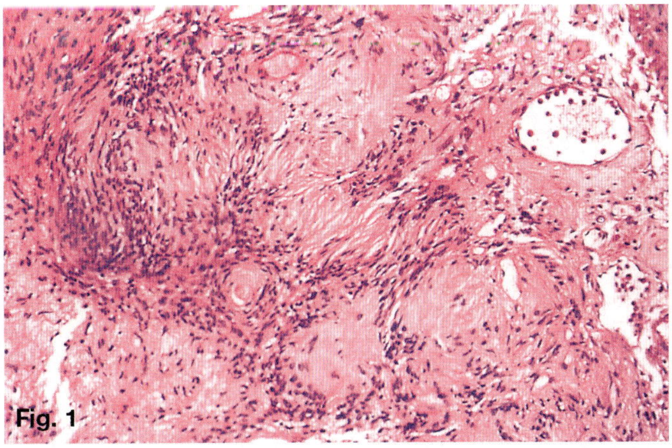

Fig. 1

A. Leiomyoma
B. Melanoma
C. Neurofibroma
D. Perineurioma
E. Schwannoma

24. What is the most likely diagnosis for the slowly growing cytokeratin-positive soft tissue mass, shown in Figure 1, on the hand of a 34-year-old female?

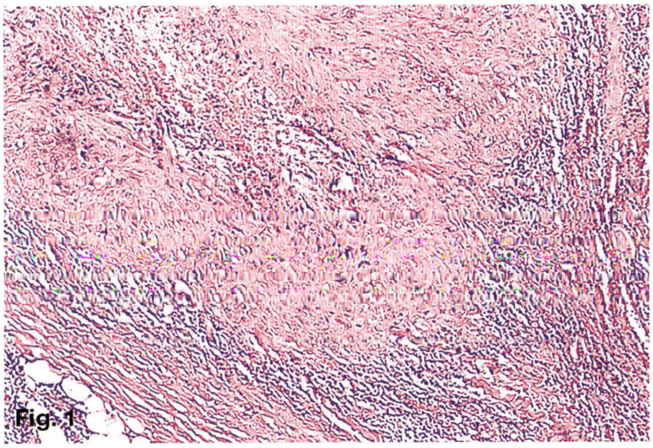

Fig. 1

A. Epithelioid angiosarcoma
B. Epithelioid sarcoma
C. Metastatic carcinoma
D. Myoepithelial carcinoma
E. Rheumatoid nodule

25. Which of the following immunohistochemical stains is most useful to establish the diagnosis of the slowly growing cytokeratin-positive soft tissue mass, shown in Figure 1, on the hand of a 34-year-old female?

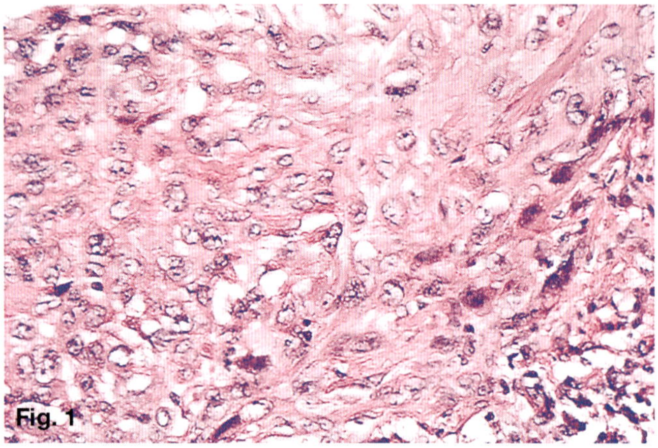

Fig. 1

A. DDIT3
B. PRKAR1A
C. SMARCA4
D. SMARCA5
E. SMARCB1

26. Which gene fusion is most often associated with clear cell sarcoma?

A. *EWSR1-ATF1*
B. *EWSR1-FLI1*
C. *EWSR1-NR4A3*
D. *EWSR1/SMAD3*
E. *EWSR1-WT1*

27. Which gene fusion is associated with Ewing sarcoma?

A. *EWSR1-ATF1*
B. *EWSR1-CREB1*
C. *EWSR1-FLI1*
D. *EWSR1-NR4A3*
E. *EWSR1-WT1*

28. Which gene fusion is associated with desmoplastic small round cell tumor?

A. *EWSR1-ATF1*
B. *EWSR1-CREB1*
C. *EWSR1-FLI1*
D. *EWSR1-NR4A3*
E. *EWSR1-WT1*

29. Which gene fusion is associated with extraskeletal myxoid chondrosarcoma?

A. *EWSR1-ATF1*
B. *EWSR1-CREB1*
C. *EWSR1-FLI1*
D. *EWSR1-NR4A3*
E. *EWSR1-WT1*

30. The intra-abdominal soft tissue mass from a 34-year-old female, shown in Figure 1, harbors a *TFE3* rearrangement. What is the most likely diagnosis?

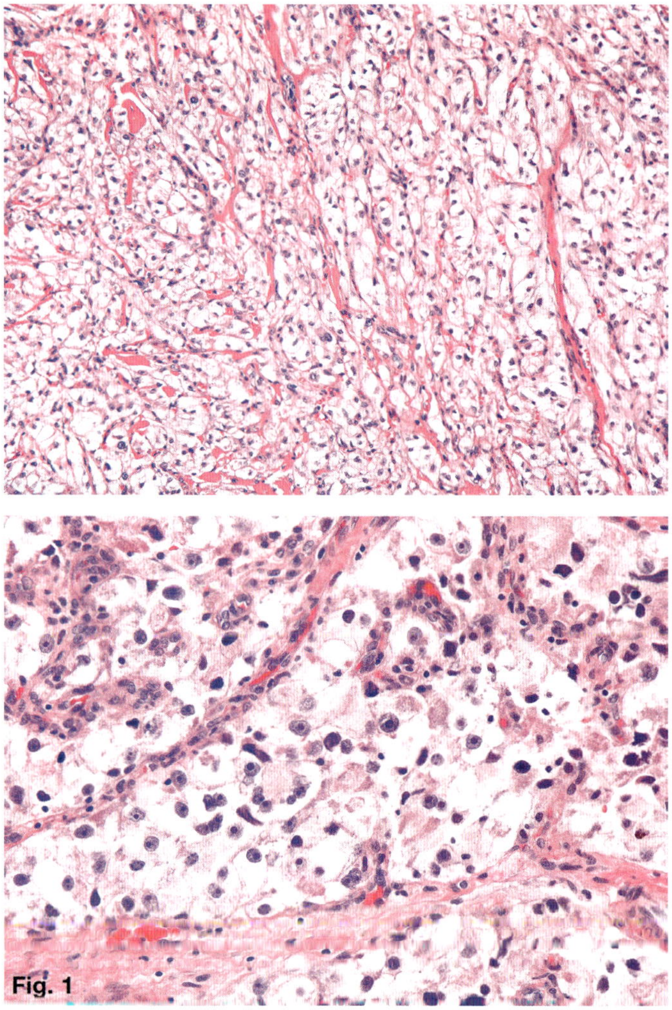

Fig. 1

A. Alveolar soft part sarcoma
B. Extraskeletal myxoid chondrosarcoma
C. Metastatic malignant melanoma
D. Myoepithelial carcinoma of soft tissue
E. Perivascular epithelioid cell tumor

31. Which of the following neoplasms is considered the soft tissue equivalent of melanoma?

A. Alveolar soft part sarcoma
B. Clear cell sarcoma
C. Epithelioid sarcoma
D. Granular cell tumor
E. Perivascular epithelioid cell tumor

32. What is the best diagnosis for the rapidly growing soft tissue tumor, shown in Figure 1, from the thigh of a 54-year-old man?

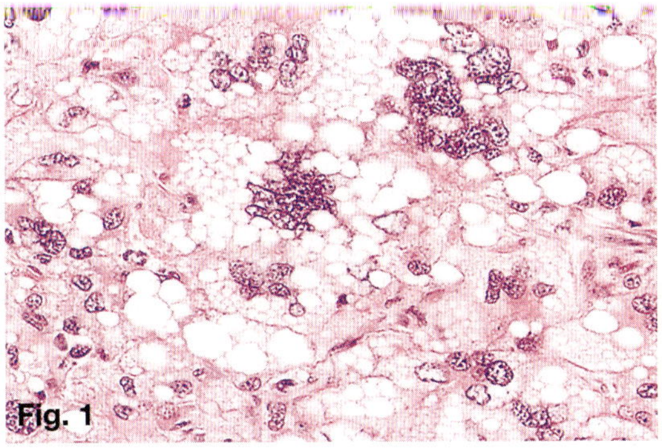
Fig. 1

A. Atypical lipomatous tumor
B. Dedifferentiated liposarcoma
C. Myxoid liposarcoma
D. Myxoid pleomorphic liposarcoma
E. Pleomorphic liposarcoma

33. What is the best diagnosis for the deep soft tissue tumor, shown in Figure 1, from the thigh of a 44-year-old man?

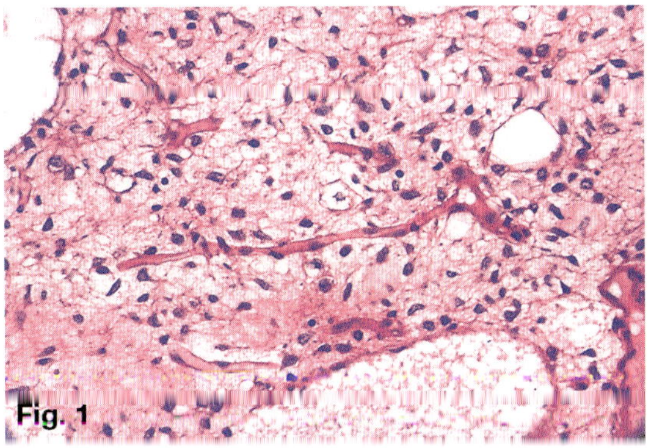
Fig. 1

A. Atypical lipomatous tumor
B. Dedifferentiated liposarcoma
C. Myxoid liposarcoma
D. Myxoid pleomorphic liposarcoma
E. Pleomorphic liposarcoma

34. The tumor, shown in Figure 1, from the deep soft tissue of the arm in a 32-year-old female harbors a t(X;18) chromosomal translocation. What is the most likely diagnosis?

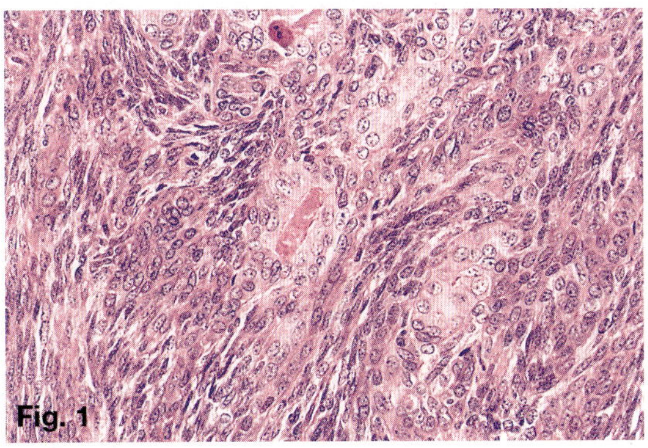
Fig. 1

A. Cellular schwannoma
B. Fibrosarcoma
C. Leiomyosarcoma
D. Solitary fibrous tumor
E. Synovial sarcoma

35. The soft tissue tumor from a 28 year old female, shown in Figure 1, expresses CD99 and NKX2.2. What is the most likely diagnosis?

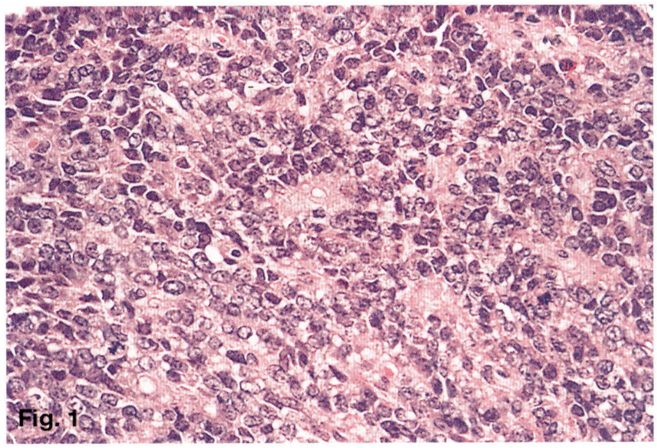
Fig. 1

A. Alveolar rhabdomyosarcoma
B. Extraskeletal Ewing sarcoma
C. Large cell lymphoma
D. Myeloid sarcoma
E. Poorly differentiated synovial sarcoma

36. What is the best diagnosis for the thigh mass, shown in Figure 1, in a 48-year-old man?

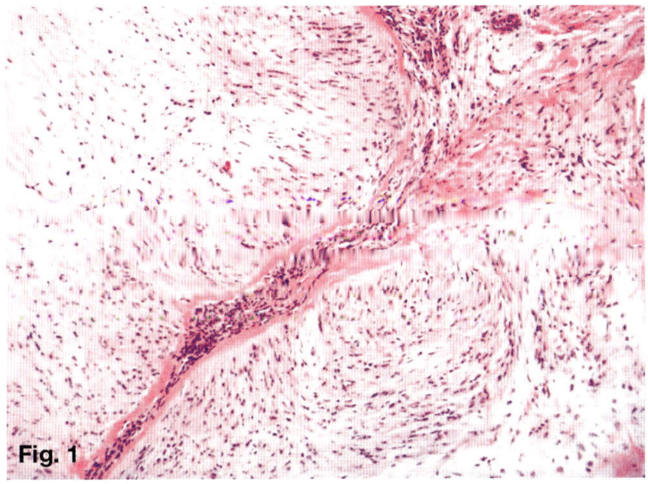
Fig. 1

A. Epithelioid myxofibrosarcoma
B. Extraskeletal myxoid chondrosarcoma
C. Myxoinflammatory fibrosarcoma
D. Ossifying fibromyxoid tumor
E. Soft tissue myoepithelioma

37. Which of the following tumors is often positive for CD99 and NKX2.2?

A. Alveolar rhabdomyosarcoma and Ewing sarcoma
B. Ewing sarcoma and extraskeletal myxoid chondrosarcoma
C. Ewing sarcoma and mesenchymal chondrosarcoma
D. Myeloid sarcoma and mesenchymal chondrosarcoma
E. Synovial sarcoma and mesenchymal chondrosarcoma

38. What is the best diagnosis for the poorly circumscribed, firm, rubbery, plaque-like soft tissue mass, shown in Figure 1, in the right forearm of an 18-year-old male?

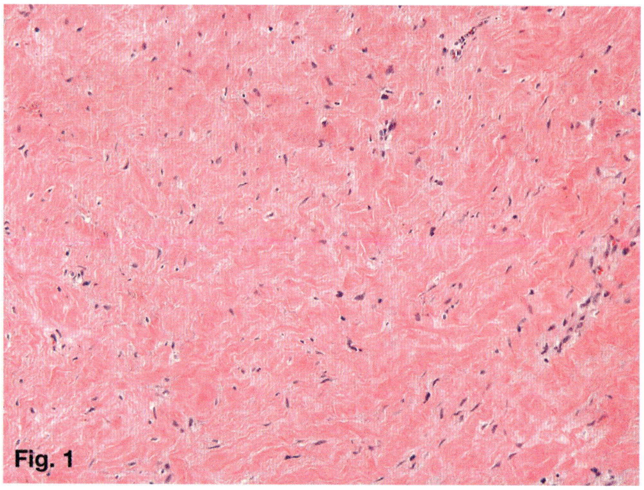

Fig. 1

A. Desmoid fibromatosis
B. Desmoplastic fibroblastoma
C. Fibroma of tendon sheath
D. Gardner fibroma
E. Nuchal fibroma

39. The soft tissue mass, shown in Figure 1, in a 20-year-old male harbors a *PAX3-FOXO1A* gene fusion. What is the most likely diagnosis?

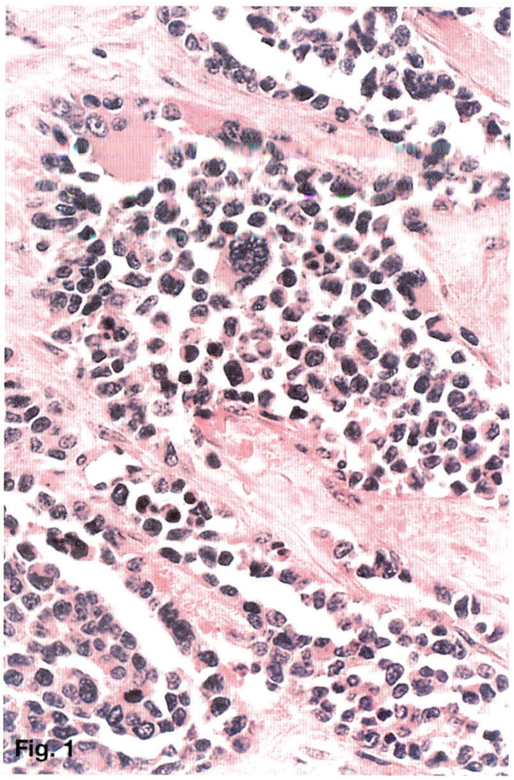

Fig. 1

A. Alveolar rhabdomyoblastoma
B. Alveolar soft part sarcoma
C. Desmoplastic round cell tumor
D. Embryonal rhabdomyoblastoma
E. Pleomorphic rhabdomyoblastoma

40. A 22-year-old male has a right pelvis mass. The tumor is surgically resected. The tumor cells, shown in Figure 1, are immunoreactive for desmin, which is expressed in a dotlike perinuclear pattern. The tumor cells are also positive for keratin. Which of the following is the most likely diagnosis?

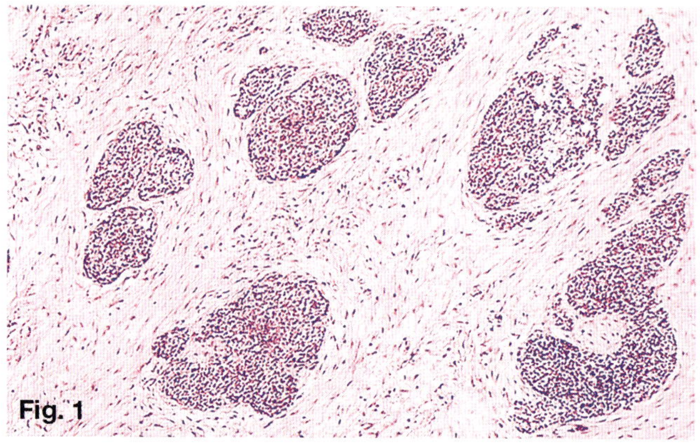

Fig. 1

A. Alveolar rhabdomyosarcoma
B. *CIC-DUX4* rearranged sarcoma
C. Desmoplastic small round cell tumor
D. Embryonal rhabdomyosarcoma
E. Extraskeletal Ewing sarcoma

41. Which of the following vascular lesions is thought to arise as a florid form of organized and recanalized thrombus?

A. Capillary hemangioma
B. Intravascular papillary endothelial hyperplasia
C. Malignant endovascular papillary angioendothelioma
D. Spindle cell hemangioendothelioma
E. Symplastic hemangioma

42. What is the most likely diagnosis for the CD34-positive, keratin AE1/AE3-positive, circumscribed tumor, shown in Figure 1, in the dermis and subcutaneous tissue of the thigh in a 28-year-old male?

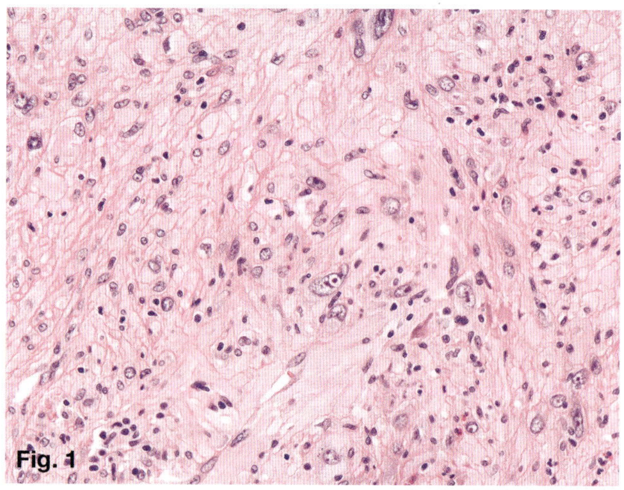

Fig. 1

A. Dermatofibrosarcoma protuberans
B. Epithelioid sarcoma
C. Malignant granular cell tumor
D. Superficial CD34-positive fibroblastic tumor
E. Undifferentiated pleomorphic sarcoma

43. A small subcutaneous nodule removed from the wrist of a 13-year-old male consists of spindly, fibroblast-like cells with spotty calcifications. The cells surrounding the calcific foci resemble chondrocytes. There is no cytologic atypia. Peripheral infiltration of muscle is seen. Which of the following is the most likely diagnosis?

A. Calcifying aponeurotic fibroma
B. Fibroma of the tendon sheath
C. Fibromatosis
D. Rheumatoid nodule
E. Schwannoma

44. What is the most likely diagnosis for the anaplastic lymphoma kinase (ALK)-positive intra-abdominal mass, shown in Figure 1, in a 44-year-old female?

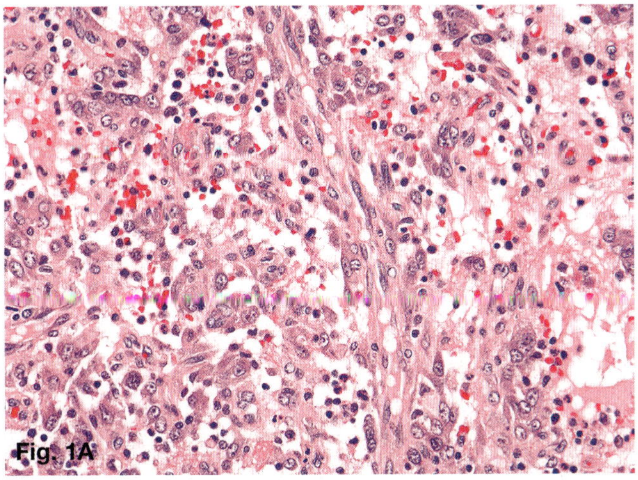
Fig. 1A

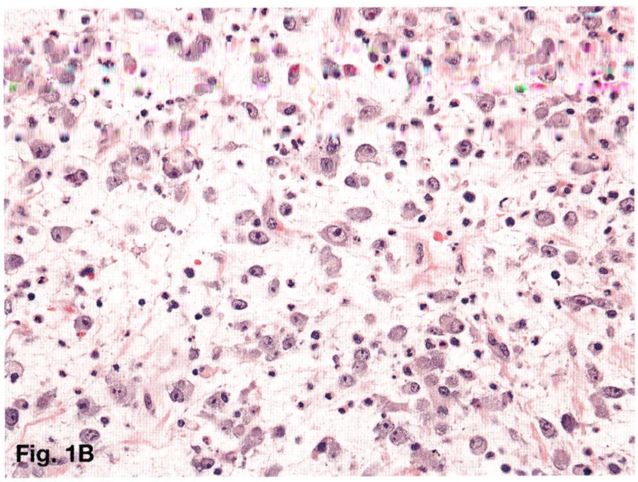
Fig. 1B

A. Desmoid fibromatosis
B. Inflammatory myofibroblastic tumor
C. Low-grade myofibroblastic sarcoma
D. *NTRK*-rearranged spindle cell neoplasm
E. Pleomorphic rhabdomyosarcoma

45. Which of the following microscopic patterns is most characteristic of dermatofibrosarcoma protuberans?

A. Cartwheel/storiform pattern with no significant atypia
B. Long spindle cell fascicles in a herringbone pattern
C. Parallel strands of keloid-like collagen
D. Spindle cell tumor with giant rosettes
E. Zonal architecture entrapping adipose tissue

46. A 48-year-old woman undergoes excision of a retroperitoneal tumor whose typical histology is shown in Figure 1. What is the most likely diagnosis?

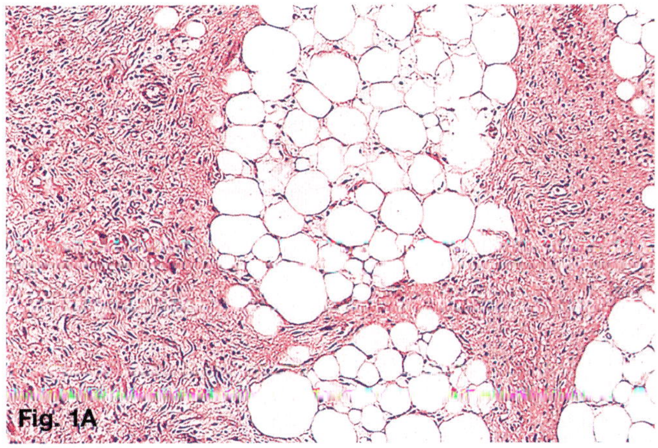
Fig. 1A

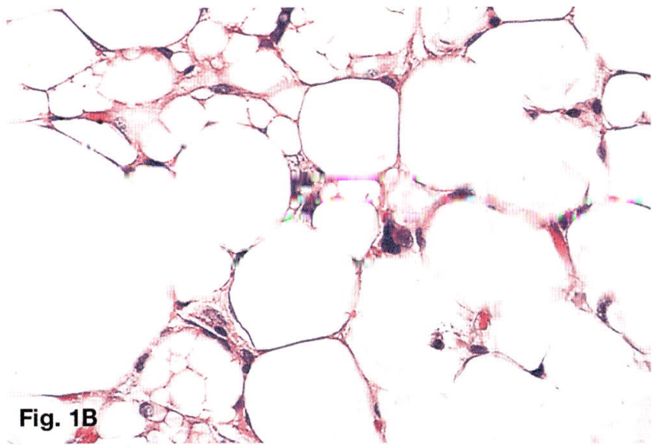
Fig. 1B

A. Atypical lipomatous tumor
B. Lipoblastoma
C. Myxoid liposarcoma
D. Pleomorphic lipoma
E. Pleomorphic liposarcoma

47. Which of the following is most characteristic of fibrosarcoma?

A. Herringbone pattern
B. Palisading of cells
C. Storiform pattern
D. Sweeping fascicles
E. Tuft and weave pattern

48. A 15-cm soft tissue mass is removed from the thigh of a 56-year-old man. The tumor cells, shown in Figure 1, are immunoreactive for vimentin but negative for cytokeratin, S100 protein, desmin, myoglobin, smooth muscle actin, and CD34. Which of the following diagnoses is most likely?

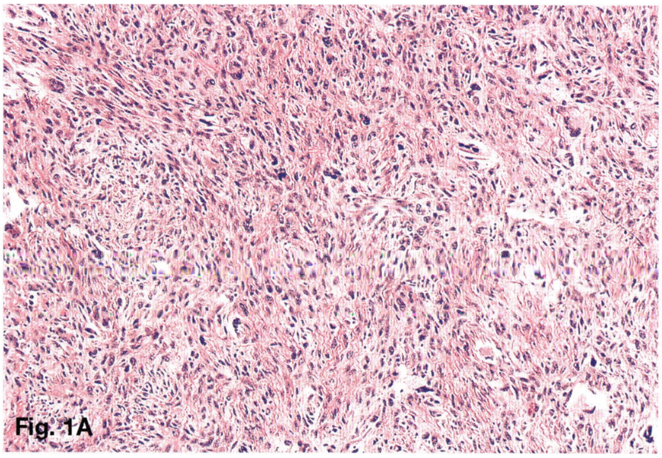
Fig. 1A

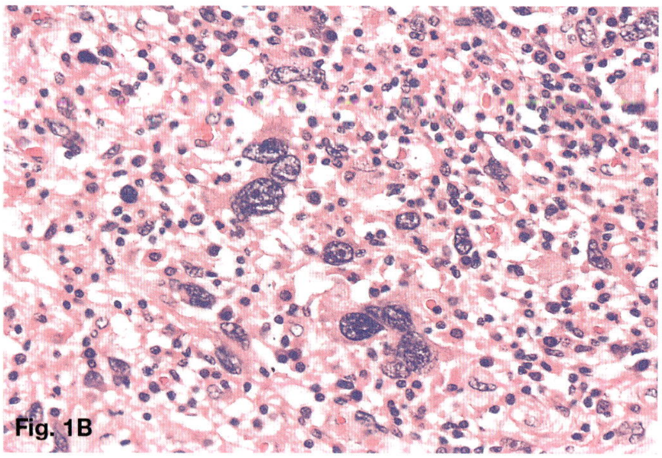
Fig. 1B

A. Dermatofibrosarcoma protuberans
B. Fibromatosis
C. Fibrosarcoma
D. Poorly differentiated rhabdomyosarcoma
E. Undifferentiated pleomorphic sarcoma

49. A highly anaplastic soft tissue neoplasm from a 5-year-old child consists of undifferentiated small cells with no distinctive features. Neoplastic cells tend to gather in dense aggregates beneath epithelial surfaces and around blood vessels, as seen in Figure 1. Which of the following is the most likely diagnosis?

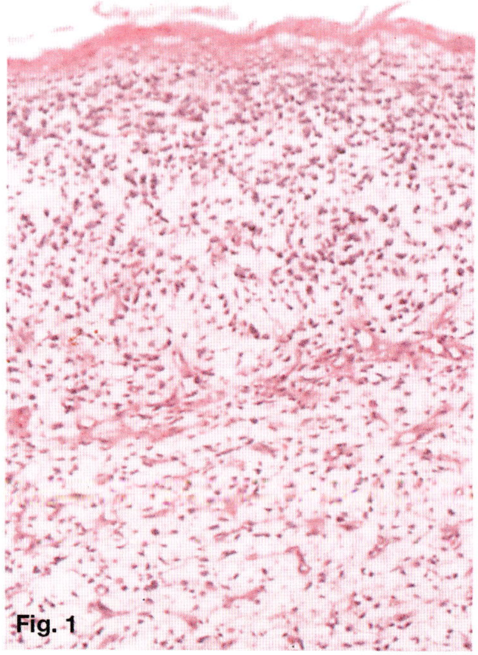
Fig. 1

A. Desmoplastic small cell tumor
B. Embryonal rhabdomyosarcoma
C. Extraskeletal Ewing sarcoma
D. Lymphoblastic lymphoma
E. Neuroblastoma

50. A 2-cm poorly circumscribed tumor is excised from the forearm of a 34-year-old female. The granular cells, shown in Figure 1, are immunoreactive for S100 protein and SOX10. Which of the following is the most likely diagnosis?

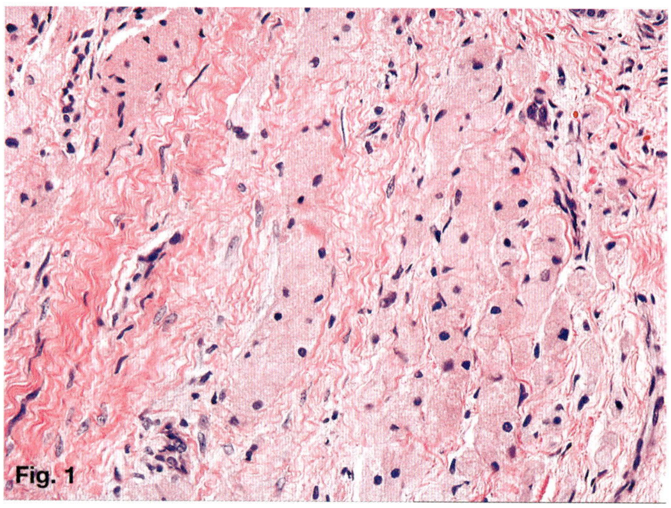
Fig. 1

A. Granular cell tumor
B. Langerhans cell histiocytosis
C. Malignant melanoma
D. Myoepithelioma
E. Perivascular epithelioid tumor

# ANSWERS AND EXPLANATIONS

**1. Correct choice: C.**

Solitary fibrous tumor is positive for STAT6. STAT6 immunohistochemistry is a highly sensitive and specific surrogate for *NAB2-STAT6* gene fusion. The fusion arises as a result of paracentric inversion involving chromosome 12q. *NAB2-STAT6* fusions convert NAB2 from a transcriptional repressor to an activator. Altered NAB2 function leads to constitutive expression of early growth response 1 (EGR1) target genes, including *IGF2* and *FGFR1*. Typically, CD34 is also strong and diffuse in solitary fibrous tumors, but it is nonspecific.

**2. Correct choice: E.**

Nodular fasciitis is a fibroblastic/myofibroblastic neoplasm that is typically benign and self-limited. It occurs in a wide range of ages and anatomic distribution. It most commonly originates in the subcutis but may also arise in the dermis, fascia, and skeletal muscle. It is generally small (<3 cm) and forms a mass that may be tender, mildly painful, or asymptomatic. Rapid growth may be clinically concerning for malignancy. Almost all cases contain recurrent gene fusions; *MYH9-USP6* is the most common fusion product, although many other *USP6* partners have been identified in nodular fasciitis and related entities (eg, cranial fasciitis, fibroma of tendon sheath, myositis ossificans, aneurysmal bone cyst). Microscopically, there is variable cellularity with an extracellular myxoid to collagenous matrix. Older lesions may be more collagenous and there may be foci of cystic degeneration. The constituent stellate spindle cells form a loose fascicular to storiform pattern (the so-called tissue culture-like and feathery growth). Nuclei are bland and ovoid, but there may be numerous mitotic figures. Scattered lymphocytes, histiocytes, and osteoclast-type giant cells are often present. The stellate cells are positive for smooth muscle actin, muscle-specific actin, and calponin. Fibrous histiocytoma contains a mixed population of foamy macrophages and spindle cells with peripheral collagen entrapment and variable expression of factor XIIIa. Desmoid-type fibromatosis exhibits a predominant fascicular pattern and expresses nuclear β-catenin. Lipoblastoma is a benign, rapidly growing neoplasm composed of embryonal white fat with variable degrees of myxoid change. It occurs predominantly in infancy and early childhood, and very rarely in adulthood. It is a superficial, localized, well-circumscribed lesion. Although myxoid liposarcoma typically occurs in the extremities (proximal thigh in particular) and exhibits prominent myxoid stroma, it is characterized by a prominent branching vasculature (the so-called chicken-wire vasculature).

**3. Correct choice: E.**

Spindle cell lipoma is a benign superficial soft tissue neoplasm. 80% of spindle cell lipomas arise in the subcutaneous tissue of the posterior neck, back, and shoulders in middle-aged to older men (45-70 years). It is rare in patients younger than 20 years. Less than 10% of cases occur in women and when they do, they tend to arise in atypical locations. Histologically, spindle cell lipoma contains a varying mixture of mature adipocytes, bland spindle cells, and ropy collagen fibers. Spindle cell lipoma is associated with breakpoint clusters around 13q14 where the *RB1* gene resides, leading to loss of RB1 on immunohistochemistry. It is part of the 13q/*RB1* family of tumors, which includes myofibroblastoma and cellular angiofibroma. Pleomorphic lipoma is a histologic variant of spindle cell lipoma characterized by large, pleomorphic, and floret-type giant cells. It arises in the same clinical setting and is also characterized by loss of RB1 on immunohistochemistry. Angiolipoma is a benign, soft tissue tumor consisting of mature adipose tissue and clusters of thin-walled vessels, often containing intraluminal fibrin thrombi. It is relatively common in young adults, typically appearing in the forearm, trunk, and upper arm during the late second to early third decade of life. The clinical presentation is often characterized by multiple subcutaneous small nodules, which are tender or painful. There is a male predominance. Chondrolipoma is a rare, slow-growing, painless variant of lipoma that affects the proximal extremities and limb girdles of adult women. Clinically, it is a lobulated, circumscribed, deep-seated tumor composed of nests and cords of uni- and multivacuolated lipoblasts with variable adipose tissue in a myxochondroid matrix. Intramuscular myxoma arises in the thigh, shoulder, and upper arm of adults, aged 40 to 70 years. On biopsy, it is a hypocellular lesion composed of bland cells set in a myxoid matrix; there are no lipoblasts.

**4. Correct choice: B.**

Intramuscular myxoma arises in the thigh, shoulder, and upper arm of adults, aged 4 to 70 years. There is a slight female predominance. It is typically solitary but may be multiple when associated with the Carney complex. On biopsy, it is a paucicellular lesion composed of bland spindle cells set in a finely granular myxoid matrix with scattered macrophages; there are no lipoblasts. It is often slightly more cellular with a collagenized capsule at the periphery.

There may be infiltration into striated muscle at the periphery, associated with muscle atrophy. GNAS1 mutations occur in 61% of intramuscular myxomas. Intramuscular lipoma is composed of mature adipocytes diffusely infiltrating the skeletal muscle. The involved muscle fibers may show some atrophy; however, there are no lipoblasts or cells with atypical nuclei. Myxofibrosarcoma is the most common sarcoma of older patients. It presents as a painless, superficial, subcutaneous mass in the extremities. Grossly, it is a multinodular, gelatinous, lobulated tumor with infiltrative margins. Microscopically, it is composed of spindle-to-stellate cells in a myxoid stroma with curvilinear vessels. Extraskeletal myxoid chondrosarcoma is a malignant mesenchymal neoplasm of uncertain differentiation with abundant myxoid matrix, multilobular architecture, and uniform cells arranged in cords, clusters, and reticular networks.

Myxoid liposarcoma arises in the deep soft tissue and is characterized by hypocellularity, chicken-wire capillary network, and myxoid matrix.

**5. Correct choice: B.**

Fetal rhabdomyoma, which is occasionally confused with well differentiated rhabdomyosarcoma, occurs predominantly in the head and neck of toddlers and is characterized by small parallel bundles of spindled skeletal muscle cells separated by thin strands of collagen and vascular tissue. Their nuclei are bland and lack mitoses.

**6. Correct choice: A.**

Elastofibroma often develops at the apex of the scapula, deep into the muscle layer. The presence of cylindrical structures composed of immature elastic fibers is characteristic. The etiology is unknown, but it is probably a reactive process. Surgical excision is curative.

**7. Correct choice: C.**

Myxoinflammatory fibroblastic sarcoma is a rare, low-grade sarcoma of the distal extremities with prominent myxoid stroma, mixed inflammation, virocyte-like cells, pseudolipoblasts, and emperipolesis. This sarcoma occurs in the hands and feet. It is a multinodular tumor consisting of fibrotic areas containing chronic inflammation intermixed with myxoid areas containing spindly and epithelioid cells. Peculiar cells in the tumor are virocytes, which resemble Reed-Sternberg cells, and cells filled with a basophilic substance similar to the extracellular matrix in myxoid areas. The constituent cells express vimentin, focal cytokeratin (CK), and focal CD68. Multiple local recurrences are not uncommon, but distant metastases are rare. Low-grade fibromyxoid sarcoma is a malignant tumor resembling fibromatosis. Myxofibrosarcoma is the most common sarcoma of older patients. It is a multinodular, gelatinous, lobulated tumor with infiltrative margins. Microscopically, it is composed of spindle-to-stellate cells in a myxoid stroma with curvilinear vessels. Sclerosing epithelioid fibrosarcoma is also an aggressive tumor composed of nests and cords of round cells with scanty cytoplasm and brisk mitotic activity, surrounded by sclerosing hyaline bands. Superficial angiomyxoma occurs in the head and neck, trunk, and genital area in children and adults. It exhibits a multilobulated growth pattern in the dermis and subcutis that is composed of bland spindle-to-stellate cells in a myxoid stroma. The vessels are thin walled and arranged in an arborizing pattern. Stromal neutrophils are seen in 50% of cases. Nests of epithelial cells may also be present related to a hair follicle.

**8. Correct choice: D.**

Low-grade fibromyxoid sarcoma occurs in the proximal extremities and trunk of young adults. There is a slight male predominance. It features alternating collagenous hypocellular areas with cellular myxoid nodules characterized by bland fusiform or spindled cells with focal to diffuse whirling in the heavily collagenized stroma with abrupt transition to myxoid areas; 45% have epithelioid areas and 40% contain poorly formed but large collagen rosettes. The hypocellular myxoid component contains arcades of thin-walled vessels. It often infiltrates adjacent skeletal muscle. Despite the bland sarcoma, this tumor can metastasize years to decades after initial diagnosis. It is EMA (epithelial membrane antigen) and MUC4 (mucin 4) positive. The *FUS-CREB3L2* gene fusion is common. Desmoid-type fibromatosis (although typically lacking myxoid areas) may be myxoid, but the fibrous cells are aligned in broad sweeping, straighter fascicles and are positive for nuclear β-catenin. Desmoplastic fibroblastoma (also called collagenous fibroma) arises in the subcutis; it is hypocellular with dense collagenous stroma and scattered stellate spindle cells. It does not recur. Giant cell fibroblastoma is a rare cutaneous tumor that occurs in boys younger than 10 years of age. Tumor cells, including multinucleated forms, are scattered within a collagenous stroma. Up to 50% of patients develop recurrences. Sclerosing epithelioid fibrosarcoma is composed of nests and cords of round cells with scanty cytoplasm and brisk mitotic activity surrounded by sclerosing hyaline bands.

**9. Correct choice: D.**

Pseudomyogenic hemangioendothelioma (epithelioid sarcoma-like hemangioendothelioma, fibroma-like variant of epithelioid sarcoma) is a locally aggressive but rarely metastasizing vascular tumor occurring most commonly in adults younger than 40 years. There is a male predominance. The most common location is the lower extremities, followed by the upper limbs and trunk. It is often multifocal (two-thirds of reported cases). It may present as painful or painless nodules. More than 50% of patients develop local recurrence; metastases are rare. It may arise in the dermis, subcutaneous tissue, muscle, or bone. Microscopically, it is characterized by fascicles or sheets of plump spindled to epithelioid cells with vesicular nuclei, variably prominent nucleoli, and bright eosinophilic cytoplasm arranged in a vaguely nodular or plexiform pattern. The constituent cells may resemble rhabdomyofibroblasts. A desmoplastic reaction may be seen, and there may be a variably prominent inflammatory (usually neutrophilic) infiltrate. The neoplastic cells are positive for AE1/AE3, ERG (erythroblast transformation specific-related gene), FLI1 (Friend leukemia integration 1), CD31, and nuclear FOSB (FBJ murine osteosarcoma viral oncogene homolog B) on immunohistochemistry. SMARCB1 (INI1) (SWI/SNF related, matrix associated, actin dependent regulator of chromatin, subfamily B, member 1 [integrase interactor 1]) is retained. The tumor is driven by overexpression of FOSB, a protein involved in the AP-1 transcription complex that plays a role in cell growth and proliferation, cellular differentiation, and apoptosis. This tumor harbors *FOSB* gene rearrangements, either due to *SERPINE1-FOSB* or *ACTB-FOSB* fusions. Epithelioid hemangioendothelioma typically has intracytoplasmic lumina with red blood cells and a prominent myxohyaline background; it lacks bright eosinophilic cytoplasm. Also, it is negative for FOSB but positive for CAMTA1 (calmodulin binding transcription activator 1). Epithelioid sarcoma shares overlapping features with pseudomyogenic hemangioendothelioma, including positivity for ERG (depending on the antibody) and CD34, but it is typically negative for CD31 and FLI1, and SMARCB1 (INI1) is lost. Kaposiform hemangioendothelioma is a rare and locally aggressive endothelial neoplasm that often involves the entire dermis and extends into the subcutaneous tissue. It occurs in children, often at birth or shortly after birth, and is characterized by proliferation of spindle-shaped endothelial cells and associated capillary hemangioma-like lymphatic vessels. Retiform hemangioendothelioma is a locally aggressive, infiltrating vascular neoplasm composed of elongated arborizing vascular channels lined by endothelial cells with prominent hobnail nuclei with hyperchromasia but no atypia and rare mitotic activity. It presents as plaque-like areas of discoloration in young adults and has a high rate of local recurrence after incomplete excision.

**10. Correct choice: D.**

Solitary fibrous tumor features a haphazard arrangement of spindled to ovoid cells with indistinct cell borders arranged around branching and dilated ("staghorn") vasculature within variably hyalinized to collagenous stroma. The cells may stream between collagen fibers. It occurs at any anatomic site, in superficial and deep soft tissues, visceral organs, and bone. Deep soft tissue is more common. CD34 is usually strong and diffuse but nonspecific. STAT6 is a highly sensitive and specific surrogate for *NAB2-STAT6* gene fusion. Myxoid changes can be prominent. A lipomatous variant contains variable amount of fat. The giant cell–rich variant, formerly known as giant cell angiofibroma, shows admixed multinucleated giant cells lining pseudovascular spaces. Fibrosarcoma is a rare malignant tumor that may arise from superficial or deep sites. The most characteristic architectural feature is a herringbone pattern, in which fascicles of neoplastic fibroblast-like cells with oval nuclei intersect at acute angles. Reticulin staining demonstrates reticulin fibers investing each cell. Dermatofibrosarcoma protuberans may resemble a subset of solitary fibrous tumors, which lack obvious hemangiopericytoma-like vasculature and appear densely cellular and monomorphic. Dermatofibrosarcoma protuberans is positive for CD34 but negative for STAT6. Also, it harbors *COLIA1-PDGFB* gene fusions. Leiomyosarcoma has a fascicular architecture and cells with blunt-ended cigar-shaped nuclei and bright pink eosinophilic cytoplasm. It is positive for smooth muscle actin, desmin, and h-caldesmon. Synovial sarcoma can exhibit hemangiopericytoma-like vasculature, but it is negative for CD34 and STAT6. Also, it harbors *SS18-SSX* gene fusions.

**11. Correct choice: B.**

Alveolar soft part sarcoma is a rare malignant mesenchymal neoplasm frequently composed of large, polygonal cells with abundant eosinophilic cytoplasm, a nested or pseudoalveolar growth pattern, and PAS/D (periodic acid-Schiff stain with diastase)-positive intracytoplasmic rhomboid or rod-shaped crystals. It predominantly affects the deep soft tissues of the extremities (thigh and buttock) in young adults and head and neck region (tongue and orbit) in children. There is a well-documented female predominance, which is less pronounced in patients greater than 30 years. It is characterized by the *ASPSCR1-TFE3* gene fusion. Alveolar rhabdomyosarcoma occurs in older children and is the most frequent type of rhabdomyosarcoma of the extremities and trunk. The characteristic microscopic appearance results from the fibrous septa that divide the tumor into alveolar-like spaces, where tumor cells at the periphery cling to the septa, while the cells in the center are discohesive. The tumor cells show strong nuclear immunoreactivity for myogenin. Epithelioid sarcoma is a malignant epithelioid tumor occurring in pediatric and adult populations. It has an unpredictable clinical course. There are two morphologic types: the classic type with epithelioid to spindled cells with central pseudogranulomatous architecture and the proximal type with predominant epithelioid and rhabdoid cells. Both types are positive for pancytokeratin and often, CD34. SMARA4 (INI1) (SWI/SNF related, matrix associated, actin dependent regulator of chromatin, subfamily A, member 4 [integrase interactor 1]) is lost. Granular cell tumor is a neoplasm composed of epithelioid to spindle cells with eosinophilic cytoplasmic granules. It has been reported in a variety of locations, most often the tongue. Ultrastructural studies have shown that the granules are modified lysosomes containing hydrolytic enzymes such as acid phosphatase. Granular cell tumors are positive for S100, inhibin, and calretinin. Malignant melanoma can be positive for S100, SOX10, HMB45, and other melanocytic markers.

**12. Correct choice: E.**

Palisaded myofibroblastoma (intranodal hemorrhagic spindle cell tumor with amianthoid fibers) occurs almost exclusively in inguinal lymph nodes. Intersecting bundles of uniform bland spindle cells with myofibroblastic or smooth muscle differentiation, interstitial hemorrhage, and hemosiderin replace nodal tissue. The constituent cells have scant eosinophilic cytoplasm, perinuclear vacuoles, and bland fusiform nuclei. Focal nuclear palisading is often present. A rim of compressed normal tissue may be seen. Amianthoid fibers (strongly eosinophilic, stellate, extracellular matrix deposits composed of crystalline fibers) may also be present with variable calcification. Mitotic figures are rare to absent; there is no atypia, slit-like vascular spaces, or extravasated red blood cells. Palisaded myofibroblastoma harbors *CTNNB1* mutations and exhibits nuclear β-catenin expression on immunohistochemistry. Benign metastasizing leiomyoma is composed of smooth muscle cells with more prominent eosinophilic cytoplasm; there is no hemorrhage or amianthoid fibers. Benign metastasizing leiomyoma positive for desmin and negative for nuclear β-catenin expression. Dendritic cell sarcoma is characterized by nests or whorls of plump cells with scattered inflammatory cells; the constituent cells are positive for CD21 and CD35. Intranodal schwannoma typically has a distinct biphasic pattern and is positive for S100 protein. Metastatic leiomyosarcoma exhibits more cytologic atypia and mitotic figures; desmin is often positive.

**13. Correct choice: B.**

Low-grade fibromyxoid sarcoma harbors a translocation t(7;16)(q34;p11) or t(11;16)(p11;p11), resulting in *FUS-CREB3L2* (>90%) or *FUS-CREB3L1*.

**14. Correct choice: B.**

MUC4 (mucin 4) expression is a useful confirmatory immunohistochemical marker for the diagnosis of low-grade fibromyxoid sarcoma, especially in distinguishing soft tissue perineurioma, since both tumors can express EMA (epithelial membrane antigen).

**15. Correct choice: D.**

Sclerosing epithelioid fibrosarcoma is a rare, malignant mesenchymal tumor that occurs in adults with median age of 45 years. These tumors are deep seated and arise in the lower extremities and limb girdles, followed by the trunk, upper limb girdles, and the head and neck. They are characterized by cords, nests, or sheets of uniform, small, round to ovoid epithelioid cells set within a dense collagenous background. The hyalinized sclerotic stroma may resemble osteoid or cartilage. Areas with pseudoalveolar patterns may be present. Focal ectatic staghorn vessels may also be present. Mitotic figures are generally rare to absent. A subset of cases contains areas morphologically similar to low-grade fibromyxoid sarcoma. Most cases are positive for MUC4 (mucin 4); EMA (epithelial membrane antigen) and smooth muscle actin may also be positive. The most common gene fusion is *EWSR1-CREB3L1*, but cases with areas of low-grade fibromyxoid sarcoma often harbor *EWSR1-CREB3L2* fusions. Metastatic signet-ring carcinoma from the breast or stomach may form cords, nests, and chains of small- to medium-sized epithelial cells, but they exhibit strong cytokeratin expression and densely sclerotic stroma is uncommon. In addition, there is often clinical evidence of a primary tumor. Ossifying fibromyxoid tumors typically have a peripheral shell of lamellar bone and express CD10, S100 protein, and desmin (70% of cases). Most cases have a *PHF1* gene rearrangement. Parosteal osteosarcoma is a low-grade, well-differentiated osteosarcoma that occurs on the surface of the metaphysis of long bones. Integration of clinical and radiologic data is the cornerstone of diagnosis. Sclerosing rhabdomyosarcoma features occasional rhabdomyoblasts. The tumor is positive for MyoD1 (myogenic differentiation 1) expression with variable desmin and myogenin expression. It is negative for MUC4. None of these latter tumors harbor *EWSR1* and *CREB3L1* rearrangements.

**16. Correct choice: B.**

Myofibroblastoma is a benign spindle cell tumor composed of fibroblasts and myofibroblasts with recurrent monoallelic loss of 13q14 region including *RB1*. It is a well-circumscribed spindle cell tumor composed of short fascicles of bland spindled cells and dense hyalinized collagen bundles. Histologic variants include collagenized or fibrous, cellular, infiltrative, myxoid, deciduoid, epithelioid, and lipomatous. It is positive for desmin and CD34. It occurs predominantly in the inguinal soft tissue in men (median age 55 years). It is part of the 13q/*RB1* family of tumors, which includes spindle cell lipoma and cellular angiofibroma. Desmoid-type fibromatosis expresses nuclear β-catenin. Nodular fasciitis is characterized by variable cellularity with an extracellular myxoid to collagenous matrix. Older lesions may be more collagenous. The constituent stellate spindle cells form a loose fascicular to storiform pattern (the so-called tissue culture-like and feathery growth). Solitary fibrous tumor features a haphazard arrangement of spindled to ovoid cells with indistinct cell borders arranged around branching and dilated ("staghorn") vasculature within variably hyalinized to collagenous stroma. Although it is CD34 positive, it is also STAT6 positive, the latter being negative in myofibroblastoma. Spindle cell lipoma arises in the subcutaneous tissue of the posterior neck, back, and shoulders in middle-aged to older men (45-70 years). Although it is CD34 positive, it is desmin negative.

**17. Correct choice: B.**

Desmoplastic fibroblastoma (collagenous fibroma) is a well-circumscribed fibroblastic lesion centered in the subcutaneous tissue of the upper extremities, back, and feet. It is characterized by a paucicellular proliferation of bland spindled (stellate) and reactive appearing fibroblasts and myofibroblasts separated by abundant collagen with a variable myxoid stroma. The fibroblasts have amphophilic cytoplasm, vesicular nuclei, and distinct nucleoli. The spindle cells are positive for smooth muscle actin. It is benign, even though about 25% extend into skeletal muscle. Desmoid-type fibromatosis is not circumscribed and is more cellular, with a fascicular architecture. It is positive for nuclear β-catenin. Fibroma of tendon sheath is a benign, well-circumscribed fibroblastic/myofibroblastic nodular proliferation usually attached to a tendon or tendon sheath. The tumor exhibits variable cellularity, with the cellularity higher at tumor edges. The constituent cells are bland and set within a collagenous background. Thin-walled slit-like vessels are characteristic and degenerative myxoid and cystic changes may be present. Occasionally, there is osseous or chondroid metaplasia. Gardner fibroma is an uncommon, benign soft tissue lesion occurring in infants, children, and teenagers. It is characterized by the presence of thick, haphazard collagen and bland fibroblasts that entrap adjacent tissue. Approximately 90% are associated with familial adenomatous polyposis or Gardner syndrome. It may be the initial diagnostic clue to Gardner syndrome and *APC* mutations. Hypertrophic scar (keloid) is composed of excessive scar tissue that extends beyond the boundaries of the initial injury. It is characterized by broad, pink bands of collagen (keloidal collagen). Hypertrophic scars are very common in dark-skinned people. Recurrence after excision is common.

**18. Correct choice: C.**

Lipoblastoma is a benign, rapidly growing neoplasm composed of embryonal white fat with variable degrees of myxoid changes. It occurs in the trunk and extremities in infancy, early childhood, and very rarely, in adulthood. Up to 90% of lipoblastomas are seen before the age of 3 years; there is a male predilection (male-to-female, 2.8:1). It is characterized by a lobular architecture with intersecting fibrovascular septa, myxoid changes, and a spectrum of fat cell maturation. It is positive for S100 protein, CD34 (adipocytes and vascular network), and desmin (mesenchymal cells). It is typically associated with *PLAG1* rearrangement. The more common lipoblastoma is superficial, localized, and well circumscribed; it is easily excised. In contrast, the rarer lipoblastomatosis is deep, diffuse, and has irregular borders; complete excision is difficult. Chondroid lipoma contains areas of chondroid matrix. Hibernoma is a rare, benign, adipocytic tumor composed of variable proportions of brown fat cells admixed with white adipose tissue.

It occurs in a wide age range (2-75 years); 60% are present in the third and fourth decades of life. Lipoma is composed of mature adipocytes with paucicellular fibrous septa. Fat necrosis may be present, but immature adipocytes are not present. Although it is typically well-circumscribed, skeletal muscle fibers are often infiltrated in intramuscular lipoma. Spindle cell lipoma arises in the subcutaneous tissue of the posterior neck, back, and shoulders in middle-aged to older men (45-70 years).

**19. Correct choice: A.**

Myxofibrosarcoma includes a range of malignant fibroblastic tumors with myxoid stroma, variable pleomorphism, and characteristic curvilinear vasculature. It is the most common sarcoma of older patients. It presents as a painless, superficial, subcutaneous mass in the limbs. More than 50% arise in a dermal or subcutaneous location. About one-third arise in the deep soft tissue. It typically forms a multinodular, gelatinous, lobulated mass with infiltrative margins. Histologically, it is composed of spindle-to-stellate cells within a myxoid stroma with curvilinear vessels and scattered pleomorphic cells. Hypercellularity and severe pleomorphism are seen in high-grade tumors. A rare epithelioid variant is characterized by nests and sheets of epithelioid cells interspersed with focal areas of more conventional myxofibrosarcoma. It is graded on a 3-tier system using the FNCLCC (Fédération Nationale des Centres de Lutte Contre le Cancer) grading system. In general, the lesser the myxoid area, the poorer the prognosis. Tumor grade affects metastasis and tumor-related mortality. The prognosis is good when the tumor is superficial and low grade. Low-grade tumors usually do not metastasize (<5%), whereas high-grade tumors have a metastatic rate of 20% to 35%. Despite the risk for metastases, myxofibrosarcoma has a better prognosis than undifferentiated pleomorphic sarcoma. Myxoid liposarcoma is characterized by hypocellularity, chicken-wire capillary network, and a myxoid matrix. Myxoinflammatory fibroblastic sarcoma is a rare, low-grade sarcoma of the distal extremities with prominent myxoid stroma, mixed inflammation, virocyte-like cells, pseudolipoblasts, and emperipolesis. It occurs in the hands and feet. Myxoid pleomorphic liposarcoma is an aggressive soft tissue tumor with poor overall survival that typically affects young patients (<30 years old). It arises in the mediastinum. Most cases consist of a variable mixture of myxoid liposarcoma and pleomorphic liposarcoma-like areas. It is more aggressive than usual myxoliposarcoma. Undifferentiated pleomorphic sarcoma is a pleomorphic sarcoma composed of fibroblasts, myofibroblasts, and histiocyte-like cells. The diagnosis is essentially based on the exclusion of specific differentiation other than fibroblasts or myofibroblasts or evidence of dedifferentiation of another soft tissue. Undifferentiated pleomorphic sarcoma has a worse prognosis than myxoliposarcoma.

**20. Correct choice: B.**

Angiomatoid fibrous histiocytoma harbors an *EWSR1-CREB1* fusion. Occasional cases harbor *FUS-ATF1* or *EWSR1-ATF1* fusion genes. Angiomatoid fibrous histiocytoma is a rare mesenchymal tumor of borderline malignant potential and uncertain histogenesis, characterized by solid nodules of epithelioid to spindled cells, blood-filled pseudoangiomatous spaces, a fibrous pseudocapsule, and a lymphoplasmacytic cuff toward the periphery. Interspersed inflammatory cells are commonly seen, and hemosiderin deposition may be prominent. Mitotic activity is usually low. Although it has been reported in a wide age range, it is more common in the first two decades of life without any sex predilection. It typically presents as a slow-growing, nontender, superficial, subcutaneous nodule in extremities, followed by the trunk and the head and neck. In the extremities, almost two-thirds of these tumors affect lymph-node bearing regions, such as popliteal fossa, antecubital fossa, axilla, and inguinal area. Most behave in an indolent fashion, but local recurrences have been reported in up to 15% of cases. Less than 5% metastasize, mostly to lymph nodes and rarely, to lung, liver, and brain.

**21. Correct choice: C.**

Myxoid pleomorphic liposarcoma is an aggressive soft tissue tumor with poor overall survival that typically affects young patients (<30 years old). It arises in the mediastinum. Most cases consist of a variable mixture of myxoid liposarcoma and pleomorphic liposarcoma-like areas. The myxoid liposarcoma-like areas are poorly to moderately cellular and composed of spindle cells with scant cytoplasm and round to oval hyperchromatic nuclei, embedded in a myxoid matrix with abundant ramified capillaries. In these areas, the nuclear atypia and pleomorphism are low but usually are more prominent than in classic myxoid liposarcoma. Myxoid pools may be seen. The pleomorphic liposarcoma-like areas are highly cellular and composed of pleomorphic cells with irregular hyperchromatic nuclei. Adipocytic differentiation is variable with scattered lipoblasts. Mitotic activity is high. *FUS/EWSR1-DDIT3* fusions and *MDM2* amplification are absent. Losses of chromosome 13, including the *RB1* loci, are frequent and have been postulated as an important factor in myxoid pleomorphic liposarcoma tumorigenesis.

**22. Correct choice: B.**

Epithelioid hemangioendothelioma is considered to be a low-grade angiosarcoma composed of tumor cells with eosinophilic cytoplasm dispersed in rows in a sclerotic background. It most frequently occurs in the soft tissues, liver, lungs, and bone. Vascular channels are inconspicuous, and the endothelial nature of the neoplasm manifests with *intracytoplasmic lumina* (the so-called "blister cells"), which may impart a "signet ring" appearance (hence the differential diagnosis with metastatic signet-ring cell carcinoma). The mitotic rate is low. Immunohistochemistry for endothelial markers (CD31 and ERG [erythroblast transformation specific-related gene]) is helpful in supporting the diagnosis. Soft tissue epithelioid hemangioendothelioma recurs in 10% of cases and in 20% of cases, metastasizes to lymph nodes, liver, and lungs. The typical epithelioid hemangioendothelioma harbors a *WWTR1-CAMTA1* rearrangement and is CAMTA1 (calmodulin binding transcription activator 1) positive. The less common *YAP1-TFE3* rearranged tumors are composed of epithelioid cells arranged in solid nests or pseudoalveolar formations enmeshed in a fibrous stroma and are positive for TFE3 (transcription factor E3).

**23. Correct choice: E.**

Schwannoma is characterized by alternating cellular Antoni A and hypocellular Antoni B areas with parallel cellular palisades of Verocay bodies. Variants include ancient schwannoma, which features hyalinization, nuclear atypia, and hemosiderin deposition; cellular schwannoma, which is composed entirely of Antoni A tissue without Verocay bodies; epithelioid schwannoma, which features single or small groups of epithelioid Schwann cells with moderate amphophilic cytoplasm and occasional nuclear pseudoinclusions and myxoid to hyalinized stroma; microcystic/reticular variant, which is composed of strands of bland spindle cells within a myxoid background, with various proportions of microcystic structures; neuroblastoma-like variant, which is defined by large, collagenous, rosette-like structures surrounded by small, round, hyperchromatic Schwann cells; and plexiform schwannoma. S100 protein and/or SOX10 immunoreactivity are usually sufficient for diagnosis. Leiomyoma is composed of elongated cells with eosinophilic or occasional fibrillar cytoplasm with distinct cell membranes and is negative for S100 protein and SOX10 but positive for desmin. Melanoma can be a challenging differential diagnosis, especially if spindled or desmoplastic, but the usual melanoma is also positive for HMB45 and melan-A. Neurofibroma is formed of spindle cells and features shredded carrot collagen and mast cells; it also tends to be more uniformly hypocellular with myxoid areas, but no hypercellular areas. Although Schwann cells constitute the predominant cell component, neurofibromas consist of all the histologic elements of a peripheral nerve, including fibroblasts and axons. Schwann cells and axons can be identified by S100 and neurofilament immunoreactivity, respectively. Neurofibromas are commonly positive for CD34 and focally for EMA (epithelial membrane antigen) as well. Schwannomas are entirely composed of neoplastic Schwann cells and do not contain axons. Perineurioma is a soft tissue neoplasm almost exclusively composed of cells resembling normal perineurium; it is positive for EMA, GLUT1 (glucose transporter 1), and claudin1.

**24. Correct choice: B.**

Epithelioid sarcoma is a malignant epithelioid tumor occurring in both the pediatric and adult populations. The clinical course is unpredictable but is typically better in pediatric patients. There are two typical morphologies, including the classic (distal) type with epithelioid to spindled cells with central pseudogranulomatous architecture; and the proximal type with predominant epithelioid and rhabdoid cells. The classic type epithelioid sarcoma is more common than the proximal type epithelioid sarcoma and occurs most commonly in adolescents and young adults, between ages 10 and 40 years. The proximal type occurs in middle-aged to older adults, with greater than 80% presenting between the ages of 20 and 65 years. The classic, distal type presents as solitary or multiple, slowly growing, usually painless, firm nodules in the extremities. It may simulate a granulomatous process, with or without necrosis (pseudogranulomatous morphology). It is composed of uniform, plump, small- to medium-sized cells with eosinophilic cytoplasm and a mixed chronic inflammatory infiltrate, with more spindle cells at the periphery. There is mild nuclear atypia and variable mitotic activity. Dystrophic calcification and metaplastic bone formation may be seen. The proximal type is characterized by multiple large nodules composed of large polygonal cells with abundant eosinophilic cytoplasm and vesicular nuclei with prominent macronucleoli. Rhabdoid morphology is common, as are frequent mitoses, necrosis, and hemorrhage. These tumors are positive for pancytokeratin, EMA (epithelial membrane antigen), vimentin, and CD34. They may also be positive for ERG (erythroblast transformation specific-related gene). INI1 (integrase interactor 1) is lost, as these tumors harbor mutations in *SMARCB1*. Epithelioid angiosarcoma usually has areas of vasoformation and expresses other vascular markers, such as CD31 and FLI1 (Friend leukemia integration 1), which are generally absent in most epithelioid sarcomas. Metastatic carcinoma is usually CD34 negative and has retained nuclear INI1. Myoepithelial carcinoma expresses cytokeratin and often EMA, but in contrast to epithelioid sarcoma, typically coexpress S100 protein and is variably positive for smooth muscle actin, calponin, CD10, and glial fibrillary acidic protein. *EWSR1* rearrangements are seen in about 50% of cases. Rheumatoid nodules are negative for cytokeratin, EMA, and CD34; they express CD68.

**25. Correct choice: E.**

Loss of nuclear SMARCB1/INI1 (SWI/SNF related, matrix associated, actin dependent regulator of chromatin, subfamily B, member 1/integrase interactor 1) is seen in over 90% of epithelioid sarcomas. SMARCB1/INI1 is part of the SWI/SNF (SWItch/sucrose nonfermentable) complex that coordinates gene expression, cell proliferation, and differentiation. Rarely, inactivation of an alternate but biologically equivalent key regulator can occur in epithelioid sarcoma, that is, *SMARCA4* inactivation in cases of SMARCB1-retained epithelioid sarcoma. Most SWI/SNF-deficient tumors share common "rhabdoid" cytomorphology. SMARCB1-INI1 loss is seen in malignant rhabdoid tumors, poorly differentiated chordoma, and in subsets of myoepithelial carcinoma (10%-40%), extraskeletal myxoid chondrosarcoma (20%), epithelioid schwannoma (40%), and epithelioid malignant peripheral nerve sheath tumor (70%).

**26. Correct choice: A.**

Clear cell sarcoma is characterized by reciprocal translocations in *EWSR1-ATF1* or *EWSR1/CREB1*, resulting in expression of the chimeric EWSR1-ATF1 (Ewing sarcoma breakpoint region 1-activating transcription factor 1) or EWSR1-CREB1 (Ewing sarcoma breakpoint region 1-cAMP response element binding protein 1) fusion proteins, respectively. One or both of these gene fusions may also be seen in angiomatoid fibrous histiocytoma, clear cell sarcoma-like tumor of the gastrointestinal tract, hyalinizing clear cell carcinoma of the salivary gland, and primary pulmonary myxoid sarcoma.

**27. Correct choice: C.**

More than 90% of Ewing sarcoma harbor a gene fusion in *EWSR1-FLI1*. The second most common fusion is in *EWSR1-ERG*. Beyond Ewing sarcoma, *EWSR1* rearrangements are now known to be the most frequent among all soft tissue neoplasms that have recurrent chromosomal translocations. *EWSR1* fusion genes may also be seen in some carcinomas and a subset of mesothelioma.

**28. Correct choice: E.**

Desmoplastic small round cell tumor is a rare soft tissue sarcoma arising in the abdomen of adolescents and young adults that is driven by a single genomic rearrangement, resulting in the expression of the *EWSR1-WT1* fusion gene.

**29. Correct choice: D.**

Approximately 70% of extraskeletal myxoid chondrosarcoma are characterized by a chromosomal rearrangement involving the *NR4A3* gene on chromosome 9 with *EWSR1* on chromosome 22, t(9;22), resulting in *EWSR1-NR4A3* gene fusion. Rearrangements of *NRA4A3* with *TAF15, TCF12, TFG,* and *HSPA8* have also been described and are associated with poorer outcomes.

**30. Correct choice: E.**

Perivascular epithelioid cell tumor is characterized by sheets or nests of epithelioid cells with clear to eosinophilic and granular cytoplasm, surrounded by delicate vasculature. Considered to be a tumor of myomelanocytic differentiation, it typically coexpresses melanoma (HMB45, melan-A, tyrosinase, and microphthalmia transcription factor) and smooth muscle markers (SMA [smooth muscle actin], MSA [muscle-specific actin], calponin, and desmin), with variable staining intensity and distribution. Focal immunoreactivity for S100 is detected in a minority of cases. It is classified as a tumor of uncertain malignant potential since recurrences may arise years after initial diagnosis. There are two main molecular subgroups: those with *TSC1/TSC2* alterations and those with *TFE3* fusions.

Somatic or germline mutations in *TSC1/TSC2* inactivate the tuberous sclerosis complex protein, leading to activation of mTOR (mammalian target of rapamycin) kinase. Approximately 10% are associated with tuberous sclerosis complex. The tumors may be well circumscribed or infiltrative. A variety of growth patterns may be seen. Sheets and nests of noncohesive epithelioid cells with clear to eosinophilic granular cytoplasm with or without a minor component of spindled cells are most common. A subset has dense eosinophilic (rhabdoid) or foamy cytoplasm. Cytologic atypia and mitoses are variable.

Melanoma-like nucleoli, intranuclear pseudoinclusions, multinucleated cells, Touton giant cells, and rare melanin pigment may be present. The vasculature varies from thin and delicate vessels to thick-walled (generally peripherally located) and staghorn vessels. A radial perivascular distribution of tumor cells is seen in about 25% of cases. Stromal hyalinization is common. There is a sclerosing variant that occurs in the pelvic region but is uncommon in the gynecologic tract. Perivascular epithelioid cell tumor belongs to a family of tumors that includes angiomyolipoma, lymphangiomyoma/lymphangiomyomatosis, and clear cell "sugar" tumors of the lungs. Angiomyolipoma and lymphangiomyoma/lymphangiomyomatosis may be associated with tuberous sclerosis.

**31. Correct choice: B.**

Clear cell sarcoma, also called *melanoma of soft parts*, develops from tendons or aponeuroses, most commonly in the feet of young adults. It is characterized by sheets and nests of monotonous epithelioid spindle cells with clear to eosinophilic cytoplasm separated by a delicate framework of fibrocollagenous stroma. The tumor cells have conspicuous nucleoli and contain both iron and melanin. Scattered Touton-type or wreath-like multinucleated giant cells may be seen. A nesting or fascicular pattern is common. Immunoreactivity for S100 protein,

SOX10, and HMB45 is consistently present, analogous to cutaneous melanomas. Clear cell sarcoma harbors *EWSR1-ATF1* or *EWSR1-CREB1* gene fusions.

**32. Correct choice: E.**

Pleomorphic liposarcoma is a high-grade, rapidly growing sarcoma with variable numbers of pleomorphic lipoblasts set within a background of a high-grade, usually pleomorphic, undifferentiated sarcoma. This example contains giant cells containing grapelike clusters of cytoplasmic vacuoles. Two-thirds occur on the extremities (lower limbs > upper). Atypical lipomatous tumors and dedifferentiated liposarcoma occur more often in the retroperitoneum. Although dedifferentiated liposarcoma may show a high-grade component with pleomorphic features, there is often a well-differentiated area. Amplification of 12q13-15 region (*MDM2* and *CDK4* genes) is present in both atypical lipomatous tumors and dedifferentiated liposarcoma. There is no pathognomonic recurrent molecular alteration in pleomorphic liposarcoma. Myxoid pleomorphic liposarcoma is an aggressive soft tissue tumor with poor overall survival that typically affects young patients (<30 years old). It arises in the mediastinum. Most cases consist of a variable mixture of myxoid liposarcoma and pleomorphic liposarcoma-like areas.

**33. Correct choice: C.**

Myxoid liposarcoma is a malignant tumor composed of primitive nonlipogenic mesenchymal cells, signet ring lipoblasts, and prominent myxoid stroma with a highly characteristic branching vascular pattern (the so-called chicken-wire vasculature). The majority of the tumor may be nonlipogenic with only scattered lipoblasts that often have a characteristic signet ring morphology. Although myxoid liposarcoma and round cell liposarcoma were initially described separately, both tumors have identical molecular alterations (either *FUS-DDIT3* or very rarely *EWSR1-DDIT3* rearrangements), and clear evidence of cases with transition between the two morphologic patterns are easily found. Both tumors are now classified as myxoid liposarcoma with a secondary designation of low grade or high grade. The percentage of round cell components needed for this distinction is debated; the WHO currently recommends that greater than 5% indicates a high-grade lesion. It typically arises in the extremities (proximal thigh is common) and has a propensity to present with a first metastasis to another soft tissue or bony site (such as from one leg to the contralateral leg or to the retroperitoneum or spine). Primary retroperitoneal involvement is rare, although metastasis to the retroperitoneal soft tissue is not uncommon. Low-grade myxoid liposarcoma is paucicellular with monomorphic, stellate- or fusiform-shaped cells without atypia associated with a prominent plexiform vasculature (delicate thin-walled arborizing and curving capillaries that form a network reminiscent of chicken-wire fencing). Signet ring lipoblasts can be seen, particularly at the periphery of lobules. There is a prominent mucoid matrix that is rich in hyaluronic acid and may form large mucoid pools (the so-called pulmonary edema pattern). High-grade myxoid liposarcoma is characterized by hypercellular solid sheets of back-to-back cells with round cells or primitive cytomorphology in greater than 5% of the sampled tumor.

**34. Correct choice: E.**

Synovial sarcoma preferentially develops *around* (but not *within*) the knee and ankle joints of young adults but may arise at any site. Characterized by a distinctive *biphasic* pattern, it consists of epithelial cells arranged in glandular formation scattered within a sarcomatous spindle cell component. The *monophasic* variant, which consists exclusively of the mesenchymal component, has been gradually recognized as being the most frequent form of synovial sarcoma. Monophasic synovial sarcoma may mimic fibrosarcoma, malignant peripheral nerve sheath tumors, and mesenchymal chondrosarcoma. The *poorly differentiated* variant, which is characterized by small, round, blue cell morphology with frequent mitoses and necrosis can mimic a variety of small blue cell tumors, including lymphoma, small cell osteosarcoma, Ewing sarcoma, rhabdomyosarcoma, and neuroblastoma. The vast majority of cases harbor a translocation between chromosomes X and 18, involving two genes of unknown function, SSX1 (synovial sarcoma, X breakpoint 1) or 2 (on chromosome X) and SYT (synovial sarcoma, translocated to chromosome 18) (on chromosome18). Immunohistochemistry can be helpful in the differential diagnosis. Synovial sarcoma is positive for cytokeratin (specifically CK7) and/or EMA (epithelial membrane antigen), at least focally. Nuclear expression of TLE1 (transducin-like enhancer of split 1) is seen in 90% of cases; BCL-2 (B-cell lymphoma 2) and CD99 occur in 60%; 30% may express S100 protein. It is negative for CD31.

**35. Correct choice: B.**

Extraskeletal Ewing sarcoma is composed of uniform small round cells that are 1 − 2*x* the size of lymphocytes that are often arranged in a sheet-like growth pattern. The cells have scant clear to eosinophilic cytoplasm, indistinct cytoplasmic membranes, round nuclei, finely stippled chromatin, and inconspicuous nucleoli. A subset exhibits neuroectodermal differentiation (Homer-Wright pseudorosettes). Atypical Ewing sarcoma shows nuclear enlargement, irregular nuclear contours, and prominent nucleoli. Strong, diffuse membranous expression for CD99 is seen in 90% to 95% of cases. NKX2.2 is highly specific. More than 90% of Ewing sarcoma harbor a gene fusion in *EWSR1 FLI1*. The second most common fusion is in *EWSR1-ERG*.

**36. Correct choice: B.**

Extraskeletal myxoid chondrosarcoma is a rare malignant mesenchymal neoplasm composed of bland cells with eosinophilic cytoplasm and round to oval nuclei with evenly distributed chromatin and inconspicuous nucleolus. The tumor cells exhibit a very characteristic architecture consisting of interconnected cords and small clusters and complex trabecular or cribriform arrays. Despite the name, there is no evidence of cartilaginous differentiation. It occurs in adults, mainly in the fourth to seventh decades. Most arise in the deep soft tissues of the proximal extremities and limb girdles, with the thigh being the most common site. It tends to metastasize to the lung. It is positive for INSM1 (insulinoma-associated protein 1), NSE (neuron-specific enolase), synaptophysin, and S100 protein (50%). About 70% of extraskeletal myxoid chondrosarcoma are characterized by a chromosomal rearrangement involving the *NR4A3* gene on chromosome 9 with *EWSR1* on chromosome 22, t(9;22), resulting in *EWSR1-NR4A3* gene fusion. Rearrangements of *NRA4A3* with *TAF15*, *TCF12*, *TFG*, and *HSPA8* have also been described and are associated with poorer outcomes.

**37. Correct choice: C.**

Ewing sarcoma and mesenchymal chondrosarcoma each can express CD99 and NKX2.2. Mesenchymal chondrosarcoma does not harbor EWSR1-FLI1 (Ewing sarcoma breakpoint region 1-Friend leukemia integration 1) gene fusion and lacks FLI1 immunoreactivity.

**38. Correct choice: D.**

Gardner fibroma is a benign soft tissue lesion that occurs in infants and children and is characterized by thick, haphazard collagen and bland fibroblasts that entrap adjacent tissue. Almost 90% are associated with familial adenomatous polyposis/Gardner syndrome and may be the initial diagnostic clue to Gardner syndrome and *APC* mutations. It is positive for CD34, CD34, cyclin D1, vimentin, and nuclear β-catenin. A significant proportion of affected patients subsequently develop desmoid-type fibromatosis, which is also positive for nuclear β-catenin. Although the histology is similar to nuchal fibroma, nuchal fibroma occurs in the posterior neck, more commonly in men (mean age, 40 years). It is CD34 positive but does not express nuclear β-catenin. Desmoplastic fibroblastoma occurs in adult men and is characterized by paucicellular, bland spindled, and reactive appearing fibroblasts and myofibroblasts separated by abundant collagen with variable myxoid stroma.

**39. Correct choice: A.**

Alveolar rhabdomyoblastoma is the second most common type of rhabdomyosarcoma. It affects adolescents and young adults (peak age range 10-25 years), often presenting in the deep soft tissue of lower extremities but can occur in the head and neck, trunk, paraspinal, pelvic, genitourinary regions, and retroperitoneum. It may also present with widespread involvement, including bone marrow infiltration (leukemia-like presentation) and lymphadenopathy. It is a high-grade sarcoma composed of nests and sheets of monomorphic cells with evidence of skeletal muscle differentiation, often arranged in a pseudoalveolar pattern. The tumor cells exhibit diffuse strong myogenin expression as well as more heterogeneous expression of desmin and MyoD1 (myogenic differentiation 1), but negative for TFE3 (transcription factor E3). It is characterized by *PAX3-FOXO1* (60%) or *PAX7-FOXO1* (20%) gene fusions. Alveolar soft part sarcoma may also exhibit a pseudoalveolar growth pattern, but it is negative for myogenin. It is characterized by the *ASPSCR1-TFE3* gene fusion and expresses TFE3. Pleomorphic rhabdomyosarcoma occurs in older adults (6th-7th decades) and is characterized by large, atypical, and frequently multinucleated bizarre eosinophilic, round, and spindle cells. Cross striations may not be apparent. Desmin expression is usually strong, while myogenin and MyoD1 staining can be more focal.

**40. Correct choice: C.**

Desmoplastic small round cell tumor chiefly affects young adult males, but may also be seen in females. The cytologic features are those of a small blue cell tumor, with scant cytoplasm, uniform nuclei, and inconspicuous nucleoli. The tumor cells are typically arranged in a nesting or jig-saw pattern with prominent desmoplasia (hence the designation). The characteristic immunohistochemical profile includes reactivity for desmin (in a dotlike perinuclear pattern), epithelial markers, and neuronal markers. It is characterized by a translocation t(11;22)(p13;q12), which gives rise to an *EWSR1-WT1* gene fusion. The prognosis is very poor. *CIC-DUX4* rearranged sarcoma is also an aggressive sarcoma arising predominantly in the soft tissues of children and young adults. Most patients present with a rapidly growing, solitary mass. Metastases may be present at the initial presentation. On biopsy, the tumor exhibits a solid and often nodular proliferation of small round or ovoid cells with amphophilic or lightly eosinophilic cytoplasm with a high nuclear to cytoplasmic ratio. The cells are positive for CD99, WT1 (Wilms tumor 1), DUX4 (double homeobox 4), and ETV4 (ETS variant 4). There is a *CIC-DUX4* gene fusion that arises from either a t(4;19)(q35;q13) or a t(10;19)(q26;q13) translocation.

**41. Correct choice: B.**

Intravascular papillary endothelial hyperplasia (Masson tumor) is a benign proliferation of reactive endothelial cells, forming numerous papillae most often lined by a single layer of plump endothelial cells. There are three types: primary arising in a dilated vessel, secondary (mixed form) arising in a preexisting vascular lesion, and rare extravascular form typically arising in a hematoma. It presents as a small, well-circumscribed lesion without necrosis, marked cytologic atypia, or infiltrative growth pattern, most commonly in the subcutaneous tissue of fingers, followed by the subcutaneous tissue in the head, neck, and upper extremities. It is considered to be an exuberant form of organizing thrombus rather than a primary tumor, arising in the context of venous stasis. Associated thrombotic material is frequently present.

**42. Correct choice: D.**

Superficial CD34-positive fibroblastic tumor is a low-grade neoplasm arising in the skin and subcutaneous tissue composed of spindle cells containing moderate to abundant granular to glassy eosinophilic cytoplasm and vesicular nuclei with distinct nucleoli and intranuclear pseudoinclusions, with interspersed pleomorphic giant cells. Tumor cells are arranged in fascicular or sheet-like patterns. Neither necrosis nor mitotic activity is identified. The tumor cells are positive for CD34 and in up to 70 of cases, keratin AE1/AE3, while all of the following are negative: MUC4 (mucin 4), smooth muscle actin, desmin, S100, and STAT6 (signal transducer and activator of transcription 6). INI1 (integrase interactor 1) is retained. Most tumors occur in middle-aged adults (range 20-76 years) with slight male predominance. Superficial CD34-positive fibroblastic tumor is associated with an indolent clinical behavior with little or no risk for disease recurrence.

**43. Correct choice: A.**

Calcifying aponeurotic fibroma occurs in the dorsal hand or wrist of children/adolescents and is considered of chondroid origin. It can be thought of as the cartilaginous equivalent of fibromatosis. Morphologically, fibromatosis, rheumatoid nodule, and schwannoma are the main differential diagnoses. Other fibrous proliferations that develop in pediatric patients include fibrous hamartoma of infancy, infantile digital fibromatosis, and fibromatosis colli.

**44. Correct choice: B.**

Inflammatory myofibroblastic tumor is a neoplasm that arises in the lung, retroperitoneum, and abdominal cavity, but it may occur in many other locations. It is associated with recurrences in 35% of cases and metastasizes in 5%. The spindly cells are neoplastic myofibroblasts expressing smooth muscle actin and vimentin. In 50% of cases, inflammatory myofibroblastic tumor harbors a fusion of the *ALK* gene with other genes, leading to overexpression of the *ALK* gene product, which can be detected on immunohistochemistry with ALK (anaplastic lymphoma kinase) antibodies. These tumors can be treated with ALK tyrosine kinase inhibitors.

**45. Correct choice: A.**

A cartwheel/storiform pattern with no significant atypia is highly characteristic of dermatofibrosarcoma prutuberans. This pattern may be seen focally in a number of other tumors (eg, peripheral nerve sheath tumors, fibromatosis, and nodular fasciitis); however, in dermatofibrosarcoma prutuberans, this pattern is present in each and every field. Local recurrence is frequent, but this tumor does not metastasize. The typical immunohistochemical profile of dermatofibrosarcoma prutuberans is positive for CD34 and negative for factor XIIIa (vice versa in fibrous histiocytoma).

**46. Correct choice: A.**

Atypical lipomatous tumor, also known as *well-differentiated liposarcoma*, is the preferred designation when applied to retroperitoneal tumors. It accounts for 45% of liposarcomas. It consists of fatty lobules separated by thick and cellular fibrous septa. Lipoblasts, characterized by vacuoles indenting the nucleus, are present. There are two histologic variants: (1) *sclerosing*, found in the retroperitoneum and spermatic cord, consisting of pleomorphic cells within a collagenous stroma and little or no adipocytic differentiation and (2) *inflammatory* variant, also found in the retroperitoneum, with a rich chronic inflammatory infiltrate. Often, two or all three patterns may be seen in any single tumor. Atypical lipomatous tumors may undergo dedifferentiation. Atypical lipomatous tumor harbors ring or giant marker chromosomes derived from amplified material from 12q13-15 in almost all cases including the genes *MDM2* and *CDK4*. This can be demonstrated by FISH (fluorescence in situ hybridization) for *MDM2* amplification or by immunohistochemistry for MDM2 (mouse double-minute 2) and CDK4 (cyclin-dependent kinase 4). Lipoblastoma occurs in children age 3 or younger. A lobular growth pattern with delicate branching vessels and myxoid change are characteristic. It is negative for 12q13-15 amplification and harbors *PLAG1* rearrangements. Pleomorphic lipoma occurs in older men in the back of the neck or shoulders and is encapsulated.

**47. Correct choice: A.**

Fibrosarcoma is a rare, malignant tumor of fibroblasts with herringbone architecture (cells in columns of short parallel lines with all the lines in one column sloping one way and lines in adjacent columns sloping the other way) and variable collagen, that can range from keloid-like (thick hyalinized collagen fibers), to loose fascicular, to focally myxoid. Usually arising in the deep soft tissue of the lower extremities or trunk, it is associated with a 50% recurrence rate and a 25% rate of metastasis (typically, lung and bone). Diagnosis of fibrosarcoma requires exclusion of dedifferentiated liposarcoma, fibromatosis, fibrosarcomatous dermatofibrosarcoma protuberans, low-grade fibromyxoid sarcoma, malignant peripheral nerve sheath tumor, and synovial sarcoma.

**48. Correct choice: E.**

Undifferentiated pleomorphic sarcoma is a high-grade sarcoma composed of fibroblasts, myofibroblasts, and histiocyte like cells. It is seen in older adults with slight male predominance, arising more commonly in the deep soft tissue of the lower extremities. A variety of patterns may be seen including storiform pattern (cells emanate from a central focus) and irregular fascicular. Pleomorphic and bizarre tumor cells with foamy cytoplasm and marked atypia are often present. Multinucleated giant cells may be seen. Numerous mitotic figures, including atypical forms, are almost always present. Rarely there may be metaplastic (not neoplastic) bone or cartilage. Undifferentiated pleomorphic sarcoma is a diagnosis of exclusion; before rendering a diagnosis, the tumor should be generously sampled and searched for other components to rule out a dedifferentiated tumor or evidence of specific differentiation other than fibroblasts or myofibroblasts.

**49. Correct choice: B.**

Embryonal rhabdomyosarcoma is the most common type of rhabdomyosarcoma. It arises in children and adolescents, commonly in the head and neck and genitourinary system, and only rarely in the extremities. It typically exhibits alternate areas of dense and loosely cellular round and spindle-to-stellate to tadpole-like cells with rhabdomyoblasts (including strap cells) in different stages of differentiation. Perivascular condensations of tumor cells in the less cellular regions are common. Some degree of myogenic differentiation (desmin, myogenin, and MyoD1 [myogenic differentiation 1]) is typically present. Botryoid embryonal rhabdomyosarcoma (sarcoma botryoides) occurs in specific locations, specifically beneath mucosal epithelial lined viscera, such as the bladder, biliary tract, vagina or upper respiratory tract, and extrahepatic bile ducts. This variant often has a grapelike (botryoid) growth pattern and comprises 10% of all embryonal rhabdomyosarcoma.

The botryoid variant frequently shows a cambium layer a hypercellular zone immediately beneath the epithelial surface. Embryonal rhabdomyosarcoma may be associated with a variety of syndromes including Costello syndrome (*HRAS*), neurofibromatosis type 1 (*NF1*), Noonan syndrome (*PTPN11* and others), Beckwith-Wiedemann syndrome (changes to 11p15), Dicer syndrome (*DICER1*), Li-Fraumeni syndrome (*TP53*), and Gorlin syndrome (*PTCH1*).

**50. Correct choice: A.**

Granular cell tumor is a soft tissue tumor that shows neural differentiation and can involve a wide variety of sites, including the tongue, larynx, and esophagus. In 5% to 15% of cases, there may be multiple lesions. It occurs over a wide age range (most commonly, 30-50 years of age). Histologically, it is composed of large, round, and polygonal to slightly spindled cells with eosinophilic, granular cytoplasm. Intracytoplasmic coarse granules, representing phagolysosomes, are positive for PAS/D (periodic acid-Schiff with diastase). In sites with overlying squamous epithelium, there may be pseudoepitheliomatous hyperplasia. The granular cells are positive for S100 protein, SOX10, CD68, inhibin, calretinin, and TFE3 (transcription factor E3). Most granular cell tumors are benign, but occasionally metastases occur. A variety of other tumors may show granular cell change, including leiomyoma, leiomyosarcoma, melanoma, dermatofibroma, and ameloblastoma. Melanoma should be positive for HMB45, which is not seen in granular cell tumors.

# 6 Joints

1. What is the best diagnosis for the femoral head, shown in Figure 1, removed from a 69-year-old male?

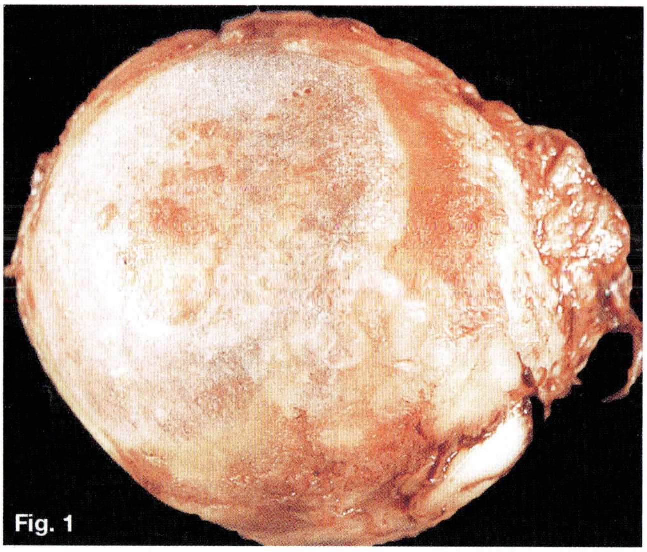

Fig. 1

A. Charcot arthropathy
B. Insufficiency fracture
C. Osteoarthritis
D. Osteonecrosis
E. Rheumatoid arthritis

2. What is the best diagnosis for the femoral head, shown in Figure 1, removed from a 72-year-old female with osteoporosis?

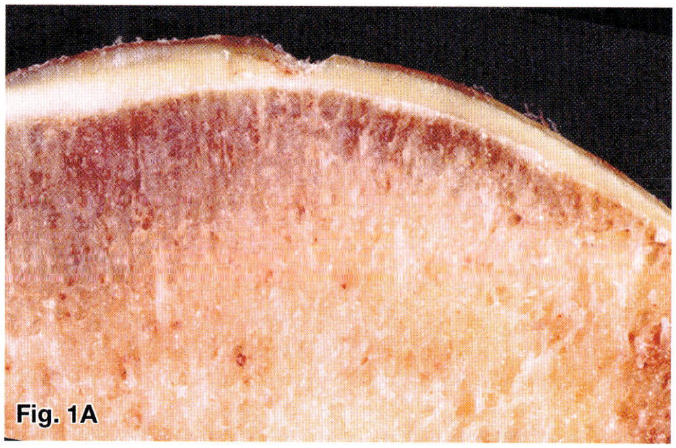

Fig. 1A

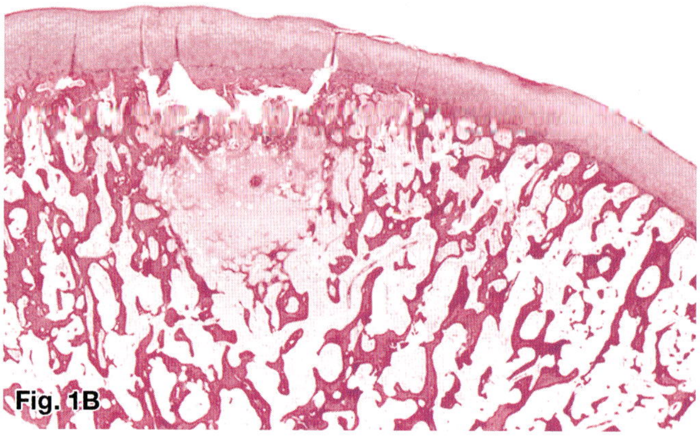

Fig. 1B

A. Avascular necrosis
B. Charcot arthropathy
C. Insufficiency fracture
D. Osteoarthritis
E. Rheumatoid arthritis

3. Which of the following histologic changes in the articular cartilage of osteoarthritic joints represents a regenerative process?

A. Clusters of cloned chondrocytes
B. Fibrillation of superficial layers
C. Ghost chondrocytes
D. Irregularity of tidemark
E. Reduced basophilic staining on H&E (hematoxylin and eosin)

All figures in this chapter are from Longacre TA, Greenson JK, Hornick JL, Reuter VE, eds. *Mills and Sternberg's Diagnostic Surgical Pathology.* 7th ed. Wolters Kluwer; 2022 except for those noted at the end of this book.

4. What is the best diagnosis for the femoral head, shown in Figure 1, removed from a 42-year-old female on corticosteroids for a connective tissue disease?

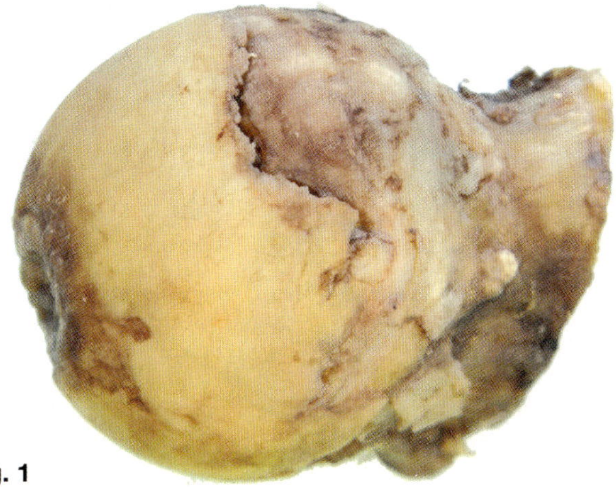
Fig. 1

A. Charcot arthropathy
B. Insufficiency fracture
C. Osteoarthritis
D. Osteonecrosis
E. Rheumatoid arthritis

5. What is the best diagnosis for the synovial tissue, shown in Figure 1, from a 45-year-old female?

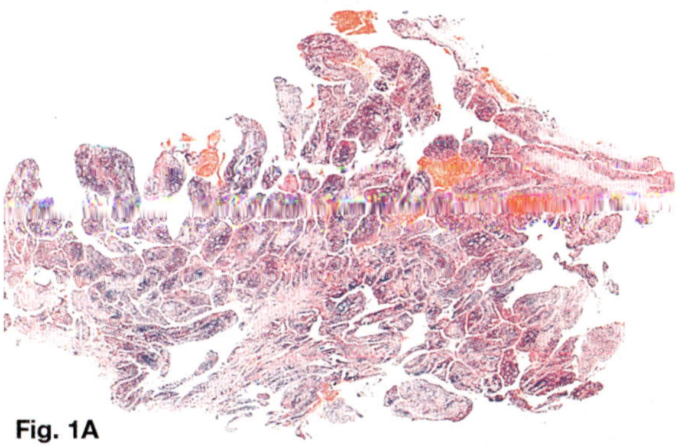
Fig. 1A

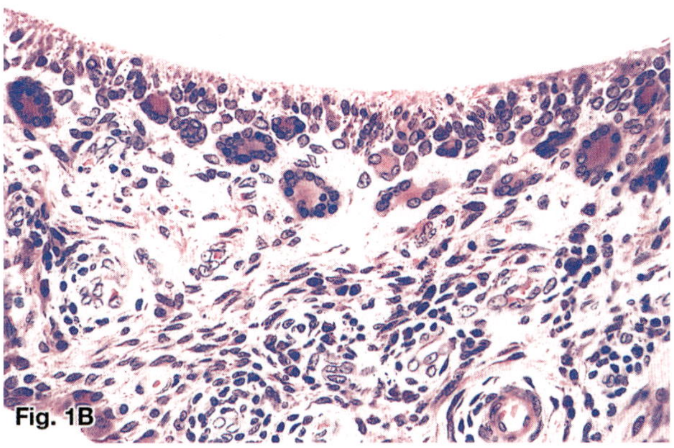
Fig. 1B

A. Hemosiderotic synovitis
B. Rheumatoid arthritis
C. Synovial chondromatosis
D. Synovial lipomatosis
E. Tenosynovial giant cell tumor

6. What is the best diagnosis for the nodule, shown in Figures 1 and 2, removed from the left index finger of a 32-year-old female?

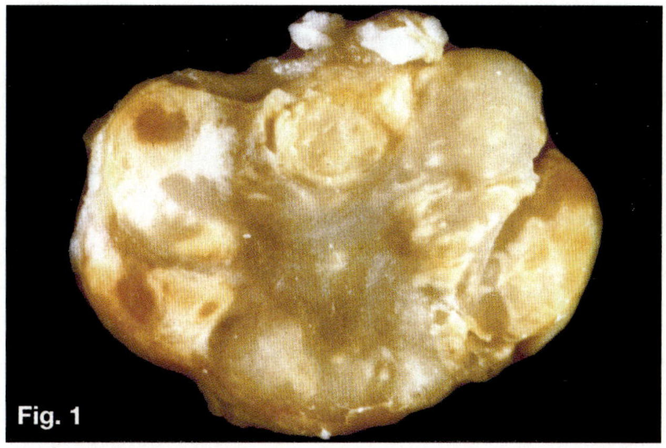
Fig. 1

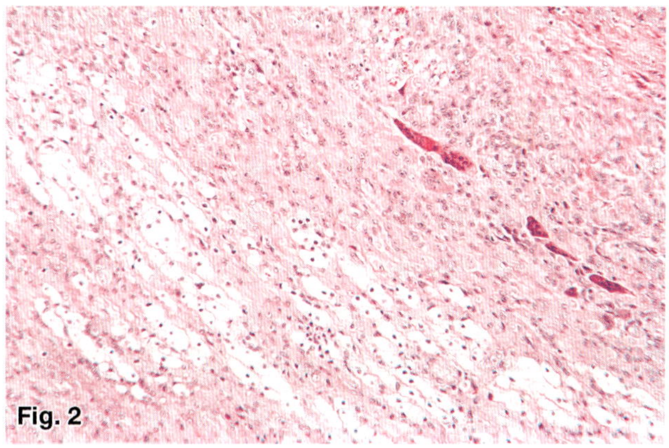
Fig. 2

A. Hemosiderotic synovitis
B. Rheumatoid arthritis
C. Synovial chondromatosis
D. Synovial lipomatosis
E. Tenosynovial giant cell tumor

7. What is the best diagnosis for tissue obtained from the knee joint, shown in Figure 1, of a 41-year-old male with a history of degenerative joint disease?

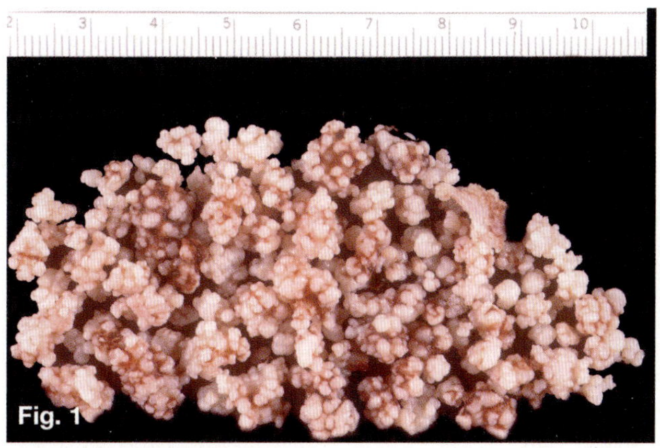
Fig. 1

A. Hemosiderotic synovitis
B. Rheumatoid arthritis
C. Synovial chondromatosis
D. Synovial lipomatosis
E. Tenosynovial giant cell tumor

8. In Hoffa disease, the most characteristic pathologic alteration is

   A. degeneration of the cartilage matrix.
   B. detachment of a piece of bone with overlying cartilage.
   C. enlargement of the infrapatellar fat pad.
   D. formation of pannus over the articular surface.
   E. presence of paraarticular chondromas.

9. A 48-year-old patient develops acute swelling and pain in the knee. A synovial aspirate from the affected joint exhibits crystals, which are blue when parallel and yellow when perpendicular to the axis of a red compensator. These crystals are composed of

   A. calcium oxalate.
   B. calcium pyrophosphate.
   C. homogentisic acid.
   D. hydroxyapatite.
   E. monosodium urate.

10. What is the most likely diagnosis for the nodule removed from the extensor surface of the forearm, shown in Figure 1, of a 48-year-old female?

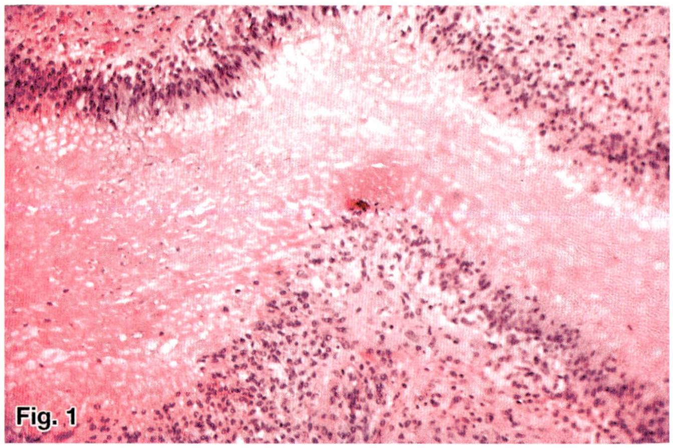
Fig. 1

   A. Acute gouty arthritis
   B. Epithelioid sarcoma
   C. Rheumatoid nodule
   D. Sarcoidosis
   E. Tuberculosis

# ANSWERS AND EXPLANATIONS

**1. Correct choice: C.**

Osteoarthritis is a degenerative disease of cartilage, where degenerative changes are accompanied by regenerative processes. Similarly, the bone underneath the articular cartilage (subchondral bone) displays both degenerative and regenerative changes. In addition to alterations of cartilage and bone, the synovial lining becomes hyperplastic and inflamed. Loose bodies, detached pieces of cartilage, or cartilage and bone may float within the joint space and may "jam" the joint.

**2. Correct choice: C.**

Subchondral insufficiency fracture is relatively common in older osteoporotic women or renal transplant recipients. It usually resolves after conservative therapy, without surgery. Many cases are misdiagnosed as osteonecrosis on magnetic resonance imaging, prompting surgical intervention. However, on gross examination, there is no evidence of osteonecrosis. The characteristic histologic features are the presence of a fracture callus and granulation tissue along both edges of a fracture line, in parallel with the articular surface.

**3. Correct choice: A.**

Osteoarthritis is a degenerative disease of cartilage, where degenerative changes are accompanied by regenerative processes. The bone underneath the articular cartilage (subchondral bone) also displays both degenerative and regenerative changes. In addition to alterations of cartilage and bone, the synovial lining becomes hyperplastic and inflamed. Loose bodies are detached pieces of cartilage or cartilage and bone that lie free within the joint space and may "jam" the joint. Regenerative changes in the cartilage include proliferation of chondrocytes that form large clusters or clones and formation of new cartilage from the underlying bone and from the periphery of the joint (fibrocartilaginous metaplasia), with increased proteoglycan synthesis.

Fibrillation of the superficial layers refers to the splitting of collagen bundles, with the formation of clefts, ghost (necrotic) chondrocyte, and irregularity of the tidemark due to altered calcification, resulting in an irregular and granular tidemark (the junction between noncalcified and calcified cartilage). Reduced basophilic staining on H&E due to loss of matrix proteoglycans in the superficial cartilage is also a degenerative process.

**4. Correct choice: D.**

The femoral head is the most common site of osteonecrosis. Risk factors include corticosteroid use and traumatic as well as other nontraumatic causes. It is characterized by necrosis of bone due to ischemia. On cross section of the affected bone, there is a characteristic wedge-shaped area of pallor or yellow discoloration corresponding to the area of infarct covered by intact cartilage. In avascular osteonecrosis, there is necrosis of bone and bone marrow. Accurate distinction between osteonecrosis and subchondral insufficiency fracture is important due to the different management and outcomes for these processes.

**5. Correct choice: B.**

The joints in rheumatoid arthritis have edematous, thick, hyperplastic synovium, covered by delicate and bulbous fronds. The synovium is hyperplastic and hypertrophied. A dense perivascular inflammatory infiltrate of T lymphocytes, plasma cells (often with eosinophilic cytoplasmic inclusions called Russell bodies), and macrophages is often present. A lymphoplasmacytic infiltrate with variable germinal centers, necrobiotic nodules, and fibrosis may also be seen. There may be increased vascularity with hemosiderin deposition but that is not the dominant finding. Organizing fibrin floating in joint space forms the so-called rice bodies. Osteophytes and new bone formation are not prominent.

**6. Correct choice: E.**

Tenosynovial giant cell tumor encompasses a group of lesions that most often arise from the synovium of joints, bursae, and tendon sheaths and show synovial differentiation.

There are three types: localized, diffuse, and malignant. The localized type is the second most common tumor of the hand (after ganglion cyst). It is well circumscribed and lobulated, usually in close association with a tendon. Histologically, it is composed of variable proportions of large epithelioid mononuclear cells, macrophages, and osteoclast-like giant cells. The diffuse type forms intra-articular tumors within large joints. The malignant type is rare, contains a definite sarcomatous area, and arises de novo or following multiple recurrences of a conventional tenosynovial giant cell tumor. Treatment of the localized type is local excision.

**7. Correct choice: C.**

Synovial chondromatosis is a locally aggressive neoplasm characterized by multiple hyaline cartilaginous nodules involving joint spaces, subsynovial tissue, or tenosynovium. Multiple, grayish-white, smooth or irregular, uniform or variably sized nodules are present as intra-articular loose bodies or embedded within or attached to synovium. It is characterized by formation of hyaline cartilaginous nodules within the synovium or free within joint spaces. It involves large joints: 60% to 70% of cases affect the knee, followed by hip, shoulder, elbow, ankle, and wrist. It occurs in the third to fifth decade and is more common in men than women. Recurrences develop in 15% to 20% of patients, more commonly in tenosynovial cases. Malignant transformation is uncommon. Synovial chondromatosis may be primary (monoarticular) or secondary (may be multiarticular). Primary synovial chondromatosis is a self-limited process that occurs in an otherwise normal joint. Secondary chondromatosis occurs in a joint previously afflicted with disease, often posttraumatic or degenerative osteoarthritis.

**8. Correct choice: C.**

Hoffa disease is a rare condition characterized by extensive enlargement of the infrapatellar fat pad, located between the joint capsule externally and the synovial-lined joint space internally. It manifests with pain in the anterior knee. Degenerative changes due to repetitive microtraumas lead to chondro-osseous metaplasia, which could be misinterpreted as paraarticular chondroma. Synovial lipomatosis is an analogous condition, leading to the expansion of subsynovial adipose tissue in any joint. Detachment of a piece of bone with overlying cartilage is the hallmark of osteochondritis dissecans, which most often affects the medial femoral condyle of young people.

**9. Correct choice: B.**

Calcium pyrophosphate crystal deposition disease (pseudogout) manifests with symptoms and signs similar to degenerative osteoarthritis, usually beginning in the fourth decade of life. Calcium pyrophosphate crystals are needle shaped and have a color pattern under a red compensator opposite to that of urate crystals. Deposition of calcium pyrophosphate in the articular cartilage results in degenerative joint disease. The term "pseudogout" is commonly reserved for cases manifesting acutely with joint swelling and pain similar to gout. Familial cases are associated with *ANKH* mutations. Calcium pyrophosphate crystal deposition disease may occur in association with conditions characterized by increased concentration of divalent ions that inhibit pyrophosphatase (hyperparathyroidism, hemochromatosis, Wilson disease). Calcium pyrophosphate crystal deposition disease is typically associated with signs and symptoms similar to degenerative osteoarthritis, usually beginning in the fourth decade of life.

**10. Correct choice: C.**

Rheumatoid arthritis is the most common inflammatory arthritis; it affects 0.5% to 1.0% of the population. About 30% to 40% of all patients with rheumatoid arthritis develop nodules, which are clinical predictors of more severe arthritis, seropositivity, joint erosions, and rheumatoid vasculitis. Rheumatoid nodules are the most common extra-articular manifestation of rheumatoid arthritis. The subcutaneous rheumatoid nodules are firm, nontender, and movable within the subcutaneous tissue; however, they could also be attached to underlying structures, such as the periosteum, fascia, and tendons. They most commonly occur on pressure points (such as the olecranon process); however, they may occur at other sites, including within the lung and other internal organs. Histologically, they exhibit a central area of fibrinoid necrosis surrounded by palisading macrophages and lymphocytes. Granulomas are typically identified in the subcutis but occasionally may involve the dermis. Mucin deposition is characteristically absent.

# 7 Nonneoplastic Diseases of Bones

1. Which of the following categories of bone disorders is due to abnormal mineralization of bone?

   A. Hyperparathyroidism, hypophosphatasia, osteogenesis imperfecta, Paget disease
   B. Hyperparathyroidism, osteopetrosis, osteoporosis, Paget disease
   C. Hypophosphatasia, metal toxicity, osteomalacia, rickets
   D. Hypophosphatemia, osteopetrosis, osteomalacia, rickets
   E. Osteogenesis imperfecta, osteomalacia, osteopetrosis, osteoporosis

2. The x-ray of the femur from a 12-year-old boy, shown in Figure 1, shows marked expansion of the distal end with numerous dense, round calcified inclusions resembling a bag of popcorn. What is the most likely diagnosis?

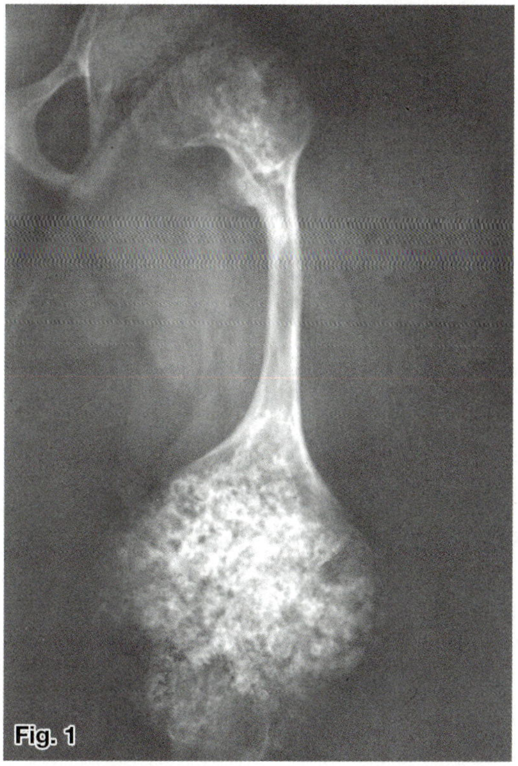

Fig. 1

   A. Achondroplasia
   B. Osteogenesis imperfecta
   C. Osteopetrosis
   D. Paget disease
   E. Rickets disease

3. The pathologic correlate of the radiologic finding shown in Figure 1 is

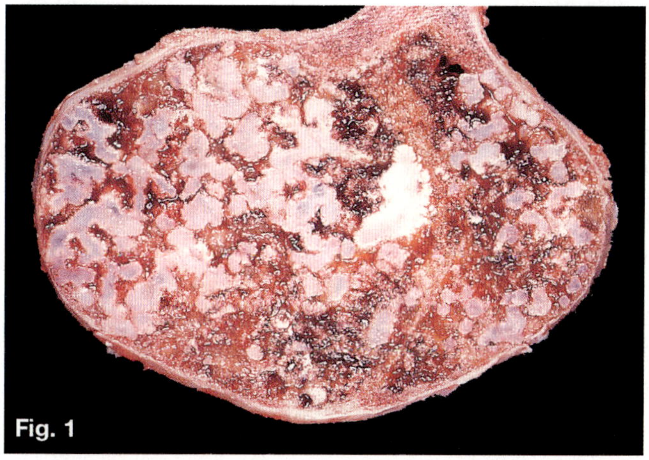

Fig. 1

   A. abnormal mineralization of growth plate.
   B. fragmentation of growth plate.
   C. increased density of bone.
   D. premature fusion of growth plate.
   E. thinning of bone trabecula.

4. What is the most likely diagnosis for the bone biopsy, shown in Figure 1, from the pelvis of a 49-year-old male with pelvic pain?

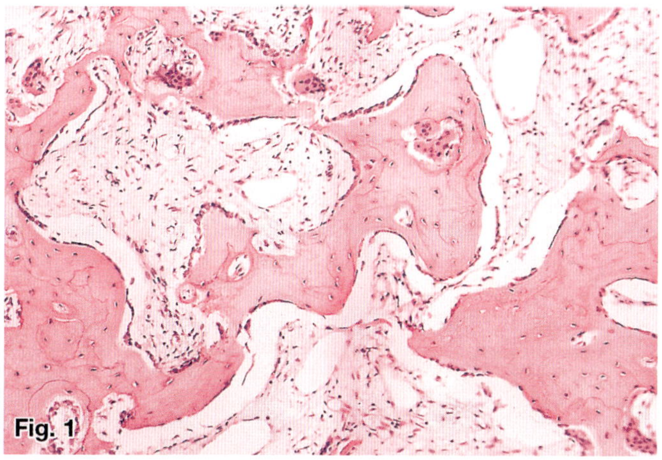

Fig. 1

   A. Aluminum toxicity
   B. Fracture callus
   C. Hypophosphatasia
   D. Osteopetrosis
   E. Paget disease

All figures in this chapter are from Longacre TA, Greenson JK, Hornick JL, Reuter VE, eds. *Mills and Sternberg's Diagnostic Surgical Pathology*. 7th ed. Wolters Kluwer; 2022 except for those noted at the end of this book.

5. What is the best diagnosis for the lumbar spine, shown in Figure 1, removed at autopsy from a 67-year-old female?

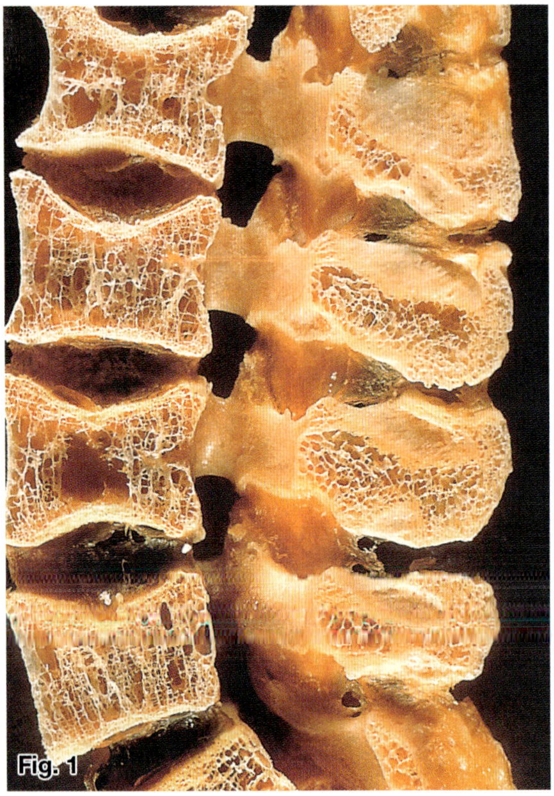
Fig. 1

A. Osteomalacia
B. Osteomyelitis
C. Osteopetrosis
D. Osteoporosis
E. Osteosclerosis

6. What is the best diagnosis for the biopsy, shown in Figures 1 and 2, obtained from the femur of a 22-year-old female with an Erlenmeyer flask deformity on x-ray?

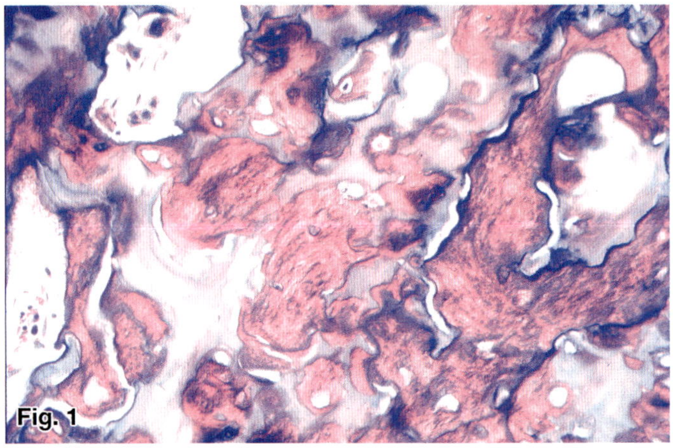
Fig. 1

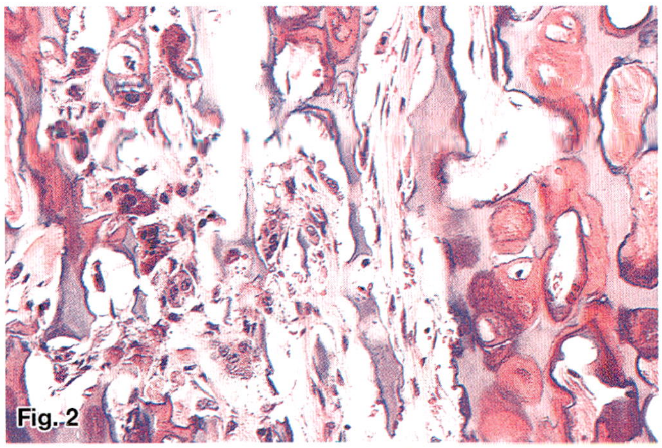
Fig. 2

A. Osteomalacia
B. Osteomyelitis
C. Osteopetrosis
D. Osteoporosis
E. Osteosclerosis

7. A 38-year-old slips on black ice and lands on his right shoulder. He notes no pain but presents to the emergency department the following week for weakness in his golf swing. An x-ray is inconclusive, and a biopsy of the right humerus (shown in Figures 1 and 2) is performed. What is the best diagnosis?

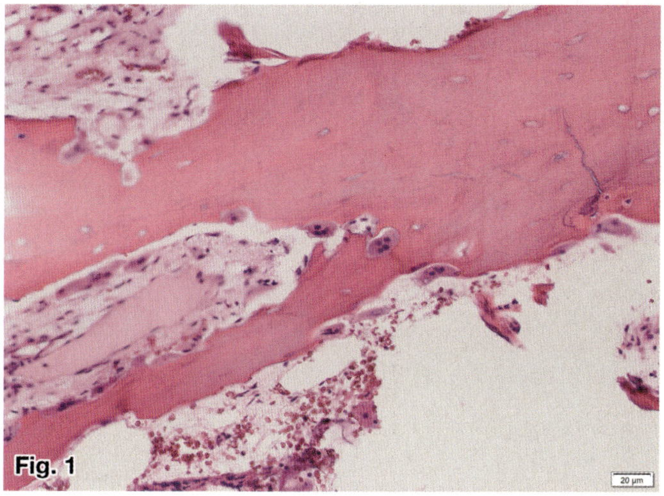
Fig. 1

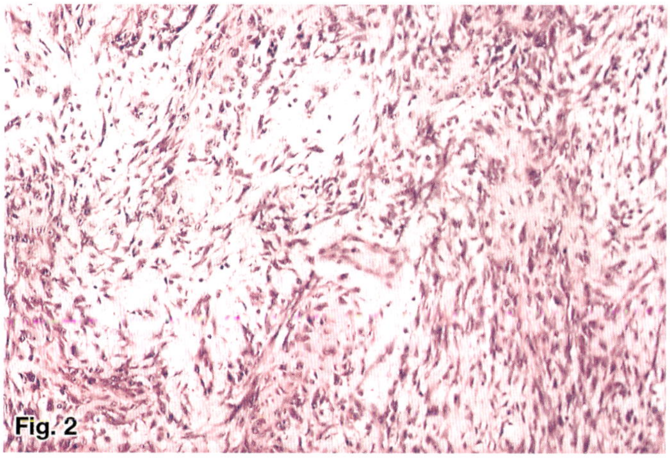
Fig. 2

A. Avascular necrosis
B. Fracture callus
C. Nodular fasciitis
D. Osteomyelitis
E. Reactive periostitis

8. A 32-year-old football player presents with a somewhat painful lump in his thigh that has been present for several months. A radiograph of the area depicts an area of poorly defined opacification. The mass is removed to reveal a well-circumscribed mass with peripheral ossification, shown in Figure 1. Sections through the center of the mass, shown in Figure 2, show immature bone and cellular fibrous stroma. What is the most likely diagnosis?

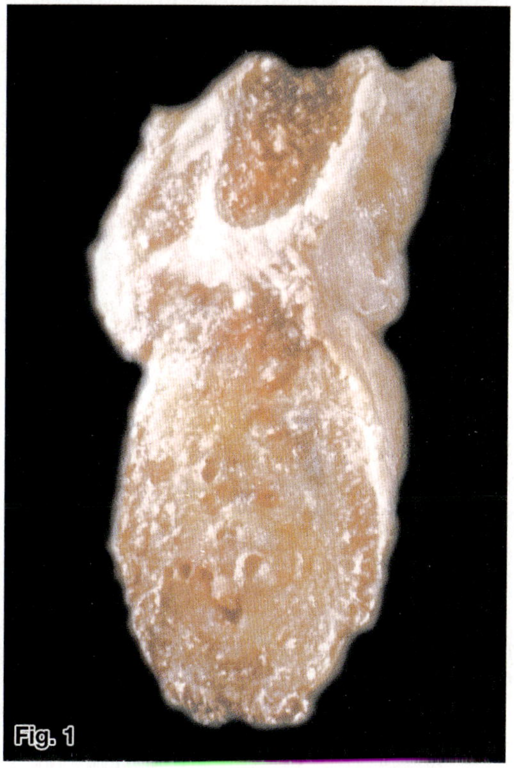
Fig. 1

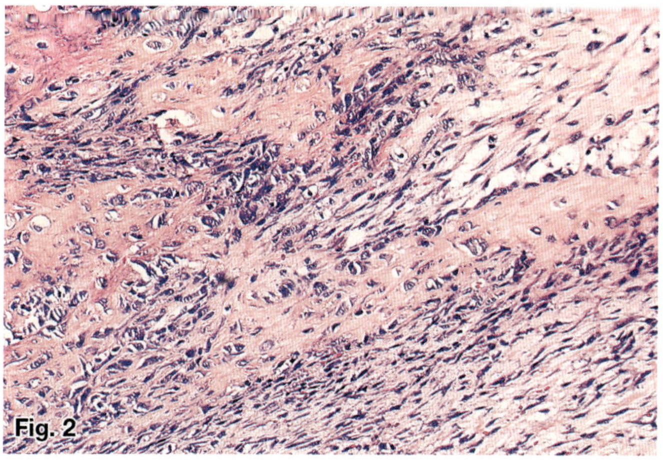
Fig. 2

A. Extraskeletal osteosarcoma
B. Myositis ossificans
C. Parosteal osteosarcoma
D. Periosteal osteosarcoma
E. Synovial sarcoma

9. Which of the following statements on infectious osteomyelitis is correct?
   A. Bacterial biofilms play a key role in chronic osteomyelitis.
   B. Brodie abscess is an acute form of osteomyelitis.
   C. Chronic osteomyelitis develops in fewer than 5% of cases.
   D. Hematogenous osteomyelitis is most common in adults.
   E. Mortality rate is approximately 50%.

10. A 54-year-old patient under treatment with hemodialysis for chronic renal failure undergoes a biopsy of a large lytic bone lesion. What is the most likely diagnosis?
   A. Brown tumor
   B. Fracture
   C. Giant cell tumor
   D. Granuloma
   E. Paget disease

# ANSWERS AND EXPLANATIONS

**1. Correct choice: C.**

Abnormal mineralization of bone can be caused by vitamin D deficiency (rickets in children, osteomalacia in adults), hereditary deficiency in alkaline phosphatase (hypophosphatasia), and certain metals (aluminum, iron, fluoride). Each is characterized by an increase in the amount of unmineralized osteoid bone, a feature known as hyperosteoidosis. Conditions characterized by abnormal mineralization will be missed on decalcified specimens. Diagnosis can be made on undecalcified sections embedded in plastic. Hyperparathyroidism, Paget disease, osteoporosis, and osteopetrosis are all due to abnormalities in bone resorption. Osteogenesis imperfecta is a condition characterized by congenital defective synthesis of collagen.

**2. Correct choice: B.**

Osteogenesis imperfecta comprises several distinct syndromes which may be due to autosomal dominant mutations, autosomal recessive mutations, or spontaneous mutations. All are due to collagen mutations, primarily *COL1A1* and *COL1A2*. Affected patients have short stature and recurrent fractures in childhood, combined with characteristic blue sclerae, small, misshapen teeth, and disproportionately shortened limbs. The fractures often involve the growth plates around the knees. This process leads to the enlargement of bone epiphysis, which becomes filled with nodules of cartilage, producing the classic bag of popcorn appearance on x-rays. Biopsies show a disrupted trabecular pattern, with crowding of osteocytes and the presence of excessive osteoid (unmineralized) bone.

**3. Correct choice: B.**

Fractures in osteogenesis imperfecta often involve the growth plates around the knees, leading to fragmentation of the growth plate and disorganized proliferation of cartilage fragments. Abnormal mineralization of the growth plate occurs in osteomalacia/rickets, hypophosphatasia, and aluminum toxicity. Increased density of bone is characteristic of osteopetrosis, an inherited disorder due to altered osteoclastic bone resorption that causes shortening of long bones and propensity to fractures. Premature fusion of growth plate happens in achondroplasia, an inherited disorder manifesting with dwarfism secondary to premature sealing of growth plates and due to mutations of fibroblast growth factor receptor-3 (FGFR-3). Thinning of trabeculae is characteristic of osteoporosis.

**4. Correct choice: E.**

This biopsy demonstrates the typical microscopic findings of Paget disease, with an increased number of osteoclasts and disorganized trabeculae lined by plump osteoblasts. The osteoclasts contain many nuclei. Paget disease is found in up to 10% of the general population in some European countries and the United States. It has declined in incidence in recent decades. Most patients are asymptomatic, but bone pain or symptoms related to one of the complications of the disease (eg, arthritis or fracture) are not uncommon. The disease may be monostotic or polyostotic. Paget disease most frequently affects the spine, pelvis, and skull. Histologically, active resorption is coupled to osteoblastic deposition of new bone. In late stages (osteosclerotic or burn-out phase), the normal bone is entirely replaced by sclerotic, structurally disorganized bone. Increased bone turnover leads to the formation of numerous haphazardly interconnecting cement lines, producing a mosaic-like appearance. The bone is mostly of the woven type, thus more fragile than mature bone. Fractures and deformities are the consequences of such alterations. Osteosarcoma develops in 1% to 2% of patients with widespread Paget disease.

**5. Correct choice: D.**

Osteoporosis reflects a reduction in bone mass due to increased bone porosity, which predisposes bones to fracture. It typically occurs in postmenopausal women. It affects the entire skeleton and is usually due to increased bone resorption, with normal levels of bone formation. Flattening of vertebral bodies, with widening and swelling of intervertebral discs (the so called fish-mouth appearance), is seen in the thoracic and upper lumbar spine.

**6. Correct choice: C.**

Osteopetrosis, also called marble bone disease, is a rare, hereditary, diffuse, and symmetric skeletal sclerosis (increased bone density) caused by osteoclast dysfunction. The bones have a "stone-like" quality but are abnormally brittle and fracture like chalk. There are two types: a severe autosomal recessive disorder that usually causes death in utero or in early childhood and a less severe autosomal dominant disorder that may not be diagnosed until adulthood when the affected patient develops fractures, or a characteristic Erlenmeyer flask deformity (loss of the normal metaphyseal flare) is detected on x-ray as an incidental finding. Long bones are typically shortened and there is uniform opacity of pelvis and peripheral bones alternating with normal bone causing a striped appearance on radiologic examination. Biopsies demonstrate extremely irregular and thickened bone trabeculae and cores of basophilic calcified cartilage as well as numerous osteoclast-like cells. Anemia is often present due to the reduction in marrow space.

Spinal involvement may result in spondylolisthesis. The differential diagnosis includes myelosclerosis/osteosclerosis, a rare condition in which replacement of the marrow by fibrous tissue (myelofibrosis) or bone (osteosclerosis), often in conjunction with a myeloproliferative disorder is associated with extramedullary hematopoiesis and the appearance in the peripheral blood of immature white cells and red cells; osteoblastic metastases, caused by cancer cells that stimulate osteoblastic cell proliferation resulting in dense sclerotic bone (most often associated with metastatic prostatic carcinoma); and Paget disease.

**7. Correct choice: B.**

At the early stage of fracture healing (1-2 weeks), fracture callus consists of hypercellular, hypervascular tissue, often with brisk mitotic activity, resembling sarcoma but without atypia or atypical mitotic figures. The presence of necrotic bone (empty lacunae, poorly staining bone matrix) can delay healing. Nodular fasciitis is another reactive process resembling sarcoma that may be associated with prior trauma, but it should not be associated with necrotic bone. Reactive periostitis (fibro-osseous pseudotumor of digits) is a rare, self-limited calcifying and ossifying soft tissue neoplasm that occurs in the hands and less often, the feet. There may be a history of trauma. Biopsy also shows a disordered fibroblastic proliferation and increased mitoses, with immature bone formation. Maturation is present at the periphery of the lesion, while the opposite is true of osteosarcoma. Osteomyelitis is associated with necrotic bone but there is also a prominent neutrophilic response.

**8. Correct choice: B.**

Myositis ossificans circumscripta is a benign, reactive, ossifying soft tissue lesion that often develops close to a bone. It usually occurs in the anterior muscle groups of the thigh and arm in physically active young males (second and third decade) with reports of a rapid growth. Up to 75% have a history of trauma in the preceding 4 to 6 weeks. It is divided into three clinical phases: early (days to a few weeks), there is diffuse, tender soft tissue swelling with decreased range of motion; intermediate (1-2 months), there is a circumscribed, indurated, firm to stony hard soft tissue mass with persistent pain and decreased range of motion; and late (>2 months), there is a stony hard soft tissue mass with decreased pain and improved range of motion. Histologically, it is characterized by a zonal pattern with different degrees of cellular differentiation (inner zone, intermediate zone, and peripheral zone). The inner central zone is composed of a fibroblastic/myofibroblastic proliferation, which is highly vascular, rich in inflammatory cells, and resembles nodular fasciitis; some multinucleated giant cells may also be seen. Areas of hemorrhage, fibrin, and entrapped atrophic muscle fibers may be seen. The intermediate zone contains a mixture of fibroblasts and osteoblasts along with osteoids separated by small-sized vessels, while the peripheral zone contains osteoid that undergoes calcification leading to lamellar bone formation. Myositis ossificans circumscripta harbors *USP6* gene rearrangements, mostly with *COL1A1*. Treatment is conservative. Extraskeletal osteosarcoma occurs in sixth or seventh decade and exhibits backward zonation (ie, most mature bone in the center with woven bone at the periphery). Parosteal osteosarcoma may mimic myositis ossificans if the latter is located near the surface of a major long tubular bone. However, radiology shows central heavy mineralization and connection with the underlying bone. Parosteal osteosarcoma consists of well-developed tumor bone, unlike the zonal pattern of myositis ossificans. Similarly, periosteal osteosarcoma exhibits connection with the bone surface with a periosteal reaction and there is no zonal pattern. Synovial sarcoma can become extensively calcified with secondary bone formation, but it also lacks a zoning pattern.

**9. Correct choice: A.**

Acute osteomyelitis may arise by hematogenous spread or direct inoculation/spread. Hematogenous osteomyelitis is typical of children (rare in adults with the exception of debilitated patients) and localizes in the metaphysis close to the growth plate. Osteomyelitis due to direct spread/inoculation is usually posttraumatic, resulting from traffic accidents, puncture wounds, or surgery. The mortality rate of acute osteomyelitis is close to 0. Chronic osteomyelitis develops in 15% to 30% of cases, usually because of inadequate antibiotic treatment or incomplete debridement. In children, chronic osteomyelitis may produce a round radiolucent lesion surrounded by a sclerotic rim (Brodie abscess). Two factors are important in the pathogenesis of chronic osteomyelitis: (a) bacteria find protection from antibiotics in the sequestrum (necrotic bone) and (b) development of bacterial colonies resistant to antibiotics, the so-called bacterial biofilms. Biofilms act as a reservoir of persistent infection so that chronic osteomyelitis will not resolve unless the biofilm is eliminated. Etiologic agents include (a) *Staphylococcus aureus*, *Streptococcus pyogenes*, *Haemophilus influenzae*, most common in hematogenous osteomyelitis; (b) gram-negative bacteria and fungi that may occur in intravenous drug users; (c) *Pseudomonas aeruginosa* in spine infections of older patients with genitourinary infections; (d) *Salmonella* in patients with sickle cell disease; (e) group B streptococci and coliform bacteria in neonatal period, (f) *Kingella kingae* in children less than 3 years; and (g) *Bartonella henselae* in cat scratch disease spreading to the spine or pelvis.

**10. Correct choice: A.**

Brown tumor arises secondary to hyperparathyroidism, a condition that enhances bone resorption. Primary (parathyroid adenoma) and secondary (chronic renal failure) hyperparathyroidism cause the same radiologic and pathologic picture. The most characteristic radiographic changes are found in the phalanges, which exhibit erosions of their tufts and subperiosteal resorption on the radial sides. Rarely, bone resorption results in large lytic lesions filled with hemosiderin-laden macrophages and reparative granulation tissue, brown tumors. Osteitis fibrosa cystica (von Recklinghausen disease) is the most severe presentation and consists of multiple brown tumors. Microscopically, the characteristic finding in brown tumors is increased osteoclastic activity due to burrowing of the osteoclasts into the bone matrix, imparting a tunnel appearance. The photomicrograph depicted here shows a lesion composed of bony trabeculae showing resorption along with scattered osteoclast-like giant cells set within a vascularized spindled stroma. A fracture shows necrotic bone and callus. Granulomas show an organized proliferation of multinucleated histiocytes with admixed lymphocytes. Giant cell tumor shows a much more uniform and dense distribution of osteoclast-type giant cells admixed with mononuclear cells exhibiting similar nuclear features. In Paget disease, the osteoclasts are usually at the surface of the bone trabeculae and contain many more nuclei. Clinical presentation and biochemical findings are important in establishing the correct diagnosis.

# 8 Bone Tumors

1. An x-ray reveals a bone mass in the right femur of a 15-year-old male. The film depicts a mushroom-like exostosis projecting away from the epiphysis at the diaphysis-metaphysis junction. The lesion, shown in Figure 1, is removed. What is the most likely diagnosis?

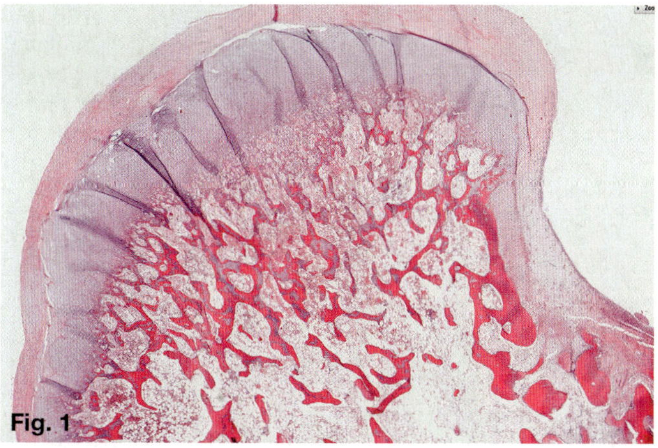

Fig. 1

A. Chondroblastoma
B. Chondromyxoid fibroma
C. Enchondroma
D. Osteochondroma
E. Periosteal chondroma

2. A tumor is removed from the second proximal phalanx of a 24-year-old man who presented with pain. The tumor expands the metaphyseal bone and produces thinning of the cortex but does not penetrate surrounding soft tissues (see Figures 1 and 2). A condition characterized by numerous tumors as this one and soft tissue hemangioma is known as

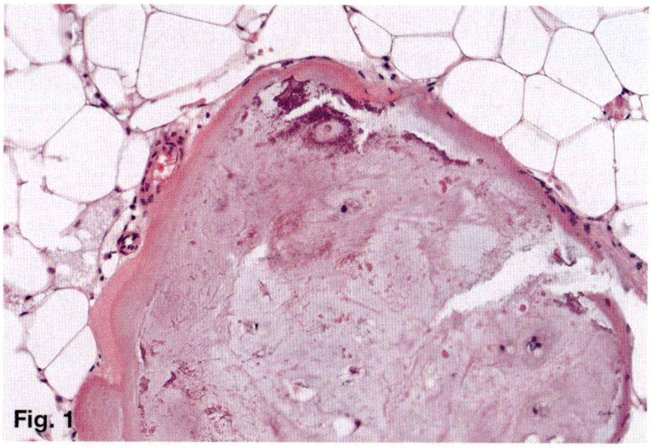

Fig. 1

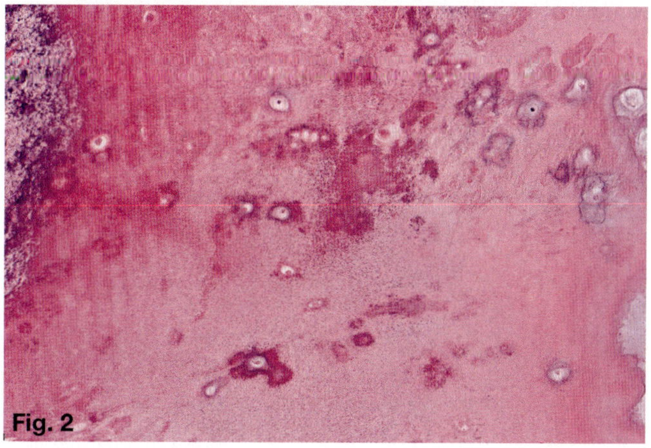

Fig. 2

A. Albright syndrome.
B. Gardner syndrome.
C. Maffucci syndrome.
D. Ollier disease.
E. osteochondromatosis.

All figures in this chapter are from Longacre TA, Greenson JK, Hornick JL, Reuter VE, eds. *Mills and Sternberg's Diagnostic Surgical Pathology.* 7th ed. Wolters Kluwer; 2022 except for those noted at the end of this book.

3. A 20-year-old woman presents with an enlarging mass on the medial surface of the distal left great toe, accompanied by pain. A radiograph demonstrates a pedunculated radiopaque mass on the dorsomedial aspect of the distal toe that is not continuous with the medullary cavity of the bone. The mass is removed. The clinical, radiographic, and pathologic features of the lesion, shown in Figure 1, are most compatible with which of the following?

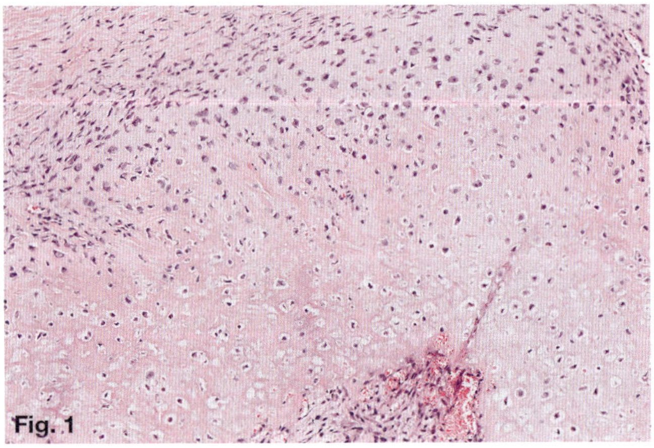

Fig. 1

A. Bizarre parosteal osteochondromatous proliferation
B. Florid reactive periostitis
C. Osteochondroma
D. Parosteal osteosarcoma
E. Subungual exostosis

4. A 14-year-old boy comes to medical attention because of persistent dull pain in the lower right thigh, not relieved by anti-inflammatory drugs. A radiograph reveals a well-demarcated peripheral lytic defect in the distal femur. The lesion, shown in Figure 1, is excised. Which of the following is the best diagnosis?

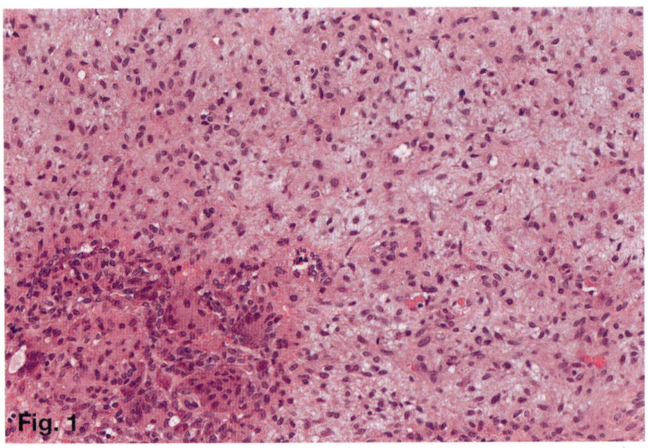

Fig. 1

A. Chondroblastoma
B. Chondromyxoid fibroma
C. Chondrosarcoma
D. Giant cell tumor
E. Osteoid osteoma

5. A 15-year-old male presents with a history of pain in the right leg that manifests at night and is promptly relieved by aspirin. A 1.5-cm radiolucent focus surrounded by an osteosclerotic rim, shown in Figure 1, is identified in the right tibia and excised. Which of the following is the most likely diagnosis?

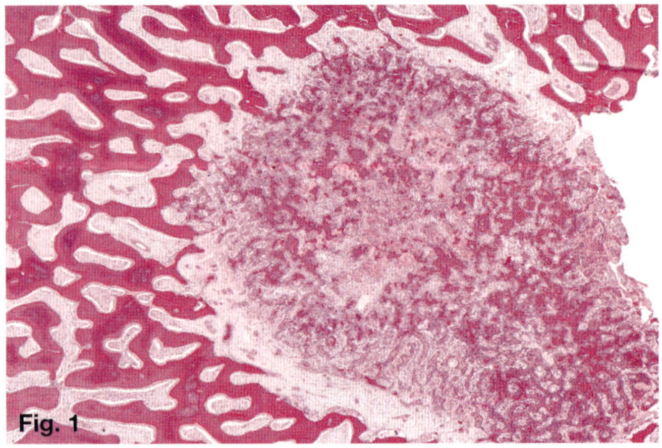

Fig. 1

A. Fibrous dysplasia
B. Osteoblastoma
C. Osteochondroma
D. Osteoid osteoma
E. Osteosarcoma

6. A 16-year-old male has a bone lesion in the distal epiphysis of his right femur. The lesion appears as a well-demarcated area of radiolucency, rimmed by sclerotic bone and extending to the articular cartilage. A biopsy is performed (see Figure 1). Given the clinical, radiographic, and pathologic features, what is the most likely diagnosis?

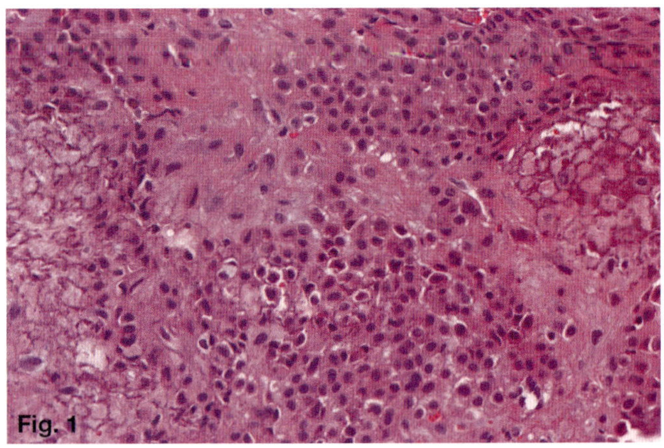

Fig. 1

A. Aneurysmal bone cyst
B. Chondroblastoma
C. Chondroma
D. Chondrosarcoma
E. Giant cell tumor of bone

7. A 15-year-old male presents with a pathologic fracture of the distal fibula. A spongy hemorrhagic mass is excised. Provided the photomicrograph, shown in Figure 1, is representative of the entire lesion, the most likely diagnosis is

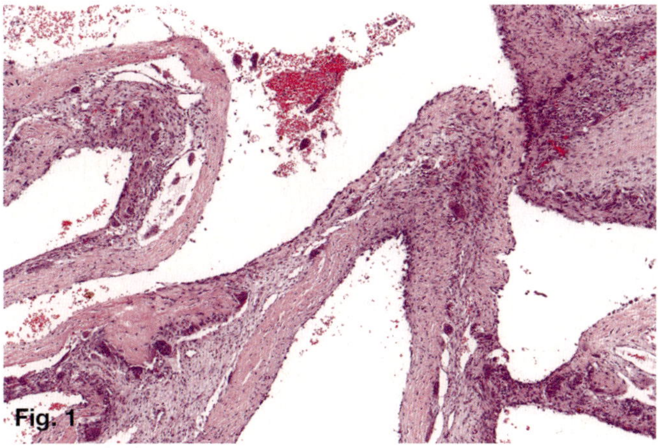
Fig. 1

A. aneurysmal bone cyst.
B. brown tumor of hyperparathyroidism.
C. central giant cell tumor.
D. hemangioma.
E. telangiectatic osteosarcoma.

8. Secondary central and secondary peripheral chondrosarcomas are morphologically identical to which of the following chondrosarcoma types?

A. Clear cell
B. Conventional
C. Dedifferentiated
D. Mesenchymal
E. Periosteal

9. Which of the following is/are the most characteristic genetic alterations associated with enchondroma and chondrosarcomas?

A. Mutations of the EXT1 or EXT2 genes
B. Mutations of the H3F3A gene coding H3.3 histone
C. Mutations of the H3F3B gene coding H3.3 histone
D. Mutations of the IDH1 or IDH2 gene
E. Rearrangement of chromosome 6 causing overexpression of GRM1

10. A 35-year-old patient presents with a 6-cm lobulated mass on the cortex of the proximal metaphysis of the right humerus, shown in Figure 1. It infiltrates the soft tissue and penetrates into the cortex of the bone without reaching the medullary cavity. Histologic examination, shown in Figure 2, reveals a lobulated tumor morphologically similar to conventional chondrosarcoma invading into underlying cortex (asterisk). What is the best diagnosis?

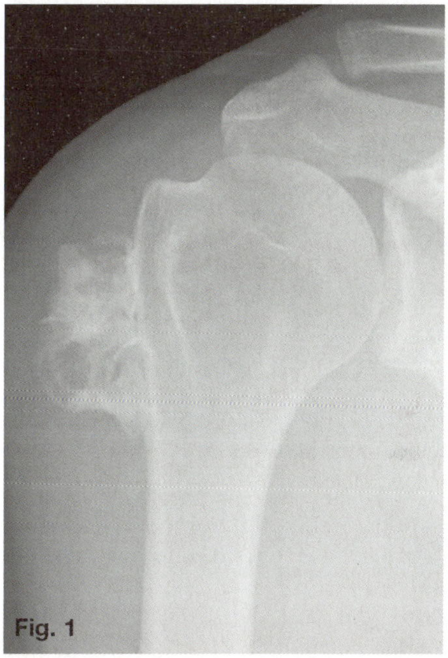
Fig. 1

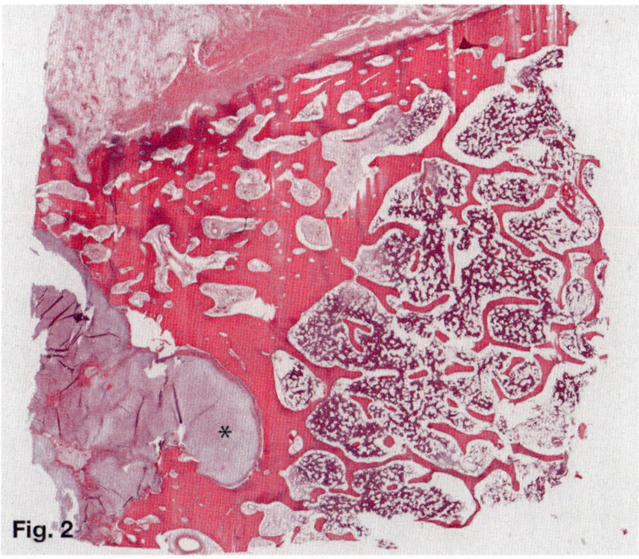

Fig. 2

A. Clear cell chondrosarcoma
B. Conventional chondrosarcoma
C. Dedifferentiated chondrosarcoma
D. Mesenchymal chondrosarcoma
E. Periosteal chondrosarcoma

11. A 60-year-old woman has a large lytic mass in the pelvis. Biopsy, shown in Figure 1, shows a biphasic morphologic pattern owing to the presence of two distinct tumor cell populations. What is the most likely diagnosis?

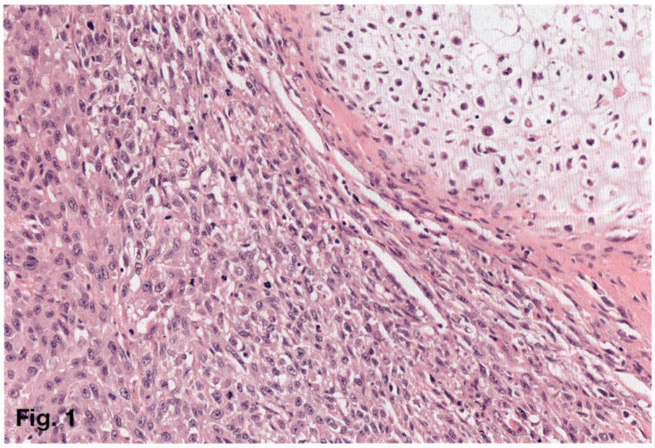

Fig. 1

A. Clear cell chondrosarcoma
B. Conventional chondrosarcoma
C. Dedifferentiated chondrosarcoma
D. Mesenchymal chondrosarcoma
E. Periosteal chondrosarcoma

12. A 22-year-old man presents with a rapidly growing soft tissue mass in the right lower extremity (see Figure 1). The mass is excised. Which of the following is the most likely diagnosis?

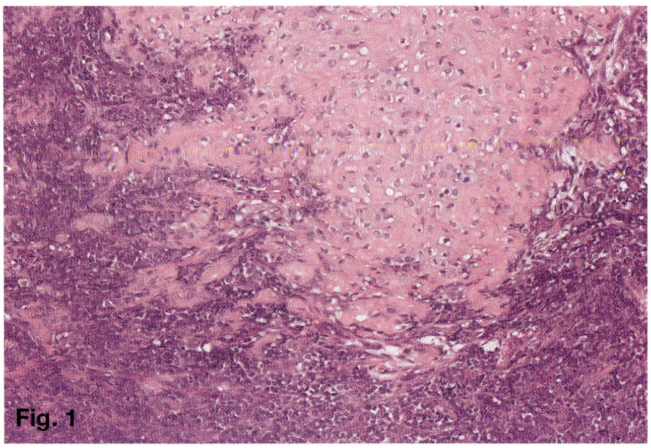

Fig. 1

A. Clear cell chondrosarcoma
B. Conventional chondrosarcoma
C. Dedifferentiated chondrosarcoma
D. Mesenchymal chondrosarcoma
E. Periosteal chondrosarcoma

13. A 34-year-old woman has a well-demarcated lytic mass in the proximal epiphysis of her right femur (see Figure 1). The mass is resected. Molecular analysis on the resected tumor does not reveal *IDH* mutations. After resection, the tumor recurred 1 year later, and the patient underwent a second resection. Five years after diagnosis, the patient is tumor free. Which of the following is the most likely diagnosis?

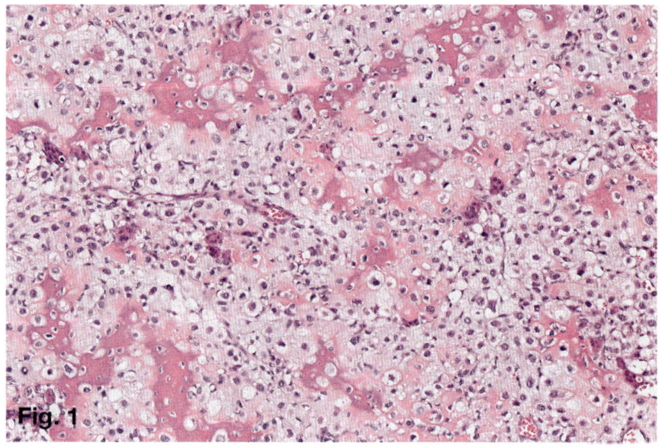

Fig. 1

A. Clear cell chondrosarcoma
B. Conventional chondrosarcoma
C. Dedifferentiated chondrosarcoma
D. Mesenchymal chondrosarcoma
E. Periosteal chondrosarcoma

14. Multiple osteomas are associated with which of the following syndromes?

A. Familial adenomatous polyposis
B. Gardner syndrome
C. Maffucci syndrome
D. McCune Albright syndrome
E. Ollier disease

15. Which of the following features is most important in establishing a diagnosis of osteosarcoma in an otherwise poorly differentiated mesenchymal tumor?

A. Fibroblastic components
B. Foci of cartilage
C. Necrotic areas
D. Osteoclast-like giant cells
E. Osteoid production

16. Most osteosarcomas arise de novo in patients older than 45 years. When the de novo cases are excluded, what is the most common underlying etiology of osteosarcoma in this age group?

A. Fibrous dysplasia
B. Infections
C. Paget disease
D. Prior radiation
E. Trauma

17. Which of the following immunohistochemical stains would be most helpful in differentiating low-grade central osteosarcoma from conventional osteosarcoma, fibrous dysplasia, and desmoplastic fibroma?

A. Keratin and EMA (epithelial membrane antigen)
B. MDM2 (mouse double-minute 2) and CDK4 (cyclin-dependent kinase 4)
C. Osteocalcin and osteonectin
D. S100 and MDM2
E. Vimentin and EMA

18. What is the most likely diagnosis for the slow-growing, extracortical, lobulated mass, shown in Figures 1 and 2, arising from the metaphasis of the distal posterior femur in a 23-year-old female?

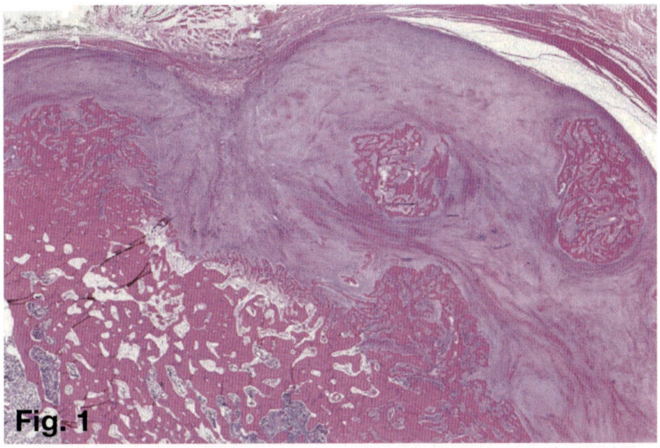
Fig. 1

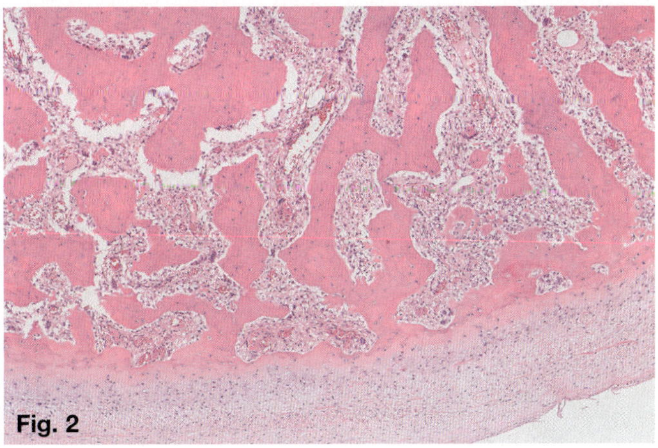
Fig. 2

A. Conventional osteosarcoma
B. High-grade surface osteosarcoma
C. Low-grade central osteosarcoma
D. Parosteal osteosarcoma
E. Periosteal osteosarcoma

19. A patient with osteosarcoma receives neoadjuvant chemotherapy before undergoing tumor resection. Which of the following parameters is the most important prognostic indicator in the resected tumor?

A. Degree of cellular atypia
B. Extent of necrosis
C. Invasion of soft tissues
D. Proliferative index
E. Vascular invasion

20. The biopsy shown in Figure 1 is from a broad-based, lucent fusiform mass on the surface of the diaphysis of the femur of a 29-year-old male. The tumor is accompanied by focal clumps of calcification and partially encircles the bone. Of the following variants/types of osteosarcoma, which is the most likely diagnosis?

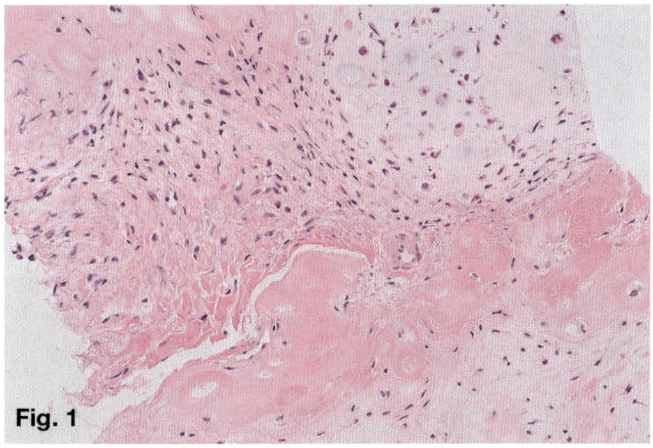
Fig. 1

A. Osteoblastic
B. Parosteal
C. Periosteal
D. Small cell
E. Telangiectatic

21. Among the histologic types of conventional osteosarcoma is a variant characterized by an increase in tumor matrix accompanied by "normalization" of cells (decreased atypia). Which of the following is it?

A. Chondroblastic
B. Fibroblastic
C. Sclerosing
D. Small cell
E. Telangiectatic

22. Which of the following histologic types of conventional osteosarcoma is depicted in the photomicrograph shown in Figure 1?

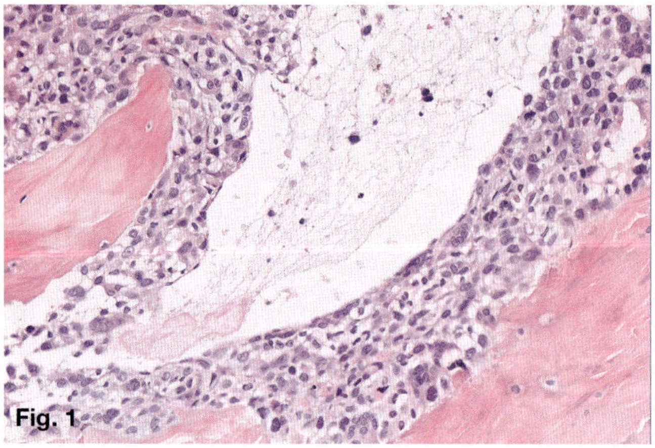

Fig. 1

A. Chondroblastic
B. Fibroblastic
C. Sclerosing
D. Small cell
E. Telangiectatic

23. Which of the following histologic types of conventional osteosarcoma is depicted in the photomicrograph shown in Figure 1?

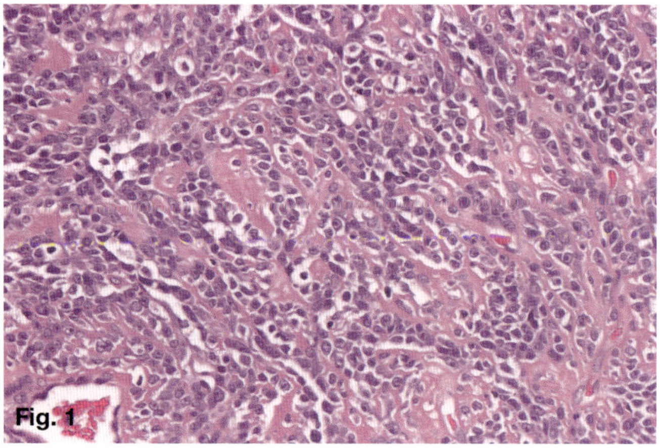

Fig. 1

A. Chondroblastic
B. Fibroblastic
C. Sclerosing
D. Small cell
E. Telangiectatic

24. A 12-year-old boy complains of pain in the right thigh. X-ray studies show a radiolucent defect in the distal metaphysis of the right femur, as seen in Figure 1. The biopsy, shown in Figure 2, demonstrates a fibroblastic population arranged in a storiform pattern. Hemosiderin-laden macrophages and clusters of giant cells are also found. These features are most consistent with

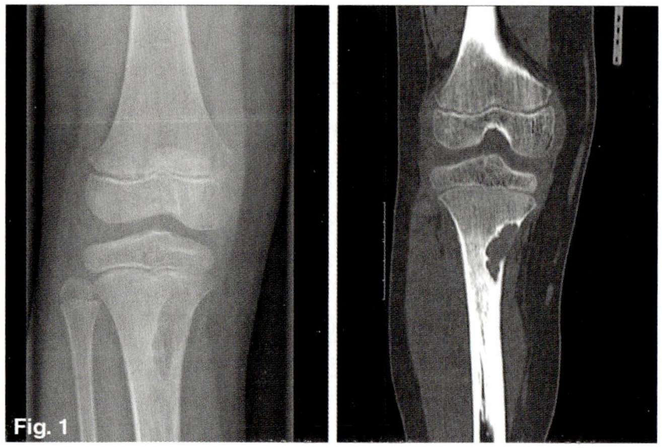

Fig. 1

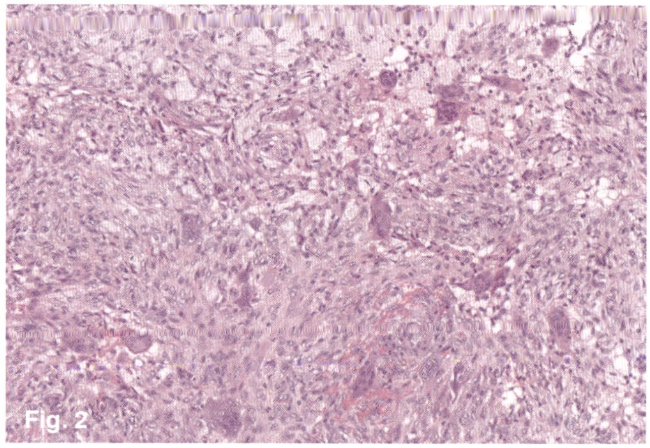

Fig. 2

A. benign fibrous histiocytoma.
B. desmoplastic fibroma.
C. fibroblastic osteosarcoma.
D. fibrosarcoma.
E. nonossifying fibroma.

25. The photomicrograph, shown in Figure 1, demonstrates the cytologic appearance of bone lesions detected in the skull and vertebral bones of a 60-year-old patient. The cells are immunoreactive for CD138 and MUM1. Which of the following is the most typical radiographic presentation of this condition?

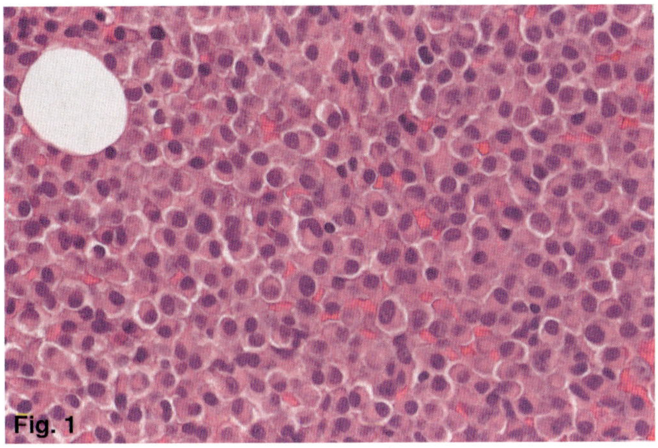
Fig. 1

A. Codman triangle
B. Expansion of bone
C. Onionskin appearance
D. Punched-out osteolytic lesions
E. Radiolucent nidus and sclerotic rim

26. A 37-year-old female undergoes resection of an osteolytic mass in the distal epiphysis of the right femur. Grossly, the mass is soft and contains multiple blood-filled cysts and brown deposits. Histologically, it has the appearance shown in Figure 1. These features are most consistent with

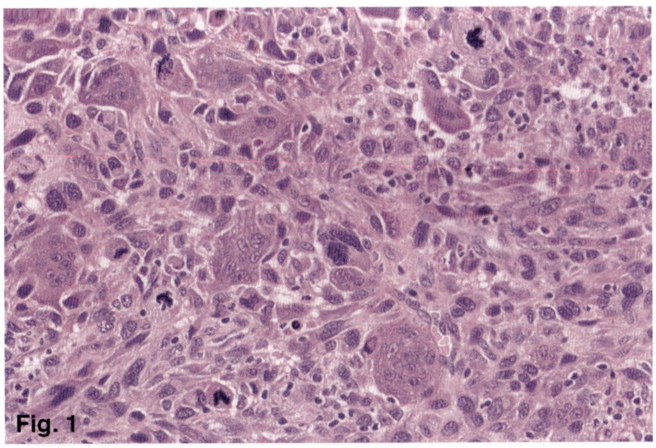
Fig. 1

A. brown tumor of hyperparathyroidism.
B. central giant cell granuloma.
C. chondroblastoma.
D. giant cell tumor.
E. tenosynovial giant cell tumor.

27. A 58-year-old man undergoes resection of an osteolytic tumor located in the clivus. The histologic appearance of the tumor is shown in Figure 1. Which of the following markers is most specific to this neoplasm?

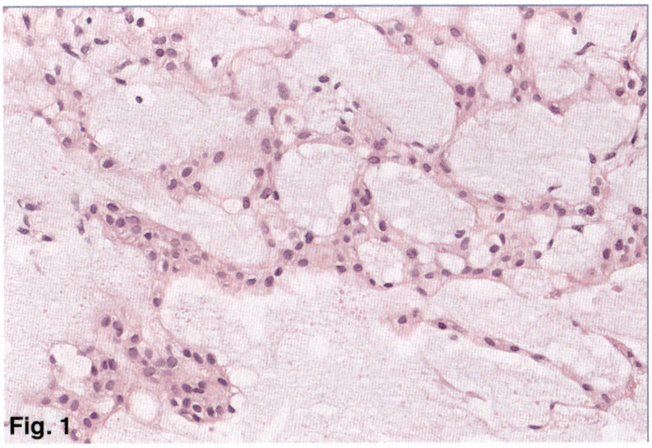
Fig. 1

A. Brachyury
B. CD10
C. CD99
D. EMA (epithelial membrane antigen)
E. S100

28. What is the best diagnosis for the mass, shown in Figure 1, removed from the distal pelvis in a 54-year-old female?

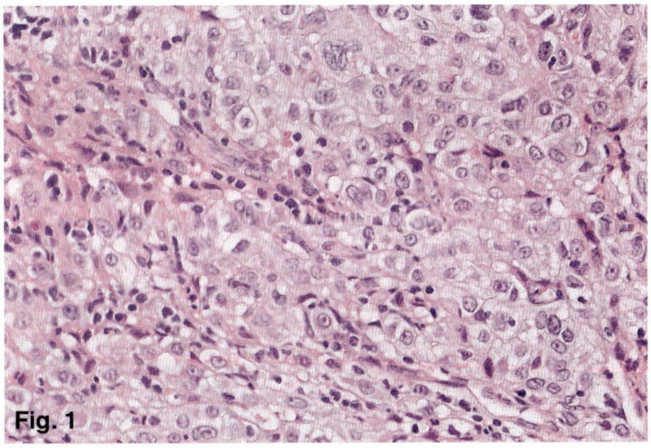
Fig. 1

A. Clear cell chondrosarcoma
B. Conventional chordoma
C. Dedifferentiated chordoma
D. Mesenchymal chondrosarcoma
E. Poorly differentiated chordoma

29. Poorly differentiated chordoma is characterized by loss of expression for which of the following immunohistochemical markers?

A. Brachyury
B. Cytokeratin
C. S100 protein
D. SMARCA4
E. SMARCB1

30. A well-demarcated osteolytic lesion in the parietal bone of a 23-year-old female is biopsied, revealing the mixed cell population shown in Figure 1. Ultrastructural studies reveal rodlike, tubular structures with expanded tennis racket-shaped ends. The diagnosis is

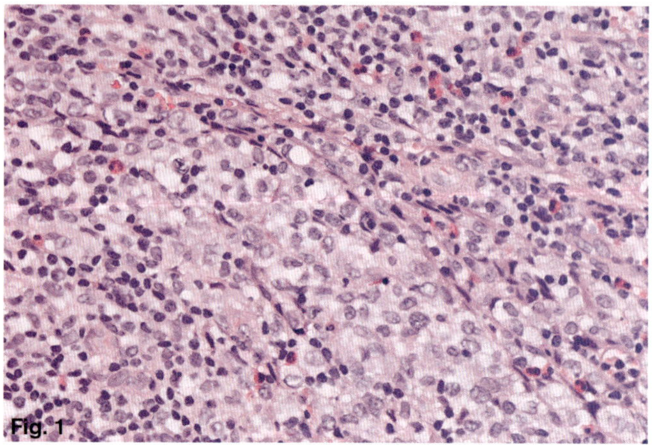
Fig. 1

A. chronic osteomyelitis.
B. infectious granuloma.
C. Langerhans cell histiocytosis.
D. metastatic carcinoma.
E. sinus histiocytosis with massive lymphadenopathy.

31. A 16-year-old male presents with swelling and pain in the right arm and fever. A mass expanding the right humerus with an onionskin pattern is identified on x-rays. A biopsy is performed (see Figure 1). Special stains demonstrate intracytoplasmic glycogen and immunoreactivity of tumor cells for CD99; TdT (terminal deoxynucleotidyl transferase) and CD45 are negative. Which of the following is the best diagnosis?

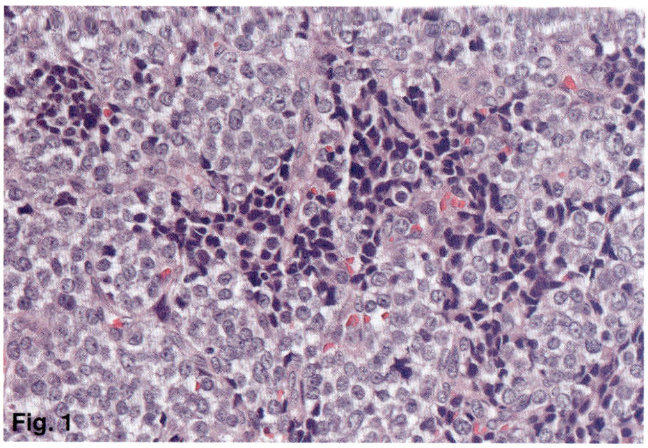
Fig. 1

A. Ewing sarcoma
B. Lymphoblastic lymphoma
C. Metastatic neuroblastoma
D. Poorly differentiated synovial sarcoma
E. Small cell osteosarcoma

32. Which of the following bone lesions is thought to be a precursor of adamantinoma?

A. Aneurysmal bone cyst
B. Fibrous dysplasia
C. Nonossifying fibroma
D. Osteofibrous dysplasia
E. Paget disease of bone

33. A 45-year-old man presents with gradually progressive leg pain. A radiograph of his left tibia reveals several variably sized lytic lesions with sclerotic borders (soap bubble appearance) involving the diaphysis. A biopsy, shown in Figure 1, is performed. What is the most likely diagnosis?

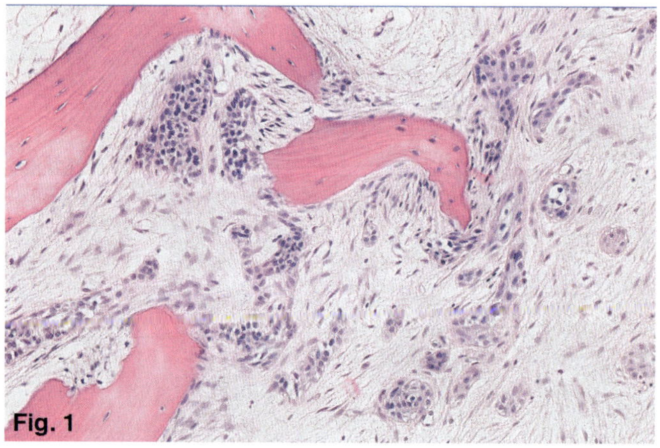
Fig. 1

A. Adamantinoma
B. Epithelioid hemangioma
C. Ewing sarcoma
D. Metastatic carcinoma
E. Osteofibrous dysplasia

34. X-ray studies reveal a unicameral cystic lesion in the proximal metaphysis of the humerus of a 14-year-old male. It contains brown fluid, and the wall is composed of vascular fibrous tissue with hemosiderin-laden macrophages and cholesterol clefts (see Figure 1). These features are consistent with

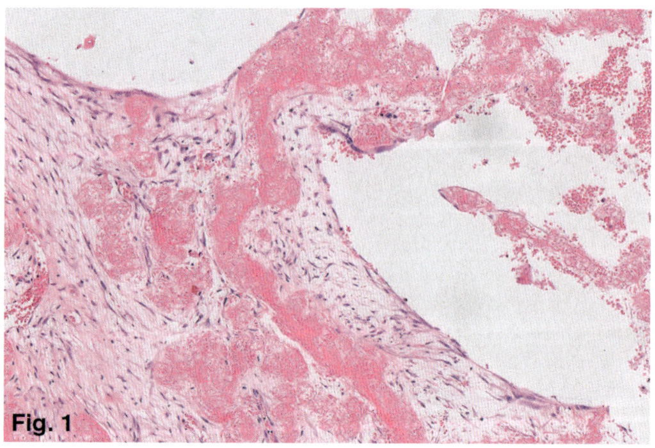
Fig. 1

A. aneurysmal bone cyst.
B. ganglion cyst of bone.
C. massive osteolysis (Gorham disease).
D. metaphyseal fibrous defect.
E. simple bone cyst.

35. A 30-year-old man presents with swelling of the right mandible. X-ray studies demonstrate an ill-defined sclerotic focus with a ground-glass appearance. Histologic examination, shown in Figure 1, reveals irregularly shaped trabeculae of immature (woven) bone within moderately cellular fibrous stroma. The bone trabeculae are not surrounded by osteoblasts or psammoma-like structures. This lesion is most consistent with

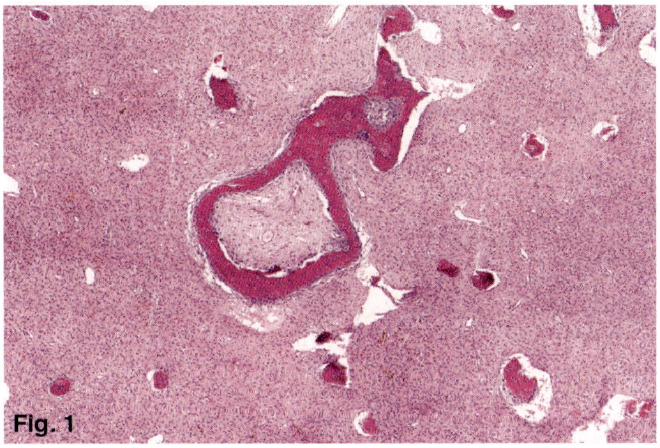
Fig. 1

A. cementifying fibroma.
B. cementoossifying fibroma.
C. fibrous dysplasia.
D. juvenile ossifying fibroma.
E. ossifying fibroma.

36. What is the best diagnosis for the tumor, shown in Figure 1, from the clivus in a 42-year-old man?

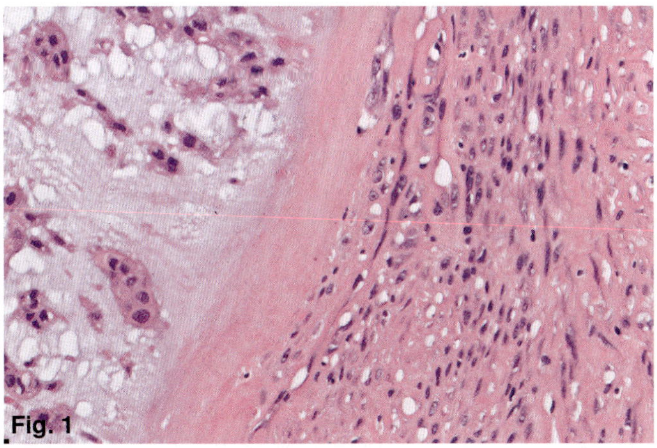
Fig. 1

A. Clear cell chondrosarcoma
B. Conventional chordoma
C. Dedifferentiated chordoma
D. Mesenchymal chondrosarcoma
E. Poorly differentiated chordoma

37. A 41-year-old female presents with right arm pain. She reports no history of trauma. An x-ray demonstrates a radiolucent lesion within the right humerus with well-defined, expansile margins. The lesion, shown in Figure 1, is removed by curettage. Which of the following is the most likely diagnosis?

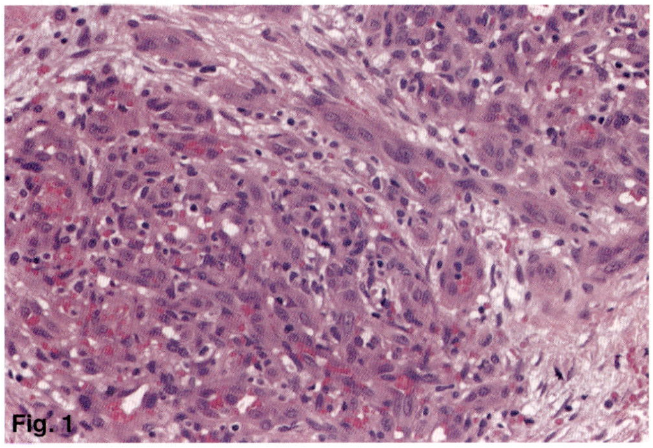
Fig. 1

A. Epithelioid angiosarcoma
B. Epithelioid hemangioendothelioma
C. Epithelioid hemangioma
D. Hemangioma
E. Skeletal angiomatosis

38. A 42-year-old man dies in a motorcycle accident. An autopsy is performed. What is the most likely diagnosis for the lesion in the distal axial skeleton, shown in Figure 1?

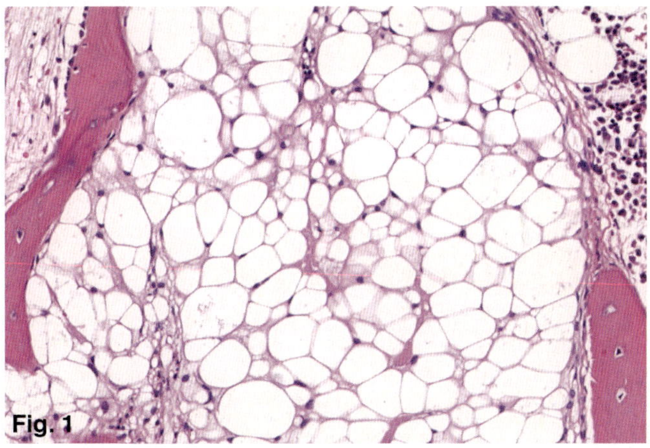
Fig. 1

A. Benign notochordal cell tumor
B. Conventional chordoma
C. Metastatic renal cell carcinoma
D. Normal fatty bone marrow
E. Traumatic fat emboli

# ANSWERS AND EXPLANATIONS

**1. Correct choice: D.**

Osteochondroma is the most frequent benign bone tumor. It probably originates from the abnormal (nonneoplastic) growth of superficial chondroid foci. It develops at the transition zone between the diaphysis and metaphysis of long bones, especially the distal femur, proximal tibia, and proximal humerus. Radiologically, it appears as a sessile or pedunculated mass growing away from the joint. The histopathologic appearance is characteristic: a nidus of mature bone surrounded by a well-differentiated cap of mature cartilage. In fact, it is the peripheral rim of cartilage that matures into the central core of the bone. The medullary cavity is in direct continuity with the stalk. Usually asymptomatic; it may produce deformities or impinge on adjacent tendons, nerves, or vessels. The rate of malignant transformation into secondary chondrosarcoma is 1% to 5%.

**2. Correct choice: C.**

Enchondromas are benign lesions composed of mature hyaline cartilage organized in a lobular pattern and surrounded by a rim of reactive bone (the so-called encasement). Enchondromas arise in long bones, 50% of cases in the hands and feet. Because the distinction between enchondroma and low-grade chondrosarcoma is difficult both radiologically and histologically, all available parameters (radiology, morphology, patient's age, location, etc) must be considered in the differential diagnosis. Malignant transformation of osteochondromas to chondrosarcoma happens rarely (<1% of cases). Innumerable chondromas are found in Maffucci syndrome and Ollier disease, caused by mutations in *IDH1* or *IDH2* (IDH: isocitrate dehydrogenase). In Maffucci syndrome, chondromas are associated with multiple soft tissue hemangiomas. In these conditions, malignant transformation occurs in up to 47% of cases. Periosteal chondroma is histologically related to enchondroma. It arises on fingers or the proximal humerus and consists of hyaline cartilage exhibiting binucleated cells, hyperchromatic and pleomorphic nuclei, and myxoid change. These features are normal in periosteal chondromas but would be interpreted as supporting a diagnosis of chondrosarcoma if the lesion were growing outside the periosteal region. In addition, periosteal chondrosarcoma causes cortical destruction and is usually much larger than periosteal chondromas.

**3. Correct choice: E.**

Subungual exostosis is a benign osteochondromatous proliferation located in the distal phalanx below the nail bed. Toes are most frequently involved (80% involve the great toe). Most common clinical presentations include long-standing pain (77%) followed by a mass or swelling in the nail which is associated with erythema and deformity of the nail bed. The lesion may develop over a course of several months to years. Histologically, the lesion consists of hypercellular cartilage with a fibrocollagenous extracellular matrix displaying a gradual transition into the cellular fibroblastic stroma. Subungual exostosis is associated with a recurrent chromosomal translocation t(x;6), rearranging the *COL12A1* and *COL4A5* genes, and upregulating expression of the *IRS4* gene. Bizarre parosteal osteochondromatous proliferation, also known as Nora lesion, affects the small bones of the hands and feet. Patients are usually in their third and fourth decades. Histologically, bizarre parosteal osteochondromatous proliferation also exhibits hypercellular cartilage, but with a less orderly maturation than is seen in subungual exostosis which is associated with irregular areas of bone with a strikingly dark blue color ("blue bone"), and haphazardly arranged spindle cells between bone trabeculae. Florid reactive periostitis affects the long bones of the hands and feet and consists of a population of spindle cells with bone trabeculae lined by osteoblasts. Osteochondromas are uncommon in the distal extremities and do not exhibit cytologic atypia. Parosteal osteosarcoma is rare in the hands and feet and infiltrates into surrounding soft tissues.

**4. Correct choice: B.**

Chondromyxoid fibroma is a rare benign tumor of cartilaginous origin that usually develops in the metaphysis of long bones, most commonly in the feet, and preferentially between 10 and 25 years of age. Its cellular pleomorphism may suggest a diagnosis of chondrosarcoma. Important features favoring a diagnosis of chondromyxoid fibroma include a well-circumscribed lesion composed of lobules of myxoid or chondroid matrix with numerous spindle or stellate cells. There is increased cellularity at the edge of the lobules where the cells are more rounded and admixed with multinucleated osteoclastic giant cells. The cells in chondromyxoid fibroma express CD166, cyclin D1, and p16. Of note, the cells within the lobules express S100, while cells at the periphery are positive for muscle-specific actin and smooth muscle actin, reflecting their myofibroblastic nature. Upregulation of the *GRM1* (metabotropic glutamate receptor 1) gene has been shown to be specific to this tumor. Chondroblastoma arises mostly in the epiphysis in young patients with immature skeletons and is composed of islands of mononuclear cells with distinct cell borders and characteristic grooved nuclei. Chicken wire–like calcifications are characteristic. Chondrosarcoma is a destructive, osteolytic lesion with invasion into adjacent bone and soft tissue. Histologically, it demonstrates infiltrative lobules of cartilage with variable degrees of cellularity and nuclear atypia. Giant cell tumor arises in the epiphyses of long bones in adults and exhibits a uniform distribution of osteoclast-type giant cells among mononuclear cells.

**5. Correct choice: D.**

The clinical history (nocturnal pain relieved by aspirin), radiography (radiolucent nidus surrounded by osteosclerotic reaction), and pathology are diagnostic of osteoid osteoma. The prototypical appearance of a well-demarcated nidus surrounded by reactive bone formation and loose fibrous tissue is depicted in this photomicrography. Osteoblastoma is histologically identical to osteoid osteoma, but it usually develops in the spinal skeleton and, by definition, is larger than 2.0 cm in diameter. Patients present with back pain, but unlike osteoid osteoma, the pain is not worse at night and is less consistently relieved by anti-inflammatory medications. Also, osteoblastoma recurs more frequently than osteoid osteoma.

**6. Correct choice: B.**

Chondroblastoma is a benign tumor that develops before the age of 20, usually in the distal femur, proximal tibia, or proximal humerus. The picture demonstrates the typical *chicken-wire* pattern of calcification. Chondroblastomas show great morphologic variability. Occasionally, the prevalence of giant cells or high cellular density leads to a mistaken diagnosis of giant cell tumor or, respectively, chondrosarcoma. The chicken-wire pattern of calcification and morphology of mononuclear cells are helpful features. The tumor manifests with pain and needs ample surgical debridement and bone grafting. Aneurysmal bone cyst may be primary or secondary to another lesion. Primary aneurysmal bone cyst is a multiloculated, blood-filled, destructive, cystic lesion and is associated with *USP6* gene rearrangements. Secondary aneurysmal bone cysts can be associated with chondroblastoma, giant cell tumor, osteoblastoma, and osteosarcoma. Aneurysmal bone cysts develop within approximately 15% of chondroblastomas. Giant cell tumor occurs in patients with a closed epiphysis (third decade of life) and demonstrates clustered giant cells that are larger and more numerous and uniformly distributed than chondroblastoma; no chondroid matrix or chicken-wire calcifications are seen.

**7. Correct choice: A.**

Aneurysmal bone cysts develop most often in vertebrae and flat bones but also in the shaft of long bones. Radiologically, it appears as an eccentric, expansile, radiolucent, cystic mass. It is composed of spaces separated by septa that lack endothelial lining and consist of a mixed fibroblastic/myofibroblastic/histiocytic population. Aneurysmal bone cyst may be primary or secondary to another lesion. Aneurysmal bone cyst can be associated with several tumors, such as chondroblastoma, giant cell tumor, osteoblastoma, and osteosarcoma. Therefore, diagnosis of a primary aneurysmal bone cyst requires a complete evaluation of the entire lesion to exclude the possibility of another tumor. When located in the mandible, the main differential diagnosis is with central giant cell granuloma. The remaining choices include the conditions most important in the differential diagnosis of a cystic hemorrhagic bone lesion.

**8. Correct choice: B.**

Chondrosarcoma is a malignant mesenchymal neoplasm-producing chondroid matrix, that arises preferentially in the third to sixth decade of life and affects usually thoracic, pelvic, and long bones. Chondrosarcomas are treated surgically since they are highly resistant to chemotherapy and radiation. There are several types:

- Conventional, subdivided into
  - *Primary central chondrosarcoma*, arising in previously normal bone, at skeletal locations characterized by endochondral ossification. It accounts for 75% of all chondrosarcomas.
  - *Secondary central chondrosarcoma*, developing from a preexisting enchondroma, usually in the setting of Maffucci or Ollier.
  - *Secondary peripheral chondrosarcoma*, developing from a preexisting osteochondroma.
- Mesenchymal
- Clear cell
- Periosteal
- Dedifferentiated

All types of conventional chondrosarcoma, whether primary or secondary, are morphologically identical and are graded the same way.

**9. Correct choice: D.**

Mutations in the genes encoding isocitrate dehydrogenase 1 and 2 (*IDH1* and *IDH2*) are found in enchondromas developing in patients with Ollier and Maffucci syndromes and a high percentage of chondrosarcomas, whether primary or secondary. Multiple osteochondroma syndrome, characterized by numerous osteochondromas, is due to mutations of the *EXT1* or *EXT2* genes, which encode exostosin-1 and exostosin-2, glycosyltransferases involved in the synthesis of heparan sulfate. Interestingly, secondary peripheral chondrosarcomas do not have mutations in *EXT1* or *EXT2*. Mutations of two genes coding for the histone H3.3 are associated with two different tumors: *H3F3A* with giant cell tumor of bone and *H3F3B* with chondroblastoma. Variable rearrangements of chromosome 6 are characteristic of chondromyxoid fibroma and lead to overexpression of GRM1, a metabotropic glutamate receptor.

**10. Correct choice: E.**

Periosteal chondrosarcoma originates from the periosteum and thus is located on the surface of cortical bone. It accounts for less than 1% of all chondrosarcomas. It is usually seen in the metaphysis of the femur or humerus, in young adults, with a peak incidence in the fourth decade. The tumor is morphologically similar to conventional chondrosarcoma. The features that distinguish this variant from periosteal chondroma include its large size (>5 cm) and the presence of infiltration into the cortex of the bone and surrounding soft tissues. In contrast to conventional secondary peripheral chondrosarcoma (arising from osteochondroma), periosteal chondrosarcoma does not have a connection with the medullary cavity.

**11. Correct choice: C.**

Dedifferentiated chondrosarcoma is characterized by the coexistence of two histologic components: a well-differentiated cartilaginous tumor (enchondroma, atypical cartilaginous tumor/chondrosarcoma grade 1, or chondrosarcoma grade 2) along with a high-grade noncartilaginous sarcoma (undifferentiated pleomorphic sarcoma, osteosarcoma, fibrosarcoma, leiomyosarcoma, rhabdomyosarcoma, or angiosarcoma). The transition between the two components is abrupt. Dedifferentiated chondrosarcoma accounts for 10% of all chondrosarcomas. The tumor is located centrally, in the pelvis, proximal or distal femur, proximal humerus, and ribs. This variant is highly aggressive. About 50% have *IDH1* or *IDH2* mutations, which are present in both components.

**12. Correct choice: D.**

Mesenchymal chondrosarcoma is a rare variant (<2% of all chondrosarcomas) consisting of poorly differentiated small cells and islands of hyaline cartilage. Some areas are highly vascular, with a hemangiopericytoma-like vascular pattern. The tumor has a peak incidence in the second and third decades and is more often located in the lower extremities, facial bones, and pelvis. Up to one-third of cases are extraosseous, arising in the meninges and low extremities. The radiologic appearance is similar to that of conventional chondrosarcoma, that is, a lytic lesion with spotty, popcorn-like calcifications. Mesenchymal chondrosarcoma harbors a recurrent *HEY1-NCOA2* gene fusion. Mesenchymal chondrosarcoma is highly aggressive, but when the cellular, undifferentiated component predominates, the tumor can be sensitive to chemotherapy and radiation.

**13. Correct choice: A.**

Clear cell chondrosarcoma accounts for 2% of chondrosarcomas. This is a low-grade variant characterized by clear cells reminiscent of the hypertrophic cells in the growth plate. Tumor cells are round, with a central nucleolus, clear cytoplasm, and sharp cell borders. The tumor is usually located in the proximal epiphyses of the femur, humerus, or tibia and manifests radiologically as a lytic but well-circumscribed lesion. Peak incidence is in the third and fourth decades. *IDH* mutations are absent in this variant. Recurrence is not infrequent after simple curettage, but metastases are rare, reflecting the low-grade nature of this tumor.

**14. Correct choice: B.**

Osteomas are rare benign tumors composed of well-developed lamellar bone that develops from the surface of a bone. They arise in bones that form by membranous ossification (mostly craniofacial bones), most frequently around the paranasal sinuses. They are probably a hamartomatous rather than a neoplastic lesion. Gardner syndrome is characterized by intestinal polyposis, multiple osteomas, epidermal cysts, and fibromatosis. The condition is autosomal dominant (like familial adenomatous polyposis), and intestinal polyps are identical to those associated with familial adenomatous polyposis. With the exception of the Gardner syndrome associated osteomas, osteomas are usually solitary and asymptomatic. Radiologically, osteoma presents as a sharply demarcated radiopaque mass projecting from a bony surface.

**15. Correct choice: E.**

Production of variably calcified osteoid is the histologic hallmark of osteosarcoma. Care should be taken to distinguish between bone entrapped by the neoplastic growth and bone/osteoid produced by tumor cells. Fibroblastic or chondroblastic components are often present and may be predominant. Giant cells are present in one-third of cases and may be extremely numerous (giant cell variant). Most tumors are resected after chemotherapy and thus contain necrotic areas.

**16. Correct choice: C.**

Osteosarcoma has two peaks of incidence, one in childhood/adolescence and the second in middle/older age. The majority of the latter cases develop in association with Paget disease. Other recognized risk factors include radiation exposure, chemotherapy, foreign bodies, and various bone conditions (ie, fibrous dysplasia and chondromatosis). Also, hereditary retinoblastoma leads to an increased risk of osteosarcoma. De novo cases outnumber the tumors arising as a complication of radiation therapy or in association with Paget disease and fibrous dysplasia.

**17. Correct choice: B.**

Low-grade central osteosarcoma accounts for less than 2% of osteosarcomas. It arises within the medullary cavity of long bones, especially around the knee. The lesion may appear aggressive radiographically, but the tumor has an excellent prognosis. The main differential diagnosis is with similar spindle cell lesions such as fibrous dysplasia and desmoplastic fibroma. Osteoid is not present in the latter lesions. Low-grade central osteosarcoma has an infiltrating border, but this feature cannot be appreciated in biopsies. Immunohistochemistry can help in this instance. Tumor cells in low-grade central osteosarcoma have supernumerary ring chromosomes that lead to amplification of *CDK4* (cyclin-dependent kinase 4) and *MDM2* (murine double-minute type 2). Thus, immunohistochemical stains with these antibodies will show enhanced expression of CDK4 and MDM2 in low-grade central osteosarcoma, but not in benign fibrous and fibro-osseous lesions such as fibrous dysplasia and desmoplastic fibroma. There is no single specific molecular marker for conventional osteosarcoma. Up to 36% of low-grade central osteosarcomas progress to high-grade sarcoma.

**18. Correct choice: D.**

Parosteal osteosarcoma comprises 4% of osteosarcomas. The tumor originates from the metaphysis, grows outward as a lobulated mass, and eventually may surround the whole bone. The indolent tumor growth is associated with a good prognosis. Histologically, it is similar to low-grade central osteosarcoma. It is composed of a spindle cell population with slender bone trabeculae that are evenly scattered and oriented in a parallel fashion. The fact that chondroid tissue is present in 50% of cases raises the differential diagnosis with osteochondroma. Moreover, if the cartilage takes up more than 50% of the tumor mass, periosteal osteosarcoma enters the differential diagnosis. Other lesions to consider in the differential diagnosis: bizarre parosteal osteochondromatous proliferation, myositis ossificans, fracture callus, and fibromatosis. Like low-grade central osteosarcoma, parosteal osteosarcoma has extra ring chromosomes leading to amplification of *CDK4* and *MDM2*, which can be demonstrated by FISH or immunohistochemistry. Up to 25% of cases progress to high-grade sarcomas.

**19. Correct choice: B.**

Patients with conventional osteosarcoma usually receive chemotherapeutic treatment before the tumor is surgically removed. The extent of necrosis reflects a response to chemotherapy and represents the best predictor of overall and disease-free survival. To assess the extent of necrosis, one must study a full cross section of the tumor at its largest diameter. A good response to therapy is defined as necrosis involving more than 90% of the tumor.

**20. Correct choice: C.**

Periosteal osteosarcoma accounts for 2% of all osteosarcomas. It originates from the inner germinative layer of the periosteum and arises from the diaphysis of the femur or tibia. Radiographically, it appears as a broad-based mass eroding into the underlying diaphyseal cortex and extending into adjacent soft tissues. Bone reaction manifests with thickened spicules of bone oriented perpendicularly to the surface. Histologically, the tumor contains nodules of atypical chondroid tissue intermixed with a malignant spindle cell population, along with lace-like osteoid deposition. Presence of such an abundant chondroid component explains why this tumor was once classified as a periosteal chondrosarcoma. However, periosteal chondrosarcoma has a better prognosis. Morphologically, this variant is considered grade 2 and is associated with a 5-year survival rate of 89%. All subtypes of conventional osteosarcoma are grade 3. Parosteal osteosarcoma is considered to be grade 1.

**21. Correct choice: C.**

Due to its bland cytologic appearance, sclerosing osteosarcoma can be mistaken for a low-grade sarcoma, while it is indeed as aggressive as all other histologic types of osteosarcoma.

**22. Correct choice: E.**

The telangiectatic type of osteosarcoma has a distinctive gross and microscopic appearance consisting of large blood-filled spaces separated by septa. Microscopically, highly pleomorphic sarcomatous cells are found within the septa and in the vascular spaces. Osteoclast-like giant cells are often seen, and atypical mitoses are frequent. Osteoid, by definition, is present but often inconspicuous. The main diagnostic challenge is distinguishing this entity from aneurysmal bone cysts in small biopsies. Presence of a translocation involving the *USP6* gene is diagnostic of aneurysmal bone cyst and excludes telangiectatic osteosarcoma.

**23. Correct choice: D.**

Small cell osteosarcoma is composed of sheets of small cells with a high nucleocytoplasmic ratio. Deposition of osteoid between tumor cells has a lace-like pattern mimicking fibrin deposition in Ewing sarcoma. In the differential diagnosis with Ewing sarcoma, keep in mind that CD99 can also be positive in small cell osteosarcoma. However, immunoreactivity for FLI1 (Friend leukemia integration 1) and EWSR1 (Ewing sarcoma breakpoint region 1) rearrangements is detected in Ewing sarcoma but not in small cell osteosarcoma. All histologic types of conventional osteosarcoma are high-grade tumors with no appreciable difference in prognosis or response to therapy.

**24. Correct choice: E.**

The clinical presentation, age, and microscopic features are consistent with a nonossifying fibroma, which is called metaphyseal fibrous defect when limited to the cortex. This condition of uncertain etiology is most often seen in male adolescents in the proximal tibia or distal femur. A storiform pattern is the most important clue to histologic diagnosis. Other features, such as hemosiderin deposits and collections of multinucleated giant cells, are nonspecific. Since this lesion is usually asymptomatic and the radiologic appearance highly distinctive, it is rarely biopsied. Radiographs typically show a well-demarcated lytic cortical lesion with sclerotic borders. Benign fibrous histiocytoma of bone is very rare and involves the nonmetaphyseal region of long bones or the pelvis. Desmoplastic fibroma is also a very rare, locally aggressive lesion morphologically analogous to aggressive fibromatosis of soft tissues. Conventional osteosarcoma, fibroblastic type requires the presence of osteoid and does not exhibit a prominent storiform pattern. Fibrosarcoma of bone is a malignant tumor of intermediate to high grade, histologically characterized (like the soft tissue counterpart) by a herringbone pattern.

**25. Correct choice: D.**

Each bone lesion of multiple myeloma characteristically appears on x-rays as sharply circumscribed punched-out areas of osteolysis. This is by no means pathognomonic of multiple myeloma, but it suggests the diagnosis in the presence of typical laboratory findings, for example, monoclonal spike in the $\gamma$ region of the serum protein electrophoresis. Codman triangle is often associated with (though not specific of) osteosarcoma. Expansion of bone and thickening of cortex is highly characteristic of chondrosarcoma. Onionskin appearance is often associated with Ewing sarcoma. Osteoid osteoma manifests with a radiolucent nidus surrounded by a sclerotic rim.

**26. Correct choice: D.**

Giant cell tumor is a locally aggressive tumor occurring in patients between 25 and 40 years of age, usually in the proximal tibia, distal radius, distal femur, and sacrum (any other site should suggest some other giant cell–rich tumor). It appears as a lytic expansile mass that extends into the subchondral bone plate. In contrast to most bone tumors, giant cell tumors are more common in females. Metastatic spread is rare, and histopathologic grading is not predictive of clinical behavior. The giant cells are reactive, while the mononuclear cells represent the true neoplastic population. These cells express receptor activators of nuclear factor kappa-B ligand, or RANKL, which is involved in the differentiation and survival of osteoclasts. A monoclonal antibody binding RANKL (denosumab) is effective in blocking tumor growth. Tumors treated with denosumab may consist entirely of woven bone and fibrous tissue and be devoid of mononuclear and giant cell components. Almost all cases of giant cell tumors harbor mutations of one of the two genes coding histone H3.3. The *H3F3A* gene is mutated in giant cell tumors, while the *H3F3B* gene is mutated in chondroblastoma. Central giant cell granuloma is located in the mandible or maxilla and affects females younger than 30 years of age. Microscopically, it is identical to giant cell lesions of the small bones (found in hands and feet) and brown tumors of hyperparathyroidism. Bilateral central giant cell granuloma in children is characteristic of cherubism, an autosomal dominant hereditary condition due to mutations of the *SH3BP2* gene.

**27. Correct choice: A.**

The photomicrograph shows the classic microscopic appearance of conventional chordoma, a malignant tumor of notochordal origin. It is located along the primitive notochord, from the base of the cranium (especially in the clivus) to the sacrum. The brachyury gene (*T* gene) encodes a transcription factor involved in notochordal development and appears to be important in the genesis of chordoma. Conventional chordomas show amplification of the brachyury gene in 7% of sporadic cases, while germline duplication is associated with an increased risk for chordomas. Brachyury has been shown to be a highly sensitive and specific marker of chordomas, which also express cytokeratin, EMA (epithelial membrane antigen), and S100 protein. Note that decalcification may result in a loss or decrease in brachyury immunoreactivity. The differential diagnosis of conventional chordoma includes chondrosarcoma (cytokeratin negative), choroid meningioma (brachyury negative), and renal cell carcinoma (CD10 positive).

**28. Correct choice: E.**

Poorly differentiated chordoma is a very rare and aggressive subtype of chordoma composed of sheets of cohesive epithelioid cells with eosinophilic cytoplasm and scattered intracytoplasmic vacuoles (signet ring-like). Focal rhabdoid morphology is often seen. Mitotic figures are numerous and necrosis is common. Physaliphorous cells and myxoid stroma are usually absent (occasional cases have focal myxoid stroma).

**29. Correct choice: E.**

Poorly differentiated chordoma is a very rare and aggressive subtype of chordoma composed of sheets of cohesive epithelioid cells with eosinophilic cytoplasm and scattered intracytoplasmic vacuoles (signet ring-like). Focal rhabdoid morphology is often seen. Mitotic figures are numerous and necrosis is common. Physaliphorous cells and myxoid stroma are usually absent (occasional cases have focal myxoid stroma). The cells are positive for brachyury and to a variable extent, S100 protein and cytokeratin, but there is a loss of SMARCB1/INI1 (SWI/SNF related, matrix associated, actin dependent regulator of chromatin, subfamily B, member 1/integrase interactor 1) staining. SMARCA4/BRG (SWI/SNF related, matrix associated, actin dependent regulator of chromatin, subfamily A, member 4/Brahma-related gene 1) is usually intact.

**30. Correct choice: C.**

Langerhans cell histiocytosis (also called eosinophilic granuloma or histiocytosis X) is a clonal proliferation of cells that morphologically and immunophenotypically resemble Langerhans cells. It is more common in childhood (1-3 years old) and involves nodal and extranodal sites (the most common site is bone). The lesional cells show prominent nuclear grooves with admixed eosinophils. Langerhans cells are positive for CD1a, langerin (CD207), and S100 protein. Most cases harbor *BRAF* V600E mutations and other RAS/MAPK (rat sarcoma/mitogen-activated protein kinase) pathway-activating mutations.

The presence of Birbeck granules on electron microscopy is pathognomonic. When it involves bone, x-rays demonstrate a well-circumscribed osteolytic lesion mimicking a metastatic carcinoma, with the differential diagnosis of osteomyelitis or infection and sinus histiocytosis with massive lymphadenopathy (Rosai-Dorfman disease). In the latter, the predominance of plasma cells and histiocytes is the salient diagnostic feature.

**31. Correct choice: A.**

Ewing sarcoma is a small blue cell tumor with a predilection for young people and preferred localization in the shaft of long bones. The onionskin pattern, detectable on x-rays, results from progressive periosteal bone apposition. CD99 expression, although characteristic of this tumor, is also detected in other neoplasms, such as lymphoblastic lymphoma and other sarcomas (eg, osteosarcoma and synovial sarcoma). Absence of CD45 and TdT (terminal deoxynucleotidyl transferase) helps rule out lymphomas. About 85% of Ewing sarcomas have the t(11;22) (q24;q12) translocation, leading to an *EWSR1-FLI1* fusion product that functions as an aberrant transcription factor. Other translocations cause the fusion of *EWSR1* with other genes of the ETS (E-twenty-six) family of transcription factors, resulting in similar effects. Recently, translocations fusing *EWSR1* to non-ETS family members or translocations not involving *EWSR1* have been reported in Ewing sarcoma. Since there are other mesenchymal tumors that harbor *EWSR1* rearrangements (myoepithelial tumors, myxoid liposarcoma, extraskeletal myxoid chondrosarcoma), demonstration of *EWSR1-FLI1* or *EWSR1-ERG* fusion products by reverse transcription polymerase chain reaction (RT-PCR) is more specific than FISH (fluorescence in situ hybridization) analysis. Poorly differentiated synovial sarcoma harbors the *SS18-SSX* gene fusion. Metastatic neuroblastoma is negative for CD99 and has an amplification of the *N-MYC* gene. The constituent cells in small cell osteosarcoma are virtually identical to the cells in Ewing sarcoma. In addition, in the absence of mineralization, true osteoid of small cell osteosarcoma can be very difficult to differentiate from collagen or fibrin which can be seen in Ewing sarcoma. To further compound the difficulty in distinguishing these two tumors, small cell osteosarcoma may express CD99. The t(11;22) (q24;q12) translocation, if present, is diagnostic for Ewing sarcoma. However, in the absence of osteoid, it may not be possible to definitively diagnose small cell osteosarcoma in limited material.

**32. Correct choice: D.**

Osteofibrous dysplasia may progress to adamantinoma so that these lesions are now considered as a spectrum. Both lesions develop in the cortex of the tibia, usually in the anterior midshaft. Osteofibrous dysplasia affects infants and children; osteofibrous dysplasia-like adamantinoma manifests at a later age in children and adolescents, while the classic adamantinoma type affects adults. Osteofibrous dysplasia-like adamantinoma has indolent growth; the classic form is more aggressive. Histologically, osteofibrous dysplasia resembles fibrous dysplasia, consisting of trabeculae of woven bone embedded in a bland spindle cell population that includes scattered keratin-positive cells. Fibrous dysplasia, however, is located in the medulla of bone and does not contain keratin-positive cells. Osteofibrous dysplasia-like adamantinoma is very similar to osteofibrous dysplasia. Classic adamantinoma consists of an epithelial component (basaloid, tubular, spindle cell, or squamous) variably admixed with an osteofibrous component that looks similar to osteofibrous dysplasia.

**33. Correct choice: A.**

Adamantinoma is a rare tumor that accounts for less than 1% of all primary bone tumors. It occurs in a wide age range. In 85% to 90% of cases, the tumor is localized to the median third of the diaphysis of the tibia. Onset is insidious and its course shows a slow, progressive character. On x-ray, single or multiple variably sized lytic lesions with sclerotic borders (soap bubble appearance) involve the diaphyseal and less commonly, the metaphyseal cortex. Despite the advances in imaging techniques, the definitive diagnosis is established by biopsy and histopathologic examination. The classic adamantinoma contains obvious epithelial elements embedded in fibro-osseous stroma. There is a high rate of recurrence with incomplete excision and recurrent potential correlates with a high epithelial to stroma ratio. The prognosis is excellent with complete radical excision. Epithelioid hemangioma is more cellular and has a lobulated growth pattern and organoid architecture. The constituent tumor cells are large polyhedrals, have eosinophilic cytoplasm, frequently contain intracytoplasmic vacuoles, and are surrounded by loose connective tissue. They are keratin positive but express a variety of vascular markers including CD31, CD34, and ERG (erythroblast transformation specific-related gene). Ewing sarcomas may exhibit overt epithelial differentiation in the form of diffuse cytokeratin and p63 expression, resembling adamantinoma of a long bone, but it is positive for CD99, NKX2.2 (NK2 homeobox 2), and FLI1 (Friend leukemia integration 1). Metastatic carcinoma is unusual below the knee and tends to occur in older patients. There is no associated osteofibrous dysplasia-like stroma and the constituent cells are typically more malignant. Clusters of keratin-positive epithelial cells are not seen in osteofibrous dysplasia.

**34. Correct choice: E.**

Simple bone cyst occurs predominantly in children and adolescents. The proximal humerus and proximal femur are the most common sites of this cystic lesion. It is characterized by a unilocular pseudocyst filled with clear or hemorrhagic fluid and lined by vascular fibrous tissue. Hemosiderin-laden macrophages, cholesterol clefts, and scattered multinucleated giant cells are additional features. It may manifest with pathologic fractures. Except in the case of fracture, it is unusual to receive a surgical specimen of simple cysts for pathologic evaluation, as the treatment of choice consists of intracystic injection of methylprednisolone or cartilage/bone grafting.

**35. Correct choice: C.**

Fibrous dysplasia is most often localized in the ribs, craniofacial bones, and femur (but any bone can be affected) and tends to occur in young adults. It is usually asymptomatic but may cause pain or pathologic fractures. It arises in the medulla of the bone and may affect one (monostotic) or more (polyostotic) bones. The monostotic form is 6 times as frequent as the polyostotic form. McCune-Albright syndrome is defined as a nonhereditary condition characterized by polyostotic fibrous dysplasia, café au lait spots, and endocrine abnormalities. Irregularly shaped (C-shaped or Chinese letter–shaped) trabeculae of woven bone *not* rimmed by osteoblasts and immersed in a fibrous stroma are the histologic hallmarks. Genetically, activating mutations in the Gs $\alpha$ (*GNAS*) gene are found in a large number (45%-93%) of cases. A postzygotic somatic activating *GNAS* mutation is the cause of McCune-Albright syndrome. Ossifying fibromas occur preferentially in the jaws and the trabeculae are contoured by osteoblasts and in cementoossifying fibromas, the trabeculae also exhibit mineralization. Juvenile ossifying fibroma occurs in young females, shows highly cellular stroma, and has an aggressive behavior. Lesions classified in the fibroma category tend to be well circumscribed, in contrast to fibrous dysplasia.

**36. Correct choice: C.**

Dedifferentiated chordoma is a biphasic tumor with two juxtaposed components (de novo) consisting of a conventional chordoma component and a high-grade sarcomatous component (high-grade undifferentiated pleomorphic sarcoma or osteosarcoma). There may only be a posttreatment sarcomatous component at a site of previously treated chordoma. The dedifferentiated component may lose brachyury, EMA (epithelial membrane antigen), or S100 protein immunoreactivity.

**37. Correct choice: C.**

Epithelioid hemangioma of bone is a benign neoplasm composed of plump, epithelioid cells of endothelial cell differentiation. It occurs in all age groups, most commonly in the fourth decade, and frequently arises in long tubular bones (40%), followed by flat bones (18%), vertebrae (16%), and the small bones of the hand and feet (8%). In about 20% of cases, multiple bones are involved. On imaging, lesions are well defined and lucent but can show soft tissue extension. Histologically, the tumor exhibits a lobulated growth pattern and is composed of epithelioid endothelial cells and numerous inflammatory cells, including eosinophils and plasma cells organized in an organoid architecture. There is no hyalinized or myxoid matrix. The individual tumor cells are large, polyhedral, eosinophilic, and frequently contain intracytoplasmic vacuoles. Mitoses may be present. Well-formed vessels are present and tumor cell cytoplasm may bulge into the lumen in a tombstone or hobnail-like pattern. The tumor cells express vascular markers (CD31, CD34, ERG [erythroblast transformation specific-related gene], and FLI1 [Friend leukemia integration 1]). Approximately 50% also express EMA (epithelial membrane antigen) and cytokeratins AE1/AE3. About 70% of osseous hemangiomas harbor either a *FOS* or *FOSB* gene fusion. Symptomatic tumors are treated with curettage. Epithelioid angiosarcoma exhibits more severe cytologic atypia with prominent nucleoli and atypical mitotic figures. It is not associated with FOS/FOSB fusions. Epithelioid hemangioendothelioma also exhibits more cytologic atypia, and the tumor cells are set within hyalinized or chondroid stroma. The cells in epithelioid hemangioendothelioma are positive for CAMTA1 (calmodulin binding transcription activator 1) or TFE3 (transcription factor E3) on immunohistochemistry. Hemangioma is the most common vascular tumor (it may actually be a vascular malformation) of bone. It is usually an incidental finding and is seen in ages 20 to 50 years, with no gender preference. It is seen in the vertebrae in 12% of autopsies. About one-third are multiple. It is composed of a thick-walled lattice-like pattern of vessels, which may be capillary or cavernous.

There is no endothelial atypia. Skeletal angiomatosis is extremely rare and characterized by thin-walled blood vessel proliferations with bone destruction.

**38. Correct choice: A.**

Benign notochordal cell tumor is an intraosseous tumor; it is not a notochordal rest or hamartoma. It is found in 14% of spinal columns and 11.5% of clivi at autopsy, usually ages 40 or more years. It may be multiple. It is typically well demarcated but unencapsulated and composed of sheets of adipocyte-like vacuolated or eosinophilic cells with fewer vacuoles. Cytoplasmic eosinophilic PAS (periodic acid-Schiff)-positive hyaline globules are often present. The nuclei are round nuclei with mild pleomorphism. The bone trabeculae are often sclerotic but there is no bony destruction. It has the same immunohistochemical profile as conventional chordoma with strong expression of S100 protein, cytokeratin, EMA (epithelial membrane antigen), and brachyury. Benign notochordal cell tumor may undergo malignant transformation to conventional chordoma. Conventional chordoma is osteolytic and composed of lobules containing cords, strands, or sheets of physaliphorous cells with myxoid matrix that are separated by thin fibrous septa. Metastatic renal cell clear carcinoma is typically lytic and exhibits an alveolar or nested pattern with vascular fibrous septa; it is usually positive for PAX8. Normal fatty marrow is negative for cytokeratin and EMA. Traumatic fat emboli are also negative for cytokeratin and EMA.

# 9 Breast

1. What is the best diagnosis for the biopsy, shown in Figure 1, of a breast nodule from a 28-year-old pregnant woman?

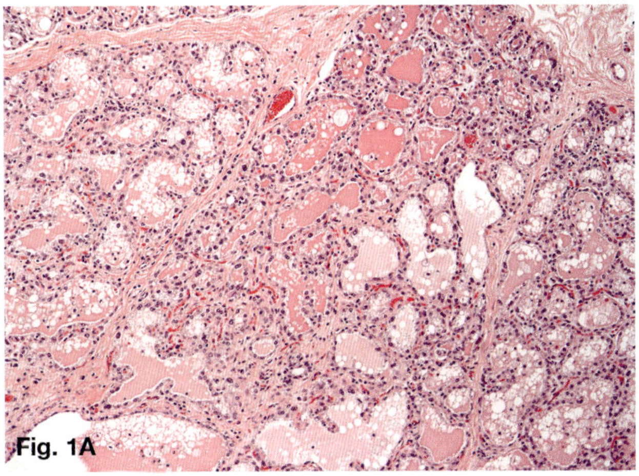

Fig. 1A

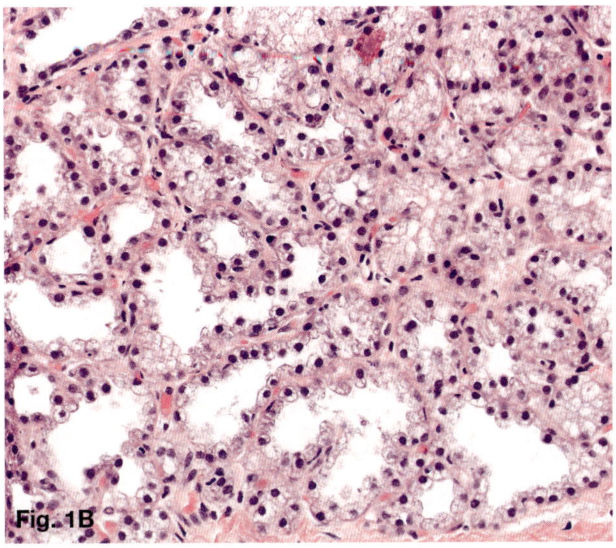

Fig. 1B

A. Apocrine adenosis metaplasia
B. Apocrine metaplasia
C. Collagenous spherulosis
D. Lactational changes
E. Usual ductal hyperplasia

2. Mammographic and gross examination of a breast mass reveals a stellate-shaped lesion containing a central core of fibrosis, shown in Figure 1. What is the best diagnosis?

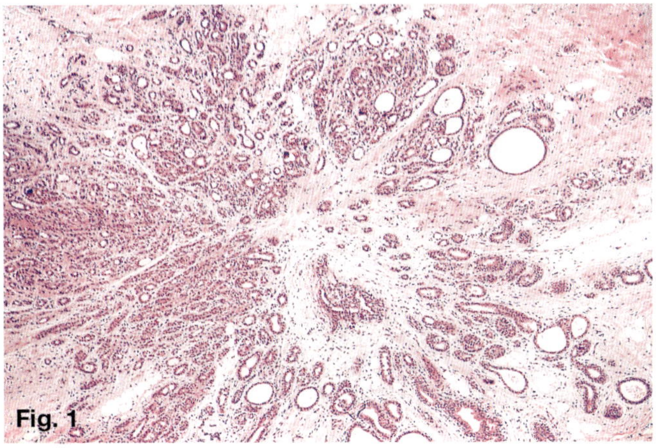

Fig. 1

A. Atypical ductal hyperplasia
B. Microglandular adenosis
C. Radial scar
D. Sclerosing adenosis
E. Tubular carcinoma

---

All figures in this chapter are from Longacre TA, Greenson JK, Hornick JL, Reuter VE, eds. *Mills and Sternberg's Diagnostic Surgical Pathology*. 7th ed. Wolters Kluwer; 2022 except for those noted at the end of this book.

3. What is the best diagnosis for the breast lesion, shown in Figures 1 and 2, in a 35-year-old woman?

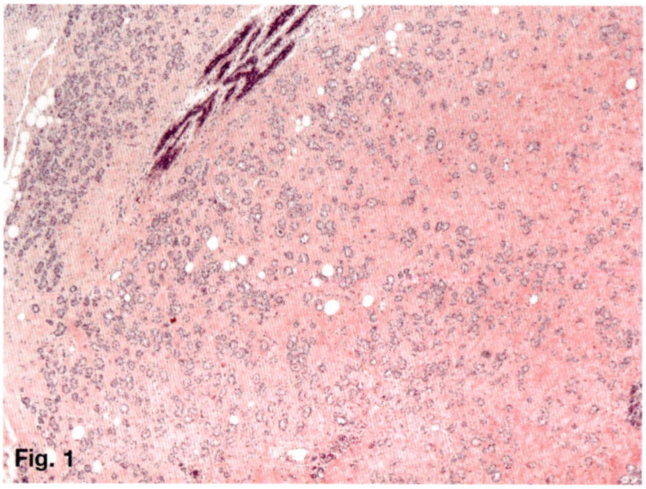

Fig. 1

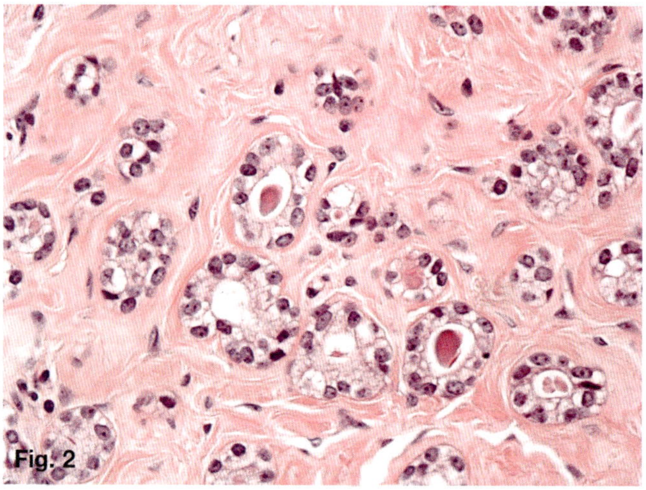

Fig. 2

A. Intraductal papilloma
B. Microglandular adenosis
C. Radial scar
D. Sclerosing adenosis
E. Tubular adenoma

4. What is the best diagnosis for the biopsy of a breast nodule, shown in Figures 1 and 2, from a 32-year-old woman?

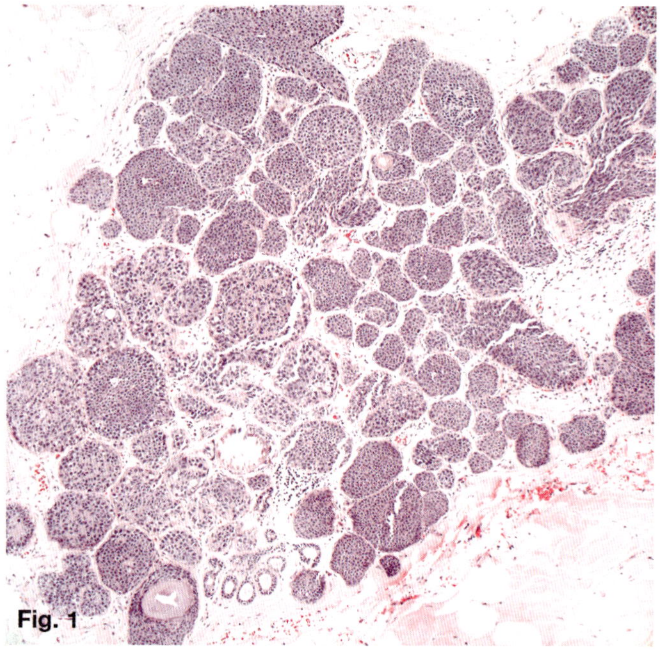

Fig. 1

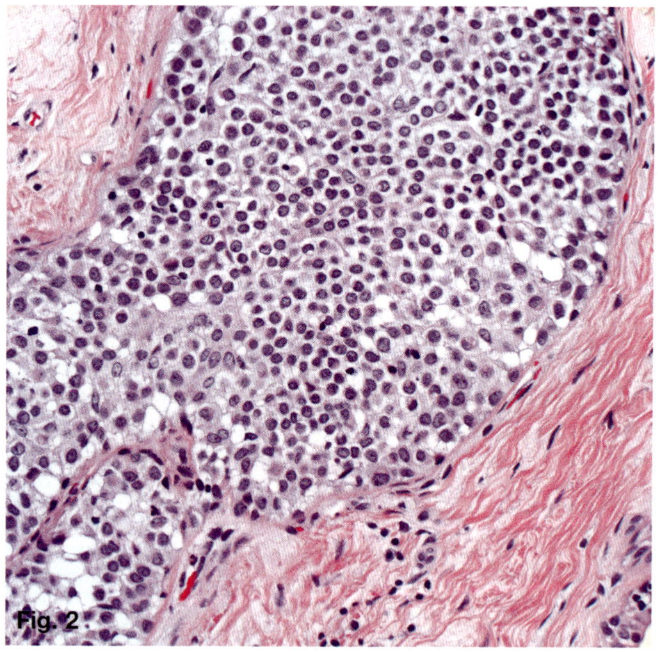

Fig. 2

A. Atypical ductal hyperplasia
B. Atypical lobular hyperplasia
C. Ductal carcinoma in situ, low grade
D. Lobular carcinoma in situ
E. Pleomorphic lobular carcinoma in situ

5. What is the best diagnosis for the biopsy of a breast nodule, shown in Figure 1, from a 42-year-old woman?

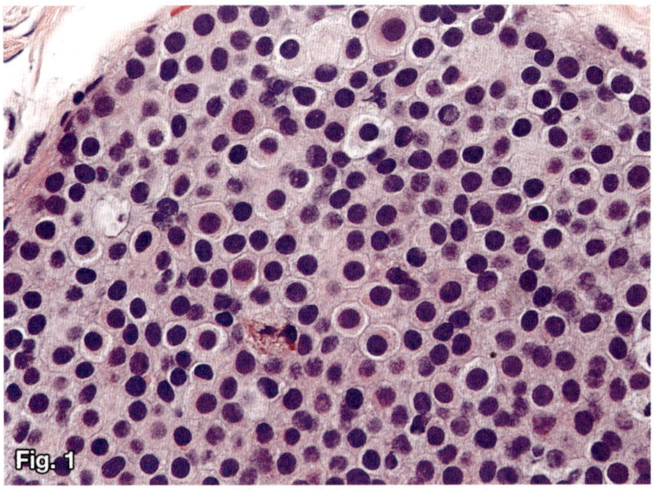
Fig. 1

A. Atypical ductal hyperplasia
B. Atypical lobular hyperplasia
C. Ductal carcinoma in situ, low grade
D. Lobular carcinoma in situ
E. Pleomorphic lobular carcinoma in situ

6. What is the best diagnosis for the biopsy of a breast nodule, shown in Figure 1, from a 42-year-old woman?

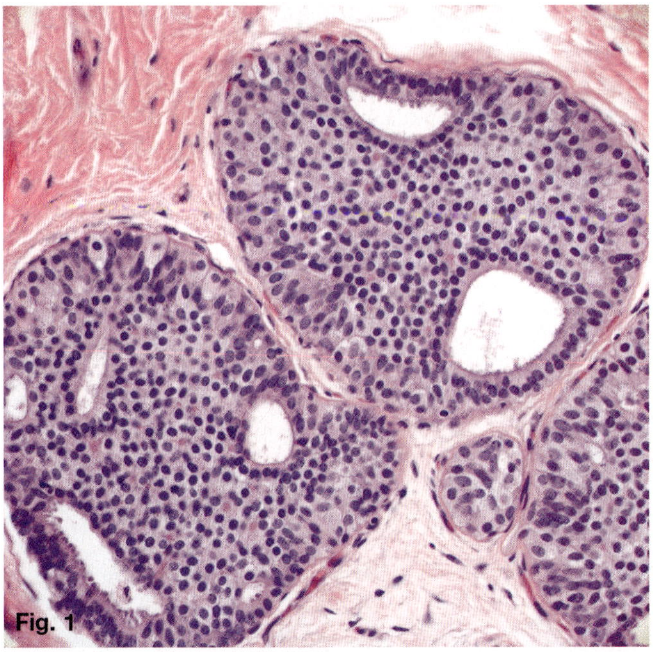
Fig. 1

A. Atypical ductal hyperplasia
B. Atypical lobular hyperplasia
C. Ductal carcinoma in situ, low grade
D. Lobular carcinoma in situ
E. Pleomorphic lobular carcinoma in situ

7. What is the best diagnosis for the biopsy of a right breast nodule, shown in Figure 1, from a 38-year-old woman?

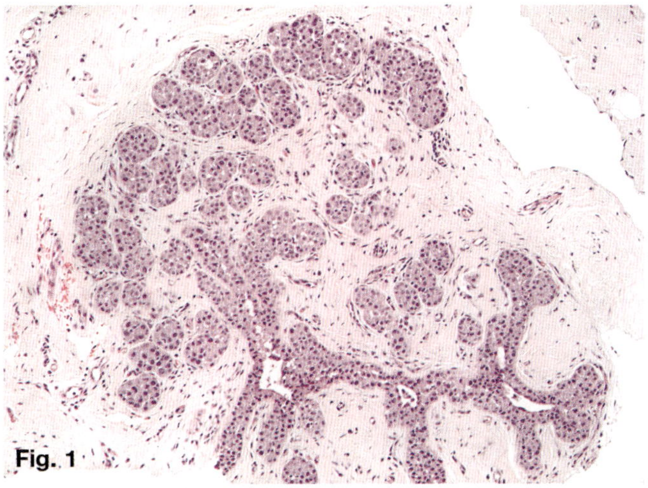
Fig. 1

A. Atypical ductal hyperplasia
B. Atypical lobular hyperplasia
C. Ductal carcinoma in situ, low grade
D. Lobular carcinoma in situ
E. Pleomorphic lobular carcinoma in situ

8. What is the best diagnosis for the biopsy of a breast nodule, shown in Figure 1, from a 42-year-old woman?

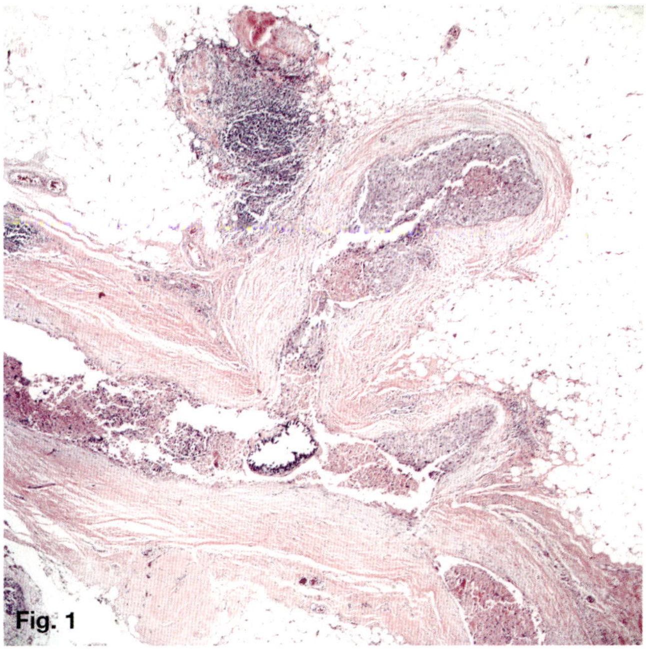
Fig. 1

A. Ductal carcinoma in situ, high grade
B. Ductal carcinoma in situ, low grade
C. Invasive ductal carcinoma
D. Pleomorphic lobular carcinoma in situ
E. Radial scar/complex sclerosing lesion

9. What is the best diagnosis for the changes shown in the bottom of Figure 1?

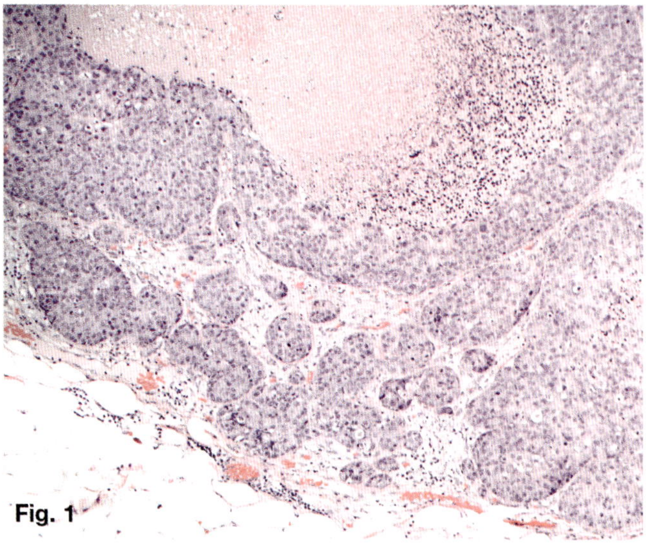

Fig. 1

A. Cancerization of lobules
B. Ductal carcinoma in situ, low grade
C. Invasive ductal carcinoma
D. Lobular carcinoma in situ
E. Pleomorphic lobular carcinoma in situ

10. What is the best diagnosis for the right breast lesion, shown in Figure 1, from this 54-year-old woman with an ill-defined lesion on routine screening mammography?

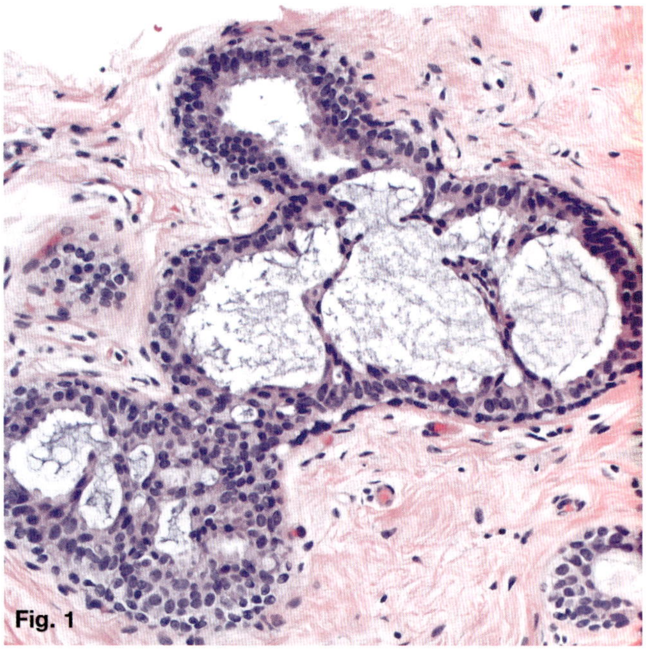

Fig. 1

A. Atypical ductal hyperplasia
B. Collagenous spherulosis
C. Ductal carcinoma in situ, low grade
D. Nipple duct adenoma
E. Usual ductal hyperplasia

11. What is the best diagnosis for the right breast lesion, shown in Figure 1, from this 44-year-old woman with an ill-defined lesion on routine screening mammography?

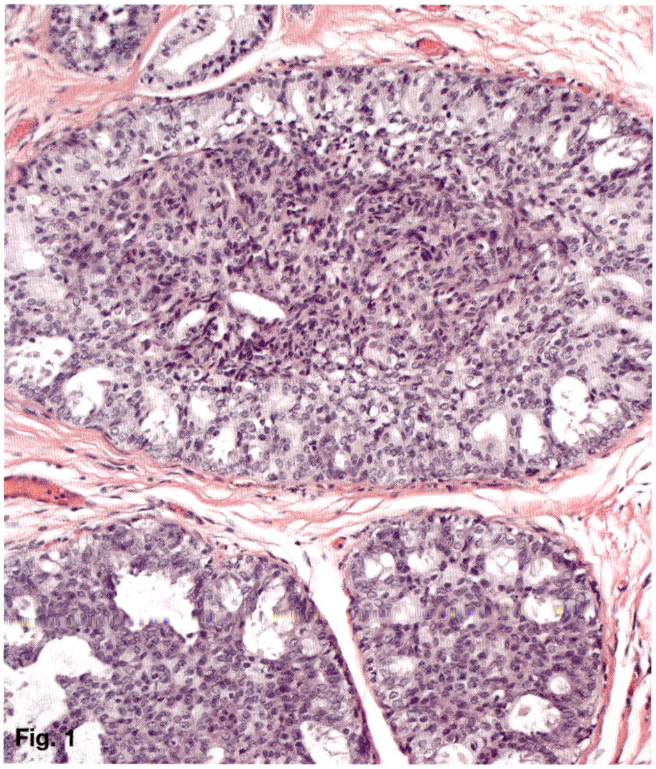

Fig. 1

A. Atypical ductal hyperplasia
B. Collagenous spherulosis
C. Ductal carcinoma in situ, low grade
D. Nipple duct adenoma
E. Usual ductal hyperplasia

12. What is the best diagnosis for the left breast lesion, shown in Figure 1, in a 34-year-old female?

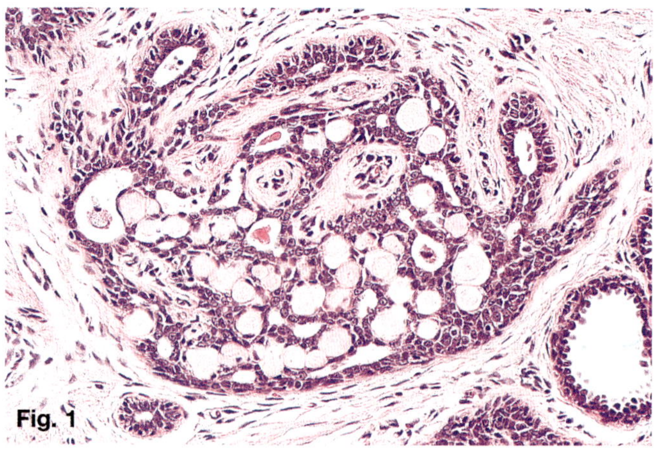

Fig. 1

A. Atypical ductal hyperplasia
B. Collagenous spherulosis
C. Ductal carcinoma in situ, low grade
D. Nipple duct adenoma
E. Usual ductal hyperplasia

13. Which of the following breast changes is associated with a relative risk of developing cancer 4 to 5 times that of the general population?

    A. Atypical ductal hyperplasia
    B. Atypical lobular hyperplasia
    C. Benign intraductal papilloma
    D. Sclerosing adenosis
    E. Usual ductal hyperplasia

14. Figure 1 depicts CK5/6 immunohistochemical stain on a lesion in a right biopsy from a 42-year-old woman. What is the best diagnosis?

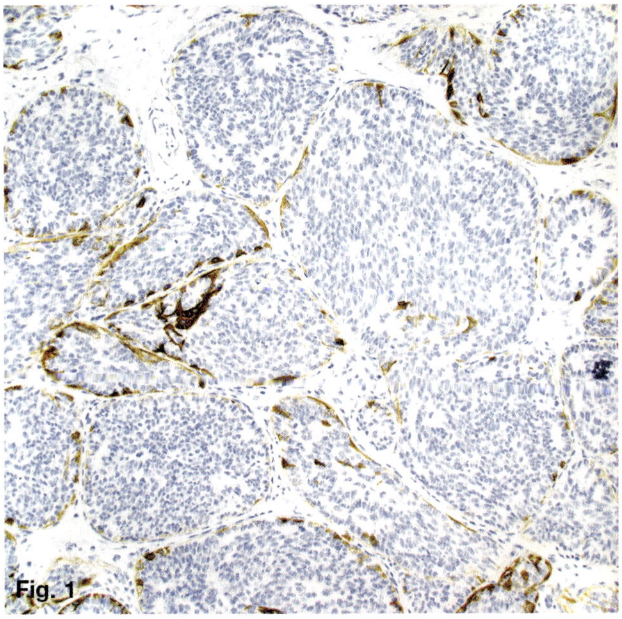
Fig. 1

    A. Atypical ductal hyperplasia
    B. Collagenous spherulosis
    C. Ductal carcinoma in situ, low grade
    D. Nipple duct adenoma
    E. Usual ductal hyperplasia

15. What is the best diagnosis for the breast lesion, shown in Figure 1, in a 35-year-old female with bloody nipple discharge and an ill-defined retroareolar mass?

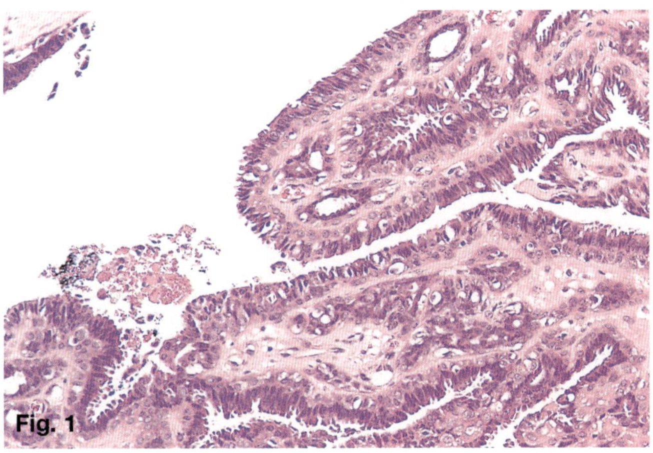
Fig. 1

    A. Apocrine metaplasia
    B. Atypical ductal hyperplasia
    C. Intraductal papilloma
    D. Tubular adenoma
    E. Usual ductal hyperplasia

16. What is the best diagnosis for the lobulated right breast lesion, shown in Figures 1 and 2, in a 66-year-old woman?

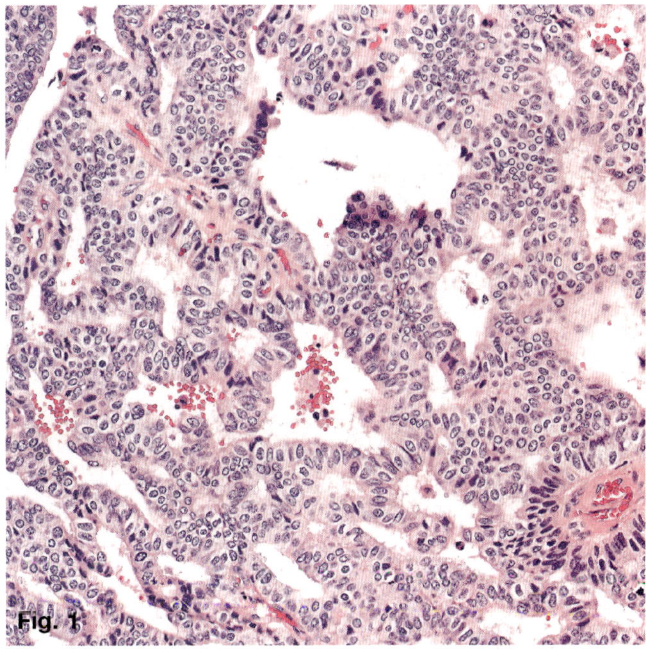
Fig. 1

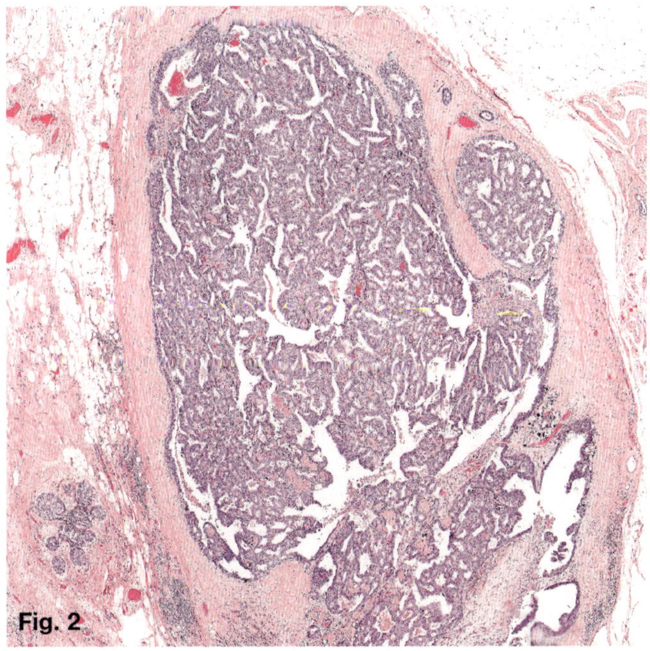
Fig. 2

    A. Encapsulated papillary carcinoma
    B. Intraductal papilloma
    C. Invasive papillary carcinoma
    D. Papillary ductal carcinoma in situ
    E. Solid papillary carcinoma

17. What is the best diagnosis for the subareolar mass lesion, shown in Figures 1 and 2, in a 75-year-old woman?

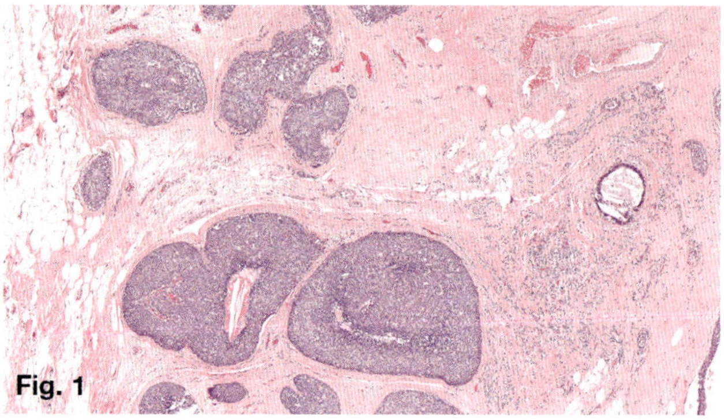
Fig. 1

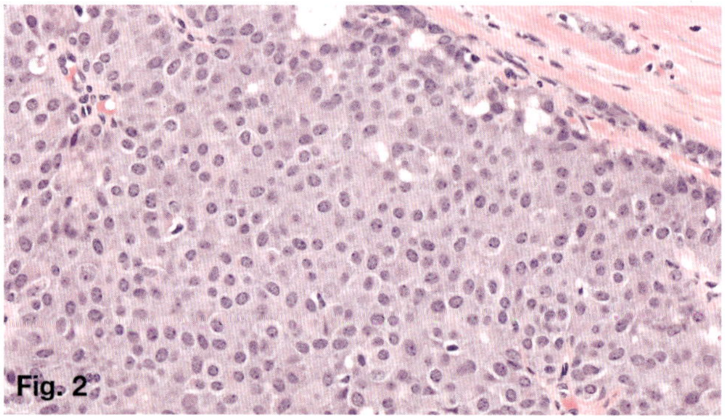
Fig. 2

A. Encapsulated papillary carcinoma
B. Intraductal papilloma
C. Invasive papillary carcinoma
D. Papillary ductal carcinoma in situ
E. Solid papillary carcinoma

18. What is the best diagnosis for the triple-negative breast mass, shown in Figure 1, in a 46-year-old woman?

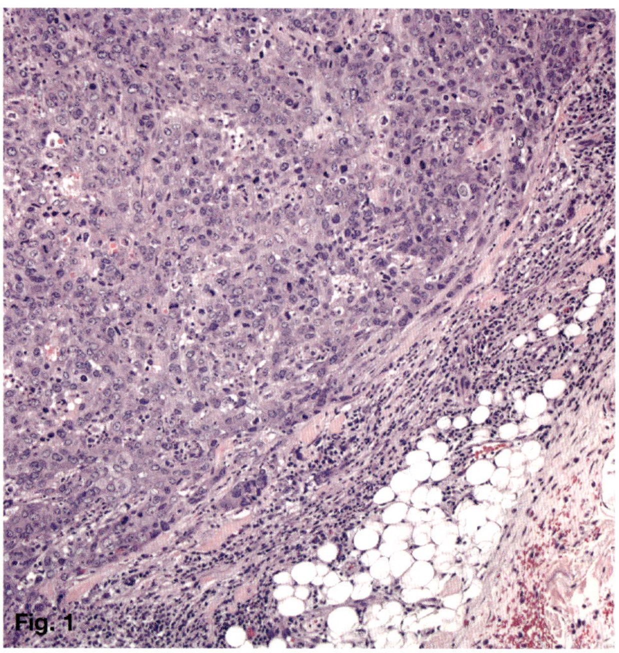
Fig. 1

A. Encapsulated papillary carcinoma
B. Invasive ductal carcinoma, medullary pattern
C. Invasive ductal carcinoma, no special type
D. Invasive papillary carcinoma
E. Invasive solid papillary carcinoma

19. What is the best diagnosis for the indurated, subcutaneous left chest wall mass, shown in Figure 1, in a 43-year-old woman?

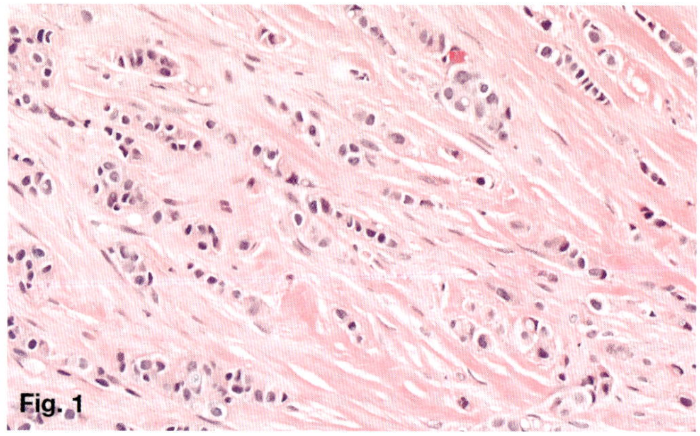
Fig. 1

A. Inflammatory breast carcinoma
B. Invasive lobular carcinoma
C. Leukemia cutis
D. Malignant melanoma
E. Small lymphocytic leukemia

20. What is the best diagnosis for the circumscribed mass in the right breast, shown in Figure 1, of a 66-year-old woman?

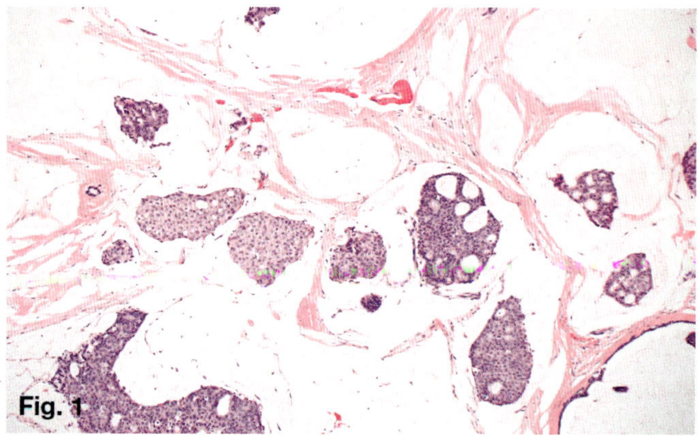
Fig. 1

A. Invasive ductal carcinoma with mucinous features
B. Invasive micropapillary carcinoma
C. Invasive mucinous carcinoma
D. Metastatic lung carcinoma
E. Mucocele-like lesion

21. A 32-year-old woman undergoes biopsy of a left breast lesion exhibiting polymorphous, grouped microcalcifications on mammography. Which of the following statements is true about the entity depicted in Figure 1?

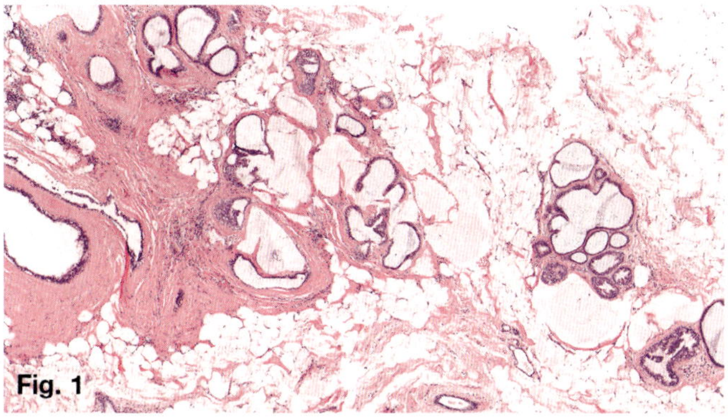

Fig. 1

A. CK5/6 and p63 are negative.
B. It typically occurs in older women.
C. Likelihood of carcinoma is high.
D. Mucicarmine staining is negative.
E. When there is stromal mucin, mucinous carcinoma must be considered.

22. What is the best diagnosis for the 2.0-cm left breast mass, shown in Figure 1, in a 55-year-old woman?

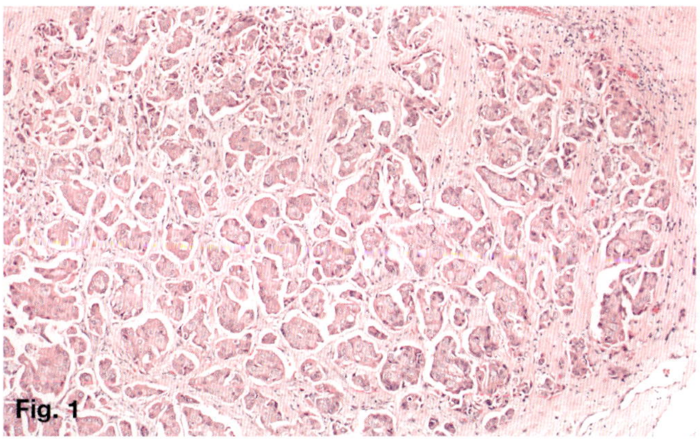

Fig. 1

A. Extensive lymph-vascular involvement by carcinoma
B. Invasive micropapillary carcinoma
C. Metastatic ovarian serous carcinoma
D. Metastatic urothelial carcinoma
E. Mucinous carcinoma with micropapillary pattern

23. Which of the following statements is true regarding the breast biopsy in Figure 1?

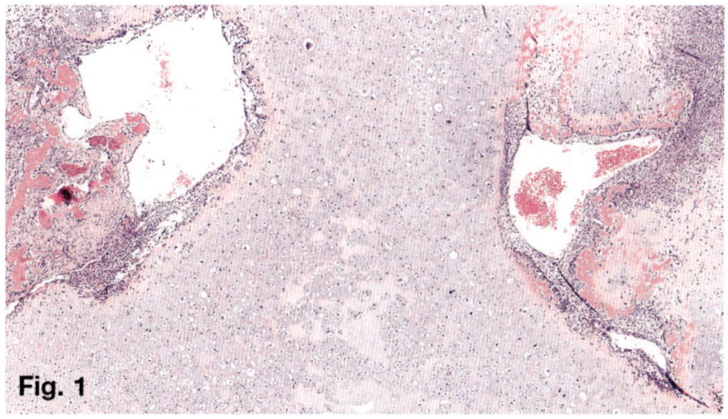

Fig. 1

A. Better prognosis than fibromatosis-like metaplastic carcinoma
B. Mesenchymal components are typically high grade
C. Metaplastic carcinoma subtype associated with worse prognosis
D. Multiple sarcomatous elements correlate with worse prognosis
E. Rhabdomyosarcomatous elements are most common

24. Which of the following statements is true regarding the breast biopsy depicted in Figure 1?

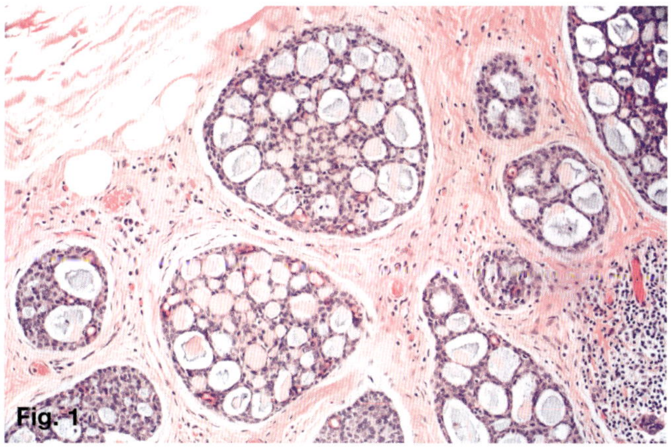

Fig. 1

A. CKIT (CD117) strongly positive in luminal cells
B. Does not harbor *MYB-NFIB* gene fusion
C. Prognosis similar to salivary gland counterpart
D. Usually ER+, PR+, HER2+
E. Usually ER+, PR+, HER2–

25. What is the best diagnosis for the left breast mass, shown in Figure 1, in a 66-year-old woman?

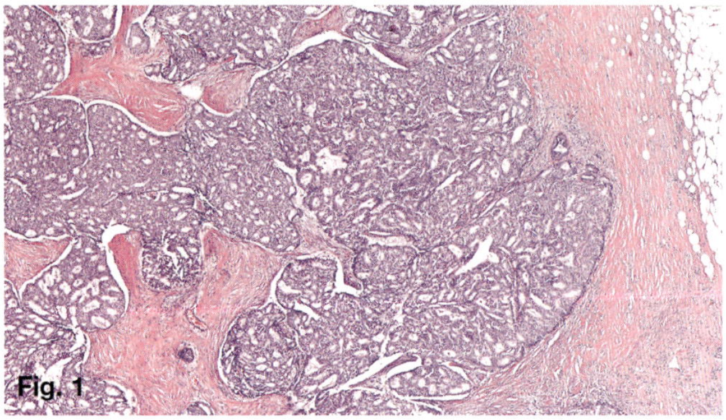

Fig. 1

A. Encapsulated papillary carcinoma
B. Invasive micropapillary carcinoma
C. Invasive papillary carcinoma
D. Invasive solid papillary carcinoma
E. Tall cell carcinoma with reversed polarity

26. What is the best diagnosis for the left breast retroareolar mass, shown in Figure 1, in a 28-year-old male-to-female transgender patient?

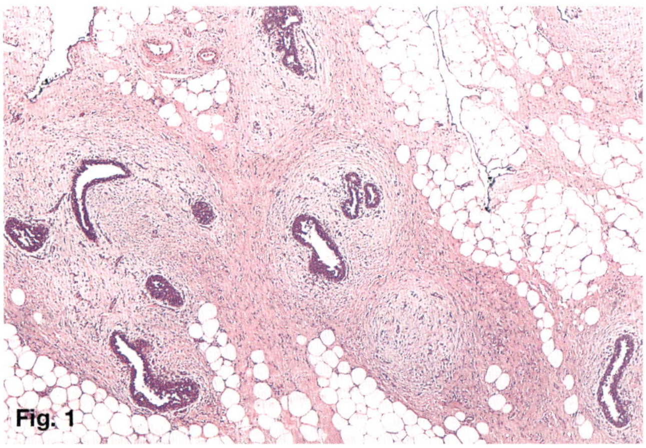

Fig. 1

A. Atypical ductal hyperplasia
B. Fibroadenoma
C. Flat epithelial atypia
D. Gynecomastia
E. Usual ductal hyperplasia

27. A 48-year-old woman presents with an erythematous, partially encrusted left nipple. On physical examination, a small, palpable dermal nodule is identified beneath the nipple. A biopsy is performed (see Figures 1 and 2). What is the best diagnosis?

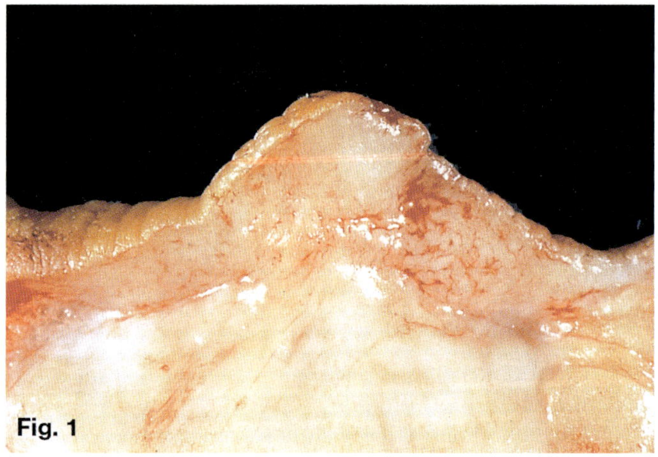

Fig. 1

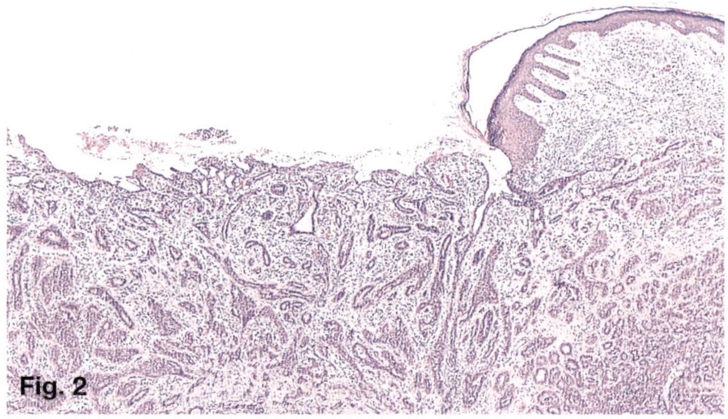

Fig. 2

A. Intraductal papilloma
B. Invasive ductal carcinoma
C. Nipple adenoma
D. Syringomatous tumor
E. Tubular adenoma

28. What is the most likely diagnosis for the biopsy of an encrusted, erythematous nipple lesion, shown in Figure 1, from a 42-year-old woman?

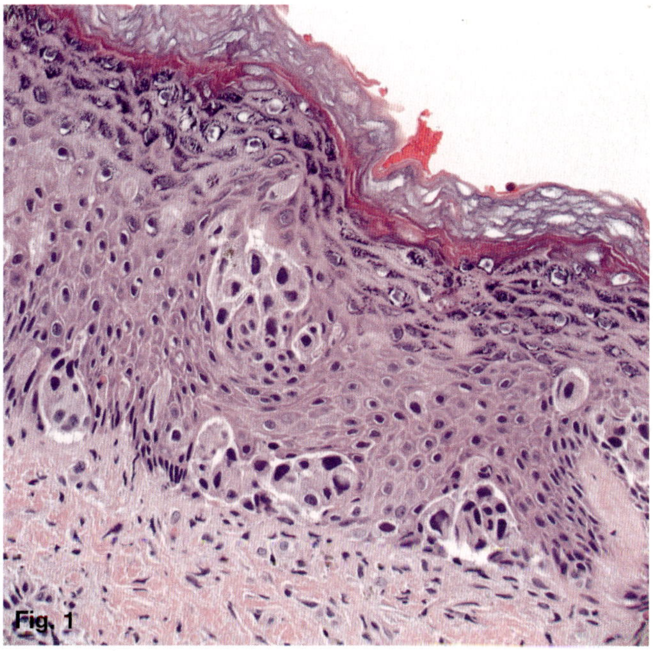

A. Bowen disease
B. Melanoma
C. Paget disease
D. Toker cell hyperplasia

29. What is the best diagnosis for the firm, mobile 2.8-cm mass in the left upper quadrant, shown in Figure 1, of a 28-year-old woman?

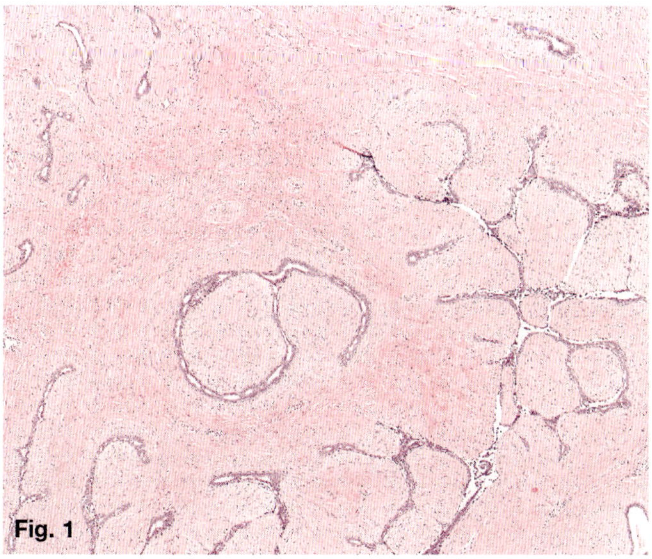

A. Breast hamartoma
B. Fibroadenoma
C. Periductal stromal tumor
D. Phyllodes tumor
E. Tubular adenoma

30. What is the best diagnosis for this firm, mobile 1.5-cm mass in the left upper quadrant, shown in Figure 1, of a 24-year-old woman?

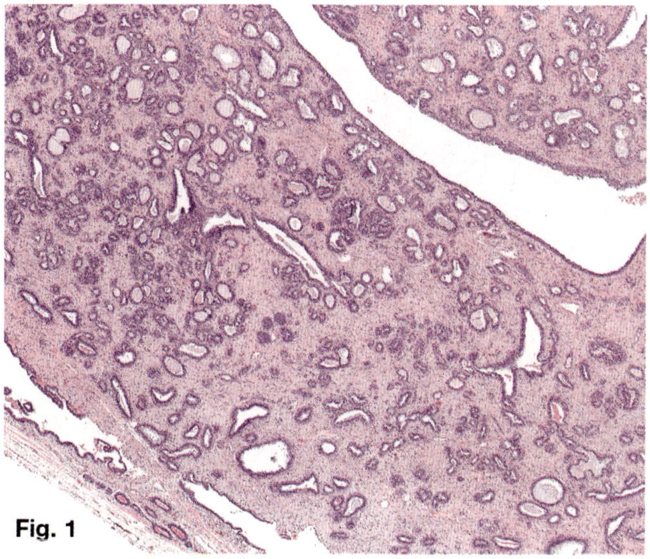

A. Cellular fibroadenoma
B. Complex fibroadenoma
C. Juvenile fibroadenoma
D. Phyllodes tumor
E. Tubular adenoma

31. What is the best diagnosis for this firm, mobile 2-cm mass in the right upper quadrant, shown in Figure 1, of a 32-year-old woman?

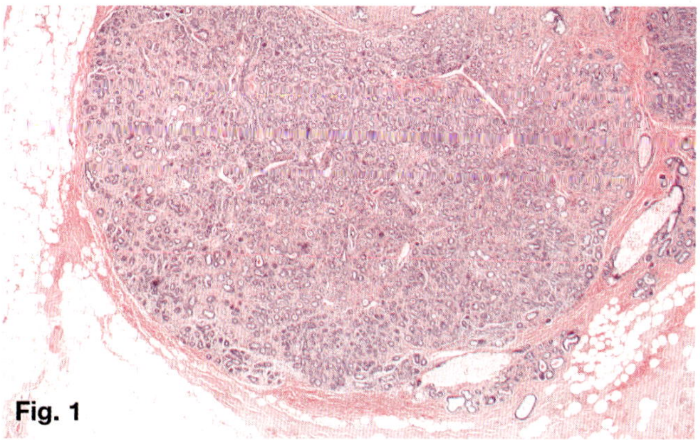

A. Cellular fibroadenoma
B. Complex fibroadenoma
C. Juvenile fibroadenoma
D. Phyllodes tumor
E. Tubular adenoma

32. What is the best diagnosis for the 4-cm mass in the upper outer quadrant, shown in Figure 1, of a 45-year-old woman?

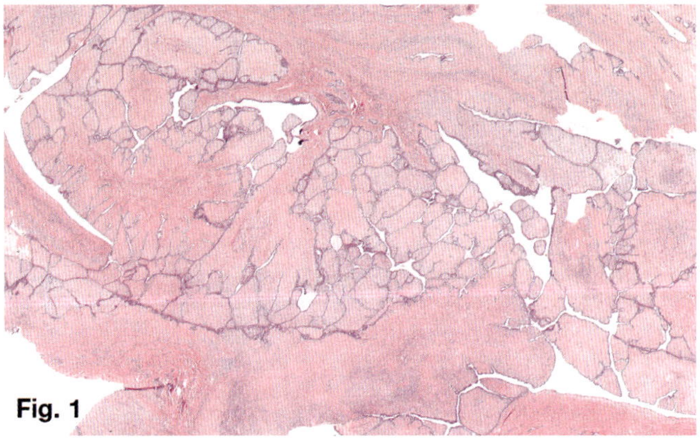
Fig. 1

A. Cellular fibroadenoma
B. Complex fibroadenoma
C. Juvenile fibroadenoma
D. Phyllodes tumor
E. Tubular adenoma

33. What is the best diagnosis for the ill-defined, enhanced right breast lesion, shown in Figure 1, discovered on magnetic resonance imaging (MRI) in a 38-year-old woman?

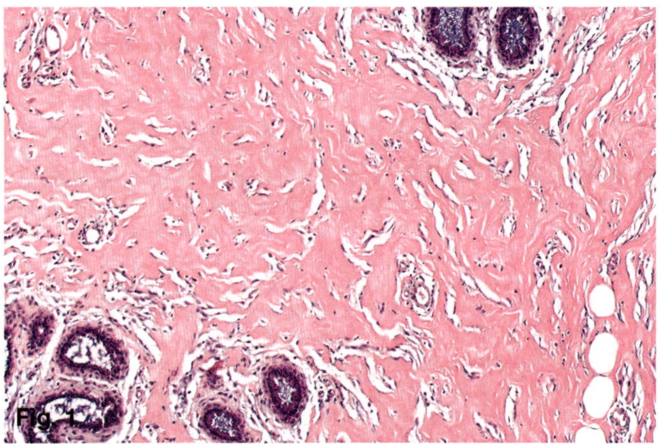
Fig. 1

A. Benign phyllodes tumor
B. Fibromatosis of the breast
C. Low-grade angiosarcoma
D. Normal breast parenchyma
E. Pseudoangiomatous hyperplasia

34. What is the best diagnosis for the slow-growing, palpable left breast mass, shown in Figure 1, in a 54-year-old woman?

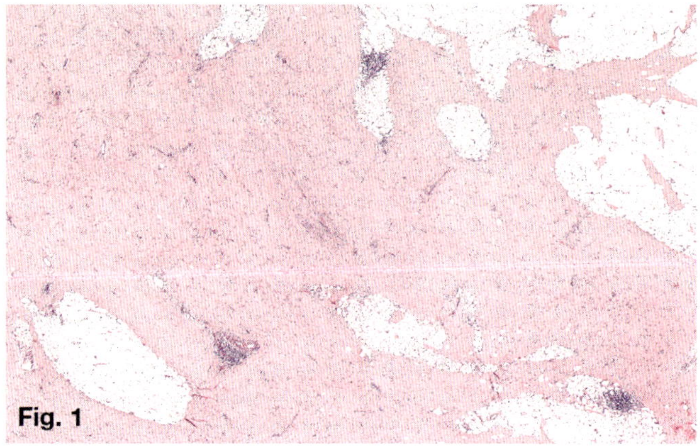
Fig. 1

A. Benign phyllodes tumor
B. Cicatrix (scar)
C. Fibromatosis of the breast
D. Metaplastic carcinoma
E. Nodular fasciitis

35. Foci of mucinous differentiation are not infrequent in infiltrating ductal carcinoma, no special type. Which of the following percentages of mucinous pattern should be present for a breast carcinoma to have a good prognosis?

A. 50%
B. 60%
C. 70%
D. 80%
E. 100%

36. What is the most likely diagnosis for the firm, ill-defined breast mass, shown in Figure 1, in a 42-year-old woman with a history of long-standing type 1 diabetes?

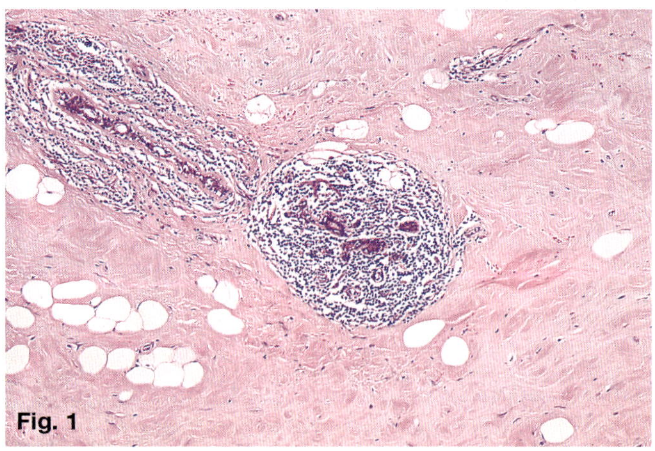
Fig. 1

A. Chronic granulomatous mastitis
B. Lymphocytic (diabetic) mastopathy
C. Mammary duct ectasia
D. Postsurgical changes/trauma
E. Small lymphocytic lymphoma

37. What is the most likely diagnosis for the breast biopsy, shown in Figure 1, obtained in a 32-year-old pregnant woman with a palpable left breast mass, pain, and nipple retraction?

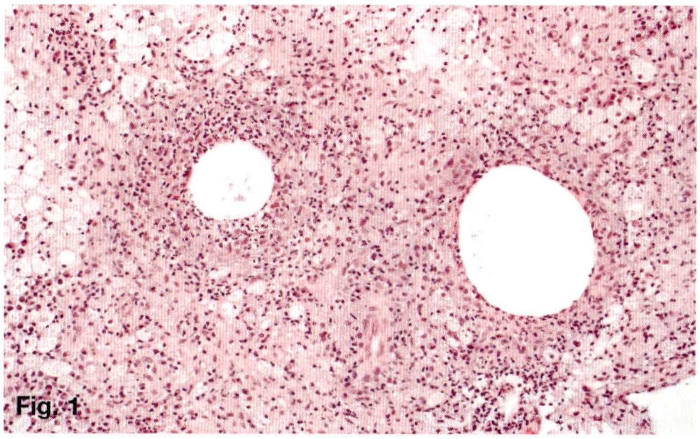

Fig. 1

A. Cystic neutrophilic granulomatous mastitis
B. Idiopathic granulomatous mastitis
C. Mammary duct ectasia
D. Postsurgical changes/trauma
E. Sarcoidosis

38. What is the best diagnosis for the core needle biopsy, shown in Figure 1, of the left breast of a 32-year-old woman?

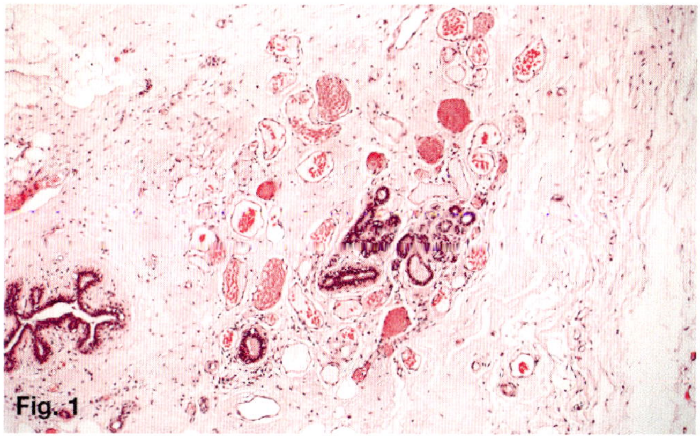

Fig. 1

A. Angiolipoma
B. Angiomatosis
C. Angiosarcoma
D. Lymphangioma
E. Perilobular hemangioma

39. Which of the following is true regarding the radiation-induced breast lesion, shown in Figure 1?

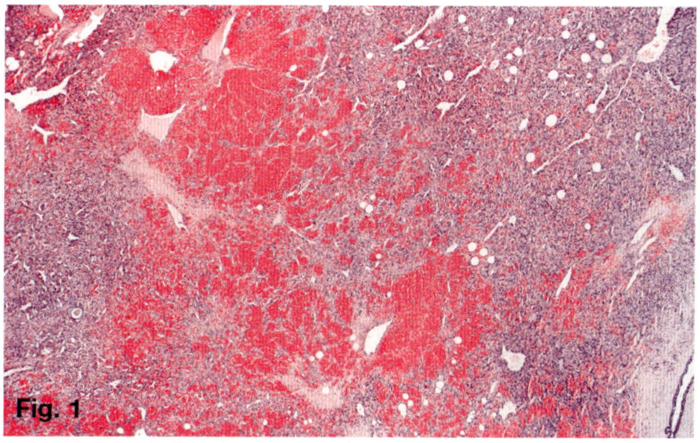

Fig. 1

A. Amplification of *MYC* is present.
B. Most often arises in the breast parenchyma and then secondarily involves the skin.
C. Patients have a median age of 40 years.
D. The majority are low grade.
E. Tumor grade is associated with prognosis

40. What is the best diagnosis for this 1.5-cm mass in the upper outer quadrant of the left breast, shown in Figure 1, in a 34-year-old woman?

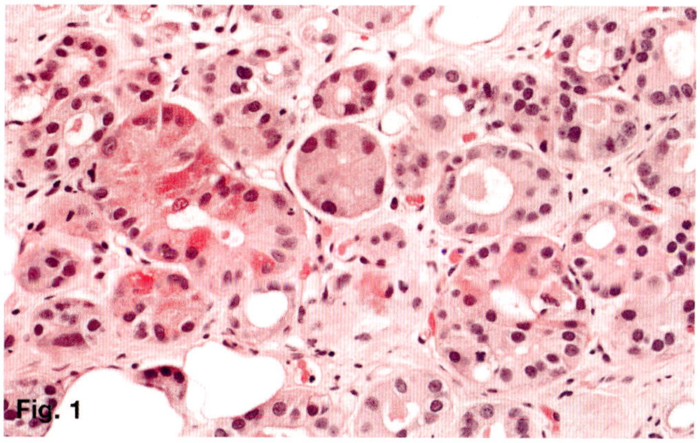

Fig. 1

A. Acinic cell carcinoma
B. Apocrine carcinoma
C. Apocrine metaplasia
D. Lactational change
E. Microglandular adenosis

41. Which of the following biologic markers is most consistent with low-grade (well-differentiated) ductal carcinoma in situ?

A. Expression for androgen receptor
B. Expression of HER2
C. Expression of p53
D. High proliferative index
E. Positivity for estrogen/progesterone receptors

42. Which of the following breast lesions lacks a myoepithelial lining in spite of its benign nature?

A. Intraductal papilloma
B. Microglandular adenosis
C. Radial scar
D. Sclerosing adenosis
E. Tubular adenoma

43. Which of the following statements applies to carcinoma of the male breast?

A. Accounts for at least 10% of all breast cancers
B. Gynecomastia is the most common risk factor
C. Klinefelter syndrome is a predisposing condition
D. Occurs in young males
E. Usually negative for estrogen/progesterone receptors

44. What is the most common clinical setting for breast abscesses?

A. Adolescence
B. Gynecomastia
C. Oral contraceptive use
D. Postpartum
E. Trauma

45. A 45-year-old woman presents with nipple discharge and retraction in the right breast. An ill-defined nodule is biopsied. It shows ducts filled with inspissated fluid and surrounded by a plasma cell–rich chronic inflammatory infiltrate and fibrosis. Which of the following is the most likely diagnosis?

A. Abscess
B. Fat necrosis
C. Invasive ductal carcinoma
D. Mammary duct ectasia
E. Paget disease

46. Inflammatory breast carcinoma is characterized by which of the following on biopsy?

A. Abscess formation in ductal carcinoma
B. Chronic inflammatory infiltration
C. Epidermal extension of neoplastic growth
D. Florid neovascular proliferation
E. Involvement of dermal lymphatic vessels

47. Which of the following is the most significant predictive factor in breast carcinoma?

A. Lymph node status
B. Lymphatic invasion
C. Tumor grade
D. Tumor size
E. Tumor type

48. Mucinous carcinoma of the breast is characterized by

A. absence of hormone receptor expression.
B. better prognosis than ductal carcinoma of no special type.
C. more frequent occurrence in younger women.
D. similar prognosis to ductal carcinoma of no special type.
E. worse prognosis than ductal carcinoma of no special type.

49. Which of the following breast carcinoma subtypes is associated with a pronounced tendency for lymphatic invasion and a poor prognosis?

A. Apocrine
B. Metaplastic
C. Micropapillary
D. Mucinous
E. Tubular

50. Which of the following is the most common predisposing factor for breast angiosarcoma?

A. Chronic lymphedema
B. Foreign bodies
C. Polyvinyl chloride
D. Radiation
E. Thorotrast

51. What is the best diagnosis for the ill-defined left breast mass with spiculated, irregular margins, shown in Figure 1, in a 63-year-old woman?

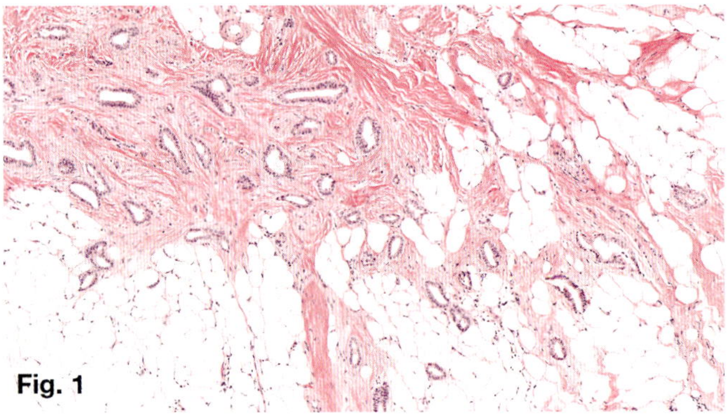

Fig. 1

A. Invasive ductal carcinoma
B. Microglandular adenosis
C. Radial scar
D. Sclerosing adenosis
E. Tubular carcinoma

52. What is the best diagnosis for the palpable right breast mass, shown in Figure 1, in a 67-year-old woman?

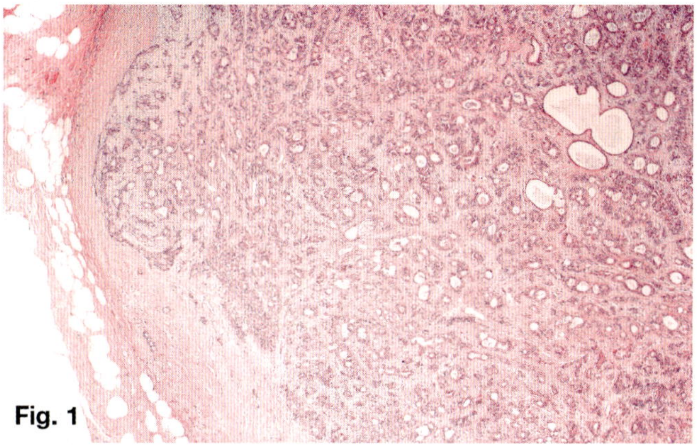

Fig. 1

A. Adenomyoepithelioma
B. Intraductal papilloma
C. Nipple adenoma
D. Sclerosing adenosis
E. Tubular adenoma

53. What is the best diagnosis for the ill-defined irregular mass, shown in Figure 1, in the left breast of a 64-year-old woman with a history of left breast carcinoma treated with local excision and radiation therapy?

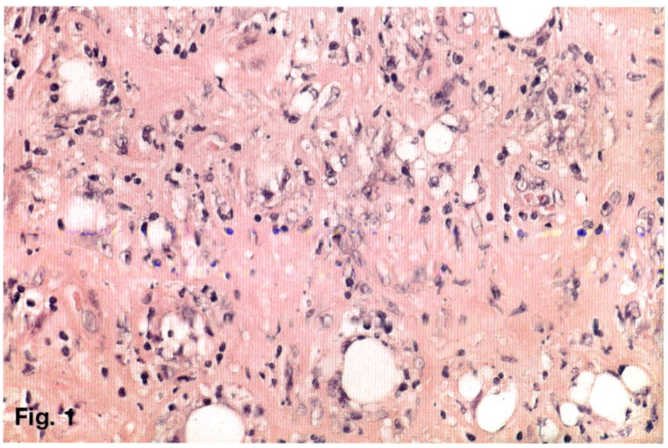

Fig. 1

A. Breast abscess carcinoma
B. Breast carcinoma
C. Fat necrosis
D. Hamartoma
E. Silicone reaction

54. What is the best diagnosis for the ill-defined area of firmness, shown in Figure 1, in the right breast of a 44-year-old woman with a history of breast implant?

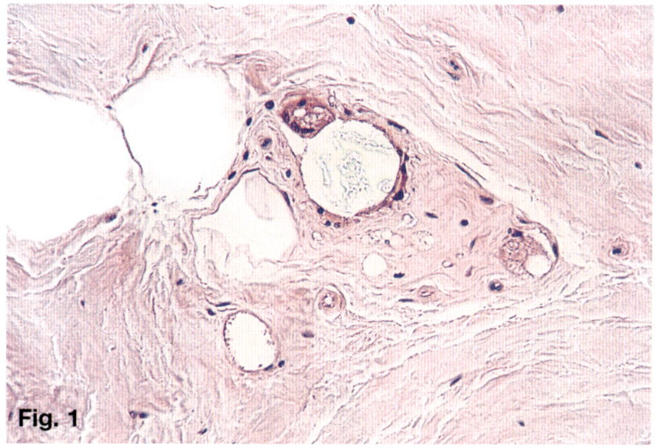

Fig. 1

A. Breast abscess carcinoma
B. Breast carcinoma
C. Fat necrosis
D. Hamartoma
E. Silicone reaction

55. Which of the following germline mutations is associated with an increased risk of developing lobular carcinoma of the breast?

A. *APC*
B. *BRCA1*
C. *BRCA2*
D. *CDH1*
E. *TP53*

56. Which subtype of breast cancer is typically associated with androgen receptor expression?

A. Acinic
B. Apocrine
C. Mucinous
D. Papillary
E. Tubular

57. What is the best diagnosis for the biopsy, shown in Figure 1, from a 32-year-old woman with palpable cysts in her left breast?

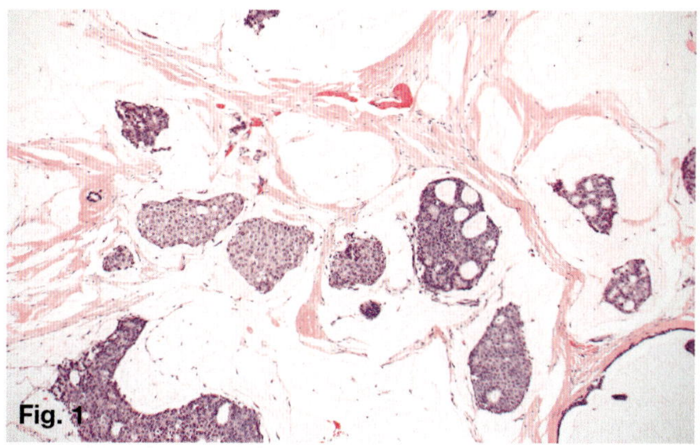

Fig. 1

A. Apocrine ductal carcinoma in situ
B. Apocrine metaplasia
C. Intraductal papilloma
D. Mammary duct ectasia
E. Pseudolactational change

58. What is the best diagnosis for the solitary right breast mass on imaging studies, shown in Figure 1, in a 63-year-old woman?

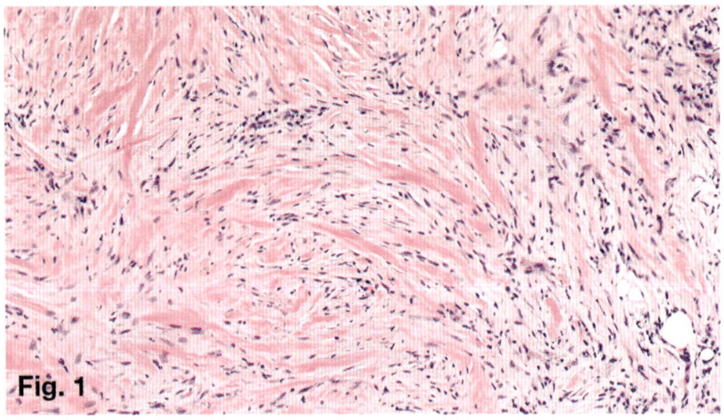

Fig. 1

A. Breast fibromatosis
B. Cicatrix (scar)
C. Fibromatosis-like metaplastic carcinoma
D. Phyllodes tumor
E. Pseudoangiomatous stromal hyperplasia

59. Salivary gland type breast carcinoma is typically

A. ER–, PR– HER2–.
B. ER+ PR+ HER2+.
C. ER+ PR+ HER2–.
D. ER-PR-HER2+.
E. None of the above.

60. Which is the best diagnosis for the salivary gland type breast carcinoma, shown in Figure 1?

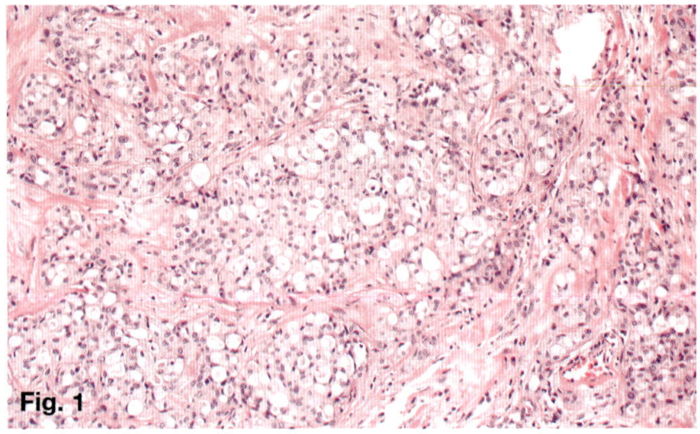

Fig. 1

A. Acinic cell carcinoma
B. Adenoid cystic carcinoma, classic type
C. Adenoid cystic carcinoma, solid type
D. Mucoepidermoid carcinoma
E. Secretory breast carcinoma

# ANSWERS AND EXPLANATIONS

**1. Correct choice: D.**

Pregnancy changes in the breast are due to the combined effects of estrogens, progesterone, prolactin, and growth hormone. They consist of marked enlargement/dilatation of lobules, due to increased number of acini, and cytoplasmic vacuolization of luminal cells reflecting increased secretory activity. The cells vary from columnar to cuboidal.

**2. Correct choice: C.**

Radial scar/complex sclerosing lesion resembles the head of a flower on low-power examination. The central fibrotic core contains distorted tubules and lobules and is surrounded by glandular elements exhibiting varying degrees of dilatation, hyperplasia, adenosis, and occasional papillomatous formations. Radial scar/complex sclerosing lesion is composed of two-cell types: luminal and myoepithelial. Microglandular adenosis is composed of only one cell type. Sclerosing adenosis is also composed of two-cell types but retains a lobular outline. Radial scar/complex sclerosing lesion may generate confusion with tubular carcinoma on high-power examination because of its disorganized, poorly circumscribed, seemingly infiltrative pattern on high power. Because of this, a low-power view is often more informative than a closer examination.

**3. Correct choice: B.**

Microglandular adenosis is a form of adenosis that lacks the two-layer lining (epithelial-myoepithelial) typical of benign lesions. It consists of tubules containing periodic acid-Schiff (PAS)-positive material. The lack of myoepithelial lining is most evident when compared to normal adjacent lobular units. Staining for myoepithelial markers confirms this feature. Myoepithelial cells, in contrast, are present in intraductal papilloma, radial scar, sclerosing adenosis, and tubular adenoma, in which the myoepithelial layer of the lesions may not be readily apparent on H&E (hematoxylin and eosin) stain.

**4. Correct choice: D.**

Lobular carcinoma in situ, classical type, is characterized by uniform, loosely cohesive, and evenly spaced cells (marbles in a bag) that fill and distend the acini. The constituent cells are slightly larger than normal, with indistinct cell borders and pale cytoplasm, small uniform nuclei, evenly distributed chromatin, and inconspicuous nucleoli. Intracytoplasmic vacuoles and pagetoid ductal involvement may be present. Lobular distention is defined as the presence of eight or more cells in the cross-sectional diameter of an acinus; if there is only partial involvement without significant distention (<50% of acini in a lobule are involved or all the acini are involved but are not distended), the lesion is diagnosed as atypical lobular hyperplasia. Pleomorphic lobular carcinoma in situ has large cells with enlarged pleomorphic nuclei; central necrosis and apocrine features can also be present. Atypical ductal hyperplasia and ductal carcinoma in situ, low grade are composed of more cohesive cells that often form microacini with polarization around microlumen. They do not have intracytoplasmic vacuoles and there is pagetoid ductal involvement. Lobular carcinoma in situ loses expression of E-cadherin, whereas E-cadherin is retained in ductal carcinoma in situ. Lobular carcinoma in situ constitutes both a risk factor and a nonobligate precursor of invasive breast cancer. Lobular carcinoma in situ is often bilateral (up to 6% of patients) and multifocal.

**5. Correct choice: C.**

Ductal carcinoma in situ, low grade is characterized by a cribriform, micropapillary, papillary, or solid intraductal proliferation of cells with monotonous, small round nuclei with smooth contours; the chromatin is fine, nucleoli are absent or indistinct, and mitotic figures are rare or absent. The constituent cells are more cohesive than the cells in lobular carcinoma in situ, and they often form microacini with polarization around microlumen. In atypical ductal hyperplasia, the architectural and cytologic features are suggestive of, but not diagnostic of, low-grade ductal carcinoma in situ due to partial involvement of ducts and limited quantitative extent.

**6. Correct choice: A.**

Atypical ductal hyperplasia is defined as an intraductal clonal epithelial cell proliferation with similar histologic features to low-grade ductal carcinoma in situ (DCIS), but with insufficient involvement or volume. It is differentiated from low-grade ductal carcinoma in situ by size (≤2 mm) or space occupied by clonal cells (≥2 spaces or only a portion of involved space).

**7. Correct choice: B.**

Atypical lobular hyperplasia is defined as a solid, discohesive proliferation of small, monomorphic cells with pale pink cytoplasm and uniform oval nuclei that distends less than 50% of lobules (resembling lobular carcinoma in situ) but is not uniformly present throughout entire lobule *or* involves all acini in a terminal duct lobular unit and so resembles lobular carcinoma in situ but does not distend the acini (ie, caliber of the involved acini is similar to that of uninvolved acini). The proliferation can involve ducts, appearing as outpouchings producing a cloverleaf pattern.

**8. Correct choice: A.**

Ductal carcinoma in situ, high grade is defined as a neoplastic proliferation of mammary ductal epithelial cells with prominent pleomorphism and large nuclei (>2.5 size of normal ductal epithelial cell) confined to the ductal-lobular system. The nuclei have vesicular chromatin with irregular distribution, prominent nucleoli, and frequent mitotic figures. Comedo necrosis is often present but not required. There may be a prominent associated stromal reaction (chronic inflammatory infiltrate, fibrosis/sclerosis) surrounding areas of high-grade ductal carcinoma in situ that can simulate invasion. In addition, there may be cancerization of lobules, secondary to extension into acini of the terminal duct lobular units.

**9. Correct choice: A.**

The image depicts comedo-type ductal carcinoma in situ with cancerization of the lobules, which results from the spread of a ductal carcinoma into the lobular component. Malignant cells usually expand and distort the lobular unit, often accompanied by fibrosis and lymphocytic infiltrate. A diagnostic error of invasion is particularly likely to occur if lobular cancerization involves an area of sclerosing adenosis, which exaggerates the distortion of the acinar architecture.

**10. Correct choice: E.**

The constituent cells of usual ductal hyperplasia show mild variation in cellular and nuclear size and shape. Small ovoid nuclei are frequently elongated or asymmetrically tapered (pear shaped). When bridges are formed, they are thin and tapering, with the nuclei arranged in a parallel configuration (as opposed to the broad and more rigid "Roman bridges" in ductal carcinoma in situ).

**11. Correct choice: E.**

Usual ductal hyperplasia is a component of fibrocystic changes and is characterized by a mammary ductal epithelial proliferation that exhibits a streaming growth pattern with fenestrated spaces and a lack of cellular polarity. The constituent cells show mild variation in cellular and nuclear size and shape. Small ovoid nuclei are frequently elongated or asymmetrically tapered (pear shaped). Many examples demonstrate cellular maturation, where the cells shrink as they progress from a basal location to the center of the proliferation, becoming small and nearly pyknotic. In addition, peripheral, irregular, and often slit-like spaces are formed.

**12. Correct choice: B.**

Collagenous spherulosis is a benign lesion composed of round spaces filled with acellular pink basement membrane material (spherules). The center of the spherules may be transparent but a thin rim of basement membrane material is always present. Spherules are surrounded by small oval or spindle myoepithelial cells with interspersed cuboidal luminal cells. Most cases are associated with benign proliferative lesions, mostly intraductal papilloma. Ductal carcinoma in situ, low grade often has a cribriform pattern which may resemble collagenous spherulosis, but the spaces are rounder and more regular (cookie cutter appearance) and they are surrounded by luminal cells, not myoepithelial cells. No pink material is present in the cribriform spaces.

**13. Correct choice: A.**

Severe (florid) ductal epithelial hyperplasia is associated with only slightly increased risk of cancer (up to 2 times). If cellular atypia is present (atypical ductal hyperplasia), breast cancer risk increases substantially, up to 4 to 5 times. This risk relates to both breasts.

**14. Correct choice: C.**

The proliferating neoplastic luminal cells in ductal carcinoma in situ are negative for CK5/6 with patchy preservation of staining in peripheral areas of the myoepithelium or residual nontumor cells, whereas CK5/6 expression is variably retained or shows a mosaic pattern in usual ductal hyperplasia or atypical ductal hyperplasia. CK5/6 is also preserved in the luminal cells of collagenous spherulosis and nipple duct adenoma.

**15. Correct choice: C.**

Intraductal papilloma is a circumscribed intraductal proliferation composed of arborizing fibrovascular cores lined by an outer layer of luminal cells and an inner layer of myoepithelial cells. Myoepithelial cells are also present at the periphery of the involved duct. This lesion usually manifests with nipple discharge. It arises from large lactiferous ducts and is composed of branching papillary fronds that fill the lumen. Monoclonality of the lesion has been demonstrated. A fibrovascular core and two-cell type lining (epithelial-myoepithelial) are the two most important criteria for distinguishing a benign papillary lesion from papillary carcinoma. Apocrine metaplasia is common in intraductal papilloma. An intraductal papilloma may be secondarily involved by usual ductal hyperplasia or atypical ductal hyperplasia.

**16. Correct choice: A.**

Encapsulated papillary carcinoma is a papillary lesion characterized by delicate papillary fronds with fibrovascular cores lined by cuboidal to columnar epithelial cells with low- to intermediate-grade atypia in the absence of a myoepithelial layer. This differentiates encapsulated papillary carcinoma from intraductal papilloma. It often has pushing borders and may arise within a cystically dilated duct, surrounded by a thick fibrous capsule. Cribriform and solid architecture may be present. A myoepithelial layer is also absent in invasive papillary carcinoma, but it exhibits a frankly infiltrative pattern without a surrounding fibrous capsule. Papillary ductal carcinoma in situ typically involves multiple ducts and may coexist with other patterns of ductal carcinoma in situ. Myoepithelium is present at the periphery. Solid papillary carcinoma is characterized by single or multiple nodules with solid architecture and rudimentary, delicate fibrovascular cores; it lacks an encircling dense fibrous capsule. The cells may be spindled, produce mucin, and have neuroendocrine features. Similar to encapsulated papillary carcinoma, it lacks myoepithelium within tumor nests and around the periphery.

**17. Correct choice: E.**

Solid papillary carcinoma is characterized by a circumscribed solid growth pattern composed of interspersed delicate fibrovascular cores with low- or intermediate-grade nuclear atypia. The constituent cells often have a plasmacytoid appearance. Neuroendocrine differentiation is common. In situ carcinoma is diagnosed when the tumor is composed of well-circumscribed solid nests in a distribution pattern consistent with an intraductal process; myoepithelial cells may or may not be demonstrable at the periphery. Invasive carcinoma is diagnosed when there is a lack of myoepithelium and a convincing pattern of infiltrative growth.

**18. Correct choice: B.**

Invasive ductal carcinoma, medullary pattern is a subtype of invasive ductal carcinoma with high-grade nuclei and prominent lymphoid infiltrate exhibiting a syncytial growth pattern and pushing border. This subtype is typically negative for ER (estrogen receptor), PR (progesterone receptor), and HER2 (human epidermal growth factor receptor 2). The majority of these tumors fall within the basal-like molecular profile.

**19. Correct choice: B.**

Invasive lobular carcinoma, classic type is composed of discohesive, small, monomorphic tumor cells arranged in single files, cords, and single cells. The cells can also be arranged concentrically around normal ducts, imparting a targetoid appearance. The constituent cells are round or ovoid with scant cytoplasm and/or intracytoplasmic lumens. The nuclei are bland, usually grade 1 or 2. Mitoses are infrequent and a desmoplastic reaction is uncommon. Inflammatory breast carcinoma is characterized by intralymphatic or intravascular carcinoma. Malignant melanoma typically exhibits more marked nuclear atypia and prominent nucleoli. Distinction from a lymphocytic, histiocytic, or myelomonocytic infiltrate can be difficult even in the presence of an associated lobular carcinoma in situ component and may require immunohistochemistry.

**20. Correct choice: C.**

Invasive mucinous carcinoma is characterized by clusters of tumor cells suspended in pools of extracellular mucin. Invasive mucinous carcinoma has been divided into two histologic groups: clusters that lie within secreted mucin (type A) or large sheets of tumor cells with neuroendocrine features and mucin production (type B). Mucinous component must be greater than 90% of tumor to be pure and have a favorable prognosis. They are ER and PR hormone receptor positive and HER2 negative (luminal A subtype). This tumor tends to occur in older women. Invasive ductal carcinoma with mucinous features exhibits histologic features of pure mucinous carcinoma but the mucinous component does not fulfill greater than 90% criteria. Because invasive mucinous carcinoma may be initially misdiagnosed on core needle biopsy due to limited sampling, the amount of mucinous component, and hence the diagnosis, is more reliably assessed on excision specimens. Invasive micropapillary carcinoma also features nests of tumor cells floating in spaces, but mucin is absent. Metastases should always be considered and are excluded on the basis of clinical history, imaging, and in some instances, site-specific immunohistochemical profiles. Mucocele-like lesion is characterized by a ruptured cyst with detached strips of bland epithelium lined by myoepithelial cells floating within extravasated mucin.

**21. Correct choice: E.**

Mucocele-like lesion is characterized by extravasated acellular mucin in periductal stroma associated with benign epithelium. Pure mucocele-like lesions without atypia typically have benign behavior. Although there may be associated hyperplasia of the cyst lining in mucocele-like lesions, there are no epithelial cells floating within the luminal or extravasated mucin, which is a critical finding in distinguishing mucocele-like lesions from mucinous carcinoma of the breast. Originally described as a benign lesion, associations with atypical ductal hyperplasia (ADH), ductal carcinoma in situ (DCIS), and invasive carcinoma have been reported in several studies. Therefore, searching for atypia when a mucocele-like lesion is present is important to exclude the possibility of ADH, DCIS, or invasive carcinoma. The diagnosis can be made on core biopsy or surgical specimen but careful evaluation of excised tissue, multiple H&E (hematoxylin and eosin) levels, and clinicopathologic correlation may be helpful to rule out in situ lesions and invasive mucinous carcinoma. Calcifications are often present (but not depicted in this image).

**22. Correct choice: B.**

Invasive micropapillary carcinoma is characterized as densely cellular groups of cells with eosinophilic cytoplasm arranged in pseudopapillae, hollow tubules, and morula that are surrounded by empty clear spaces set within a fibrocollagenous stroma. The constituent cells show characteristic reverse polarity (inside-out pattern) with the apical surface abutting the epithelial stromal interface. The nuclei around the periphery bulge with knobby appearance. Extensive true angiolymphatic invasion is typically present. The tumor cells express EMA (epithelial membrane antigen), E-cadherin, and p120 catenin in an inside-out pattern, that is, EMA exhibits membranous staining of tumor cells abutting stroma and E-cadherin, and p120 catenin exhibit cup-shaped basolateral membranous staining with sparing of the apical surface. Tumor clusters do not demonstrate reverse polarity in the context of extensive lymphovascular invasion by a primary or metastatic carcinoma. Metastatic ovarian serous carcinoma is PAX8+, WT1+, GATA3−, and GCDFP-15−. Often there is a clinical history of ovarian cancer. Mucinous carcinoma with micropapillary pattern shows micropapillary epithelium floating in mucin pools.

**23. Correct choice: D.**

The image depicts metaplastic carcinoma with heterologous mesenchymal differentiation (matrix-producing carcinoma). The mesenchymal component ranges from bland and differentiated to frankly malignant. With the exception of fibromatosis-like metaplastic carcinoma (which has a better prognosis), matrix-producing carcinomas are associated with a better prognosis when compared to other metaplastic carcinomas. Osseous and cartilaginous elements are more common than rhabdomyosarcomatous elements. Multiple sarcomatous elements correlate with a worse prognosis.

**24. Correct choice: A.**

Adenoid cystic carcinoma exhibits glandular lumina along with pseudocysts containing basement membrane–like (glassy and eosinophilic) material. The large pseudocystic spaces contain Alcian blue positive, PAS-negative material (hyaluronic acid), whereas the true glandular lumina contains PAS-positive, Alcian blue–negative material (neutral mucin). The pseudocystic spaces are immunoreactive with antibodies to basement membrane components. CKIT (CD117) is strongly positive in luminal cells. Similar to the salivary gland adenoid cystic carcinoma, breast adenoid cystic carcinoma typically harbors the *MYB-NFIB* gene fusion. This tumor is usually ER−, PR−, HER2−. In contrast to the salivary gland tumor, breast adenoid cystic carcinoma has a good prognosis.

**25. Correct choice: C.**

Invasive papillary carcinoma is a rare, invasive breast carcinoma characterized by arborizing fibrovascular stalks lined by epithelial cells (>90% papillary architecture) without a surrounding fibrous capsule. Encapsulated papillary carcinoma has a rounded pushing border and is surrounded by a fibrous capsule. Invasive micropapillary carcinoma exhibits dense clusters of morula-like epithelial structures surrounded by empty spaces, devoid of fibrovascular cores and shows reverse polarity. Invasive solid papillary carcinoma consists of expansile nodules with a solid pattern and delicate fibrovascular cores. Tall cell carcinoma with reversed polarity features cells arranged in solid, papillary, and glandular structures, resembling thyroid follicles. The constituent glands contain colloid-like material. The tumor cells are columnar or cuboidal and their nuclei are positioned near the luminal (apical) surfaces, as opposed to the base. These tumors are ER−, PR−, and HER2−.

**26. Correct choice: D.**

Gynecomastia is characterized by increased number of ducts with a three-layer epithelium consisting of luminal epithelium expressing CK5/6; intermediate cuboidal to columnar epithelium expressing ER (estrogen receptor), PR (progesterone receptor), and AR (androgen receptor); and an outer myoepithelium expressing CK5/6. Three patterns of proliferative changes can be seen: (1) florid pattern consisting of irregular branching ducts, mild-to-moderate epithelial hyperplasia, and cellular, myxoid, and/or edematous stroma cuffing around ducts, which may simulate papillary usual ductal hyperplasia or atypical ductal hyperplasia; (2) intermediate pattern consisting of a mixture of florid and fibrous patterns, which may simulate flat epithelial atypia, and (3) fibrous pattern consisting of quiescent epithelium within a hyalinized hypocellular stroma, which may simulate fibroadenoma.

**27. Correct choice: C.**

Nipple adenoma is a benign epithelial proliferation with a variety of morphologic patterns that arises near the collecting ducts of the nipple and may be continuous with the overlying epidermis. Histologically, it consists of a florid epithelial proliferation of the lactiferous ducts of the nipple with a papillary hyperplasia, adenosis, sclerosing, or mixed pattern. The epithelium is cytologically bland. There may be erosion or ulceration of the overlying skin or nipple if it is continuous with the skin surface. Intraductal papilloma is similar to nipple adenoma, but arises below the skin surface, and involves lactiferous ducts within deeper breast parenchyma, and is unlikely to be a palpable subdermal mass. Invasive ductal carcinoma has a more infiltrative growth pattern and is negative for myoepithelial cell markers. Syringomatous tumor is characterized by teardrop, comma, and branching-shaped ducts with an infiltrative growth with desmoplastic stroma; it does not involve the epidermis. Tubular adenoma is a well-circumscribed proliferation of uniform glands with scant stroma.

**28. Correct choice: C.**

Paget disease of the breast refers to the spread of an underlying breast carcinoma to the epidermis of the nipple. Up to two-thirds of cases are associated with an underlying carcinoma, which may be in situ or invasive. Prognosis depends on the extent of the underlying carcinoma. Paget cells have abundant slightly eosinophilic vacuolated cytoplasm and prominent nucleoli. They are immunoreactive for EMA (epithelial membrane antigen), low-molecular-weight keratin, and typically for HER2 (human epidermal growth factor receptor 2), but not for S100 protein or HMB45. Melanoma and Bowen disease should be considered in the differential diagnosis and are excluded on the basis of immunohistochemical stains. Clinically, the condition manifests with crusted erythema of the nipple and areola. Paget cells should not be confused with Toker clear cells or Toker cell hyperplasia, normally found in the nipple epidermis. Toker cells have a benign cytologic appearance and usually do not form clusters.

**29. Correct choice: B.**

Fibroadenoma typically occurs in young women and manifests as a well-demarcated mobile nodule within the breast parenchyma. As the designation implies, histologically the lesion is composed of both a stromal and an epithelial component. The stromal component appears to be the true neoplastic element. Breast hamartoma is a well-circumscribed, often encapsulated mass composed of normal but disorganized components of breast tissue. Phyllodes tumor exhibits a well-developed leaflike architecture with accompanied increased stromal cellularity and prominent mitotic activity (≥3/10 high-power fields) or the finding of three or more characteristic histologic features (stromal overgrowth, fat infiltration, stromal fragmentation, subepithelial stromal condensation, stromal nuclear pleomorphism). Periductal stromal tumor is a phyllodes tumor that lacks the characteristic frond-like architecture.

**30. Correct choice: C.**

Juvenile fibroadenoma is characterized by three features: the young patient's age, large size, and hypercellularity of the stromal and epithelial components. A characteristic tufted or gynecomastoid pattern is seen in the tubular component, in which tufts of epithelial cells protrude into the lumen. Complex fibroadenoma refers to fibroadenomas containing cystic change, sclerosing adenosis, papillary apocrine metaplasia, or epithelial calcifications; they may be associated with a slightly higher risk of subsequent carcinoma.

**31. Correct choice: E.**

Tubular adenoma is a variant of fibroadenoma that exhibits an adenosis-like pericanalicular proliferation of tightly packed ductules with small lumina that may contain scant secretions.

**32. Correct choice: D.**

Phyllodes tumor originates from intralobular stroma and is accompanied by a nonneoplastic glandular component. Nodules of proliferating stroma are lined by epithelium in a leaflike configuration. This tumor affects older women (45 years is the median age of incidence) and has a propensity to recur and occasionally metastasize. Metastatic potential is in direct relation to the degree of cellular anaplasia. Thus, cellular density of stroma, cytologic atypia, and mitotic activity are prognostically relevant factors. High-grade lesions are similar to poorly differentiated sarcomas. Extensive sampling is recommended to assess malignant features because histologic heterogeneity in phyllodes tumors is common.

**33. Correct choice: E.**

Pseudoangiomatous hyperplasia (PASH) is a benign lesion consisting of complex interanastomosing spaces within the dense collagenous, keloid-like stroma, simulating vascular structures. The spindle cells are positive for ER (estrogen receptor), PR (progesterone receptor), and CD34 but negative for other vascular markers. It is usually an incidental finding but may present as a palpable mass or as an area of nonmass enhancement on magnetic resonance imaging (MRI).

**34. Correct choice: C.**

Fibromatosis of the breast is composed of long intersecting fascicles of bland spindle cells with indistinct borders and hyperchromatic nuclei with occasional nucleoli. The cells infiltrate normal ducts and lobules, adipose tissue, and skeletal muscle, thus mimicking invasive process. The background stroma often has thickened collagen resembling keloid. It is positive for β-catenin, calponin, and smooth muscle actin. Up to 80% of cases are positive for β-catenin (nuclear). Benign phyllodes tumor is a well-circumscribed mass with hyperplastic epithelium within a hypercellular stroma composed of spindle cells with mild atypia and low mitotic activity. Cicatrix (scar) is a localized lesion composed of bland spindle cells with associated histiocytes, foreign body giant cell reaction, and lymphocytes. Fibromatosis-like metaplastic carcinoma may simulate fibromatosis on limited biopsies, but it is positive for CK5/6 and negative for nuclear β-catenin staining. Nodular fasciitis is rarely encountered in the breast but can present as a focally infiltrative lesion composed of spindle cells forming short fascicles or storiform pattern with increased mitotic activity; it is negative for nuclear β-catenin staining.

**35. Correct choice: E.**

It is generally agreed that a specific type of breast cancer may be diagnosed if at least 90% of the tumor shows that given pattern. However, mucinous tumors are an exception, because a favorable prognosis applies only to those cases in which the *entire* tumor is composed of mucinous carcinoma.

**36. Correct choice: B.**

Lymphocytic (diabetic) mastopathy is a breast condition that is morphologically equivalent to lymphocytic lobulitis. It occurs predominantly in women with type 1 diabetes and is characterized by periductal, perilobular, and perivascular lymphocytic infiltrate leading to lobular atrophy and dense, keloid-like fibrosis. Lesions may be multiple and bilateral. Multifocal painful nodules represent the most usual clinical presentation. Chronic granulomatous mastitis, a lesion of uncertain pathogenesis, is associated with a granulomatous reaction centering on lobules. Mammary duct ectasia is characterized by periductal chronic inflammation in association with marked dilatation of ducts. Postsurgical changes/trauma may exhibit areas of dense fibrosis, but foci of fat necrosis, foamy histiocytes, and multinucleated giant cells, as well as organizing hemorrhage, are also present. Extranodal small lymphocytic lymphoma is characterized by a monomorphous population of neoplastic lymphocytes that express CD20, CD5, CD23, PAX5, and BCL2.

**37. Correct choice: A.**

Cystic neutrophilic granulomatous mastitis is characterized by granulomas composed of epithelioid histiocytes and giant cells with central lipid vacuoles containing gram-positive bacteria and rimmed by neutrophils. It is associated with *Corynebacterium* species, although microbiologic evidence can be difficult to obtain. Patients commonly present with a unilateral, painful breast mass with nipple inversion or discharge. There may be associated fever and leukocytosis. Lobular (idiopathic) granulomatous mastitis, an entity of unknown etiology, is a diagnosis of exclusion. It is characterized by a lobulocentric granulomatous inflammatory process which typically contains neutrophils, which may create microabscesses, simulating cystic neutrophilic granulomatous mastitis. Multinucleated giant cells, lymphocytes, plasma cells, and eosinophils are distributed within and around lobules, but with extensive inflammation, the lobulocentric distribution may be obliterated. Sarcoidosis is characterized by non-necrotizing epithelioid granulomas, asteroid bodies, and Schaumann bodies.

**38. Correct choice: E.**

Perilobular hemangioma is a benign proliferation of well-differentiated, nonanastomosing small, thin-walled capillary vessels involving the intralobular stroma. No cytologic atypia, hemorrhage, mitotic activity, or necrosis is present. Most are 2 mm or more and found incidentally on core needle biopsy.

**39. Correct choice: A.**

Breast angiosarcoma may be primary or secondary (most commonly secondary to radiation). Radiation-induced breast angiosarcoma occurs in older women, is often high grade, and arises in the skin and then secondarily involves the breast parenchyma. Most harbor mutations in *MYC*. Although the tumors are often graded, the grade does not predict prognosis.

**40. Correct choice: A.**

Acinic cell carcinoma is a rare form of breast carcinoma that resembles its salivary gland counterpart. The tumor is composed of a monotonous, diffuse infiltration of cells with abundant finely granular, weakly eosinophilic or clear vacuolated cytoplasm and central round nuclei with prominent nucleoli. Cytoplasmic dark eosinophilic coarse PAS (periodic acid-Schiff) diastase-resistant granules (resembling Paneth cells) can be seen. A microglandular pattern may also be seen. Apocrine metaplasia of the breast is characterized by enlarged epithelial cells with abundant granular eosinophilic cytoplasm that can show apical snouts, eccentric nuclei, and prominent nucleoli. Apocrine carcinoma shows a more extensive proliferation and nuclear pleomorphism as well as architectural complexity such as well-formed "Roman" bridges or rigid cribriform structures. Lactational change is typically confined to a single lobule or several lobules without an infiltrative pattern. Microglandular adenosis does not exhibit granular cytoplasm.

**41. Correct choice: E.**

Low-grade ductal carcinoma in situ is more often ER/PR positive, HER2 negative, and has a lower proliferation rate. In contrast, high-grade ductal carcinoma in situ is frequently HER2 positive, harbors mutations in *TP53*, and exhibits a high-proliferation index. Expression for androgen receptors can be seen in both low-grade and high-grade ductal carcinoma in situ.

**42. Correct choice: B.**

Microglandular adenosis is a form of adenosis that lacks the two-layer lining (epithelial-myoepithelial) typical of benign lesions. It consists of tubules containing PAS (periodic acid-Schiff)-positive material. The lack of myoepithelial lining is evident when compared to normal adjacent lobular units and staining for myoepithelial markers confirms this feature. In contrast, myoepithelial cells are present in intraductal papilloma, radial scar, sclerosing adenosis, and tubular adenoma.

**43. Correct choice: C.**

Patients with Klinefelter syndrome have an increased risk for breast carcinoma. Male breast cancer accounts for less than 1% of all cases of breast cancer. It usually develops in older men, and gynecomastia is *not* a risk factor. The majority of cases express hormone receptors.

**44. Correct choice: D.**

Breast abscesses develop almost exclusively in the lactating breast and are generally due to *Staphylococcus aureus.*

**45. Correct choice: D.**

Mammary duct ectasia (also known as periductal mastitis) presents in multiparous women in their 40s or 50s as a poorly circumscribed subareolar nodule, often accompanied by nipple retraction. Because of these features, it is often biopsied to rule out malignancy. Histologically, it consists of dilated ducts filled with inspissated secretion and surrounded by florid chronic inflammation. Plasma cells are numerous, justifying the old designation of plasma cell mastitis. A granulomatous reaction and fibrosis may develop, resulting in nipple retraction.

**46. Correct choice: E.**

Inflammatory breast carcinoma is associated with a rapidly growing cancer that infiltrates dermal lymphatics. This leads to swelling and erythema of the breast, simulating an inflammatory condition (hence the clinical designation). Inflammatory breast carcinoma is not a specific histopathologic subtype of breast cancer. Rather, it is a clinical manifestation that may be seen in association with different types of invasive breast carcinoma. It implies a poor prognosis.

**47. Correct choice: A.**

Prognostic factors are used to assess the prognosis at the time of diagnosis, whereas predictive factors correlate with response to a specific treatment. Of all the prognostic factors listed, lymph node status is the most significant. The absence of axillary lymph node metastases is associated with 80% survival at 10 years. With up to 3 nodes involved, the survival rate is approximately 40%, and 15% with more than 10 nodes involved.

**48. Correct choice: B.**

Mucinous carcinoma is characterized by abundant extracellular mucin production so that neoplastic cells seem to float in a sea of mucin. This variant (<5% of all breast cancer) occurs predominantly in older women and is associated with a lower rate of nodal metastasis and longer survival. Grossly, mucinous carcinomas are well circumscribed. Tumor cells frequently express hormone receptors.

**49. Correct choice: C.**

Micropapillary carcinoma is a rare form of breast cancer characterized histologically by tubuloalveolar or micropapillary formations lacking fibrovascular cores and surrounded by a clear space. Lymphatic and/or vascular invasion is observed in 33% to 67% of cases. Most cases of micropapillary carcinoma are found in association with infiltrating ductal carcinoma of no special type or mucinous carcinoma. Presence of a micropapillary pattern is a negative prognostic indicator.

**50. Correct choice: D.**

Breast angiosarcoma is rare (0.05% of malignant breast tumors), but it is the most common type of mammary sarcoma. It most frequently arises after radiation treatment for breast cancer at a median age of 70 years. It typically arises within the radiation field 6 to 7 years following radiation but may develop within a shorter latency period of 1 to 2 years. Cutaneous angiosarcoma of the upper limb arises in the setting of chronic lymphedema, typically occurring after mastectomy and axillary dissection but may secondarily extend to the breast and/or chest wall. Thorotrast and polyvinyl chloride (PVC) exposure have been associated with angiosarcomas of the liver.

**51. Correct choice: E.**

Tubular carcinoma is a special subtype of invasive breast carcinoma with a favorable prognosis. It is composed of well-differentiated, angular tubular structures (>90%) with open lumina lined by a single layer of low-grade malignant epithelial cells, within a fibrous/desmoplastic stroma. The tumor cells are cuboidal to columnar with uniform, small- to intermediate-sized nuclei and often have apical cytoplasmic tufting or snouts. There is no significant cytologic atypia, multilayering, or high mitotic activity (the presence of these would rule out tubular carcinoma). Luminal secretions or calcifications may be present. The tumor cells are ER positive and HER2 negative. If mixed with invasive ductal carcinoma of no special type, the tumor has a worse prognosis. Invasive low-grade ductal carcinoma has similar low-grade cytologic features to tubular carcinoma, with or without prominent apical cytoplasmic tufting but with more complex architecture. There is multilayering, stratification, glandular fusion or branching, and greater than 10% ribbons or cords. Microglandular adenosis has more rounded (not angulated) tubules with intraluminal colloid-like secretory material; although it lacks myoepithelium, the basement membrane material is present. Also, it is ER negative. Radial scar does not infiltrate at the periphery and is often intermixed with fibrocystic changes; myoepithelium is present. Sclerosing adenosis retains an overall lobular architecture but exhibits compression of glands and the glands contain two layers (inner epithelial and outer myoepithelial).

**52. Correct choice: A.**

Adenomyoepithelioma is a benign well circumscribed, biphasic proliferation of epithelial and myoepithelial cells. The epithelial cells usually form glandular spaces and can show apocrine, sebaceous, or squamous metaplasia, or exhibit a papillary configuration. Myoepithelial cells are usually dominant and may be spindled, tubular, or lobulated. Intraductal papilloma is predominantly a papillary lesion composed of papillary structures with fibrovascular cores; myoepithelium is present but it is not prominent. Nipple adenoma arises in the collecting ducts of the nipple. Tubular adenoma is very well circumscribed and is characterized by a proliferation of tubules with only a single layer of myoepithelial cells surrounding the epithelial component.

**53. Correct choice: C.**

Fat necrosis is a nonneoplastic inflammatory reaction that is commonly secondary to adipose tissue injury characterized by necrotic adipose tissue with foamy histiocytes, chronic inflammatory cells, and multinucleated giant cells. It may simulate carcinoma both clinically and radiologically. Breast abscesses typically occur in postpartum. Breast hamartoma is a well-circumscribed, often encapsulated mass composed of normal but disorganized components of breast tissue. Silicone reaction may not only feature areas of fat necrosis but also contains spaces with refractile material.

**54. Correct choice: E.**

Silicone foreign body inflammatory reaction is induced by silicone leakage or rupture of silicone-containing breast prosthesis or as a reaction to silicone injection. When diffuse in the breast, it may be referred to as silicone mastitis. When nodular in the breast, it forms silicone granulomas. If there is leakage to regional lymph nodes, it can cause silicone lymphadenitis. Although many of the features are not specific (ie, chronic inflammatory cells, foreign body giant cell reaction, and fibrosis with fat necrosis), the presence of histiocytes containing clear, refractile, nonpolarizable material within cytoplasmic vacuoles and/or extracellular silicone (nonbirefringent crystals or particles within empty spaces) are diagnostic. Long-standing reactions include a well-defined band of collagenized fibrous tissue forming a fibrous capsule or bursa with calcifications and/or bone.

**55. Correct choice: D.**

Germline mutations in *CDH1* (which encodes E-cadherin) result in hereditary diffuse gastric cancer syndrome which may also be associated with increased risk for developing lobular carcinoma in situ and invasive lobular carcinoma in the breast. No increased risk of developing lobular carcinoma of the breast is associated with germline *BRCA1* and *BRCA2* mutations. Germline *TP53* and *APC* mutations result in Li-Fraumeni syndrome and familial adenomatous polyposis, respectively, which are not associated with lobular carcinoma of the breast.

**56. Correct choice: B.**

Carcinomas with apocrine differentiation are composed of tumor cells with apocrine cytology: large atypical epithelial cells with abundant eosinophilic and granular cytoplasm, enlarged nuclei, and prominent nucleoli. Apocrine morphology must be present in greater than 90% of the tumor. Carcinomas with apocrine differentiation are usually triple negative (ER–, PR–, and HER2–); however, HER2 (human epidermal growth factor receptor 2) amplification and/or overexpression has been reported in 30% to 60% of tumors. Carcinomas with apocrine differentiation typically demonstrate diffuse and strong AR (androgen receptor) immunoreactivity. Focal AR immunoreactivity may be seen in up to 60% of invasive breast carcinomas, with no special type.

**57. Correct choice: B.**

Apocrine metaplasia of the breast is characterized by enlarged epithelial cells with abundant granular eosinophilic cytoplasm that can show apical snouts, eccentric nuclei, and prominent nucleoli. Apocrine ductal carcinoma in situ shows more extensive proliferation and nuclear pleomorphism as well as architectural complexity such as well-formed "Roman" bridges or rigid cribriform structures.

**58. Correct choice: C.**

Fibromatosis-like spindle cell metaplastic carcinoma is a variant of metaplastic carcinoma with low-grade, bland spindle cells histologically resembling fibromatosis. It is characterized by a proliferation of spindle-shaped, fibroblast-like, and myofibroblast-like cells arranged in interlacing fascicles with irregular infiltrative margins into surrounding breast parenchyma. Mitotic figures are absent or rare. The background stroma can be fibrotic, sclerotic, or collagenized, and there is often an associated stromal lymphocytic infiltrate at the periphery. The constituent cells are positive for CK5/6 and p63 as well as broad-spectrum keratins. Fibromatosis-like spindle cell metaplastic carcinoma has a propensity for local recurrence but lymph node and distant metastases are rare. Fibromatosis and scar tissue are negative for cytokeratins. Phyllodes tumor has a leaflike growth pattern and is negative for CK5/6 and high-molecular-weight keratin. Pseudoangiomatous stromal hyperplasia is also negative for keratins and is positive for CD34.

**59. Correct choice: A.**

Salivary gland type breast carcinoma is typically ER–, PR–, HER2– (triple negative) but is considered an indolent tumor with low rates of distant metastasis and excellent long-term survival, despite the triple-negative phenotype.

**60. Correct choice: E.**

Secretory breast carcinoma is a rare subtype of low-grade, circumscribed invasive breast carcinoma composed of vacuolated tumor cells producing intracellular and extracellular PAS+ secretions forming a microcystic, solid, and tubular architecture. It is the most common primary pediatric breast cancer but can occur at any age. Most tumors have a translocation yielding an *ETV6-NTRK3* fusion gene. Like other salivary gland type breast cancers, it is typically triple negative for estrogen receptor, progesterone receptor, and HER2 (human epidermal growth factor receptor 2). Acinic cell carcinoma is composed of cells with clear cytoplasm (hypernephroid pattern) and expresses proteins of its salivary gland counterpart (eg, $\alpha$-1-chymotrypsin, salivary gland amylase).

# 10 Brain, Spinal Cord, and Meninges

1. Which of the following is true about gliosis?

    A. Associated with a Ki-67 labeling index higher than 5%
    B. Expands the brain region where it develops
    C. Glial cells are uniformly distributed
    D. Positive for mutations of IDH1 or p53
    E. Presence of gemistocytes favors glioma

2. Rosenthal fibers may be found in

    A. Alexander disease.
    B. pilocytic astrocytoma.
    C. reactive astrocytosis around infarcts.
    D. reactive astrocytosis around tumors.
    E. all of the above.

3. At autopsy, the brain of a 35-year-old man with a history of AIDS shows diffuse edema and opacification of the leptomeninges. On histologic examination, the subarachnoid space is filled with the organisms seen in the GMS (Grocott methenamine silver stain)-stained section, shown in Figure 1, and a scanty mononuclear infiltrate. Which of the following is the etiologic agent?

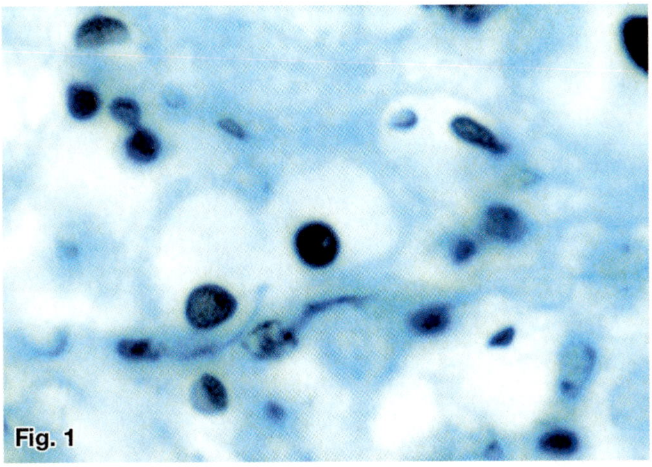

Fig. 1

    A. *Candida*
    B. *Coccidioides*
    C. *Cryptococcus*
    D. *Histoplasma*
    E. *Tropheryma whipplei*

4. A 54-year-old woman treated with immunosuppression for lupus develops clumsiness and difficulty speaking. Brain biopsy of a deep white matter lesion shows atypical astrocytes and foamy macrophages that contain blue balls of myelin as depicted in Figure 1. What is the most likely diagnosis?

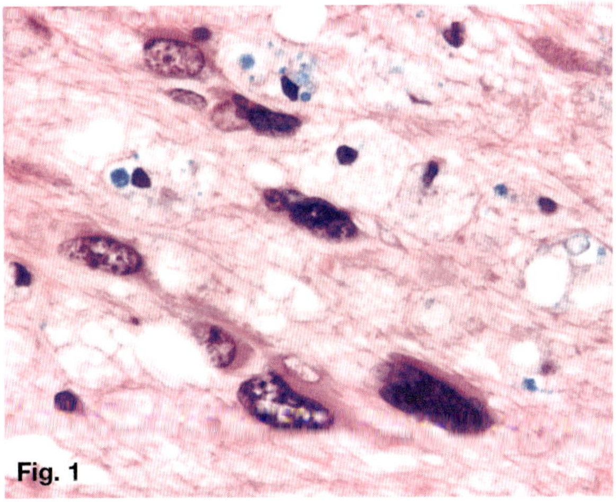

Fig. 1

    A. CMV encephalitis
    B. Creutzfeldt-Jakob disease
    C. Multiple sclerosis
    D. Progressive multifocal leukoencephalopathy
    E. Vasculitis secondary to lupus

5. Progressive multifocal leukoencephalopathy (PML) is most common in patients who are immunocompromised, especially those with AIDS. Which of the following is the etiologic agent of this condition?

    A. Arbovirus
    B. Cytomegalovirus (CMV)
    C. Herpes simplex virus (HSV)
    D. Herpes zoster
    E. Papovavirus

All figures in this chapter are from Longacre TA, Greenson JK, Hornick JL, Reuter VE, eds. *Mills and Sternberg's Diagnostic Surgical Pathology*. 7th ed. Wolters Kluwer; 2022 except for those noted at the end of this book.

6. Biopsy of the cerebral frontal lobe from a 57-year-old man with suspected Alzheimer disease reveals coalescing round vacuoles and gliosis involving all six cortical layers as shown in Figure 1. Which of the following is the most likely diagnosis?

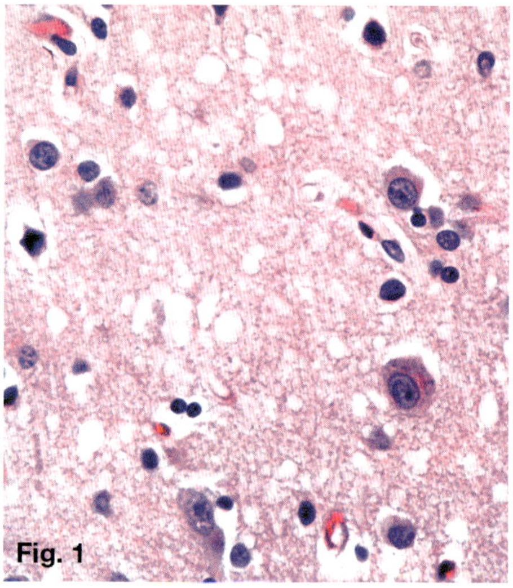
Fig. 1

A. Creutzfeldt-Jakob disease
B. Neurocysticercosis
C. Parkinson disease
D. Subacute sclerosing panencephalitis
E. Toxoplasmosis

7. Which of the following is true regarding prion disease?

A. Brain biopsy/autopsy is the gold standard for diagnosis
B. Can be transmitted by plasma products
C. Cannot be transmitted by corneal transplants
D. Caused by PRION virus
E. Rarely occurs sporadically

8. Which of the following is the most frequent primary malignant tumor of the central nervous system?

A. Anaplastic oligodendroglioma
B. Ependymoma
C. Glioblastoma multiforme
D. Lymphoma
E. Medulloblastoma

9. Which of the following gliomas occurring in adults is not typically associated with *IDH* mutations?

A. Astrocytoma
B. Gemistocytic astrocytoma
C. Oligodendroglioma
D. Primary glioblastoma
E. Secondary glioblastoma

10. What is the best diagnosis for the brain tumor, shown in Figures 1 and 2, from a 43-year-old woman with recent onset seizures and an expansile, poorly defined mass of low density on a computed tomography (CT) scan?

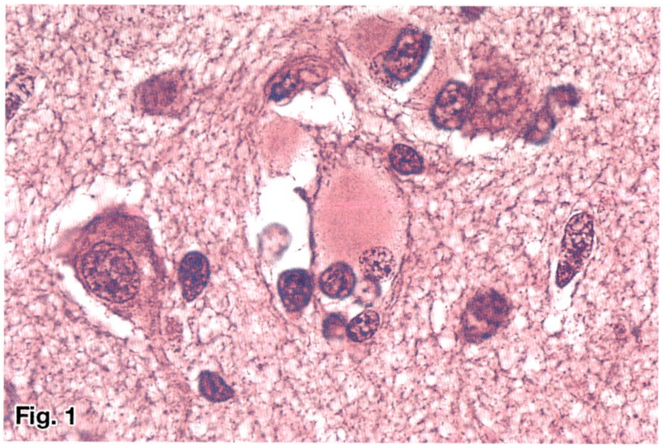
Fig. 1

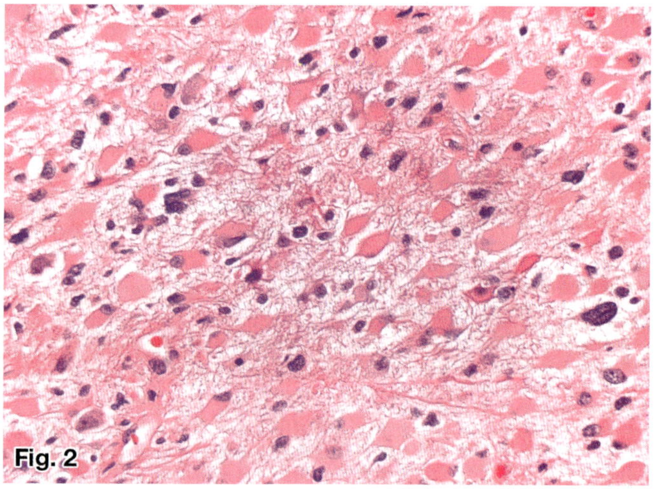
Fig. 2

A. Astroblastoma
B. Gemistocytic astrocytoma
C. Pilomyxoid astrocytoma
D. Protoplasmic astrocytoma
E. Subependymal giant cell astrocytoma

11. A cystic tumor is resected from the right cerebellar hemisphere of a 15-year-old patient. Histologically, it is composed of spindly cells, as shown in Figure 1. The neoplasm has a biphasic pattern, with alternating compact and microcystic areas. Rosenthal fibers are numerous in the compact areas. Cells are immunoreactive for glial fibrillary acidic protein (GFAP) but not IDH1. What is the most likely diagnosis?

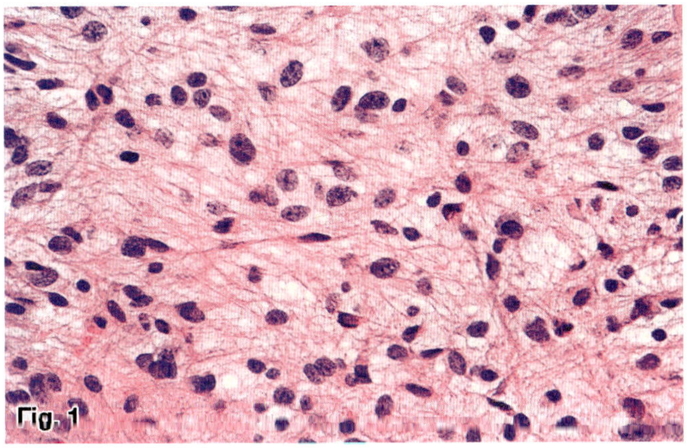


A. Astroblastoma
B. Pilocytic astrocytoma
C. Pilomyxoid astrocytoma
D. Protoplasmic astrocytoma
E. Subependymal giant cell astrocytoma

12. A biopsy of a mass growing from the floor of the lateral ventricle reveals a glial tumor composed of highly pleomorphic, giant astrocytes with large nuclei and prominent nucleoli, as shown in Figure 1. Some tumor cells express glial fibrillary acidic protein (GFAP), while others express neurofilaments. The patient is affected by

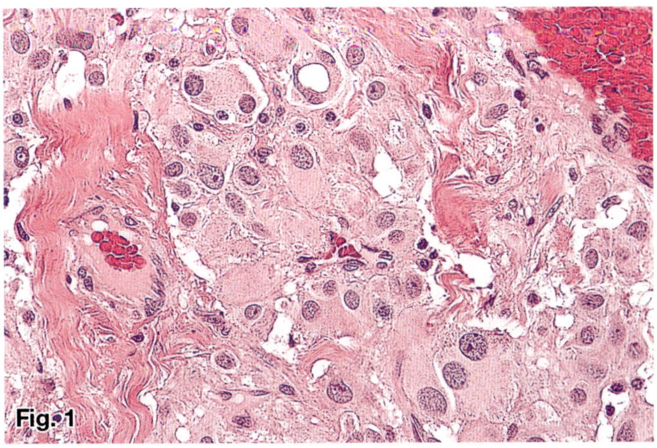


A. neurofibromatosis type 1.
B. neurofibromatosis type 2.
C. Sturge-Weber syndrome.
D. tuberous sclerosis.
E. von Hippel-Lindau syndrome.

13. What is the best diagnosis for the left temporal lobe mass, shown in Figure 1, attached to the dura in a 46-year-old man?

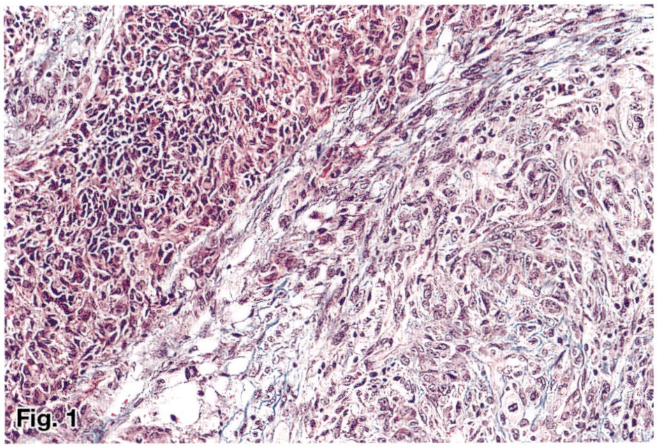


A. Fibrous meningioma
B. Glioblastoma
C. Gliosarcoma
D. Metastatic carcinoma
E. Primary sarcoma

14. A biopsy of a brain tumor reveals a homogeneous cellular composition, which is shown in Figure 1. The neoplastic cells are negative for glial fibrillary acidic protein (GFAP) immunohistochemistry. These features are most consistent with

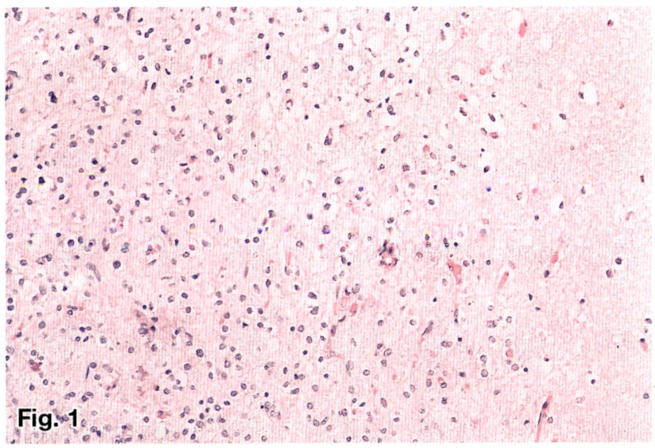


A. central neurocytoma.
B. clear cell ependymoma.
C. germinoma.
D. low-grade astrocytoma.
E. oligodendroglioma.

15. Which of the following genetic alterations is pathognomonic of oligodendrogliomas?

A. Deletions of 1p-19q and mutations in *IDH1* and *IDH2*
B. Inactivation of INI1 and mutations in *IDH1* and *IDH2*
C. Loss of chromosome 22 and mutations in *IDH1* and *IDH2*
D. Mutations of *BRAF* and *IDH1* and *IDH2*
E. Mutations of *BRAF* and *TP53*

16. The biopsy of a ring-enhancing tumor in the left parietal lobe of a 60-year-old patient reveals an astrocytic tumor (GFAP [glial fibrillary acidic protein] positive) displaying the features shown in Figure 1. What is the best diagnosis?

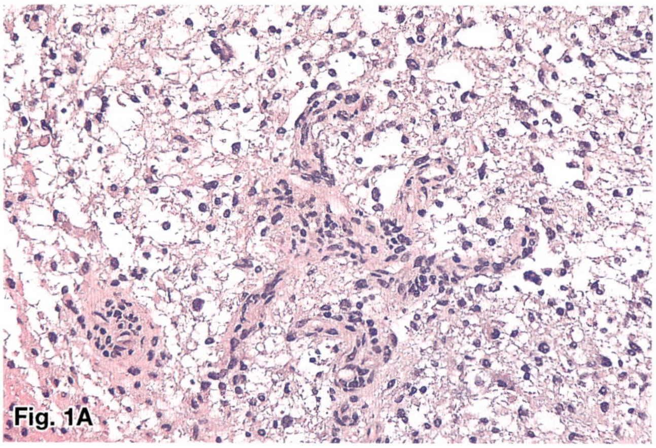
Fig. 1A

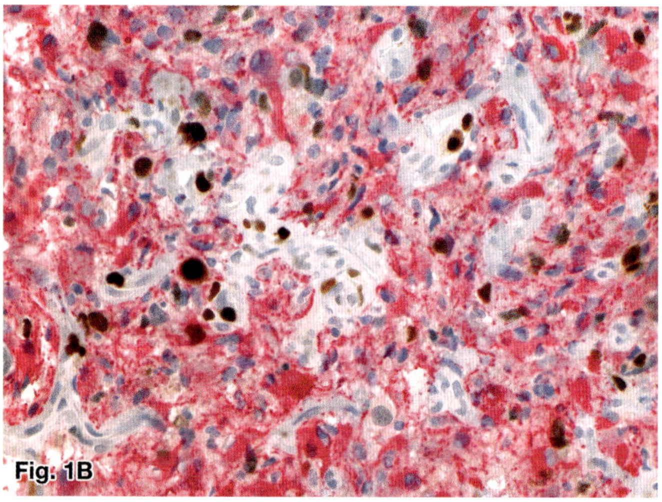
Fig. 1B

A. Astrocytoma, IDH mutant, grade 3
B. Astrocytoma, IDH mutant, grade 4
C. Astrocytoma, IDH mutant, WHO grade 2
D. Glioblastoma, IDH-wild type, WHO grade 4
E. Pleomorphic xanthoastrocytoma

17. Histologic examination of a well-circumscribed mass involving the cerebellum and fourth ventricle of an 18-year-old female reveals a tumor whose histologic appearance is shown in Figure 1. Which of the following is the most likely diagnosis?

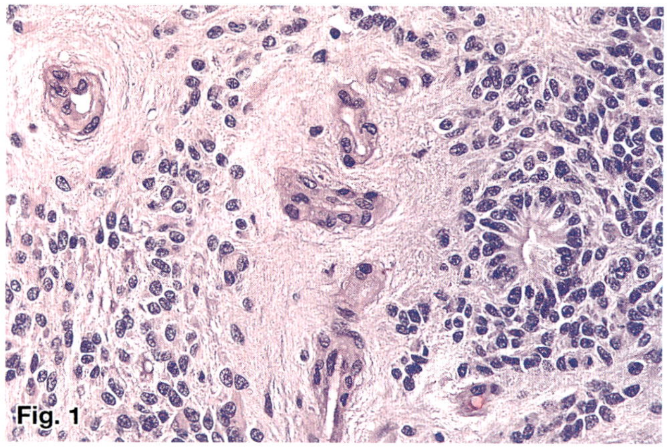
Fig. 1

A. Astroblastoma
B. Ependymoma
C. Hemangioblastoma
D. Medulloblastoma
E. Pilocytic astrocytoma

18. What is the best diagnosis for the tumor, shown in Figures 1 and 2, in the cauda equina of a 48-year-old man?

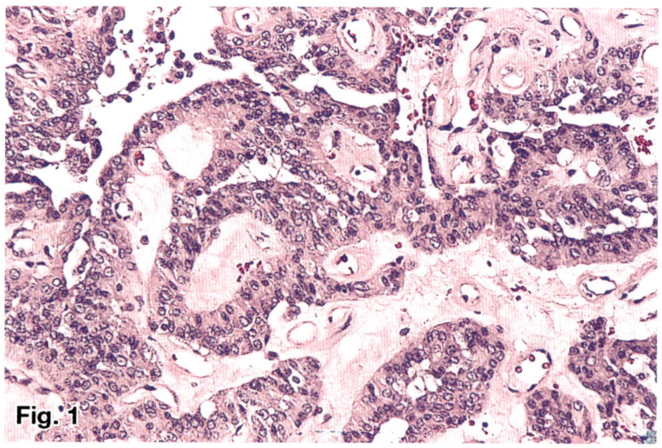
Fig. 1

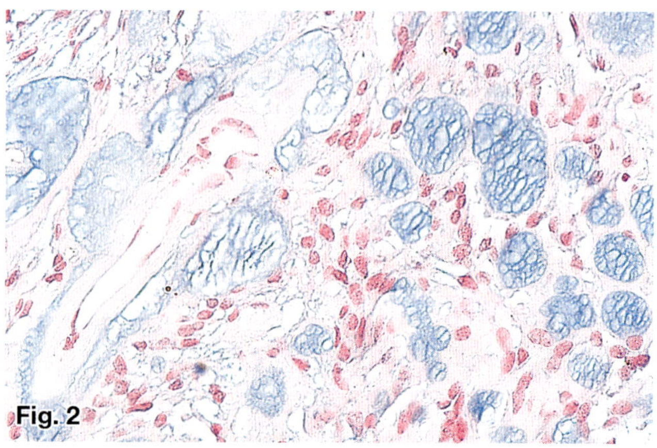
Fig. 2

A. Fibrous meningioma
B. Metastatic carcinoma
C. Myxopapillary ependymoma
D. Paraganglioma
E. Schwannoma

19. Which of the following is correct about ganglioglioma?

    A. Composed exclusively of neoplastic neuronal cells
    B. Dysplastic neuronal cells are evenly scattered throughout the tumor
    C. Not a true neoplasm but a hamartomatous lesion
    D. Occurs most commonly in the cerebellum
    E. Presents most frequently as a cyst with a mural nodule

20. Histologic examination of a midline (vermis) cerebellar tumor from a 5-year-old child shows sheets of monotonous small cells with a high nucleocytoplasmic ratio, as seen in Figure 1. There is mitotic activity as well as numerous apoptotic bodies. Neoplastic cells are glial fibrillary acidic protein (GFAP) negative but show multifocal immunoreactivity for synaptophysin. Which of the following is the most likely diagnosis?

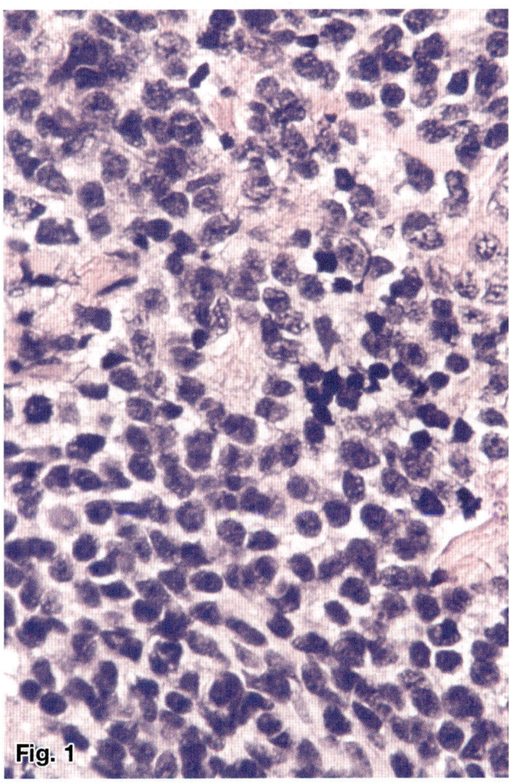


    A. Ependymoblastoma
    B. Ependymoma
    C. Medulloblastoma
    D. Pilocytic astrocytoma
    E. Pineoblastoma

21. A primary brain tumor arises in the lateral ventricle of a 4-year-old boy that has been stained for CAM5.2 cytokeratin (Figure 1) and for transthyretin (Figure 2). What is the diagnosis?

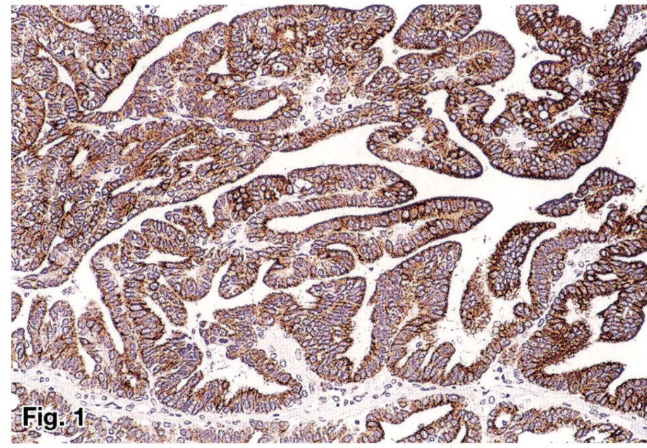


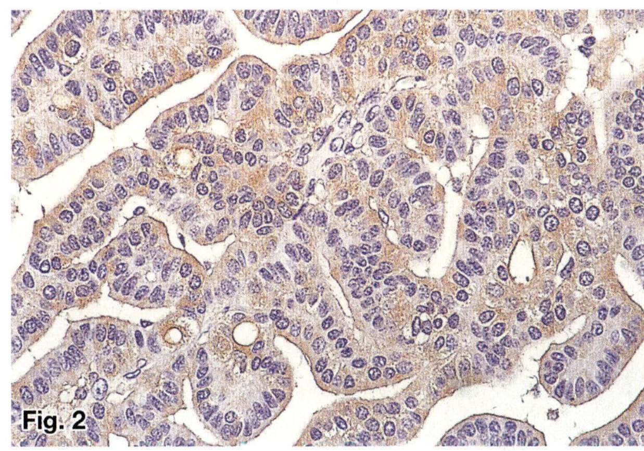


    A. Choroid plexus papilloma
    B. Ependymoma
    C. Metastatic carcinoma
    D. Papillary meningioma
    E. Papillary neoplasm of the endolymphatic sac

22. What is the most likely diagnosis for the cerebellar tumor, shown in Figure 1, from a 47-year-old female with a history of bilateral renal cell carcinoma (clear cell type)?

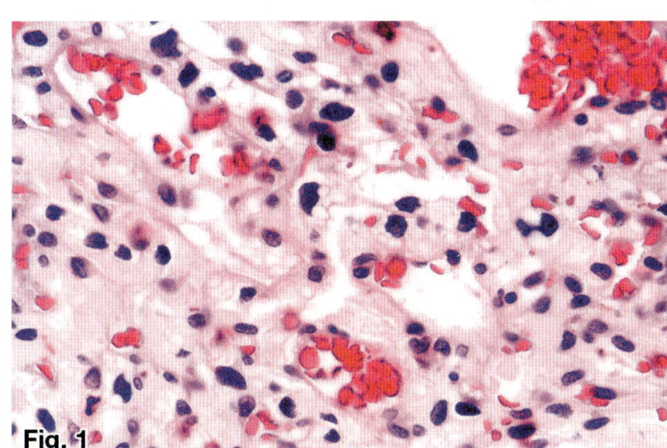


    A. Angiomatous meningioma
    B. Ependymoma
    C. Hemangioblastoma
    D. Paraganglioma
    E. Pilocytic astrocytoma

23. A 58-year-old woman presents with headaches. Magnetic resonance imaging (MRI) reveals a contrast-enhancing dural-based tumor in the left parietal region. Light microscopic features of the resected tumor are shown in Figure 1. The neoplastic cells are immunoreactive for epithelial membrane antigen (EMA) and negative for S100 protein. Which of the following is the best diagnosis?

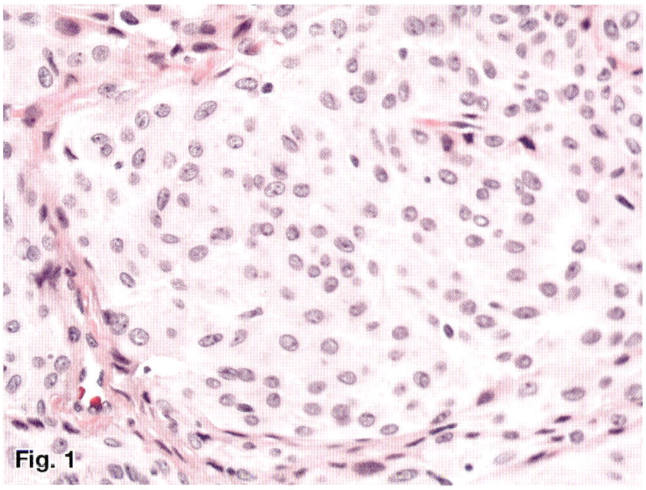

Fig. 1

A. Chordoid meningioma
B. Clear cell meningioma
C. Fibrous meningioma
D. Meningothelial meningioma
E. Transitional meningioma

24. Which of the following histologic types are classified as grade 3 meningiomas?

A. Angiomatous, microcystic
B. Clear cell, secretory
C. Lymphoplasmacyte rich, metaplastic
D. Meningothelial, fibroblastic
E. Papillary, rhabdoid

25. Which of the following histologic types are classified as grade 2 meningiomas?

A. Angiomatous, psammomatous
B. Chordoid, clear cell
C. Lymphoplasmacyte rich, secretory
D. Meningothelial, fibroblastic
E. Papillary, rhabdoid

26. What is the best diagnosis for the tumor, shown in Figure 1, in the cerebellar pontine angle in a 42-year-old woman?

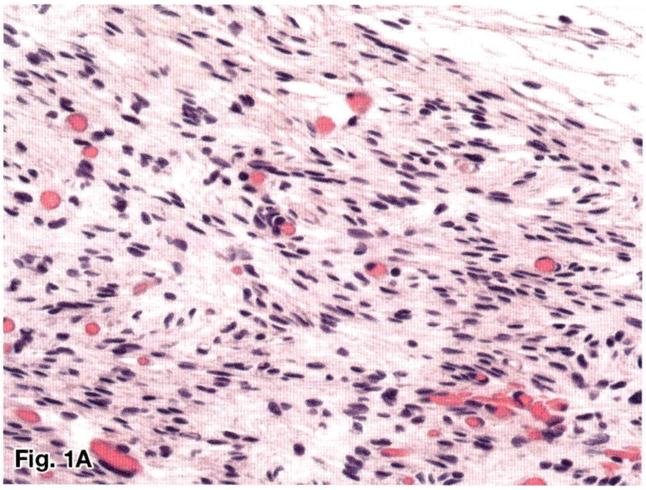

Fig. 1A

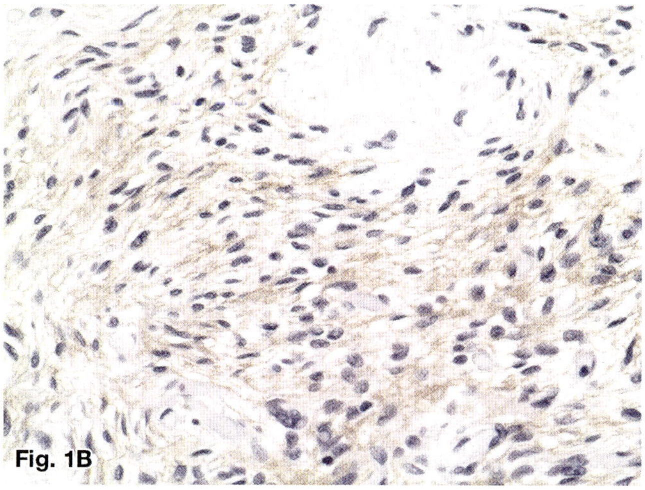

Fig. 1B

A. Fibrillary astrocytoma
B. Fibroblastic meningioma
C. Pilocytic astrocytoma
D. Schwannoma
E. Solitary fibrous tumor

27. Which of the following meningiomas commonly occurs in the spinal region?

A. Chordoid meningioma
B. Clear cell meningioma
C. Fibrous meningioma
D. Meningothelial meningioma
E. Psammomatous meningioma

28. What is the best diagnosis for the extra-axial clivus tumor, shown in Figure 1, in a 42-year-old man?

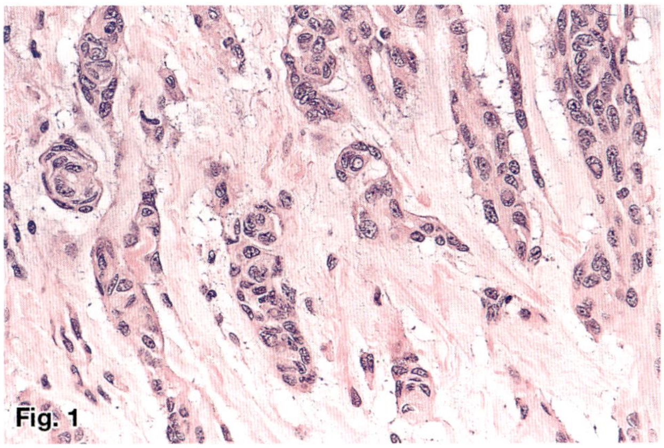
Fig. 1

A. Chondrosarcoma
B. Chordoid glioma
C. Chordoid meningioma
D. Chordoma
E. Metastatic carcinoma

29. A 44-year-old man undergoes surgery for excision of an osteolytic tumor, shown in Figure 1, located in the clivus. The tumor cells are immunoreactive for cytokeratin (see Figure 2), epithelial membrane antigen (EMA), and S100. Which of the following is the most likely diagnosis?

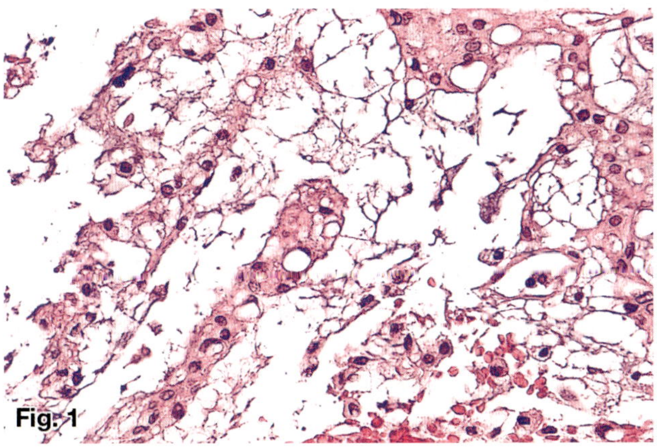
Fig. 1

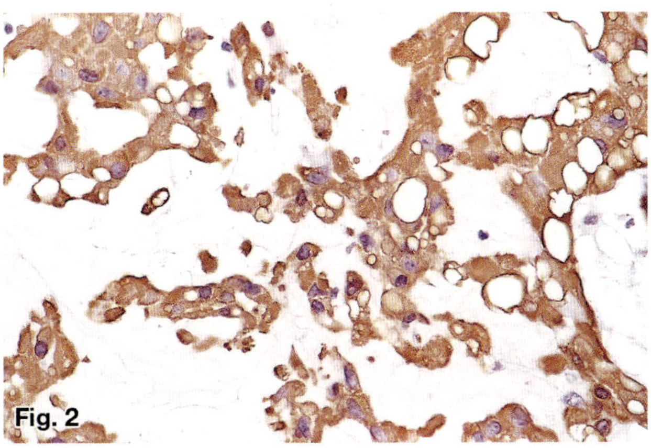
Fig. 2

A. Astrocytoma
B. Chondrosarcoma
C. Chordoma
D. Hemangioblastoma
E. Metastatic carcinoma

30. What is the best diagnosis for the tumor, shown in Figures 1 and 2, arising in the cauda equina of a 55-year-old man?

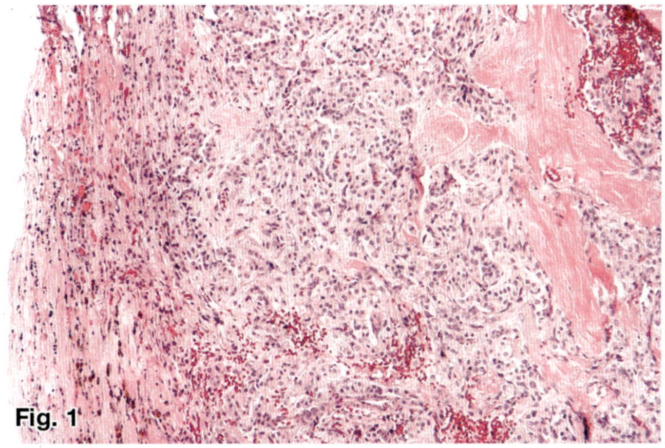
Fig. 1

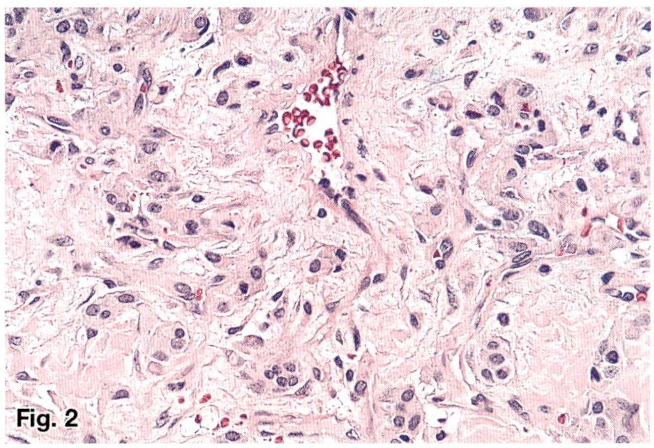
Fig. 2

A. Angiomatous meningioma
B. Chordoma
C. Hemangioblastoma
D. Myxopapillary ependymoma
E. Paraganglioma

31. What is the best diagnosis for the extra-axial lesion, shown in Figure 1, at the base of the skull in a 43-year-old man?

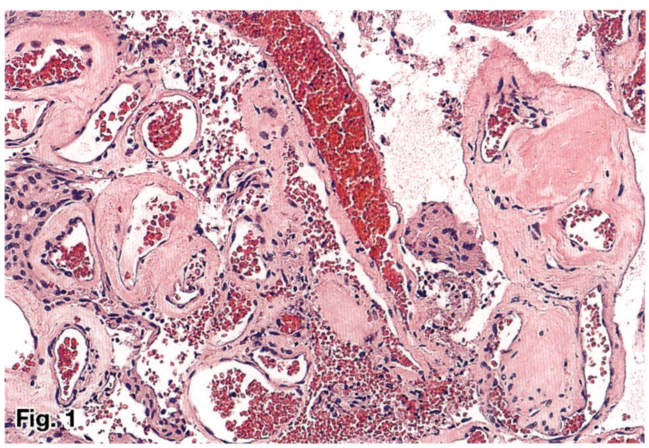
Fig. 1

A. Amyloid angiopathy
B. Angiomatous meningioma
C. Arteriovenous malformation
D. Hemangioblastoma
E. Treatment (radiation) effect

32. Which of the following vascular lesions is shown in Figure 1 (elastic stain)?

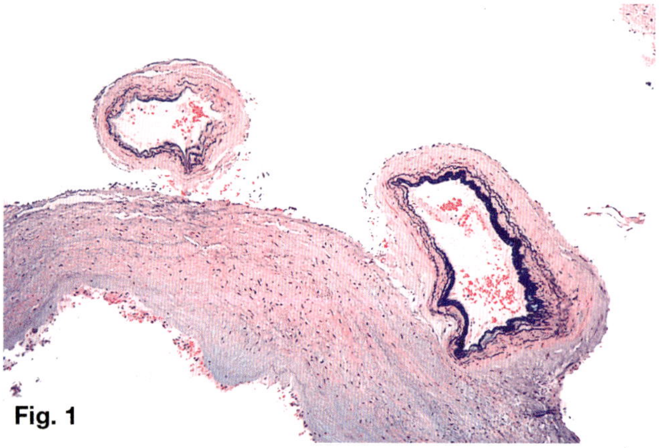

Fig. 1

A. Arteriovenous malformation
B. Capillary telangiectasia
C. Cavernous angioma
D. Cerebral amyloid angiopathy
E. Venous malformation

33. Which of the following vascular changes is expected to be seen by light microscopy in a skin biopsy from a patient with cerebral autosomal dominant angiopathy with subcortical infarcts and leukoencephalopathy (CADASIL)?

A. Congo red–positive material in the media
B. Hyalinization and thickening of media
C. Leukocytoclastic vasculitis
D. Microaneurysms
E. Periodic acid-Schiff (PAS)-positive granular material in the media of small arteries and arterioles

34. A 45-year-old woman with new onset headaches presents with a cystic lesion in the third ventricular wall, close to the foramen of Monro. The cyst is excised (Figure 1). Which of the following is the most likely diagnosis?

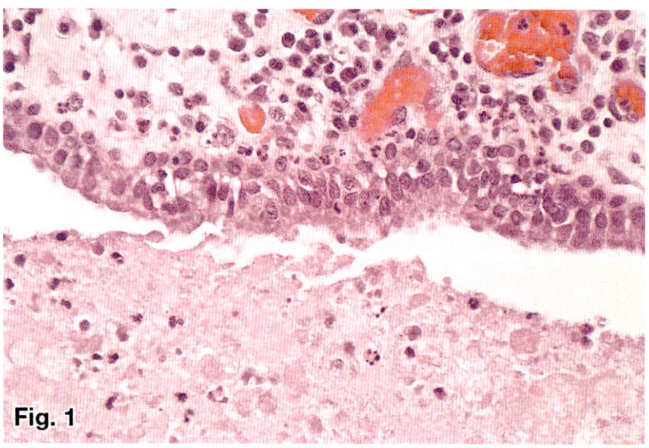

Fig. 1

A. Colloid cyst
B. Craniopharyngioma
C. Cysticercus
D. Ependymal cyst
E. Rathke cleft cyst

35. Which of the following brain neoplasms is characterized by a gross appearance of cyst with a mural nodule?

A. Chordoma, dysgerminoma, lymphoma
B. Ependymoma, schwannoma, epidermoid cyst
C. Hemangioblastoma, ganglioglioma, pilocytic astrocytoma
D. Medulloblastoma, pineoblastoma, retinoblastoma
E. Oligodendroglioma, low-grade astrocytoma, glioblastoma

36. Which of the following is the most common location of central nervous system (CNS) germinomas?

A. Cerebellopontine angle
B. Pineal region
C. Posterior fossa
D. Sacral region
E. Spinal cord

37. Which of the following accounts for the great majority of primary central nervous system (CNS) lymphomas?

A. Diffuse large B-cell lymphoma
B. Follicular lymphoma
C. Hodgkin lymphoma
D. Lymphomatoid granulomatosis
E. T-cell lymphoma

38. Dysplastic gangliocytoma of the cerebellum is associated with which of the following syndromes?

A. Cowden
B. Li-Fraumeni
C. Nevoid basal cell carcinoma
D. Turcot
E. von Hippel-Lindau

39. A computed tomography (CT) scan shows an intracerebral hemorrhage located superficially within the right frontal lobe of a 75-year-old man. After surgical evacuation of the hematoma, a β-amyloid immunohistochemical stain reveals cortical and leptomeningeal arterioles similar to that shown in this photomicrograph. Which of the following is the most likely underlying cause of the hemorrhage?

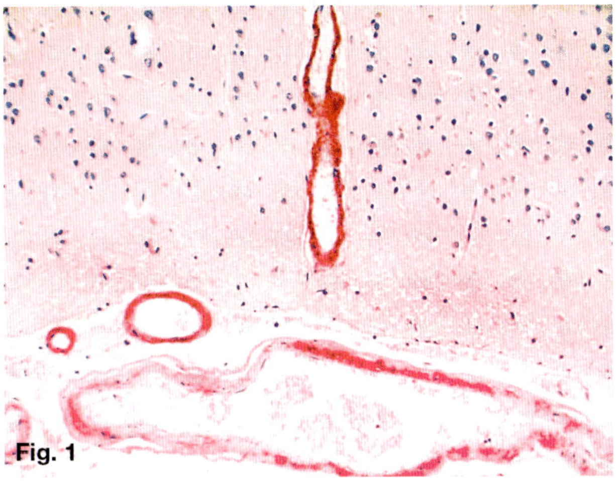
Fig. 1

A. Amyloid angiopathy
B. CADASIL (cerebral autosomal dominant angiopathy with subcortical infarcts and leukoencephalopathy)
C. Coagulopathy
D. Hypertension
E. Trauma

40. What is the best diagnosis for the mass, shown in Figure 1, arising in the anterior lateral ventricle of a 30-year-old man?

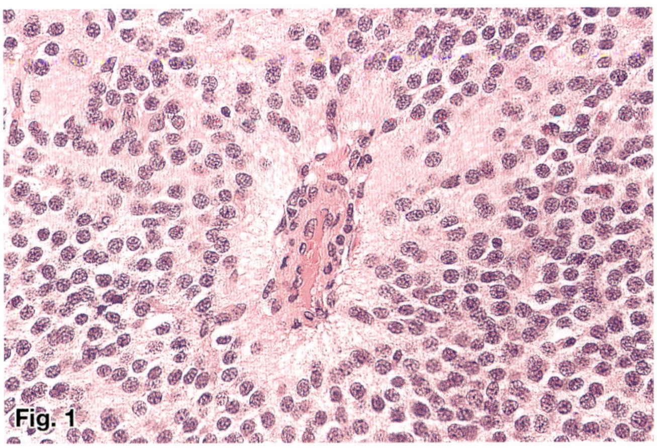
Fig. 1

A. Central neurocytoma
B. Ependymoma
C. Ganglioneuroma
D. Oligodendroglioma
E. Pineocytoma

41. What is the best diagnosis for the pineal gland tumor, shown in Figure 1, in a 20-year-old male?

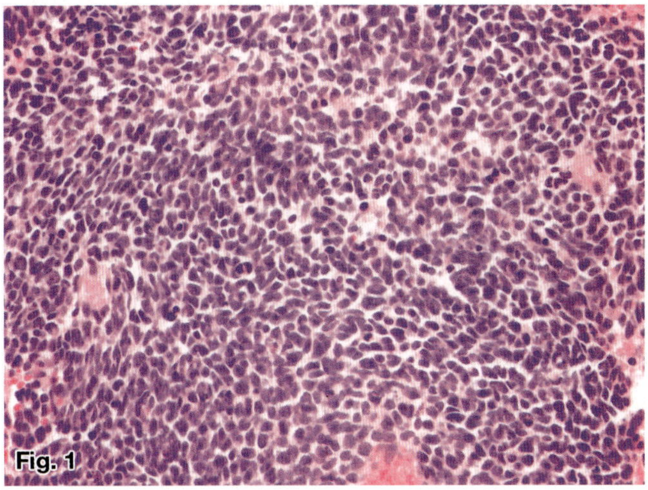
Fig. 1

A. Atypical teratoid/rhabdoid tumor
B. Germinoma
C. Medulloblastoma
D. Metastatic small cell carcinoma
E. Pineoblastoma

# ANSWERS AND EXPLANATIONS

**1. Correct choice: C.**

Distinguishing between gliosis and glioma may be difficult. Gliosis is a nonspecific reaction of the central nervous system (CNS) to a variety of injuries, neoplastic and nonneoplastic. It is defined as increased number of astrocytes and/or increased number and length of astrocytic processes. It often includes gemistocytes, which are hypertrophic astrocytes with abundant eosinophilic glial fibrillary acidic protein (GFAP)-filled cytoplasm and peripherally placed nucleus. Gliosis does not expand brain parenchyma, in contrast to gliomas. The Ki-67 labeling index in gliosis is well below 5%. No mutations are found in purely gliotic tissue, while diffuse astrocytomas are characterized by mutations of IDH1 or p53.

**2. Correct choice: E.**

Rosenthal fibers result from the accumulation of αB-crystallin and glial fibrillary acidic protein (GFAP) in hypertrophic processes of reactive astrocytes. They may develop in any form of reactive gliosis, as well as within certain tumors (particularly pilocytic astrocytomas) and around brain neoplasms (especially craniopharyngioma and hemangioblastoma). Some nonneoplastic conditions, such as hemangiomas and old infarcts, may elicit florid reactive gliosis containing Rosenthal fibers. Alexander disease is a rare form of hereditary leukodystrophy due to GFAP gene mutations: It is associated with innumerable Rosenthal fibers in the white matter, perivascular, and subpial regions.

**3. Correct choice: C.**

The figure shows the typical morphology of *Cryptococcus neoformans*, a 5-μm yeast surrounded by a thick polysaccharide capsule that stains for mucicarmine and periodic acid Schiff (PAS). It is the most common cause of fungal meningitis in patients with AIDS. Typically, the infection is associated with abundant gelatinous edema, produced by the mucoid fungal capsule, and scanty inflammatory response. Fungal infections involving the central nervous system (CNS) include (a) *yeast forms*, for example, cryptococcosis, coccidioidomycosis, histoplasmosis, candidiasis, and blastomycosis, and (b) hyphal forms, for example, zygomycetes (*Rhizopus*, *Mucor*), *Aspergillus*, and *Pseudallescheria*.

**4. Correct choice: D.**

Progressive multifocal encephalopathy (PML) affects oligodendroglia, causing widespread and multifocal white matter destruction mimicking multiple sclerosis. Histologically, it is characterized by multifocal myelin degeneration, bizarre astrocytes, and oligodendroglia with intranuclear inclusions. Sometimes, a biopsy of PML lesions may be erroneously interpreted as high-grade glioma because of bizarre astrocytes. Knowledge of the clinical history (immunosuppression) and magnetic resonance imaging (MRI) findings (multifocal white matter lesions) assists in the diagnosis. Cerebral vasculopathy secondary to lupus is associated with microthrombi and microinfarcts.

**5. Correct choice: E.**

Progressive multifocal encephalopathy (PML) is due to a papovavirus known as JC (John Cunningham) virus (from the initials of the first patient in whom the virus was identified). The virus affects oligodendroglia, causing widespread and multifocal white matter destruction mimicking multiple sclerosis. Histologically, it is characterized by multifocal myelin degeneration, bizarre astrocytes, and oligodendroglia with intranuclear inclusions. Sometimes, a biopsy of progressive multifocal leukoencephalopathy (PML) lesions may be erroneously interpreted as high-grade glioma because of bizarre astrocytes. Knowledge of the clinical history (immune depression) and magnetic resonance imaging (MRI) findings (multifocal white matter lesions) assist in the diagnosis.

**6. Correct choice: A.**

Creutzfeldt-Jakob disease occurs in three forms: sporadic (most common), hereditary, and acquired, including kuru, variant Creutzfeldt-Jakob disease, and iatrogenic Creutzfeldt-Jakob disease (contaminated surgical equipment or contaminated transplanted tissue (cornea, dura). Neuropil vacuolation involves all six layers of the cerebral cortex, reactive gliosis, and occasional plaques of amyloid-like material in the neocortex in variant Creutzfeldt-Jakob disease. Diffuse cortical vacuolization can be seen in advanced Alzheimer disease and is a diagnostic pitfall. Molecular diagnosis of prions is needed to confirm the diagnosis of Creutzfeldt-Jakob disease.

**7. Correct choice: A.**

Prion disease results from the benign form of a prion protein changing to an insoluble protease-resistant form leading to the formation of plaques in the brain. The prion protein assumes an abnormal configuration, which promotes change to the abnormal configuration of other proteins. Most cases are sporadic (85%). Less common cases are hereditary or acquired (through corneal transplants, pituitary gland-derived growth hormone, dura mater transplants, inadequately sterilized brain electrodes, and transfusion of blood components, but not plasma). Brain biopsy/autopsy and molecular studies of the tissue are the gold standard for diagnosis.

**8. Correct choice: C.**

Approximately 50% of brain tumors are metastatic. Gliomas account for 50% of primary brain tumors; of these, glioblastoma is the most common.

**9. Correct choice: D.**

Adult-type diffuse gliomas are now classified into three groups: glioblastoma, *IDH* wildtype, WHO grade 4; astrocytoma, *IDH* mutant, WHO grade 2-4; and oligodendroglioma, *IDH* mutant and 1p/19q codeleted, WHO grade 2-3. Gemistocytic astrocytoma is a variant of *IDH*-mutant astrocytoma. Glioblastoma, *IDH* wildtype, WHO grade 4 is considered to be a primary glioblastoma, while secondary glioblastoma arises from low-grade diffuse astrocytoma or anaplastic astrocytoma and harbors mutations in *IDH*.

**10. Correct choice: B.**

The word *gemistocyte* describes a hypertrophic astrocyte with a plump cytoplasm and long processes. Gemistocytes (nonneoplastic) are commonly found in florid long-standing gliosis. A small portion of diffuse astrocytomas are composed of neoplastic gemistocytes, and this variant is thus named gemistocytic astrocytoma. Gemistocytic astrocytomas are graded the same way as conventional diffuse astrocytomas. However, grade 2 gemistocytic astrocytomas tend to behave more aggressively than conventional grade 2 astrocytomas.

**11. Correct choice: B.**

Pilocytic astrocytoma occurs predominantly in children and young adults. The cerebellar hemisphere is the most common location, followed by the hypothalamic/suprasellar region. Its most common radiologic appearance is that of a cyst with a mural nodule. The neoplasm is composed of elongated cells with long hairlike (pilocytic) processes. The biphasic pattern of alternating densely fibrillar and loosely structured areas and the presence of Rosenthal fibers are the most characteristic features. Like all astrocytomas, pilocytic astrocytomas are immunoreactive for glial fibrillary acidic protein (GFAP) but lack *IDH1* or *IDH2* mutations. Nuclear pleomorphism may be marked, and some mitotic activity may be found, but the tumor is usually well circumscribed and slow growing. Surgical resection is usually curative. Thus, pilocytic astrocytomas are considered to be grade 1 in the WHO system. Tumors in a diencephalic location, however, may be less amenable to total resection and have a worse prognosis.

**12. Correct choice: D.**

Subependymal giant cell astrocytoma is a tumor that grows from the medial portion of the floor of the lateral ventricles, near the foramen of Monro. It is pathognomonic of tuberous sclerosis, which is due to mutations of *TSC1* or *TSC2* genes. Tuberous sclerosis manifests with multiple hamartomatous lesions in the skin, central nervous system (CNS), and visceral organs. Cortical tubers are malformative (hamartomatous) nodules, probably resulting from faulty cortical development. Other lesions include shagreen patches and ash-leaf patches of the skin, cardiac myomas, and renal angiomyolipomas. It is a benign tumor, but its cellular pleomorphism, sometimes associated with necrosis, mitoses, and microvascular hyperplasia, may be misleading.

**13. Correct choice: C.**

The figure shows the classic architecture of gliosarcoma, which consists of a mixture of sarcoma and glioblastoma. The sarcomatous component is reticulin rich and glial fibrillary acidic protein (GFAP) negative. Gliosarcomas usually have a gross appearance of a desmoplastic metastasis or fibrous meningioma, rather than a glioma. Awareness of this variant is important for diagnostic purposes, but the prognosis of gliosarcoma is the same as glioblastoma, WHO grade 4. Meningiomas, sarcomas, and metastatic carcinomas lack glial elements.

**14. Correct choice: E.**

Oligodendroglioma are characterized by round uniform nuclei and perinuclear halos (similar to normal oligodendroglia) imparting a *fried egg* appearance. Another characteristic feature of oligodendrogliomas is their vascularity, consisting of delicate branching capillaries arranged in a *chicken-wire* pattern. Oligodendrogliomas are slowly growing tumors located in the subcortical white matter of the cerebral hemispheres. Calcifications are frequent. Although slowly growing, oligodendrogliomas ultimately have a poor prognosis. Their infiltrative behavior prevents complete surgical resection. Oligodendrogliomas are graded as 2 or 3. Grade 3 oligodendrogliomas have nuclear pleomorphism, mitotic activity, necrosis, and microvascular hyperplasia in various combinations. Oligodendrogliomas have a better prognosis than astrocytomas of the same grade.

**15. Correct choice: A.**

Deletions of 1p and 19q and mutations in *IDH1* and *IDH2* define glial tumors of oligodendroglial lineage and are associated with a better prognosis and better response to chemotherapy. Mutations in the genes encoding isocitrate dehydrogenase *IDH1* are particularly common in adult astrocytomas and oligodendrogliomas.

**16. Correct choice: D.**

Glioblastoma, IDH-wild type, WHO grade 4 is an aggressive, infiltrating, astrocytic glioma that lacks mutations in *IDH1* or *IDH2* genes and is histologically defined by brisk mitotic activity and microvascular proliferation or necrosis. It is molecularly defined by the presence of *TERT* promoter mutation, *EGFR* gene amplification, or copy number changes in the form of combined gain of chromosome 7 and loss of chromosome 10. Microvascular proliferation (visible in the right lower corner of the first picture) consists of hyperplasia of endothelial/perithelial cells in capillary vessels, often leading to glomeruloid formations.

**17. Correct choice: B.**

Ependymomas are derived from ependymal cells and thus develop in proximity to cerebral ventricles. Neoplastic cells tend to arrange themselves around small vessels as perivascular pseudorosettes or around a small lumen as ependymal rosettes. Ependymomas are grade 2/3 tumors according to the WHO classification. Although slowly growing and well demarcated, the tumor has a propensity to recur as a progressively more malignant, less differentiated glioma. Ependymomas are positive for S100, GFAP (glial fibrillary acidic protein), and vimentin and show a perinuclear dotlike pattern of EMA (epithelial membrane antigen).

**18. Correct choice: C.**

Myxopapillary ependymoma is a variant of ependymoma characterized by spindly ependymal cells arranged in a fascicular and papillary pattern within a myxoid intercellular matrix. It usually occurs in the distal segment of the spinal cord, that is, the conus medullaris. A definitive cure is usually achieved by total excision.

**19. Correct choice: E.**

Ganglioglioma is characterized by a dual cell composition: neoplastic glial cells (usually of astrocytic phenotype) admixed with neoplastic cells with a neuronal (ganglion-like) morphology. Dysplastic ganglion cells display atypical features and are usually grouped in disorganized clusters. The temporal lobe is the most common site, and seizures are the most frequent manifestation. Gangliogliomas (like pilocytic astrocytoma and pleomorphic xanthoastrocytoma) often present as a cyst with a mural nodule. Gangliocytoma is a very rare tumor composed exclusively of neoplastic ganglion cells. Dysembryoplastic neuroepithelial tumor is a mixed neuronal–glial lesion of hamartomatous nature that occurs in the temporal lobe and also manifests with seizures. Dysplastic gangliocytoma of the cerebellum (AKA Lhermitte-Duclos disease) is a true neoplasm consisting of granular cell neurons. Central neurocytoma is a tumor of neuronal lineage that develops within the ventricles, resembles oligodendroglioma by light microscopy, and expresses neuronal markers (eg, synaptophysin).

**20. Correct choice: C.**

Medulloblastoma is composed of uniform small cells with high nucleocytoplasmic ratios and molding nuclei. A helpful morphologic feature is the presence of Homer-Wright rosettes (there is one in the figure), consisting of a fibrillary core surrounded by tumor cells. Medulloblastoma is the most common central nervous system embryonal tumor of childhood and is second only to pilocytic astrocytoma for all intracranial neoplasms. There are four histologic groups: classic, desmoplastic/nodular, medulloblastoma with extensive nodularity, and large cell/anaplastic medulloblastoma. Classic medulloblastoma is characterized by a syncytial arrangement of densely packed undifferentiated cells (embryonal cells). Desmoplastic/nodular medulloblastoma is composed of densely packed, undifferentiated cells with hyperchromatic and pleomorphic nuclei that produce dense intercellular reticulin fiber networks with nodular reticulin-free zones. Medulloblastoma with extensive nodularity exhibits an expanded lobular architecture due to reticulin-free nodular zones becoming enlarged and rich in neuropil-like tissue. Large cell/anaplastic medulloblastoma features anaplasia with marked nuclear pleomorphism, high mitotic count, and high apoptotic count with nuclear molding. The desmoplastic and medulloblastoma with extensive nodularity variants have a better prognosis.

**21. Correct choice: A.**

Choroid plexus papilloma accounts for 0.5% of primary brain tumors. It grows within the ventricles. Most cases affect children, but they may occur in adults or older people. Choroid plexus tumors in children tend to occur in the lateral and third ventricles, while those in adults are more often located in the fourth ventricle. Histologically, choroid plexus papilloma resembles normal choroid plexus, but the cells are elongated instead of having the characteristic hobnail appearance of normal choroid plexus. Choroid plexus papilloma is WHO grade 1, atypical choroid plexus papilloma is grade 2, and choroid plexus carcinoma is grade 3.

**22. Correct choice: C.**

Hemangioblastoma is a benign neoplasm that develops most frequently in the posterior fossa but may occur in supratentorial and spinal regions. It is composed of foamy, vacuolated cells (the true neoplastic elements) amid a rich vascular network. Patients with von Hippel-Lindau syndrome frequently develop cerebellar and retinal hemangioblastomas as well as renal cell carcinoma. In these patients, it is important to differentiate hemangioblastomas from metastatic renal cell carcinoma, which exhibits similar morphologic features. Inhibin immunoreactivity is seen in hemangioblastomas but not in renal cell carcinomas.

**23. Correct choice: D.**

Meningioma is the most common benign primary intracranial tumor. It originates from the arachnoid cap cells and is attached to the dura. As it grows, it pushes the underlying brain, without infiltrating the parenchyma. Most sporadic meningiomas show monosomy of chromosome 22. Meningiomas exhibit a wide range of morphologic patterns, the most frequent being meningothelial (as in Figure 10.23), transitional, and fibrous. Diagnostic features include a syncytial appearance of tumor cells, whorl formation, intranuclear pseudoinclusions, and psammoma bodies. The most common variants are grade 1. Meningioma expresses epithelial membrane antigen (EMA) and progesterone receptors.

**24. Correct choice: E.**

The most common meningioma variants are WHO grade 1. Papillary and rhabdoid variants are grade 3.

**25. Correct choice: B.**

The most common meningioma variants are WHO grade 1. The chordoid and clear cell variants are grade 2.

**26. Correct choice: B.**

Fibroblastic meningioma (fibrous meningioma) is a predominantly spindle cell neoplasm with few or no meningothelial nests or whorls; it often has thick bundles of collagen. Schwannoma has a biphasic pattern and is positive for SOX10 and S100 protein. Solitary fibrous tumor is positive for STAT6. Fibrillary and pilocytic astrocytomas are negative for epithelial membrane antigen (EMA) and are typically not associated with thick bundles of collagen.

**27. Correct choice: E.**

Psammomatous meningioma is typically found in the spinal cord. It is characterized by numerous psammoma bodies with a paucity of intervening meningothelial cells.

**28. Correct choice: C.**

Chordoid meningioma is characterized by epithelioid cells or spindle cells (often partly vacuolated) that are arranged in cords within a pale basophilic myxoid matrix. Often there are interspersed areas of more typical meningioma, but pure chordoid cases may be seen. Chordoid morphology must be the predominant pattern for diagnosis of chordoid meningioma and WHO grade 2 designation. Chondrosarcoma may be meningeal, but it is positive for S100 protein and negative for epithelial membrane antigen (EMA). Chordoid glioma typically occurs in the third ventricle and is positive for glial fibrillary acidic protein (GFAP). Chordoma may arise in the clivus, although it is usually bone invasive; it is positive for brachyury, S100 protein, and cytokeratin, as well as EMA. Metastatic carcinoma may be meningeal, but are usually diffusely positive for cytokeratin, while chordoid meningiomas exhibit more limited cytokeratin expression.

**29. Correct choice: C.**

Chordoma arises from notochordal remnants distributed along the midline, from the base of the skull (clivus) to the sacrum.

The clivus and sacrum are the first and second most common sites, accounting for 85% of cases. Tumor cells are called physaliphorous and exhibit cytoplasm filled with large vacuoles. The constituent cells are arranged in chords and nests within a mucinous background. Positivity for epithelial markers (EMA [epithelial membrane antigen] and keratin) is typically coexistent with immunoreactivity for S100, which allows differentiation from chondrosarcoma, the main differential diagnostic consideration. Chondrosarcomas are immunoreactive for S100 but not for EMA or cytokeratin. Chordoma is bone destructive and usually recurs after surgical resection. Occasionally, it may give rise to lung, lymph node, or skin metastases. Brachyury is a specific immunohistochemical marker of chordomas and is useful in confirming the diagnosis and excluding the other differential diagnostic entities.

**30. Correct choice: E.**

Paraganglioma in the central nervous system is a low-grade, well-circumscribed neuroendocrine neoplasm of the cauda equina/filum terminale region. It exhibits the typical organoid (zellballen) architecture comprising nests or lobules of chief cells surrounded by sustentacular cells with intervening delicate capillary and reticulin networks. Ganglion cell metaplasia (gangliocytic neuroendocrine tumors) and Schwann cell (ganglioneuromatous) differentiation may be seen in up to 25% of cases. Meningioma is epithelial membrane antigen (EMA) positive. Chordoma is positive for EMA, S100 protein, cytokeratin, and brachyury. Myxopapillary ependymoma is positive for glial fibrillary acidic protein (GFAP), and hemangioblastoma is positive for inhibin.

**31. Correct choice: B.**

Angiomatous meningioma is a type of meningioma with a prominent vascular component (should exceed 50% of the total tumor area). The macrovascular variant can mimic a vascular malformation, whereas the microvascular variant can mimic hemangioblastoma.

**32. Correct choice: A.**

Arteriovenous malformation originates as an abnormal direct shunt between arteries and veins, which leads to arterialization of venous channels. Thus, the malformation comprises a mixture of arteries, veins, and vessels with intermediate features. Stains for elastin reveal irregular duplication or discontinuity of the elastic lamina. Arteriovenous malformations usually manifest with acute hemorrhage, sometimes with seizures and occasionally are discovered by chance. The risk of hemorrhage is up to 4.0% per year. Capillary telangiectasia is usually asymptomatic and found incidentally at autopsy. Venous malformation refers to abnormal dilatation of a vein, the most common example of which is the great vein of Galen malformation.

**33. Correct choice: E.**

CADASIL (cerebral autosomal dominant angiopathy with subcortical infarcts and leukoencephalopathy) presents with migraine headaches and recurrent subcortical leading to progressive neurologic impairment and dementia. The condition is caused by autosomal dominant mutations of the *Notch3* gene (chromosome 19). The diagnosis can be made by genetic testing on DNA from white blood cells. Skin biopsies are also used for diagnosis. By light microscopy, small arteries and arterioles show thickening of the media secondary to accumulation of basophilic, granular material. Immunohistochemistry for Notch3 protein is a highly sensitive and specific diagnostic tool. Congo red–positive material in the media is characteristic of amyloid angiopathy. Hyalinization and thickening of media are found in arteriolosclerosis due to hypertension.

**34. Correct choice: A.**

Colloid cyst is a benign, unilocular, epithelium-lined cyst that contains mucinous or protein-rich fluid and is typically located in the midline of the third ventricle. It probably develops from endodermal remnants, accounting for its respiratory-type epithelium. This lesion is usually asymptomatic, but patients may present with headaches.

**35. Correct choice: C.**

Gross or radiologic presentation of a cyst with a mural nodule is characteristic of at least four tumors, all of which are WHO grade 2-3: pilocytic astrocytoma, hemangioblastoma, ganglioglioma, and pleomorphic xanthoastrocytoma. The mural nodule is contrast enhancing in all of these tumors. Metastases may also be partially cystic. Craniopharyngioma often contains multiple cysts. Epidermoid tumor is usually composed of a unilocular cyst with uniform thin walls and keratin-filled lumen. Medulloblastoma and pineoblastoma have a solid pattern. Oligodendroglioma and low-grade astrocytomas are intraparenchymal tumors with diffuse, mostly solid growth. Glioblastoma characteristically shows a variegated gross appearance with areas of hemorrhage and necrosis.

**36. Correct choice: C.**

The two most common germ cell tumors in the central nervous system (CNS) are germinomas and teratomas. A great majority of germ cell tumors develop in the sellar/suprasellar region: most of them are germinomas and teratomas. Germinomas develop in the pineal or sellar region, sometimes in both at the same time. Mature teratoma is the most common type of sacrococcygeal germ cell tumor. Up to 90% of them occur in females. If present at birth, they are most often benign; if the tumor becomes clinically apparent after 2 months of age, it is usually malignant. The most common malignant sacrococcygeal germ cell tumor is the yolk sac tumor.

**37. Correct choice: A.**

The great majority of primary central nervous system (CNS) lymphomas are diffuse large B-cell lymphomas (DLBCL). DLBCL affects immunocompetent people in their 50s to 60s and patients who are immunocompromised (usually AIDS). In immunocompetent patients, the location is periventricular, and there is no association with Epstein-Barr virus (EBV). In patients who are immunocompromised, DLBCL is usually associated with EBV infection and presents as a ring-enhancing mass on magnetic resonance imaging (MRI). All other types of lymphoma are rare. Hodgkin lymphoma may spread to the intracranial cavity, where it seeds the dura. Lymphomatoid granulomatosis (LG) is an EBV-induced lymphoproliferative disorder characterized by angiocentric and angiodestructive inflammation. Primary and secondary T-cell lymphoma is rare in the CNS.

**38. Correct choice: A.**

Dysplastic gangliocytoma of the cerebellum is a hamartomatous cerebellar lesion characterized by enlarged cerebellar folia and replacement of the internal granular layer by dysplastic ganglion cells. The treatment is surgical resection. It has a favorable prognosis although recurrences may be seen in up to 25% of cases. It is associated with Cowden disease, an autosomal dominant disorder with trichilemmomas, hamartomas, intestinal polyposis, palmoplantar keratoses, and oral papillomas. Patients have an increased incidence of breast, genitourinary, central nervous system (CNS), and thyroid tumors due to a germline mutation in *PTEN.*

**39. Correct choice: A.**

Cerebral amyloid angiopathy (CAA) is a common cause of intracerebral hemorrhage in older patients, with or without associated Alzheimer dementia (AD). Since CAA involves cortical and leptomeningeal vessels, hemorrhage is cortical based and thus defined as "*lobar.*" It is due to the accumulation of *amyloid-β* (the same amyloid found in senile plaques of AD) within the vascular walls. Congo red staining and/or immunohistochemistry for amyloid-β confirms the diagnosis. The causes of intracerebral bleeding in decreasing order of frequency are:

1. Hypertension
2. CAA
3. Anticoagulants
4. Tumors
5. Drugs, licit and illicit
6. Vascular malformations: arteriovenous malformation (AVM) and berry aneurysm
7. Others: septic emboli, trauma, and hematologic disorders

**40. Correct choice: A.**

Central neurocytoma is a rare, well-differentiated, intraventricular neoplasm with neuroepithelial differentiation, typically arising near the foramen of Monro, and usually involving the lateral or third ventricle(s). It is characterized by sheets of uniform, small to medium, round cells with fine chromatin stippling (salt and pepper) and occasional perinuclear clearing, interspersed with patches of fibrillary matrix. Perinuclear clearing may be prominent, similar to oligodendrogliomas. Central neurocytoma is positive for synaptophysin and Neu-N, but typically negative for glial fibrillary acidic protein (GFAP). It is classified as a WHO grade 2 tumor. Oligodendroglioma is more infiltrative and harbors an *IDH1/2* mutation and chromosome 1p/19q codeletion. Ependymoma is strongly positive for GFAP. Ganglioneuroma is characterized by mixed neuronal (ganglion cells) and glial neoplastic components. Pineocytoma arises in the pineal region.

**41. Correct choice: E.**

Pineoblastoma is characterized by sheets of densely packed cells with high-grade (anaplastic/undifferentiated) features including a high N/C (nuclear-to-cytoplasmic) ratio with minimal cytoplasm and large hyperchromatic nuclei. It is the second most common pineal gland tumor after germ cell tumor. It often exhibits focal nuclear molding and Homer-Wright or Flexner-Wintersteiner rosettes. It is an aggressive tumor (WHO grade 4) with a 5% 5-year survival rate.

# 11 Neuroendocrine and Paracrine Systems

1. Which of the following are most likely to be seen in multiple endocrine neoplasia type 1 (MEN1)?
   A. Angiomyolipoma, lymphangioleiomyomatosis, pancreatic neuroendocrine tumor
   B. Hemangioblastoma, pancreatic neuroendocrine tumor, pheochromocytoma
   C. Hyperparathyroidism, medullary carcinoma of the thyroid, paroxysmal hypertension
   D. Hyperparathyroidism, pituitary adenoma, pancreatic neuroendocrine tumor
   E. Medullary carcinoma of the thyroid, mucosal neuromas, paroxysmal hypertension

2. Which of the following are most likely to be seen in multiple endocrine neoplasia type 2A (MEN2A)?
   A. Angiomyolipoma, lymphangioleiomyomatosis, pancreatic neuroendocrine tumor
   B. Hemangioblastoma, pancreatic neuroendocrine tumor, pheochromocytoma
   C. Hyperparathyroidism, medullary carcinoma of the thyroid, pheochromocytoma
   D. Hyperparathyroidism, prolactin-secreting pituitary adenoma, Zollinger-Ellison syndrome
   E. Medullary carcinoma of the thyroid, mucosal neuromas, paroxysmal hypertension

3. Which of the following are most likely to be seen in multiple endocrine neoplasia type 2B (MEN2B)?
   A. Angiomyolipoma, lymphangioleiomyomatosis, pancreatic neuroendocrine tumor
   B. Hemangioblastoma, pancreatic neuroendocrine tumor, pheochromocytoma
   C. Hyperparathyroidism, medullary carcinoma of the thyroid, paroxysmal hypertension
   D. Hyperparathyroidism, prolactin-secreting pituitary adenoma, Zollinger-Ellison syndrome
   E. Medullary carcinoma of the thyroid, mucosal neuromas, paroxysmal hypertension

4. Which of the following are most likely to be seen in Von Hippel-Lindau disease?
   A. Angiomyolipoma, lymphangioleiomyomatosis, pancreatic neuroendocrine tumor
   B. Hemangioblastoma, pancreatic neuroendocrine tumor, pheochromocytoma
   C. Hyperparathyroidism, medullary carcinoma of the thyroid, paroxysmal hypertension
   D. Hyperparathyroidism, prolactin-secreting pituitary adenoma, Zollinger-Ellison syndrome
   E. Medullary carcinoma of the thyroid, mucosal neuromas, paroxysmal hypertension

5. Which of the following are most likely to be seen in tuberous sclerosis complex?
   A. Angiomyolipoma, lymphangioleiomyomatosis, retinal hamartoma
   B. Hemangioblastoma, pancreatic neuroendocrine tumor, pheochromocytoma
   C. Hyperparathyroidism, medullary carcinoma of the thyroid, paroxysmal hypertension
   D. Hyperparathyroidism, prolactin-secreting pituitary adenoma, Zollinger-Ellison syndrome
   E. Medullary carcinoma of the thyroid, mucosal neuromas, paroxysmal hypertension

6. Which of the following are most likely to be seen in neurofibromatosis type 1?
   A. Acoustic neuromas, café au lait spots, plexiform neurofibroma
   B. Acoustic neuromas, optic glioma, pheochromocytoma
   C. Café au lait spots, Lisch nodules, pheochromocytoma
   D. Café au lait spots, plexiform neurofibroma, optic glioma
   E. Café au lait spots, plexiform neurofibroma, pheochromocytoma

All figures in this chapter are from Longacre TA, Greenson JK, Hornick JL, Reuter VE, eds. *Mills and Sternberg's Diagnostic Surgical Pathology*. 7th ed. Wolters Kluwer; 2022 except for those noted at the end of this book.

7. In which two anatomic sites can paragangliomas be mistaken for epithelial neuroendocrine tumors?

   A. Bladder and duodenum
   B. Bladder and lung
   C. Bladder and pancreas
   D. Duodenum and lung
   E. Duodenum and pancreas

8. What percent of paragangliomas is associated with a hereditary syndrome?

   A. 10% to 20%
   B. 20% to 30%
   C. 30% to 40%
   D. 40% to 50%
   E. 50% to 60%

9. Which site is most common for gangliocytic paraganglioma?

   A. Ampulla/duodenum
   B. Large intestine
   C. Retroperitoneum
   D. Salivary gland
   E. Urinary bladder

10. What is the most likely diagnosis for the small blue cell tumor with loss of RB1 and SSTR2, shown in Figure 1?

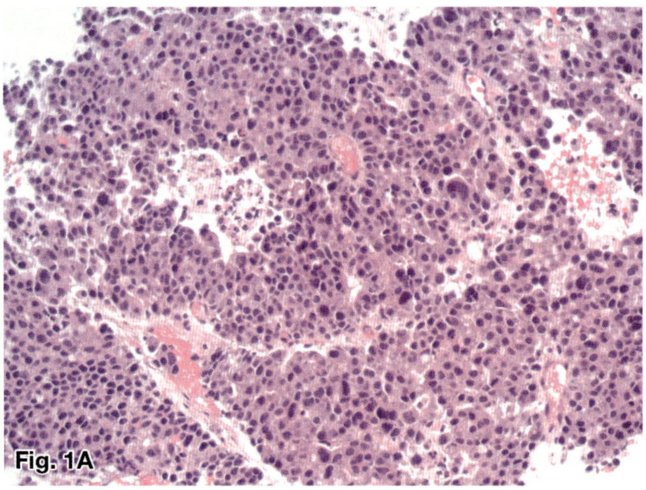

Fig. 1A

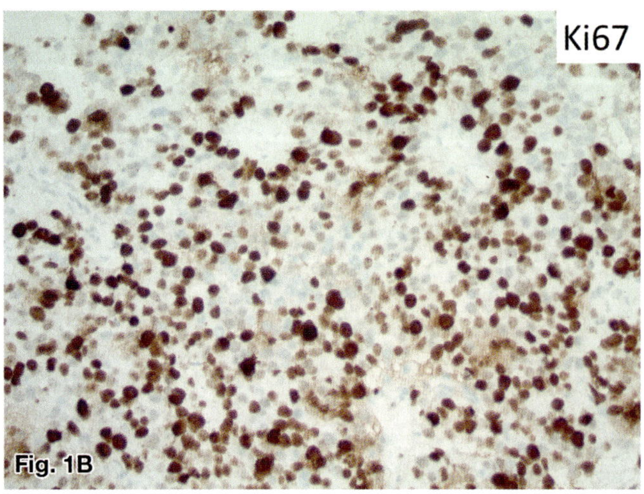


Fig. 1B

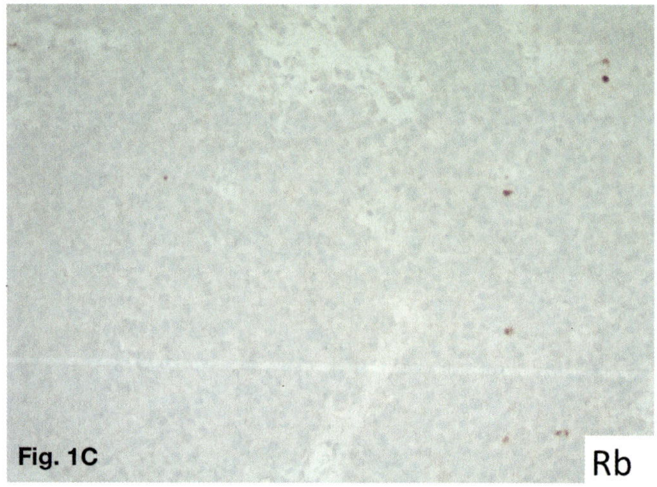


Fig. 1C

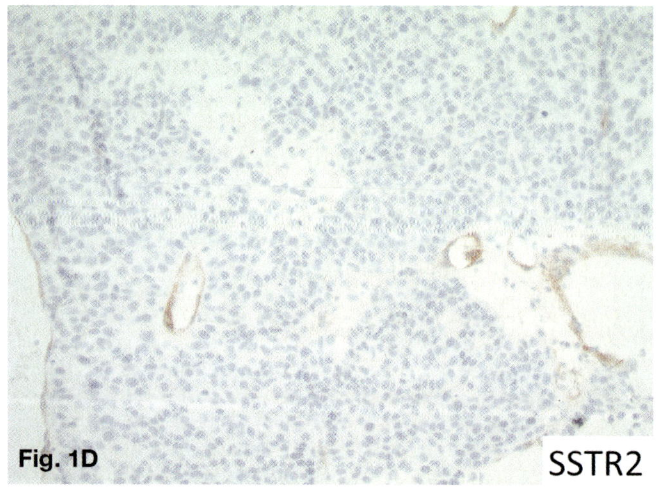


Fig. 1D

   A. Embryonal rhabdomyosarcoma
   B. Extraskeletal Ewing sarcoma
   C. Neuroendocrine carcinoma
   D. Nuclear protein in testis carcinoma
   E. Sinonasal undifferentiated carcinoma

# ANSWERS AND EXPLANATIONS

**1. Correct choice: D.**

Multiple endocrine neoplasia type 1 (MEN1) is a syndrome characterized by mutations in the *MEN1* gene on chromosome 11q13 and development of multiple endocrine tumors (and other tumor types). It exhibits an autosomal dominant inheritance pattern and the classic constellation of pituitary, parathyroid, and pancreatic tumors (the three Ps). The pancreatic tumors are often multifocal and associated with nesidiodysplasia and nesidioblastosis. A variety of nonendocrine tumors are also part of *MEN1* (meningioma, ependymoma, angiofibroma). The penetrance is 100%, with all patients developing parathyroid adenomas by age 50. Patients with gastrinomas, typically found in the duodenum, may have Zollinger-Ellison syndrome.

**2. Correct choice: C.**

Multiple endocrine neoplasia type 2A (MEN2A) is an autosomal dominate syndrome associated with mutations in the *RET* oncogene on chromosome 10 and characterized by medullary carcinoma of the thyroid, pheochromocytoma, and parathyroid hyperplasia or adenomas. Almost all patients have medullary thyroid carcinoma, which is frequently multicentric and begins with thyroid parafollicular C-cell hyperplasia. The pheochromocytomas usually produce epinephrine disproportionately to norepinephrine, in contrast to sporadic cases, and hypertensive crisis secondary to pheochromocytoma is a common manifestation. Hypertension in patients with MEN2A with pheochromocytoma is more often paroxysmal than sustained, in contrast to the usual sporadic case. Up to 20% of patients have evidence of hyperparathyroidism (which may be long standing), with hypercalcemia, nephrolithiasis, nephrocalcinosis, or renal failure. Hyperparathyroidism frequently involves multiple glands as either diffuse hyperplasia or multiple adenomas. Variants of MEN2A include MEN2A with cutaneous lichen amyloidosis, MEN2A with Hirschsprung disease, and familial medullary carcinoma.

**3. Correct choice: E.**

Multiple endocrine neoplasia type 2B (MEN2B) is an autosomal dominant disorder associated with mutations in the *RET* oncogene characterized by medullary thyroid carcinoma, pheochromocytoma, multiple facial neuromas, and a "marfanoid" habitus. Hypertension in patients with MEN2B with pheochromocytoma is more often paroxysmal than sustained, in contrast to the usual sporadic case.

**4. Correct choice: B.**

Von Hippel-Lindau syndrome is an autosomal dominant hereditary condition associated with tumors arising in multiple organs. These include hemangioblastomas, which are blood vessel tumors of the brain, spinal cord, and retina. The retinal tumors are also called retinal angiomas, which can lead to blindness if not treated in a timely manner. Other characteristic tumors are pancreatic neuroendocrine tumor and pheochromocytoma as well as clear cell renal cell carcinoma. The pancreatic tumors are often multifocal and associated with nesidiodysplasia and nesidioblastosis. Other features include renal cysts, pancreatic cysts, epididymal cystadenomas, broad ligament cystadenomas, and endolymphatic sac tumors, which are tumors of the inner ear that may cause hearing loss.

**5. Correct choice: A.**

Tuberous sclerosis complex is an autosomal dominant genetic disorder characterized by an increased predisposition to hamartoma formation affecting multiple systems. It results from mutations in the genes *TSC1* and *TSC2*. The hamartomatous lesions include angiomyolipoma, lymphangioleiomyomas, retinal hamartomas, and cardiac rhabdomyomas, as well as skin and nail lesions. Tumors of the brain often cause seizures or developmental delays. Pulmonary cysts and lymphangioleiomyomatosis can affect the lungs and are the most common cause of fatality for patients who exhibit evidence of lymphangioleiomyomatosis.

**6. Correct choice: D.**

Neurofibromatosis type 1 is an autosomal dominant hereditary multisystem disorder characterized by multiple café au lait macules, intertriginous freckling, multiple cutaneous neurofibromas, and learning disability or behavior problems. About 50% have plexiform neurofibromas, but most are internal and not suspected clinically. Plexiform neurofibromas can cause pain, neurologic deficits, and abnormalities of involved or adjacent structures. Less common but potentially more serious manifestations include optic nerve gliomas, other central nervous system gliomas, and malignant peripheral nerve sheath tumors. Approximately 50% of affected individuals have neurofibromatosis type 1 as the result of a de novo *NF1* disease-causing variant.

**7. Correct choice: D.**

The duodenum and lung are two sites, where paragangliomas are likely to be misdiagnosed as epithelial neuroendocrine tumors. It is important to distinguish these two tumors due to their different circulating biomarkers and their associated genetic syndromes.

**8. Correct choice: C.**

About 30% to 40% of paragangliomas may be hereditary and patients who present with a paraganglioma should be evaluated for a possible hereditary syndrome.

**9. Correct choice: A.**

Gangliocytic paraganglioma is a rare triphasic neoplasm that arises in the second part of the duodenum and ampullary region. It is usually benign but may rarely (<10%) metastasize. The triphasic histology consists of epithelioid, spindle, ganglion-type cells. It is seen in a wide age range (15-84 years). It may resemble a well-differentiated neuroendocrine tumor, paraganglioma, or ganglioneuroma. The epithelioid cells are positive for chromogranin, synaptophysin, progesterone receptor, and somatostatin. The ganglion cells are positive for S100 protein, chromogranin, synaptophysin, and somatostatin, while the spindle cells are positive for S100 protein and BCL2 (B-cell lymphoma 2). Similar tumors may rarely be seen outside the ampulla/duodenum.

**10. Correct choice: C.**

Loss of RB1 and/or SSTR2 in conjunction with expression of neuroendocrine markers (chromogranin, synaptophysin, and INSM1, among others) can be helpful in establishing a diagnosis of neuroendocrine carcinoma. Embryonal rhabdomyosarcoma expresses myogenin and MyoD1, but not neuroendocrine markers. Extraskeletal Ewing sarcoma may express synaptophysin and other neuroendocrine markers, but is positive for CD99 and NKX2.2. Nuclear protein in testis (NUT) carcinoma is usually negative for neuroendocrine markers and is positive for NUTM1. Sinonasal undifferentiated carcinomas do not express neuroendocrine markers.

# 12 Pituitary and Sellar Region

1. A reticulin-stained section of a 0.8-cm pituitary tumor removed by transsphenoidal resection is shown in Figure 1. If functioning, which of the following is the most common clinical presentation of this tumor?

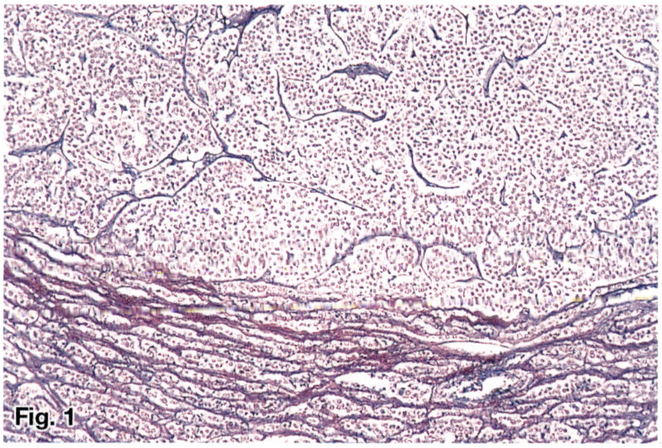

Fig. 1

   A. Acromegaly/gigantism
   B. Cushing syndrome
   C. Hyperprolactinemia
   D. Panhypopituitarism
   E. Visual field deficits

2. A 23-year-old female undergoes transsphenoidal resection of a prolactinoma after receiving prolonged treatment with bromocriptine. Which of the following are morphologic effects of bromocriptine on the pituitary tumor?

   A. Apoplexy
   B. Chronic inflammation
   C. Increase in cellular atypia
   D. Necrosis of pituitary parenchyma
   E. Shrinkage and fibrosis

3. An intracranial tumor characteristic of childhood is shown in Figure 1. This tumor is most likely to arise in which of the following regions?

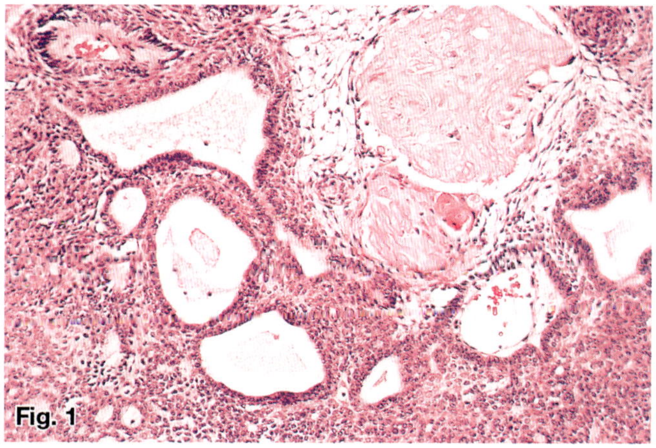

Fig. 1

   A. Cribriform lamina of ethmoid
   B. Petrous portion of temporal bone
   C. Posterior fossa
   D. Suprasellar region
   E. Temporal lobe

All figures in this chapter are from Longacre TA, Greenson JK, Hornick JL, Reuter VE, eds. *Mills and Sternberg's Diagnostic Surgical Pathology.* 7th ed. Wolters Kluwer; 2022 except for those noted at the end of this book.

4. A 9-year-old girl is diagnosed with central diabetes insipidus. A magnetic resonance imaging (MRI) of the head reveals a nodular lesion in the suprasellar region. Biopsy reveals the changes shown in Figure 1. The abnormal cells in the epithelioid clusters are immunoreactive for CD1a and S100. Which of the following is the most likely diagnosis?

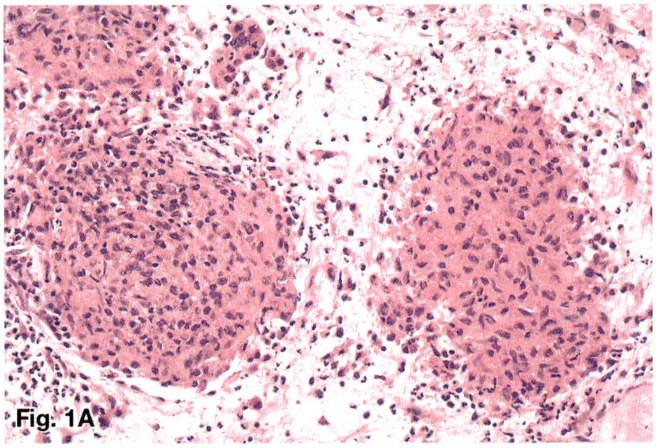

Fig. 1A

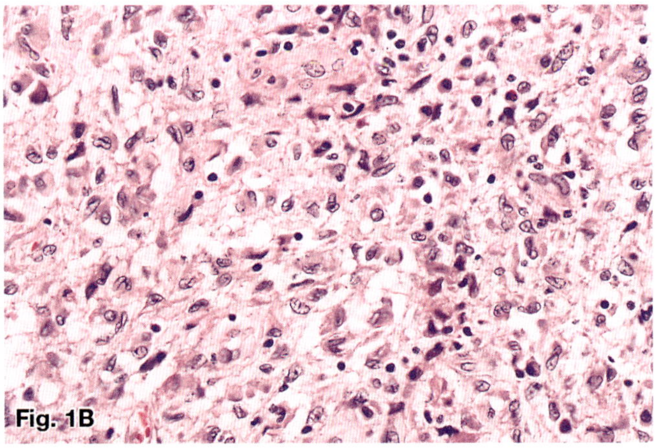

Fig. 1B

A. Granular cell tumor
B. Langerhans cell histiocytosis
C. Lymphocytic hypophysitis
D. Mycobacterial infection
E. Sarcoidosis

5. Three months after an uncomplicated delivery, a 35-year-old woman presents with signs and symptoms of pituitary insufficiency. Magnetic resonance imaging (MRI) reveals a pituitary mass, which is biopsied. The biopsy findings are shown in this photomicrograph. Which of the following is the most likely diagnosis?

A. Granulomatous hypophysitis
B. Ischemic necrosis (Sheehan syndrome)
C. Lymphocytic hypophysitis
D. Pituicytoma
E. Pituitary adenoma

6. Which of the following factors accounts for the primary form of empty sella syndrome?

A. Compression by herniated arachnoid
B. Irradiation to sellar tumors
C. Pituitary apoplexy
D. Postpartum pituitary necrosis
E. Surgical intervention

7. What is the most common cause of Cushing syndrome?

A. Adrenal adenoma
B. Adrenal carcinoma
C. Glucocorticoid use
D. Lung carcinoma
E. Pituitary adenoma

8. A 34-year-old man with enlarged hands and feet as well as enlarged facial features presents with hypertension. What type of pituitary adenoma is most likely present?

A. Corticotroph
B. Gonadotroph
C. Lactotroph
D. Null
E. Somatotroph

9. What is the most likely clinical presentation for this type of pituitary adenoma?

A. Acromegaly
B. Amenorrhea
C. Hypercortisolism
D. Hypogonadism
E. Hypothyroidism

10. What is the most likely diagnosis for the patchy glial fibrillary acidic protein (GFAP)-positive sellar biopsy, shown in Figure 1, in a 55-year-old woman with headaches and visual disturbance?

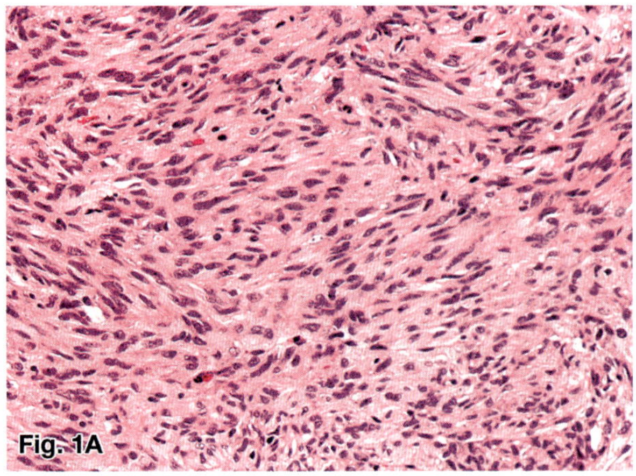

Fig. 1A

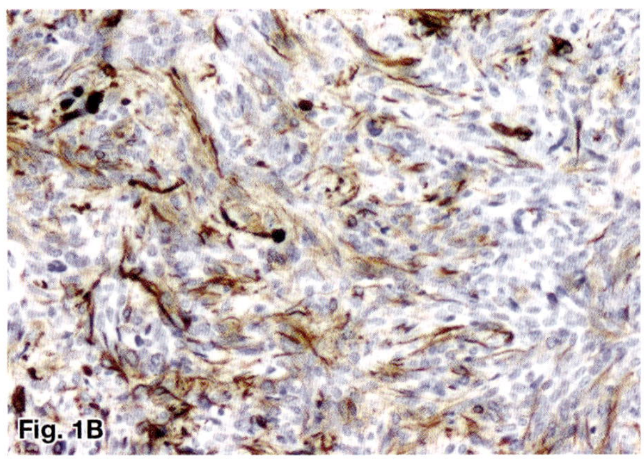

Fig. 1B

A. Meningioma
B. Normal neurohypophysis
C. Pilocytic astrocytoma
D. Pituicytoma
E. Sellar schwannoma

# ANSWERS AND EXPLANATIONS

**1. Correct choice: C.**

Pituitary adenomas exhibit loss of the reticulin network of the normal adenohypophysis, as depicted in the figure, which also demonstrates a peripheral rim of compressed pituitary gland with intact reticulin. A pituitary adenoma may have sheet-like, papillary, and trabecular patterns. Pituitary adenomas account for approximately 10% of intracranial neoplasms. Microadenomas measure less than 1 cm, and macroadenomas measure more than 1 cm. Functioning adenomas are usually microadenomas and become clinically apparent with an endocrine syndrome related to the specific hormone produced. In contrast, macroadenomas are usually hormonally inactive and manifest by compression of nearby structures, most commonly the optic chiasm, causing bitemporal hemianopsia ("tunnel vision"). Prolactinomas are the most frequent of functioning adenomas. Hyperprolactinemia manifests with amenorrhea-galactorrhea syndrome in women, with subtle and easily overlooked symptoms in men.

**2. Correct choice: E.**

Almost 50% of all functioning pituitary adenomas secrete prolactin (growth hormone [GH] and adrenocorticotropic hormone [ACTH] follow in order of frequency). Prolactinomas can be treated with dopamine agonists such as bromocriptine, which inhibits prolactin secretion. Bromocriptine results in gradual shrinkage of the tumor with diffuse interstitial fibrosis, without evidence of tumor necrosis or degeneration.

Because bromocriptine is not tumoricidal, the treatment is not curative. Bromocriptine has serious side effects and has been replaced by *cabergoline*, a well-tolerated selective D2 agonist with a long half-life. Apoplexy refers to hemorrhage within a pituitary adenoma or hypertrophic pituitary (eg, in pregnancy), which results in the rapid expansion of the pituitary gland.

**3. Correct choice: D.**

Craniopharyngioma is a histologically benign tumor that is thought to arise from misplaced odontogenic epithelium and is morphologically similar to adamantinoma (ameloblastoma). It develops in the suprasellar region and often contains cystic spaces and abundant calcium deposits. Children are most often affected. Histologically, it contains tongues of well-differentiated epithelium with peripheral palisading and central stellate reticulum, multifocal deposits of wet keratin (ie, with ghost keratinized cells), and abundant calcifications. A papillary variant of craniopharyngioma tends to develop in adults and middle-aged persons. Craniopharyngiomas do not metastasize but recur frequently after surgery.

**4. Correct choice: B.**

The pituitary/hypothalamic region is the most frequent site of central nervous system involvement by Langerhans cell histiocytosis, and diabetes insipidus is the most common clinical presentation. Langerhans cells form granuloma-like collections and express S100, CD1a, and langerin (not CD68 as macrophages). Granular cell tumors are usually clinically silent and located in the pituitary stalk; they are composed of polygonal cells with round, peripheral nuclei and granular cytoplasm. Cerebral tuberculosis and sarcoidosis tend to affect the basal surface of the brain, producing caseating granulomas and non-necrotizing granulomas, respectively.

**5. Correct choice: C.**

Lymphocytic hypophysitis is a complication of pregnancy that usually manifests in the postpartum period with pituitary hypofunction. Neuroimaging may suggest a pituitary adenoma.

Histologically, it is characterized by florid lymphocytic and plasmacytic infiltration, sometimes with germinal center formation, but without necrosis or granulomas. The lymphocytic population is mixed and polyclonal. Postpartum pituitary insufficiency may be caused by Sheehan syndrome, which is an ischemic infarction of the pituitary gland due to prolonged hypotension during delivery. Pituicytomas are rare benign glial tumors arising from pituicytes (the specialized glial cells of the neurohypophysis). Granulomatous hypophysitis is a very rare condition that affects the anterior pituitary in adult men or women (no association with pregnancy); it is distinct from sarcoidosis, which preferentially involves the neurohypophysis and hypothalamus.

**6. Correct choice: A.**

The primary form of empty sella syndrome is due to an arachnoidal diverticulum that herniates through a defect of the sellar diaphragm and exerts compression on the pituitary gland. About 50% of adults have an incompetent sellar diaphragm, and 5% have an empty sella. Irradiation to sellar tumors, pituitary apoplexy, postpartum pituitary necrosis, and surgical intervention are the most common causes of the secondary form. Clinical manifestations include visual deficits due to chiasmal prolapse and impaired endocrine function secondary to traction on the pituitary stalk.

**7. Correct choice: C.**

Long-term, high-dose use of glucocorticoids is the most common cause of Cushing syndrome. The most common cause of Cushing disease is excess secretion of adrenocorticotropin hormone (ACTH) by a pituitary adenoma. The remainder of the endogenous cases are caused by ectopic ACTH-secreting tumors and primary adrenal neoplasms.

**8. Correct choice: E.**

Acromegaly is most commonly caused by a somatotroph pituitary adenoma that secretes growth hormone (GH). Acromegaly can develop at any age after puberty, but it is most often diagnosed during the fourth and fifth decades of life (middle age). In adults, excess GH causes bones, cartilage, and other tissues to increase in size. Characteristic changes include larger hands, feet, ears, lips, and nose. The jaw and forehead are more prominent. High levels of GH can result in increased insulin-like growth factor, which may lead to type 2 diabetes, hypertension, and heart disease.

**9. Correct choice: C.**

Crooke hyaline change is characterized by large chromophobic or eosinophilic cells with a glassy hyaline appearance (due to accumulation of keratin filaments); it can be seen in neoplastic and nonneoplastic corticotrophs.

**10. Correct choice: D.**

Pituicytomas are tumors that arise from the pituicytes of the neurohypophysis and pituitary infundibulum. In addition to the classic pituicytoma, oncocytic, granular, and ependymal variants may be seen. Pituicytoma belongs to the group of thyroid transcription factor 1 (TTF1)-expressing tumors of the neurohypophysis and infundibulum. Characteristic features include fascicles of spindle cells or epithelioid cells expressing TTF1, S100 protein, and glial fibrillary acidic protein (GFAP). Surgical resection is curative. Meningioma is characterized by whorls, psammoma bodies, nuclear inclusions, and collagen deposition. It is epithelial membrane antigen (EMA) positive but negative for TTF1, but the fibrous variant may be positive for S100 protein. Normal neurohypophysis and infundibulum contain axons and Herring bodies and is positive for vasopressin. Pilocytic astrocytoma has Rosenthal fibers and granular bodies. Sellar schwannoma is TTF1 negative.

# 13 Pathology of Thyroid and Parathyroid

1. Which of the following lymph nodes should the finding of thyroid tissue be considered bona fide evidence of metastatic papillary carcinoma?

   A. Lateral jugular
   B. Paratracheal
   C. Prelaryngeal
   D. Pretracheal
   E. Thyroid

2. Which of the following forms of thyroiditis is thought to be caused by a viral infection?

   A. Graves disease
   B. Hashimoto thyroiditis
   C. Lymphocytic thyroiditis
   D. Riedel thyroiditis
   E. Subacute (granulomatous) thyroiditis

3. A thyroid specimen reveals the histopathologic changes shown in Figures 1 and 2. Which of the following is the most likely diagnosis?

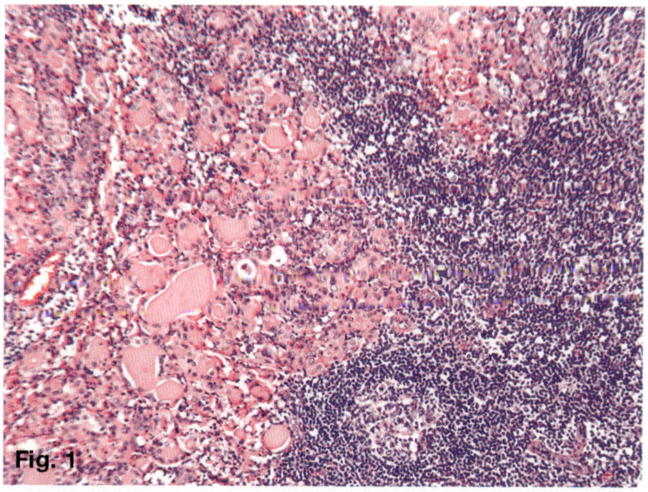
Fig. 1

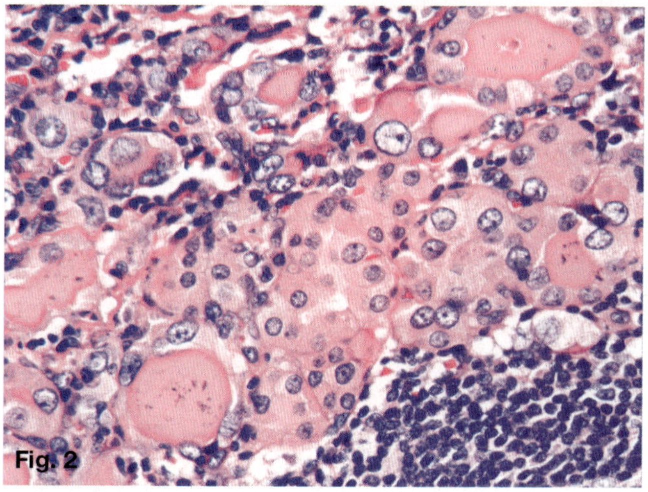
Fig. 2

   A. de Quervain (subacute) thyroiditis
   B. Hashimoto thyroiditis
   C. Papillary carcinoma
   D. Riedel thyroiditis
   E. Subacute lymphocytic (painless) thyroiditis

All figures in this chapter are from Longacre TA, Greenson JK, Hornick JL, Reuter VE, eds. *Mills and Sternberg's Diagnostic Surgical Pathology*. 7th ed. Wolters Kluwer; 2022 except for those noted at the end of this book.

4. A patient with Graves disease receives antithyroid drugs and propranolol before subtotal thyroidectomy. Which of the following histopathologic aspects will regress with treatment?

   A. Follicular hyperplasia
   B. Glandular enlargement
   C. Lymphocytic infiltration
   D. Presence of Hürthle cells
   E. Presence of lymphoid follicles

5. Riedel thyroiditis is considered to be similar to which of the following disorders?

   A. Amyloidosis
   B. de Quervain thyroiditis
   C. Hashimoto thyroiditis
   D. Progressive systemic sclerosis
   E. Retroperitoneal fibrosis

6. Figure 1 shows the external surface and cut surface of a very enlarged thyroid that was surgically removed. Histologic examination reveals nodules consisting of colloid-filled follicles of varying size. The nodules are separated by scar tissue containing hemosiderin-laden macrophages. Which of the following is the most likely diagnosis?

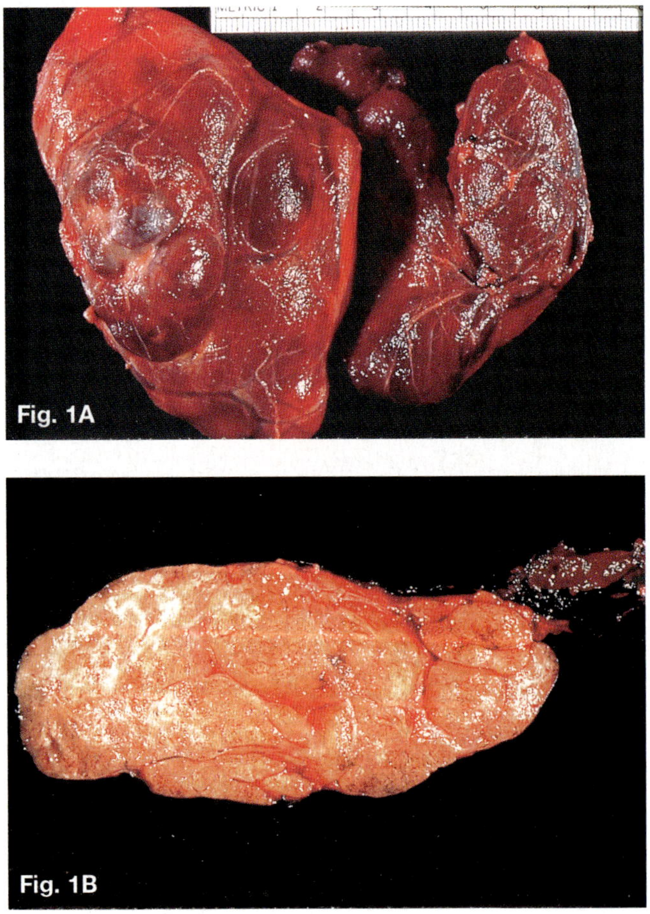


   A. Diffuse simple goiter
   B. Multinodular goiter
   C. Subacute thyroiditis
   D. Thyroid adenoma
   E. Thyroid cyst

7. A thyroid nodule is excised and demonstrates the histology shown in Figure 1. Which of the following is the most common gene mutation in this lesion?

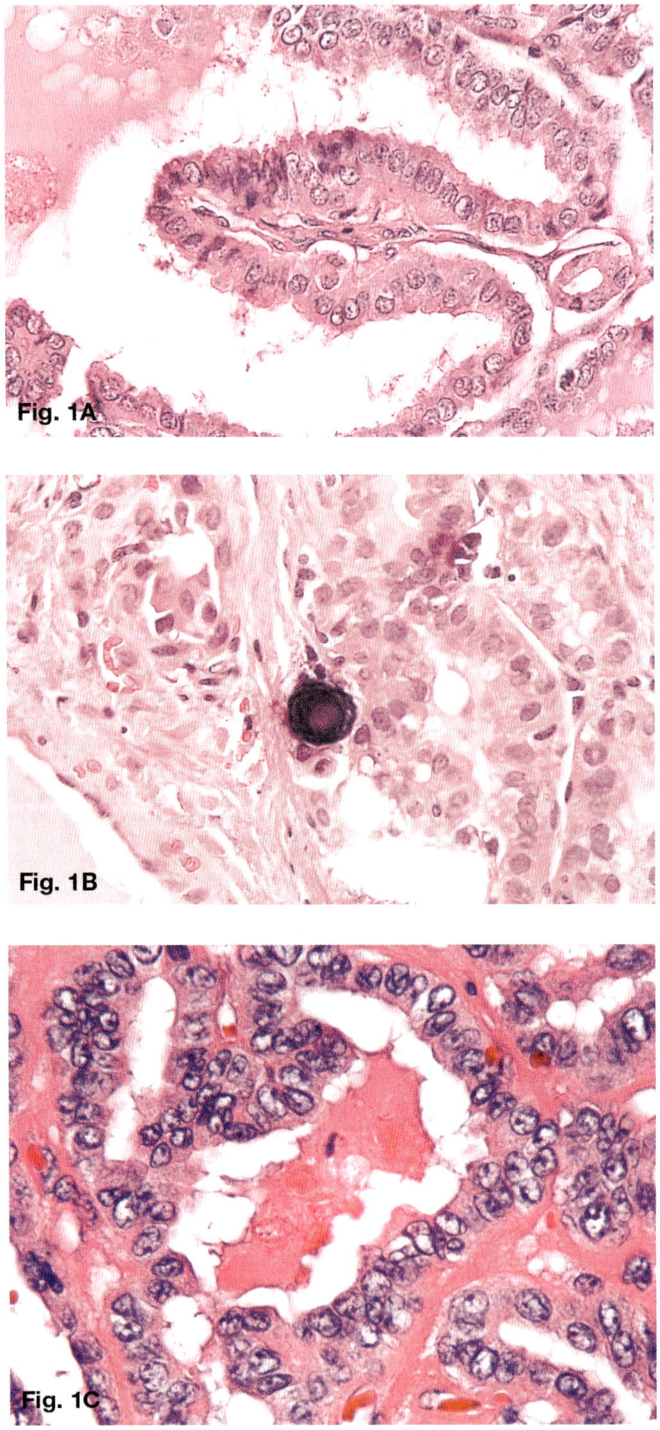


   A. *BRAF*
   B. *HRAS*
   C. *KRAS*
   D. *NRAS*
   E. *RET*

8. Which variant of papillary thyroid carcinoma is shown in Figure 1?

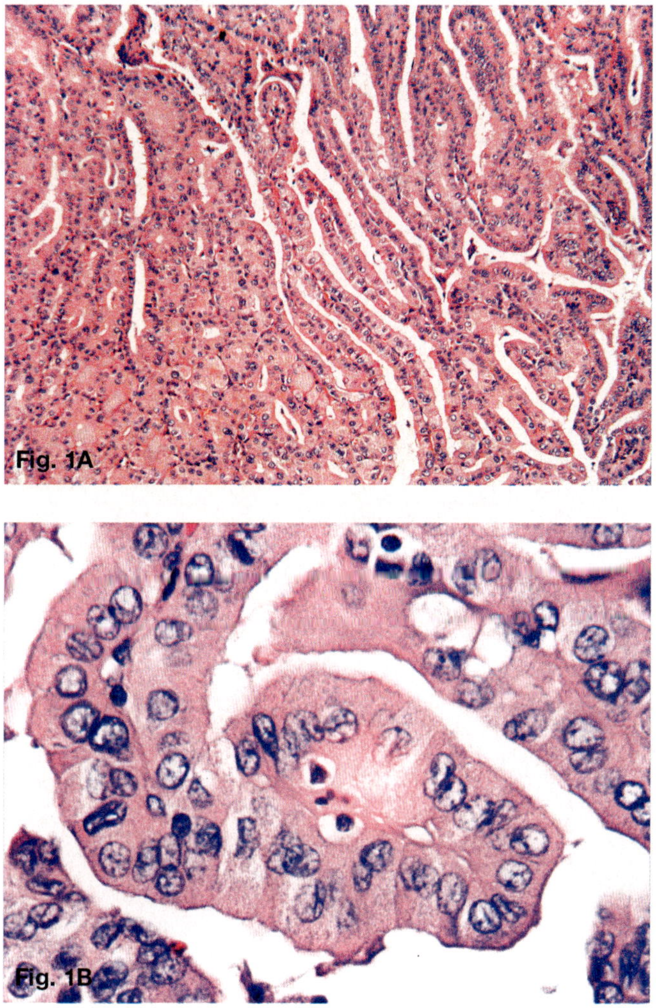

Fig. 1A

Fig. 1B

A. Diffuse sclerosing
B. Follicular
C. Microcarcinoma
D. Tall cell
E. Warthin-like

9. A thyroid tumor removed from a 7-year-old male is depicted in Figure 1. Which variant of papillary thyroid carcinoma is this?

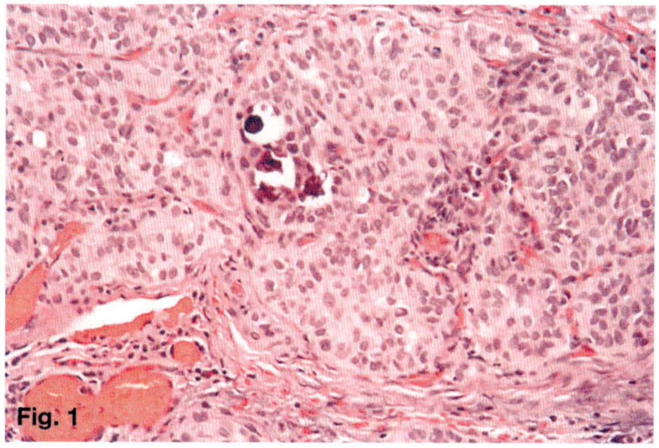

Fig. 1

A. Columnar cell
B. Diffuse sclerosing
C. Follicular
D. Oxyphilic
E. Solid/trabecular

10. Figure 1 shows an invasive thyroid tumor. Which of the following is true?

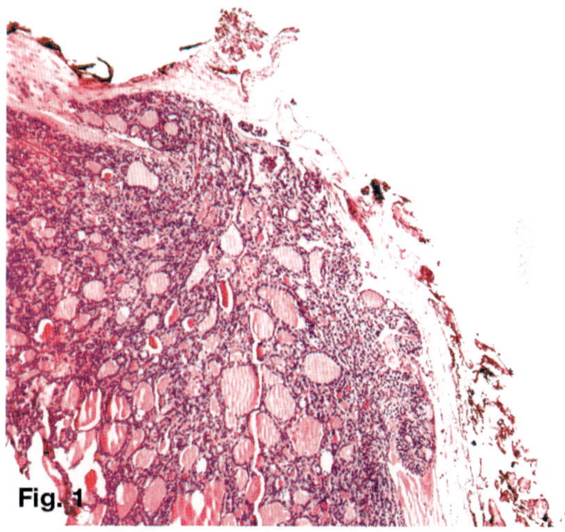

Fig. 1

A. It is most commonly multiple and occult.
B. Lymphatic metastasis is the usual route of spread.
C. Prognosis is related to capsular and vascular invasion.
D. Prognosis is related to the presence of RAS (rat sarcoma) mutations.
E. The brain is the most common target of hematogenous metastasis.

11. What is the best diagnosis for the focal finding, shown in Figure 1, in a thyroid removed for a diagnosis of follicular carcinoma?

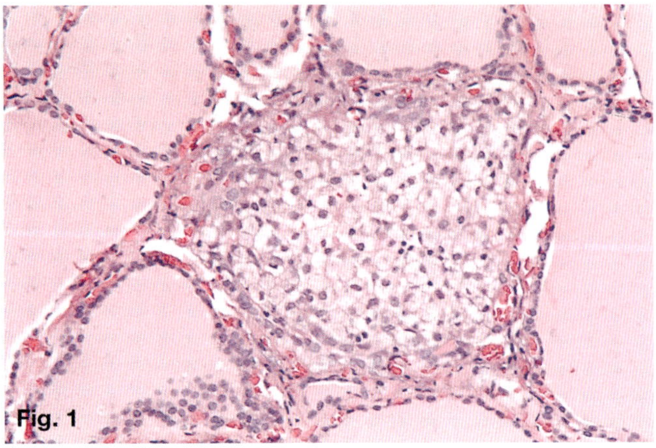
Fig. 1

A. C cell nodular proliferation
B. Focal nonspecific thyroiditis
C. Painless/silent thyroiditis
D. Palpation thyroiditis
E. Toxic nodular goiter

12. Which familial syndrome is associated with the thyroid neoplasm depicted in Figure 1?

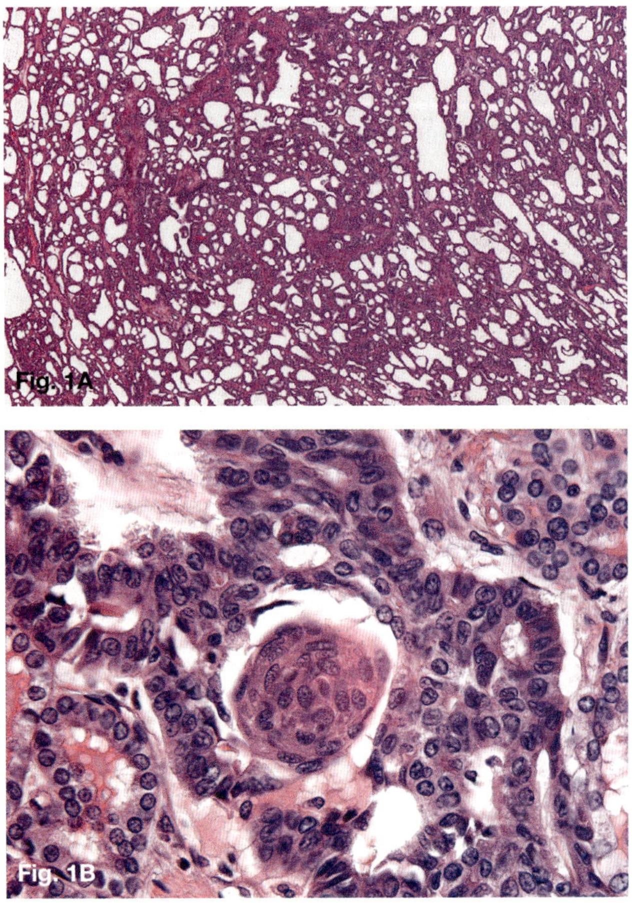
Fig. 1A
Fig. 1B

A. Familial adenomatous polyposis
B. Multiple endocrine neoplasia 1 (MEN1)
C. Multiple endocrine neoplasia 2A (MEN2A)
D. Multiple endocrine neoplasia 2B (MEN2B)
E. Neurofibromatosis 1

13. The photomicrograph shown in Figure 1 demonstrates the histologic features of an isolated thyroid nodule. The most important step in pathologic examination of this specimen is

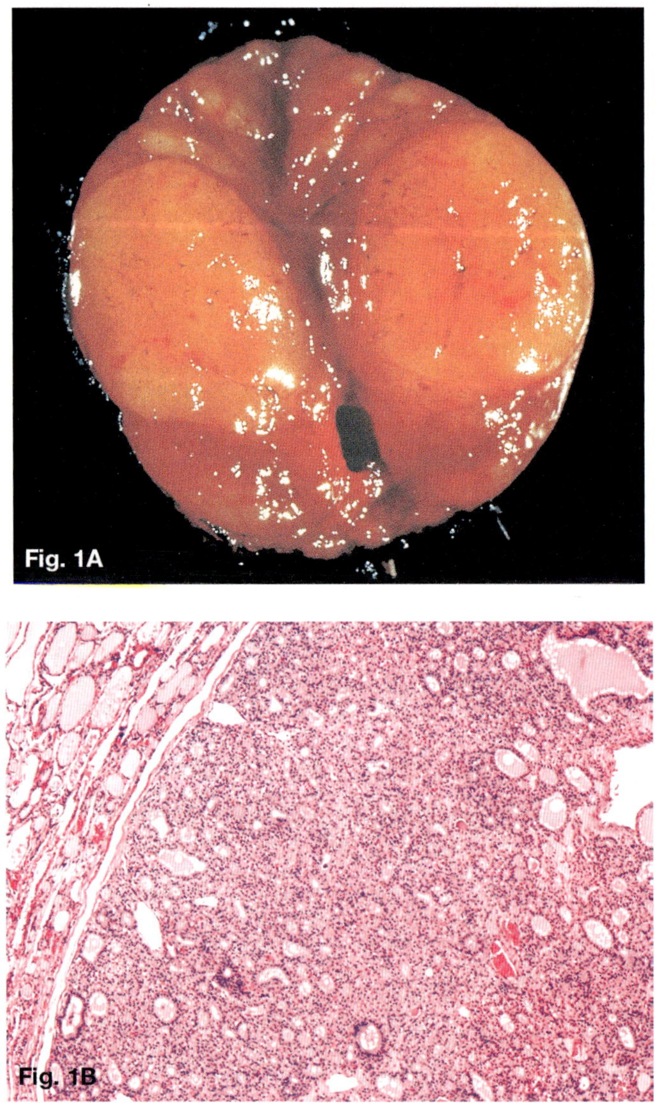
Fig. 1A
Fig. 1B

A. determination of Ki-67 labeling index.
B. DNA ploidy analysis.
C. identification of areas of oncocytic change.
D. measurement of main diameter.
E. microscopic evaluation of capsule.

14. What is the best diagnosis for the thyroid nodule, shown in Figure 1, discovered on routine physical examination of a 54-year-old female?

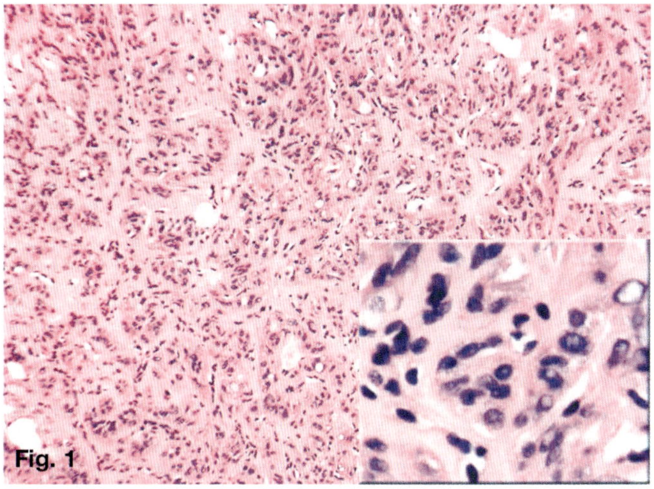


A. Extra-adrenal pheochromocytoma
B. Hyalinizing trabecular neoplasm
C. Medullary thyroid carcinoma
D. Sclerosing papillary thyroid cancer
E. Trabecular adenoma

15. The thyroid tumor shown in the gross photograph in Figure 1 is composed of large cells with well-defined cell borders, abundant granular cytoplasm, and large nucleus with prominent nucleolus. The cytoplasm of such cells is filled with

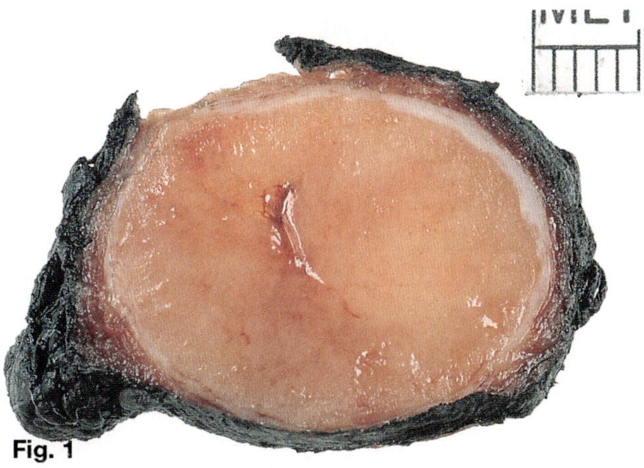


A. glycogen.
B. lipids.
C. lysosomes.
D. mitochondria.
E. thyroglobulin.

16. A thyroid biopsy reveals the tumor shown in the photomicrograph in Figure 1. Which of the following immunohistochemical stains is likely to be positive in the eosinophilic material present in the stroma?

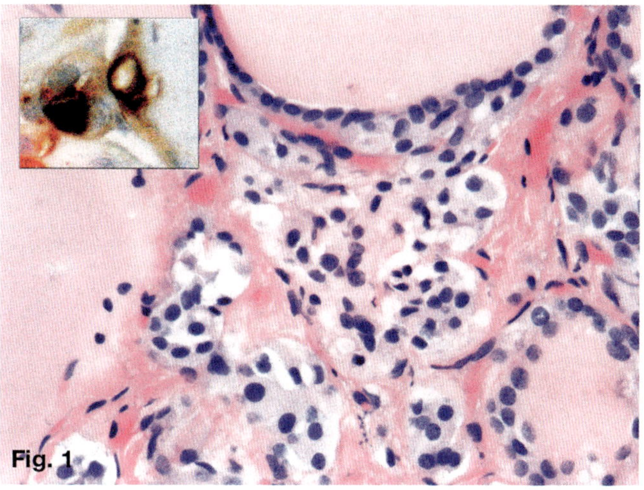


A. Calcitonin
B. Carcinoembryonic antigen (CEA)
C. Cytokeratin
D. Synaptophysin
E. Thyroglobulin

17. A 30-year-old man with a diagnosis of multiple endocrine neoplasia (MEN) type 2A undergoes prophylactic total thyroidectomy (see Figure 1). Which of the following is the most likely diagnosis?

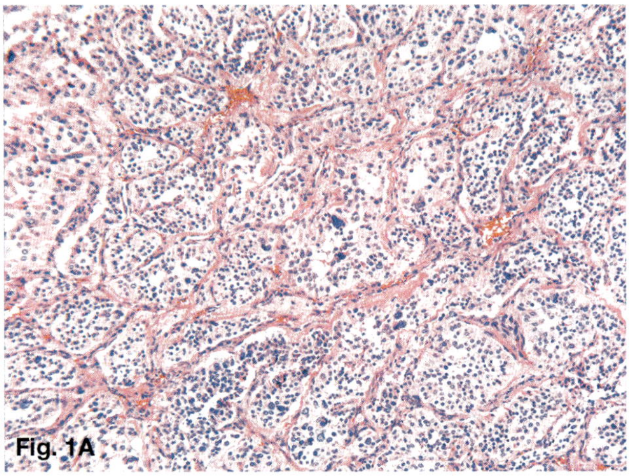
Fig. 1A

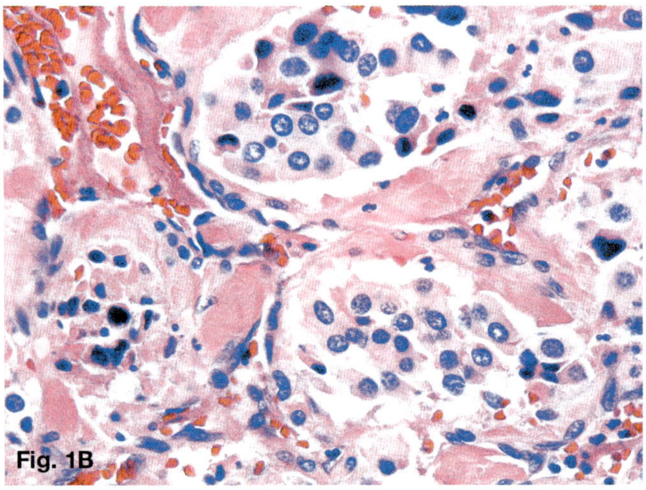
Fig. 1B

A. Anaplastic carcinoma
B. Follicular carcinoma
C. Medullary carcinoma
D. Papillary carcinoma
E. Paraganglioma

18. A 70-year-old woman undergoes thyroidectomy for removal of a large infiltrative tumor. Local lymph node metastases are found. The microscopic features of the mass are shown in Figure 1. Which of the following is the most likely diagnosis?

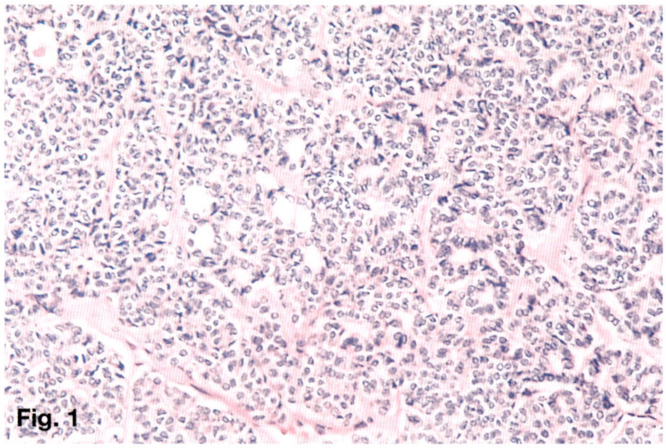
Fig. 1

A. Anaplastic carcinoma
B. Follicular carcinoma
C. Medullary carcinoma
D. Papillary carcinoma
E. Poorly differentiated carcinoma

19. An older patient undergoes surgery for the removal of a thyroid mass. The surgical specimen reveals a poorly circumscribed hemorrhagic tumor extending beyond the thyroid into adjacent tissues. The histologic appearance of the tumor is demonstrated in Figure 1. The tumor also contains regions with a spindle cell morphology and areas of increased vascularity. The tumor shows diffuse vimentin and focal keratin immunoreactivity. Which of the following is the most likely diagnosis?

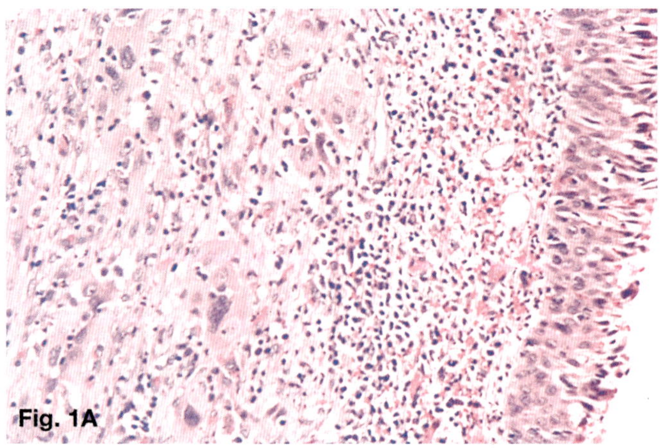
Fig. 1A

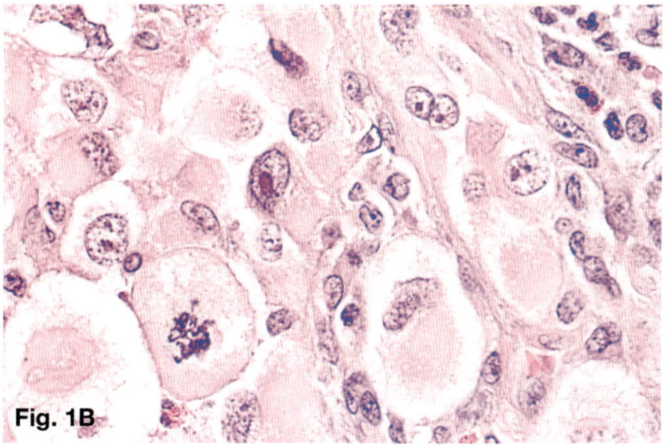

Fig. 1B

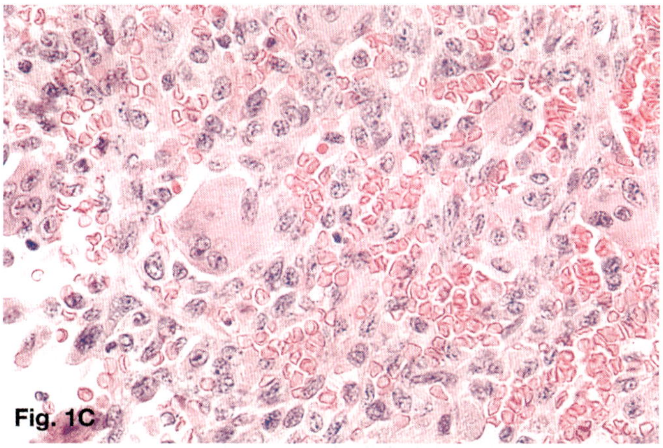

Fig. 1C

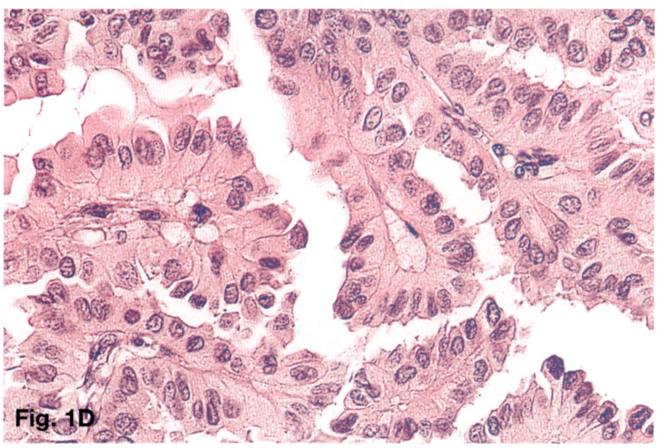

Fig. 1D

A. Anaplastic carcinoma
B. Angiosarcoma
C. Giant cell tumor
D. Hemangiopericytoma
E. Metastatic carcinoma

20. Which of the following criteria is most useful in differentiating parathyroid adenoma from hyperplasia?

A. DNA ploidy studies
B. Identification of at least one normal gland
C. Proliferative indices such as Ki-57
D. Proportion of cell types
E. Size of lesion

21. Which of the following parathyroid lesions may lead to massive enlargement of the superior parathyroid glands?

A. Chief cell hyperplasia
B. Lipoadenoma
C. Oxyphil adenoma
D. Oxyphil cell hyperplasia
E. Water-clear cell hyperplasia

22. A 45-year-old woman with hypercalcemia (15 mg/dL) undergoes surgical resection of a large neck tumor adherent to adjacent structures. The tumor weighs 13 g and histologically is composed of pleomorphic epithelial cells arranged in a trabecular fashion, as shown in this picture. Intranuclear pseudoinclusions are noted. Mitotic activity is high. Which of the following is the most likely diagnosis?

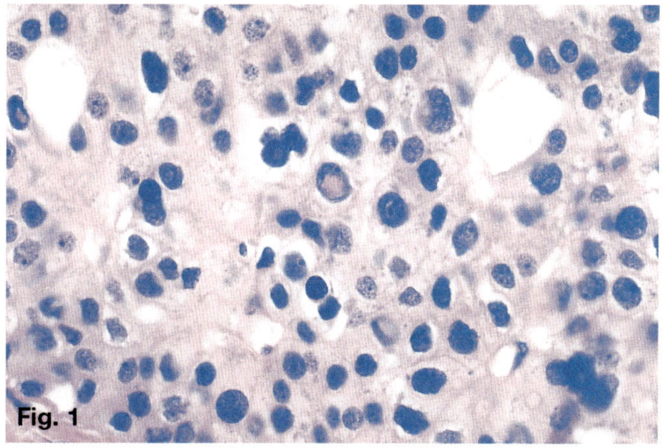

Fig. 1

A. Medullary thyroid carcinoma
B. Papillary thyroid carcinoma
C. Parathyroid adenoma
D. Parathyroid carcinoma
E. Parathyroid chief cell hyperplasia

23. With the availability of intraoperative rapid parathyroid hormone (PTH) assay, the role of the pathologist during parathyroid surgery is to

A. distinguish between adenoma and hyperplasia on H&E (hematoxylin and eosin)-stained frozen section.
B. document the presence, cellularity, and weight of parathyroid tissue.
C. perform intraoperative fat stain to distinguish between hyperplastic and normal gland.
D. request a biopsy of at least one more gland if the first one is negative for adenoma.

24. Which of the following statements is correct regarding the fine-needle aspiration (FNA) of the thyroid gland?

A. Accuracy of FNA is operator independent.
B. Aspirate is nondiagnostic if it has fewer than 6 clusters of 15 follicular cells.
C. FNA has doubled the number of patients undergoing thyroid surgery.
D. Thyroid FNA is diagnostic but not therapeutic.
E. Ultrasound guidance does not affect specimen adequacy.

25. Figure 1 shows a fine-needle aspirate from a symmetrically enlarged thyroid. Which of the following is the most likely diagnosis?

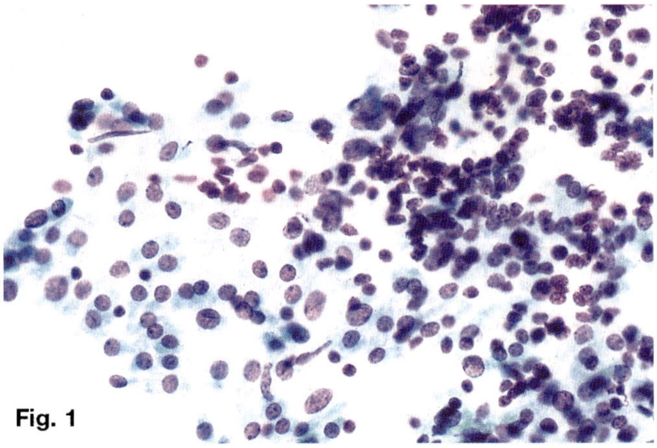

Fig. 1

A. Chronic lymphocytic thyroiditis
B. Hürthle cell neoplasm
C. Lymphoma
D. Nodular goiter
E. Papillary carcinoma

26. Figure 1 shows a fine-needle aspirate from a well-circumscribed thyroid nodule. Which of the following is the most likely diagnosis?

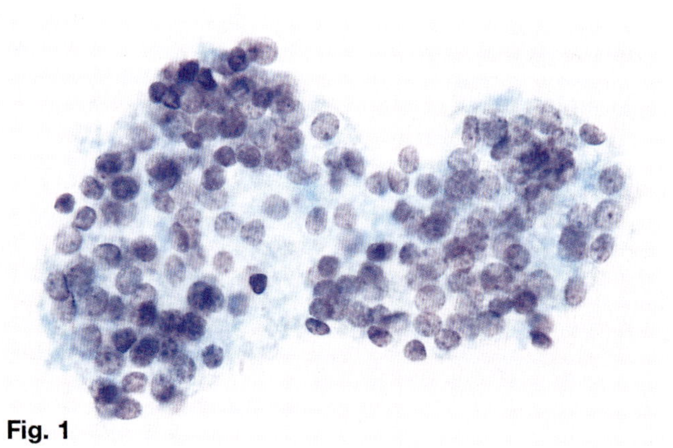

Fig. 1

A. Chronic lymphocytic thyroiditis
B. Follicular neoplasm
C. Hürthle cell neoplasm
D. Medullary carcinoma
E. Papillary carcinoma

27. Figure 1 shows a fine-needle aspirate from a well-circumscribed thyroid nodule. Which of the following is the most likely diagnosis?

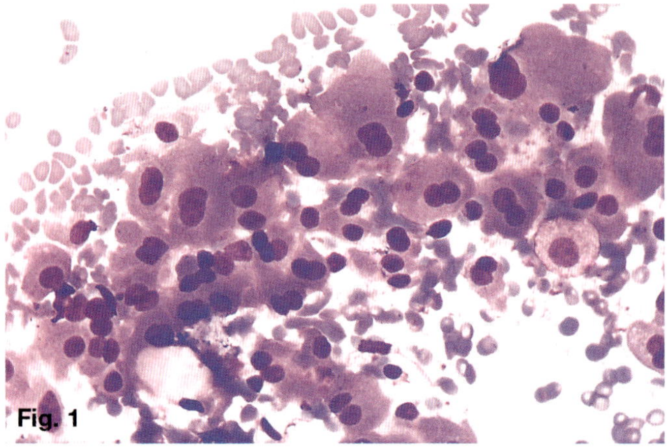

Fig. 1

A. Chronic lymphocytic thyroiditis
B. Follicular neoplasm
C. Hürthle cell adenoma
D. Nodular goiter
E. Papillary carcinoma

28. Which of the following thyroid lesions is present in the thyroid fine-needle aspirate (FNA) shown in Figure 1?

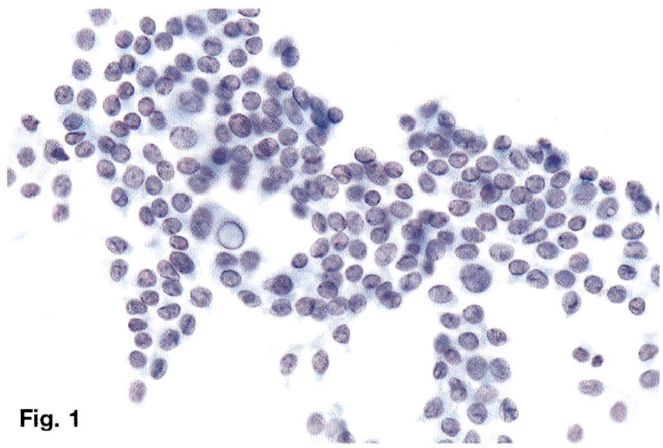

Fig. 1

A. Chronic lymphocytic thyroiditis
B. Follicular neoplasm
C. Hürthle cell adenoma
D. Nodular goiter
E. Papillary carcinoma

29. The thyroid fine-needle aspirate (FNA), shown in Figure 1, is most consistent with

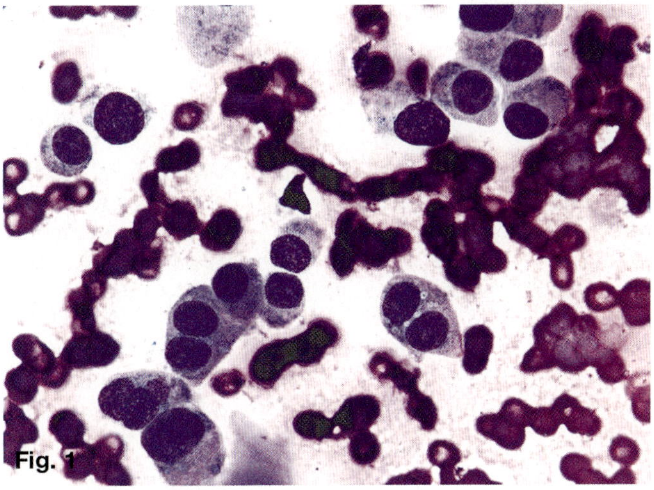


A. chronic lymphocytic thyroiditis.
B. follicular neoplasm.
C. Hürthle cell neoplasm.
D. medullary carcinoma.
E. papillary carcinoma.

30. The thyroid fine-needle aspirate (FNA), shown in Figure 1, is most consistent with

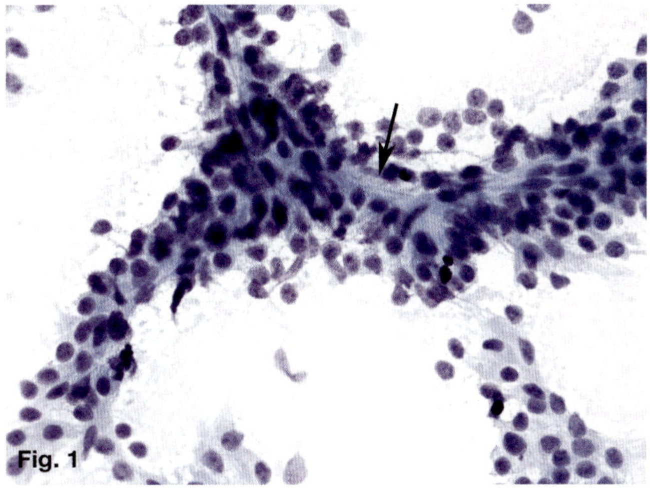


A. follicular adenoma.
B. follicular carcinoma.
C. Hürthle cell neoplasm.
D. papillary carcinoma.
E. parathyroid adenoma.

# ANSWERS AND EXPLANATIONS

**1. Correct choice: A.**

Heterotopic thyroid tissue can be found anywhere in the region of the thyroglossal duct and below the thyroid in the substernal region, the so-called Wölfler triangle, with the base at the mandible and the apex at the aortic arch. Thyroid tissue may be found in lymph nodes, esophagus, larynx, trachea, heart, and great vessels, but the most frequent location is the posterior tongue close to the foramen cecum. Conversely, parathyroid, salivary gland, thymus, adipose, and muscle tissue may be found in the thyroid. Thyroid tissue found in lymph nodes medial to the jugular vein is considered benign as long as it is contained within the lymph node capsule and does not exhibit atypical features (nuclear clearing, psammoma bodies). Thyroid tissue in nodes lateral to the jugular vein is metastatic papillary carcinoma regardless of its morphology.

**2. Correct choice: E.**

Subacute (granulomatous) thyroiditis (de Quervain thyroiditis) is an autoimmune process triggered by viral infections such as measles, mumps, adenovirus, or coxsackievirus. It affects mostly women aged 30 to 50, usually in summertime. Nonnecrotizing granulomas constitute the histopathologic hallmark of de Quervain thyroiditis. Histiocytes and multinucleated giant cells often contain colloid material. Patients present with neck pain exacerbated by swallowing, thyroid enlargement, transient hyperthyroidism, and flu-like symptoms. The clinical picture resolves spontaneously. The majority of patients return to a euthyroid state within a couple of months.

**3. Correct choice: B.**

Hashimoto thyroiditis is characterized by extensive lymphocytic inflammation with germinal centers and Hürthle cells. Hürthle cells are follicular cells with abundant eosinophilic granular (oncocytic) cytoplasm. Follicular cells may show nuclear clearing (see Figure 2), which can be mistaken for papillary carcinoma. The condition manifests with thyroid enlargement and symptoms of hyperthyroidism, and later on (the burnout phase) with hypothyroidism. Hashimoto thyroiditis is the most frequent cause of hypothyroidism in Western countries. The mechanism is autoimmune, principally mediated by a type 2 hypersensitivity reaction. Autoantibodies to a variety of fixed thyroid antigens are produced, triggering inflammation and destruction of thyroid tissue. Subacute lymphocytic thyroiditis (silent or painless thyroiditis) represents a less severe form of Hashimoto and is characterized by multifocal lymphocytic infiltration without germinal centers or Hürthle cells. It produces transient hyperthyroidism and is self-limited.

It is referred to as postpartum thyroiditis when occurring in the postpartum period.

**4. Correct choice: A.**

Graves disease is characterized by hyperplasia/hypertrophy of follicular cells associated with lymphocytic infiltration. Grossly, the thyroid is symmetrically enlarged (50-150 g, normal: 14-18 g). Follicular cells become columnar and have large nuclei. Papillary fronds grow within the follicles, and the colloid exhibits a characteristic "scalloping." Such hyperplastic changes regress after antithyroid treatment. Thus, thyroidectomy specimens show only lymphocytic infiltration, occasional Hürthle cells, and lymphoid follicles with germinal centers. Graves disease may be considered as part of a spectrum of autoimmune thyroid disease. It shares features with Hashimoto thyroiditis, such as a genetic defect in suppressor T cells that leads to a proliferation of B cells producing antithyroid autoantibodies. These thyroid receptor antibodies (TRAbs) are directed against thyrotropin receptors, thus stimulating growth and function.

**5. Correct choice: E.**

Riedel thyroiditis is characterized by diffuse yet asymmetric fibrosis of the thyroid. Fibrotic areas have a stony hard consistency. Fibrosis extends beyond the thyroid parenchyma, resulting in fixation of the organ to adjacent tissues and thus mimicking an infiltrative neoplasm. The thyroid parenchyma is replaced by keloid-like fibrous tissue containing a sparse lymphohistiocytic infiltrate with plasma cells. This process is sometimes associated with other, similar fibrosclerosing conditions, such as retroperitoneal fibrosis, mediastinal fibrosis, and sclerosing cholangitis. Riedel thyroiditis is part of the spectrum of IgG4 (immunoglobulin G subclass 4)-related disease, characterized by a lymphoplasmacytic infiltrate enriched in IgG4-positive plasma cells, accompanied by fibrosis and elevated serum IgG4 levels.

**6. Correct choice: B.**

Multinodular goiter is typically an asymmetrically enlarged gland with a distinct multinodular architecture. The nodularity is due to uneven response of thyroid follicles to thyroid-stimulating hormone (TSH) stimulation. The nodules can cause vascular compression and rupture of follicles, leading to necrosis, scarring, hemosiderin deposits, calcification, and cyst formation. Clinical manifestations are due to compression of nearby structures, with dysphagia, breathing difficulty, and superior vena cava syndrome. The nodules are polyclonal, but over time a nodule may become monoclonal and function autonomously. In a small number of cases, a hyperfunctioning nodule may lead to hyperthyroidism (Plummer syndrome). Diffuse simple goiter refers to a diffuse enlargement of the thyroid without nodules. It is most frequently endemic, due to iodine deficiency in specific areas of the world. Most patients are euthyroid.

**7. Correct choice: D.**

Papillary thyroid carcinoma is the most common thyroid malignancy and *BRAF* mutations are the most common mutations in classic papillary thyroid cancer, occurring in up to 60% of cases. Mutations in *RAS* (*HRAS, NRAS,* and *KRAS*) occur in 13%, particularly in the follicular variant.

The *RET* gene is expressed in C cells but not in normal follicular cells. Rearrangements of *RET* gene, known as *RET/PTC,* are found not only in papillary thyroid cancer (about 30% of cases) but also in other benign and malignant thyroid lesions.

Characteristic microscopic features include a papillary architecture, nuclear clearing with pseudoinclusions (the so-called Orphan Annie-eyed nuclei), nuclear crowding, and psammoma bodies. The presence of psammoma bodies in tissue sections or cytologic preparations from the head and neck region suggests the presence of a papillary carcinoma.

**8. Correct choice: D.**

The rare tall-cell variant of papillary thyroid cancer is associated with a more aggressive clinical course than the other subtypes. This variant is defined as the presence of neoplastic cells lining papillary projections that have a height at least 3 times their width. The diffuse sclerosing type involves the thyroid parenchyma in a diffuse fashion and is characterized by fibrosis and abundant psammoma bodies. This variant has a poorer prognosis than does the classic type, but the prognosis is not as poor as the tall-cell variant. The follicular variant consists of follicles, but neoplastic cells have the nuclear features of classic papillary thyroid cancer; the prognosis is the same as conventional papillary carcinoma. Papillary microcarcinoma is, by definition, less than 1 cm in greatest diameter and is a common incidental finding. The Warthin-like variant has a morphology similar to Warthin cell tumors of the salivary gland and develops in a background of lymphocytic thyroiditis.

**9. Correct choice: E.**

A solid growth pattern is present in many cases of papillary thyroid cancer. A diagnosis of solid variant is made when the solid growth exceeds 50% of the tumor. Nuclear features are the same as those of classic papillary thyroid carcinoma (PTC). This variant is most frequent in children and has been reported in 30% of patients who developed papillary carcinoma after being exposed to radiation in the Chernobyl nuclear accident. Care should be taken not to confuse this variant with the more aggressive insular carcinoma.

**10. Correct choice: C.**

The figure demonstrates a follicular neoplasm with capsular and vascular invasion. Follicular carcinoma refers to all thyroid carcinomas displaying a follicular pattern, excluding the follicular variant of papillary carcinoma, Hürthle cell carcinoma, and other rare tumors. Assessment of capsular and vascular invasion is the most crucial step with regard to prognosis. Based on this parameter, follicular cancers are subclassified into *minimally invasive* (good prognosis) and *widely invasive* (poor prognosis). Blood-borne metastasis is the preferred route of spread, with lungs and bones the most frequent targets. *RAS* mutations are more frequent in follicular than in papillary neoplasms but are not definitively correlated with prognosis. Lymphatic metastases are characteristic of papillary carcinoma. Loss of heterozygosity (LOH) on chromosomes 10q and 3p is seen in follicular carcinoma and suggests a role of tumor suppressor genes. The *t*(2;3) translocation leading to the expression of PAX8 peroxisome proliferator-activated receptor γ (PPAR-γ) chimeric protein is specific for follicular carcinoma.

**11. Correct choice: D.**

Palpation thyroiditis is a common finding in thyroidectomy specimens and can be seen in over 85% of surgically resected thyroids. It is thought to be due to minor trauma, such as vigorous physical examinations. Histologically, it is characterized by single or multiple small granulomas centered in disrupted follicles, composed of lymphocytes (usually T cells), macrophages (some foamy), and occasional multinucleated giant cells associated with colloid breakdown. No necrosis or neutrophils are present. It is a clinically insignificant finding.

**12. Correct choice: A.**

The cribriform-morular variant of papillary thyroid cancer is an uncommon thyroid carcinoma characterized by a complex architecture that includes areas of cribriform, papillary, trabecular, or solid growth with squamoid morules. Colloid is scant or absent. Classical nuclear features of papillary thyroid carcinoma (nuclear enlargement, elongation, overlapping, grooves, membrane irregularity, pseudoinclusions, clearing, chromatic marginalization) are also rare or absent in this tumor. Although it was traditionally considered to be a variant of papillary thyroid carcinoma, recent studies demonstrate that the tumor is driven by Wnt/β-catenin pathway activation. Germline *APC* gene mutation is seen in cases of familial adenomatous polyposis (FAP). Diffuse nuclear and cytoplasmic positivity for β-catenin is the hallmark of both FAP-associated or non–FAP-associated cases. It occurs almost exclusively in women; the mean age is 26 to 33 years (range of 8-61). It is associated with an indolent clinical course with a good prognosis but some aggressive cases have been reported.

**13. Correct choice: E.**

Follicular adenoma is a common benign, but monoclonal, lesion and appears as a solitary encapsulated mass. Mitotic figures are usually rare. Follicular adenoma is the most common, but trabecular, colloid, atypical, and papillary forms are rare morphologic variants. Dysregulation of thyroid-stimulating hormone (TSH) receptor function is crucial in the pathogenesis of these tumors. Somatic mutations in one of the TSH receptor units result in increased cyclic adenosine monophosphate (cAMP) levels and clonal expansion. DNA ploidy has no prognostic relevance. Careful microscopic evaluation should be performed to rule out capsular invasion, the single most important predictor of malignant behavior.

**14. Correct choice: B.**

Hyalinizing trabecular neoplasm of the thyroid is composed of follicular cells showing a trabecular growth pattern of large cells with pale to eosinophilic cytoplasm embedded in stromal hyaline material. The nuclei exhibit grooves and intranuclear inclusions. More than one-half of tumors also show intracytoplasmic 2- to 5-μm yellow perinuclear inclusions (yellow bodies) with surrounding clear halo. They represent lysosomes. Stromal calcifications are frequent. There is no vascular or capsular invasion. Most are clinically benign. To date, hyalinizing trabecular neoplasm of the thyroid is the only thyroid tumor to demonstrate rearrangement of *GLIS* (*PAX8-GLIS1* and *PAX8-GLIS3*). Mutations in *BRAF* are absent. Medullary thyroid carcinoma stains for calcitonin and chromogranin, and the nuclei show neuroendocrine features (coarse and fine chromatin). Stromal amyloid is seen in 75%. The cells in extra-adrenal paraganglioma are also positive for chromogranin, and intermixed S100 positive sustentacular cells may be present. Sclerosing papillary thyroid carcinoma exhibits an invasive growth pattern and occurs predominately in children and young adults. Trabecular adenoma is a variant of follicular adenoma.

**15. Correct choice: D.**

Oncocytic follicular (Hürthle cell) lesions are characterized by prominent oncocytic changes. The constituent cells contain eosinophilic granular cytoplasm, which is packed with large mitochondria. Oncocytic cells are found in nodular goiter, nonspecific thyroiditis, long-standing hyperthyroidism, Hashimoto thyroiditis, and neoplasms, so they are not specific to any disease. True oncocytic (Hürthle cell) tumors are usually encapsulated and have a characteristic tan-brown cut surface. Most of them have a follicular architecture, but others exhibit papillary or solid patterns. Whether an oncocytic thyroid tumor should be diagnosed as adenoma or carcinoma depends on the presence of capsular/vascular invasion, and it has been reported that capsular/vascular invasion is more frequent in nodules with oncocytic morphology compared to classic follicular lesions. Clear cell change may occur in thyroid neoplasms (including Hürthle cell tumors) due to the accumulation of lipids, glycogen, or thyroglobulin (signet-ring neoplasm).

**16. Correct choice: A.**

Medullary thyroid carcinoma arises from calcitonin-secreting C cells. Amyloid accumulates in the stroma surrounding cell nests. This form of amyloid derives from precalcitonin, and thus immunohistochemistry for calcitonin will often stain amyloid as well. Cells of papillary thyroid carcinoma (PTC) express carcinoembryonic antigen (CEA) and neuroendocrine markers, such as synaptophysin and chromogranin, but not thyroglobulin. The H&E (hematoxylin and eosin) features of these tumors may be extremely diverse. The classic pattern is that of a tumor composed of cells with amphophilic cytoplasm arranged in nests separated by fibrous septa. However, other histologic patterns may be seen, including an oncocytic subtype that mimics the Hürthle cell tumor.

**17. Correct choice: C.**

Medullary thyroid carcinoma occurs in multiple endocrine neoplasia (MEN) 2A, MEN 2B, and familial medullary thyroid carcinoma (FMTC). Hyperplasia of C cells is now recognized to be the precursor of this tumor. Stage is the primary prognostic factor.

**18. Correct choice: E.**

Poorly differentiated carcinoma is of follicular origin that has a prognosis intermediate between follicular/papillary carcinomas and anaplastic carcinomas. An interesting aspect of this neoplasm is its unique geographic distribution, being more frequent in some parts of Europe and South America. The alternate designation of insular carcinoma refers to its architecture, characterized by solid nests of small cells with occasional follicles, but solid and trabecular patterns may also be seen. Although poorly differentiated, this neoplasm displays immunoreactivity for thyroglobulin (common to both follicular and papillary carcinomas). The presence (10% or more) of poorly differentiated carcinoma in a well-differentiated follicular carcinoma is associated with more aggressive clinical behavior.

**19. Correct choice: A.**

Anaplastic carcinoma, also referred to as undifferentiated carcinoma, is a highly malignant tumor that may exhibit several patterns, including squamous-like, spindle cell, and giant cell types, and individual tumors are usually composed of multiple cell types. Immunohistochemical and ultrastructural studies have confirmed the epithelial nature of this highly undifferentiated neoplasm. Thyroglobulin immunoreactivity is usually absent, and thyroid transcription factor-1 (TTF-1) is expressed in less than 50% of cases. The prognosis is extremely poor, with the majority of patients dying within 6 months after diagnosis.

**20. Correct choice: B.**

Chief cell hyperplasia is the second most common cause of primary hyperparathyroidism after adenoma. Differentiating adenoma from chief cell hyperplasia is crucial to clinical management. There are no specific morphologic features (size of lesion, cell types, etc) that permit a definitive diagnosis, except for the finding of a rim of compressed but normal parathyroid tissue around an adenoma and/or identification of a normal parathyroid gland during surgery. The intraoperative approach to this problem used to rely on frozen section examination of the largest parathyroid gland resected in toto followed by biopsy of at least one normal-appearing gland. This historical approach has been radically changed by the introduction of intraoperative parathyroid hormone assay.

**21. Correct choice: E.**

Water-clear cell hyperplasia is a rare form of parathyroid hyperplasia composed of water-clear cells with distinct borders. It may produce massive glandular enlargement, especially of the superior parathyroid glands. It manifests with hyperparathyroidism. Chief cell hyperplasia is the most common form of parathyroid hyperplasia. A lipoadenoma is an adenoma with abundant adipose tissue.

**22. Correct choice: D.**

Parathyroid carcinomas are rare and account for 1% to 2% of primary hyperparathyroidism. They are usually large tumors (average weight: 12 g) that adhere to adjacent anatomic structures. Clinically, they may be mistaken for thyroid cancer. Nuclear pleomorphism and mitotic activity are features of parathyroid carcinomas, although occasional mitotic figures may be found in parathyroid adenomas. Large adenomas may develop focal hemorrhage, which results in areas of fibrosis entrapping tumor cells and producing a picture of capsular invasion. However, frank invasion of surrounding tissues is only found in carcinomas.

**23. Correct choice: B.**

The availability of the intraoperative rapid parathyroid hormone (PTH) assay has greatly simplified the pathologist's role in evaluating parathyroid histology during surgery. Blood samples for rapid PTH assay are taken from thyroid veins before and after excision of an enlarged gland. Fall in PTH blood levels indicates successful removal of the abnormal gland. The pathologist is expected to document the weight of the specimen and report on its histologic nature and cellularity. There is no more need to engage in the challenging task of distinguishing between parathyroid adenoma, hyperplastic parathyroid, and normal parathyroid gland on frozen sections.

**24. Correct choice: B.**

Fine-needle aspiration (FNA) as a first step in the diagnostic assessment of thyroid lesions has reduced the number of patients undergoing surgery and increased the percentage of thyroid surgical specimens that contain malignancy. It has therapeutic value in cystic lesions. Ultrasound guidance improves the adequacy of aspirates and is recommended for nodules that are nonpalpable, posteriorly located, or predominantly cystic or if a previous FNA yields inadequate specimens. The accuracy of FNA is estimated at 75% to 97%, and this wide range is mostly due to operator's experience. By the Bethesda system, a thyroid FNA is considered nondiagnostic (inadequate) if it contains fewer than 6 clusters of follicular cells, each cluster consisting of at least 10 cells.

**25. Correct choice: A.**

Fine-needle aspirate (FNA) of chronic lymphocytic thyroiditis contains mature and transformed lymphocytes, plasma cells, macrophages including tingible-body macrophages, and clusters of follicular cells and Hürthle cells. The main differential diagnoses are lymphoma (whose risk is increased in Hashimoto disease) and Hürthle cell neoplasms. Aspirates of nodular goiter usually yield abundant colloid with scanty cells (follicular and reactive), but cellular density and composition depend on whether a hyperplastic nodule or a cyst is aspirated.

**26. Correct choice: B.**

Fine-needle aspirate (FNA) of follicular neoplasms tends to be highly cellular and has little colloid. The diagnostic finding is that of syncytial aggregates of follicular cells with nuclear crowding. In practice, it is not feasible to distinguish between adenoma and carcinoma based on cytologic atypia. The same morphology can also be seen in aspirates of hyperplastic nodules from nodular goiters.

**27. Correct choice: C.**

Fine-needle aspirate (FNA) of Hürthle cell neoplasms consists of a monotonous population of loosely cohesive cells with abundant granular cytoplasm. The uniformity of nuclear features in Hürthle cell neoplasm is in contrast with the nuclear variability and enlargement of Hürthle cells found in aspirates of chronic lymphocytic thyroiditis.

**28. Correct choice: E.**

Fine-needle aspirate (FNA) of papillary thyroid carcinoma exhibits a wide range of morphologic features including: (a) papillary fragments or branched sheets, (b) follicular structures in the follicular variant, (c) nuclear crowding and pleomorphism, (d) nuclear grooves, (e) intranuclear (cytoplasmic) pseudoinclusions, (f) multinucleated giant cells, and (g) psammoma bodies. Since each of these features may be encountered in other lesions, the FNA diagnosis rests on a set of criteria rather than isolated findings.

**29. Correct choice: D.**

Fine-needle aspirate (FNA) of medullary thyroid carcinoma is usually highly cellular. The tumor cells have a plasmacytoid look imparted by their peripherally located nucleus. The cytoplasm is granular. Amyloid is present in a minority of cases, and immunohistochemistry for calcitonin is positive in fewer than 60%.

**30. Correct choice: E.**

Fine-needle aspirate (FNA) of intrathyroid parathyroid adenoma may be mistaken for a thyroid neoplasm. The presence of a monotonous population of cells arranged around vascular cores (arrow). Parathyroid chief cells contain uniform round nuclei. The presence of oxyphilic cells may also suggest the diagnosis.

# 14 Adrenal Glands

1. An autopsy of a stillborn baby boy reveals very large cells in the adrenal cortex, as shown in Figure 1. This finding is most likely associated with which of the following conditions?

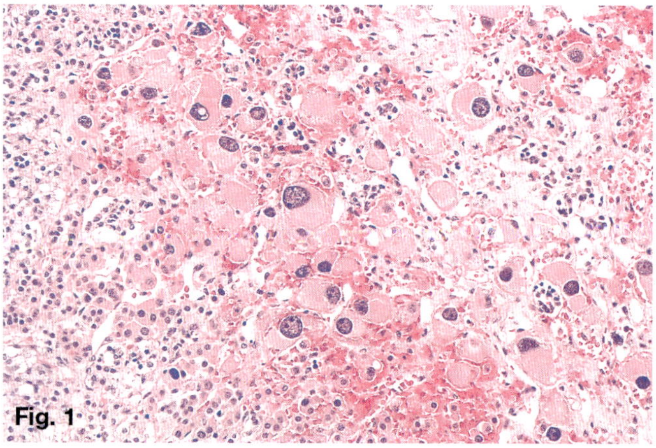

Fig. 1

   A. Adrenoleukodystrophy
   B. Beckwith-Wiedemann syndrome
   C. Carney complex
   D. Multiple endocrine neoplasia 2 (MEN2)
   E. von Hippel-Lindau disease

2. The deficient activity of which of the following enzymes leads to the most frequent form of congenital adrenal hyperplasia?

   A. 3-β-Hydroxysteroid dehydrogenase
   B. 11-β-Hydroxylase
   C. 17-α-Hydroxylase
   D. 21-Hydroxylase
   E. Steroid acute regulatory (STAR) gene product

3. Which of the following is the most common of adrenal hypofunction in the United States?

   A. Amyloidosis
   B. Autoimmune adrenalitis
   C. Bilateral metastases
   D. Hemorrhage
   E. Tuberculosis

4. The condition depicted in Figure 1 represents the most common form of adrenocorticotropic hormone (ACTH)-independent Cushing syndrome and is often associated with which of the following?

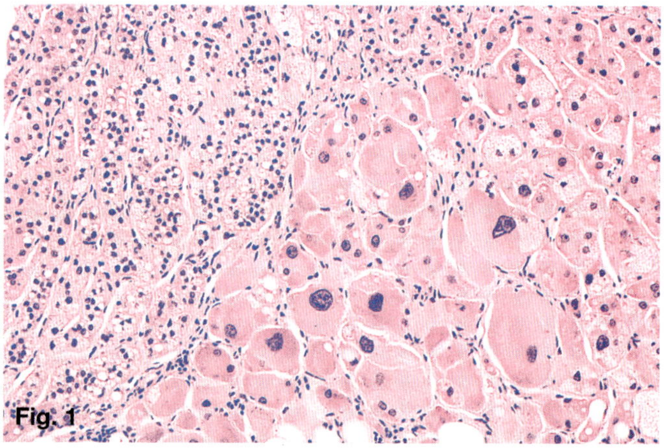

Fig. 1

   A. Adrenoleukodystrophy
   B. Beckwith-Wiedemann syndrome
   C. Carney complex
   D. Multiple endocrine neoplasia 2 (MEN2)
   E. von Hippel-Lindau disease

---

All figures in this chapter are from Longacre TA, Greenson JK, Hornick JL, Reuter VE, eds. *Mills and Sternberg's Diagnostic Surgical Pathology*. 7th ed. Wolters Kluwer; 2022 except for those noted at the end of this book.

5. Surgical excision of a 1.5-cm adrenal gland is performed in a 32-year-old man with hyperaldosteronism (Figure 1). A section of the nodule is provided in Figure 2. Large bizarre nuclei are scattered throughout the tumor, but mitotic figures are not appreciated. No capsular or capsular invasion is present. The cells are immunoreactive for low-molecular-weight keratin and vimentin, but not epithelial membrane antigen (EMA). Which of the following is the most likely diagnosis?

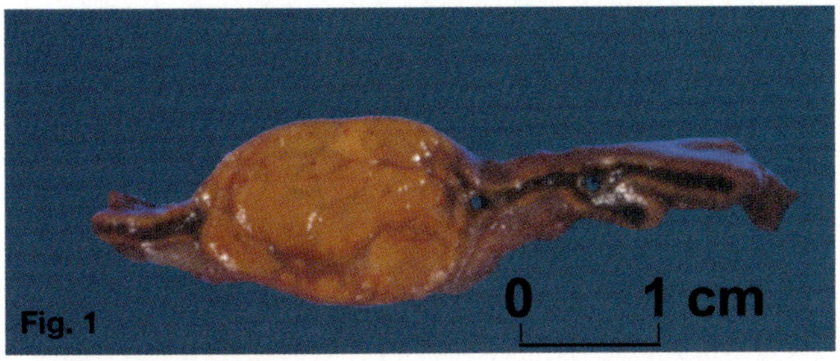

Fig. 1

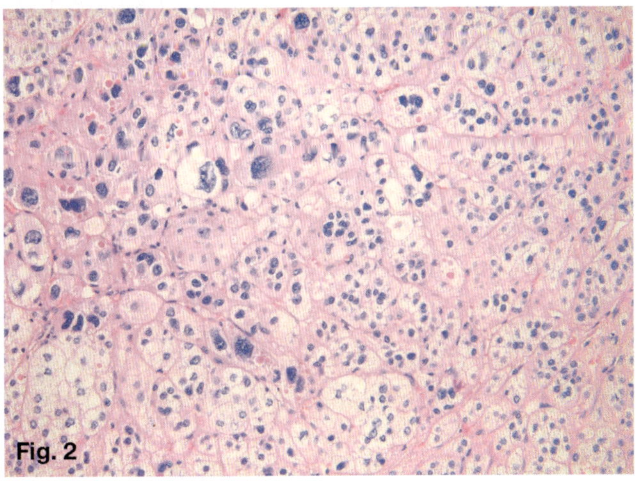
Fig. 2

A. Adrenal cytomegaly
B. Adrenocortical adenoma
C. Adrenocortical carcinoma
D. Metastatic renal cell carcinoma
E. Pheochromocytoma

6. A patient suffering from hypertension undergoes surgical excision of an adrenal tumor. Histologic examination reveals intracytoplasmic eosinophilic inclusions such as the ones seen in Figure 1. On closer examination, these bodies consist of concentric laminations. The presence of such inclusions indicates

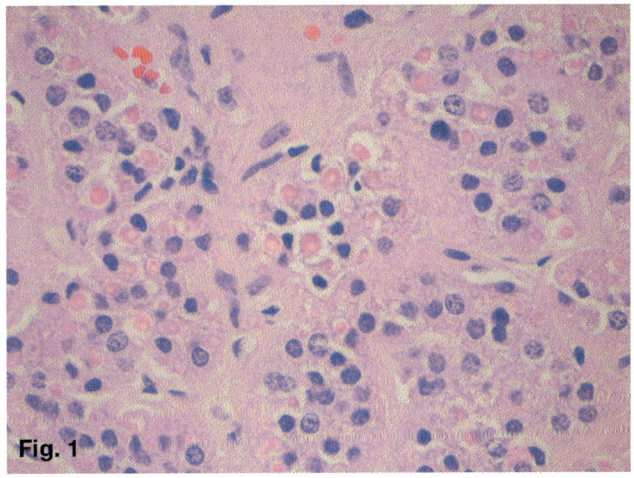
Fig. 1

A. aggressive behavior of tumor,
B. hyperproduction of androgens.
C. hyperproduction of cortisol.
D. nonfunctioning adenoma.
E. prior treatment with spironolactone.

7. Which of the following features is characteristic of adrenocortical carcinoma?

A. Approximately 80% of tumors produce hormones
B. Homogeneous cut surface without necrosis or hemorrhage
C. Paucity of mitotic figures or atypical mitoses
D. Presence of glandular formations
E. Small size (<100 g) at clinical presentation

8. A 2.5-cm unilateral nonfunctioning left adrenal mass is found on imaging studies performed for an unrelated disorder. The adrenal gland is removed to reveal a dark orange to brown discrete mass. Only rare mitotic figures are seen, and there are no atypical mitoses (see Figure 1). There is no necrosis, sinusoidal or capsular invasion or angioinvasion. The constituent cells are positive for melan-A and synaptophysin, but not for chromogranin (see Figure 2). PAX8 is negative. The Ki-67 proliferation index is 2%. What is the most likely diagnosis?

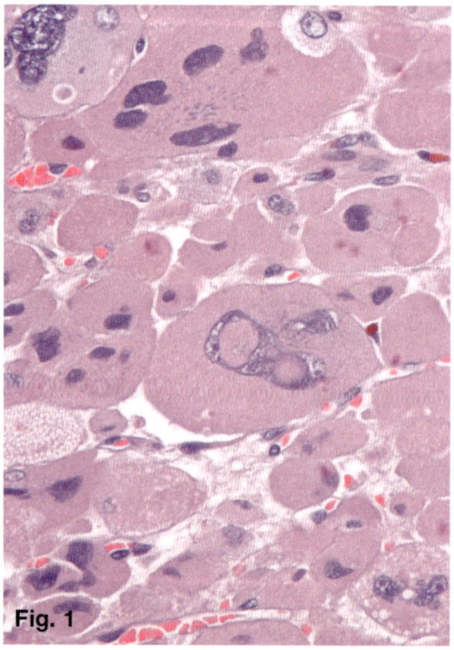
Fig. 1

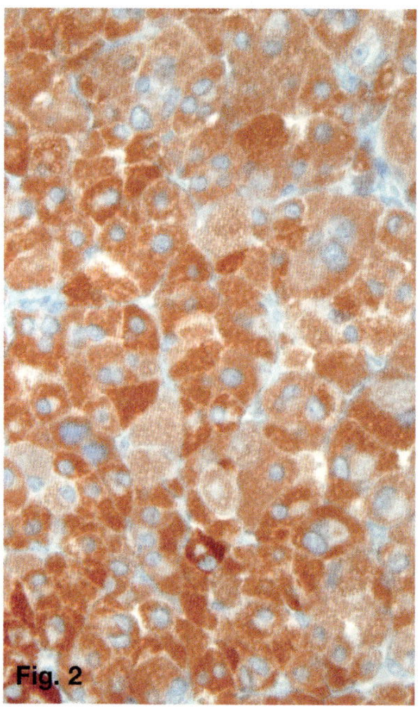
Fig. 2

A. Adrenal cortical carcinoma
B. Hepatocellular carcinoma
C. Oncocytic adenoma (oncocytoma)
D. Pheochromocytoma
E. Renal cell carcinoma

9. A large suprarenal mass is removed from a 56-year-old woman. Its histologic appearance is shown in Figure 1. The tumor displays diffuse immunoreactivity for vimentin, inhibin, calretinin, melan-A, and D2-40. It is negative for S100, epithelial membrane antigen (EMA), α-fetoprotein (AFP), synaptophysin, chromogranin, and cytokeratin. Which of the following is the most likely diagnosis?

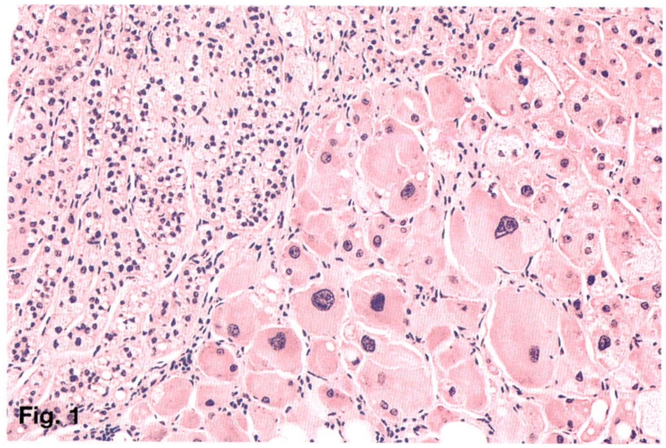
Fig. 1

A. Adrenocortical carcinoma
B. Hepatocellular carcinoma
C. Metastatic adenocarcinoma
D. Pheochromocytoma
E. Renal cell carcinoma

10. A surgically resected adrenal gland has a circumscribed, but nonencapsulated, tumor measuring 5 cm in greatest dimension. The cut surface is yellow with areas of brown color. The tumor has the microscopic features shown in Figure 1. Which of the following is the most likely diagnosis?

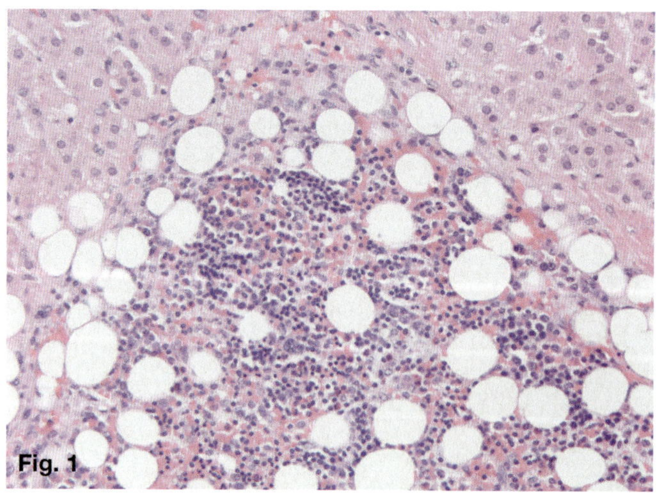
Fig. 1

A. Adrenal lipoma
B. Adrenoleukodystrophy
C. Angiomyolipoma
D. Hemangioma
E. Myelolipoma

11. A 2-year-old child undergoes resection of an adrenal mass whose histologic appearance is shown in Figure 1. A fibrillary (neuropil-like) background is appreciated. Fewer than 5% of tumor cells display evidence of ganglionic differentiation. Immunohistochemistry for synaptophysin shows granular cytoplasmic staining and highlights Homer-Wright rosettes. Based on these features, this neuroblastic tumor should be classified as

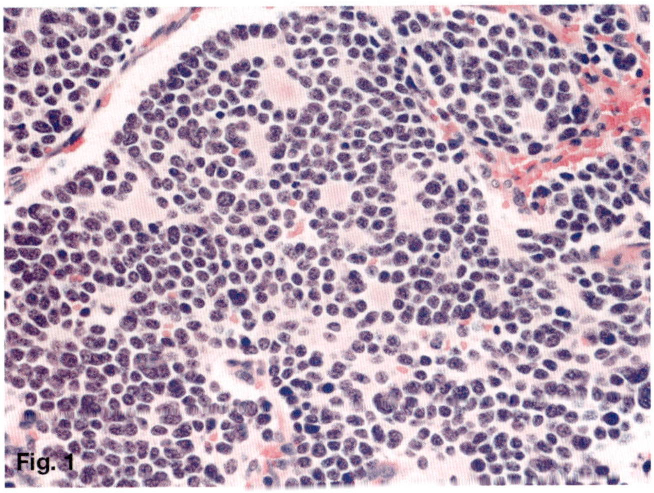


A. differentiating neuroblastoma.
B. ganglioneuroblastoma, intermixed.
C. ganglioneuroblastoma, nodular.
D. poorly differentiated neuroblastoma.
E. undifferentiated neuroblastoma.

12. Which of the following factors has a positive prognostic impact on neuroblastomas?

A. Age older than 3 years
B. Deletion of chromosome 1p
C. Diploid karyotype
D. Low levels of nerve growth factor (NGF) receptor TRK (tropomyosin receptor kinase)-A
E. Mitosis-karyorrhexis index (MKI) less than 2%

13. Which of the following is the most reliable criterion for distinguishing benign from malignant pheochromocytomas?

A. Metastasis
B. Mitotic rate
C. Number of sustentacular cells
D. Tumor size
E. Vascular and capsular invasion

14. In which of the following familial syndromes do pheochromocytomas most commonly develop?

A. Li-Fraumeni syndrome
B. Multiple endocrine neoplasia (MEN) type 1
C. Multiple endocrine neoplasia (MEN) type 2
D. von Hippel-Lindau syndrome (VHL)
E. von Recklinghausen disease

15. What is the most likely diagnosis for the adrenal medullary tumor shown in Figure 1 in a 45-year-old woman with a history of neurofibromatosis 1?

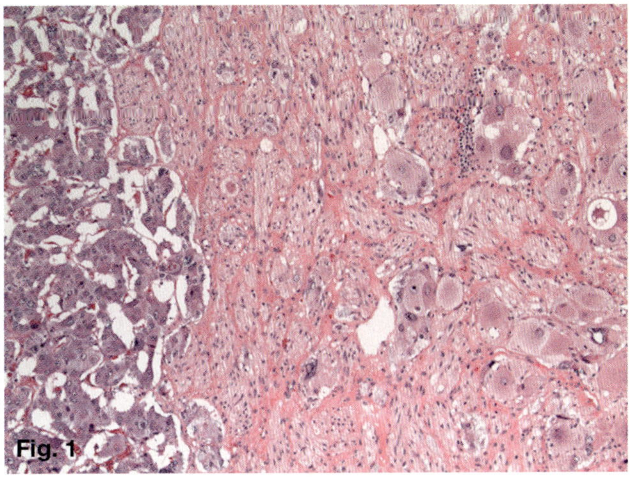


A. Composite pheochromocytoma
B. Ganglioneuroblastoma, intermixed
C. Ganglioneuroblastoma, nodular
D. Ganglioneuroma
E. Plexiform neurofibroma

# ANSWERS AND EXPLANATIONS

**1. Correct choice: B.**

The photomicrograph shows adrenal cytomegaly. Cytomegalic cells can measure up to 150 μm in diameter and are normally found in the fetal adrenal gland and 3% of stillborn infants. Cytomegalic cells are numerous in infants with Beckwith-Wiedemann syndrome, which is an overgrowth syndrome characterized by macroglossia, visceromegaly, asymmetric macrosomia, and a propensity to develop several neoplasms, including Wilms tumor, adrenocortical carcinoma, hepatoblastoma, and rhabdomyosarcoma. Beckwith-Wiedemann syndrome is reported in 1 out of 12,000 newborns. Beckwith-Wiedemann syndrome is subtyped based on different alterations on chromosome 11. It is sporadic in 85% of cases and autosomal dominant in the remaining cases.

**2. Correct choice: D.**

Congenital adrenal hyperplasia is a group of disorders due to autosomal recessive mutations of genes that encode for enzymes involved in the synthesis of steroid hormones. About 95% of cases are due to deficiency of 21-hydroxylase (1 in 14,500 births), which results in defective production of cortisol and aldosterone. The resultant accumulation of 17-hydroxypregnenolone leads to increased synthesis of adrenal androgens.

**3. Correct choice: B.**

Approximately 75% of cases of deficient adrenocortical function are due to Addison disease, which is an immune-mediated destruction of the adrenal cortex associated with autoantibodies to adrenal antigens (P450, the most frequent target). The adrenal cortex is markedly atrophic and infiltrated by a florid chronic inflammatory population. The medulla is unaffected. All the other conditions listed are rare causes of adrenal insufficiency.

**4. Correct choice: C.**

Primary pigmented nodular adrenocortical disease (PPNAD) is a rare form of adrenocortical hyperplasia but the most common form of adrenocorticotropic hormone (ACTH)-independent Cushing syndrome. PPNAD occurs sporadically or in association with the Carney complex, which is an inherited, autosomal dominant disorder characterized by myxomas in the heart and skin, pigmented skin lesions, and a variety of endocrine and nonendocrine neoplasms. PPNAD in the Carney complex manifests with Cushing syndrome and may degenerate into adrenocortical carcinoma. On gross examination, PPNAD consists of multiple pigmented nodules of cortical cells (1-3 mm), while the intervening cortex is atrophic. Microscopically, the nodules are composed of large, granular eosinophilic cells that often contain large hyperchromatic nuclei with prominent nucleoli (the so-called "micronodular dysplasia"). The cells are usually filled with lipofuscin. In general, the majority of cases of adrenocortical hyperfunction are caused by a pituitary adenoma, while bronchial carcinoids and small cell carcinomas account for most cases of cortical hyperplasia due to ectopic production of ACTH or corticotropin-like factors.

**5. Correct choice: B.**

Adrenocortical adenoma is a benign lesion that is usually of small size, rarely exceeding 5 cm. It is composed of well-differentiated cells closely resembling the zona fasciculata. Adrenal adenomas are usually asymptomatic but may give rise to Cushing, Conn, or adrenogenital syndromes. In this case, the adenoma is associated with Conn syndrome (hyperaldosteronism). The differential diagnosis between adenoma and carcinoma favors adenoma when the size is small, mitotic activity is absent or minimal, and vascular and capsular invasion are absent. Combined cytokeratin and vimentin expression is characteristic of adenoma, whereas cytokeratin expression is often focal or absent in carcinoma.

**6. Correct choice: E.**

Spironolactone bodies are often detected in aldosterone-secreting adrenal adenomas excised from patients previously treated with spironolactone. Ultrastructurally, they are composed of a concentric arrangement of membranes. By immunohistochemistry, aldosterone has been found in spironolactone bodies. The clinical diagnosis of primary hyperaldosteronism (Conn syndrome) is based on clinical and laboratory findings (ie, hypertension combined with hypokalemia, hyperkaluria, and increased plasma renin activity). Adenomas are responsible for over two-thirds of cases of hyperaldosteronism.

**7. Correct choice: A.**

Eighty percent of adrenal cortical carcinomas are functional and produce cortisol, aldosterone, androgenic steroids, or both. By the time of diagnosis, most tumors are large in size and have often spread to regional lymph nodes, liver, lungs, and other organs, which accounts for its dismal prognosis. The cut surface is characteristically variegated, with multifocal hemorrhage and necrosis. Mitotic figures are frequent, including atypical mitoses (in contrast to cortical adenoma), but glandular formations are absent (in contrast to most renal cell carcinomas). There are two peaks of incidence: one in the fourth decade and a smaller one in childhood. A variety of histologic features have been proposed to be of use in distinguishing malignant adrenal cortical tumors from their benign counterparts. These include high nuclear grade, greater than 5 mitotic figures/50 high-power fields, diffuse architecture (>33% of tumor), clear or vacuolated cytoplasm (<25% of tumor), necrosis, venous invasion, sinusoidal invasion, and capsular invasion. The reticulin network is retained in adenoma but disrupted in carcinoma.

**8. Correct choice: C.**

Oncocytic adenoma (oncocytoma) is uncommon but is characterized by eosinophilic (oncocytic) cells, diffuse architecture, and high-grade nuclear atypia, three features that are useful in distinguishing usual adrenal cortical carcinoma from adenoma. Therefore, oncocytic adenoma (oncocytoma) is best distinguished from oncocytic adrenal cortical carcinoma on the basis of a combination of major criteria and minor criteria. The major criteria for malignancy are high mitotic rate, atypical mitotic figures, and venous invasion. The minor criteria for malignancy are large size (>10 cm) and weight (>200 g), necrosis, capsular invasion, and sinusoidal invasion. The presence of one major criterion indicates malignancy, while one to four minor criteria indicate tumors of uncertain malignant potential (borderline tumors). The absence of all criteria indicates benignancy. The reticulin network is retained in adenoma but disrupted in carcinoma. Ki-67 proliferation index is less than 5% in adenomas. Oncocytic adrenal cortical carcinoma is the most common adrenal cortical carcinoma histologic variant, but only 24% of all adrenocortical oncocytic tumors are malignant. A common deletion in mitochondrial DNA (mtDNA 4,977 bp) can be seen in benign, borderline, and malignant oncocytic adrenocortical tumors.

**9. Correct choice: A.**

The list of choices corresponds to those malignancies that enter the differential diagnosis with adrenal cortical carcinoma. Keratin has been found to be positive, although focally, in up to 60% of cases if antigen retrieval is employed, while vimentin is positive in most cases. Markers that have been recently shown to be positive in most adrenal cortical carcinomas include inhibin, calretinin, melan-A, and D2-40. A marker of steroid-producing tumors is steroidogenic factor 1 (SF-1), which has a nuclear expression. Of note, adrenal glands are involved by metastases in 30% of patients with metastatic tumors, and 50% of these cases are bilateral.

**10. Correct choice: E.**

Myelolipoma is a benign lesion consisting of mature adipose tissue with scattered islands of hematopoietic tissue. The size may be from minuscule to extremely large. Average age at diagnosis is 50 years. Most cases are asymptomatic and discovered accidentally. It is not clear whether this is a neoplasm or a reactive lesion. Adrenal lipoma is composed of mature fat cells but no hematopoietic elements. Adrenoleukodystrophy is a rare genetic disease leading to the accumulation of very long-chain fatty acids in the adrenals and demyelination of central nervous system (CNS) and peripheral nerves. Angiomyolipoma is a tumor most commonly found in the kidney and composed of a mixture of adipose tissue, vascular structures, and smooth muscle. Adrenal hemangioma is a benign vascular proliferation.

**11. Correct choice: D.**

Poorly differentiated neuroblastoma is characterized by the presence of a neuropil background with less than 5% differentiating neuroblasts (ganglionic cells). Neuroblastic tumors are divided into neuroblastoma; ganglioneuroblastoma, intermixed; ganglioneuroma and ganglioneuroblastoma, nodular. Neuroblastoma is further divided into three grades: undifferentiated, poorly differentiated, and differentiating. See Table 1 for classification and grading of neuroplastic tumors.

**12. Correct choice: E.**

Mitosis-karyorrhexis index (MKI) less than 2% is associated with a positive prognosis in neuroblastomas. Numerous independent as well as interrelated factors have been found to influence the prognosis of neuroblastomas. Hyperdiploidy and high levels of nerve growth factor (NGF) receptor TRK (tropomyosin receptor kinase)-A are considered to be positive prognostic indicators. Older age, deletion of chromosome 1p, deletion of chromosome 11q, and *MYCN* amplification are associated with a poorer prognosis. Figure 1 depicts the age-linked prognostic groups for neuroblastoma.

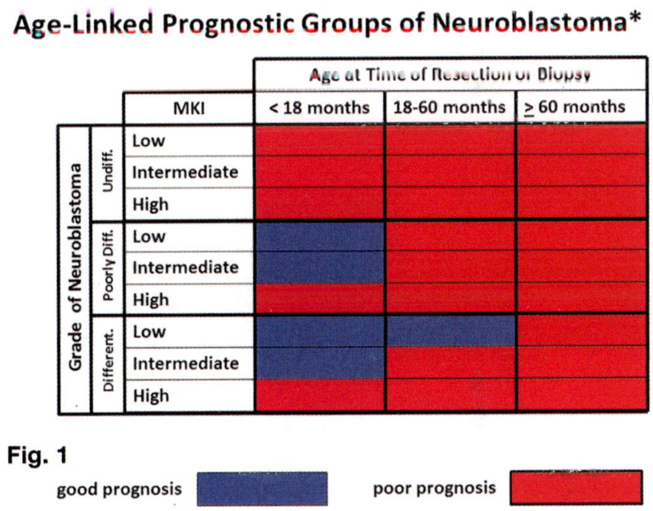


**Fig. 1**

* Applies to neuroblastic nodules for prognostic subsets of ganglioneuroblastoma nodular

**TABLE 1 Classification and Grading of Neuroblastic Tumors**

| International Neuroblastoma Pathology Committee (1999) | |
|---|---|
| Neuroblastoma (Schwannian stroma-poor NT) | |
| Undifferentiated | Absence of neuropil and <5% ganglionic differentiation[a] |
| Poorly differentiated | Neuropil present and <5% ganglionic differentiation |
| Differentiating | Neuropil present, >5% ganglionic differentiation, and <50% Schwannian stroma |
| Ganglioneuroblastoma, intermixed (Schwannian stroma-rich NT) | Nests of neuroblasts and neuropil intermixed with ganglion cells and >50% Schwannian stroma |
| Ganglioneuroma (Schwannian stroma-dominant NT | |
| Maturing | Mature ganglion cells and Schwannian stroma with intermixed individual neuroblasts without formation of nests of neuroblasts |
| Mature | Mature ganglion cells and Schwannian stroma without neuroblasts |
| Ganglioneuroblastoma, nodular (composite Schwannian stromarich/stroma-dominant and stroma-poor NT) | Composite tumor of neuroblastoma nodule in a background of either ganglioneuroblastoma intermixed or ganglioneuroma |

NT, neuroblastic tumor.
[a]Ganglionic differentiation is defined as the cell diameter being equal to or greater than 2 times the nuclear diameter.

**13. Correct choice: A.**

There is no reliable morphologic or clinical method for distinguishing between benign and malignant pheochromocytomas except metastatic spread. Capsular and vascular invasion is seen in both benign and malignant cases. However, greater tumor size, extensive necrosis, and lack of cytoplasmic hyaline globules tend to be more frequent in malignant than in benign pheochromocytomas.

**14. Correct choice: C.**

Familial pheochromocytomas are often bilateral and multicentric and occur at an earlier age than sporadic forms. Up to 50% of patients with multiple endocrine neoplasia (MEN) type 2 (A or B) develop pheochromocytomas. This tumor is also seen in up to 20% of patients with von Hippel-Lindau syndrome (VHL) and up to 5% of patients with von Recklinghausen disease. Genetic screening of sporadic pheochromocytomas shows that one-fifth of cases occur in carriers of familial syndromes. The condition known as familial paraganglioma/pheochromocytoma is an inherited, autosomal dominant condition caused by mutations in the genes for succinate dehydrogenase subunits D, B, or C.

**15. Correct choice: A.**

Composite pheochromocytomas are rare composite tumors with neuroblastoma, ganglioneuroma, ganglioneuroblastoma, or malignant peripheral nerve sheath tumor. They may be associated with neurofibromatosis 1. Ganglioneuroma is the most common component. Since pheochromocytomas may contain ganglion cells, the presence of a Schwann cell component is essential for the diagnosis of a ganglioneuromatous component. Many composite tumors are associated with the signs and symptoms typical of pheochromocytomas.

# 15 Paragangliomas

1. Which of the following is considered the single most reliable marker of malignancy in a paraganglioma?

   A. Presence of dense sclerosis with distortion of zellballen
   B. Presence of large eosinophilic cytoplasmic inclusions
   C. Scattered nuclear hyperchromasia and pleomorphism
   D. Spindle and cellular pseudosarcomatous component
   E. Tumor where paraganglionic tissue is not normally present

2. A 50-year-old man presents with bradycardia and a slowly growing, painless mass near the angle of the left mandible. A well-demarcated, rubbery tumor measuring 4.5 cm is excised and a representative section is obtained for processing and review (Figure 1). What is the best diagnosis?

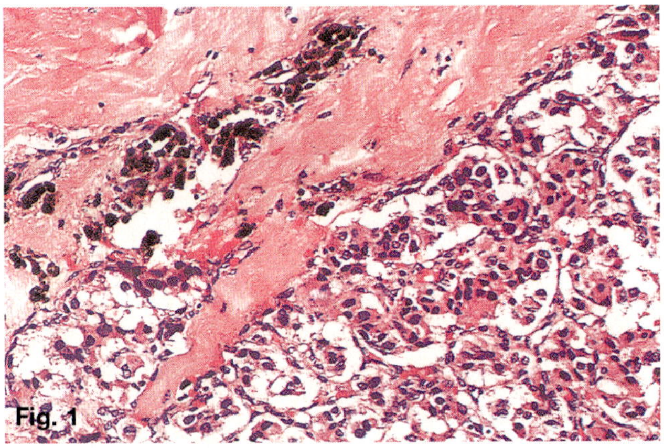

Fig. 1

   A. Carotid body paraganglioma
   B. Jugulotympanic paraganglioma
   C. Pheochromocytoma
   D. Soft tissue glomus tumor
   E. Vagal paraganglioma

3. The photomicrograph shown in Figure 1 depicts a section of a neck paraganglioma stained with an antibody that identifies a marker for sustentacular cells. This marker is

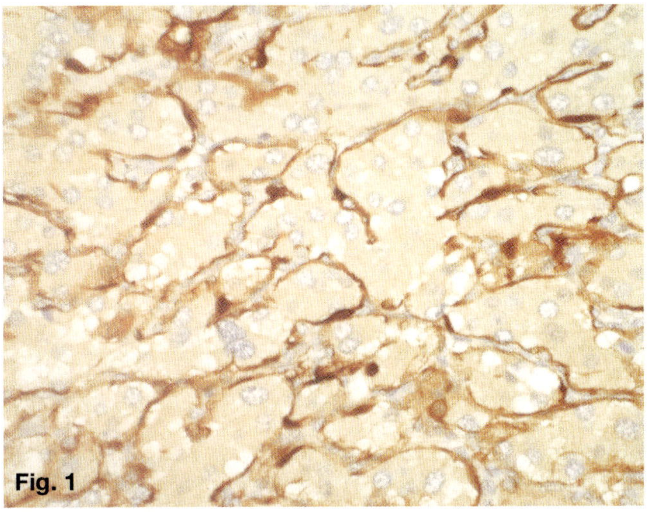

Fig. 1

   A. chromogranin.
   B. GATA3.
   C. OCT4.
   D. S100.
   E. synaptophysin.

All figures in this chapter are from Longacre TA, Greenson JK, Hornick JL, Reuter VE, eds. *Mills and Sternberg's Diagnostic Surgical Pathology.* 7th ed. Wolters Kluwer; 2022 except for those noted at the end of this book.

4. The nodule, shown in Figure 1, was found in the coccygeal region. Which of the following is the most likely diagnosis?

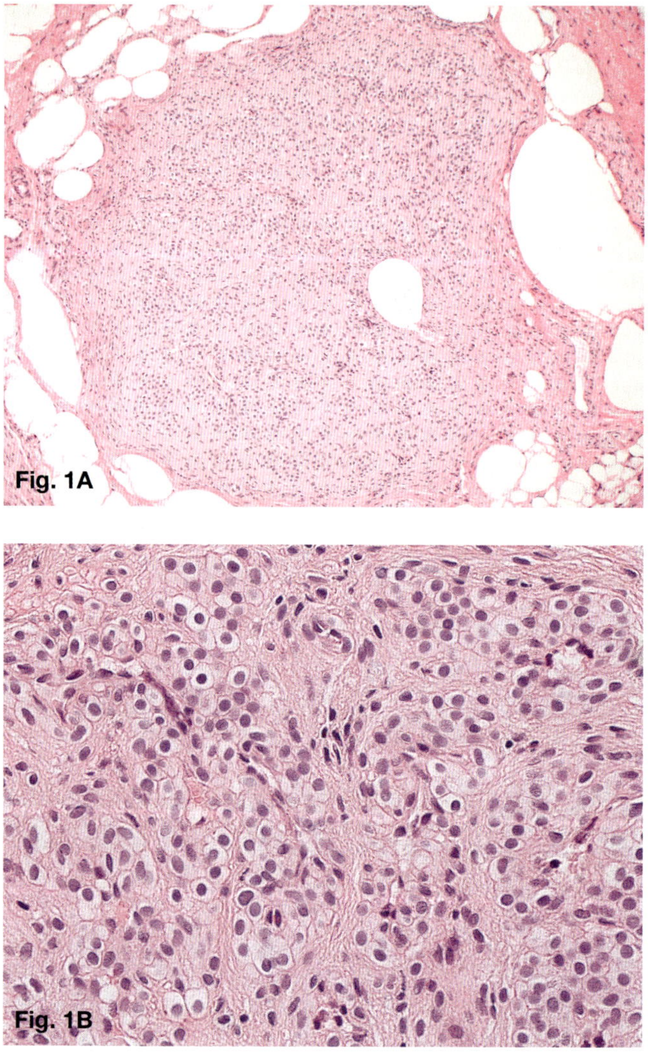

Fig. 1A

Fig. 1B

A. Gangliocytic paraganglioma
B. Glomus coccygeum
C. Glomus tumor of the coccyx
D. Paraganglioma of the cauda equina
E. Paraganglioma of the coccyx

5. Which antibody can be used to detect succinate dehydrogenase (SDH) deficiency in extra-adrenal paragangliomas?

A. SDHA
B. SDHAF2
C. SDHB
D. SDHC
E. SDHD

6. A 50-year-old woman presents with tinnitus and hearing loss. A polypoid mass measuring 1.5 cm is removed from her left middle ear (see Figure 1). What is the best diagnosis?

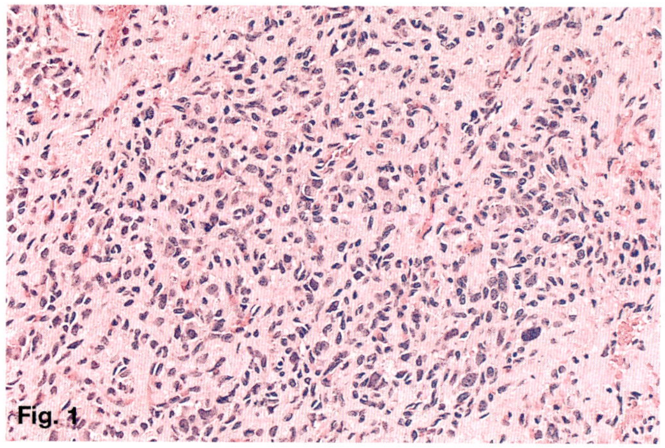

Fig. 1

A. Carotid body paraganglioma
B. Jugulotympanic paraganglioma
C. Pheochromocytoma
D. Soft tissue glomus tumor
E. Vagal paraganglioma

7. What is the most common location for the paraganglioma depicted in the photomicrograph shown in Figure 1?

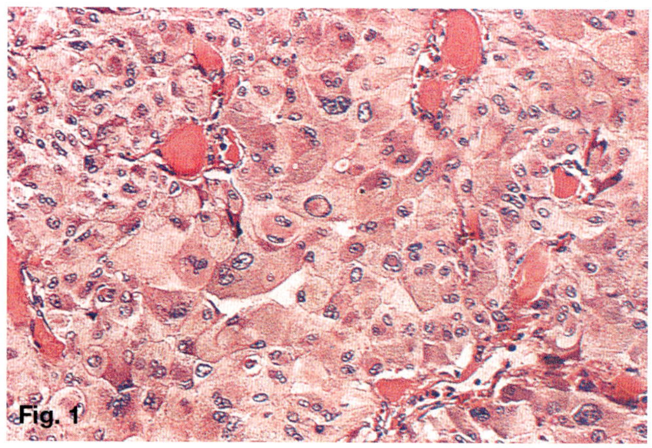

Fig. 1

A. Abdomen
B. Base of skull
C. Neck
D. Pelvis
E. Thorax

8. Which succinate dehydrogenase (SDH) gene mutation is typically associated with SDH-deficient gastrointestinal stromal tumor?

   A. *SDHA*
   B. *SDHAF2*
   C. *SDHB*
   D. *SDHC*
   E. *SDHD*

9. Which of the following constitute the Carney triad?

   A. Atrial myxoma, ephelides (freckles), myxoid neurofibroma
   B. Atrial myxoma, lentigines, peripheral nerve sheath tumors
   C. Gastrointestinal stromal tumor, paraganglioma, pituitary adenoma
   D. Gastrointestinal stromal tumor, paraganglioma, pulmonary chondroma
   E. Paraganglioma, pituitary adenoma, pulmonary chondroma

10. A 54-year-old female presents with painless hematuria and a recent onset of syncopal episodes during urination. Ultrasound scan demonstrated a mass in the trigone of the bladder, measuring 1.5 cm. A transurethral resection of the mass was performed (see Figure 1). During the procedure, the patient developed severe hypertension. What is the best diagnosis?

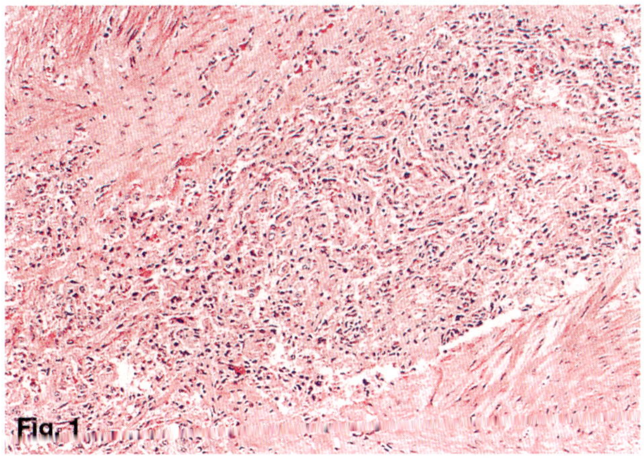


   A. Bladder paraganglioma
   B. Neuroendocrine tumor
   C. Normal paraganglion
   D. Pheochromocytoma
   E. Urothelial carcinoma

# ANSWERS AND EXPLANATIONS

**1. Correct choice: E.**

It is important to understand the anatomic distribution of normal paraganglion tissue because a key criterion for the diagnosis of malignant paraganglioma is spread to a site that does not normally have nonneoplastic paraganglion tissue. A variety of changes may be seen in paragangliomas, but as in epithelial neuroendocrine neoplasms, these changes are not associated with an increased risk of metastases. These changes include dense sclerosis, eosinophilic cytoplasmic inclusions, nuclear hyperchromasia and pleomorphism, spindled foci imparting a pseudosarcomatous appearance, and occasionally, melanin-like pigmentation. Tumor cell necrosis, vascular invasion, and markedly increased mitotic index are rarely seen but may herald more aggressive clinical behavior.

**2. Correct choice: A.**

This is the typical clinical, gross, and histologic presentation of a carotid body paraganglioma (chemodectoma). Paragangliomas may arise from parasympathetic paraganglia of the head and neck or from the sympathetic ganglia in the abdominal/pelvic cavities. Carotid body paraganglioma is the most common paraganglioma in the head and neck. In some patients, there may be signs or symptoms of cranial nerve palsy. Bradycardia and syncopal episodes are uncommon but reported. The carotid body tumors are rarely functional. Approximately 10% metastasize, usually to lymph nodes, lung, and bone. Nevertheless, the possibility of multicentric paragangliomas in the syndromic setting should be considered before diagnosing a metastasis. A key criterion for the diagnosis of metastasis is spread to a site that does not normally have nonneoplastic paraganglion tissue. Paragangliomas of the head and neck are morphologically similar, regardless of their location, and feature a nesting, zellballen-like arrangement.

**3. Correct choice: D.**

Chief cells form the nests of paragangliomas and express neuroendocrine markers, such as synaptophysin, chromogranin, and INSM1. Sustentacular cells encircle the nests and express S100. OCT4 is a sensitive marker of adrenal medullary and extra-adrenal medullary tissue. GATA3 is positive in the urinary bladder and pelvic paragangliomas. An array of other markers can be demonstrated in paragangliomas, most of which are related to the production of hormonal substances by paraganglionic tissue. Only rarely, such production results in clinical manifestations, as in the case of Cushing syndrome, due to adrenocorticotropic hormone (ACTH) secretion or watery diarrhea due to vasoactive intestinal peptide (VIP) secretion by sympathoadrenal paragangliomas.

**4. Correct choice: B.**

Glomus coccygeum is a normal structure of unknown function located at the tip of the coccyx. It consists of small epithelial-like cells, immunoreactive for vimentin and smooth muscle actin, layered around small vessels. It can be mistaken for a coccygeal glomus tumor or a paraganglioma in rectal or uterine resections performed for any reason. Paragangliomas of the cauda equina are located in the cauda equina, in connection with the filum terminale, thus within the dural sac; the differential diagnosis includes myxopapillary ependymoma. Gangliocytic paraganglioma is a tumor with a mixed paraganglioma/ganglioneuroma appearance arising in the duodenal wall.

**5. Correct choice: C.**

The succinate dehydrogenase (SDH) genes *SDHA*, *SDHB*, *SDHC*, and *SDHD* are encoded by autosomal nuclear DNA, but the SDH proteins are assembled at the inner mitochondrial membrane to form the mitochondrial complex 2, also known as the SDH complex, with the accessory factor SDHAF2 being necessary for flavination of SDHA. When any component of the SDH complex undergoes double hit inactivation, the entire complex becomes unstable, resulting in the degradation of the SDHB subunit. Therefore, immunohistochemistry for SDHB is negative in neoplastic cells whenever there is a double hit by mutation/inactivation of *SDHA*, *SDHB*, *SDHC*, *SDHD*, or *SDHAF2*.

**6. Correct choice: B.**

Jugulotympanic paraganglioma, also called glomus jugulare tumor, is the most common tumor of the middle ear. It typically occurs in women, aged 40 to 69 years. Most arise in the jugular bulb causing a mass in the middle ear or external auditory canal; 10% to 15% arise from the tympanic branch of the glossopharyngeal nerve (Jacobson nerve) causing a middle ear mass; and less than 5% arise from the posterior auricular branch of the vagus nerve (Arnold nerve) causing an external auditory canal mass. Patients with tympanic paragangliomas present with conductive hearing loss or tinnitus, while those with jugular paragangliomas often present with cranial nerve palsies. The differential diagnosis includes acoustic neuroma, meningioma, and middle ear adenoma. Soft tissue glomus tumor is not to be confused with glomus jugulare tumor, as the former is composed of cells resembling modified smooth muscle cells of the normal glomus body. The glomus body, a thermoregulator, is a specialized form of arteriovenous anastomosis localized in dermal and precoccygeal soft tissue.

**7. Correct choice: A.**

The photomicrograph depicts the typical microscopic features of extra-adrenal paragangliomas. These tumors arise from sympathetic paraganglia, which are histologically and functionally analogous to the adrenal medulla. Extra-adrenal paragangliomas typically have a broad anastomosing trabecular architecture similar to carcinoid tumors; however, an alveolar or zellballen pattern characteristic of head-and-neck paragangliomas can occasionally be seen. The highest concentration of extra-adrenal paraganglia is found in the retroperitoneal para-aortic regions from the origin of the inferior mesenteric arteries to the aortic bifurcation. They are known as organs of Zuckerkandl. Therefore, extra-adrenal paragangliomas are most commonly found in the retroperitoneal region of the abdomen. Abdominal extra-adrenal paragangliomas are malignant in 25% to 50% of cases.

**8. Correct choice: A.**

There is some correlation, albeit inconsistent, between the individual succinate dehydrogenase (SDH) subunit that is mutated/epimutated and some of the nonparaganglioma-related neoplasms. *SDHA* mutation is particularly associated with SDH-deficient gastrointestinal stromal tumors, whereas *SDHB* is more likely to be associated with SDH-deficient renal cell carcinoma.

**9. Correct choice: D.**

Carney triad is commonly associated with epimutation in *SDHC*. The triad consists of gastrointestinal stromal tumors, paraganglioma, and pulmonary chondroma. Not to be confused with Carney complex, which is a rare genetic disorder characterized by multiple benign tumors affecting the heart, skin, and endocrine system. Carney complex is due to mutations in *PRKAR1A*. Several acronyms for the Carney complex have been proposed. The LAMN acronym refers to lentigines, atrial myxomas, and blue nevi. The NAME acronym refers to nevi, atrial myxoma, neurofibromas, and ephelides (freckles).

**10. Correct choice: A.**

Bladder paraganglioma is an extra-adrenal paraganglioma arising from paraganglion cells that are normally present in the bladder. The median age is around 4 years, with an age range of 10 to 88 years. Young women are often affected. About 50% have hematuria and about 50% have a history of a "micturition attack" during urination with a full bladder, consisting of bursting headache, pounding sensation, anxiety, sweating, syncope, hypertension, or hematuria. Many cases are hereditary and associated with familial paraganglioma, neurofibromatosis Type 1, von Hippel-Lindau disease, Carney triad, or rarely multiple endocrine neoplasia 2 (MEN2). About 5% to 15% are malignant, but this cannot be predicted from histology. Bladder paragangliomas resemble paragangliomas elsewhere, with zellballen (diffuse patterns of large polygonal cells in clusters separated by a delicate fibrovascular stroma); cells have abundant eosinophilic granular cytoplasm, fairly uniform nuclei with smooth chromatin. Frequently involvement of the muscularis propria is present, but there is no desmoplastic reaction. In addition to the usual immunohistochemical profile of extra-adrenal paragangliomas, bladder paragangliomas may express GATA3. Neuroendocrine tumors may have a focal nesting pattern but are positive for cytokeratin. Pheochromocytoma arises in the adrenal medulla. Urothelial carcinoma may have a nesting pattern but more atypia; although it is positive for GATA3, it is also positive for cytokeratin and usually associated with carcinoma in situ or noninvasive papillary carcinoma.

# 16 Bone Marrow

1. The bone marrow biopsy shown in Figure 1 is most consistent with which of the following clinical conditions?

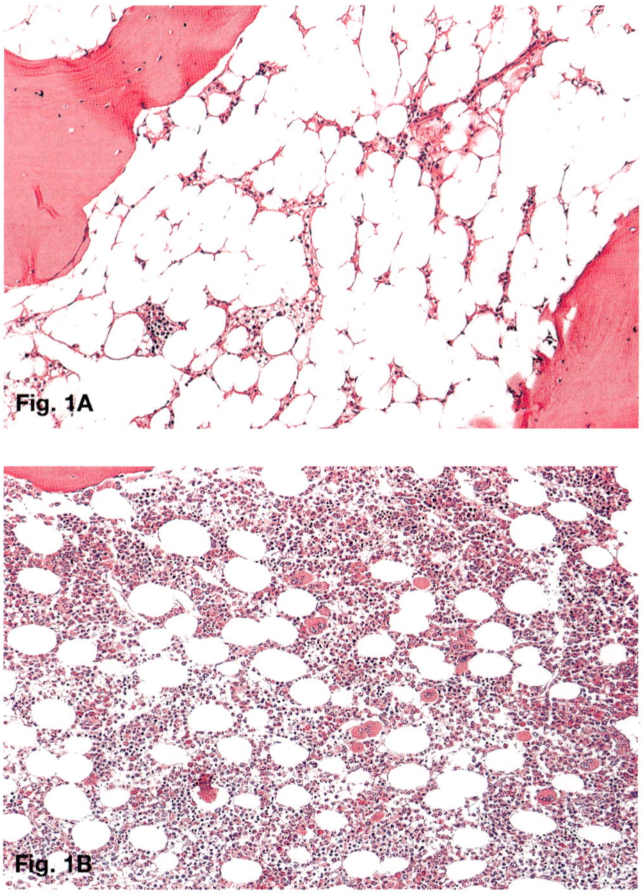


A. Acute leukemia
B. Blood loss
C. Bone marrow transplantation following normalization of blood counts
D. Ineffective hematopoiesis
E. Pancytopenia

2. The bone marrow smear and biopsy shown in Figure 1 is associated with positive parvovirus B19 immunoglobulin M (IgM) antibodies and negative IgG antibodies. These findings are most consistent with which of the following clinical presentations?

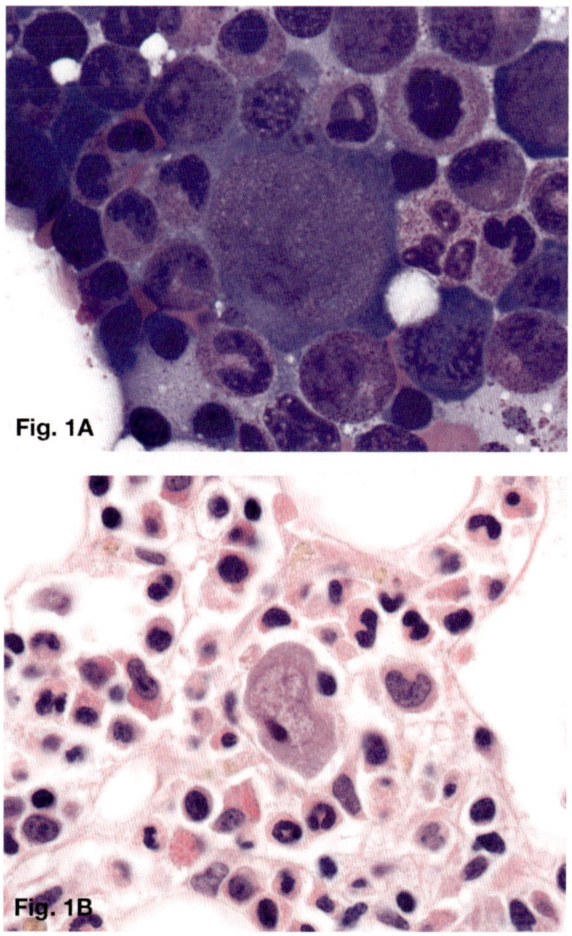


A. Acute myeloid leukemia
B. Immune thrombocytopenic purpura
C. Myelodysplastic syndrome
D. Neutropenia
E. Sudden, severe aplastic anemia

All figures in this chapter are from Longacre TA, Greenson JK, Hornick JL, Reuter VE, eds. *Mills and Sternberg's Diagnostic Surgical Pathology*. 7th ed. Wolters Kluwer; 2022 except for those noted at the end of this book.

3. The microscopic findings of a bone marrow biopsy from a 40-year-old patient with AIDS are shown in Figure 1. Besides AIDS, this characteristic change is associated most commonly with

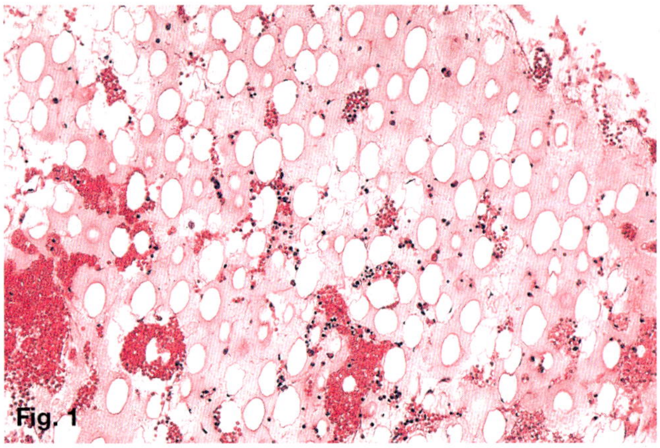


A. bone marrow transplantation.
B. cachexia.
C. drug toxicity.
D. parvovirus B19 infection.
E. rheumatoid arthritis.

4. A bone marrow biopsy from a 30-year-old male with fever of unknown origin reveals several lesions such as the one shown in Figure 1. Culture studies and special stains for infectious organisms are negative. What is the most common etiology of this lesion in a bone marrow biopsy?

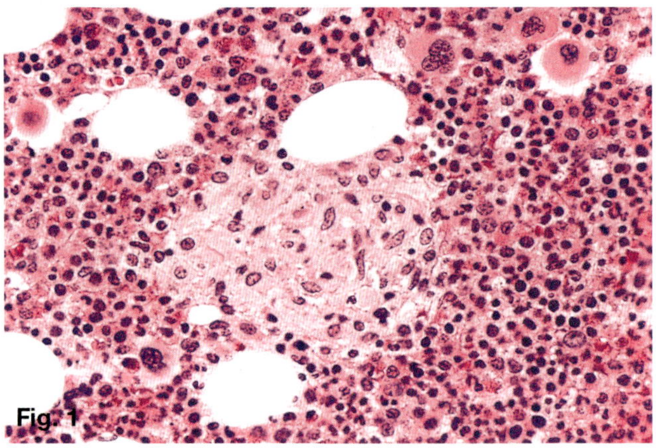


A. Idiopathic
B. Infectious
C. Non-Hodgkin lymphoma
D. Q fever
E. Sarcoidosis

5. A bone marrow biopsy is performed in a patient with clinical and hematologic findings suggestive of acute leukemia. Which of the following morphologic features allows distinguishing acute myeloid leukemia (AML) from acute lymphoblastic leukemia (ALL)?

A. Auer rods
B. Blast size
C. Chromatin pattern
D. Cytoplasmic features
E. Presence and number of nucleoli

6. Which of the following studies provides the most important prognostic indicators in acute leukemias?

A. Cytochemistry
B. Cytogenetics
C. Immunophenotyping
D. Molecular analysis
E. Morphology

7. A 12-year-old boy presents with fatigue, easy bruising, and a markedly elevated white blood count. A bone marrow aspirate and biopsy are performed. The smear shows myelomonocytic blasts and abnormal eosinophils with basophilic granules as depicted in Figure 1. Which of the following statements reflects this type of leukemia?

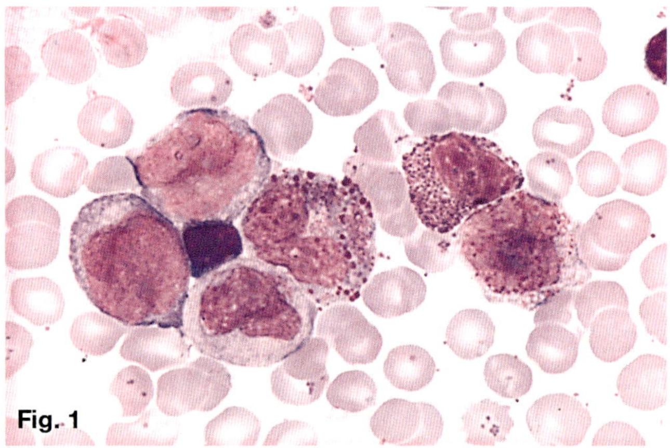


A. Associated with inv(16)(p13;q22)
B. Diagnosis requires 20% blasts
C. Eosinophils increased in peripheral smear
D. Has poorer prognosis than other acute myeloid leukemia (AML)
E. Low incidence of extramedullary disease

8. A 32-year-old woman presents with severe fatigue and weakness with pancytopenia and leukopenia. A bone marrow biopsy and aspiration are performed and representative morphology is shown in Figure 1. Soon after the biopsy, she develops disseminated intravascular coagulation. This leukemia is associated with which cytogenetic abnormality?

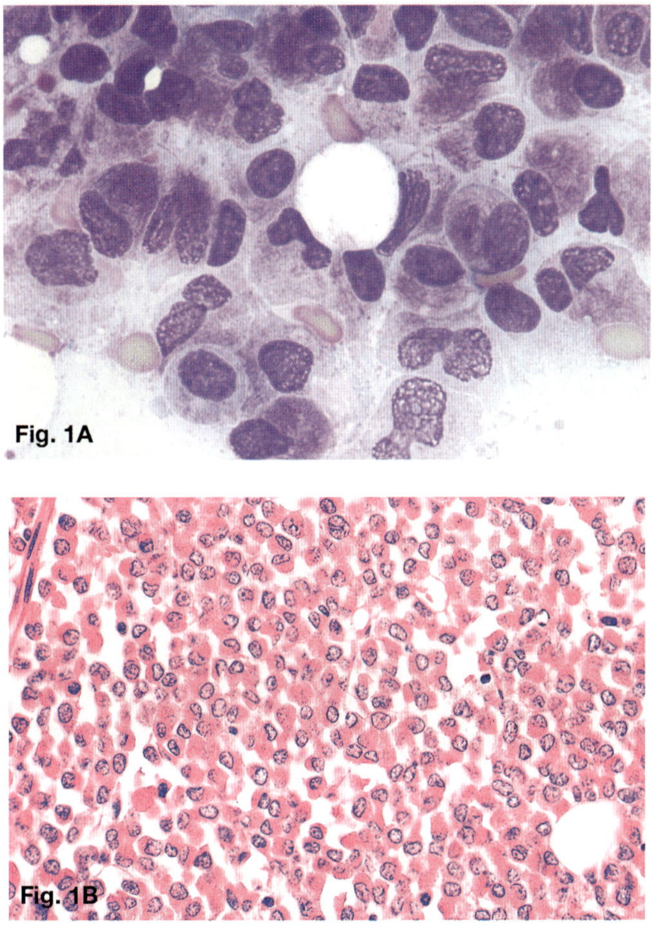

Fig. 1A

Fig. 1B

   A. t(1;22)(p13;q13)
   B. t(6;9)(p23;q34)
   C. t(8;21)(q22;q22)
   D. t(9;11)(p22;q23)
   E. t(15;17)(q22;q21)

9. Which is the most common type of acute myeloid leukemia, not otherwise specified?

   A. Acute megakaryoblastic leukemia
   B. Acute monoblastic and monocytic leukemia
   C. Acute myeloid leukemia with maturation
   D. Acute myeloid leukemia without maturation
   E. Acute myelomonocytic leukemia

10. A 58-year-old woman undergoes bone marrow examination because of blood cytopenia without apparent cause. The peripheral blood smear shows pancytopenia with pseudo-Pelger-Huët neutrophils (Figure 1). The aspirate contains abnormally segmented neutrophils and dysmorphic erythroid precursors (Figure 2) and small, hypolobated megakaryocytes (Figure 3), but blasts are not increased. The bone marrow biopsy shows clusters of immature myeloid precursors in an abnormal location, far from bone trabeculae. Which of the following is the most likely diagnosis?

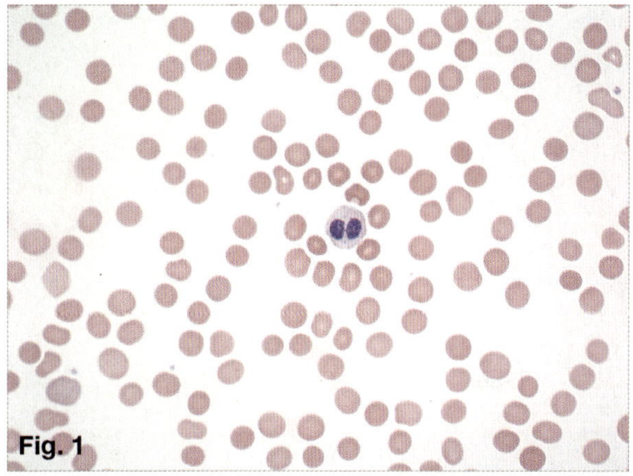

Fig. 1

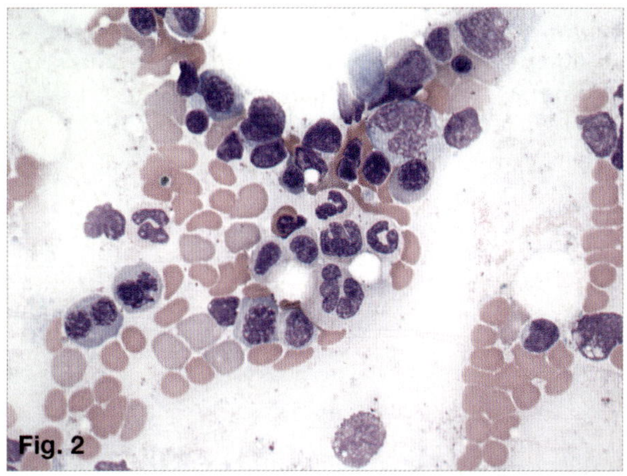

Fig. 2

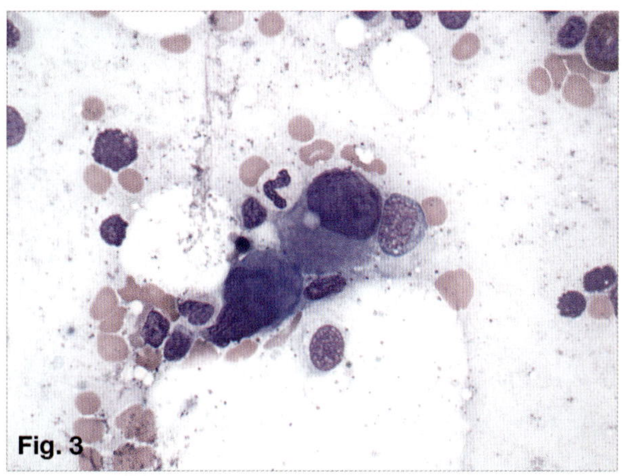

Fig. 3

   A. Chronic idiopathic myelofibrosis
   B. Chronic myeloid leukemia
   C. Essential thrombocythemia
   D. Myelodysplastic syndrome
   E. Polycythemia vera

11. A 60-year-old woman presents with headache, dizziness, vertigo, and visual disturbances. She has a markedly elevated hematocrit and hemoglobin as well as increased platelet count. A bone marrow biopsy (Figure 1) is markedly hypercellular with a striking increase in erythroid precursors and megakaryocytes. What is the most likely diagnosis?

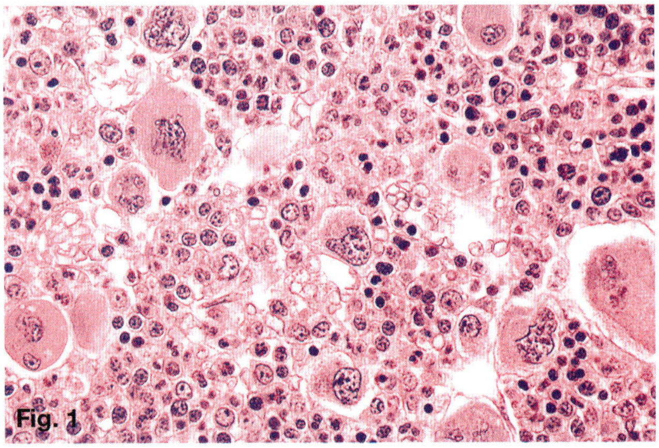


A. Chronic myeloid leukemia
B. Essential thrombocythemia
C. Polycythemia vera
D. Primary myelofibrosis
E. Secondary erythrocytosis

12. A 62-year-old African American woman has moderate-to-marked thrombocytosis on a routine complete blood count. Her peripheral smear shows platelet anisocytosis and abnormally large platelets. A bone marrow biopsy is performed (Figure 1). What is the most likely diagnosis?

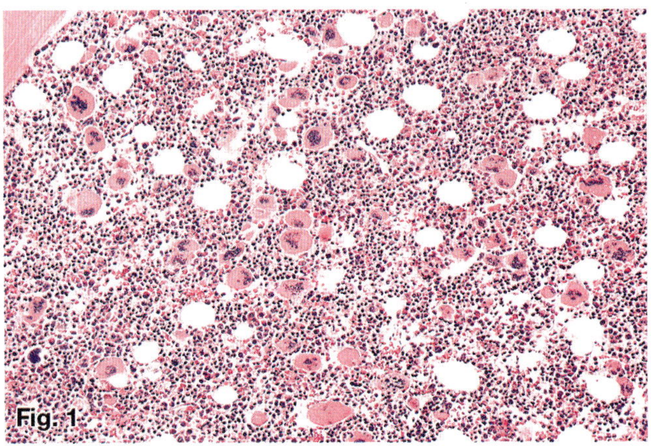


A. Chronic myeloid leukemia
B. Essential thrombocythemia
C. Mastocytosis
D. Polycythemia vera
E. Primary myelofibrosis

13. A 70-year-old man has anemia, thrombocytopenia, and splenomegaly. His peripheral blood smear shows a leukoerythroblastic pattern and teardrop erythrocytes. A bone marrow biopsy shows features depicted in Figure 1. What is the most likely diagnosis?

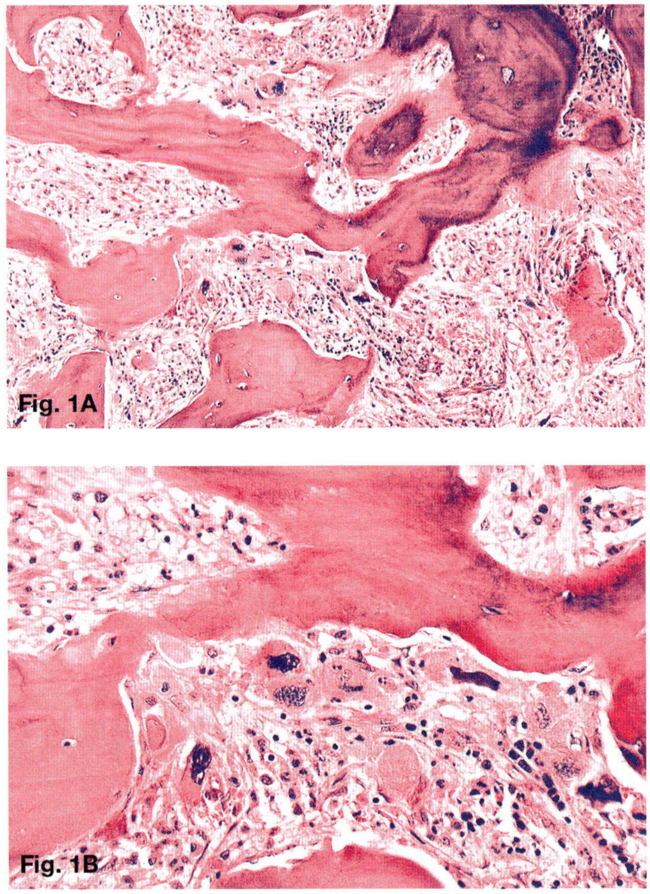


A. Chronic myeloid leukemia
B. Essential thrombocythemia
C. Mastocytosis
D. Polycythemia vera
E. Primary myelofibrosis

14. A 54-year-old man has leukocytosis with predominantly neutrophils and myelocytes on a routine blood examination. Occasional myeloblasts are present on the peripheral blood smear (Figure 1). What is the most likely diagnosis?

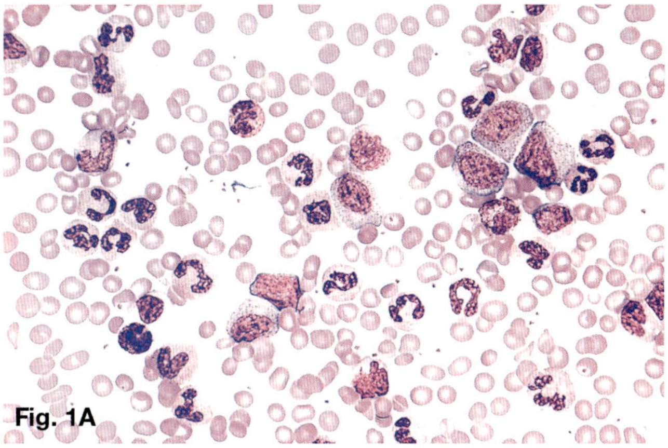
Fig. 1A

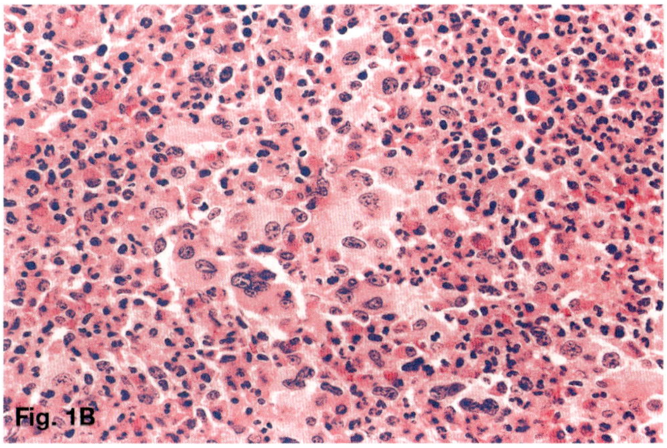
Fig. 1B

A. Chronic myeloid leukemia
B. Essential thrombocythemia
C. Mastocytosis
D. Polycythemia vera
E. Primary myelofibrosis

15. Systemic mast cell disease is clinically suspected in a 67-year-old female patient. A bone marrow biopsy reveals multiple foci of abnormal cell infiltrates such as the one shown in Figure 1. Which of the following special techniques is most useful to confirm bone marrow involvement by mast cell disease?

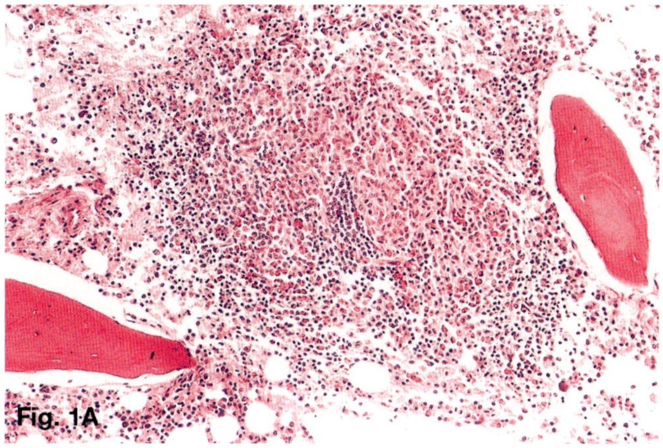
Fig. 1A

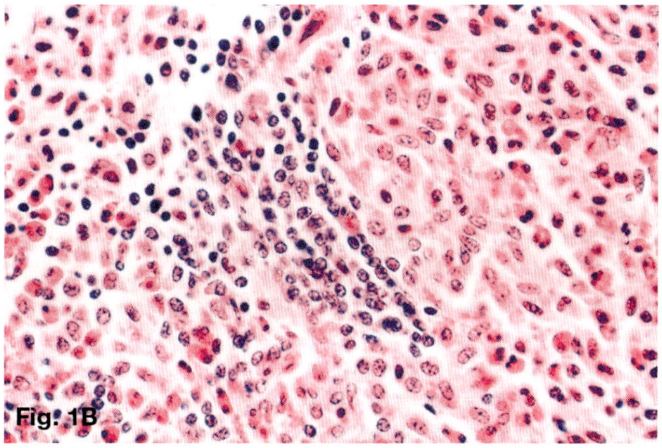
Fig. 1B

A. CD1a immunohistochemistry
B. Myeloperoxidase histochemistry
C. Tartrate-resistant acid phosphatase (TRAP) histochemistry
D. Tryptase immunohistochemistry
E. Ultrastructural studies

16. A focal paratrabecular pattern of marrow involvement by non-Hodgkin lymphoma as depicted in Figure 1 is most consistent with

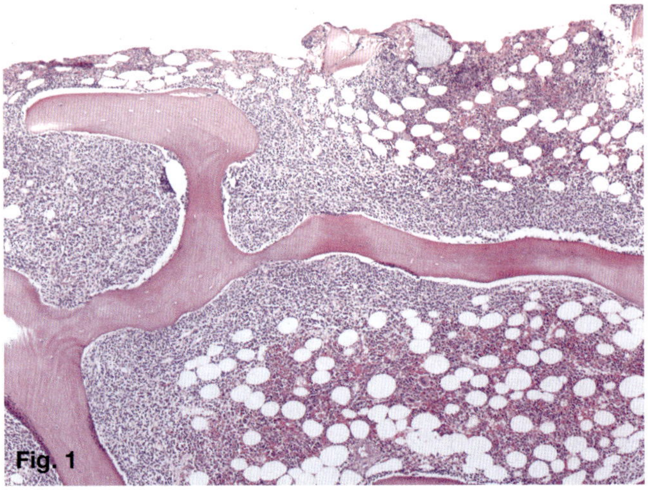

Fig. 1

A. Burkitt lymphoma.
B. follicular lymphoma.
C. hepatosplenic T-cell lymphoma.
D. mantle cell lymphoma.
E. small lymphocytic lymphoma/chronic lymphocytic leukemia.

17. A focal, random pattern of marrow involvement by non-Hodgkin lymphoma as depicted in Figure 1 is most consistent with

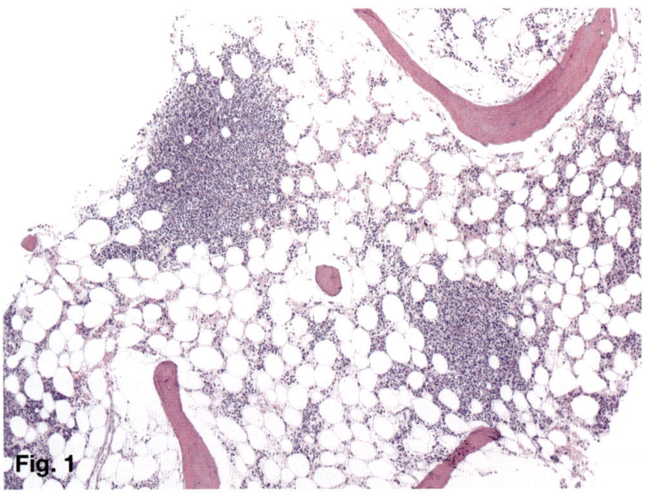

Fig. 1

A. Burkitt lymphoma.
B. follicular lymphoma.
C. hepatosplenic T-cell lymphoma.
D. mantle cell lymphoma.
E. small lymphocytic lymphoma/chronic lymphocytic leukemia.

18. With respect to evaluation of bone marrow involvement by Hodgkin lymphoma, which of the following is correct?

A. Aspirate smears are more sensitive than are trephine biopsies.
B. "Dry taps" imply a lack of bone marrow involvement.
C. Hodgkin lymphoma type can be correctly classified in the bone marrow.
D. Immunohistochemistry for CD45 is useful in identifying Reed-Sternberg cells.
E. Reed-Sternberg cells are found in a stromal reaction characteristic of Hodgkin lymphoma.

19. A bone marrow biopsy of a 60-year-old woman contains a cell cluster like the one shown in Figure 1. This finding is commonly associated with

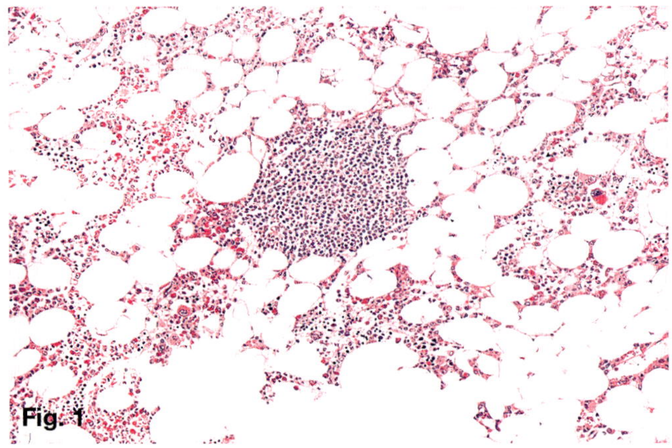

Fig. 1

A. acquired immunodeficiency syndrome.
B. no specific disorder.
C. rheumatoid arthritis.
D. small lymphocytic lymphoma.
E. splenic marginal zone lymphoma.

20. A 58-year-old man presents with a history of progressive fatigue and weight loss. A complete blood count reveals pancytopenia but no blasts. A bone marrow biopsy was performed (Figure 1) showing extensive marrow replacement by mononuclear cells with widely spaced nuclei, some of which exhibit a reniform appearance. Molecular testing detected a *BRAF* V600E mutation on the bone marrow sample. What is the most likely diagnosis?

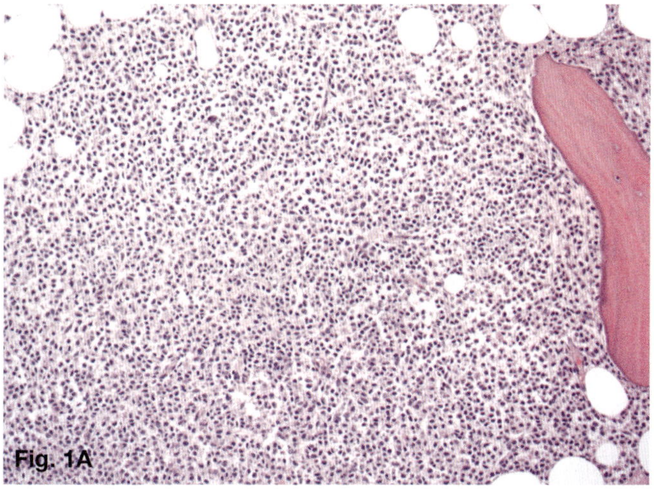
Fig. 1A

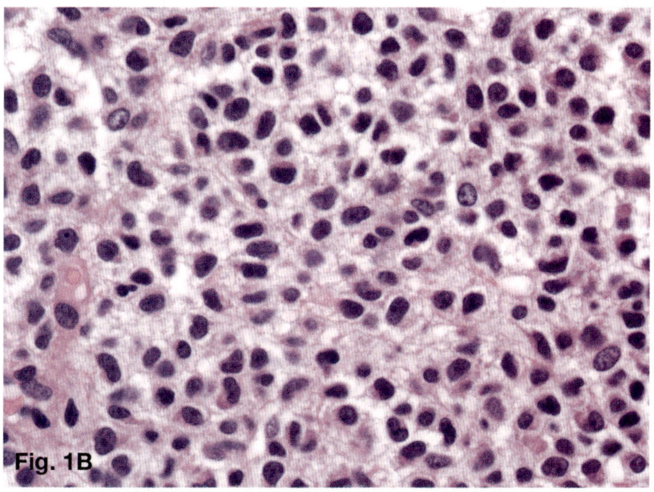
Fig. 1B

A. Chronic lymphocytic leukemia
B. Diffuse large B-cell lymphoma
C. Hairy cell leukemia
D. Mantle cell lymphoma
E. Reactive polymorphous lymphohistiocytic lesions

21. A bone marrow examination is performed in a 58-year-old man with a monoclonal spike in his serum protein electrophoresis. The smear of the marrow aspirate contains more than 10% of the cells shown in Figure 1. Immunohistochemistry for immunoglobulin (Ig) light chains shows the ratio between $\kappa$ and $\lambda$ expression to be in excess of 16:1. Which of the following is the most likely diagnosis?

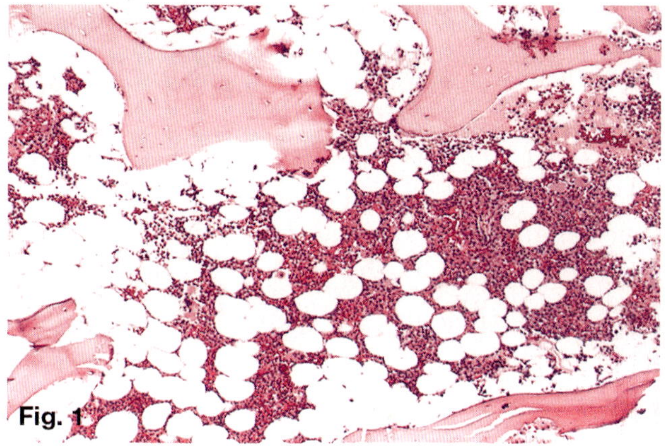
Fig. 1

A. Immunoblastic lymphoma
B. Monoclonal gammopathy of undetermined significance (MGUS)
C. Multiple myeloma
D. Plasmacytoma
E. Reactive plasmacytosis

22. A 56-year-old man presents with monoclonal gammopathy, organomegaly, polyneuropathy, and multiple bone lesions. What is the most likely diagnosis?

A. Monoclonal gammopathy of undetermined significance (MGUS)
B. Nonsecretory myeloma
C. Osteosclerotic myeloma
D. Plasma cell leukemia
E. Smoldering myeloma

23. A bone marrow aspirate from a 25-year-old woman of Jewish descent with hepatosplenomegaly and pancytopenia reveals the cells shown in Figure 1. This patient's condition is due to inherited deficiency of

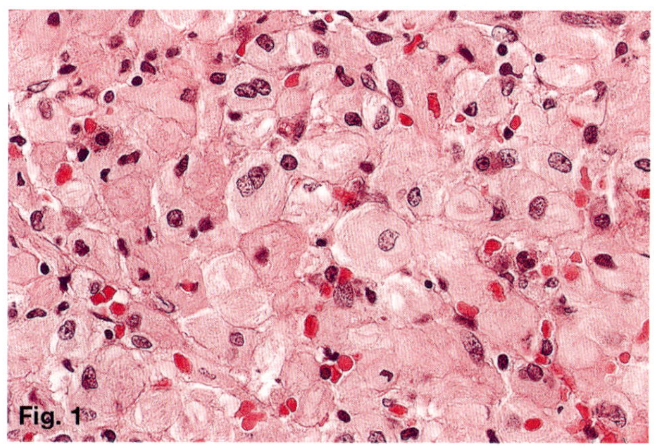
Fig. 1

A. acid maltase (acid $\alpha$-glucosidase).
B. acid sphingomyelinase.
C. $\alpha$-1-antitrypsin.
D. $\beta$-hexosaminidase A.
E. galactocerebrosidase.

24. Large numbers of normal lymphoid progenitor cells (hematogones) depicted in Figure 1 are seen in which of the following conditions?

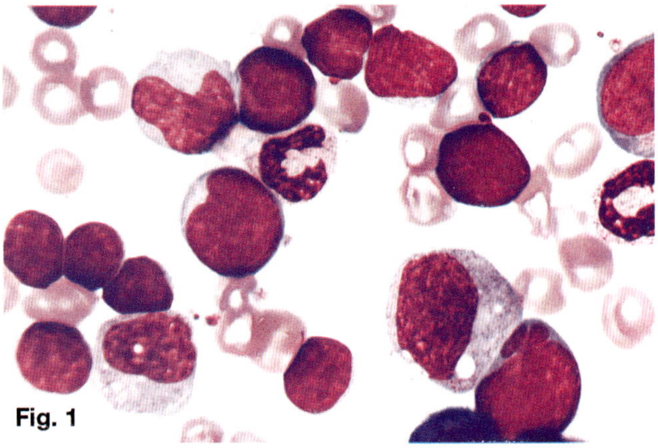

Fig. 1

A. Congenital cytopenias
B. Immune cytopenias
C. Immune thrombocytopenic purpura
D. Regenerative marrows
E. All of the above

25. A 5-year-old boy with Down syndrome has anemia, neutropenia, and thrombocytopenia on a complete blood count. He has no adenopathy and imaging studies are unremarkable. A bone marrow aspirate and biopsy are performed. Blasts with sparse cytoplasm and a high nuclear-to-cytoplasmic ratio are present on the peripheral blood smear (Figure 1). Auer rods are absent. The bone marrow biopsy is markedly hypercellular and the marrow is replaced by a uniform, diffuse proliferation of blasts with scant cytoplasm (Figure 2). Flow cytometry demonstrates the blasts express CD19, CD22, CD79a, and CD10, as well as CD34, TdT (terminal deoxynucleotidyl transferase), and CD15. What is the most likely diagnosis?

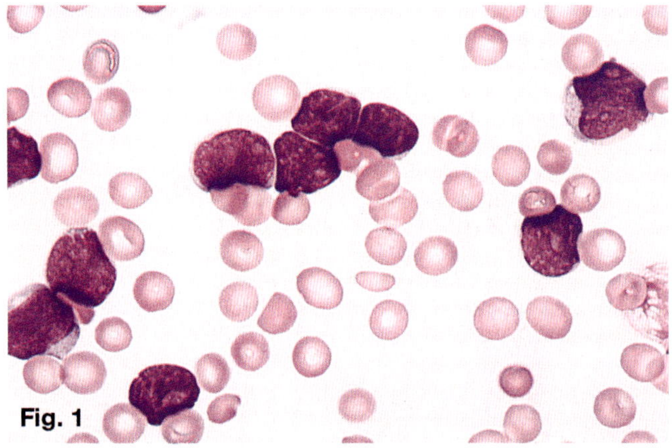

Fig. 1

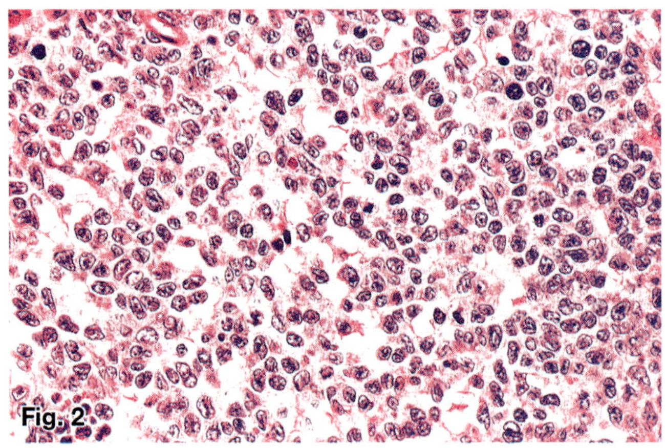

Fig. 2

A. Acute megakaryoblastic leukemia
B. Acute myeloid leukemia
C. B-lymphoblastic leukemia (B-ALL)
D. T-lymphoblastic leukemia (T-ALL)
E. Transient abnormal myelopoiesis

# ANSWERS AND EXPLANATIONS

**1. Correct choice: E.**

Severe aplastic anemia manifests with pancytopenia and is due to a marked decrease in hematopoietic marrow, associated with the expansion of fat. In the most severe cases, as the one in Figure 1, scanty hematopoietic cell clusters are found admixed with hemosiderin-laden histiocytes, lymphocytes, and plasma cells. Acute leukemia leads to hypercellular marrow. Blood loss will cause a compensatory expansion of the erythroid line. Successful bone marrow transplantation results in normocellular marrow and clinically manifests with a return of blood counts to normal levels (1-2 months after the operation, faster with autologous transplants). Ineffective hematopoiesis leads to hypercellular bone marrow.

**2. Correct choice: E.**

Parvovirus B19 infection should always be considered as one of the causes of sudden and severe aplastic anemia. Bone marrow smears show giant pronormoblasts (see Figure 1). Although it is more common in children with hematologic disorders and patients who are immunocompromised, cases have occurred in adults who are immunocompetent. The virus affects bone marrow erythroid precursors, causing marked erythroblast hypoplasia and immature giant erythroblasts with resultant sudden and severe, but transient aplastic crisis. Occasional erythroblasts may have intranuclear inclusions with a surrounding rim of residual chromatin (see Figure 2). The virus can be detected in the abnormal pronormoblasts by immunohistochemistry or in situ hybridization.

**3. Correct choice: B.**

Serous atrophy is a frequent finding in patients with AIDS as well as in patients suffering from extreme malnutrition, cachexia, and starvation. The gelatinous eosinophilic appearance of the extracellular substance and atrophy of the adipose tissue are diagnostic features.

**4. Correct choice: A.**

Each of the conditions in the provided choices is potential cause of bone marrow granulomas. However, in the majority of cases (probably up to 80%), the underlying etiology remains unclear despite all appropriate investigations, including special stains, cultures, and polymerase chain reaction (PCR) for microorganisms. Another very common form of granuloma that can be seen in the bone marrow is a lipid granuloma, which is analogous to that observed in the spleen, liver, and lymph nodes. Histiocytes in lipid granulomas contain intracytoplasmic lipid droplets.

**5. Correct choice: A.**

All of the previous morphologic features are helpful in distinguishing acute myeloid leukemia (AML) from acute lymphoblastic leukemia (ALL), but only unequivocal Auer rods (present in two-thirds of AML cases) can definitively establish a diagnosis of AML on the morphologic ground. Auer rods appear as cytoplasmic, eosinophilic, needle-like inclusions within myeloid cells. AML affects middle-aged persons and is subdivided depending on blast maturation, morphology, and cytogenetic abnormalities.

**6. Correct choice: B.**

Cytogenetic abnormalities are the most important prognostic indicators in acute leukemias and can help diagnose specific entities. Cytochemistry is useful in distinguishing acute myeloid leukemia (AML) from acute lymphoblastic leukemia (ALL). Myeloperoxidase (or Sudan Black) will be positive in AML but not ALL, and nonspecific esterase allows the identification of monocytic differentiation in AML. Immunophenotyping by flow cytometry allows distinguishing AML from ALL when morphology and cytochemistry are not conclusive and help to classify ALL. Molecular analysis can be used to establish clonality, detect chromosomal abnormalities, identify mutations or fusion genes, and identify tumor-associated viruses. Morphology is essential in the differential diagnosis between leukemias, other neoplasms, and nonneoplastic disorders, in distinguishing between AML and ALL, and in the classification of leukemias.

**7. Correct choice: A.**

Acute myeloid leukemia (AML) with inv(16)(p13;q22) or t(16;16)(p13;q22); CBFB-MYH11 (core-binding factor β-myosin heavy chain 11) is a subtype of AML characterized by myelomonocytic differentiation and presence of abnormal eosinophils. The diagnosis of AML with inv(16)(p13;q22). The abnormal eosinophils are increased in the marrow but typically not in the peripheral blood smear. The prognosis is good compared with other AMLs, even though the incidence of extramedullary disease is higher than for most types of AML.

**8. Correct choice: E.**

Promyelocytic leukemia is an acute myeloid leukemia with predominance of abnormal promyelocytes, characterized by t(15;17)(q24.1;q21.2) leading to PML-RARA (promyelocytic leukemia-retinoic acid receptor α) fusion. It occurs in young to middle-aged adults. There are two morphologic variants: hypergranular and microgranular. Early diagnosis and treatment are important due to the high risk of coagulopathy and disseminated intravascular coagulation. Leukopenia is a common presenting sign for the hypergranular variant (depicted in Figure 1). The hypergranular variant is characterized by abnormal promyelocytes varying in size and shape, frequently with kidney-shaped or bilobed nuclei. The cytoplasm is packed with large granules, staining bright pink, red, or purple. Auer rods, frequently in bundles, are often present. The microgranular variant has submicroscopic azurophilic granules and predominantly bilobed nuclei.

**9. Correct choice: C.**

Acute myeloid leukemia (AML), not otherwise specified, encompasses the cases of AML that do not fulfill the criteria for inclusion in one of the more specified AML entities. The criterion for AML, not otherwise specified, is the presence of greater than or equal to 20% myeloid blasts in the peripheral blood or bone marrow. AML with maturation is the most common type of AML, not otherwise specified. It is defined as follows: 20% or more of nonerythroid cells in peripheral blood or bone marrow are myeloblasts; monocytic precursors are less than 20% in bone marrow, and granulocytes are 10% of cells or more.

**10. Correct choice: D.**

Myelodysplastic syndrome is a heterogeneous bone marrow stem cell disorder that results in maturation defects of one or more myeloid lines leading to ineffective hematopoiesis. It usually manifests with blood cytopenia in patients older than 50 years and has a propensity to transform into acute myeloid leukemia (AML). The bone marrow is usually hypercellular. A useful diagnostic feature is the finding of abnormal, immature myeloid precursors away from their normal paratrabecular location. About one-third of patients will progress to AML within a few months.

**11. Correct choice: C.**

Polycythemia vera is a myeloproliferative disorder defined as panhyperplasia of the bone marrow accompanied by increased numbers of circulating erythrocytes, leukocytes, and platelets.

The most striking abnormality is hyperplasia of both megakaryocytes and erythroid precursors.

Hemoglobin, hematocrit, and platelet count are increased, while blood levels of erythropoietin are decreased. Diagnostic criteria include elevated gender-dependent hemoglobin or hematocrit or increased red cell mass, hypercellular marrow with panmyelosis and atypical megakaryocytes, low serum erythropoietin levels, and the presence of *JAK2* V617F or *JAK2* exon 12 mutations. Bone marrow reticulin increases progressively until the histologic picture is indistinguishable from primary myelofibrosis in the late stages. Blood levels of erythropoietin are increased, and megakaryocytic hyperplasia is absent in secondary erythrocytosis.

**12. Correct choice: B.**

Essential thrombocythemia is a myeloproliferative disorder characterized by marked hyperplasia of megakaryocytes and sustained platelet counts over $450 \times 10^9$/L (according to the WHO definition). Megakaryocytes in the bone marrow have atypical features, the most characteristic of which are described as staghorn-like, with large hyperlobated nuclei.

**13. Correct choice: E.**

Primary myelofibrosis is characterized by progressive fibrosis and obliteration of functioning marrow, with secondary development of extramedullary hematopoiesis in the spleen and liver.

In the initial hypercellular (prefibrotic) phase, the marrow is hypercellular with an increase in granulocytic precursors and megakaryocytes; fibrosis may not be readily apparent, unless reticulin staining is used; blood cell count is normal or increased. At a later patchy phase, the increase in bone marrow fibrosis is patchy and accompanied by a progressive reduction in functioning marrow; the blood cell count begins to drop; extramedullary hematopoiesis and splenomegaly develop. The advanced obliterative phase is characterized by extensive bone marrow fibrosis, teardrop erythrocytes in peripheral blood, and compensatory extramedullary hematopoiesis with massive splenomegaly. Atypical megakaryocytes are present in all phases. Factors released by megakaryocytes appear to initiate the pathologic process.

**14. Correct choice: A.**

Chronic myeloid leukemia is a myeloproliferative neoplasm characterized by clonal granulocytic proliferation. Most patients are diagnosed in the chronic phase and almost 50% of patients diagnosed in the United States are asymptomatic and diagnosed during a routine examination. The disease arises from a pluripotent stem cell with t(9;22)(q34.1;q11.2) chromosomal translocation and formation of the Philadelphia (Ph) chromosome, containing the *BCR-ABL1* fusion gene. During the chronic phase, the bone marrow is hypercellular with myeloid hyperplasia (the myeloid-to-erythroid ratio is ≥10:1) and increased basophils and eosinophils. Blasts are less than 5% in the chronic phase but increase during the accelerated phase and eventually equal or exceed 20% in the blast phase.

**15. Correct choice: D.**

Mastocytosis arises as a clonal proliferation of mast cells that may present as solitary organ involvement or widespread systemic disease. The systemic form of mast cell disease involves the bone marrow in the majority of cases, most frequently in a patchy manner. A bone marrow biopsy is usually performed to confirm the clinical diagnosis. Presence of bone marrow infiltrates of at least 15 mast cells each represents the WHO major criterion. The diagnosis is made with a combination of the major criterion plus one of the minor criteria or three minor criteria. Mast cells are spindly cells similar to histiocytes or fibroblasts. They have cytoplasmic granules that stain red with toluidine blue. Immunocytochemistry for mast cell tryptase is the most sensitive and specific method for the identification of mast cells in the bone marrow. They also express CD117, but this marker is also expressed by early myeloid precursors. An activating KIT mutation is found in 95% of cases and imparts resistance to tyrosine kinase treatment.

**16. Correct choice: B.**

Non-Hodgkin lymphoma involves the bone marrow in up to 50% of cases. Bone marrow biopsies are usually performed for staging purposes. Marrow involvement can be categorized into five patterns: focal paratrabecular, focal random, interstitial, diffuse, and intravascular/intrasinusoidal. The focal paratrabecular pattern is the most common and is typically seen in follicular lymphoma, predominantly small cell lymphoma, and mixed small and large cell lymphoma.

**17. Correct choice: E.**

Non-Hodgkin lymphoma involves the bone marrow in up to 50% of cases. Bone marrow biopsies are usually performed for staging purposes. In addition to the more common focal paratrabecular pattern, focal random, interstitial, diffuse, and intravascular/intrasinusoidal patterns can be seen. The focal random pattern is typically seen in small lymphocytic lymphoma. An interstitial and diffuse pattern of marrow involvement is seen in Burkitt and lymphoblastic lymphoma, while an intravascular/sinusoidal pattern is characteristic of splenic marginal zone lymphoma, hepatosplenic T-cell lymphoma, intravascular large B-cell lymphoma.

**18. Correct choice: E.**

Hodgkin lymphoma involves the bone marrow in 5% to 15% of cases at the time of clinical presentation. The pattern of involvement is usually diffuse. Aspiration smears are ineffective in detecting Hodgkin lymphoma in the bone marrow, in contrast to trephine iliac biopsies, especially when these are performed bilaterally. A "dry tap" is usually caused by extensive bone marrow fibrosis. Reed-Sternberg cells can be more easily detected in areas with the typical cellular background of Hodgkin lymphoma or areas of fibrosis. They are not found in areas of otherwise normal marrow. Immunostains for CD15 and CD30 are positive on Reed-Sternberg cells and may help identify them in difficult cases. Leukocyte common antigen (LCA [CD45]) is negative on Reed-Sternberg cells.

**19. Correct choice: B.**

Lymphocytic aggregates represent the most common reactive lymphoid lesions in the bone marrow. Found in up to 47% of all marrow biopsies; the frequency of lymphocytic aggregates increases with age, but they have no pathologic significance. Their small size, round configuration, and well-demarcated outline help distinguish them from lymphomas. Other reactive lymphoid infiltrates include reactive polymorphous lymphohistiocytic lesions (lymphocytes, transformed lymphocytes, plasma cells, and histiocytes), seen in AIDS and rheumatoid arthritis; lymphoid follicles with germinal centers seen in immune or inflammatory disorders; systemic polyclonal immunoblastic proliferations.

**20. Correct choice: C.**

Hairy cell leukemia is a rare, indolent lymphoproliferative neoplasm of mature B cells with a distinct clinical presentation that includes peripheral blood cytopenias, Splenomegaly is often present in more long-standing cases and there may be circulating neoplastic cells with hairlike cytoplasmic projections. The cells express CD11c bright, CD22 bright, CD25, CD103, CD123 and CD200 bright, and TRAP (tartrate resistant acid phosphatase) positive. *BRAF* V600E mutation is a hallmark genetic mutation in greater than 95% of cases. Reactive lymphoid hyperplasia of bone marrow is characterized by an increase in benign-appearing lymphocytes and can be polymorphous, comprising small- to medium-sized lymphocytes admixed with plasma cells, histiocytes, and sometimes occasional immunoblasts, eosinophils, and mast cells. It is associated with immune cytopenia, collagen vascular disease, and AIDS.

**21. Correct choice: C.**

The diagnosis of multiple myeloma relies on serum and urine protein electrophoresis and immunofixation, serum and urine protein quantification, serum-free light chain analysis, radiographic skeletal studies, and bone marrow examination. The pattern and extent of marrow infiltration are very variable. The rule of 10% of plasma cells in marrow smears as a minimum for a diagnosis is not always valid because the involvement of bone marrow may be patchy. Light chain restriction by immunohistochemistry is often useful in confirming the monoclonal nature of plasma cells. Ratios greater than 16:1 are usually associated with multiple myeloma, whereas ratios less than 16:1 are found in reactive plasmacytosis and monoclonal gammopathy of undetermined significance (MGUS). No bone lesions are present in MGUS, a condition seen in up to 3% of persons over 70. Use of CD138 immunohistochemistry is useful in evaluating the numbers of plasma cells.

**22. Correct choice: C.**

The osteosclerotic variant of multiple myeloma is associated with sclerotic bone lesions, sometimes with polyneuropathy, organomegaly, endocrinopathy, monoclonal gammopathy, and skin lesions (POEMS syndrome); the prognosis is good. Smoldering and indolent myeloma have the same features as do classic multiple myeloma in the marrow, but these conditions remain without end-organ damage for a long time, even without treatment. Monoclonal gammopathy of undetermined significance (MGUS) affects up to 3% of persons older than 70 and lacks bone lesions and light chains in the urine; it progresses to multiple myeloma in 25% of cases within 10 years. The nonsecretory variant is rare; in this variant, no monoclonal protein is detected in blood or urine, but monoclonal light chains can be demonstrated in marrow plasma cells by immunohistochemistry.

**23. Correct choice: E.**

Gaucher disease is an autosomal recessive disorder characterized by hepatosplenomegaly, painful bone lesions, pancytopenia due to bone marrow failure, and accumulation of glucocerebroside-laden histiocytes (Gaucher cells), which have a characteristic crumpled paperlike cytoplasm. It is common among Jewish people of East European descent and results from glucocerebrosidase deficiency. Pompe disease (glycogenosis type II) is associated with the accumulation of glycogen in all organs, especially the heart and due to deficiency in acid maltase (acid α-glucosidase). Niemann-Pick disease is characterized by the accumulation of sphingomyelin in the nervous system and visceral organs (liver and spleen), and death before 3 years is due to deficiency in acid sphingomyelinase. Tay-Sachs disease, characterized by accumulation of GM2 ganglioside in neurons and retina, with mental retardation and neurologic deterioration beginning in the first year of life is due to a deficiency in galactocerebrosidase.

**24. Correct choice: E.**

Increased numbers of normal lymphoid progenitor cells (hematogones) may be seen in all of the conditions mentioned in the options, as well as in some other neoplastic disorders. Hematogones express a reproducible spectrum of B-cell precursor-associated antigens including CD10, CD19, CD20, CD22, CD34, CD38, CD45, and TdT (terminal deoxynucleotidyl transferase). They are heterogeneous in their expression of these antigens and show a characteristic maturation pattern that is best identified on multicolor flow cytometry. Pathologists should be knowledgeable about the conditions in which these normal lymphoid progenitor cells are increased (sometimes dramatically, up to 70% of the marrow) to avoid misdiagnosis of B-lymphoblastic leukemia/lymphoma.

**25. Correct choice: C.**

Leukemia is the most common childhood malignancy. It accounts for almost 30% of all malignancies in children. The most common types in children are acute lymphoblastic leukemia (ALL) and acute myeloid leukemia (AML). ALL is a highly aggressive neoplasm of precursor lymphoid (blast) cells. There are two main subtypes based on lymphoid lineage: B-lymphoblastic leukemia/lymphoma (B-ALL/LBL) and T-lymphoblastic leukemia/lymphoma (T-ALL/LBL).

Immunophenotyping should be performed on all cases of ALL to differentiate it from AML and to distinguish B-ALL from T-ALL. The lymphoblasts in B-ALL express various combinations of B-lymphocyte-associated antigens CD19, CD79a, CD22, CD24, CD10, and CD9 as well as CD34, TdT (terminal deoxynucleotidyl transferase), HLA-DR (human leukocyte antigen-DR), CD38, and CD45. In about 50% of cases, the blasts coexpress myeloid antigens CD13, CD15, and CD33 which do not warrant their designation as biphenotypic. T-ALL/LBL most commonly presents as an anterior mediastinal mass with or without superior vena cava syndrome. The lymphoblasts in T-ALL express various combinations of T-lymphocyte-associated antigens Cd1a, CD2, CD3, CD4, CD5, CD7, and CD8 as well as TdT. Acute megakaryoblastic leukemia blasts may resemble lymphoblasts but variably express CD13, Cd33, HLA-DR, and CD71; most express CD36. Megakaryocytic-specific antigens CD41, CD42b, and CD61 are also expressed. Transient abnormal myelopoiesis is a clonal proliferation of myeloid blasts and other immature myeloid cells that occurs in the peripheral blood in 10% of neonates with Down syndrome. The process usually resolves without therapeutic intervention, but up to 30% of affected patients develop AML 1 to 3 years later (typically acute megakaryoblastic leukemia). Patients with Down syndrome are at risk for all the choices. In fact, there is an approximately equal distribution between AML and ALL in young children with Down syndrome.

# 17 Lymph Nodes

1. The reactive pattern seen in the H&E (hematoxylin and eosin)-stained section of an enlarged lymph node, shown in Figure 1, is most consistent with

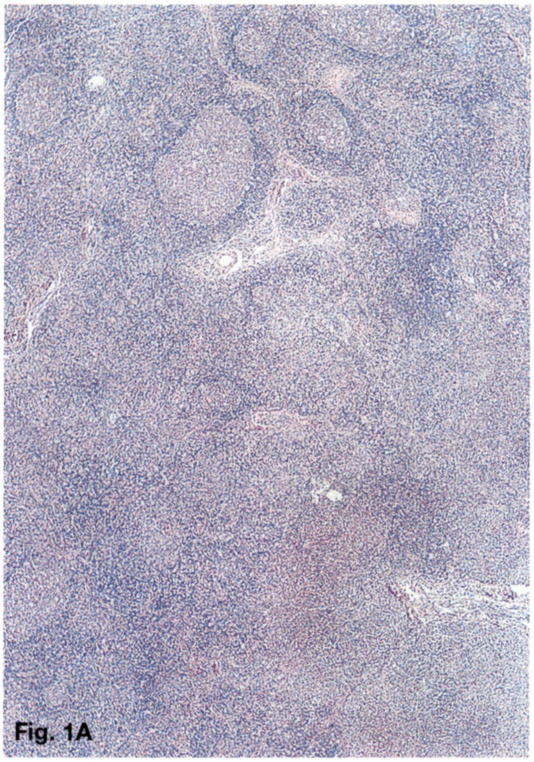

Fig. 1A

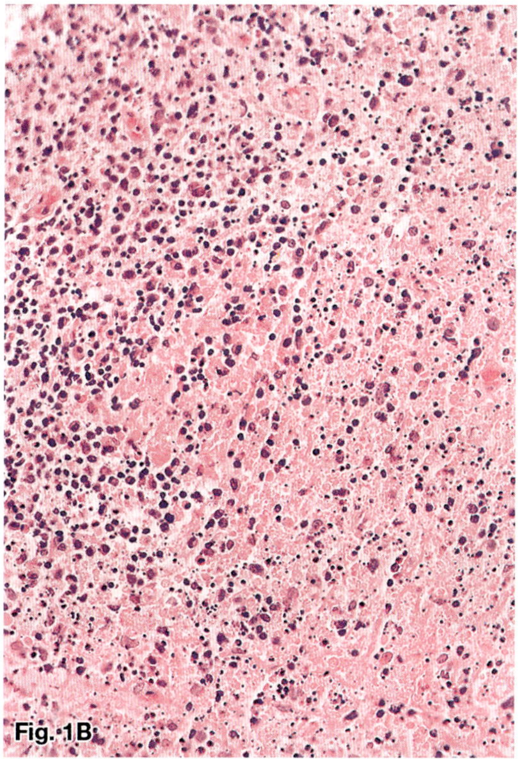

Fig. 1B

A. acquired immunodeficiency syndrome.
B. cat-scratch disease.
C. syphilis.
D. systemic lupus erythematosus.
E. toxoplasmosis.

All figures in this chapter are from Longacre TA, Greenson JK, Hornick JL, Reuter VE, eds. *Mills and Sternberg's Diagnostic Surgical Pathology*. 7th ed. Wolters Kluwer; 2022 except for those noted at the end of this book.

2. The pattern of follicular hyperplasia seen in the lymph node shown in Figure 1 is most characteristic of

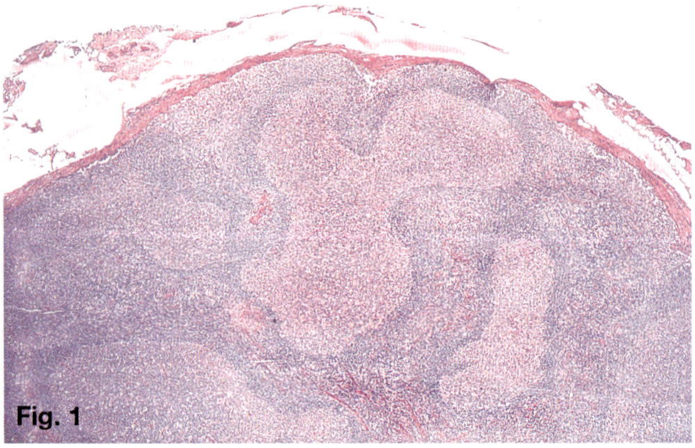
Fig. 1

A. acquired immunodeficiency syndrome.
B. cat-scratch disease.
C. syphilis.
D. systemic lupus erythematosus.
E. toxoplasmosis.

3. An 11-year-old presents with low-grade fever and left axillary lymphadenopathy. According to the report, there is a new kitten in the house. The enlarged axillary lymph node is removed (Figure 1), showing follicular hyperplasia, capsulitis, and subcapsular necrotizing granulomas. What is the most likely diagnosis?

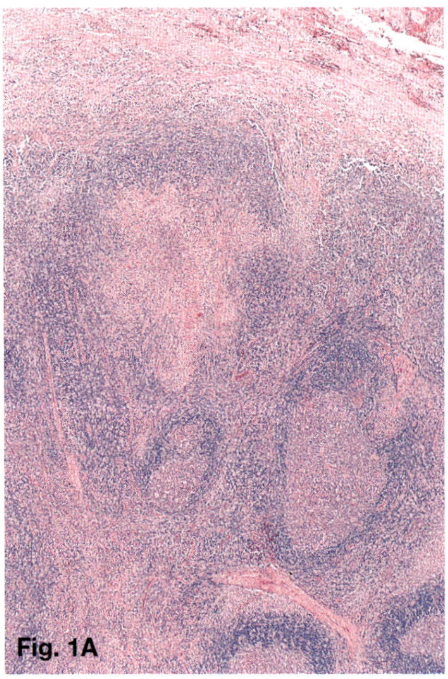
Fig. 1A

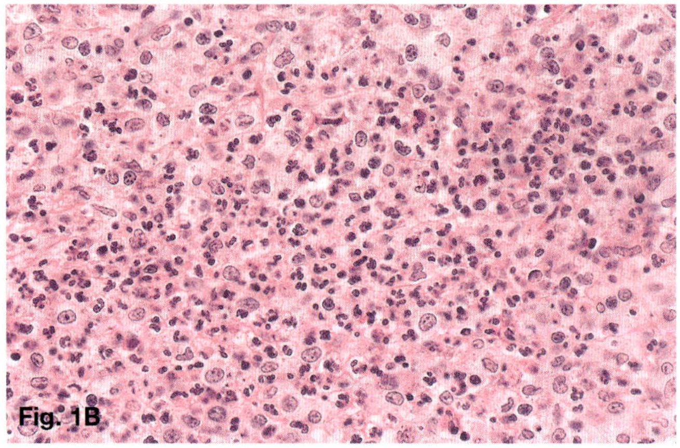
Fig. 1B

A. Acquired immunodeficiency syndrome
B. Cat-scratch disease
C. Kikuchi syndrome
D. Kimura disease
E. Toxoplasmosis

4. What is the best diagnosis for the mediastinal lymph node biopsy, shown in Figure 1, from an otherwise healthy 44-year-old man?

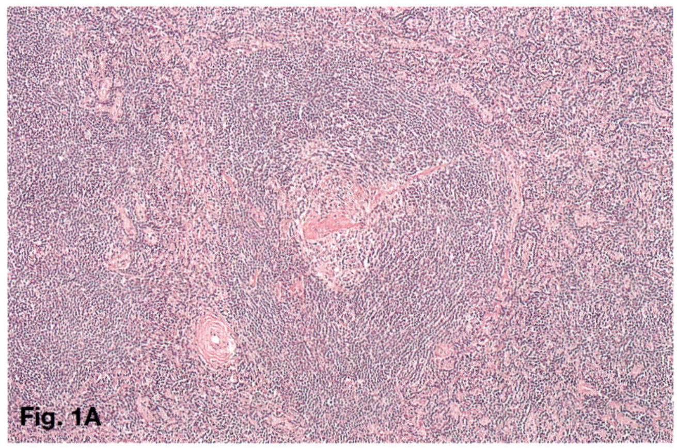
Fig. 1A

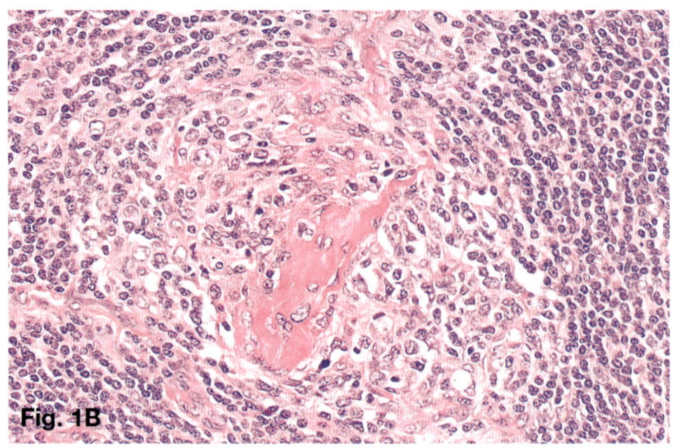
Fig. 1B

A. Castleman disease, hyaline-vascular variant
B. Follicular dendritic cell sarcoma
C. HIV-associated lymphadenitis
D. Immunoglobulin G subclass 4 (IgG4)-related disease
E. Mantle cell lymphoma

5. Which of the following statements is true with regard to Castleman disease?

   A. Human herpesvirus 8 (HHV-8) plays no pathogenetic role.
   B. Necrosis is a constant feature of lymph node involvement.
   C. Plasma cell population is monoclonal.
   D. Plasma cell variant is more likely associated with systemic involvement.
   E. Prognosis is the same for both localized and systemic forms.

6. A lymph node biopsy from a 28-year-old man with fever, cervical lymphadenopathy, and splenomegaly reveals the histopathologic changes depicted in Figure 1, which consist of marked interfollicular expansion by a mixed cellular infiltrate with numerous immunoblasts, small lymphocytes, and few plasma cells. The follicular architecture is partially preserved. Which of the following is the most likely diagnosis?

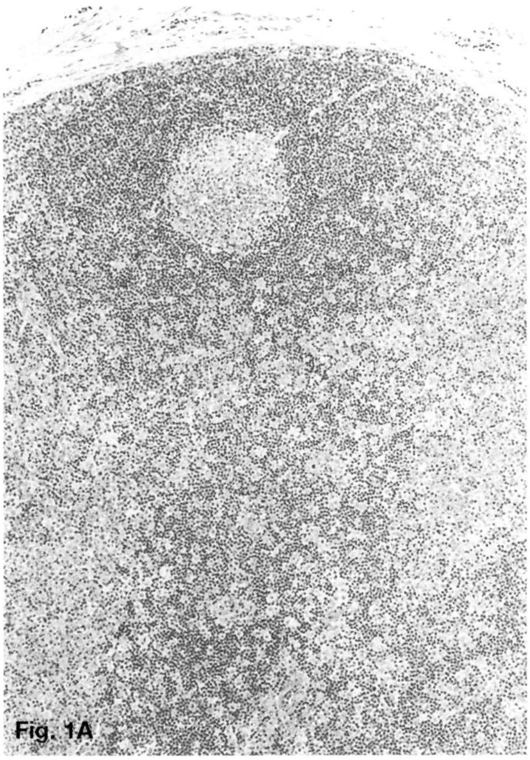

Fig. 1A

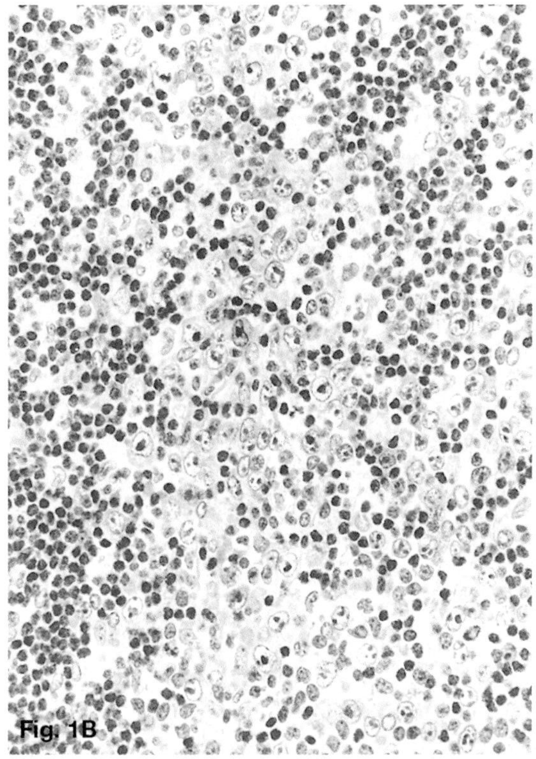

Fig. 1B

   A. Angiofollicular hyperplasia
   B. Angioimmunoblastic lymphoma
   C. Cat-scratch disease
   D. Immunoblastic lymphadenopathy
   E. Infectious mononucleosis

7. What is the most likely diagnosis of the lymph node process, shown in Figure 1, from a 22-year-old man with fever, leukocytosis, and bilateral cervical lymphadenopathy?

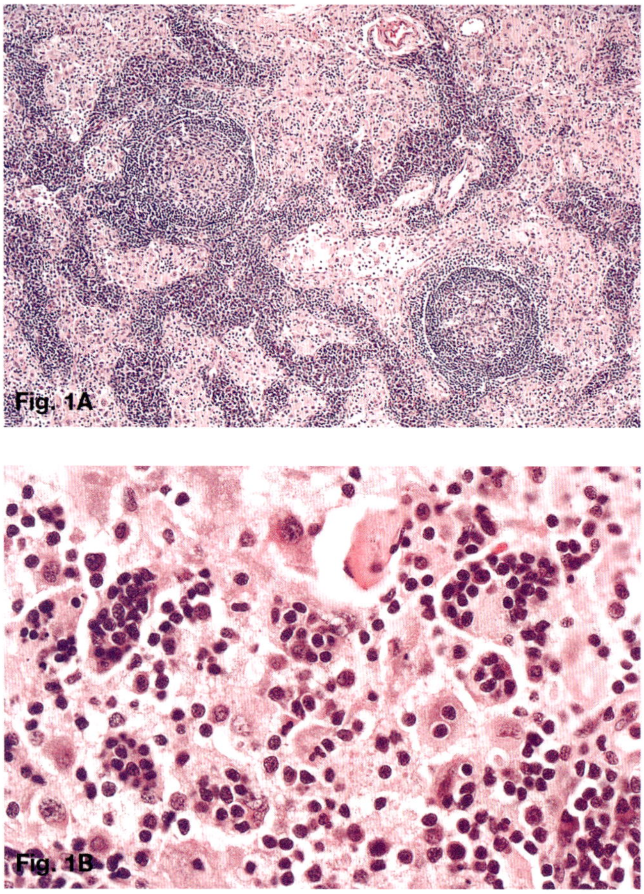


A. Castleman disease, plasma cell variant
B. Hemophagocytic lymphohistiocytosis
C. Langerhans cell histiocytosis
D. Rosai-Dorfman disease
E. Sinus histiocytosis

8. What is the most likely diagnosis for the moderately enlarged inguinal lymph node, shown in Figure 1, in a 54-year-old man with a history of atopic dermatitis and recent COVID-19 vaccination?

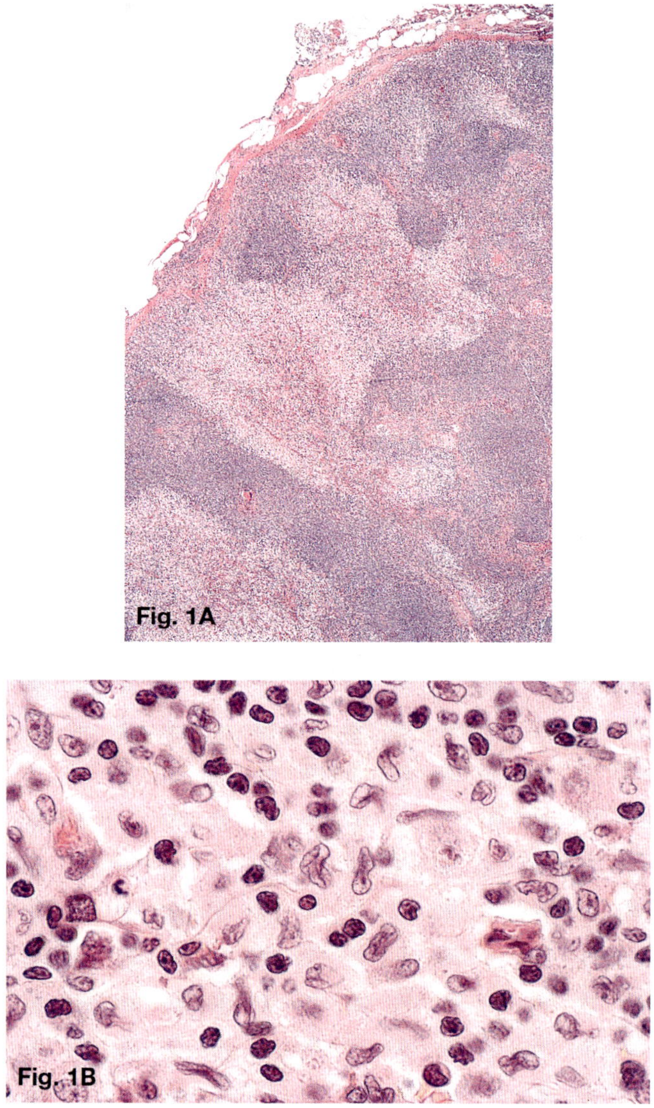


A. Dermatopathic lymphadenopathy
B. Hodgkin lymphoma
C. Langerhans histiocytosis
D. Mycosis fungoides
E. Postvaccination lymphadenopathy

9. A 25-year-old man presents with cervical node enlargement. A biopsy of an affected lymph node shows effacement of lymph node architecture by a nodular growth, a thin rim of compressed normal node, and a predominantly small lymphocytic population with admixed histiocytes and scattered large cells like those seen in Figures 1 and 2. The latter are immunoreactive for CD45, CD20, CD79a, Bcl-6, and PAX-5 and negative for CD15. Which of the following is the Hodgkin lymphoma variant in this case?

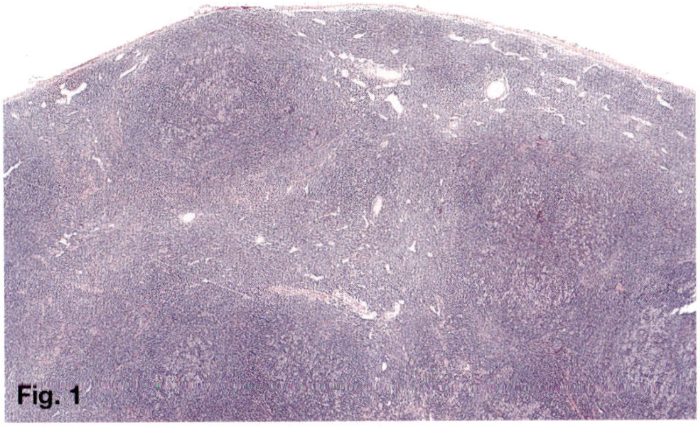
Fig. 1

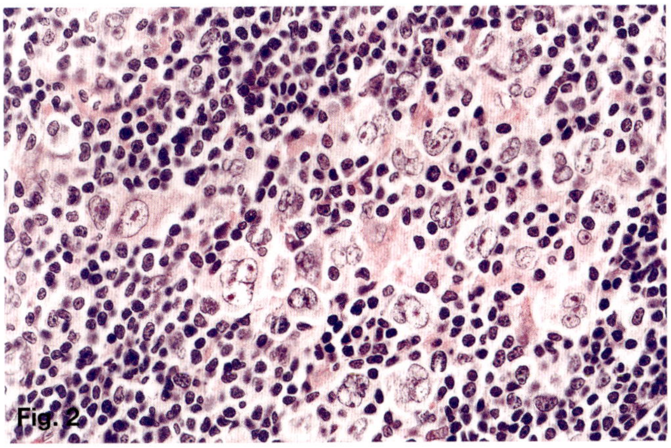
Fig. 2

A. Lymphocyte-depleted classic
B. Lymphocyte-rich classic
C. Mixed cellularity classic
D. Nodular lymphocyte-predominant
E. Nodular sclerosis classic

10. A 44-year-old man presents with an enlarged cervical lymph node. A biopsy of the lymph node reveals a nodular growth pattern that effaces the nodal architecture, sparing an attenuated rim of residual lymphoid tissue. Within a cellular background rich in small lymphocytes, classic Reed-Sternberg cells are identified (Figure 1). The latter express CD15 but not CD45. Which of the following is the Hodgkin lymphoma variant in this case?

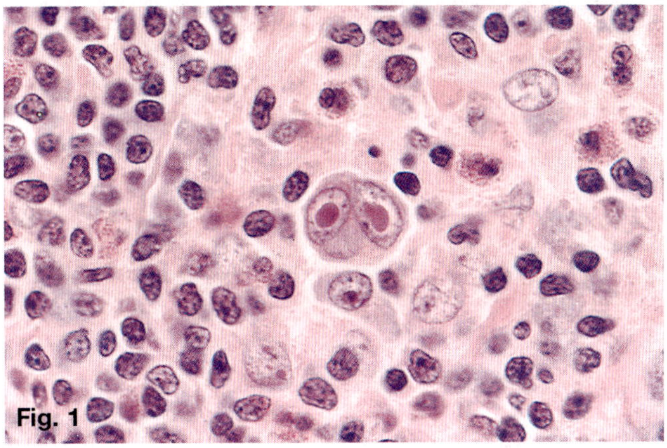
Fig. 1

A. Lymphocyte-depleted classic
B. Lymphocyte-rich classic
C. Mixed cellularity classic
D. Nodular lymphocyte-predominant
E. Nodular sclerosis classic

11. A 28-year-old woman presents with fever, night sweats, and a mediastinal mass. A biopsy of the mediastinal mass reveals a nodular pattern of growth with broad bands of collagen, as shown in this low-power photomicrograph (Figure 1). A formalin-fixed section (Figure 2) and a mercuric chloride–fixed section (Figure 3) demonstrate a mixed lymphohistiocytic, plasmacellular, and eosinophilic infiltrate, along with the cells shown in these high-power photomicrographs. These cells are CD15 and CD30 positive and CD45 negative. Which is the most likely Hodgkin lymphoma variant in this case?

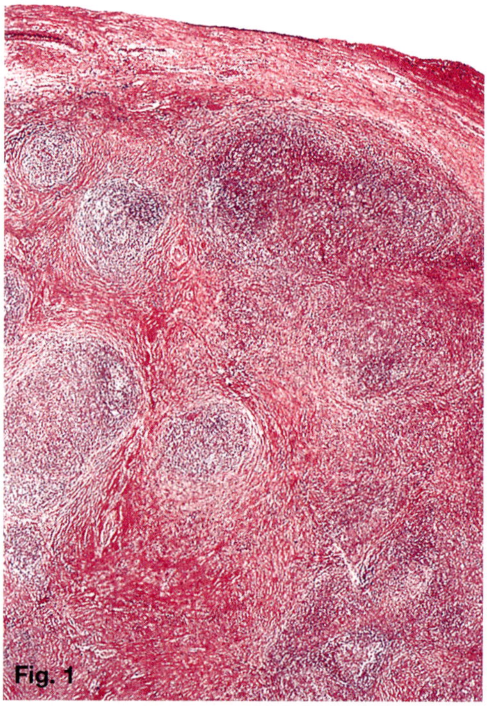
Fig. 1

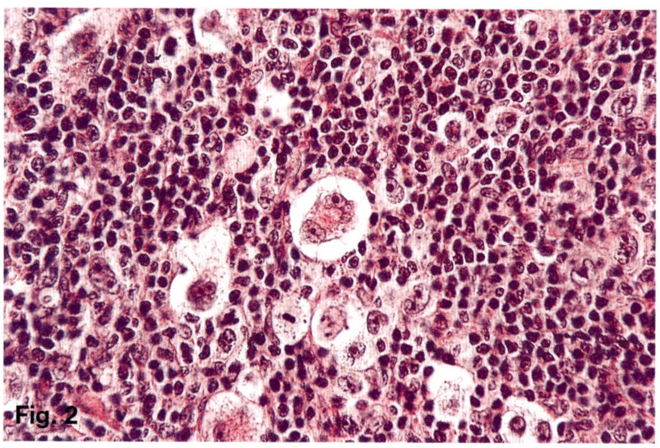
Fig. 2

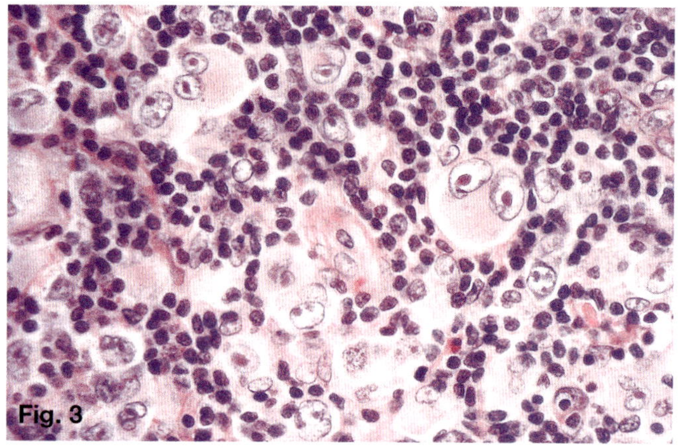
Fig. 3

A. Lymphocyte-depleted classic
B. Lymphocyte-rich classic
C. Mixed cellularity classic
D. Nodular lymphocyte-predominant
E. Nodular sclerosis classic

12. A lymph node biopsy reveals the cell population shown in Figure 1, including many classic Reed-Sternberg cells. In this case, a diagnosis of mixed cellularity classic Hodgkin lymphoma is justified if

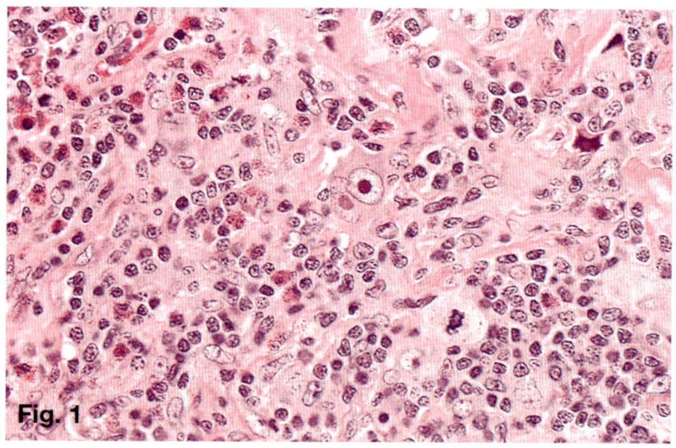
Fig. 1

A. broad bands of birefringent collagen result in a nodular pattern.
B. classic Reed-Sternberg cells are rare.
C. lacunar cells are abundant.
D. Reed-Sternberg cells are easily found within an infiltrate of lymphocytes, histiocytes, plasma cells, and eosinophils.
E. Reed-Sternberg cells are immunoreactive for CD45 but negative for CD15.

13. Figure 1 depicts a lymph node biopsy from the retroperitoneum of a 60-year-old man with liver and bone marrow involvement. Which is the most likely Hodgkin lymphoma variant in this case?

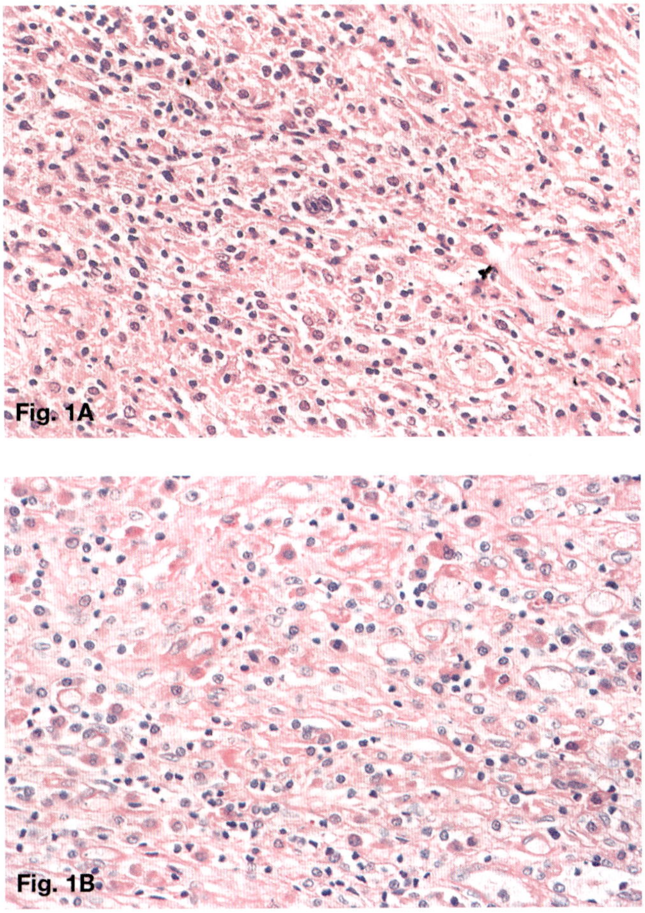

Fig. 1A

Fig. 1B

A. Lymphocyte-depleted classic
B. Lymphocyte-rich classic
C. Mixed cellularity classic
D. Nodular lymphocyte-predominant
E. Nodular sclerosis classic

14. Which of the following immunophenotypes is characteristic of classic Reed-Sternberg cells?

A. CD5− CD10+ Bcl-6+
B. CD5+ CD10− CD23+
C. CD5− CD10+ CD43+
D. CD15− CD30− CD45+
E. CD15+ CD30+ CD45−

15. A lymph node biopsy from a 60-year-old man with peripheral lymphocytosis and generalized lymphadenopathy reveals complete effacement of the nodal architecture, as shown in Figures 1 and 2. The nodal parenchyma is replaced by diffuse sheets of small lymphocytes with round nuclei and scanty cytoplasm. Pale-staining proliferation centers have irregular borders (asterisks). Mitotic figures are rare. Which of the following immunohistochemical features are most consistent with this morphology?

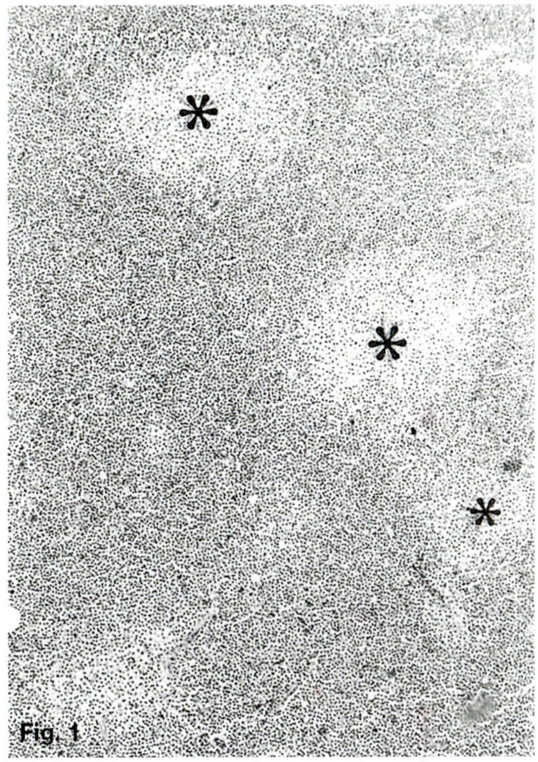

Fig. 1

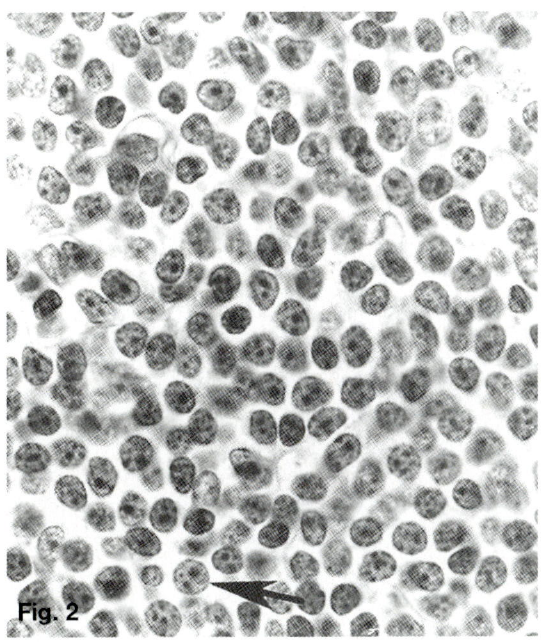

Fig. 2

A. CD5−, CD10−, CD20+
B. CD5+, CD10+, CD20+
C. CD5−, CD23+, CD43−
D. CD5+, CD23−, CD43−
E. CD5+, CD23+, CD43+

16. A 70-year-old man suffers from a lymphoma involving lymph nodes, bone marrow, spleen, and brain. Histologically, the lymph nodes display a vaguely nodular architecture, with striking expansion of the mantle zone around small residual follicles, as shown in Figure 1. Figure 2 demonstrates the cytologic features of the abnormal lymphocytic population. Which of the following genotypic abnormalities characterizes this type of lymphoma?

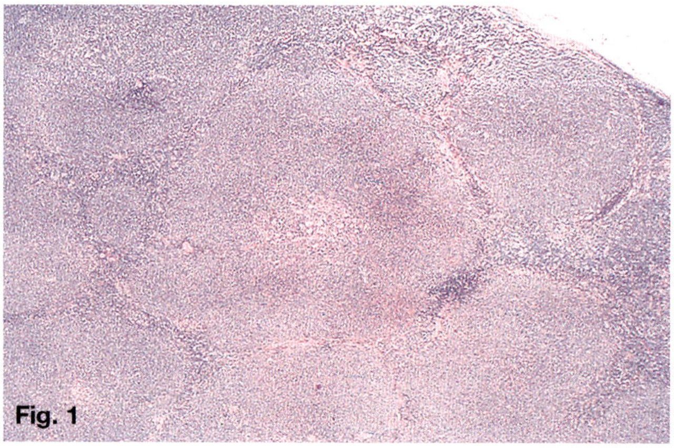

Fig. 1

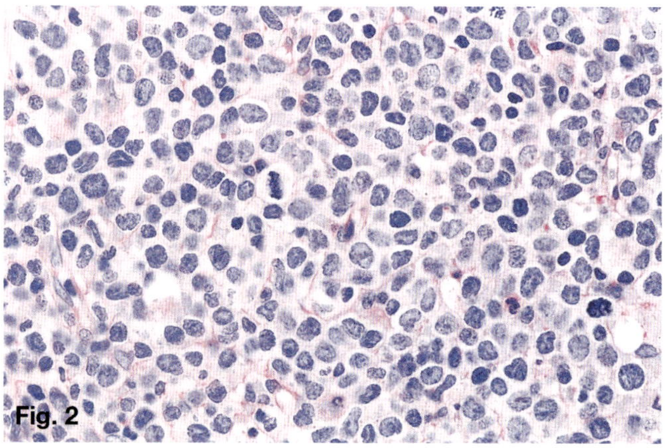

Fig. 2

A. t(8;14)
B. t(11;14)
C. t(11;18)
D. t(14;18)

17. The low-power photomicrograph in Figure 1 shows a lymphoma composed of CD10-positive and CD5-negative lymphocytes with high levels of cytoplasmic immunoglobulin G (IgG). Which of the following cytogenetic abnormalities is most likely to be present?

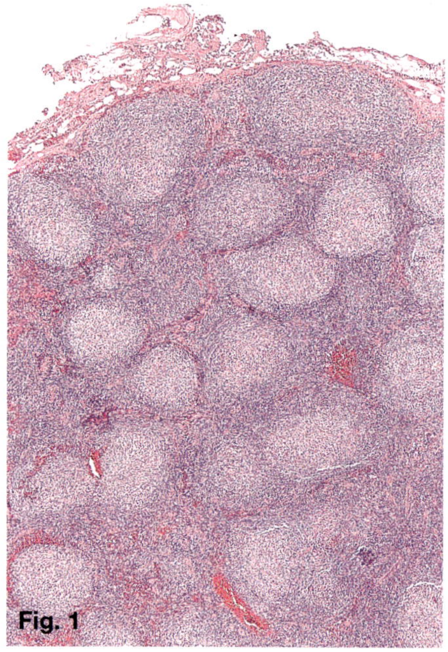

Fig. 1

A. t(8;14)
B. t(11;14)
C. t(11;18)
D. t(14;18)

18. Which of the following methods is used for grading follicular lymphomas?

A. Assessing the degree of dysplasia of centrocytes
B. Counting centroblasts in 10 high-power fields
C. Counting centrocytes in 10 high-power fields
D. Estimating the extent of follicular growth pattern
E. Estimating the proportion of large transformed cells

19. Figure 1 shows a lymphoma composed of neoplastic cells resembling monocytoid B cells. What is the most likely diagnosis?

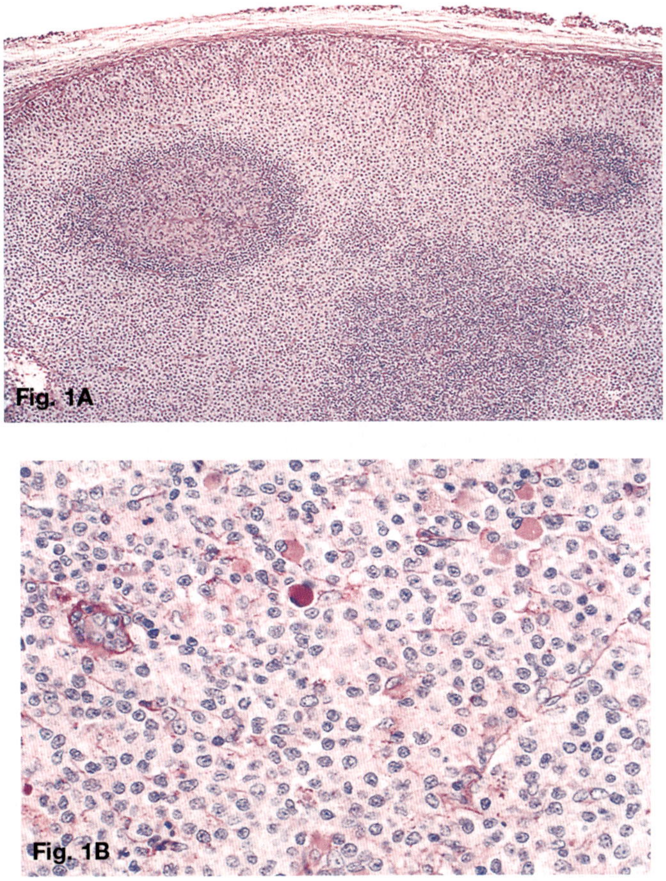

Fig. 1A

Fig. 1B

A. Follicular lymphoma
B. Hairy cell leukemia
C. Mantle cell lymphoma
D. Mastocytosis
E. Nodal marginal zone lymphoma

20. A 60-year-old man presents with rapidly enlarging axillary lymph nodes. A biopsy of one of the enlarged nodes shows the atypical lymphocytic population depicted in Figure 1. The neoplastic cells express CD19, CD20, CD22, CD79a, OCT2, BOB1, and PAX-5, while they are negative for CD5 and surface immunoglobulins. Which of the following is the most likely diagnosis?

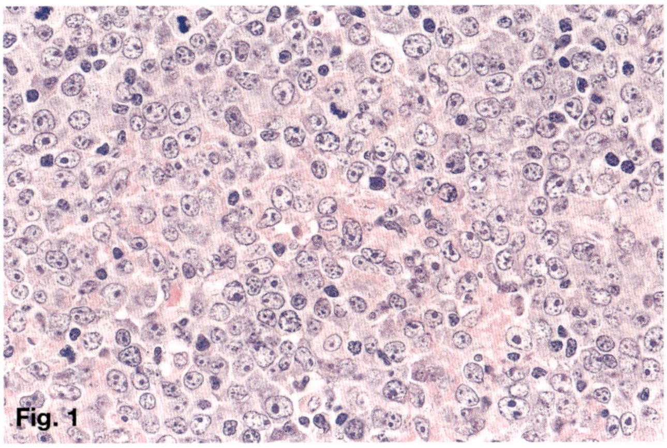

Fig. 1

A. Burkitt lymphoma
B. Diffuse large B-cell lymphoma
C. Follicular lymphoma, high grade
D. Lymphoplasmacytic lymphoma
E. T-cell lymphoblastic lymphoma

21. A 52-year-old man presents with fever, weight loss, night sweats, and axillary and cervical adenopathy. One of the lymph nodes is biopsied to show small numbers of atypical large B cells scattered singly or in clusters, with a predominance of T cells admixed with histiocytes (Figure 1). What is the most likely diagnosis?

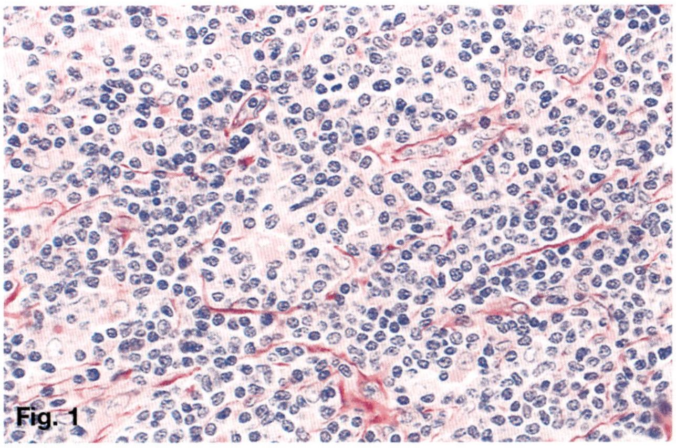

Fig. 1

A. Anaplastic lymphoma kinase (ALK)-positive large B-cell lymphoma
B. Epstein-Barr virus (EBV)-positive diffuse large B-cell lymphoma
C. Large B-cell lymphoma with IRF4 rearrangement
D. Peripheral T-cell lymphoma
E. T-cell/histiocyte-rich large B-cell lymphoma

22. A 38-year-old HIV male presents with a large pleural effusion. The pleural fluid contains immunoblastic cells with abundant basophilic cytoplasm, round nuclei, and single prominent nucleoli. Many of the cells exhibit a perinuclear halo and variable nuclear pleomorphism with binucleated cells. What is the most likely diagnosis?

    A. Anaplastic lymphoma kinase (ALK)-positive large B-cell lymphoma
    B. Epstein-Barr virus (EBV)-positive diffuse large B-cell lymphoma
    C. Large B-cell lymphoma with IRF4 rearrangement
    D. Primary effusion lymphoma
    E. T-cell/histiocyte-rich large B-cell lymphoma

23. A 24-year-old woman presents with dyspnea and is found to have an anterior mediastinal mass. The mass is biopsied and shows sclerosis and mostly large lymphoid cells that are CD-negative B cells, as depicted in Figure 1. What is the most likely diagnosis?

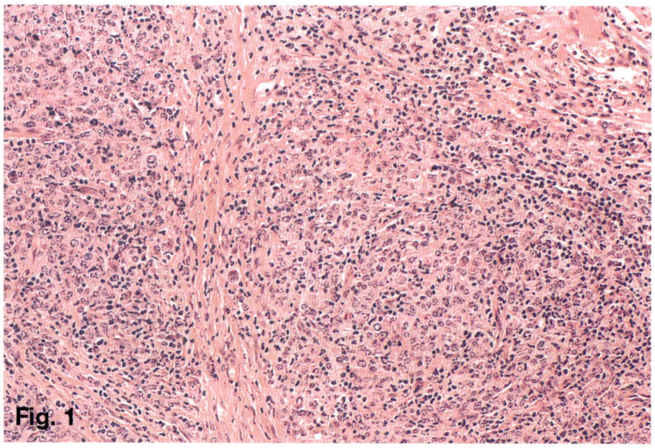

Fig. 1

    A. Anaplastic lymphoma kinase (ALK)-positive large B-cell lymphoma
    B. Classic Hodgkin lymphoma
    C. Epstein-Barr virus (EBV)-positive diffuse large B-cell lymphoma
    D. Large B-cell lymphoma with IRF4 rearrangement
    E. Primary mediastinal large B-cell lymphoma

24. Which of the following is true with respect to the lymph node depicted in Figure 1?

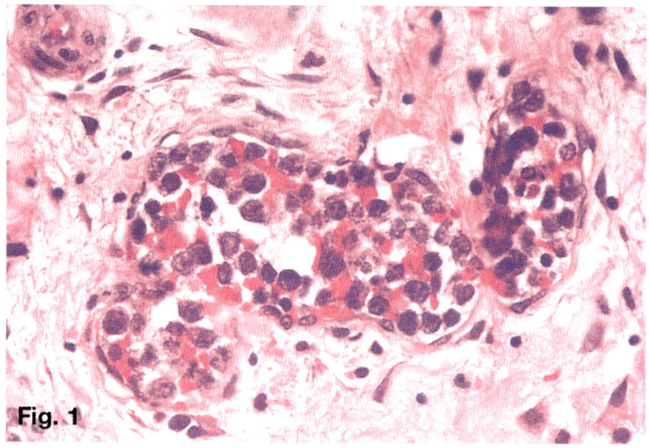

Fig. 1

    A. It is associated with aggressive disease.
    B. It is associated with T-cell lymphomas.
    C. It rarely involves skin and central nervous system.
    D. It typically occurs in younger patients.
    E. Lymph node involvement is common.

25. Histologic examination of an ileocecal mass removed from a 24-year-old woman reveals the atypical lymphoid population shown in Figure 1. The neoplastic cells are lymphocytes with amphophilic cytoplasm, round nuclei, and small nucleoli. Mitotic activity is very high. Immunohistochemistry for Ki-67 shows a labeling index close to 100%. The majority of cases of this lymphoma are associated with translocations or rearrangements involving

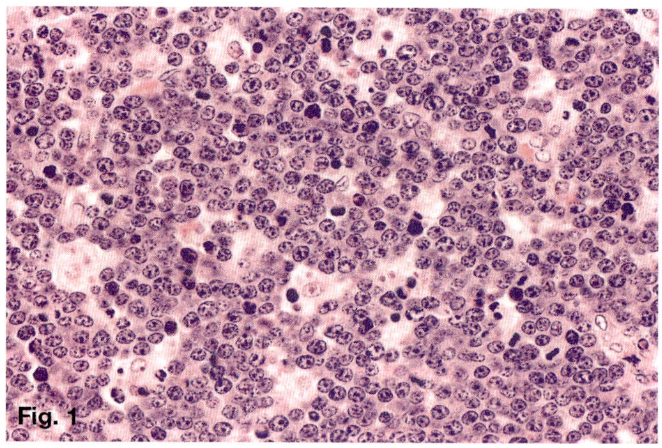

Fig. 1

    A. BCL-1.
    B. BCL-2.
    C. C-myc.
    D. PAX-5.
    E. TAL1.

26. A 20-year-old male has a large mass in the anterior mediastinum, hilar lymphadenopathy, and pleural effusion. Resection of the mass reveals a diffuse lymphomatous infiltrate as shown in Figure 1, characterized by cells with angular irregular nuclei, blast-like dispersed chromatin, and inconspicuous nucleoli (Figure 2). Mitotic figures are frequent. Immunohistochemical studies show neoplastic cells to be positive for CD3 and CD7. Which of the following markers is expressed in virtually 100% of this type of lymphoma?

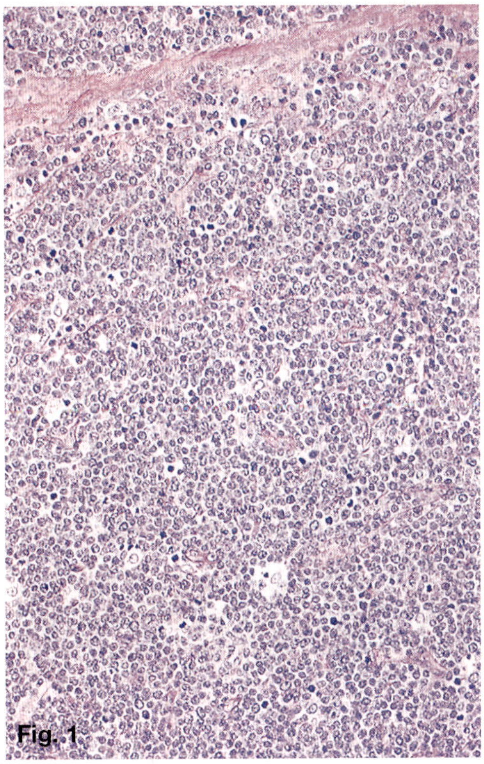
Fig. 1

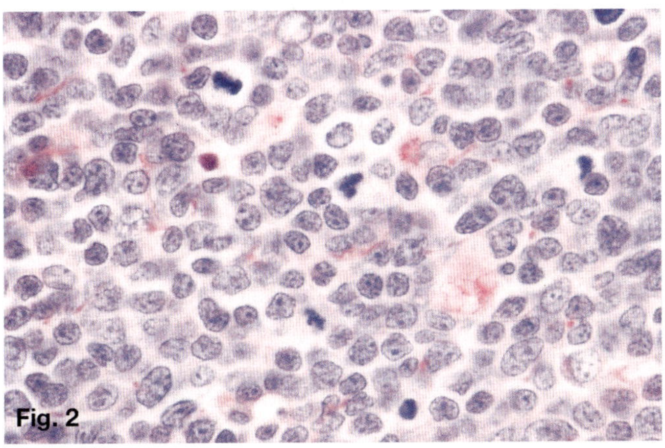
Fig. 2

A. CD10
B. CD20
C. CD30
D. HLA-DR (human leukocyte antigen-DR)
E. TdT (terminal deoxytransferase)

27. A 50-year-old woman presents with generalized lymphadenopathy, night sweats, and pruritus. A lymph node biopsy reveals a diffuse lymphomatous growth resulting in uniform effacement of nodal architecture, as shown in this low-power photomicrograph (Figure 1). The morphology of infiltrating lymphoid cells is demonstrated in this high-power picture (Figure 2). The neoplastic cells express pan-T-cell antigens, CD4, and CD8 but are negative for TdT (terminal deoxytransferase), CD1, and CD30. Which of the following is the most likely diagnosis?

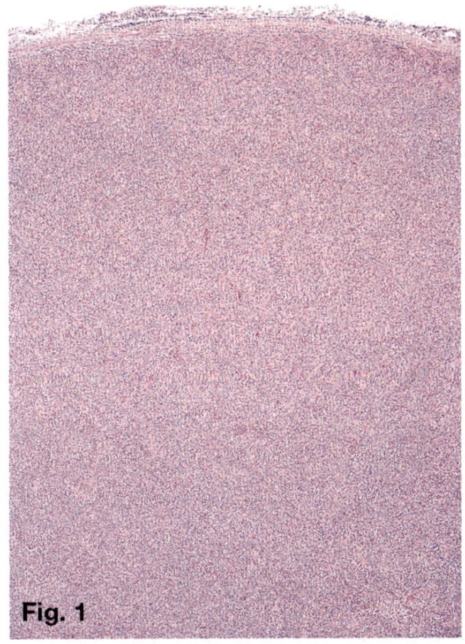
Fig. 1

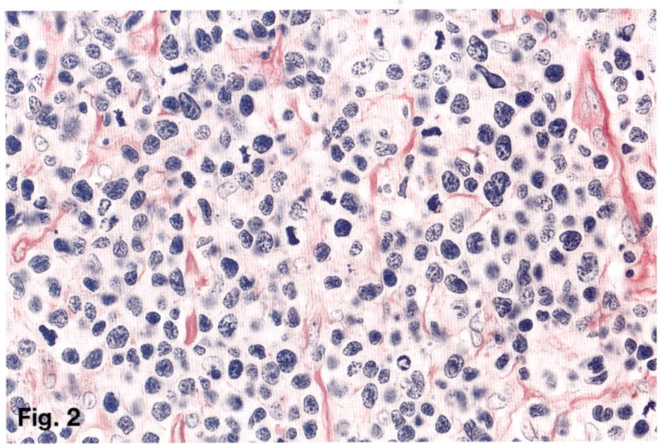
Fig. 2

A. Anaplastic large cell lymphoma
B. Angioimmunoblastic T-cell lymphoma
C. Mycosis fungoides
D. Natural killer cell lymphoma
E. Peripheral T-cell lymphoma, unspecified

28. A 55-year-old woman presents with generalized lymphadenopathy, fever, weight loss, and skin rash accompanied by pruritus. Laboratory studies reveal hypergammaglobulinemia. A lymph node biopsy reveals a polymorphous cell population amidst a florid network of small vessels, as shown in this picture (Figure 1). A section immunostained for CD21 is represented in this picture (Figure 2). Which of the following is the most likely diagnosis?

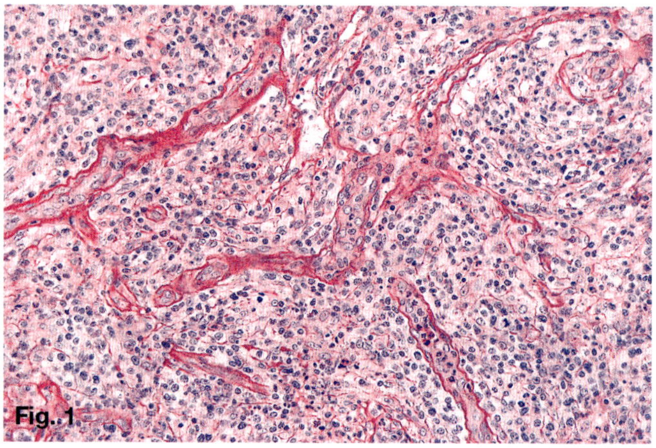
Fig. 1

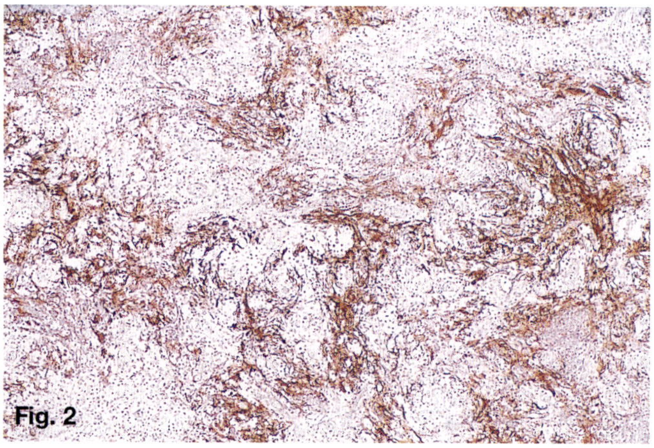
Fig. 2

A. Anaplastic large cell lymphoma
B. Angioimmunoblastic lymphoma
C. Large granular lymphocytic leukemia
D. Natural killer cell lymphoma
E. Precursor T-cell lymphoblastic lymphoma/leukemia

29. A lymph node from a 25-year-old patient with lymphadenopathy shows invasion of the subcapsular sinus by highly pleomorphic cells, as shown in Figure 1. Lymphoid follicles are spared. The neoplastic cells display cytoplasmic immunoreactivity for CD30 and epithelial membrane antigen (EMA). What is the most likely diagnosis?

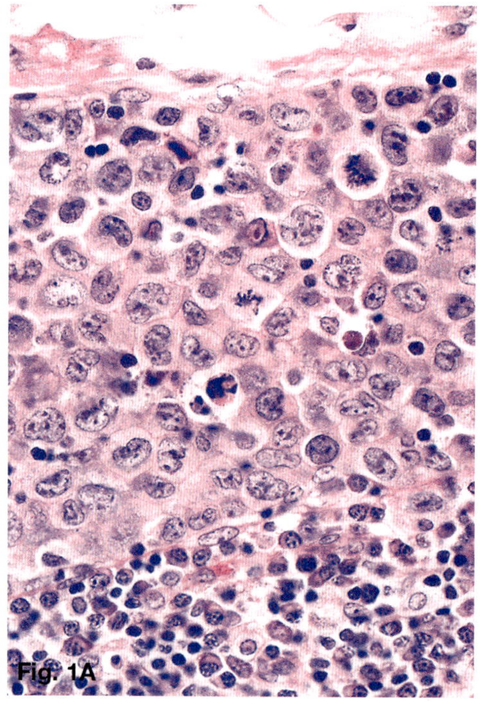
Fig. 1A

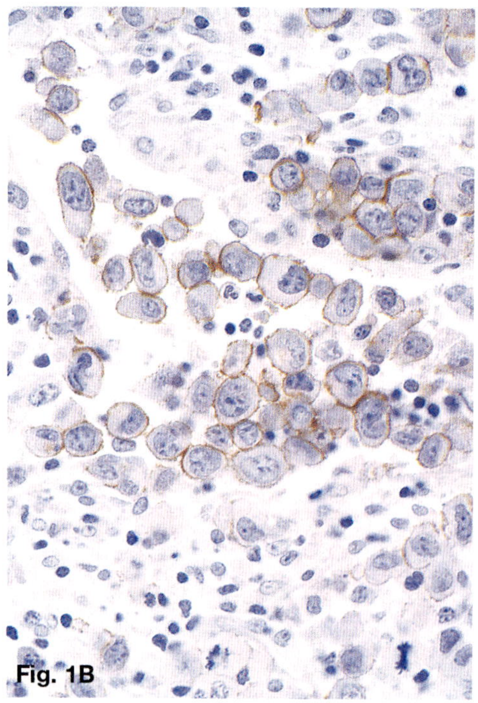
Fig. 1B

A. Anaplastic large cell lymphoma
B. Angioimmunoblastic lymphoma
C. Large granular lymphocytic leukemia
D. Natural killer cell lymphoma
E. Precursor T-cell lymphoblastic lymphoma/leukemia

30. Adult T-cell leukemia/lymphoma (ATLL) is caused by

A. Epstein-Barr virus (EBV).
B. human herpesvirus 8 (HHV-8).
C. human immunodeficiency virus (HIV).
D. human papillomavirus (HPV).
E. human T-cell lymphotropic virus type I (HTLV-I).

31. A 60-year-old man presents with raised erythematous plaques on the back and enlarged axillary and inguinal lymph nodes. Biopsy of the skin lesions reveals a band-like infiltrate of atypical medium-large-sized lymphocytes with cerebriform nuclei. The infiltrate extends to the deeper dermis and hair follicles. Figure 1 shows the findings in a node biopsy obtained from this patient. Which of the following is the cell of origin of this neoplasm?

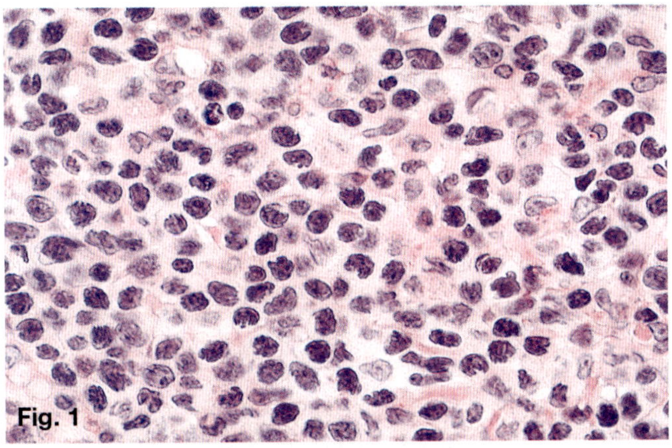
Fig. 1

A. CD4-positive T cell
B. CD8-positive T cell
C. Histiocyte
D. Langerhans cell
E. Natural killer cell

32. Posttransplant lymphoproliferative disorder (PTLD) is one of the most frequent long-term complications of solid organ or bone marrow transplantation. Which of the following viruses is thought to play a critical pathogenetic role in PTLD?

A. Cytomegalovirus
B. Epstein-Barr virus
C. Hepatitis B virus
D. Hepatitis C virus
E. Hepatitis D virus

33. Which of the following lymphoproliferative disorders is associated with Epstein-Barr virus?

A. Endemic Burkitt lymphoma
B. Extranodal natural killer (NK)/T-cell lymphoma
C. Lymphomatoid granulomatosis
D. Plasmablastic lymphoma
E. All of the above

34. A 60-year-old man presents with fever, weight loss, cervical lymphadenopathy, hepatosplenomegaly, and skin lesions. A biopsy is performed, which shows pleomorphic cells, including some multinucleated forms associated with a mixed inflammatory cell background, as shown in Figure 1. The cells are positive for CD45, CD68, and CD163. What is the most likely diagnosis for this lymph node biopsy?

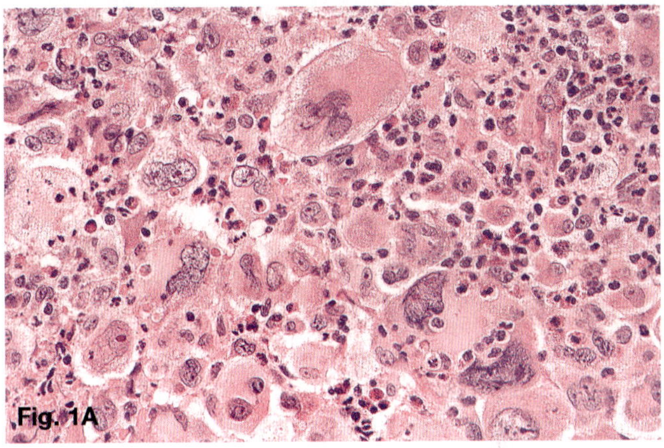
Fig. 1A

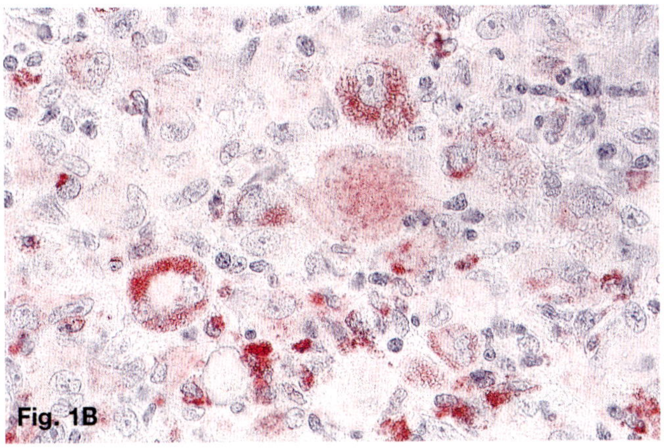
Fig. 1B

A. Anaplastic large cell lymphoma
B. Diffuse large B-cell lymphoma
C. Histiocytic sarcoma
D. Langerhans cell histiocytosis
E. Rosai-Dorfman disease

35. A 50-year-old man presents with a gradually enlarging, painless cervical lymph node. A biopsy shows effacement of the nodal architecture by oval- and spindle-shaped cells that are positive for CD21 and CD35 (Figure 1). What is the most likely diagnosis for this lymph node biopsy?

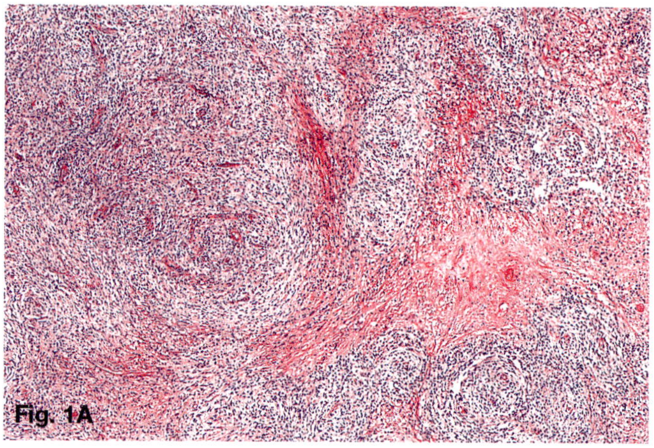

Fig. 1A

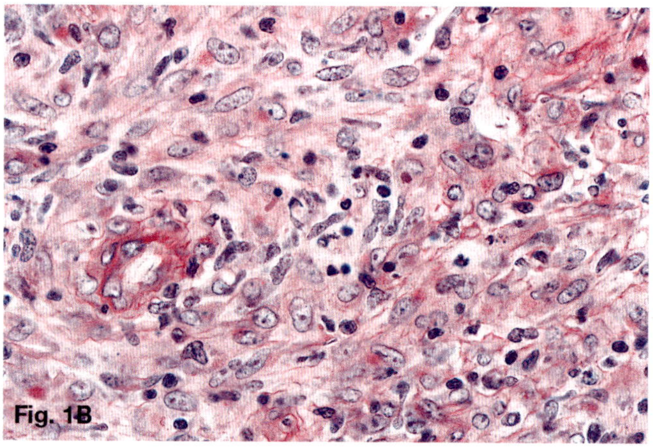

Fig. 1B

A. Inflammatory myofibroblastic tumor
B. Interdigitating reticulin cell sarcoma
C. Follicular dendritic cell sarcoma
D. Kaposi sarcoma
E. Langerhans cell histiocytosis

36. This cervical lymph node is removed from a 34-year-old male who is HIV positive (see Figure 1). What is the most likely diagnosis?

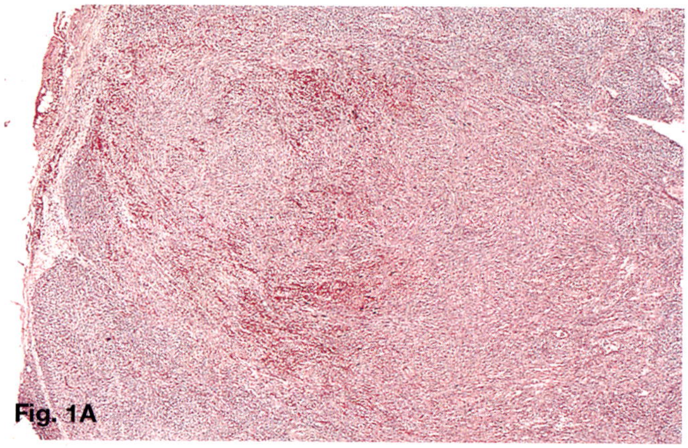

Fig. 1A

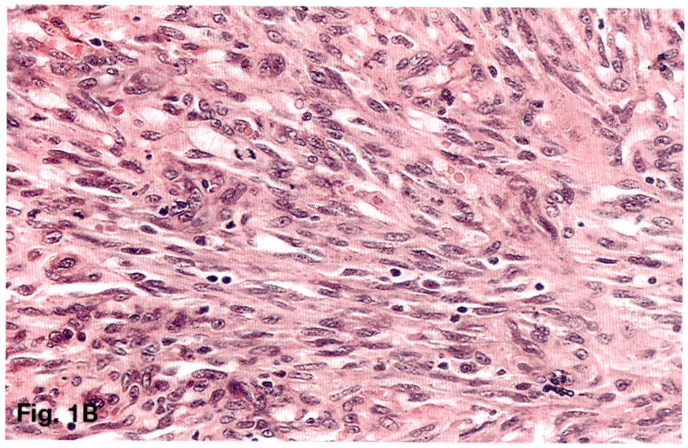

Fig. 1B

A. Bacillary angiomatosis
B. Inflammatory pseudotumor
C. Kaposi sarcoma
D. Mycobacterial spindle cell tumor
E. Vascular transformation of lymph node sinuses

37. A 44-year-old African American woman presents with persistent dry cough, weight loss, fatigue, and night sweats. An enlarged cervical lymph node is biopsied. It shows numerous epithelioid granulomas without necrosis, as shown in Figure 1. What is the most likely diagnosis for this lymph node biopsy?

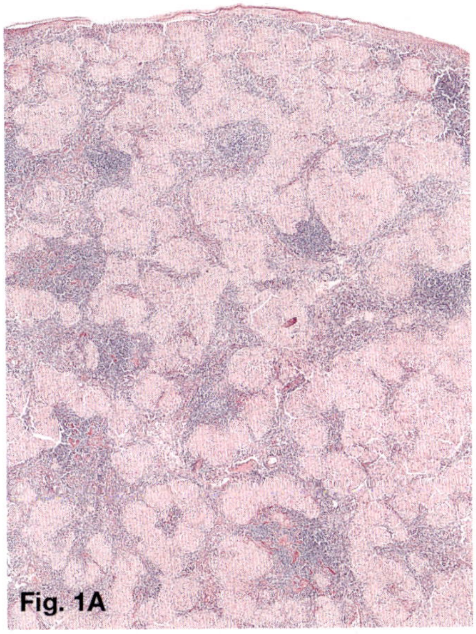
Fig. 1A

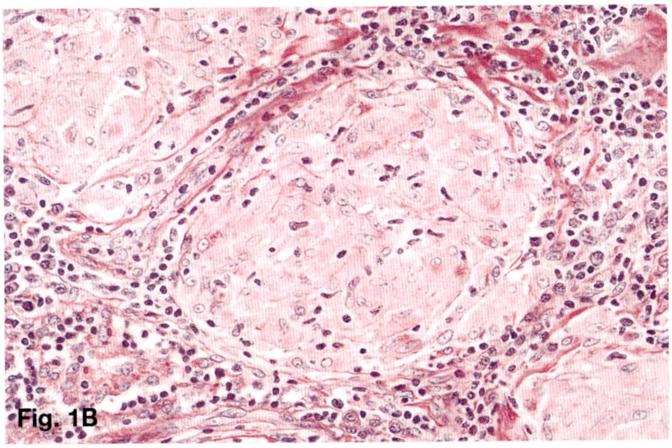
Fig. 1B

A. Inflammatory pseudotumor
B. Kikuchi-Fujimoto disease
C. Kimura disease
D. Langerhans histiocytosis
E. Sarcoidosis

38. A 28-year-old female presents with cervical lymphadenopathy, fever, and leukopenia. Biopsy of one of the involved lymph nodes shows partial effacement of the nodal architecture by histiocytes, plasmacytoid dendritic cells, immunoblasts, and large zones of necrosis with karyorrhectic debris. Neutrophils are absent and there is no associated follicular lymphoid hyperplasia. What is the most likely diagnosis?

A. Inflammatory pseudotumor
B. Kikuchi-Fujimoto disease
C. Kimura disease
D. Langerhans histiocytosis
E. Sarcoidosis

39. A 29-year-old previously healthy Asian man presents with an enlarged cervical lymph node. A biopsy of the lymph node demonstrates follicular hyperplasia associated with expansion of the interfollicular areas by abundant eosinophils, often forming eosinophilic microabscesses. Infectious and autoimmune workups are unrevealing. He is not taking any medications. Immunohistochemistry showed a mixture of CD3-positive T cells and CD20-positive B cells. Which of the following is the best diagnosis?

A. Bacillary angiomatosis
B. HIV lymphadenitis
C. Kikuchi-Fujimoto disease
D. Kimura disease
E. Langerhans cell histiocytosis

40. Which of the following infectious etiologies of hemophagocytic lymphohistiocytosis has been most commonly implicated?

A. COVID-19
B. Cytomegalovirus
C. Epstein-Barr virus
D. Influenza virus
E. Parvovirus B19

# ANSWERS AND EXPLANATIONS

**1. Correct choice: D.**

Patients with systemic lupus erythematosus often develop cervical lymphadenopathy. Enlarged nodes exhibit follicular hyperplasia with preservation of nodal architecture. In addition, there are characteristic areas of well-demarcated cortical necrosis containing hematoxylin bodies and scanty neutrophilic infiltration. Table 1 provides a summary for reactive lymphadenopathies.

**2. Correct choice: A.**

Generalized lymphadenopathy may occur before overt-acquired immunodeficiency syndrome (AIDS). Enlarged lymph nodes show follicular hyperplasia characterized by a peculiar dumbbell or serpentine shape of their germinal centers (see image). The mantle cell layer is attenuated, creating the impression of naked germinal centers. Later on, nodes acquire changes similar to hyaline-vascular or the plasma cell type of Castleman disease. Advanced stages feature the disappearance of follicles, lymphocyte depletion, and vascular hyperplasia, which mimics immunoblastic lymphoma. Syphilis lymphadenitis is characterized by striking capsulitis and plasma cell infiltration.

**3. Correct choice: B.**

Cat-scratch disease is caused by *Bartonella henselae*, a small bacillus identifiable by Warthin-Starry stain. This condition is characterized by follicular hyperplasia associated with necrosis and granulomatous inflammation. Necrotic areas are located in the subcapsular region, surrounded by palisading histiocytes and infiltrated by neutrophils. *Capsulitis* is consistently present. This pattern is not pathognomonic of cat-scratch disease, as it is found in other infectious conditions, for example, tularemia, lymphogranuloma venereum, and *Yersinia* infection. Kikuchi syndrome does not have neutrophils. Kimura disease is dominated by eosinophils. Toxoplasmosis lymphadenitis is characterized by florid follicular hyperplasia, perifollicular epithelioid histiocytes, and patches of monocytoid B cells. Mild capsular inflammation and scarring may be seen.

**4. Correct choice: A.**

Castleman disease (angiofollicular hyperplasia) is characterized by numerous regressively transformed small follicular centers organized around hyalinized vessels, scattered throughout the node like a "bag of marbles." An "onionskin" arrangement

**TABLE 1 Reactive Processes in Relation to Etiologic Factor and Architectural Distortion**

| Etiologic Factor | Architectural Distortion |
|---|---|
| Infections | Reactive states with follicular hyperplasia |
| Viral-associated adenitis (infectious mononucleosis, postvaccinal, herpes zoster, cytomegalovirus, measles, HIV) | Nonspecific follicular hyperplasia and progressive transformation of germinal center |
| Secondary syphilis | Rheumatoid arthritis |
| Toxoplasmosis | Sjögren syndrome |
| Cat-scratch disease | Adult-onset Still disease |
| Various granulomatous processes | Systemic lupus erythematosus |
| Whipple disease | Kimura disease |
| Rheumatologic/immunologic | Histiocytic necrotizing lymphadenitis (Kikuchi-Fujimoto disease) |
| Rheumatoid arthritis | Cat-scratch disease |
| Lupus erythematosus | Toxoplasmosis |
| Sjögren syndrome | Syphilis |
| Immunodeficiency states | HIV infection |
| Infarction, some cases | Castleman disease (angiofollicular hyperplasia)[a] |
| Adult-onset Still disease | IgG4-related disease |
| IgG4-related sclerosing disease | Reactive states with interfollicular hyperplasia |
| Drug induced | Whipple disease |
| Dilantin | Viral adenitis |
| Unknown cause | Posttransplant lymphoproliferative disorder |
| Sarcoidosis | Virus-associated hemophagocytic syndrome |
| Angiofollicular hyperplasia | Hemophagocytic lymphohistiocytosis |
| Inflammatory pseudotumor | Dermatopathic lymphadenopathy |
| Dermatopathic lymphadenopathy | Sinus histiocytosis with massive adenopathy |
| Sinus histiocytosis with massive adenopathy (Rosai-Dorfman disease) | Reactive states causing diffuse architectural effacement |
| Necrotizing adenitis | Drug reactions |
| Kimura disease | Sarcoidosis |
| | Infarction |
| | Vasoproliferative lesions |

HIV, human immunodeficiency virus; IgG4, immunoglobulin G subclass 4.
[a]A subset of Castleman disease cases show clonal mutational abnormalities indicating a subset of cases are neoplastic.

of lymphocytes around small vessels is a characteristic feature. There are three histologic types: hyaline-vascular variant (see image), plasma cell variant, and mixed hyaline-vascular and plasma cell variant. The plasma cell variant exhibits follicular lymphoid hyperplasia and sheets of interfollicular plasma cells, while the mixed hyaline-vascular and plasma cell variant exhibits features of both. Follicular dendritic cell sarcoma is characterized by storiform or whorled bundles of spindle cells with interspersed small lymphocytes and is positive for follicular dendritic cell markers (CD21, CD23, CD35). HIV-associated lymphadenitis is associated with clinical and serologic evidence of HIV. Lymphadenopathy in immunoglobulin G subclass 4 (IgG4)-related disease is characterized by a dense lymphoplasmacytic infiltrate containing numerous IgG4-positive plasma cells. Hyperplastic and regressed follicles, some with penetrating vessels, may be present and there are numerous plasma cells in the interfollicular area. Serologic studies may assist in establishing the diagnosis. Mantle cell lymphoma is a clonal B-cell neoplasm featuring atypical lymphocytes that express CD5 and cyclin D1; it harbors a *CCND1-IGH* translocation.

**5. Correct choice: D.**

Castleman disease (angiofollicular hyperplasia) is characterized by numerous regressively transformed small follicular centers organized around hyalinized vessels, scattered throughout the node like a "bag of marbles." An "onionskin" arrangement of lymphocytes around small vessels is a characteristic feature. The plasma cells are polyclonal. Castleman disease may be subclassified into hyaline-vascular and plasma cell variants. There are two clinical presentations: (1) unicentric (localized), occurring in patients who are HIV negative as a localized lymphadenopathy or mass lesion (commonly in the mediastinum). This form is usually of the hyaline-vascular type, not accompanied by systemic symptoms, and treated with surgical excision. (2) multicentric (systemic), manifesting with generalized lymphadenopathy and constitutional symptoms. This form is usually of the plasma cell variant and is divided into human herpesvirus 8 (HHV-8) associated, POEMS (polyneuropathy, organomegaly, endocrinopathy, M-protein, skin changes) associated, and idiopathic forms. Interleukin-6 (IL-6) appears to be an important pathogenetic factor, and serum levels correlate with systemic manifestations. Patients with multifocal (systemic) disease often develop progressive disease, complicated by infection, Kaposi sarcoma, or lymphoma.

**6. Correct choice: E.**

Infectious mononucleosis is due to Epstein-Barr virus infecting B lymphocytes. Cytotoxic (CD8+) T lymphocytes represent the majority of atypical lymphocytes in peripheral smears. This condition may lead to partial effacement of lymph node follicular architecture, with a pattern mimicking either nodular-sclerosing Hodgkin lymphoma or high-grade non-Hodgkin lymphoma. Large numbers of immunoblasts, with abundant cytoplasm and prominent nucleoli, are the hallmark of infectious mononucleosis. Immunoblasts are of both B- and T-cell lineages, but B cells predominate. Transformed immunoblasts may mimic Reed-Sternberg cells or the neoplastic lymphocytes of immunoblastic lymphoma. Clinical history and immunophenotyping are required to distinguish this reactive process from lymphoma.

**7. Correct choice: D.**

The classic presentation of nodal Rosai-Dorfman disease (sinus histiocytosis with massive lymphadenopathy) is that of a young black male with massive cervical lymphadenopathy. However, extranodal involvement presentation is seen in almost 50% of cases. The lymph node sinuses are replete with numerous histiocytes, some showing emperipolesis, that is, phagocytosis of blood elements (mostly lymphocytes). The histiocytes are positive for S100 protein, CD68, and CD14. Good prognosis is associated with localized disease and poor prognosis with extensive extranodal involvement. Castleman disease, plasma cell variant, is characterized by follicular lymphoid hyperplasia and sheets of interfollicular plasma cells, but no significant sinus histiocytosis. Hemophagocytic lymphohistiocytosis is characterized by fever, cytopenia, and hepatosplenomegaly; the lymph nodes show intact architecture with cytologically benign histiocytes filled with lymphocytes, neutrophils, and red blood cells. The histiocytes are negative for S100 protein. Langerhans cell histiocytosis is characterized by histiocytes with irregular, grooved, folded, or indented nuclei with fine chromatin, inconspicuous nucleoli, and abundant pale eosinophilic cytoplasm; they are negative for S100 protein but positive for CD1a and langerin. Sinus histiocytosis is a reactive process characterized by prominent sinuses in lymph nodes containing normal histiocytes.

**8. Correct choice: A.**

Dermatopathic lymphadenopathy is a reactive lymphadenopathy characterized by paracortical expansion with increased interdigitating dendritic cells, Langerhans cells, and histiocytes, typically including melanophages. It is classically associated with chronic skin irritation, inflammation, or infection. Classic Hodgkin lymphoma contains Reed-Sternberg or Hodgkin cells that are positive for CD30, PAX-5, and CD15. Typically, there is no increase in interdigitating dendritic cells or Langerhans cells. Langerhans histiocytosis is characterized by sinusoidal involvement with partial or total effacement of the lymph node architecture. Formation of aggregates and sheets of Langerhans cells is often seen in Langerhans cell histiocytosis, often with abundant eosinophils. Up to 50% harbor mutations in *BRAF* V600E. Mycosis fungoides is a neoplastic T lymphocytic cell disorder characterized by T cells with cerebriform nuclei that demonstrate partial loss of CD7. T-cell receptor (TCR) clonality assay may be required in patients with a history of primary cutaneous lymphoproliferative disorder where regional lymph nodes show dermatopathic changes. Postvaccination lymphadenopathy exhibits similar features to that of infectious mononucleosis, that is, partial architectural effacement due to marked sinusoidal and capsular infiltration by immunoblasts that often have Reed-Sternberg-like features and atypia. Axillary lymphadenopathy, not inguinal lymphadenopathy, is a known side effect of COVID-19 vaccination.

**9. Correct choice: D.**

Nodular lymphocyte-predominant Hodgkin lymphoma accounts for 5% of all Hodgkin lymphoma. There is complete effacement of the nodal architecture by a vaguely nodular growth, which leaves a thin rim of residual node (see Figure 1). "Popcorn cells" represent the defining cellular feature (see Figure 2). They express B-lymphocytic markers and CD45, but not CD15. The immunophenotype of this Reed-Sternberg cell variant supports the notion that it is derived from the germinal center. The prognosis is good. The vaguely nodular growth pattern of most cases of nodular lymphocyte-predominant Hodgkin lymphoma may lead to a mistaken diagnosis of follicular center cell lymphoma. The diffuse subtype is rare and characterized by increased numbers of T lymphocytes.

**10. Correct choice: B.**

Lymphocyte-rich classic Hodgkin lymphoma accounts for 2% to 3% of Hodgkin lymphoma and has a favorable prognosis. It has a nodular growth pattern and lymphocyte-rich cellularity, but in contrast to the nodular lymphocyte-predominant variant, it contains the classical type of Reed-Sternberg cell. Lymphocyte-rich classic Hodgkin lymphoma tends to occur in a slightly older patient population with more frequent mediastinal involvement than the nodular lymphocyte-predominant variant.

**11. Correct choice: E.**

Nodular sclerosis classic Hodgkin lymphoma is the most common subtype of Hodgkin lymphoma (60% of cases) and manifests in young adults with mediastinal, cervical, or supraclavicular adenopathy. It is characterized by nodularity, dense collagen bands, and a thickened capsule with the prototypical CD15+, CD30+, and CD45− lacunar variant classic Reed-Sternberg cells. Lacunar cells are characterized by a conspicuous pericellular halo, which is due to formalin fixation and is thus absent in B5-fixed tissue. Nodular sclerosis classic Hodgkin lymphoma may contain large numbers of the mononuclear variant of Reed-Sternberg cell, which exhibits a large vesicular nucleus and a prominent nucleolus, and the same immunoreactivity as the classic Reed-Sternberg cell. The British National Lymphoma Investigation has proposed a grading system of nodular sclerosis classic Hodgkin lymphoma based on the number of Reed-Sternberg cells relative to the reactive cell population, but this system is not used for clinical purposes.

**12. Correct choice: D.**

Mixed cellularity classic Hodgkin lymphoma accounts for up to 30% of all cases of Hodgkin lymphoma and tends to affect patients older than those with nodular-sclerosing classic Hodgkin lymphoma. As its designation implies, it is characterized by a mixed cellular infiltrate in which T lymphocytes are often predominant. Reed-Sternberg cells are easily found and express CD15 and CD30, but not CD45. Thin bands of fibrosis may be seen, but these are different from the broad birefringent bands of fibrosis in nodular-sclerosing classic Hodgkin lymphoma. Prognosis is generally good but worse than that of nodular-sclerosing classic Hodgkin lymphoma.

**13. Correct choice: A.**

Lymphocyte-depleted classic Hodgkin lymphoma accounts for fewer than 5% of all Hodgkin lymphoma. It affects older patients (median age: 50s), who present with diffuse disease and systemic manifestations. Lymphocyte-depleted classic Hodgkin lymphoma is characterized by a disorganized pattern of fibrosis, in which intercellular fibrinoid material is present on the periodic acid-Schiff (PAS) stain. Reed-Sternberg cells may be difficult to detect but display the usual CD45−/CD15+/CD30+ phenotype. Other cases may exhibit diffuse, sheet-like Reed-Sternberg cells with bizarre morphology which may mimic non-Hodgkin lymphoma or carcinoma. The latter variant explains the old designation of Hodgkin sarcoma. Bone marrow involvement is usually found, so diagnosis can be made by marrow biopsy. Liver involvement is frequent as well. Systemic manifestations include reduced pancytopenia and altered liver function tests.

**14. Correct choice: E.**

Classic Reed-Sternberg cells express CD15 and CD30, but not CD45. The opposite is true for the Reed-Sternberg cell found in nodular lymphocyte-predominant Hodgkin lymphoma. Chronic lymphocytic leukemia/small lymphocytic lymphoma is typically CD5+ CD10− CD23+. Burkitt lymphoma is CD5− CD10+ CD43+, and follicular lymphoma is typically CD5− CD10+ Bcl-6+.

**15. Correct choice: E.**

Chronic lymphocytic leukemia/small lymphocytic lymphoma affects predominantly older patients and has a slow clinical course. The neoplastic population is composed of monomorphic small lymphocytes of perifollicular B-cell origin. Its phenotype is as follows: CD5+, CD23+, CD43+, and BCL-2+.

**16. Correct choice: B.**

Mantle zone lymphoma is thought to originate from perifollicular B cells. It gives rise to a characteristic mantle zone expansion resulting in a nodular pattern. Mantle zone lymphoma is an aggressive malignancy that occurs predominantly in older male patients with stage III–IV disease. Patients present with lymphadenopathy and extranodal involvement (bone marrow, spleen, liver, bowel, and brain). Translocation t(11;14) involves the genes of immunoglobulin (Ig) heavy chain and cyclin D1/CCND1 (*bcl-1*), resulting in overexpression of cyclin D1. Cyclin D1 can be demonstrated in paraffin tissue by immunohistochemistry. Typical immunophenotype of mantle zone lymphoma is CD5+, BCL-2+, CD10−, CD23−. Burkitt lymphoma is associated with t(8;14). Follicular lymphoma is associated with t(14;18), while t(11;18) is associated with gastrointestinal low-grade mucosa-associated tissue lymphoma.

**17. Correct choice: D.**

Follicular lymphoma is the most common non-Hodgkin lymphoma in the United States, presenting as generalized lymphadenopathy and marrow involvement in middle-aged patients. The neoplastic lymphocytes consist of a variable mixture of centrocytes and centroblasts. The genotypic hallmark of follicular lymphoma (FL) is a translocation involving the gene of immunoglobulin heavy chain (IgH) on chromosome 14 and the gene of BCL-2 on chromosome 18, leading to overexpression of BCL-2, an apoptosis-inhibiting protein. Lymphocytes of follicular lymphoma resemble normal germinal center B cells and express pan-B-cell antigens (including CD20). Like normal germinal center cells, they express CD10 and Bcl-6 and not CD5 or CD43. In contrast to normal follicles, however, follicular lymphoma cells express BCL-2, whose immunohistochemical detection is helpful in distinguishing follicular lymphoma from normal follicles. The antiapoptotic activity of BCL-2 accounts for the slow growth of follicular lymphoma, which is, however, incurable.

**18. Correct choice: B.**

Follicular lymphoma is composed of a variable mixture of centrocytes and centroblasts. Centrocytes have clefted nuclei with clumped chromatin and no nucleoli. Centroblasts have open nuclei with nucleoli located against the nuclear membrane. Grading is based on the fact that prognosis worsens with increasing numbers of centroblasts. The most recent World Health Organization (WHO) guidelines for grading follicular lymphoma recommend counting centroblasts in 10 random but representative 40 times fields and calculating the average per field. Grade 1: 0 to 5 centroblasts per HPF (high-power field). Grade 2: 6 to 15 centroblasts per HPF. Grade 3a: greater than 15 centroblasts per HPF with admixed centrocytes. Grade 3b: greater than 15 centroblasts per HPF without admixed centrocytes. Grade 3b has the worst prognosis. Estimating the degree of follicular growth pattern is also recommended.

**19. Correct choice: E.**

The nodal form of marginal zone lymphoma features a prominent perifollicular and subcapsular pattern of growth. The neoplastic cells resemble monocytoid B cells found in reactive conditions. Monocytoid B cells are 2 to 3 times larger than small lymphocytes and display pale cytoplasm. They express surface BCL-2 (like normal marginal zone cells but unlike monocytoid cells) and immunoglobulin M (IgM) or IgG and are negative for CD5, CD10, and CD23. The nodal form of marginal zone lymphoma has an indolent clinical course. The mucosa-associated lymphoid tissue (MALT) form of marginal zone lymphoma is indistinguishable from the nodal form.

**20. Correct choice: B.**

Diffuse large B-cell lymphoma accounts for up to 30% of all non-Hodgkin lymphomas. Patients present with rapidly enlarging lymph nodes, and 30% to 40% have extranodal presentations (skin, breast, testes, bowel, thyroid, brain, liver, and spleen). Bone marrow involvement occurs in 25% of cases. The median age is 60 years, but diffuse large B-cell lymphoma may affect children. The neoplastic cells are transformed lymphocytes of B-cell origin that express pan-B-cell markers. Diffuse large B-cell lymphoma can have variable immunophenotypes, sometimes overlapping with follicular lymphoma (CD10+ and CD5–), but surface immunoglobulins are negative on diffuse large B-cell lymphoma. The neoplastic lymphocytes are large and have vesicular nuclei and prominent nucleoli. The nuclei may be multilobated and simulate Reed-Sternberg cells. Overall 5-year survival is 46%.

**21. Correct choice: E.**

T-cell/histiocyte-rich large B-cell lymphoma is a large B-cell lymphoma in which there are scattered neoplastic B cells that compose less than 10% of the total cells and are seen in a background of numerous reactive small T cells and histiocytes with no significant small B-cell component. Reactive cells compose greater than 90% of total cells with numerous small T cells and histiocytes but few reactive B cells. The neoplastic B cells are positive for pan-B-cell markers and CD45 but typically negative for CD15 and CD30. The prognosis is poor. T-cell/histiocyte-rich large B-cell lymphoma is negative for anaplastic lymphoma kinase (ALK) and Epstein-Barr virus (EBV). Large B-cell lymphoma with IRF4 rearrangement occurs in children and young adults. The lymph nodes of head and neck or Waldeyer ring are affected. On biopsy, there is a proliferation of medium to large cells arranged in a diffuse, diffuse and follicular, or follicular pattern. The cells exhibit a germinal center B-cell phenotype with diffuse IRF4/MUM1 expression. Most cases show *IRF4* rearrangement. Peripheral T-cell lymphoma has numerous small T cells, but the neoplastic atypical tumor cells often occur in aggregates (not scattered) and express one or more T-cell markers.

**22. Correct choice: D.**

Primary effusion lymphoma not only occurs most frequently in patients who are HIV positive, but also develops in patients who are non-immunosuppressed, often older. It arises in the pericardial, pleural, or peritoneal cavity. Although they are B-cell lineage, the large, transformed immunoblastic or anaplastic cells lack B- or T-cell-associated surface antigens. They are positive for human herpesvirus 8 (HHV-8) and occasionally for Epstein-Barr virus (EBV).

**23. Correct choice: E.**

Primary mediastinal large B-cell lymphoma is the most common anterior mediastinal non-Hodgkin lymphoma. Patients present with cough, dyspnea, or superior vena cava syndrome. The neoplastic cells are usually intermediate-sized lymphoid cells arranged in a diffuse or clustered distribution with associated prominent sclerosis. The nuclei are round to oval and may be hyperchromatic or vesicular. Clear cell change (abundant pale cytoplasm) is often present. Typically, a subset of the neoplastic cells is pleomorphic and may resemble Reed-Sternberg cells. Aside from direct extension into surrounding structures, extra-mediastinal involvement is unusual at the time of initial diagnosis. The main differential diagnosis is classic Hodgkin lymphoma, diffuse large B-cell lymphoma, and B-cell lymphoma unclassifiable.

**24. Correct choice: A.**

Intravascular large B-cell lymphoma is a rare large B-cell lymphoma that is characterized by lymphoma cells, predominantly within the lumina of blood vessels, especially capillaries, with the exclusion of larger arteries and veins and a few to no circulating lymphoma cells in the peripheral blood. Skin and central nervous system involvement is common. Lymph nodes may show focal or diffuse architectural effacement without prominent intravascular components. It typically occurs in older patients and is characterized by an aggressive clinical course and a poor prognosis.

**25. Correct choice: C.**

Burkitt lymphoma is a high-grade non-Hodgkin lymphoma with a Ki-67 labeling index characteristically close to 100%.

There are three clinical variants: (a) endemic, which occurs in regions of Africa and New Guinea; it involves the jaw or abdomen and 95% are Epstein-Barr virus (EBV) positive; (b) sporadic, which affects children and young adults throughout the world and is occasionally EBV positive; (c) immunodeficiency associated, which affects patients who are HIV positive and involves the distal ileum, cecum, and mesentery; 25% are EBV positive. The sporadic and HIV-associated forms involve extranodal sites, most commonly the gastrointestinal (GI) tract, presenting as an ileocecal or peritoneal mass. The African form has a predilection for the mandible. EBV is associated with all cases of the African form, 25% of HIV-associated cases, and only occasionally with sporadic cases. The characteristic translocation in Burkitt lymphoma involves immunoglobulin (Ig) loci (usually IgH [immunoglobulin heavy chain] on chromosome 14) and the c-*myc* gene: t(8;14). Choice A relates to mantle zone lymphoma (the BCL-1 protein is cyclin D), choice B to follicular lymphoma, choice D to lymphoplasmacytic lymphoma, and choice E to acute T-cell lymphoblastic leukemia/lymphoma (other T-cell receptor loci are also involved).

**26. Correct choice: E.**

T-cell lymphoblastic lymphoma/leukemia arises from immature (precursor) T cells and may have two clinical presentations: (a) T-cell acute lymphoblastic leukemia (T-ALL), with T lymphoblasts in the bone marrow and blood, and (b) T-lymphoblastic lymphoma (T-LBL), which presents in children and young adults as a mediastinal mass with involvement of supradiaphragmatic lymph nodes. If untreated, the condition spreads to the viscera and central nervous system (CNS) and gives rise to a leukemic phase indistinguishable from T-cell acute lymphoblastic leukemia. Neoplastic cells are positive for T-cell markers, including CD3 and CD7, but 25% of cases express common ALL antigen (CD10). TdT (terminal deoxytransferase) is expressed in all cases. TdT is a special DNA polymerase expressed by precursor T and B cells. Human leukocyte antigen-DR (HLA-DR) is absent in T-ALL, unlike B-cell acute lymphoblastic leukemia.

**27. Correct choice: E.**

Peripheral T-cell lymphoma, unspecified is the most common form of T-cell lymphoma. It arises from mature post-thymic T lymphocytes and typically manifests in adults with generalized lymphadenopathy and "B symptoms" (fever, weight loss, pruritus, eosinophilia, etc). Most patients have marrow involvement. The diffuse and homogeneous effacement of lymph node architecture is typical of peripheral T-cell lymphoma. The neoplastic cells have pleomorphic nuclei and clear cytoplasm. Besides pan-T-cell markers, peripheral T-cell lymphoma often expresses CD4 and CD8, but it is remarkably negative for terminal deoxytransferase (TdT) and CD1 (which are positive in T-cell acute lymphoblastic leukemia/lymphoma). T-cell receptor (TCR) gene rearrangement is detected in most cases. Frequent relapses and a 25% 5-year survival rate are expected. Some peripheral T-cell lymphomas have an expression of CD30, which raises the differential diagnosis with anaplastic lymphoma kinase (ALK)-negative anaplastic large cell lymphoma. Cases associated with immunophenotypic expression of cytotoxic or natural killer cell markers behave more aggressively. There are three morphologic variants of peripheral T-cell lymphoma: lymphoepithelioid (Lennert), follicular, and T-zone lymphoma. Lennert lymphoma is a pattern characterized by scattered histiocytic islands amidst the diffuse lymphomatous growth.

**28. Correct choice: B.**

Angioimmunoblastic T-cell lymphoma affects adults presenting with "B symptoms," generalized lymphadenopathy, and frequent polyclonal hypergammaglobulinemia. Neoplastic cells express CD4, CD10, and other markers of follicular T-helper cells. The eye-catching feature of angioimmunoblastic T-cell lymphoma is the presence of a rich small-vessel meshwork with periodic acid-Schiff (PAS)-positive vessel walls. Follicular dendritic cells are abundant around the vessels and can be identified by CD21 immunohistochemistry. T-cell receptor (TCR) gene rearrangement has been found in 75% of cases and appears to be limited to the CD10+ cells.

**29. Correct choice: A.**

The most characteristic cells composing anaplastic large cell lymphoma (the so-called hallmark cells) appear cohesive and have marked nuclear pleomorphism, prominent nucleoli, abundant cytoplasm, and brisk mitotic activity. Such cohesive growth of highly anaplastic cells can be confused with poorly differentiated carcinomas or histiocytic sarcomas. Hallmark cells express CD30, usually T-cell antigens, and often epithelial membrane antigen (EMA). Expression of cytotoxic granule–associated protein suggests an origin from cytotoxic lymphocytes. One-tenth of anaplastic large cell lymphomas express B-cell antigens such as PAX-5. Anaplastic large cell lymphoma may be primary (arising de novo) or secondary (developing from preexisting lymphoma, usually mycosis fungoides). Translocation *t(2;5)(p23;q35)* is the most characteristic chromosomal abnormality. This translocation leads to the expression of a novel protein named *NPM-ALK*, resulting from the fusion of genes coding for nucleophosmin (NPM) and anaplastic lymphoma kinase (ALK). Expression of this protein can be detected by immunohistochemically using the *ALK1* antibody.

**30. Correct choice: E.**

Adult T-cell leukemia/lymphoma is a T-cell neoplasm caused by human T-cell leukemia virus type I (HTLV-I). It is endemic in south Japan, the Caribbean islands, New Guinea, central Africa, and parts of South America. HTLV-I is transmitted like HIV, by blood transfusion, sexual intercourse, needle sharing, and mother to child via placenta or breast milk. A lifetime risk of developing leukemia is approximately 5% in individuals with seropositivity. Adult T-cell leukemia/lymphoma develops after a latency of decades following infection. It may present as an acute (most frequent), lymphomatous, chronic, or smoldering form. The acute form is rapidly fatal and involves lymph nodes, viscera, skin, and bones. Circulating leukemic cells have unique hyperlobated, cloverleaf-shaped nuclei. The neoplastic lymphocytes express CD4, the activation marker CD25, and FoxP3, a phenotype corresponding to regulatory T cells (Treg). HTLV-I provirus can be demonstrated in the neoplastic cells.

**31. Correct choice: A.**

Mycosis fungoides/Sézary syndrome (MF/SS) is a neoplasm of peripheral CD4-positive (helper) T lymphocytes. MF/SS initially involves the skin and then progresses to systemic spread. Lymph node involvement is frequent, occurring in 70% of cases, especially in the axillary and inguinal regions. Sézary syndrome refers to generalized skin involvement in the form of exfoliative erythroderma, which is associated with leukemia. The neoplastic cells have a characteristic convoluted cerebriform nucleus. Lymph node involvement may be graded according to the National Cancer Institute (NCI) classification, the Dutch system, or the International Society for Cutaneous Lymphomas and the European Organization of Research and Treatment of Cancer (ISCL/EORTC) staging system. Increasing degrees of nodal involvement as assessed by either one of these three grading schemes is correlated with increasingly poorer survival.

**32. Correct choice: B.**

Posttransplant lymphoproliferative disorder (PTLD) complicates solid organ or bone marrow transplantation in 1% to 10% of cases. B-cell proliferations account for 95% of cases; the others are T-cell lymphomas. PTLD encompasses at least three clinicopathologic forms: (1) plasmacytic hyperplasia or infectious mononucleosis-like PTLD occurs in children and young adults early after transplantation, involving lymph nodes and tonsils. It resolves with a reduction in immunosuppression; (2) polymorphic PTLD is more aggressive and consists of clonal growth of a mixed, pleomorphic population of lymphocytes, immunoblasts, and plasma cells that efface the lymph node architecture; and (3) monomorphic PTLD is a lymphoma, usually with the features of diffuse large B-cell lymphoma. Epstein-Barr virus (EBV) is detected in 80% to 85% of all PTLDs.

**33. Correct choice: E.**

In addition to posttransplant lymphoproliferative disorder (PTLD), Epstein-Barr virus is linked to a variety of lymphoproliferative disorders, including endemic Burkitt lymphoma, extranodal natural killer (NK)/T-cell lymphoma, lymphomatoid granulomatosis, plasmablastic lymphoma, lymphomas arising in patients with congenital or acquired immunodeficiencies, as well as Epstein-Barr virus-positive diffuse large B-cell lymphoma, not otherwise specified.

**34. Correct choice: C.**

Histiocytic sarcoma is a rare, malignant neoplasm of mature histiocytes. It may show highly pleomorphic or spindle cytology, mimicking pleomorphic or spindle cell sarcoma. The neoplastic cells are positive for histiocyte markers (CD68, CD163), lysozyme, and CD45, but negative for T- and B-cell markers. A subset appears to be dedifferentiated from B-cell lymphomas. It is an extremely aggressive disease and patients typically present with B symptoms, lymphadenopathy, and hepatosplenomegaly.

**35. Correct choice: C.**

Follicular dendritic cell sarcoma is a low-grade sarcoma that presents as a painless solid mass in nodal and extranodal sites. Cervical lymph nodes are most commonly affected. It is characterized by oval to spindled cells with dispersed chromatin, small nucleoli, eosinophilic and fibrillar cytoplasm with syncytial borders arranged in fascicles, whorls, or storiform patterns. Binucleate or occasional multinucleate forms and nuclear pseudoinclusions may be present. An admixed population of lymphocytes, eosinophils, plasma cells, or neutrophils may also be present. Immunohistochemistry showing expression of two or more follicular dendritic cell markers (CD21, CD23, clusterin) is essential for diagnosis.

**36. Correct choice: C.**

In patients with HIV infection, Kaposi sarcoma is typically lymphadenopathic or extracutaneous. When it involves the lymph nodes, it is characterized by nodular masses in the capsular and subcapsular regions. The nodules are formed by a proliferation of dense spindle cell fascicles forming slit-like vascular channels, extravasated red blood cells, and hemosiderin. Mitotic figures are often prominent. Polymerase chain reaction (PCR) confirms the presence of human herpesvirus 8 (HHV-8) DNA in more than 95% of cases.

**37. Correct choice: E.**

Sarcoidosis is a multisystem granulomatous disease with nonspecific clinical manifestations that commonly affect the pulmonary system and other organs including the eyes, skin, liver, spleen, and lymph nodes. Sarcoidosis usually presents with persistent dry cough, eye and skin manifestations, weight loss, fatigue, night sweats, and erythema nodosum. Sarcoidosis is more common in adults (<50 years) of African American or Scandinavian descent. Infectious agents should always be excluded by special stains and cultures. Sarcoid granulomas may coexist with Hodgkin lymphoma, non-Hodgkin lymphoma, and non-hematologic malignancies.

**38. Correct choice: B.**

Kikuchi-Fujimoto disease is a benign, self-limited lymphadenitis of unknown etiology. It predominantly affects young adults, with cervical lymphadenopathy, fever, and often leukopenia. The involved lymph nodes show histiocytes, plasmacytoid dendritic cells, immunoblasts, and necrosis with karyorrhectic debris. The transformed cells are predominantly CD8-positive T cells with a cytotoxic phenotype. The absence of neutrophils and lack of follicular hyperplasia distinguish Kikuchi-Fujimoto disease from cat-scratch disease and other bacterial infections.

**39. Correct choice: D.**

Kimura disease is a benign disorder of unknown etiology with an indolent clinical course. It predominantly affects young Asian males. There can be involvement of nodal and extranodal sites, most commonly skin, head, and neck. It is characterized by hyperplastic follicles with germinal centers associated with the expansion of the interfollicular areas by abundant eosinophils, often forming eosinophilic microabscesses. There may be disruption of follicles by the increased eosinophils causing folliculolysis. There is often an admixture of lymphocytes, plasma cells, mast cells, and histiocytes. Stromal and perivascular sclerosis may occur in late-stage lesions.

**40. Correct choice: C.**

Hemophagocytic lymphohistiocytosis is an immune activation syndrome due to congenital or acquired defective natural killer (NK)/T-cell function with uncontrolled hypercytokinemia and end-organ damage. It is characterized by histiocytic infiltration of reticuloendothelial organs with hemophagocytosis of erythrocytes, leukocytes, platelets, and their precursor cells. Patients present with sudden onset of a systemic inflammatory response syndrome with symptoms including high unremitting fevers, malaise, rash, jaundice, and myalgia, along with cytopenias, hepatosplenomegaly, and generalized lymphadenopathy. The acquired form has been linked to infection (particularly viruses that include most often, Epstein-Barr virus, but also cytomegalovirus and more recently, COVID-19), malignancy (most often NK/T-cell neoplasms, such as panniculitis-like T-cell lymphoma and nasal type extranodal NK/T-cell lymphoma), immunosuppression, and rheumatologic/autoimmune disease.

# 18 Spleen

1. A splenectomy specimen from a patient with clinically diagnosed idiopathic thrombocytopenic purpura (ITP) is submitted for pathologic examination. As shown in Figure 1, there is prominent follicular hyperplasia. Which of the following is most likely to be seen in the red pulp?

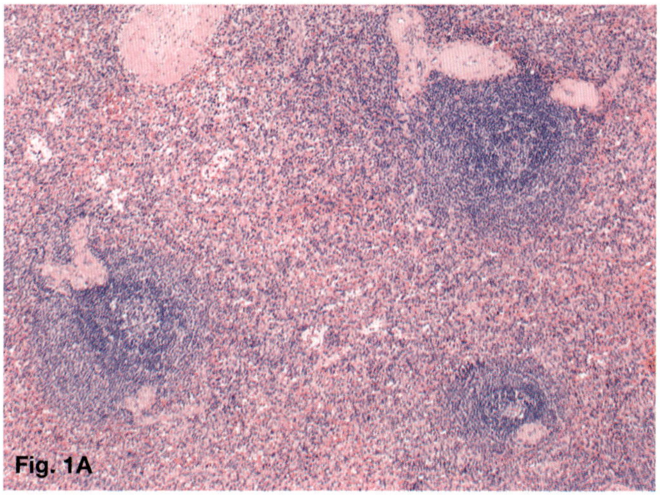

Fig. 1A

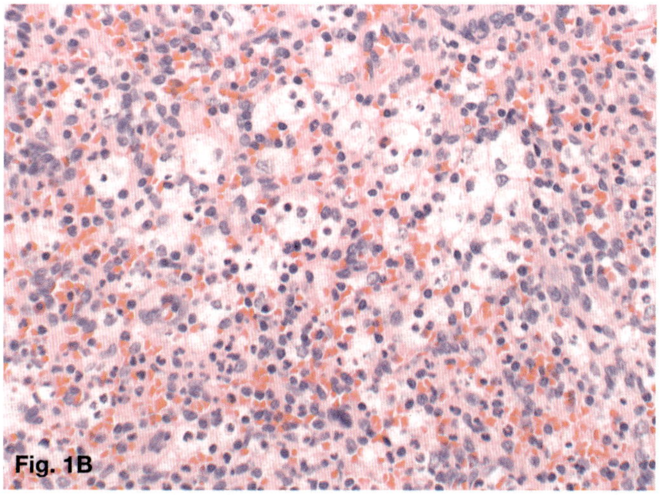

Fig. 1B

A. Arteriolar thrombi
B. Ceroid-laden histiocytes in the red pulp
C. Congested red pulp cords
D. Hemophagocytosis
E. Immunoblastic proliferation

2. A 55-year-old man with lymphoma, anemia, and thrombocytopenia underwent splenectomy (Figure 1). The white pulp is expanded and effaced by neoplastic lymphocytes that express CD5 and CD23, but not cyclin D1 or tartrate. Which of the following is the most likely diagnosis?

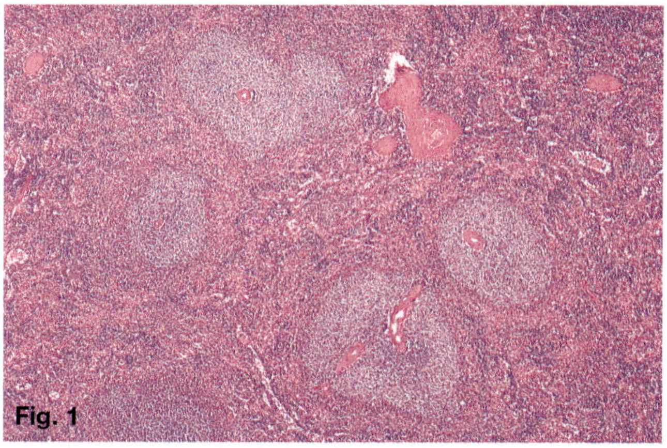

Fig. 1

A. Hairy cell leukemia
B. Lymphoplasmacytic lymphoma
C. Mantle cell lymphoma
D. Marginal zone lymphoma
E. Small lymphocytic lymphoma

All figures in this chapter are from Longacre TA, Greenson JK, Hornick JL, Reuter VE, eds. *Mills and Sternberg's Diagnostic Surgical Pathology*. 7th ed. Wolters Kluwer; 2022 except for those noted at the end of this book.

3. Figure 1 shows the characteristic infiltration pattern and cellular morphology of a splenic lymphoma bearing a *t*(11;14) chromosomal translocation. Morphologically, this lymphoma is similar to small lymphocytic lymphoma (SLL). Which of the following markers allows differentiation from SLL?

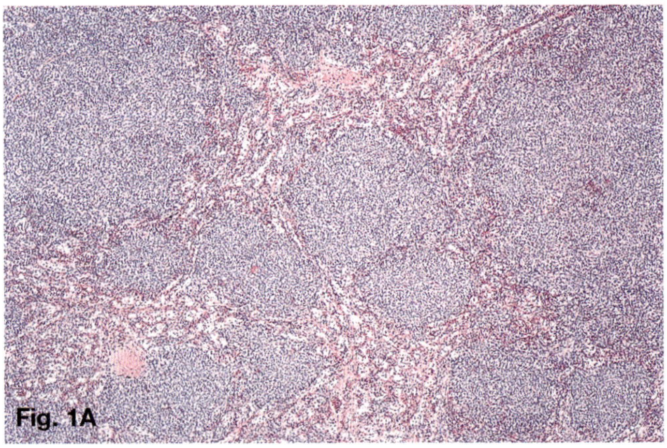

Fig. 1A

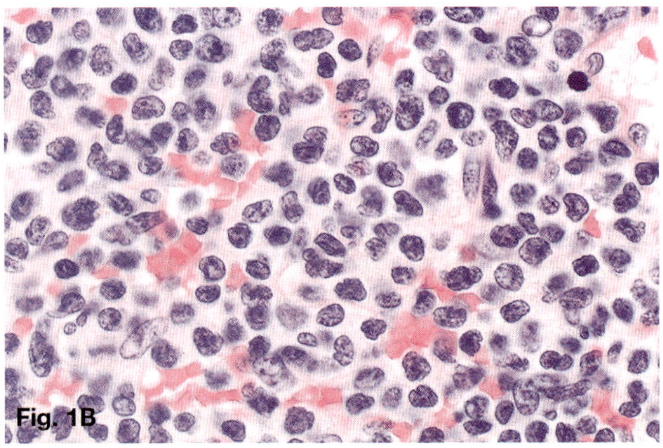

Fig. 1B

A. CD5
B. CD10
C. CD23
D. CD43
E. Cyclin D1

4. A 70-year-old man presents with abdominal pain and fullness in the left upper quadrant.

On physical examination, severe splenomegaly is found. Laboratory studies show pancytopenia and paraproteinemia. He undergoes splenectomy, which reveals white pulp expansion as shown in Figures 1 and 2. The infiltrating cells express CD19, CD20, and immunoglobulin M (IgM). They are negative for CD5, CD10, CD23, and cyclin D1. Which of the following is the most likely diagnosis?

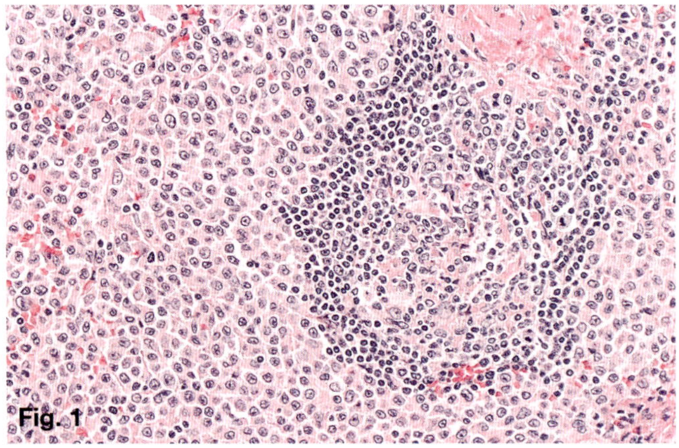

Fig. 1

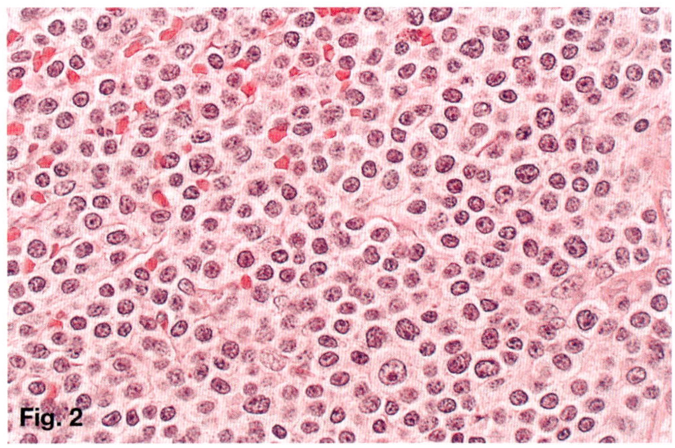

Fig. 2

A. Follicular lymphoma
B. Hairy cell leukemia
C. Mantle cell lymphoma
D. Marginal zone lymphoma
E. Small lymphocytic lymphoma

5. A 58-year-old man presents with a very large spleen and pancytopenia. A bone marrow aspirate does not yield any material (dry tap). A splenectomy is performed. The cut surface of the removed spleen is homogeneous without nodular lesions. On histologic examination, the cords and sinuses of the red pulp appear filled with numerous atypical cells, as seen in Figure 1. These cells are positive for tartrate-resistant alkaline phosphatase (TRAP) and immunoreactive for CD11c and CD22 antigens. Ultrastructural studies demonstrate cells with cytoplasmic villous projections. The most likely diagnosis is

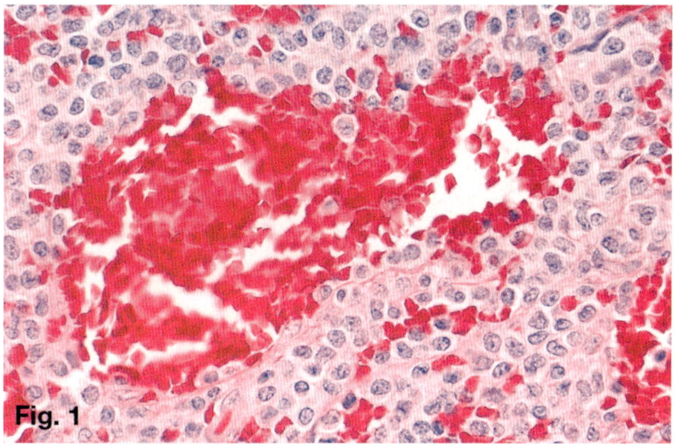
Fig. 1

A. chronic monocytic leukemia.
B. hairy cell leukemia.
C. mantle cell lymphoma.
D. marginal zone lymphoma.
E. myelofibrosis.

6. Figure 1 shows the cut surface of a very enlarged spleen. Which of the following disorders is most consistent with this gross appearance?

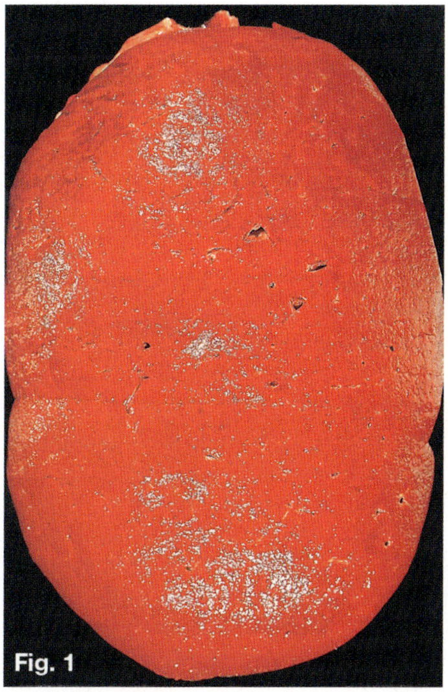
Fig. 1

A. Chronic myeloid leukemia
B. Hodgkin lymphoma
C. Large B-cell lymphoma
D. Reactive follicular hyperplasia
E. Small lymphocytic lymphoma

7. Figure 1 shows the red pulp of a massively enlarged spleen. The cell population seen here is most compatible with which of the following disorders?

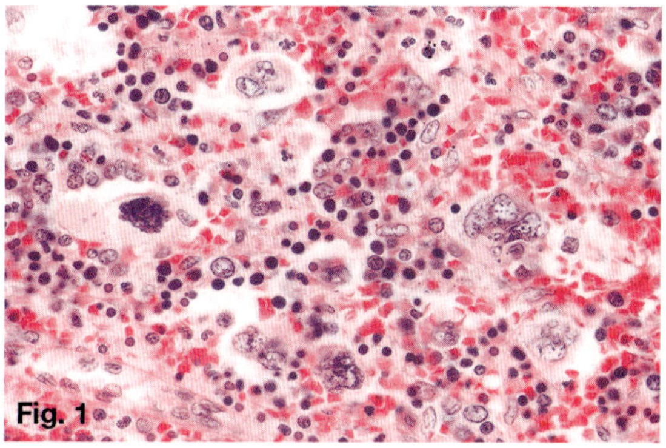
Fig. 1

A. Chronic myeloid leukemia
B. Hairy cell leukemia
C. Hereditary spherocytosis
D. Infectious mononucleosis
E. Primary myelofibrosis

8. What is the most likely diagnosis for the solitary, well-defined hypodense 3.0-cm mass, shown in Figure 1, in the spleen of a 44-year-old woman undergoing a computed tomography (CT) scan for possible appendicitis?

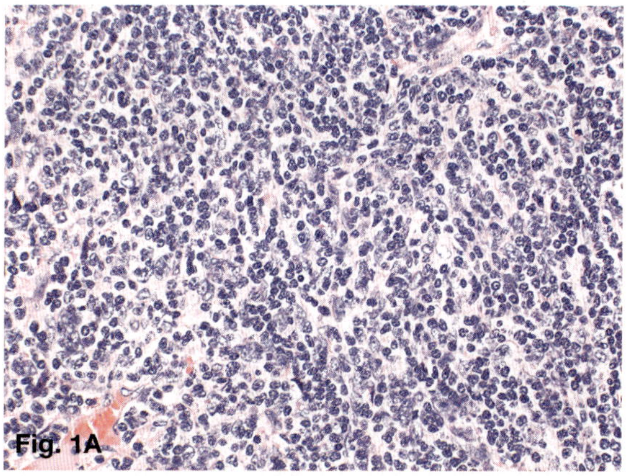
Fig. 1A

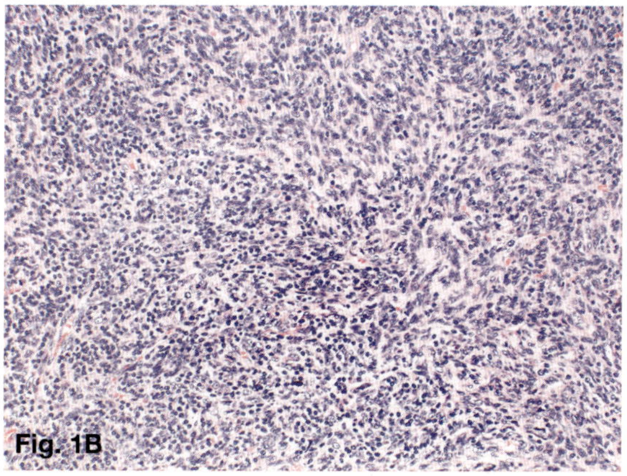
Fig. 1B

A. Epstein-Barr virus (EBV)-positive inflammatory follicular dendritic cell/fibroblastic reticular cell tumor
B. Follicular dendritic cell sarcoma
C. Inflammatory myofibroblastic tumor
D. Interdigitating dendritic cell sarcoma
E. Mycobacterial spindle cell pseudotumor

9. What is the best diagnosis for the incidental splenic mass, shown in Figure 1, in a 50-year-old man?

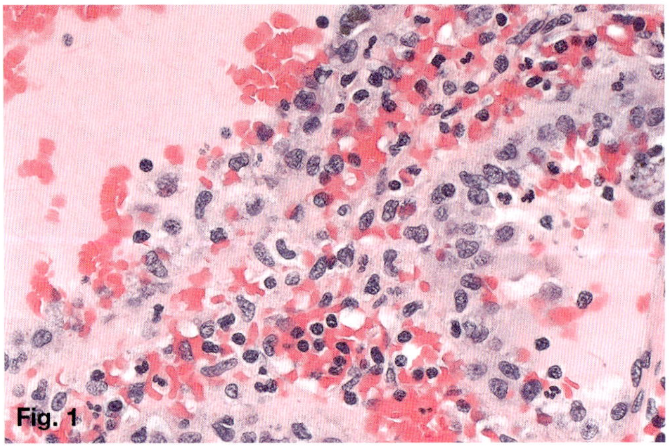

Fig. 1

A. Angiosarcoma
B. Hemangioma
C. Littoral cell angioma
D. Lymphangioma
E. Sclerosing angiomatoid nodular transformation

10. A 44-year-old woman undergoes exploratory laparotomy for suspected carcinomatosis. One of the abdominal nodules is submitted for frozen section (Figure 1) with the resultant diagnosis of calcifying fibrous tumor. The nodules are excised and she undergoes splenectomy for a coincidental splenic mass. What is the most likely diagnosis?

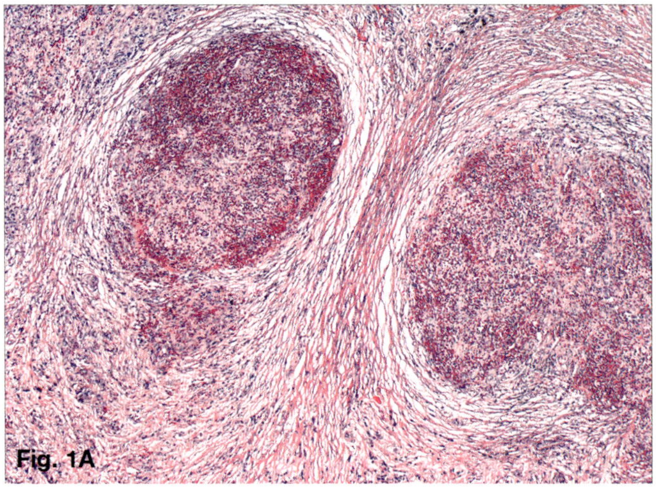

Fig. 1A

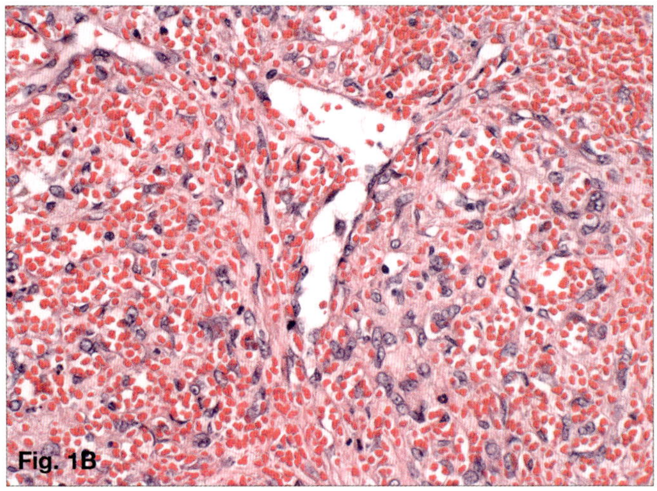

Fig. 1B

A. Angiosarcoma
B. Hamartoma
C. Hemangioma
D. Lymphangioma
E. Sclerosing angiomatoid nodular transformation

# ANSWERS AND EXPLANATIONS

**1. Correct choice: B.**

Splenic disorders may be divided into those primarily affecting white pulp or red pulp. Reactive follicular hyperplasia is a finding associated with various disorders, including idiopathic thrombocytopenic purpura, thrombotic thrombocytopenic purpura, rheumatoid arthritis, hemolytic anemias, Castleman disease, and AIDS. Idiopathic thrombocytopenic purpura (ITP) is further characterized by ceroid (lipid)-laden histiocytes in the red pulp, as evidence of active platelet phagocytosis. Arteriolar thrombi are characteristic of thrombotic thrombocytopenic purpura. Congested red pulp cords are nonspecific and may be seen, for example, in hemolytic anemias. Hemophagocytosis is related to hemophagocytic syndromes. An immunoblastic proliferation is typical of infectious mononucleosis.

**2. Correct choice: E.**

Small lymphocytic lymphoma produces a distinctive infiltrative pattern, resulting in expansion and fusion of white pulp, with extension into the red pulp by neoplastic small, round lymphocytes. The differential diagnosis includes hairy cell leukemia when there is extensive infiltration into the red pulp and higher-grade lymphomas when splenic involvement by small lymphocytic lymphoma is accompanied by proliferation centers with admixed large cells. In these cases, immunophenotyping and clonal analysis can resolve the diagnostic dilemma.

**3. Correct choice: E.**

Many patients with mantle cell lymphoma present with splenomegaly. Splenic involvement results in a marked expansion of the white pulp, with fusion of white pulp into irregularly shaped nodules, similar to small lymphocytic lymphoma/chronic lymphocytic leukemia. The neoplastic cells in mantle zone lymphoma are small lymphocytes with dense chromatin and irregular nuclear contours. Since mantle cell lymphoma and small lymphocytic lymphoma/chronic lymphocytic leukemia each express CD5 and CD43 and CD23 may be positive in mantle cell lymphoma as well as small lymphocytic lymphoma/chronic lymphocytic leukemia, their distinction is largely based on the *t*(11;14), which results in overexpression of cyclin D1.

**4. Correct choice: D.**

Splenic marginal zone lymphoma is an indolent lymphoma that often manifests with marked splenomegaly and anemia or pancytopenia due to marrow involvement. Liver and node involvement are frequent. Atypical villous lymphocytes are present in the peripheral blood, whereas a monoclonal peak is often present in serum and/or urine. The typical pattern of growth is known as marginal zone pattern. The marginal zone expands, surrounding an attenuated mantle zone (as seen in Figure 1). Marginal zone lymphocytes have abundant, pale-staining cytoplasm and are virtually identical to monocytoid B cells (seen in Figure 2). Negative immunostains for CD5, CD43, and cyclin D1 rule out small lymphocytic lymphoma and mantle cell lymphoma. Follicular lymphoma is ruled out by negative CD10.

**5. Correct choice: B.**

Patients with hairy cell leukemia (HCL) are typically in their 50s or 60s and present with massive splenomegaly and pancytopenia. The spleen is uniformly and diffusely involved. The red pulp is infiltrated by mononuclear cells with reniform or oval nuclei. Mitotic figures are rare. Red lakes are eye-catching microscopic features, consisting of erythrocyte-filled cavities lined by neoplastic cells. The villous projections seen on ultrastructural examination account for its designation. Hairy cell leukemia arises from B lymphocytes. The V600E mutation in the *BRAF* gene has been recently shown to be a genetic hallmark of HCL. Detection of this mutation is of diagnostic value in ambiguous cases. Mantle cell and marginal zone lymphomas present with a nodular pattern involving predominantly the white pulp. Erythrophagocytosis is observed in chronic monocytic leukemia.

**6. Correct choice: A.**

A wide range of pathologic processes in the spleen shows predominant red pulp involvement: congestion, infections, leukemias and myeloproliferative disorders, histiocytic proliferations, and nonhematopoietic neoplasms. As the red pulp expands, the white pulp becomes less conspicuous, until the cut surface appears uniformly red, as shown in this case of chronic myeloid leukemia. All other answer choices refer to conditions that would manifest with predominant white pulp involvement and a nodular pattern on the cut surface.

**7. Correct choice: E.**

The image here shows red pulp sinuses replete with hematopoietic elements of all three lines (megakaryocytes, and myeloid and nucleated red blood cells are present), which is most characteristic of primary myelofibrosis. Progressive fibrosis and obliteration of functioning bone marrow lead to compensatory extramedullary hematopoiesis, which involves the spleen and, less frequently, the liver. Identification of all three hematopoietic lines is a prerequisite for the diagnosis of extramedullary hematopoiesis in the spleen, as myeloid precursors and megakaryocytes can be found in chronic myeloid leukemia. Hairy cell leukemia is characterized by diffuse red pulp infiltration by mononuclear cells with reniform or oval nuclei. In hereditary spherocytosis, red pulp cords are extremely congested and packed with spherocytes. Infectious mononucleosis leads to massive expansion of the red pulp by immunoblasts.

**8. Correct choice: A.**

Epstein-Barr virus (EBV)-positive inflammatory follicular dendritic cell/fibroblastic reticular cell tumor is an extranodal EBV-positive indolent neoplasm with a phenotypic spectrum ranging from follicular dendritic cells to fibroblastic reticular cells associated with a prominent polymorphic inflammatory background. The spleen followed by the liver is the most common site of involvement. The neoplastic cells are spindled to oval, with vesicular chromatin, a small, central nucleolus, and indistinct cytoplasmic borders. A loose fascicular pattern with a storiform appearance may be seen in association with an inflammatory background composed of small lymphocytes, plasma cells, and histiocytes; eosinophils can be present. At least some of the constituent cells exhibit follicular dendritic cell markers. Anaplastic lymphoma kinase (ALK) is negative. All the other choices are EBV negative.

**9. Correct choice: C.**

Littoral cell angioma is a typically benign splenic vascular tumor that arises from littoral cells lining splenic red pulp sinuses. It is characterized by a proliferation of anastomosing, tortuous, blood-filled vascular channels lined by tall endothelial cells with variable hemophagocytosis, often with papillary projections and cystic spaces. Sloughing of endothelial cells into vascular spaces is common. There is usually no sclerosis or cytologic atypia. The constituent cells exhibit endothelial (factor VIII, CD31) and histiocytic (CD68, CD163, lysozyme) differentiation. CD34 expression is typically absent. Splenic angiosarcoma exhibits cytologic atypia, tumor necrosis, and high mitotic rate; it is CD34 positive. Splenic hemangioma is characterized by a single layer of bland endothelial cells that are CD34 positive but negative for histiocytic markers. Splenic lymphangioma is often subcapsular and composed of cystic, malformed lymphatic channels with attenuated endothelial lining; it also lacks histiocytic markers.

**10. Correct choice: E.**

Sclerosing angiomatoid nodular transformation is a benign, circumscribed nodule in the spleen composed of angiomatoid nodules set in a dense, collagenized stroma. The nodules contain a mixture of slit-like, round or irregular vascular spaces lined by cytologically bland, sometimes plump endothelial cells, lacking atypia, necrosis, and mitotic figures. Three types of vessels (as seen in the normal splenic red pulp) are present: capillaries (CD34+/CD8−/CD31+), sinusoids (CD34−/CD8+/CD31+), and small veins (CD34−/CD8−/CD31+). IgG4-positive plasma cells are occasionally numerous with increased immunoglobulin G subclass 4 (IgG4):IgG ratio; however, serum IgG4 is not elevated. The adjacent splenic tissue is unremarkable. It may be associated with abdominal disseminated calcifying fibrous tumors simulating carcinomatosis.

# 19 Jaws, Oral Cavity, and Oropharynx

1. A nodular lesion is excised from the lower gingiva of a 30-year-old female patient. Histologically, it consists of vascular stroma containing numerous osteoclast-like giant cells and hemosiderin deposits, as demonstrated in Figure 1. Which of the following is the most likely diagnosis?

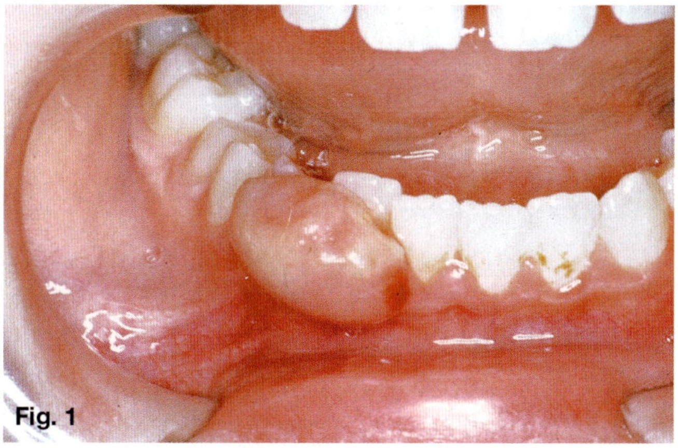

Fig. 1

A. Granular cell tumor
B. Masson hemangioma
C. Peripheral giant cell granuloma
D. Pyogenic granuloma
E. Verruciform xanthoma

2. The majority of solitary papillomas of the oral cavity are associated with

A. Frank koilocytosis.
B. human papillomavirus (HPV) types 6 and 11.
C. human papillomavirus (HPV) types 16 and 18.
D. progression to carcinoma.
E. squamous dysplasia.

3. Which of the following oral lesions is a non–human papillomavirus (HPV)-associated process?

A. Condyloma acuminatum
B. Multifocal epithelial hyperplasia
C. Oral hairy leukoplakia
D. Squamous papilloma
E. Verruca vulgaris

4. A 40-year-old man undergoes resection of a tumor located in the right palatine tonsil, which is diagnosed as a squamous cell carcinoma (SCC). The patient does not smoke or drink alcohol. Further investigations reveal the presence of human papillomavirus (HPV) DNA in the tumor. Which of the following is correct regarding this form of SCC?

A. Aberrant overexpression of p16 is usually present
B. Buccal mucosa is the most common site
C. HPV types 6 and 11 are the most common
D. It has a worse prognosis compared to smoking-related SCC
E. Its incidence is declining in the United States

5. A 55-year-old male with a 30-year smoking history presents with the oral lesion shown in Figure 1. The lesion cannot be scraped off. Which of the following is the most frequent histologic finding in this lesion?

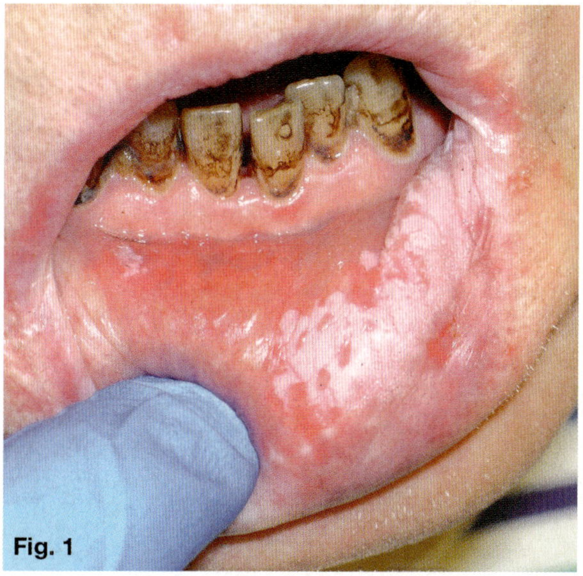

Fig. 1

A. Carcinoma in situ
B. Dysplasia
C. Hyperkeratosis
D. Parakeratosis
E. Subepithelial bandlike chronic inflammation

All figures in this chapter are from Longacre TA, Greenson JK, Hornick JL, Reuter VE, eds. *Mills and Sternberg's Diagnostic Surgical Pathology*. 7th ed. Wolters Kluwer; 2022 except for those noted at the end of this book.

6 to 10. Match the microscopic diagnosis with the corresponding oral epithelial lesion in the images.

6. Keratinizing low-grade dysplasia

7. Keratinizing high-grade dysplasia

8. Carcinoma in situ

9. Nonkeratinizing high-grade dysplasia

10. Microinvasive carcinoma

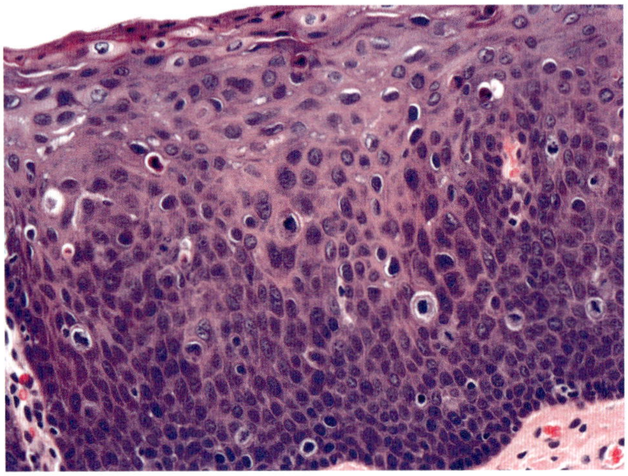

A.

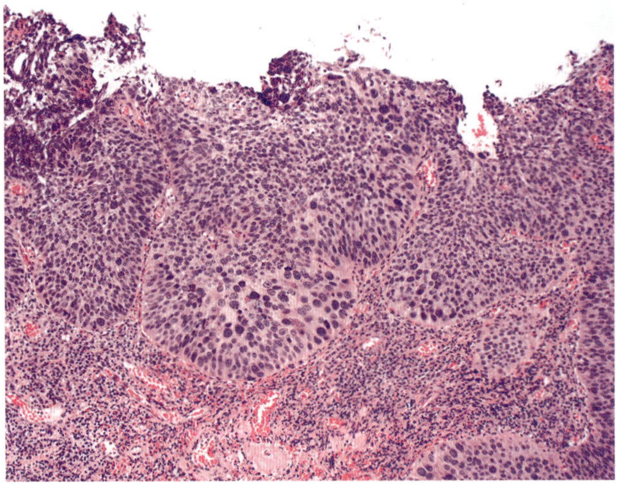

B.

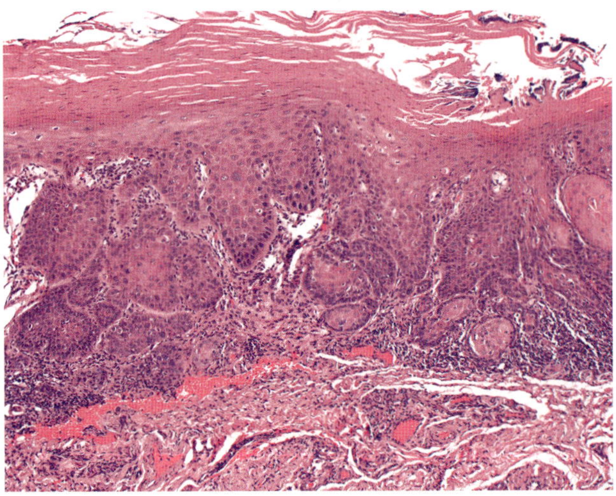

C.

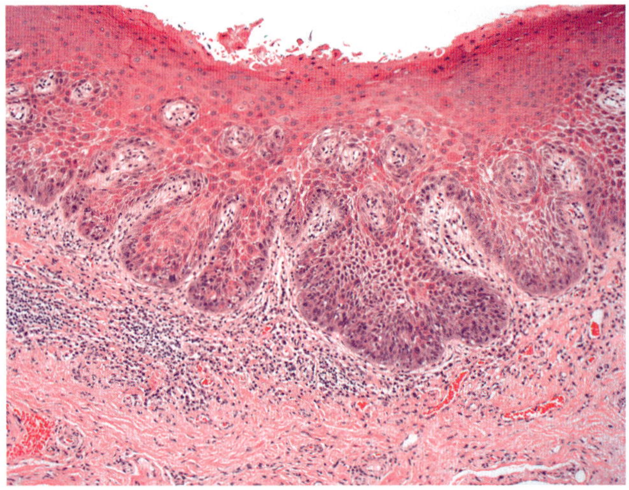

D.

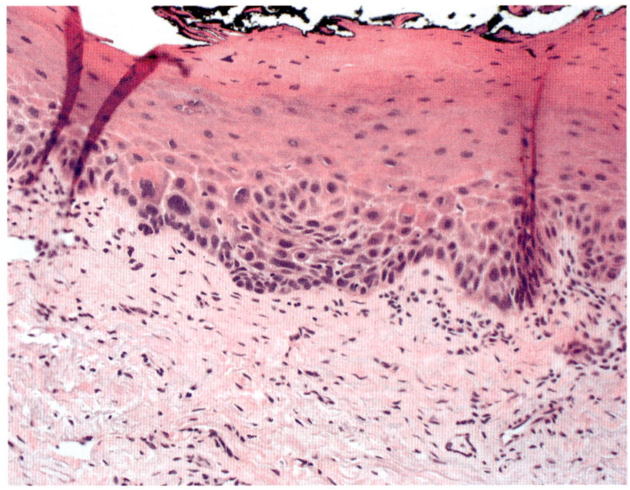

E.

11. Of the histopathologic parameters listed, which one is the most significant predictor of regional lymph node metastasis in oropharyngeal squamous cell carcinoma?

A. Host response
B. Lymph node reaction pattern
C. Pattern of invasion
D. Perineural invasion
E. Tumor grade

12. A 67-year-old male with a 40 pack-year smoking history presents with a large firm fungating mass growing from the lower lip and invading contiguous soft tissues and the mandible. Grossly, the lesion appears as a raised, plaque-like mass with white and red areas, as shown in Figure 1. Microscopically, the lesion is characterized by a bland squamous cell proliferation with uniform cells with orderly maturation lacking dysplastic features. These characteristics are most consistent with

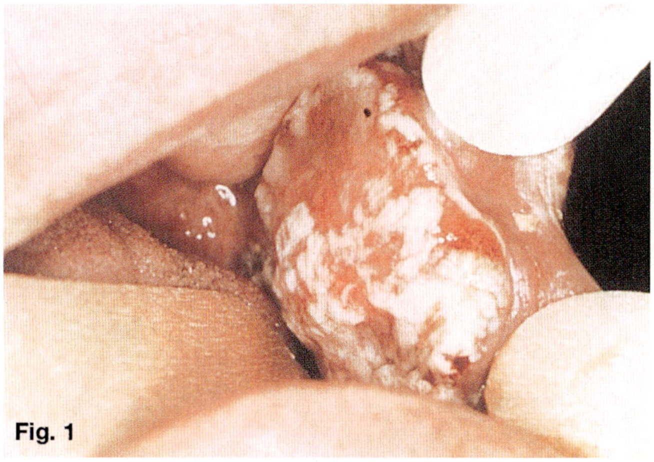
Fig. 1

A. adenosquamous cell carcinoma.
B. basaloid squamous cell carcinoma.
C. papillary squamous cell carcinoma.
D. spindle cell squamous carcinoma.
E. verrucous carcinoma.

13. A 42-year-old White male with no smoking history presents with a firm mass on the back of the tongue. A representative H&E (hematoxylin and eosin) section of the tumor is shown in Figure 1. Which of the following immunohistochemical stains would be most helpful to establish the diagnosis?

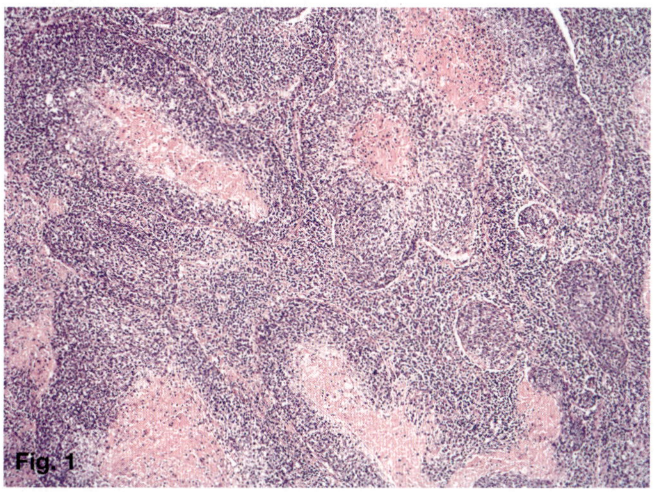
Fig. 1

A. CK5/6
B. EBV (Epstein-Barr virus)
C. p16
D. p40
E. p53

14. The image shows a representative H&E (hematoxylin and eosin) section of a base of tongue mass. The tumor cells are diffusely positive for p63. Which of the following statements is true regarding this entity?

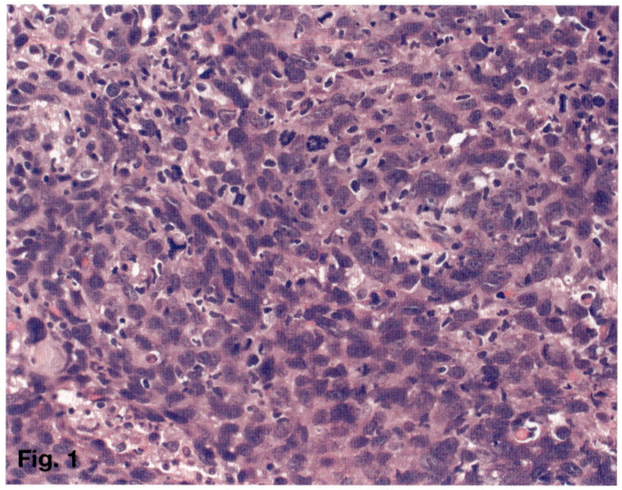
Fig. 1

A. Cancers associated with Epstein-Barr virus (EBV)
B. Commonly occurs in salivary glands, particularly the parotid gland
C. More common in and occurs most frequently in the seventh decade of life
D. Positive for low-risk human papillomavirus (HPV) in situ hybridization
E. Rare variant of nonkeratinizing squamous cell carcinoma

15. A 62-year-old male with a 50 pack-year smoking history presents with a rapidly growing neck mass. Positron emission tomography (PET) scan shows metastasis to regional lymph nodes and the brain. A biopsy was taken, and H&E (hematoxylin and eosin) sections show solid nests and cords of a poorly differentiated malignancy that is positive for AE1/AE3, Cam 5.2, and p16 and is negative for CK5/6 and p63. Ki-67 shows a proliferation index of 42%. Positive *nuclear* expression of the following immunostains is diagnostic of this malignancy?

A. INSM1
B. Melan-A
C. p40
D. SOX-10
E. Synaptophysin

16. X-rays performed during a routine dental examination on a 30-year-old woman reveal a periapical lucency of one of the maxillary incisors. The lesion is removed, and its microscopic appearance is shown in Figure 1. Which of the following is the most likely diagnosis?

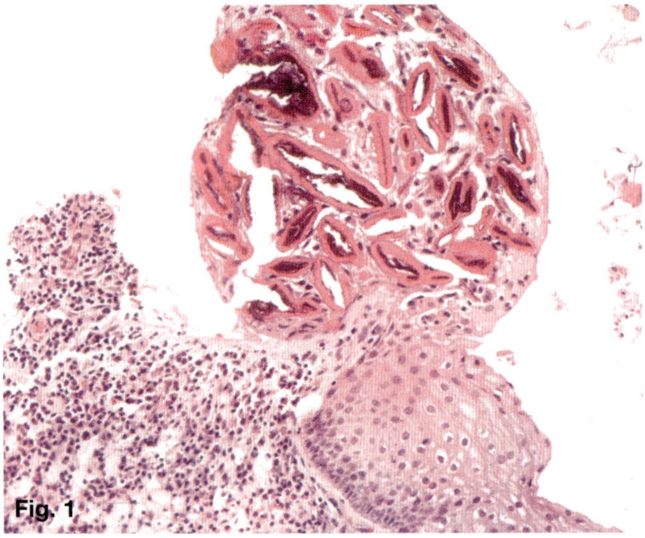


A. Calcifying odontogenic cyst
B. Dentigerous cyst
C. Eruption cyst
D. Periapical cyst
E. Radicular cyst

17. Dentigerous cysts are most commonly associated with

A. dental caries.
B. Gorlin syndrome.
C. McCune-Albright syndrome.
D. traumatic injury.
E. unerupted teeth.

18. Figure 1 shows the histologic appearance of a lesion that appeared as an expansile radiopaque mass in the jaw of a 12-year-old boy. Which of the following is the diagnosis?

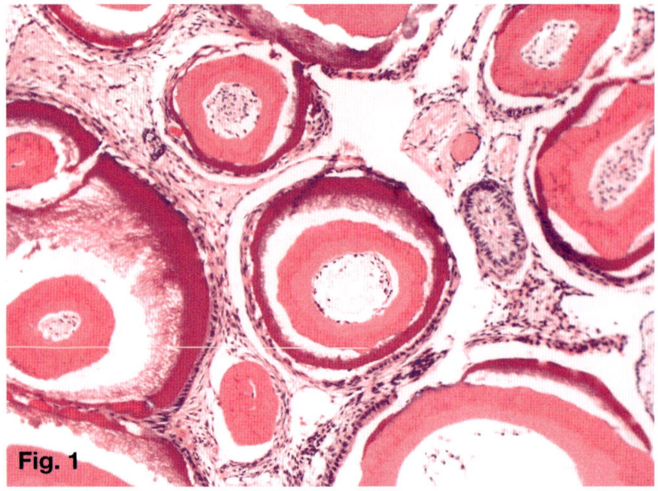


A. Adenomatoid odontogenic tumor
B. Ameloblastic fibroma
C. Ameloblastoma
D. Odontoma
E. Squamous odontogenic tumor

19. A multicystic tumor is resected from the jaw of a 40-year-old patient. The most characteristic microscopic features of this tumor are seen in Figure 1. Mitotic figures are inconspicuous, and nuclear atypia is minimal. The fibrous stroma between epithelial islands is paucicellular and without apparent mitotic activity. Which of the following is the most likely diagnosis?

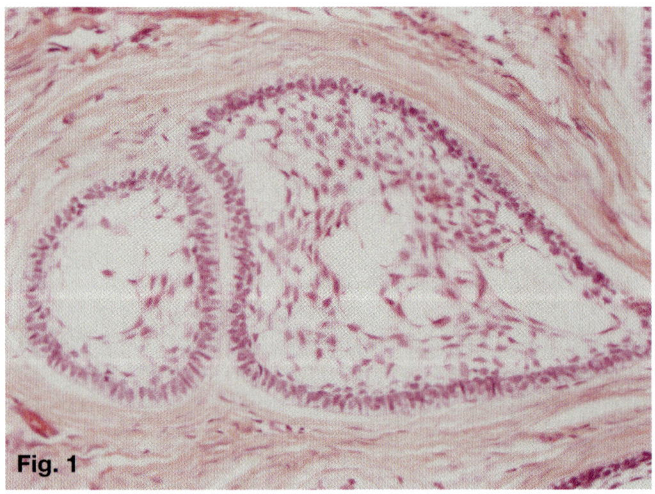


A. Ameloblastic carcinoma
B. Ameloblastic fibroma
C. Ameloblastoma
D. Calcifying epithelial odontogenic tumor
E. Odontoma

# ANSWERS AND EXPLANATIONS

**1. Correct choice: C.**

Peripheral giant cell granuloma (PGCG) is a reactive lesion that occurs most often in young women and clinically resembles pyogenic granuloma. It consists of nonencapsulated granulation tissue with numerous multinucleated giant cells. It arises in the gingiva and may erode into alveolar bone. Bilateral giant cell granulomas of the jaws are pathognomonic of cherubism (an autosomal dominant condition). PGCG is histologically identical to central giant cell granuloma (AKA reparative granuloma) of the mandible. Granular cell tumor occurs predominantly in the tongue. Masson hemangioma is also known as intravascular papillary endothelial hyperplasia. Verruciform xanthoma develops in older patients and consists of lipid-laden macrophages covered by hyperplastic epithelium.

**2. Correct choice: B.**

Oral papilloma is the most common benign epithelial neoplasm of the oral cavity, most commonly located on the hard palate, soft palate, and uvula. It is strongly associated with low-risk human papillomavirus (HPV) serotypes 6 and 11, but frank koilocytotic atypia is rarely seen. Dysplastic changes are unusual, and the lesion does not progress to carcinoma. Oral papillomas are not contagious and are cured by surgical removal.

**3. Correct choice: C.**

Oral hairy leukoplakia (OHL) is an Epstein-Barr virus (EBV)-induced verruciform hyperkeratotic lesion of the tongue typically occurring in patients with AIDS/HIV infection and patients with immunosuppressive conditions; however, OHL has been reported in patients with no evidence of immunosuppression. Histologic features of OHL include irregular epithelial hyperplasia with a dense corrugated parakeratotic layer immediately lying above a band of epithelial cells with pale clear cytoplasm (ballooned cells), which may contain koilocytes and Cowdry inclusions. All other listed lesions are associated with human papillomavirus (HPV) infection.

**4. Correct choice: A.**

The increasing incidence of oropharyngeal carcinoma (OPC) is mostly attributable to the increasing number of human papillomavirus (HPV)-associated cases. HPV-associated OPCs tend to occur in younger individuals without a history of smoking or alcohol use and are usually located at the base of the tongue or the tonsils. HPV-associated OPCs have a much better prognosis than HPV-independent tumors. Subtype 16 is the most frequently detected subtype, while types 18, 31, 33, and 35 are found infrequently. Aberrant overexpression of p16 is a characteristic molecular effect of HPV-mediated carcinogenesis so that immunohistochemistry for p16 is used to support HPV infection. In situ hybridization or polymerase chain reaction (PCR) is used to confirm the presence of HPV DNA.

**5. Correct choice: B.**

The figure depicts a patchy white thickening of oral mucosa that is clinically referred to as oral leukoplakia. This is a clinical term applied to any patch or plaque that measures at least 5 mm or greater in diameter and cannot be removed by scraping nor can it be diagnosed as a recognizable entity. The gingival gutter is the most frequently involved site. The underlying histopathologic changes with their respective prevalence are as follows: hyperkeratosis (80%), dysplasia (12%), carcinoma in situ (3%), and invasive carcinoma (5%). Malignant transformation is observed in 5% to 15% of all cases of idiopathic leukoplakia. Bandlike subepithelial chronic inflammation is a feature of oral lichen planus.

**6-10. Correct choices: 6 E; 7 D; 8 B; 9 A; 10 C.**

Oral epithelial dysplasia is broadly categorized into keratinizing and nonkeratinizing intraepithelial dysplasia. Grading of dysplasia was historically a three-tier system (low, moderate, and severe) but is moving toward a two-tier system, where low-grade dysplasia is low grade from the three-tier system and high-grade dysplasia incorporates moderate and severe from the three-tier system.

Keratinizing intraepithelial dysplasia (KIT) is most common. KIT low-grade dysplasia shows limited architectural changes, preservation of cellular maturation, and, at most, there is minimal cellular atypia, characterized by slightly increased basal and parabasal cells occupying the lower half of epithelium. KIT high-grade dysplasia is characterized by immature epithelial cells occupying at least the lower half to whole epithelial thickness with architectural changes such as elongated, widened, and downwardly projecting rete ridges with abnormal maturation. Cellular atypia is moderate to severe with loss of cell polarity, marked nuclear pleomorphism, and hyperchromasia with increased nuclear-to-cytoplasmic ratio, coarse nuclear chromatin, irregular nuclear contours, increased mitotic figures, and dyskeratosis.

Nonkeratinizing intraepithelial dysplasia (NKID) is much less common and tends to occur in anatomic areas where early lesional changes remain clinically quiescent. The histologic findings in NKID include an absence of surface keratosis and the presence of increasing gradations of dysplasia characterized by replacement of the normal cells by atypical, small, immature basaloid cells, similar to uterine cervix. NKID low-grade dysplasia shows dysplastic cells limited to the lower "third." NKID high-grade dysplasia involves the lower "two-thirds" to full thickness, which is also referred to as carcinoma in situ.

Microinvasive squamous cell carcinoma is a cancer that infiltrates into the superficial compartment of the lamina propria. There is no consensus on the definition of microinvasive carcinoma, but the preferred definition is invasive carcinoma extending into the stroma no more than 0.5 mm measured from the epithelial basement membrane and without angioinvasion. Depth of invasion has shown a good correlation with the rate of lymph node metastasis: less than 4 mm, 8.3%; 4 to 8 mm, 35%; and greater than 8 mm, 83%. There are two patterns of microinvasion: (a) the one shown in the picture consisting of irregular, discontinuous nests of dysplastic epithelium extending into underlying stroma, with a marked desmoplastic reaction;

and (b) a form analogous to actinic keratosis, where tongues of dysplastic epithelium extend into the underlying stroma while still continuous with the surface epithelium.

**11. Correct choice: C.**

The most important histopathologic prognostic factors include (1) pattern of growth/invasion, (2) depth of invasion (DOI), and (3) angiolymphatic and perineural invasion. (1) The patterns of noncohesive, irregular, jagged small cords and infiltrative, widespread single cells are associated with a higher rate of regional lymph node metastasis than are patterns composed of well-defined, blunt pushing borders or thick, rounded invasive cords of tumor. (2) DOI is an independent predictor of lymph node metastasis for cancers of numerous oral sites. Regional metastases are rare with a DOI less than 4 mm, but frequent when greater than 8 mm. (3) Angiolymphatic and perineural invasion are negative prognostic factors.

**12. Correct choice: E.**

Verrucous carcinoma (VC) is a variant of squamous cell carcinoma that is extremely well-differentiated with slow growth. Approximately 5% of all oropharyngeal squamous cell carcinomas are of the verrucous type. The most difficult challenge is identifying this lesion as a neoplasm because of the lack of cytologic markers of malignancy. VC is locally invasive but is unlikely to metastasize unless there is evidence of any component of a conventional invasive squamous cell carcinoma. The remaining choices refer to rare variants of oropharyngeal squamous cell carcinoma. Adenosquamous cell carcinoma is a rare aggressive variant originating from the minor salivary glands with a mixed glandular–squamous pattern. Basaloid squamous cell carcinoma is an aggressive subtype consisting of islands of basaloid cells with abrupt keratinization and peripheral palisading. Papillary squamous cell carcinoma is a rare form of squamous cell carcinoma that may arise all along the upper aerodigestive tract and has a papillary architecture. Spindle cell squamous carcinoma is an admixture of squamous cell carcinoma and a sarcomatous component.

**13. Correct choice: C.**

The image shows an invasive cystic and solid nonkeratinizing (basaloid) malignant neoplasm with background lymphocytic cells and the absence of associated desmoplastic stromal response. These features are characteristic of oropharyngeal high-risk human papillomavirus (HPV)-positive nonkeratinizing squamous cell carcinoma. These carcinomas are often cystic with central areas of necrosis and early lymph node metastases that are frequently cystic. These cancers may invade without associated desmoplasia, and the neoplastic cells may be obscured by the lymphocytic infiltrate. Diagnosis can be confirmed by blocklike p16 positivity and/or high-risk HPV in situ hybridization. CK5/6, p63, and p40 are all markers of squamous differentiation.

**14. Correct choice: E.**

Lymphoepithelial-like carcinoma of the oropharynx represents a rare variant of human papillomavirus (HPV)-positive nonkeratinizing squamous cell carcinoma. It tends to occur in men who are younger than 60 years and are nonsmokers. The most common site is the tonsil, followed by the base of tongue and soft palate. Although the histology is identical to that of its more common nasopharyngeal counterpart, these cancers are not associated with Epstein-Barr virus (EBV). The tumor cells are immunoreactive for p16 (diffuse and strong nuclear and cytoplasmic staining) and positive for high-risk HPV by in situ hybridization.

**15. Correct choice: A.**

Oropharyngeal poorly differentiated neuroendocrine carcinoma is rare with an aggressive clinical course. Many patients have disseminated disease at presentation with metastasis to regional lymph nodes and other distant sites. Most patients are men, mean age of 61 years, with a heavy smoking history. There is an association with high-risk human papillomavirus (HPV), but HPV status does not confer a better prognosis. Diagnosis is confirmed by immunoreactivity with keratins and at least one neuroendocrine marker, such as synaptophysin, chromogranin, or INSM1, of which, only INSM1 is a nuclear marker. Focal p40 staining can be seen in cases with a squamous differentiation (biphasic pattern).

**16. Correct choice: D.**

Cysts of the jaw are subdivided into odontogenic and nonodontogenic (developmental). The five choices in this question include the most common odontogenic cysts. Among these, periapical cysts are the most frequent and affect adults in their 20s and 30s. It develops from pulpal necrosis secondary to inflammation due to caries or trauma. Necrosis and inflammation stimulate growth of Malassez rests, which form the epithelial cyst lining. The lining epithelium also contains keratinized foci, goblet cells, and peculiar hyaline bodies known as Rushton bodies (see figure). Periapical cysts present radiologically as well-demarcated radiolucent defects around the apex of a tooth. Maxillary incisors and mandibular molars are the most common sites. Nonodontogenic cysts develop at points of embryologic junction between head and neck structures. Most odontogenic cysts have nonspecific epithelial lining so that the histologic findings must be correlated with clinical findings, particularly location and radiologic appearance, to reach a diagnosis. This diagram shows the most typical locations of the various types of jaw cysts.

**17. Correct choice: E.**

Dentigerous cyst is one of the most common dental lesions, found in approximately 1% of adults. It develops in close association with unerupted teeth. Swelling and, less frequently, pain are clinical symptoms. The cyst is usually lined by ameloblastic-type (tooth-forming) epithelium, which is stratified and keratinizing with a conspicuous basal layer. Hemorrhage, infection, or a tangential cut may impair the identification of the characteristic epithelial lining.

**18. Correct choice: D.**

Odontomas are common jaw hamartomas in which complete differentiation of ameloblasts and odontoblasts results in the formation of mature enamel, dentin, and cementum. A complex odontoma (see figure) consists of disorganized collections of dentin, enamel, and cementum and radiologically mimics osteoma. A compound odontoma, instead, is a mass of rudimentary small teeth.

**19. Correct choice: C.**

Ameloblastoma is the most common tumor arising from ameloblastic (tooth-forming) epithelium. It usually involves the jaw. In most cases, multiple cysts, whether macroscopic or microscopic, develop within the tumor. The distinguishing feature is the presence of epithelial islands with peripheral palisading and central loosely textured regions known as stellate reticulum. If cytologic atypia and mitotic activity are prominent, the tumor should be diagnosed as ameloblastic carcinoma. Ameloblastic fibroma is a biphasic tumor consisting of ameloblastic epithelium and myxoid stroma. Odontoma is a common hamartoma of the jaw, usually detected as an incidental finding in children and composed of disorganized tooth components or rudimentary small teeth.

# 20 Salivary Glands

1. Which of the following is the most common location of heterotopic salivary gland tissue?

    A. Ear
    B. Lymph node
    C. Palatine tonsil
    D. Right sternomastoid muscle
    E. Thyroid gland

2. A cystic lesion is removed from the right parotid gland of a 23-year-old man. The cyst wall is shown in Figure 1. This lesion is frequently associated with

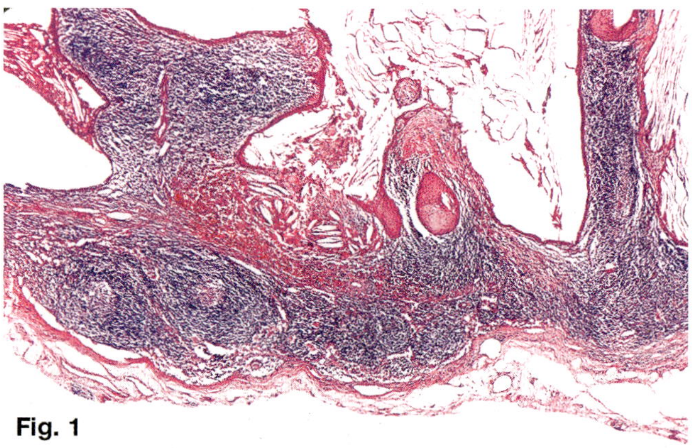

Fig. 1

    A. coxsackievirus.
    B. Epstein-Barr virus.
    C. human immunodeficiency virus.
    D. human papillomavirus.
    E. paramyxovirus.

3. A 46-year-old male presents with an ulcer on the hard palate. A biopsy reveals necrosis of salivary gland parenchyma, chronic inflammation, and foci of squamous epithelium mixed with mucous acini. Squamous cells exhibit nuclear pleomorphism and mitotic activity. The lesion displays a lobular architecture, as demonstrated in Figure 1. Which of the following is the most likely diagnosis?

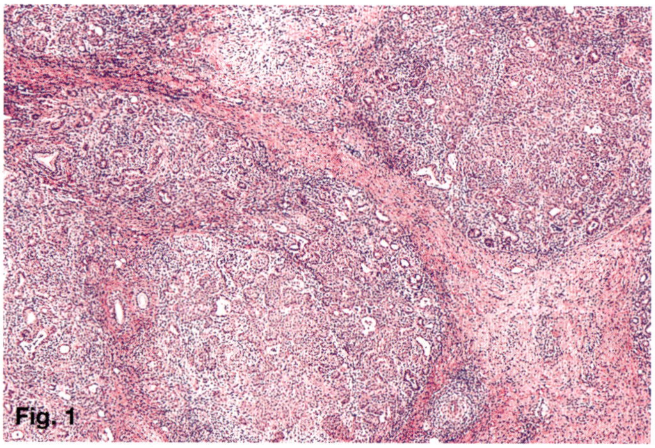

Fig. 1

    A. Acute viral sialadenitis
    B. Chronic sialadenitis
    C. Mucoepidermoid carcinoma
    D. Necrotizing sialometaplasia
    E. Squamous cell carcinoma

All figures in this chapter are from Longacre TA, Greenson JK, Hornick JL, Reuter VE, eds. *Mills and Sternberg's Diagnostic Surgical Pathology*. 7th ed. Wolters Kluwer; 2022 except for those noted at the end of this book.

4. A 40-year-old man presents with a 1-year history of swelling of the right submandibular gland. On palpation, a slightly tender, very firm mass is appreciated. Fearing a malignancy, the submandibular gland is removed exhibiting the histologic features shown in Figure 1. Which of the following is the most likely diagnosis?

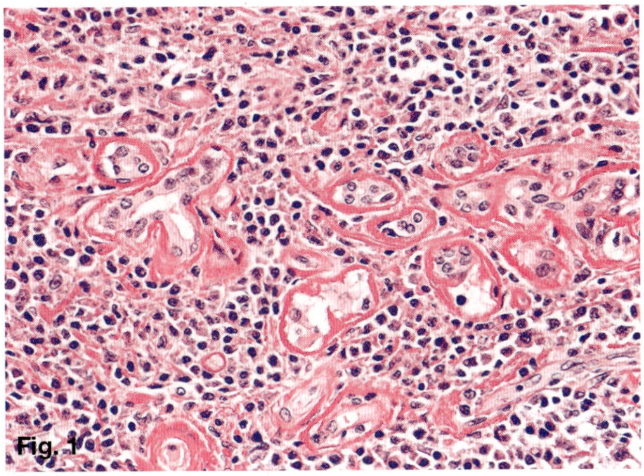

Fig. 1

A. Acute viral sialadenitis
B. Chronic sclerosing sialadenitis
C. Granulomatous sialadenitis
D. Necrotizing sialometaplasia
E. Sjögren syndrome

5. A 40-year-old woman presents with enlargement of the left parotid gland and dryness of the eyes and mouth. A biopsy of the parotid and minor salivary glands shows the histologic changes represented in Figure 1. Laboratory studies reveal high titers of circulating antibodies to ribonucleoproteins (RNP), including SS-A (Ro) and SS-B (La). This patient has an increased risk of developing which type of lymphoma?

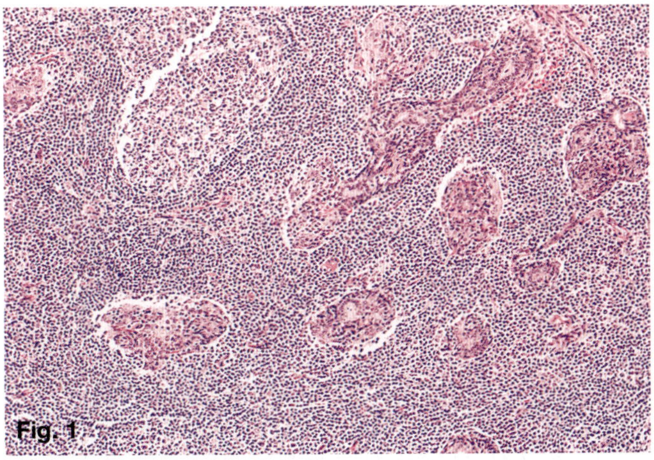

Fig. 1

A. Chronic lymphocytic leukemia/small lymphocytic lymphoma
B. Diffuse large B-cell lymphoma
C. Follicular lymphoma
D. Mantle cell lymphoma
E. Marginal zone lymphoma

6. A well-demarcated, slowly growing 4.0-cm tumor is resected from the left parotid gland of a 45-year-old female patient. Its cut surface is variegated, with myxoid and blue-gray areas. The microscopic appearance of the tumor is demonstrated in Figure 1. Which of the following is the most common molecular alteration in this entity?

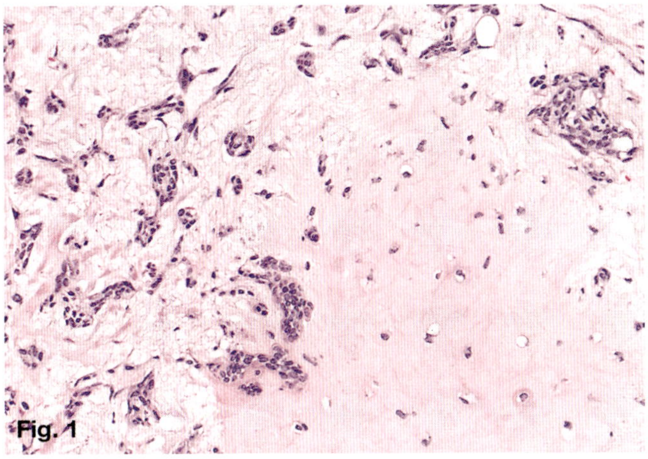

Fig. 1

A. *CTNNB1* mutation
B. *HMGA2* fusion
C. *MYB* fusion
D. *PLAG1* fusion
E. *TP53* mutation

7. A 60-year-old man presents with bilateral painless swelling of the parotid gland. Image studies reveal a 1.5-cm mass in the right parotid and a 2.0-cm mass in the left parotid. Both tumors are resected and appear to have similar microscopic appearance, which is shown in Figure 1. Which of the following is the strongest predisposing condition for the development of this tumor?

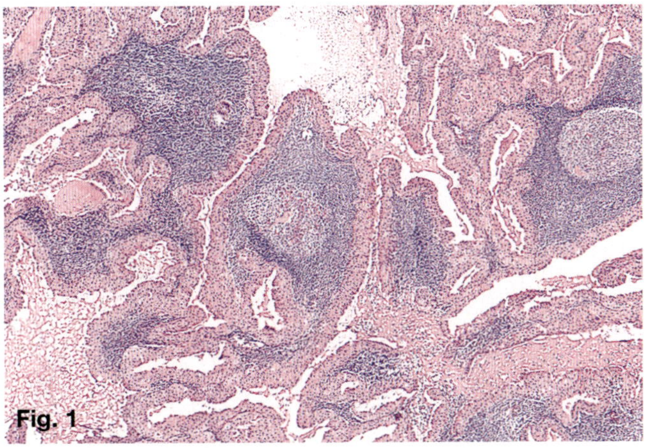

Fig. 1

A. Epstein-Barr virus infection
B. HIV infection
C. Radiation
D. Sjögren syndrome
E. Smoking

8. Figure 1 demonstrates the typical microscopic features of a well-circumscribed, encapsulated mass removed from the parotid of a 65-year-old woman. What is the most common molecular alteration in this entity?

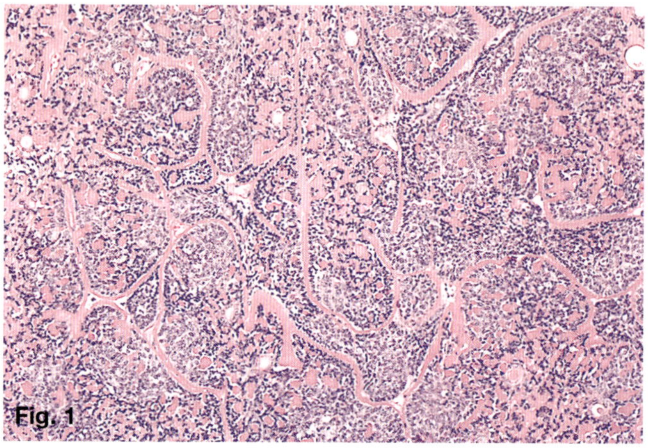

Fig. 1

A. *CTNNB1*
B. *CYLD*
C. *FLI1*
D. *MAML2*
E. *PLAG1*

9. The most common location of the salivary gland tumor depicted in Figure 1 is

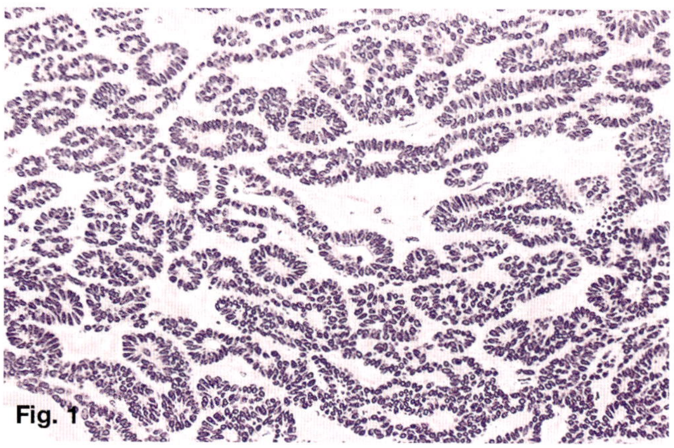

Fig. 1

A. hard palate.
B. parotid gland.
C. sublingual gland.
D. submandibular gland.
E. upper lip.

10. The tumor shown in Figure 1 was removed from the parotid gland of a 38-year-old woman. Which of the following is the most important risk factor for this neoplasm?

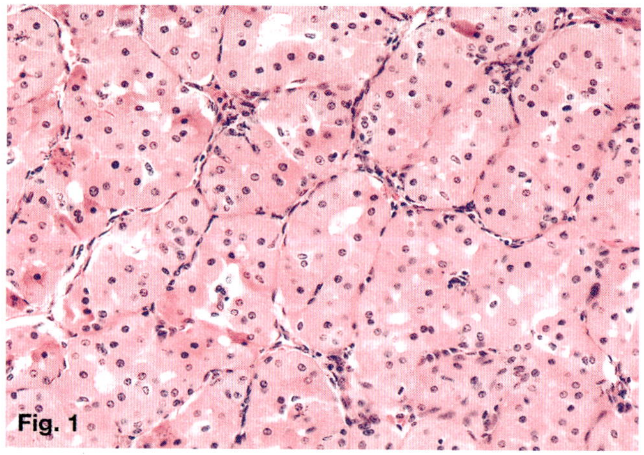

Fig. 1

A. Alcohol
B. Chronic sclerosing sialadenitis
C. Radiation
D. Sjögren syndrome
E. Smoking

11. Of the five salivary gland neoplasms shown in the figures, which one is always found in the parotid and periparotid region?

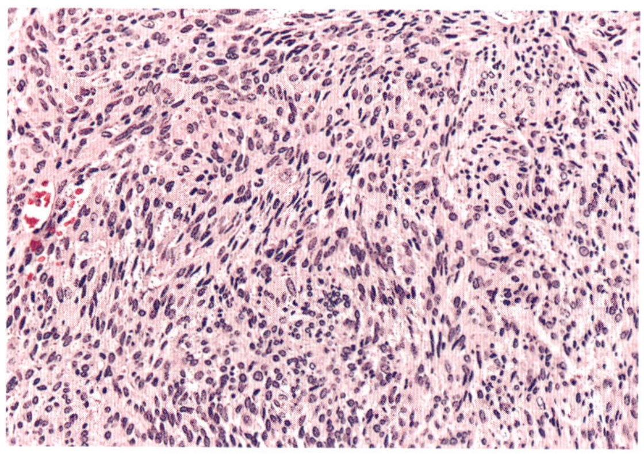

A.

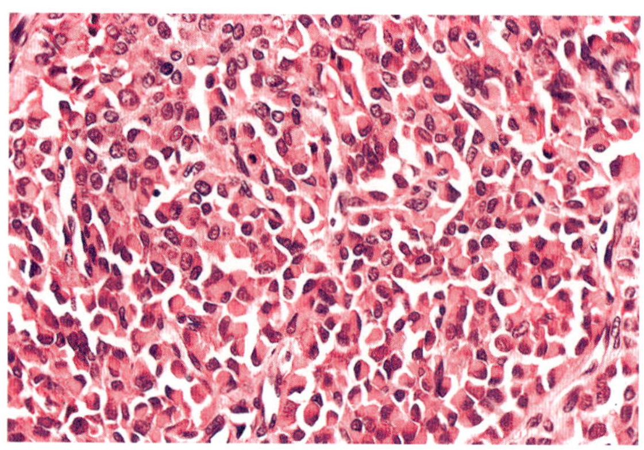

B.

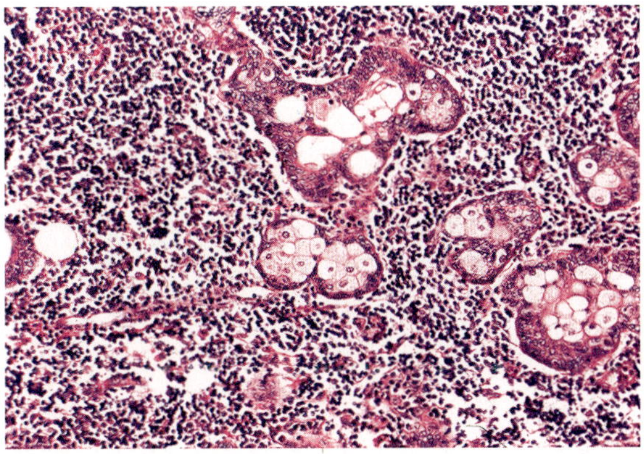

C.

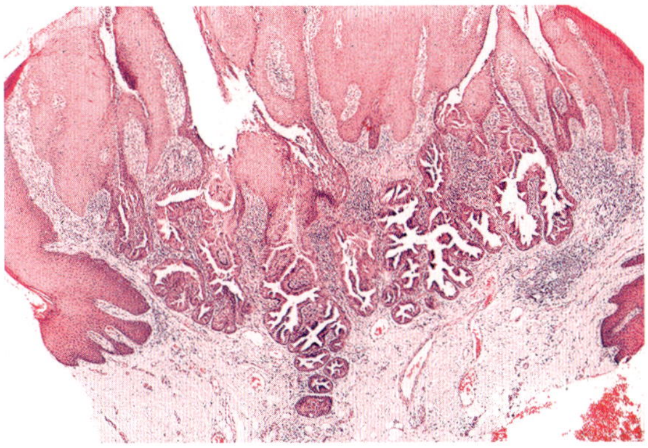

D.

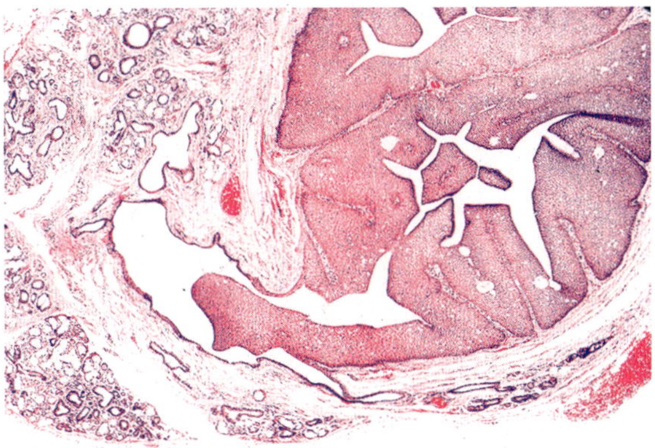

E.

12. Which of the following is true regarding the tumor depicted in Figure 1?

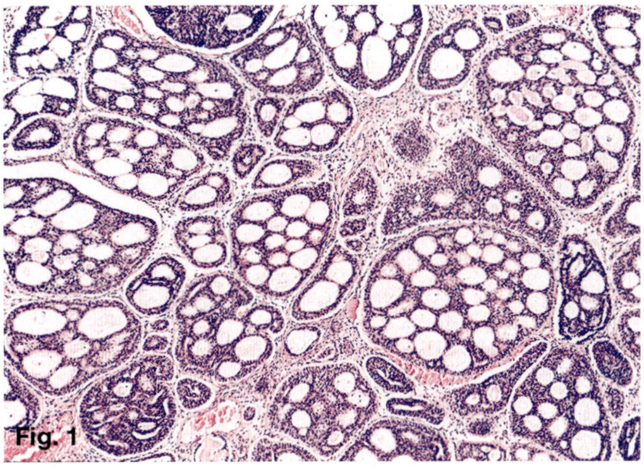

Fig. 1

A. Early and frequent lymph node metastasis
B. Highest prevalence in the parotid gland
C. Prominent perineural invasion
D. Rarely recurs after surgical intervention
E. Slow-growing and indolent neoplasm

13. What is the most common molecular alteration seen in the entity from question 12?

A. *CRTC1-MAML2* fusion
B. *ETV6-NTRK3* fusion
C. *MYB-NFIB* fusion
D. *MYBL1-NFIB* fusion
E. *NCOA4-RET* fusion

14. What is the molecular alteration seen in the most common salivary gland malignancy in childhood?

A. t(6;9)
B. t(8;11)
C. t(11;19)
D. t(12;15)
E. t(X;18)

15. A 55-year-old woman undergoes resection of a mass in the parotid gland. On gross examination, the mass is well delineated and solid gray. Histologic examination demonstrates a predominantly solid growth composed of cells with finely granular basophilic cytoplasm, as shown in Figure 1. Which of the following is the most likely diagnosis?

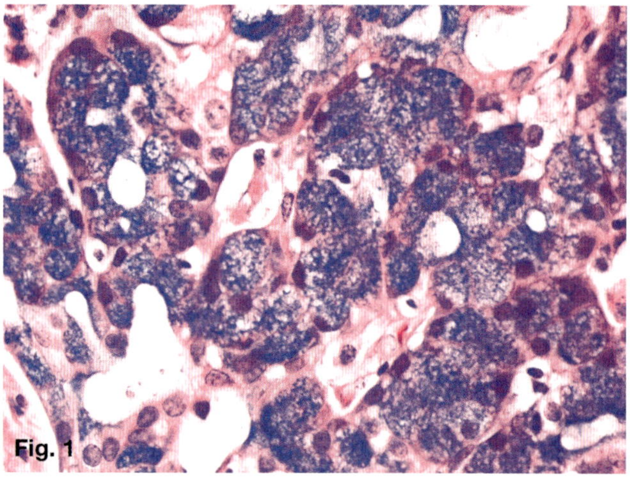


A. Acinic cell carcinoma
B. Adenoid cystic carcinoma
C. Mucoepidermoid carcinoma
D. Polymorphous low-grade adenocarcinoma
E. Secretory carcinoma

16. The parotid tumor shown in Figure 1 is positive for fluorescence in situ hybridization (FISH) break-apart probe for *ETV6*. Strong expression of which of the following pair of immunostains would be diagnostic of this tumor?

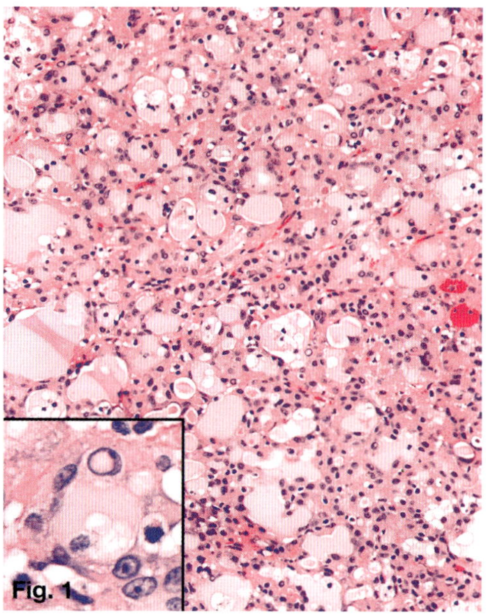


A. Calponin and CK5/6
B. Calponin and DOG1
C. PAX8 and thyroglobulin
D. S100 and mammaglobin
E. S100 and SOX10

17. A 65-year-old male presents with facial nerve pain and a rapidly growing infiltrative parotid mass. Positron emission tomography (PET) scan shows regional lymph node and liver metastases. A representative H&E (hematoxylin and eosin) section of this tumor is shown in Figure 1. The tumor is positive for mammaglobin and androgen receptor (AR) by immunohistochemistry. What is the diagnosis?

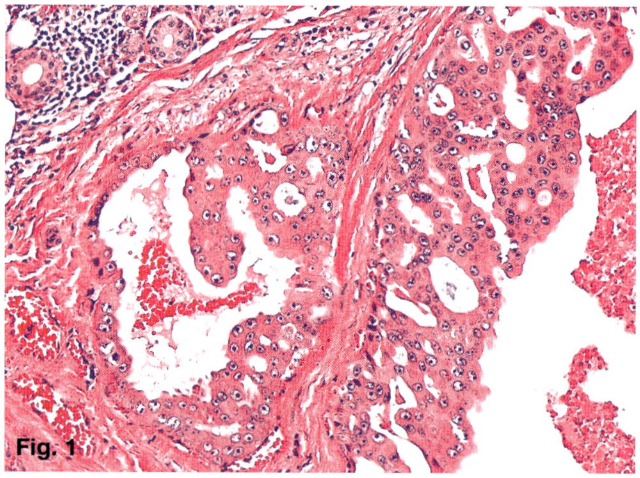


A. Adenoid cystic carcinoma
B. Intraductal carcinoma
C. Metastatic breast carcinoma
D. Mucoepidermoid carcinoma
E. Salivary duct carcinoma

# ANSWERS AND EXPLANATIONS

**1. Correct choice: B.**

Salivary gland heterotopia is most commonly found in the lymph nodes of the neck and head. Extranodal heterotopia may involve high sites, including the ear, mandible, palatine tonsil, pituitary gland, and other intracranial regions, or low sites, such as the right sternomastoid muscle and thyroid. During embryonic development, the delayed formation of a capsule around the parotid gland (compared to the other salivary glands) allows parotid buds and lymphoid tissue to intermingle, which results in the presence of lymph nodes within the parotid and of salivary gland tissue within lymph nodes. This phenomenon explains why lesions such as Warthin tumor, sebaceous lymphadenoma, and lymphoepithelial cysts, characterized by a combination of lymphoid and epithelial tissue, are found only in parotid and periparotid tissues.

**2. Correct choice: C.**

The image shows the typical histologic findings in a lymphoepithelial cyst. This lesion consists of multilocular fluid-filled cystic spaces lined by squamous or glandular epithelium; intervening solid areas contain lymphoid aggregates with germinal centers. The lesion probably develops as a result of cystic dilatation in intranodal salivary gland inclusions, with subsequent squamous metaplasia of the cyst lining. Lymphoepithelial cysts are almost exclusively found in the parotid-periparotid region because of the abovementioned intimate mixture of salivary gland and lymphoid tissue. This type of lesion is frequent in patients with AIDS, owing to the prominent lymphoid hyperplasia that occurs in the initial phase of the disease, which leads to blockage of ducts and cyst formation. The lymphoepithelial cyst associated with AIDS is called cystic lymphoid hyperplasia.

**3. Correct choice: D.**

Necrotizing sialometaplasia is due to infarction of a salivary gland and most commonly involves the small salivary glands in the hard palate. Ischemic necrosis of ducts and acini leads to acute and chronic inflammation, followed by squamous metaplasia. Admixture of viable mucous acini and squamous epithelium may be mistaken for mucoepidermoid carcinoma or squamous cell carcinoma, particularly because the metaplastic squamous epithelium shows nuclear pleomorphism and mitotic activity. Squamous metaplasia develops at the center of the salivary gland, arising from preexisting ducts, whereas necrosis with accompanying inflammation involves the periphery of the glands. Preservation of the lobular architecture is an important clue for the differential diagnosis of a malignant neoplasm.

**4. Correct choice: B.**

Chronic sclerosing sialadenitis (aka Küttner tumor) is a variant of chronic sialadenitis. It presents as a palpable mass in the submandibular gland (rarely in other salivary glands), clinically mimicking a neoplasm. It is a type of chronic sialadenitis characterized by florid lymphoplasmacytic infiltration and prominent periductal fibrosis. The latter is the most distinguishing feature. About 50% of the plasma cells express immunoglobulin G subclass 4 (IgG4), and this lesion is thought to be part of the IgG4-related disorders. The common type of chronic sialadenitis is usually due to ductal obstruction (stones), which results in chronic inflammation, progressive glandular atrophy, and fibrosis. Benign lymphoepithelial lesion is the most typical histologic feature of Sjögren syndrome. Mumps used to be the most frequent form of acute viral sialadenitis, microscopically characterized by edema, chronic inflammatory infiltration, and vacuolization of acinar cells. Any form of granulomatous condition can affect salivary glands, including sarcoidosis, mycobacterial and fungal infections, and cat scratch disease.

**5. Correct choice: E.**

Sjögren syndrome involves lacrimal and salivary glands bilaterally. Chronic inflammation of these glands is characterized by the formation of unique benign lymphoepithelial lesions (demonstrated in the picture), which consist of aggregates of epithelial/myoepithelial cells (epimyoepithelial islands) scattered in a sea of marginal zone or monocytoid-type B lymphocytes. Patients often have circulating anti-ribonucleoprotein (anti-RNP) autoantibodies (Ro and La are most frequent). The following are the San Diego criteria for the diagnosis of Sjögren syndrome:

- Keratoconjunctivitis sicca
- Xerostomia
- Extensive lymphocytic infiltration of minor salivary glands
- Laboratory evidence of autoimmune disorder

Patients with Sjögren syndrome are at greatly increased risk of developing lymphoma, usually of the marginal zone/mucosa-associated lymphoid tissue (MALT) type. Other extrasalivary manifestations include tubulointerstitial nephritis, primary biliary cirrhosis, sclerosing cholangitis, pancreatitis, interstitial lymphocytic pneumonia, and vasculitis.

**6. Correct choice: A.**

Pleomorphic adenoma comprises about 70%, 50%, and 45% of the tumors in the parotid, submandibular, and minor salivary glands, respectively. The tumor is well circumscribed, but small fingerlike transcapsular projections extend from the periphery of the mass into adjacent salivary gland tissue. The histologic pattern is highly variable based on the epithelial and stromal elements. The epithelial components may form trabeculae, tubules, ductules, nonkeratinizing squamous cell aggregates, keratinizing squamous cysts, mucous cysts, aggregates of plasmacytoid or spindled myoepithelial cells, scattered sebaceous cells, or sheets of nondescript epithelium. The stromal elements are nearly as variable as the epithelial and may include mucoid, myxoid, fibroblastic, cartilaginous, osseous, and lipogenic elements. The amount of epithelium versus stroma varies tremendously from lesion to lesion. Most pleomorphic adenomas harbor activating PLAG1 fusions. HMGA2 fusions are the second most common.

**7. Correct choice: E.**

Warthin tumor, also called papillary cystadenoma lymphomatosum, develops more frequently in males and affects almost exclusively the parotid gland. It is bilateral in 10% of cases. Smoking is a well-recognized risk factor for this tumor. Grossly, it is characterized by multiple small cysts. The histologic picture is highly characteristic (the alternative designation is virtually descriptive): cystic spaces lined by epithelium forming papillary fronds with a florid lymphocytic population forming germinal centers. Epithelial cells have a typical oncocytic appearance, being packed with mitochondria (an electron microscopy [EM] feature). Malignant transformation is rare.

**8. Correct choice: A.**

Basal cell adenoma is an infrequent benign tumor that usually develops in the parotid gland. The solid pattern is the most common and is characterized by a jigsaw-like arrangement of nests of uniform epithelial cells within a mesenchymal background. The nests show peripheral palisading and are separated by PAS (periodic acid-Schiff)-positive basement membrane–like material. This neoplasm is surrounded by a capsule, whose presence is important to distinguish it from basal cell adenocarcinoma and adenoid cystic carcinoma. The membranous pattern contains hyaline stromal around and within the cell nests. A capsule is often absent in the membranous variant, which probably accounts for its high recurrence rate. Tumor cells are immunoreactive for pan-keratin, epithelial membrane antigen (EMA), carcinoembryonic antigen (CEA), S100, and smooth muscle actin. Most basal cell adenomas show strong nuclear β-catenin immunoreactivity in correlation with *CTNNB1*-activating mutations. A tumor with these features but with cytologic atypia, mitoses, and infiltrative growth is a basal cell adenocarcinoma.

**9. Correct choice: E.**

Canalicular adenoma is closely related to basal cell adenoma and 75% occur in the seromucinous glands of the upper lip. Grossly, they may present as both well-demarcated encapsulated or unencapsulated nodule, often multifocal. Women and African Americans are more frequently affected. The microscopic pattern is highly characteristic, with budding ductular structures that appear in a canalicular (beaded) architecture. Cuboidal to columnar basaloid cells with round to oval nuclei with scant, slightly eosinophilic cytoplasm. Cells express keratins, S100, and focally glial fibrillary acidic protein (GFAP), which often shows a luminal staining pattern.

**10. Correct choice: C.**

Oncocytoma accounts for just 1% of all salivary gland tumors. While oncocytic cell change can be found in a wide variety of salivary gland neoplasms (such as Warthin tumor, mucoepidermoid carcinoma, acinic cell carcinoma, and pleomorphic adenoma), oncocytomas are entirely composed of oncocytic cells. Approximately 20% of patients with this tumor have a history of prior radiation exposure to the face or upper torso that occurred 5 years or more before tumor discovery. On gross examination, oncocytomas are usually 3 to 4 cm in size with an encapsulated, multinodular growth pattern, and have a characteristic light brown to mahogany color.

**11. Correct choice: C.**

Sebaceous lymphadenoma consists of nests of sebaceous cells within a lymphoid background. Two features unique to the parotid gland explain why such tumors occur exclusively at this location: (a) the parotid gland has a tendency to undergo sebaceous metaplasia; and (b) there is an intimate intermixture of parotid buds and lymphoid tissue during embryonic development. Choices A and B show the spindle cell and plasmacytoid variants, respectively, of the rare myoepithelioma, which may develop in the parotid (50% of cases) or minor salivary glands (40%). It is entirely composed of myoepithelial cells, which express p63, smooth muscle actin, calponin, and CD10. Choices D and E show sialadenoma papilliferum and inverted papilloma, respectively. These are two forms of ductal papilloma. Both occur in minor salivary glands, the former exhibiting an exophytic growth and the latter characterized by endophytic growth.

**12 and 13. Correct choices: 12 C; 13 A.**

Adenoid cystic carcinoma (ACC) accounts for approximately 10% of all salivary gland tumors, and it is the most common malignant tumor of the submandibular and minor salivary glands. There are three patterns of growth and multiple patterns are often seen in the same tumor. The cribriform pattern is the most common, with microcysts filled with basement membrane–like material surrounded by uniform cuboidal cells, as well as true mucus-filled glandular spaces. The combination of cystic and glandular spaces is required for diagnosis. The tubular pattern is seen in 20% to 30% of cases and is characterized by smaller ductlike arrays of basaloid epithelial cells surrounding a single central lumen-like space with fibrotic/hyalinized stroma. The solid pattern is the least frequently encountered and characterized by solid nests of basaloid cells, often in a hyalinized stroma. The tubular ACC can be confused with polymorphous adenocarcinoma (PAC), an indolent neoplasm. Immunohistochemically, ACC shows two distinct cell populations: myoepithelial cells that are positive for p40, p63, and S-100 protein, and ducts that are negative for those markers. In comparison, PAC is diffusely positive for S-100 protein and consistently positive for p63 but negative for p40. Perineural invasion is a constant feature, resulting in tumor spread well beyond the surgical margins: this accounts for recurrences 10 to 20 years following resection, with resultant poor long-term prognosis. Although ACC may involve lymph nodes by direct extension, direct lymph node metastases are rare. Approximately 40% to 70% of adenoid cystic carcinomas exhibit a t(6;9) translocation, resulting in an *MYB-NFIB* gene fusion, whereas 10% to 20% harbor *MYBL1-NFIB*.

**14. Correct choice: C.**

Mucoepidermoid carcinoma represents approximately 5% of all salivary gland tumors, with approximately 67% arising in the parotid gland and 33% in the minor salivary glands. The incidence tends to peak at approximately the fifth decade, but it is the most common salivary gland malignancy in childhood. It consists of a mixture of three different neoplastic components, including squamous nests, mucus-producing glands, and intermediate elements referred to as "basal cells." Mucicarmine staining highlights the mucinous component. This neoplasm is graded as low, intermediate, and high grade based on nuclear atypia, intracystic component, mitotic activity, perineural invasion, and necrosis. Low-grade forms show well-formed glandular or microcystic structures lined by a single layer of mucus-secreting columnar cells, and these may recur but do not metastasize. Intermediate-grade lesions show solid nests of squamous, intermediate, basaloid cells or clear cells. High-grade tumors behave aggressively and show perineural invasion, focal necrosis, increased mitotic figures, and greater pleomorphism. The genetic hallmark is translocation of the *MAML2* gene on chromosome 11, where the most common is a t(11;19) translocation resulting in *CRTC1-MAML2* fusion.

**15. Correct choice: A.**

Acinic cell carcinoma accounts for 2% of salivary gland tumors, with over 90% arising in the parotid gland. This tumor is more common in women, and the peak incidence is in the fifth and sixth decades of life. Microscopically, the tumor cells have finely granular, basophilic cytoplasm, resembling normal serous salivary gland cells. Oncocytic, basaloid, and nonspecific-appearing ductal cells are also present. These varied cell types may be arranged in equally varied growth patterns, including solid, acinar, microcystic, papillary cystic, and follicular. Acinic cell carcinoma is a well-differentiated tumor that typically lacks overt cytologic features of malignancy. The presence of prominent nuclear pleomorphism, high mitotic rate, or necrosis is uncommon and should prompt consideration of other entities. Molecularly, it is characterized by a recurrent chromosomal rearrangement (t(4; 9)(q13; q31)) that upregulates the transcription factor NR4A3. Recurrence rate is 20%; nodal metastases are found in 10% and distant metastases in 6% of cases. The 5-year survival rate is 83%.

**16. Correct choice: D.**

Secretory carcinoma of salivary glands is identical in morphology and immunophenotype to secretory carcinoma of the breast. Morphologically, these tumors have relatively uniform glandular cells with moderate eosinophilic cytoplasm and prominent eosinophilic to slightly basophilic extracellular secretory material. They lack the other cell types (serous, indeterminate, clear, etc) seen in acinic cell carcinoma. While most secretory carcinomas are indolent and low-grade, focal high-grade transformation can be seen with the presence of solid growth, infiltrative growth, brisk mitotic activity, increased nuclear atypia, and/or necrosis. Strong staining for S-100 protein and mammaglobin confirms the diagnosis without molecular studies, which frequently show *ETV6* rearrangements.

**17. Correct choice: E.**

Salivary duct carcinoma is an aggressive neoplasm occurring primarily in the parotid gland of middle-aged and older males. Its most distinguishing feature is an intraductal growth of cells showing apocrine differentiation with frequent comedo-like necrosis, a striking resemblance to intraductal carcinoma of the breast. The tumor cells often have an apocrine appearance with large nuclei and prominent nucleoli. Perineural spread along branches of the facial nerve is often extensive, making complete resection difficult or impossible. Lymph node metastases are common, and nearly two-thirds of patients develop distant metastases to the brain, liver, adrenals, and lungs. Immunohistochemically, it resembles breast carcinoma with positivity for mammaglobin and other breast markers; however, salivary duct carcinoma differs from most breast carcinomas by exhibiting positivity for androgen receptors and is less commonly reactive for estrogen and progesterone receptors. Genetically, it most frequently shows mutations in *TP53* and *KIT*, and commonly has mutations and/or amplifications in *PIK3CA*, *EGFR*, *PTEN*, *ERBB2*/4, *AR*, and *APC*.

# 21 Nose, Paranasal Sinuses, and Nasopharynx

1. A biopsy of a polypoid lesion in the nasal cavity reveals a mixed inflammatory reaction containing the microcysts seen in Figure 1. Each cyst measures up to 200 μm in diameter and contains innumerable spores. Which of the following is the most likely diagnosis?

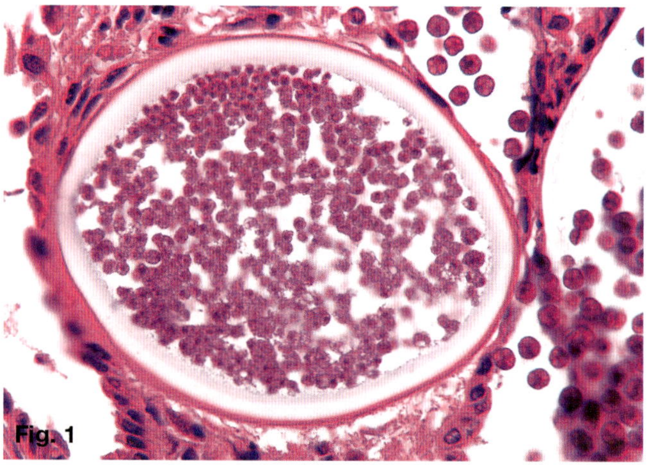
Fig. 1

A. Actinomycosis
B. Aspergillosis
C. Mucormycosis
D. Myospherulosis
E. Rhinosporidiosis

2. A 32-year-old man who recently immigrated from Egypt presents with destructive ulcerative lesions of the nasal and nasopharyngeal cavities. Biopsies show extensive chronic inflammatory infiltrates, mostly consisting of foamy macrophages and plasma cells. A Gram stain identifies pink small rods within the macrophages. Which of the following is the most likely diagnosis?

A. Leprosy
B. Rhinoscleroma
C. Rosai-Dorfman disease
D. Syphilis
E. Tuberculosis

3. A 35-year-old male undergoes resection of a nasal polyp, which reveals the histologic features shown in Figure 1. Which of the following is most likely to be associated with this kind of polyp?

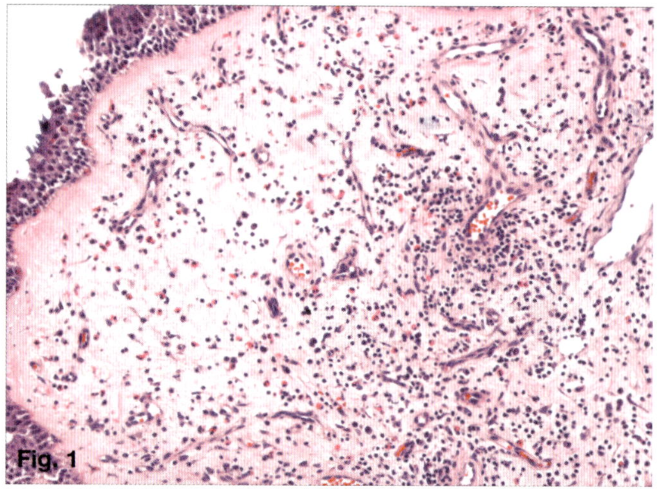
Fig. 1

A. Arise from maxillary antrum
B. Asthma and aspirin intolerance
C. Cystic fibrosis
D. Epstein-Barr virus (EBV) infection
E. Occupational risk

All figures in this chapter are from Longacre TA, Greenson JK, Hornick JL, Reuter VE, eds. *Mills and Sternberg's Diagnostic Surgical Pathology*. 7th ed. Wolters Kluwer; 2022 except for those noted at the end of this book.

4. A 35-year-old man presents with unilateral nasal obstruction. Inspection reveals an exophytic growth filling the right nasal fossa. The lesion is removed. Its microscopic appearance is shown in Figure 1. Which of the following is true about this polyp?

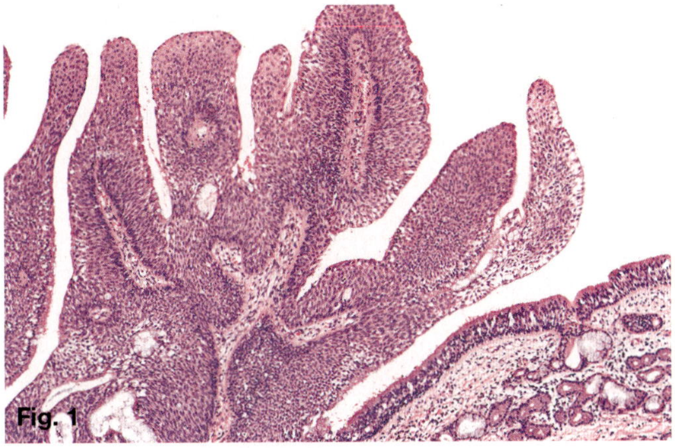


A. Associated with Epstein-Barr virus (EBV)
B. Associated with human papillomavirus (HPV)
C. Associated with 10% risk of invasive carcinoma
D. Develops on the lateral nasal wall
E. Low recurrence rate after resection

5. Figure 1 shows a papilloma removed from the nasal fossa of a 50-year-old man who presented with epistaxis. Which of the following is true about this lesion?

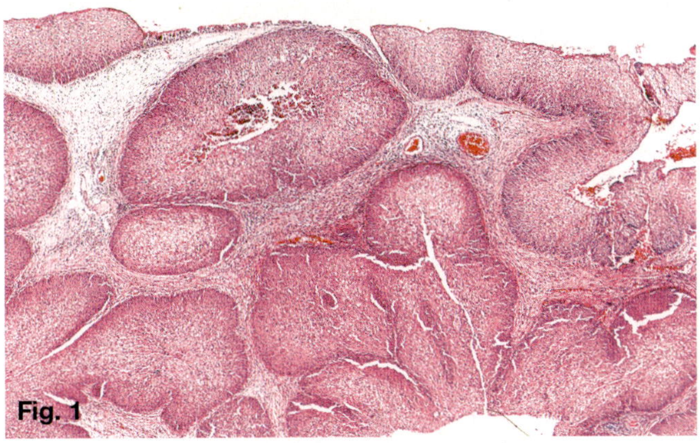


A. Develops from the lateral nasal wall
B. Human papillomavirus (HPV) found in the majority of cases
C. Not associated with risk of invasive carcinoma
D. Recurrence rate is 5% with simple excision
E. Women are more often affected than men

6. What is the underlying molecular abnormality that is usually associated with the papilloma shown in Figure 1?

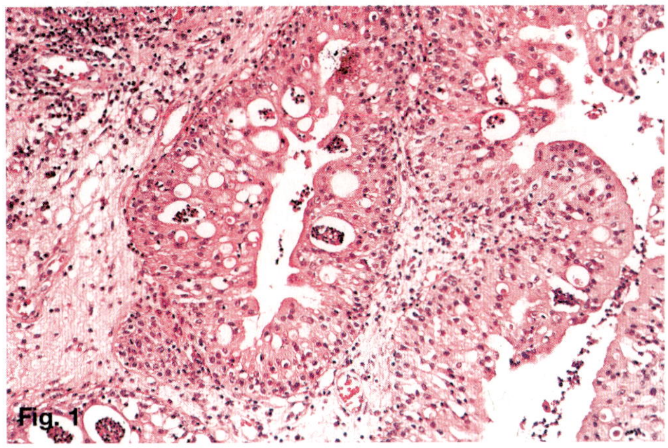


A. *EGFR*
B. *KRAS*
C. *NUT*
D. *p16*
E. *p53*

7. A 58-year-old male with a history of chronic rhinosinusitis undergoes resection of a polypoid lesion growing in the posterior nasal septum. The microscopic appearance of the lesion is demonstrated in Figure 1. On high power, the epithelium lining the glands resembles respiratory epithelium. Which of the following is the most likely diagnosis?

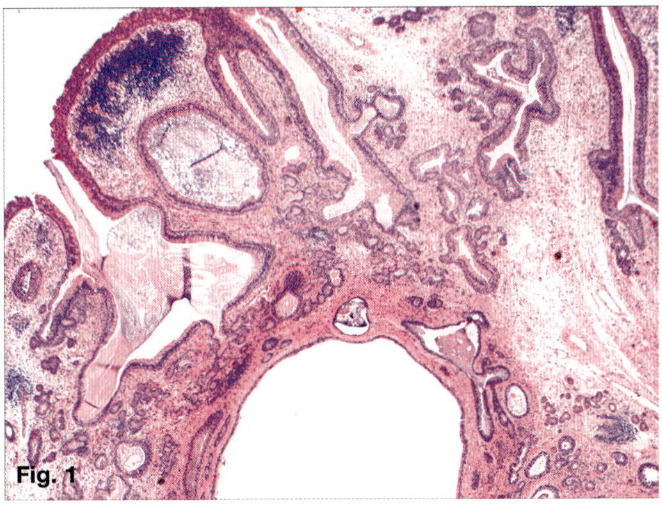


A. Chondromesenchymal hamartoma
B. Inflammatory polyp
C. Inverted papilloma
D. Low-grade adenocarcinoma
E. Respiratory epithelial adenomatoid hamartoma

8. A 14-year-old boy undergoes biopsy of a nasopharyngeal lesion near the Eustachian tube opening. The microscopic appearance of the lesion is shown in Figure 1. Which of the following is true of this entity?

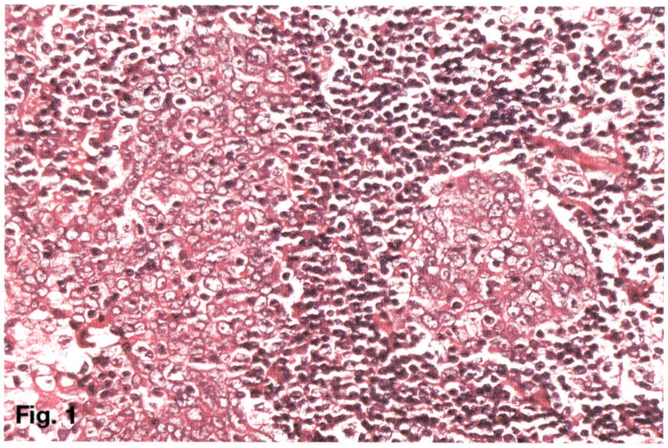

Fig. 1

A. Associated with high-risk human papillomavirus (HPV) serotypes
B. Commonly presents as cervical lymph node metastases from an occult primary
C. Distinguishing differentiated variants from lymphoma is difficult on H&E (hematoxylin and eosin) stain
D. First-line treatment is chemotherapy followed by surgical resection
E. Positive Epstein-Barr virus (EBV) by in situ hybridization (ISH) in background lymphocytes is diagnostic

9. A midline sinonasal tumor from a 25-year-old woman consists of sheets of poorly cohesive cells with scanty cytoplasm and uniform nuclei with prominent nucleoli, as shown in Figure 1. Mitotic figures and apoptotic bodies are numerous. Scattered throughout the tumor are foci of abrupt keratinization. This tumor is most likely to express

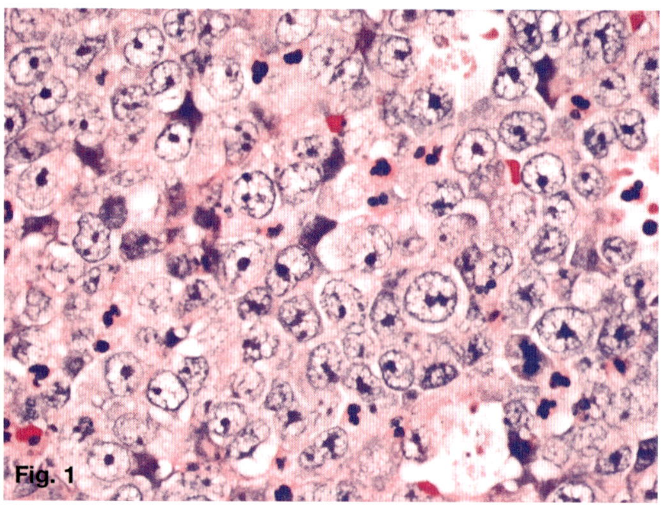

Fig. 1

A. CD45.
B. CD99.
C. HMB45.
D. NUT.
E. S100.

10. A 32-year-old male presents with a rapidly enlarging sinonasal mass. Some characteristic morphologic features are seen in Figure 1. No well-differentiated components are seen. The diagnostic immunohistochemical stain for this tumor is shown in Figure 2. Which of the following is the immunostain shown in Figure 2?

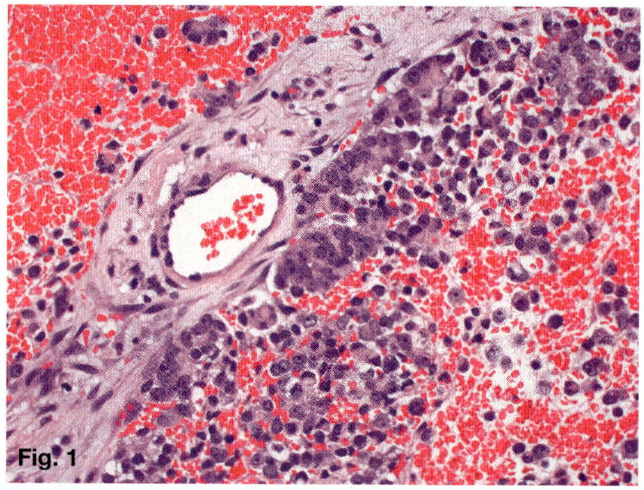

Fig. 1

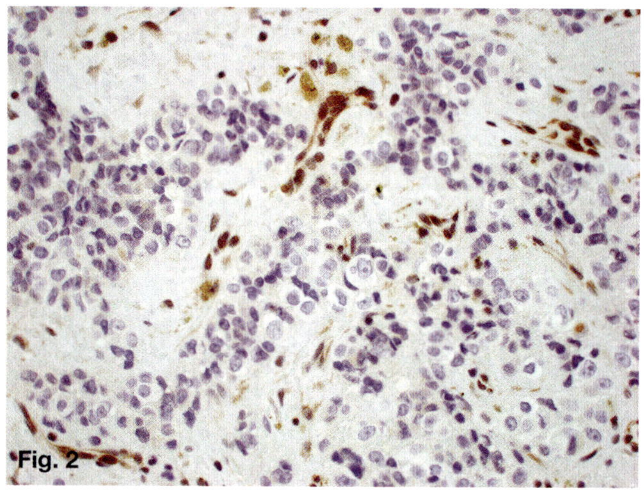

Fig. 2

A. CD34
B. Desmin
C. Pan-cytokeratins
D. S100
E. SMARCB1

11. A 54-year-old female is found to have a tumor in the left ethmoid sinus. A biopsy reveals carcinoma characterized by glandular architecture, as shown in Figure 1. Which of the following is the most likely diagnosis?

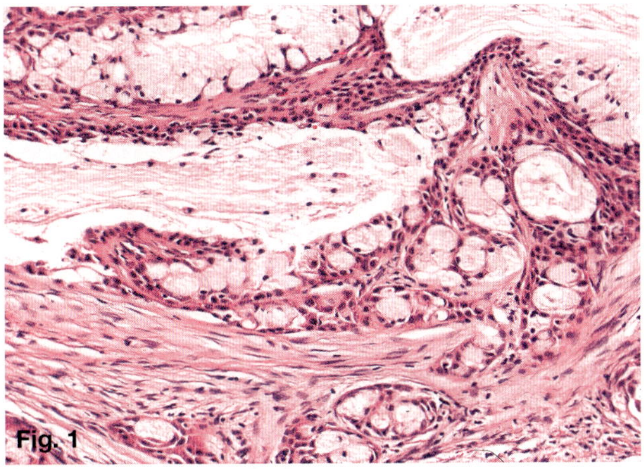
Fig. 1

A. Adenoid cystic carcinoma
B. Intestinal-type adenocarcinoma
C. Low-grade sinonasal adenocarcinoma
D. Mucoepidermoid carcinoma
E. Serous cystadenoma

12. A 40-year-old man presents with an intranasal polypoid mass arising from the roof of the nasal fossa. The mass is red and soft. Microscopic examination reveals irregular, circumscribed nests of tumor cells separated by stroma. The constituent tumor cells are uniform small cells with a high nuclear:cytoplasm ratio as seen in Figure 1. Marked capillary proliferation in a lobular pattern is also present. These features are most consistent with a lesion arising from

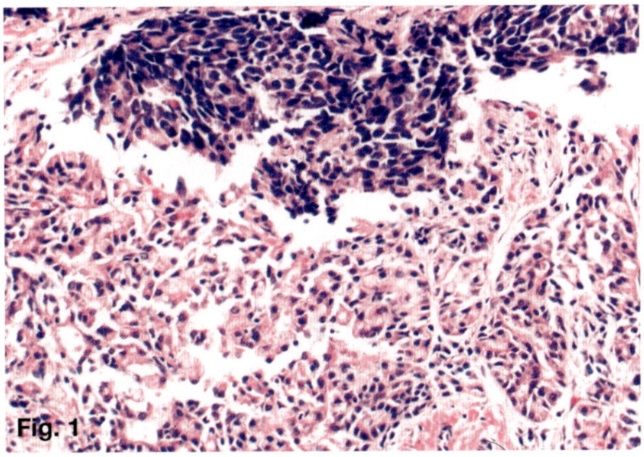
Fig. 1

A. erectile-like fibrovascular tissue.
B. lymphocytes.
C. melanocytes.
D. olfactory neuroepithelium.
E. squamous epithelium of the nasal fossa.

13. Which of the following is true of sinonasal malignant melanomas?

A. Characteristic dotlike perinuclear pan-cytokeratin staining
B. Commonly associated with mutations in *BRAF* gene
C. First-line therapy is radiation and chemotherapy
D. Majority contain intracytoplasmic melanin pigment
E. Most commonly presents in the sphenoid sinuses

14. A 24-year-old male presents with small red nodules in the nasal cavity. Figure 1 shows the morphologic features. The tumor cells show scattered weak expression of CD99 and are diffusely positive for desmin and myoD1. Pan-cytokeratins and SOX10 are negative. Which of the following is the most common cytogenetic abnormality in this entity?

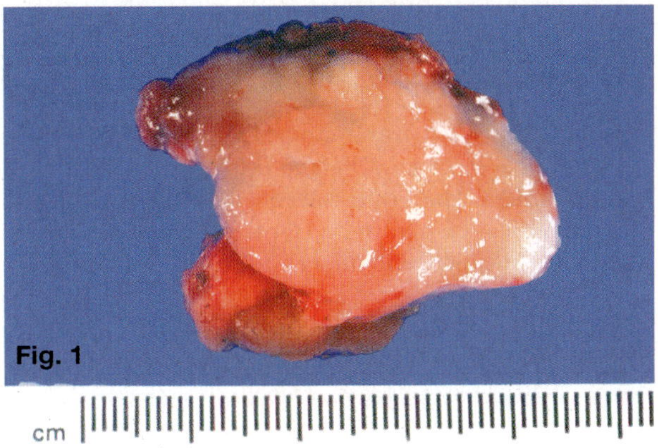

Fig. 1

A. t(1;13)
B. t(2;13)
C. t(11;22)
D. t(16;17)
E. t(X;17)

15. Which of the following lymphoplasmacytic proliferative disorders presents clinically as a "midfacial necrotizing lesion"?

A. Diffuse large B-cell lymphoma
B. Follicular dendritic cell tumor
C. Marginal zone lymphoma
D. Natural killer (NK)/T-cell lymphoma
E. Plasmacytoma

16. An 18-year-old male with a history of recurrent nasal epistaxis undergoes resection of a mass located in the posterolateral wall of the roof of the nasal fossa. Histologically, the lesion consists of a bundle of vascular structures within a stroma rich in stellate cells and mast cells, as shown in Figure 1. Which of the following hormones is thought to play a role in the pathogenesis of this lesion?

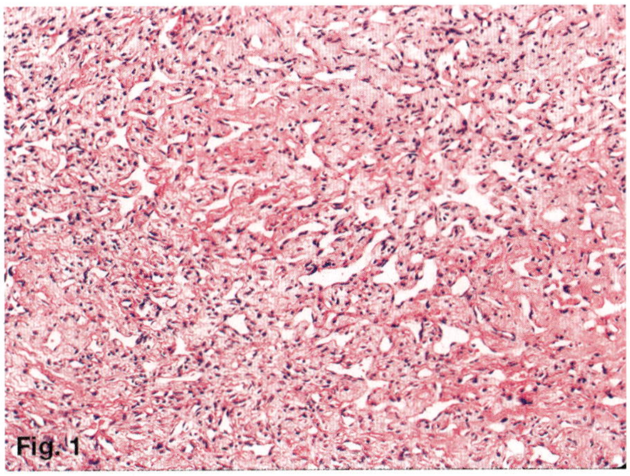
Fig. 1

A. Estradiol
B. Growth hormone
C. Progesterone
D. Serotonin
E. Testosterone

# ANSWERS AND EXPLANATIONS

**1. Correct choice: E.**

Rhinosporidiosis, which is endemic in India, Sri Lanka, and parts of South America and Africa, is occasionally seen in the United States. Rhinosporidiosis is caused by an infectious organism, probably a fungus, whose sporangia appear as thick-walled, 200-μm microcysts containing thousands of spores. Actinomycosis is a rare cause of nasal infection. Aspergillosis is a common cause of nasal/paranasal infection that can spread to the retro-orbital space, cranial vault, or parapharyngeal regions. It is commonly associated with allergic mucin, an eosinophil-rich exudate containing Charcot-Leyden crystals. Mucormycosis is most common in patients with diabetes and is due to fungi of the genus *Mucorales*, which appear as broad, irregular, nonseptate hyphae. Myospherulosis is a form of foreign body reaction to petrolatum present in preparations used for hemostatic packing. Petrolatum results in the formation of bag-like spaces within the tissue-containing spherules that come to resemble yeasts. Such spherules are denatured red blood cells.

**2. Correct choice: C.**

Rhinoscleroma is a chronic, destructive inflammatory disease of the nose that may extend to the orbit, pharynx, larynx, and gastrointestinal tract, causing extensive ulcerations. The causative agent is *Klebsiella rhinoscleromatis*, a gram-negative rod. Rhinoscleroma may be mistaken for leprosy, since both conditions are associated with sheets of foamy histiocytes (Mikulicz cells). Leprosy involves the nasal cavity in 95% of cases and is caused by *Mycobacterium leprae*, an acid-fast bacillus, which also induces foamy histiocytic response.

**3. Correct choice: B.**

Nasal polyps can be grouped into three categories: (a) inflammatory (most common), (b) associated with cystic fibrosis (CF), and (c) antrochoanal. Inflammatory polyps usually manifest in patients older than 30 years and are associated with bronchospasms on aspirin consumption in 14% of cases. They are composed of edematous lamina propria infiltrated by lymphocytes, eosinophils, and plasma cells. Since inflammatory nasal polyps are rare in childhood, nasal polyps in children should arouse suspicion of CF. Antrochoanal polyps arise from the wall of the maxillary sinus protruding into the nasal cavity through the maxillary meatus via a long slender stalk. *Note*: CF-associated polyps contain acid mucin (Alcian blue positive), whereas inflammatory polyps contain neutral mucin (PAS [periodic acid-Schiff] positive).

**4. Correct choice: B.**

Papillomas of the nose and paranasal sinuses can be divided into two types: squamous and Schneiderian. Squamous papillomas arise from the vestibule and are covered by keratinizing squamous epithelium. Schneiderian papillomas are heterogeneous. They are usually lined by nonkeratinizing squamous, intermixed with respiratory (columnar ciliated) and transitional epithelium. Three main forms are recognized: exophytic, inverted, and oncocytic. The one presented here is the exophytic type, which arises from the nasal septum and is not associated with carcinoma. Most cases are unilateral. In situ hybridization and polymerase chain reaction (PCR) studies have shown that most exophytic papillomas contain human papillomavirus (HPV), usually of the nononcogenic types 6 and 11.

**5. Correct choice: A.**

The inverted papilloma type is the most common form of Schneiderian papillomas. It usually arises from the lateral wall and grows as deeply invaginating (endophytic) nests and ribbons of benign nonkeratinizing squamous epithelium mixed with respiratory and transitional epithelium. Only a minority of them are associated with human papillomavirus (HPV). In contrast to the exophytic type, inverted papillomas carry a 10% to 15% risk of invasive carcinoma, which may be already present in the lesion at the time of resection (synchronous) or develop at a later time (metachronous). Exophytic and inverted, but not oncocytic, Schneiderian papillomas are more frequent in men. All types have a high recurrence rate (25%) if treated by excision only. Medial maxillectomy can reduce the recurrence rate to 5% for lateral papillomas.

**6. Correct choice: D.**

Oncocytic papilloma has areas of cell proliferation identical to inverted papilloma; however, the majority of the cells in oncocytic papilloma have a finely granular eosinophilic cytoplasm, less sharply defined cell borders, and inspissated mucin droplets. When the inflammatory infiltration is prominent, it may resemble inflammatory polyps, but the latter do not have oncocytic cells. Oncocytic sinonasal papillomas almost always harbor KRAS (Kirsten rat sarcoma virus) mutation, and it is not associated with human papillomavirus (HPV). Inverted papillomas usually harbor epidermal growth factor receptor (EGFR) mutations, and exophytic sinonasal papillomas are strongly associated with low-risk HPV infection. Oncocytic papilloma and inverted papilloma both carry the risk of malignancy.

**7. Correct choice: E.**

Respiratory epithelial adenomatoid hamartoma (REAH) is a rare lesion that usually develops in the posterior nasal septum. It is frequently associated with a history of chronic rhinosinusitis. The low-power appearance of edematous stroma and chronic inflammation may mimic an inflammatory polyp, but REAH contains numerous, irregularly shaped glands lined by ciliated, respiratory-like epithelium. The glandular basement membrane is unusually thick. There is no cellular atypia or mitotic activity and no risk of malignancy.

**8. Correct choice: C.**

Nonkeratinizing nasopharyngeal carcinoma (NPC) can be separated into differentiated and undifferentiated subtypes; however, there is no prognostic difference between the two, and mixtures of both patterns are common. Fifty to eighty percent of patients with nonkeratinizing NPC are initially seen with cervical lymph node metastases from an occult primary. In the differentiated form, the neoplastic cells form well-defined, cohesive cell nests and cords separated by inflammation, which allows for its ready recognition as a carcinoma, and diagnosis is straightforward. In the undifferentiated variant, the inflammatory component permeates the tumor nests and causes the separation of the carcinoma cells in a "sea" of polymorphic inflammation that is predominantly lymphoid. Such lesions may be difficult or impossible to distinguish from lymphoma on H&E (hematoxylin and eosin)-stained sections. There is a strong association with Epstein-Barr virus (EBV) infection. In situ hybridization for EBV RNA should show positivity overlying the neoplastic epithelial cells but not the smaller lymphoid component. Nasopharyngeal carcinoma is treated exclusively with radiation.

**9. Correct choice: D.**

NUT (nuclear protein in testis) carcinoma is highly aggressive with a median overall survival of 6.5 months. It is associated with translocations involving the *NUTM1* gene. It preferentially involves midline structures, including the sinonasal region, and is not associated with human papillomavirus (HPV) or Epstein-Barr virus (EBV). The typical morphology is composed of sheets of undifferentiated cells with little amphiphilic or eosinophilic cytoplasm. Nuclei have irregular contours, although they tend to be somewhat uniform in size, with fine to vesicular chromatin and prominent nucleoli. Mitotic figures and apoptotic bodies are numerous. Abrupt well-differentiated squamous differentiation may be seen. Immunohistochemical analysis is key in the differential diagnosis. NUT carcinoma expresses keratin and epithelial membrane antigen (EMA), and diagnostic evaluation can now rely on immunohistochemistry for NUT protein. The other answer choices are negative in NUT carcinoma.

**10. Correct choice: E.**

SMARCB1 (SWI/SNF-related matrix-associated actin-dependent regulator of chromatin subfamily B member 1)-deficient sinonasal carcinomas are uncommon, with fewer than 100 cases described, although it is likely underdiagnosed. Affected patients tend to present at high stage, and on average, 56% of patients have died of their disease 15 months after diagnosis. SMARCB1-deficient sinonasal carcinoma grows as nests of undifferentiated-appearing cells in the sinonasal submucosa. It is highly infiltrative, with high mitotic rates and frequent necrosis. On low power, it appears to be "blue" and basaloid, but on high power, the characteristic rhabdoid or plasmacytoid appearance can be seen. By immunohistochemistry, SMARCB1-deficient sinonasal carcinomas are consistently positive for cytokeratins and negative for SMARCB1.

**11. Correct choice: C.**

Sinonasal adenocarcinomas can be categorized into the following:

- Salivary-type adenocarcinomas: Adenoid cystic carcinoma is the most frequent type in this region, followed by mucoepidermoid carcinoma.
- Nonsalivary adenocarcinomas, nonintestinal type:
  - Low-grade adenocarcinoma is a well-differentiated adenocarcinoma composed of glands lined by cuboidal/columnar cells without nuclear stratification. Some glands are cystically dilated, and others contain papillary infoldings. Good prognosis. No known association with carcinogens.
  - High-grade adenocarcinoma has prominent cellular pleomorphism, a high mitotic rate, and often prominent necrosis and cannot be classified as either salivary or intestinal type of tumor. Solid and trabecular growth pattern with occasional small cystic spaces and are composed of neoplastic cells that have a small amount of amphiphilic cytoplasm. Negative for CD20 and CDX2. Poor prognosis. No known association with carcinogens.
- Intestinal-type adenocarcinoma is a locally aggressive neoplasm arising most commonly in the ethmoid sinus and associated with long-term exposure to fine wood dust. Morphologically, it usually resembles colonic adenocarcinoma.

**12. Correct choice: D.**

Olfactory neuroblastoma is a malignant tumor that derives from the neuroepithelial cells of the olfactory mucosa. It shows morphologic characteristics of other neuroectodermal-derived tumors, such as medulloblastoma and adrenal neuroblastoma, including evidence of neural differentiation: synaptophysin immunoreactivity, Homer-Wright rosettes, fibrillary background, and dense-core granules on electron microscopy (EM). Lobular proliferation of blood vessels is sometimes seen, which may generate confusion with a vascular neoplasm. The most important differential diagnosis is with lymphoma (when a small cell population is prevalent) or poorly differentiated carcinoma (if large cells are predominant). Olfactory neuroblastomas express neuroendocrine markers such as synaptophysin and chromogranin, and one-third is positive for keratin.

**13. Correct choice: D.**

Sinonasal malignant melanomas account for approximately 1% of all malignant melanomas. Mostly found in the nasal cavity at the anterior septum, inferior turbinate, and middle turbinate. Physical examination typically demonstrates a sessile or polypoid mass that is often pigmented. Complete excision is the treatment of choice; radiation and chemotherapy have had little or no value as adjuvant treatment. The prognosis is poor. Approximately 70% of upper respiratory tract malignant melanomas contain intracytoplasmic melanin pigment. Common morphologic patterns include (in order of decreasing frequency) small blue cell, spindle cell, epithelioid, and pleomorphic. Tumor cells show strong immunochemical reactions to melanoma markers, while rarely positive for CKs (cytokeratins). Sinonasal small cell carcinoma will often display dotlike perinuclear staining. Mutations of the *BRAF* gene are uncommon as compared to cutaneous counterparts. Mutations in NRAS (neuroblastoma RAS viral oncogene homolog) and CKIT (KIT proto-oncogene receptor tyrosine kinase) are much more common in melanomas arising in this location.

**14. Correct choice: B.**

Rhabdomyosarcoma in the head and neck arises, in descending order, in the orbit, nasopharynx, middle ear/mastoid, and nose/paranasal sinuses. Approximately 75% of the patients are 12 years of age or younger, but examples are seen in adolescents, adults, and older individuals. The most common is the embryonal subtype followed by the alveolar subtype. The image is characteristic of the alveolar rhabdomyosarcoma, which has fibrous septa lined by a single row of round tumor cells, with additional tumor cells lying free between the septa (central dyscohesion). Embryonal rhabdomyosarcoma frequently has alternating hypercellular and hypocellular fields. The stroma is sparsely collagenized or myxoid. The t(2;13) and, less commonly, t(1;13) translocations are well documented for the alveolar subtype and are distinct from the cytogenetic abnormalities seen in embryonal variants. Both are immunoreactive to desmin, myogenin, and myoD1. Ewing sarcoma would be diffusely positive for CD99.

**15. Correct choice: D.**

Natural killer (NK)/T-cell lymphoma is an extranodal lymphoma characterized by an angiocentric pattern and highly destructive behavior, with prominent necrosis. Most cases consist of neoplastic NK cells, a few of T cells. It shows a strong association with Epstein-Barr virus (EBV). Rare in U.S. and Europe, and more frequent in East Asia and Latin America. It affects the upper respiratory tract, especially midfacial structures, presenting as a midfacial necrotizing lesion. Alternative designations include lymphomatoid granulomatosis, midline malignant reticulosis, and angiocentric immunoproliferative lesion.

**16. Correct choice: E.**

Nasopharyngeal angiofibroma is a vascular lesion encountered predominantly in males between the ages of 10 and 25. The fact that it develops during adolescence suggests that the growth of this lesion is driven by androgens, which is consistent with the finding of testosterone receptors in the tumor. It arises in a well-defined region of the nasal fossa from specialized erectile fibrovascular tissue. Differentiation of angiofibroma from capillary hemangioma is important, considering their different evolution. Angiofibroma is composed of small vessels within irregularly arranged collagen fibers and stellate cells. Capillary hemangiomas consist of thin-walled vessels and lack abundant stroma. Spontaneous regression of angiofibromas may occur, but larger lesions need surgery and/or radiation therapy.

# 22 Larynx

1. A vocal cord polypoid nodule is removed from a 45-year-old enthusiastic bowler who presented with hoarseness. The nodule is located at the junction between the middle and anterior third of the right vocal cord and measures 4 mm. Histologically, it is composed of edematous stroma containing dilated blood vessels, perivascular fibrinous exudate, and hemosiderin deposits. Which of the following is the most likely diagnosis?

   A. Angioma
   B. Contact ulcer
   C. Localized amyloidosis
   D. Pyogenic granuloma
   E. Vocal cord polyp

2. A 22-year-old patient has undergone multiple resections of laryngeal papillomas since the age of 16. The lesions appear histologically as in Figure 1. Mild nuclear atypia with koilocytotic changes is observed. Which of the following is the most likely etiology of these lesions?

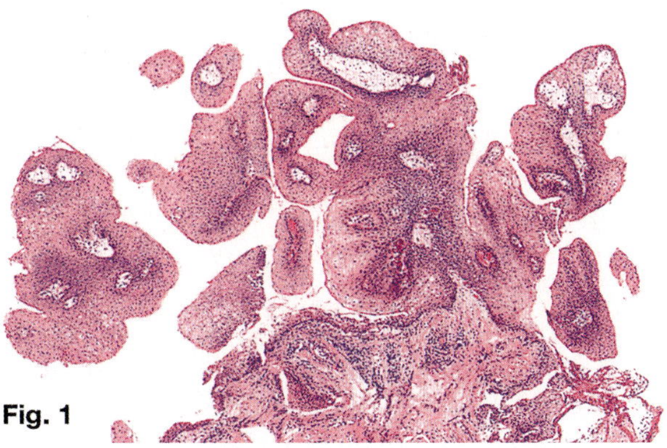

Fig. 1

   A. Exposure to alcohol
   B. Exposure to cigarette smoking
   C. Inherited mutations of the epidermal growth factor receptor gene
   D. Viral infection
   E. Voice overuse

3. Which of the following images can be classified as moderate-grade dysplasia?

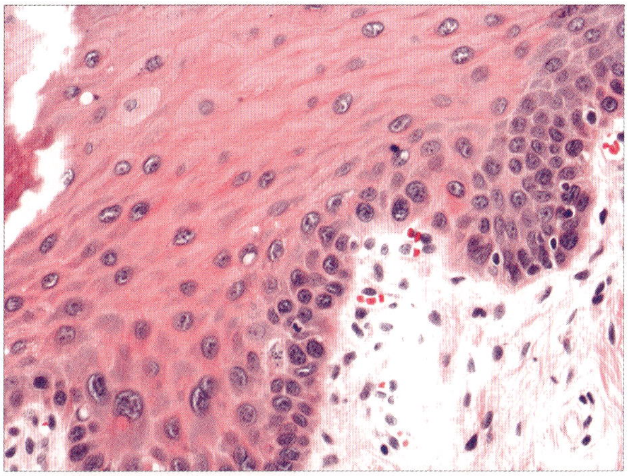

A.

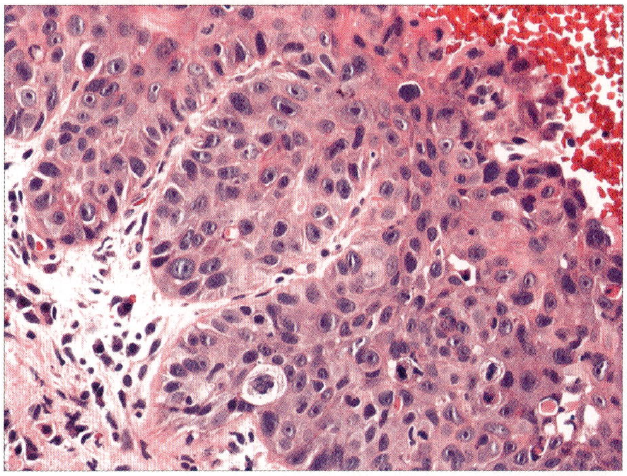

B.

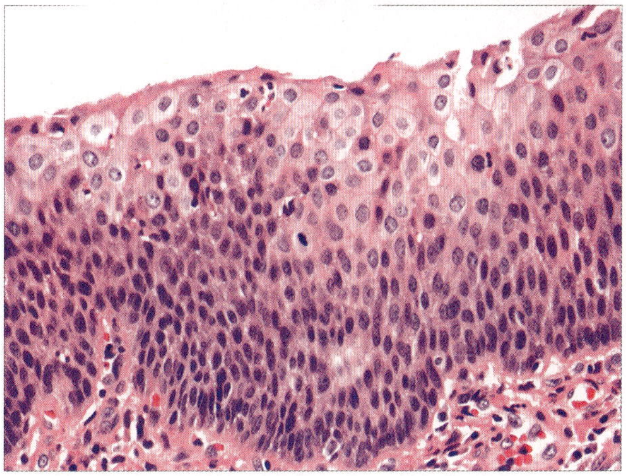

C.

All figures in this chapter are from Longacre TA, Greenson JK, Hornick JL, Reuter VE, eds. *Mills and Sternberg's Diagnostic Surgical Pathology.* 7th ed. Wolters Kluwer; 2022 except for those noted at the end of this book.

D. 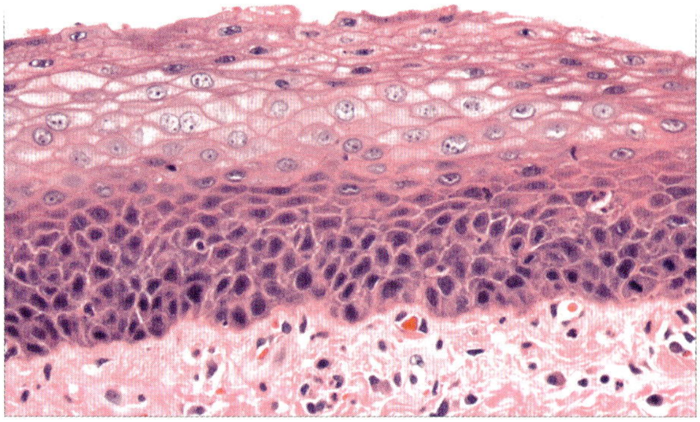

E. 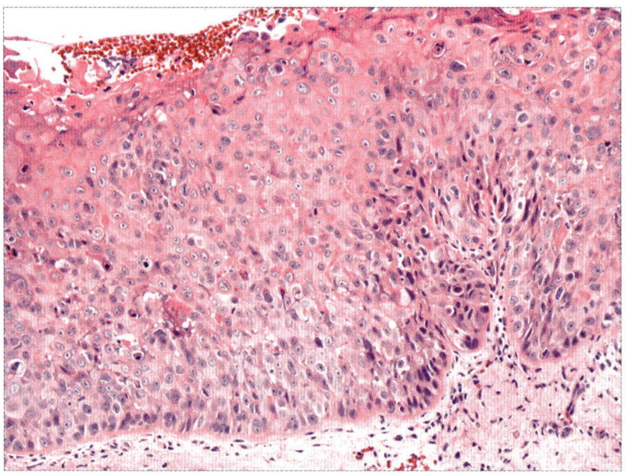

4. Which of the following is true of the tumor shown in Figure 1?

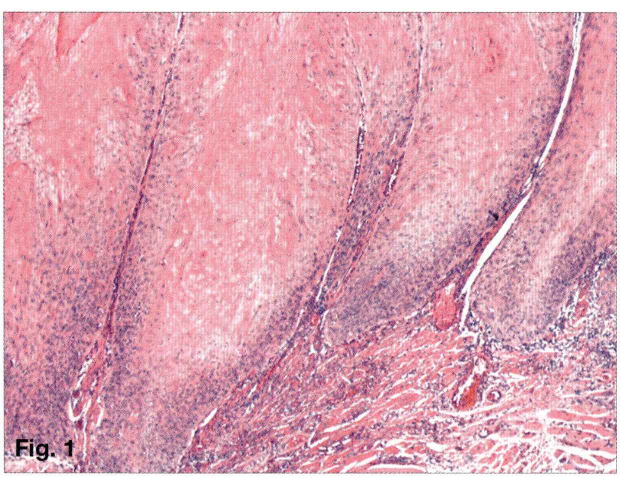


A. Associated with high-grade human papillomavirus (HPV) serotypes
B. Cytologically, shows mitotic activity limited to the basal layers
C. Frequently shows more cytologic atypia than verrucous hyperplasia
D. Typically located in the supraglottic region and more common in women
E. Usually presents with regional lymph node metastasis at time of diagnosis

5. A representative section of an ulcerated exophytic mass is shown in Figure 1. Focal areas of conventional squamous cell carcinoma are also seen. Mitotic figures are easily identifiable. Cartilage and rare giant cells are seen intermingling with the spindle cells. The tumor cells are positive for p40. Which of the following is the most likely diagnosis?

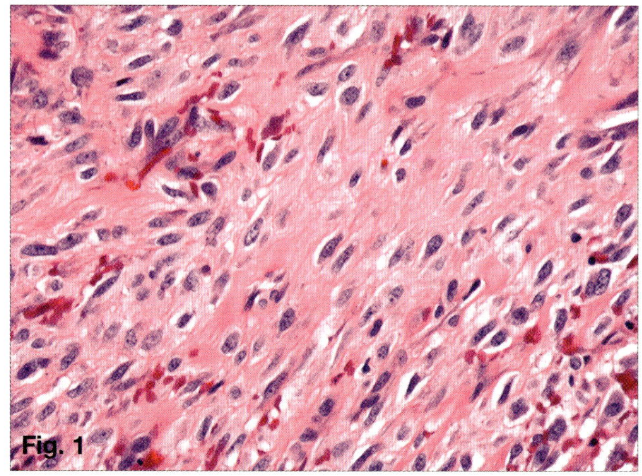


A. Chondrosarcoma
B. Fetal rhabdomyoma
C. Fibrosarcoma
D. Inflammatory myofibroblastic tumor
E. Spindle cell carcinoma

6. A representative section of a supraglottic polypoid and hemorrhagic mass is shown in Figure 1. There is tumor necrosis and easily identifiable mitotic figures. The tumor cells are positive for pan-keratin and CD56. Which of the following is the best diagnosis?

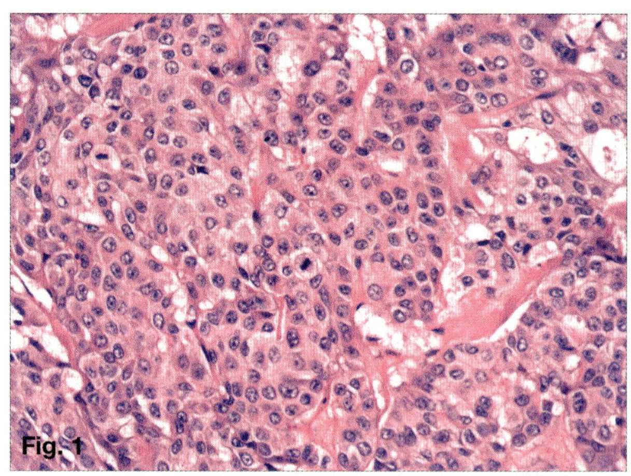


A. Adenoid cystic carcinoma
B. Basaloid squamous cell carcinoma
C. Glomus tumor
D. Neuroendocrine carcinoma
E. Undifferentiated carcinoma

7. Which of the following is the most common malignant hematolymphoid lesion of the larynx?

A. Burkitt lymphoma
B. Diffuse large B-cell lymphoma
C. Follicular lymphoma
D. Mantle cell lymphoma
E. Marginal zone lymphoma

# ANSWERS AND EXPLANATIONS

**1. Correct choice: E.**

Vocal cord polyp, also called *singer's nodule*, is a benign nodular lesion that usually develops on the anterior third of the vocal cords in people who abuse their voices. In the early stages, it is composed of edematous stroma with fibroblastic hyperplasia (*gelatinous type*). Later, hyalinization of the stroma develops (leading occasionally to a misdiagnosis of localized amyloidosis), along with vascular proliferation (prompting confusion with pyogenic granuloma or angioma). *Angiomas* develop in a supraglottic location; vessels in angiomas are thick walled, whereas singer's nodule has thin-walled vessels. *Pyogenic granuloma* (lobular capillary hemangioma) does not occur in the larynx. *Contact ulcer* (laryngeal granuloma) is ulcerated granulation tissue that may have a polypoid nodular appearance and mimic a neoplasm. It develops in the posterior vocal cord as a result of intubation, acid reflux, or vocal cord abuse.

**2. Correct choice: D.**

The microscopic features and clinical history are consistent with *laryngeal papillomatosis*, a condition associated with human papillomavirus (HPV) (usually types 6 and 11 and, occasionally, 16 and 18) and manifesting with numerous laryngeal papillomas that recur repeatedly. Mild atypical changes and koilocytosis are consistently present, but frank dysplasia is rarely seen. Those arising from the respiratory epithelium may not show an orderly pattern of maturation and thus may be mistaken for carcinoma in situ. The HPV genome is detectable in all cases by immunohistochemistry or in situ hybridization. Association with HPV 16 and 18 does not result in increased risk of malignancy. Patients with chronic disease only seldom develop squamous cell carcinomas. Exposure to alcohol, tobacco, or other irritants and voice overuse are associated with laryngitis and laryngeal keratosis.

**3. Correct choice: C.**

Laryngeal squamous cell carcinoma (SCC) develops through progressive intraepithelial lesions to invasive carcinoma in a manner analogous to other epithelial cancers such as cervical SCC. Clinically, precursor lesions are similar to those described in the mouth: leukoplakia and erythroplakia, which harbor dysplastic changes or frank carcinoma in 5% to 50% of cases. The World Health Organization (WHO) currently uses a two-tier system for the grading of intraepithelial neoplasia of the larynx and classifies these lesions as low-grade dysplasia (including squamous hyperplasia and mild squamous dysplasia) and high-grade dysplasia (including moderate and severe squamous dysplasia and carcinoma in situ).

Grading of squamous precursor lesions is based on architectural and cytologic atypia. *Architectural atypia* refers to disturbed cellular maturation: altered nuclear polarization, mitotic figures above the basal layer, dyskeratosis, and early keratinization. Drop-shaped rete ridges are also a useful indicator of dysplasia. *Cytologic atypia* refers to nuclear pleomorphism and hyperchromasia, increased nuclear size, anisocytosis, increased nucleocytoplasmic ratio, prominent nucleoli, and atypical mitotic figures.

- (D) *Squamous hyperplasia*: Increase in epithelial thickness and hyperkeratosis, without architectural or cytologic atypia. Low risk of SCC.
- (A) *Mild dysplasia*: Basal cell hyperplasia and cytologic atypia confined to the lower third of the epithelium.
- (C) *Moderate dysplasia*: Architectural and cytologic atypia extends into the middle third of the epithelium.
- (E) *Severe dysplasia*: Architectural and cytologic atypia extends to more than two-thirds of the thickness of the epithelium. Cytologic atypia is marked.
- (B) *Carcinoma in situ*: Architectural and severe cytologic atypia involving the full thickness of the epithelium. This is a malignant transformation without actual invasion.

**4. Correct choice: B.**

Verrucous carcinoma typically involves the vocal cords and is much more common in men in the sixth to seventh decades of life. Human papillomavirus (HPV) does not play a role (or only plays a minor role) in the development of these tumors. Histologically, these tumors are composed of thickened and folded squamous epithelium frequently with abundant keratosis and parakeratosis. The tumor bases are circumscribed and composed of broad tongues of squamous epithelium that extend deeper than the surrounding nonneoplastic epithelium into the subepithelium. Cytologically, little, if any, atypia should be present, with normal maturation and mitotic activity limited to the basal levels of the neoplasm. Somewhat counterintuitively, verrucous carcinoma frequently shows less cytologic atypia than verrucous hyperplasia, which often shows some degree of dysplasia. Invasive irregular nests of squamous cells should not be seen. The lesions have an excellent prognosis, and less than 10% of patients die from their tumors; none develop metastases.

**5. Correct choice: E.**

Spindle cell carcinoma (also known as sarcomatoid squamous cell carcinoma) is a poorly differentiated biphasic tumor that shows a majority mesenchymal phenotype (spindled) and minor squamous component. Most cases have mild-to-moderate cellularity and mild-to-moderate cellular pleomorphism. Necrosis is only occasionally present, although mitotic figures are frequent. A variety of growth patterns can be seen, including nodular fasciitis–like, fibromatosis-like, storiform, herringbone, and fascicular growth patterns. Furthermore, osteocartilaginous regions and giant cells, including osteoclast-like giant cells, can also be seen. Spindle cell carcinomas of the larynx can mimic any number of mesenchymal lesions. Pan-keratin and p40 are helpful immunostains to perform in the diagnostic evaluation.

**6. Correct choice: D.**

Laryngeal neuroendocrine carcinomas occur more frequently in older individuals and in men and are most often supraglottic and submucosal. The image shows a moderately differentiated neuroendocrine carcinoma. The WHO classification divides them into three categories:

- *Well-differentiated neuroendocrine carcinoma (carcinoid tumor)*: It has the same morphology as pulmonary carcinoids. Necrosis, cellular atypia, and mitotic activity are absent. They do not metastasize and have excellent prognosis.

- *Moderately differentiated neuroendocrine carcinoma (atypical carcinoid tumor)*: These are the most frequent neuroendocrine tumors in the larynx. Their morphology is similar to carcinoids but has necrosis, mitotic activity, and cytologic atypia. The 5-year survival rate is 50%.
- *Small cell carcinoma*: Very rare, it looks and behaves like small cell carcinoma of the lungs.

**7. Correct choice: B.**

Most hematolymphoid neoplasia has been reported within the larynx, including predominantly cutaneous or mucosal lymphomas such as mycosis fungoides. The most common malignant hematolymphoid lesions involving the larynx are diffuse large B-cell lymphomas and extramedullary plasmacytomas.

# 23 Ear and Temporal Bone

1. A small painful nodule excised from the upper right helix of a 28-year-old male consists of an ulcer demarcated by acanthotic epidermis on each side and granulation tissue at the base, as demonstrated in Figure 1. The chronic inflammatory infiltration at the base of the ulcer extends to the perichondrium. These features are most consistent with

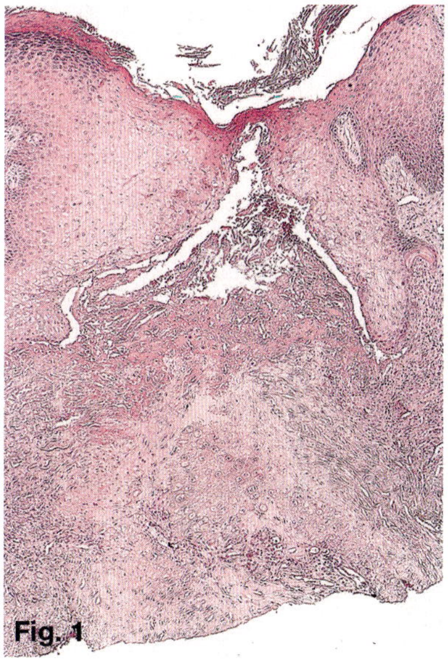

Fig. 1

A. chondrodermatitis nodularis chronica helicis.
B. gout.
C. malakoplakia.
D. ochronosis.
E. spectacle frame acanthoma.

2. A mass is removed from the middle ear of a 48-year-old woman. Figure 1 shows its histopathologic features. Which of the following is the most likely diagnosis?

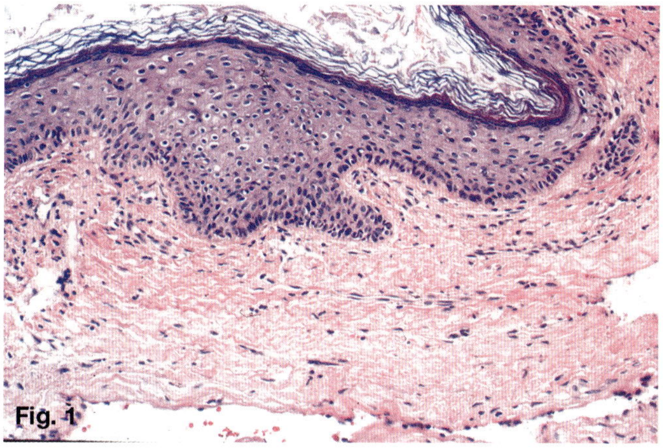

Fig. 1

A. Adenoma of the middle ear
B. Cholesteatoma
C. Cholesterol granuloma
D. Dermoid cyst
E. Squamous cell carcinoma

All figures in this chapter are from Longacre TA, Greenson JK, Hornick JL, Reuter VE, eds. *Mills and Sternberg's Diagnostic Surgical Pathology.* 7th ed. Wolters Kluwer; 2022 except for those noted at the end of this book.

3. A 47-year-old man presents with tinnitus and painful swelling of both ears. He reports past episodes of pain and swelling of the nose as well. He also complains of recurrent debilitating joint pains. On physical examination, "cauliflower" deformities of both ears and a "saddle" nose are noticed. The patient is found to have bilateral sensorineural hearing loss. A biopsy of the ear shows the histopathologic changes depicted in Figure 1. Which of the following is the most likely pathogenetic mechanism of this condition?

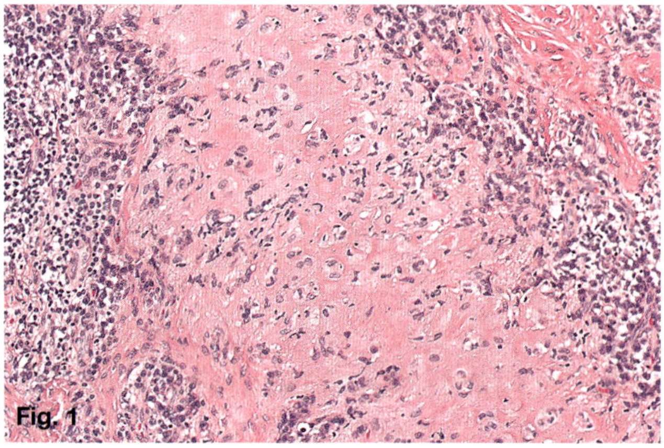
Fig. 1

A. Autoimmune
B. Genetic
C. Infectious
D. Metabolism disorder
E. Neoplastic

4. A total stapedectomy is performed for the treatment of otosclerosis in a 45-year-old male. Which of the following histologic changes is most likely to be present?

A. Extensive osteolysis of the footplate
B. New woven bone formation in the crura
C. New woven bone formation in the footplate
D. Pathologic changes limited to otic capsule
E. Spongiosis and formation of large marrow cavities

5. A 40-year-old woman undergoes excision of slow-growing, skin-covered polypoid nodule in the external auditory canal. Its morphologic appearance is shown in Figure 1. Which of the following is this tumor?

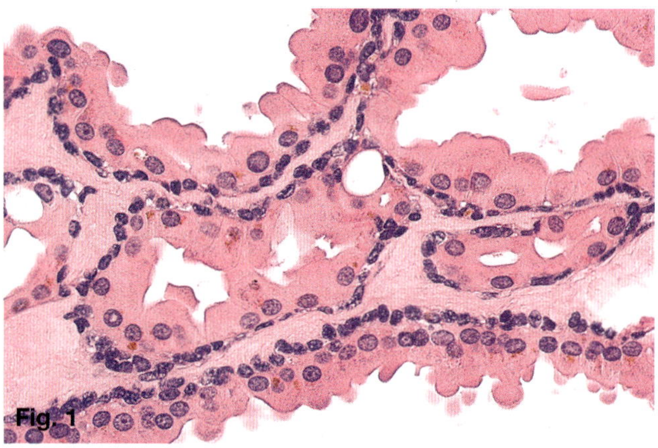
Fig. 1

A. Adenoid cystic carcinoma
B. Ceruminous gland adenocarcinoma
C. Ceruminous gland adenoma
D. Mucoepidermoid carcinoma
E. Syringocystadenoma papilliferum

6. A 30-year-old woman presents with a pruritic subcutaneous nodule in the left auricle. There is no regional lymphadenopathy. Local surgical excision is performed. The histologic appearance of the lesion is shown in Figure 1. Which of the following is true regarding this entity?

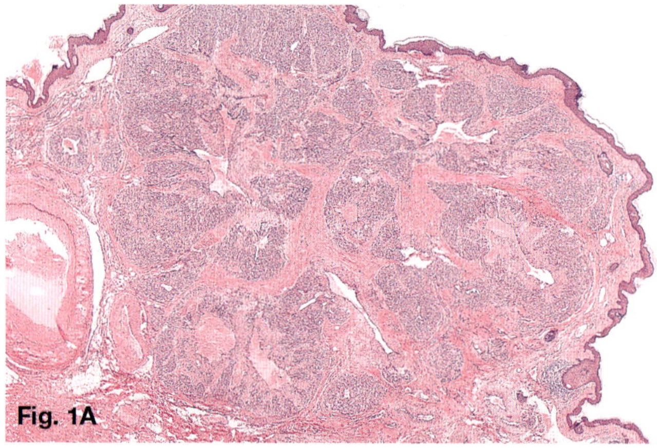
Fig. 1A

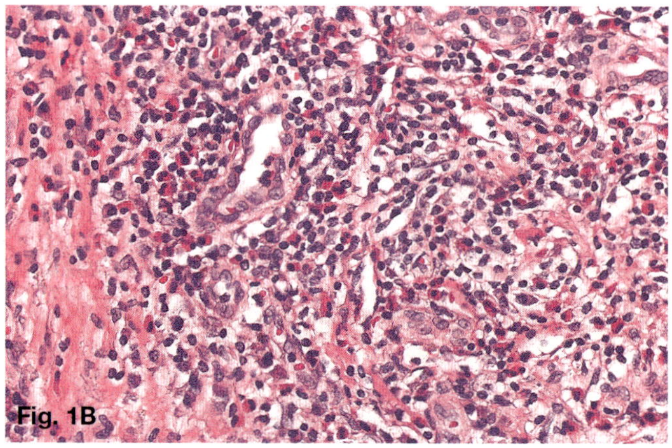
Fig. 1B

A. Associated with human herpesvirus 8 (HHV-8)
B. Endothelial cells show mild pleomorphism and nuclear hyperchromasia
C. GLUT1 (glucose transporter type 1) expression is diagnostic for this lesion
D. Lesion limited to the dermis
E. Variant of Kimura disease

7. A small tumor is removed from the middle ear of a 40-year-old man suffering from conductive hearing loss. Figure 1 demonstrates neoplastic cells with glandular and solid components. The tumor cells are diffusely positive for cytokeratin and patchy positive for synaptophysin. S100 and SMA (smooth muscle actin) are negative. Which of the following is the most likely diagnosis?

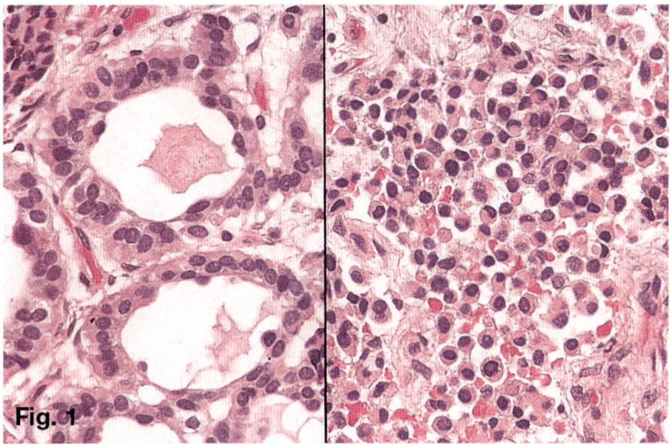
Fig. 1

A. Ceruminous adenocarcinoma
B. Meningioma
C. Middle ear adenoma
D. Neuroendocrine carcinoma
E. Paraganglioma

8. A 30-year-old woman presents with progressive hearing loss and pain in the right ear. Magnetic resonance imaging (MRI) reveals a middle ear mass, which is resected. Histologically, the tumor is composed of nests of uniform oval cells with abundant eosinophilic cytoplasm. The tumor cells are immunoreactive for synaptophysin but negative for keratin and epithelial membrane antigen (EMA). S100 and glial fibrillary acidic protein (GFAP) immunohistochemistry is negative, except for a few scattered cells. The tumor cells show a loss of expression for succinate dehydrogenase subunit B (SDHB) by immunohistochemistry. Which of the following is the most likely diagnosis?
A. Acoustic neuroma
B. Carcinoid tumor
C. Jugulotympanic paraganglioma
D. Meningioma
E. Middle ear adenoma

9. A 25-year-old woman presents with a 1-year history of unilateral conductive hearing loss. Imaging studies reveal an osteolytic tumor measuring 4.5 cm and located at the posterior medial surface of the petrous portion of the temporal bone. The tumor is resected. Its histologic appearance is shown in Figure 1. Tumor cells are positive for pan-keratin, vimentin, and glial fibrillary acidic protein (GFAP) and negative for thyroglobulin, thyroid transcription factor 1 (TTF1), and PAX8. This tumor is associated with which of the following syndromes?

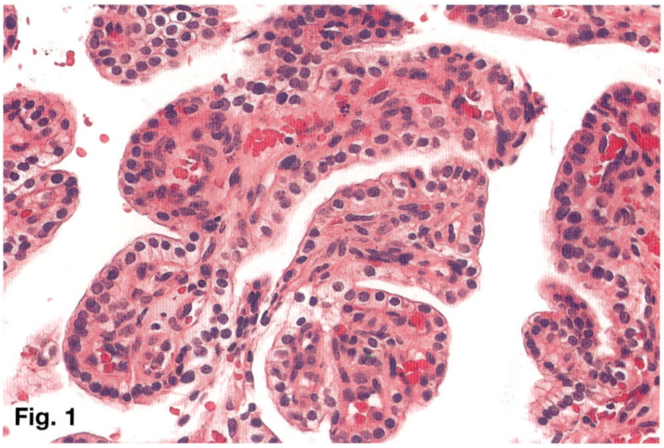
Fig. 1

A. Li-Fraumeni syndrome
B. Neurofibromatosis type 2
C. Tuberous sclerosis
D. Turcot syndrome
E. von Hippel-Lindau syndrome

# ANSWERS AND EXPLANATIONS

**1. Correct choice: A.**

Chondrodermatitis nodularis chronica helicis is an idiopathic, nonneoplastic ulcerative lesion of the auricle that presents as a unilateral reddish painful nodule of the helix (most commonly in the superior portion) in middle-aged or older men. Cold exposure, solar damage, local trauma, and pressure necrosis are suspected etiopathogenetic factors. The skin is probably the initial target, with secondary cartilage involvement. Surgical excision is curative. Gout produces urate crystal deposits (tophi) consisting of basophilic amorphous material with histiocytic and giant cell reaction. Ochronosis may manifest with darkly discolored wax or a dark bluish discoloration of the ear lobe in children, owing to the accumulation of homogentisic acid in cartilage. Malacoplakia is an inflammatory lesion usually involving the genitourinary tract and rarely the ear. It is characterized by sheets of macrophages with PAS (periodic acid-Schiff)-positive granules and Michaelis-Gutmann bodies. Spectacle frame acanthoma, AKA granuloma fissuratum, develops behind the ear or on the nose due to irritation from eyeglasses.

**2. Correct choice: B.**

Cholesteatomas are basically epidermoid cysts containing pearly keratin and lined by an epidermal layer devoid of adnexa. There are congenital and acquired forms. The congenital form is usually "closed" (ie, with intact tympanic membrane) and arises from epidermoid cell rests. The more common acquired form is "open" (ie, with perforated tympanic membrane) and develops in the context of chronic otitis media. The squamous epithelium lining the cyst wall is morphologically similar to epidermis, but shows an increased proliferative index, as shown by Ki-67 immunoreactivity. Cholesteatomas undergo progressive growth with erosion of the middle ear bones and ossicles. Pathogenetic mechanisms are still unclear but probably involve epidermal invasion from the external canal into the middle ear, retraction pockets from the tympanic membrane, or trauma.

**3. Correct choice: B.**

Relapsing polychondritis (RP) is an autoimmune disease targeting cartilage at multiple sites, including ears, nose, larynx, bronchi, and joints. It also affects the eyes, heart valves, and skin. It occurs in White people in their 40s to 60s. The ear cartilage is involved in 90% of cases. Recurrent episodes lead to scarring and deformities, that is, cauliflower ears. The same alterations develop in the nose cartilage, resulting in saddle nose deformity. RP can be diagnosed if there are at least three of the following features: (a) recurrent auricular chondritis of both auricles, (b) inflammatory arthritis, (c) nasal chondritis, (d) evidence of ocular inflammation, (e) chondritis involving larynx and/or tracheal cartilages, and (f) evidence of cochlear or vestibular damage, combined with histologic evidence of chondritis. Histologically, RP is characterized by perichondrial mixed acute/chronic inflammation. The cartilage becomes necrotic and acquires an eosinophilic appearance. Destroyed cartilage is then replaced by scar. Patients with RP often suffer from other autoimmune disorders (systemic lupus erythematosus [SLE], rheumatoid arthritis, Sjögren syndrome, autoimmune thyroid disease, etc) and have antibodies to type II collagen in the serum and immune complexes in the inflamed cartilage. No evidence supports a hereditary or familial predisposition. RP can be fatal, due to respiratory or cardiovascular system involvement.

**4. Correct choice: C.**

Otosclerosis is a common condition that affects the otic capsule and extends to the footplate of the stapes, where the characteristic changes may be observed if a whole stapedectomy is performed. Severe forms of otosclerosis manifest with conductive hearing loss. An increased amount of new woven bone and neovascularization represent the typical microscopic findings. Because these changes are limited to the footplate, partial stapedectomies (which consist of crura and head only) do not show any alterations. Spongiosis, with the formation of ample marrow cavities, occurs in the early stages. Other conditions mimicking otosclerosis include Paget disease and osteogenesis imperfecta.

**5. Correct choice: D.**

Neoplasms of ceruminous glands are rare. Benign ceruminous tumors include ceruminous gland adenoma, pleomorphic adenoma, and syringocystadenoma papilliferum. Malignant ceruminous tumors include ceruminous gland adenocarcinoma, adenoid cystic carcinoma, and mucoepidermoid carcinoma. The gross appearance of ceruminal gland neoplasms includes skin-covered, circumscribed, polypoid, or rounded masses from 1 to 4 cm in diameter. Histologically, ceruminal gland adenomas are unencapsulated but well-demarcated glandular proliferations. The glands are composed of two-cell layers. The inner or luminal epithelial cell is cuboidal or columnar with eosinophilic cytoplasm and the decapitation-type secretion (apical "snouts"), whereas the outer cell layer is of myoepithelial differentiation. Ceruminous gland adenocarcinoma displays a mixed cribriform/solid growth pattern, with prominent cellular atypia and loss of the double-cell layer.

**6. Correct choice: C.**

Epithelioid hemangioma (EH), also known as angiolymphoid hyperplasia with eosinophilia, is a benign vascular lesion. It usually arises in the head and neck, and the external ear is a frequent site. It is characterized by single or multiple, pink to red-brown indurated cutaneous papules or subcutaneous nodules. Human herpesvirus 8 (HHV-8) has not been identified in association with EH. EH consists of a nodular proliferation of vessels lined by plump endothelial cells protruding into the lumen like hobnails, admixed with a rich lymphocytic and eosinophilic infiltrate. The vascular spaces are lined by epithelioid endothelial cells with mild pleomorphism, hyperchromatic nuclei, copious eosinophilic cytoplasm, and inconspicuous nucleoli. Increased mitotic activity and moderate to marked nuclear pleomorphism are not seen. The endothelial cells in EH are immunoreactive for CD31, ETS-related gene (ERG), and, to a lesser extent, CD34. Staining for glucose transporter protein 1 (GLUT1) is typically absent. EH is morphologically akin to Kimura disease, but the latter occurs in Asian males and in locations other than head and neck. The clinical and histologic differences allow these entities to be separated and considered as distinct clinicopathologic entities.

**7. Correct choice: C.**

Middle ear adenoma (MEA) is a benign neoplasm that originates from the middle ear mucosa, at sites including the Eustachian tube, mastoid spaces, ossicles, and chorda tympani. Conductive hearing loss is the most common presentation. Histologically, MEA is a glandular tumor with varied architecture, solid, sheetlike, trabecular, cystic, or cribriform growth patterns. The glands are composed of a single layer of cuboidal-to-columnar cells with a varying amount of eosinophilic cytoplasm and a round-to-oval hyperchromatic nucleus. Cellular pleomorphism may be prominent, but mitotic figures are uncommon. The cells may have a prominent plasmacytoid appearance that is particularly evident not only in the more solid areas of growth but also in the cells forming the glandular structures. The tumor is immunoreactive for pan-keratin and CK7 (weakly for CK20), but negative for S100, smooth muscle actin, and desmin. Variable amounts of neuroendocrine differentiation may be seen.

**8. Correct choice: C.**

Jugulotympanic paraganglioma (JTP) is a locally invasive neoplasm that is specifically located in the middle ear or temporal bone region and is the most common tumor of the middle ear. The most common symptom is conductive hearing loss. The hallmark histologic feature is the presence of cell nests arranged in a "zellballen" pattern. The tumor cells are predominantly composed of chief cells, often round or oval cells with uniform nuclei; a dispersed chromatin pattern; and abundant eosinophilic, granular, or vacuolated cytoplasm. The immunohistochemical profile includes chromogranin, synaptophysin, GATA3 in the chief cells, and S100 protein and SOX10 staining localized to the peripheral sustentacular cells. Epithelial markers and mesenchymal markers are negative. Germline alterations can be identified in patients with a clinically apparent sporadic JTP, which is most commonly associated with mutations in the *SDHD* gene.

**9. Correct choice: E.**

Endolymphatic sac papillary tumor (ESPT) is an uncommon but distinct neoplasm, representing in the majority of cases a manifestation of von Hippel-Lindau (VHL) syndrome. Owing to its aggressive behavior, the current WHO Classification of Head and Neck Tumors recognized it as a low-grade epithelial malignancy. ESPT is characterized by a papillary growth pattern, and neoplastic cells vary in look from flattened- or attenuated-appearing cells to columnar-appearing cells with pale to clear cytoplasm. Cell borders may be seen, but, not infrequently, the neoplastic cells lack a distinct cell membrane. Endolymphatic sac tumors (ELSTs) are diffusely cytokeratin positive and also show variable reactivity for epithelial membrane antigen (EMA), S100 protein, vimentin, neuron-specific enolase (NSE), glial fibrillary acidic protein (GFAP), Ber-EP4, and synaptophysin. Differential diagnosis includes metastatic endometrioid adenocarcinoma (MEA), choroid plexus papilloma, and metastatic papillary carcinomas of the thyroid gland and kidney. Neurofibromatosis type 2 (central type) causes meningiomas and bilateral schwannomas. Subependymal giant cell astrocytoma is the central nervous system (CNS) tumor pathognomonic of tuberous sclerosis. Turcot syndrome and Li-Fraumeni syndrome are associated with glioblastoma and medulloblastoma.

# 24 Eye and Ocular Adnexa

1. The designation of phthisis bulbi refers to

   A. atrophic disorganized eye with ossification.
   B. chronically inflamed eye.
   C. glaucomatous eye.
   D. globe with heavy deposition of iron or copper.
   E. ruptured globe due to trauma.

2. A 25-year-old man undergoes penetrating keratoplasty (PKP) due to an advanced degenerative condition leading to thinning of the central corneal stroma. The corneal button submitted for pathologic evaluation reveals multiple breaks in the Bowman layer, as shown in Figure 1. Which of the following is the most likely diagnosis?

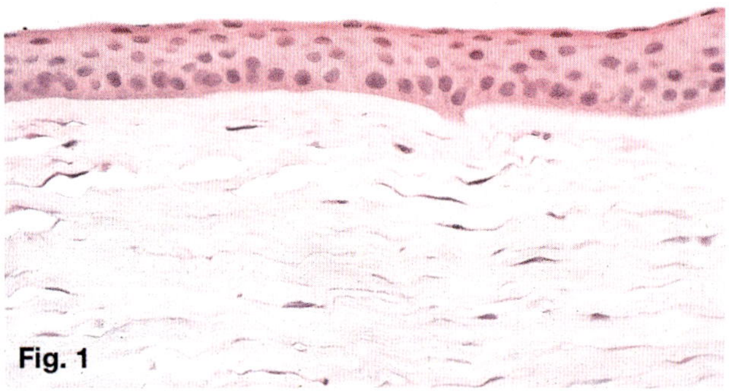

Fig. 1

   A. Bullous keratopathy
   B. Chronic actinic keratopathy
   C. Chronic herpes simplex keratitis
   D. Fuchs endothelial dystrophy
   E. Keratoconus

3. Which of the following is true regarding the type of corneal dystrophies most frequently observed in corneal specimens submitted to the pathologist in the United States?

   A. Accumulation of a keratan sulfate–related glycosaminoglycan
   B. Corneal deposits positive for transforming growth factor-β–induced protein
   C. Frequently associated with mutation in *CHST6* gene
   D. Irregular linear opacities resulting from stromal amyloid deposition
   E. Multiple wartlike excrescences on the Descemet membrane

4. A conjunctival biopsy is performed in a 50-year-old female with a history of chronic interstitial lung disease. The biopsy reveals nonnecrotizing granulomas, but stains and polymerase chain reaction (PCR) analysis for microorganisms are negative. Which of the following is the most probable cause?

   A. Cat scratch fever
   B. Rheumatoid arthritis
   C. Sarcoidosis
   D. *Treponema pallidum*
   E. Tularemia

5. Which of the following is the most common type of lymphoma affecting the conjunctiva and orbit?

   A. Burkitt lymphoma
   B. Diffuse large B-cell lymphoma
   C. Follicular lymphoma
   D. Hodgkin lymphoma
   E. Marginal zone B-cell lymphoma

6. A 50-year-old woman undergoes excision of a yellowish nodule of the upper eyelid. The specimen is submitted for histologic evaluation with a clinical diagnosis of chalazion. Figure 1 shows the microscopic appearance of the lesion. Which of the following is the correct diagnosis?

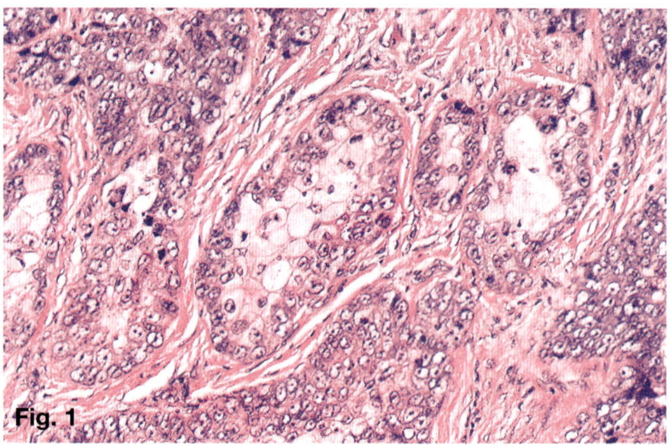

Fig. 1

   A. Basal cell carcinoma
   B. Chalazion
   C. Sebaceous cell carcinoma
   D. Squamous cell carcinoma
   E. Xanthelasma

All figures in this chapter are from Longacre TA, Greenson JK, Hornick JL, Reuter VE, eds. *Mills and Sternberg's Diagnostic Surgical Pathology.* 7th ed. Wolters Kluwer; 2022 except for those noted at the end of this book.

7. Which of the following features is most significant in the prognosis of the most common malignant tumor of the eye in childhood?

   A. Extent of necrosis
   B. Extent of optic nerve invasion
   C. Immunohistochemical features
   D. Mitotic activity
   E. Presence of calcification

8. Enucleation of the right eyeball is performed on a 42-year-old male. Gross examination reveals a mushroom-shaped mass arising from the choroid. Figure 1 shows the microscopic appearance of the lesion. The tumor cells are positive for S100 and SOX10. Which of the following is true regarding this neoplasm?

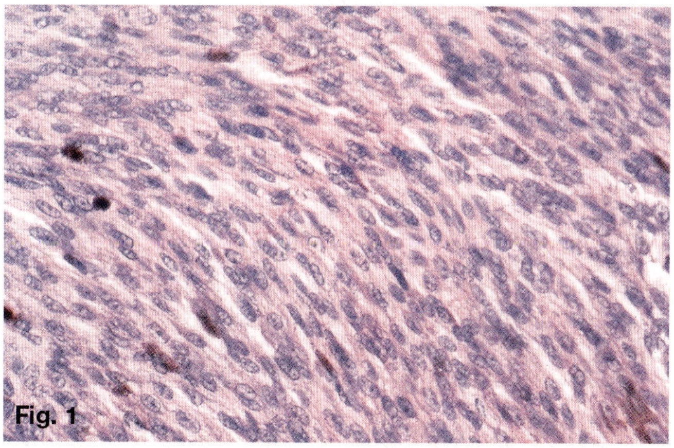

Fig. 1

   A. Best prognosis when arising from the ciliary body
   B. Frequent involvement of the optic nerve
   C. Mitotic figures are readily identifiable
   D. Monosomy 3 is associated with poor prognosis
   E. Uncommon primary intraocular malignant neoplasm in the United States

# ANSWERS AND EXPLANATIONS

**1. Correct choice: A.**

Phthisis bulbi may be defined as numerous pathologic processes that eventually culminate in an atrophic disorganized eye. Phthisical eyes usually manifest extensive scleral thickening and chronic retinal detachment, and the intraocular contents are markedly disorganized. Frequently present with intraocular ossification that usually contain marrow elements with adipose tissue.

**2. Correct choice: E.**

Keratoconus is a noninflammatory condition that leads to progressive thinning of the central cornea stroma, which bulges outward into a cone shape. The resulting astigmatism impairs visual acuity and prevents adequate refractive correction. The histopathologic features of keratoconus include thinning and fibrosis of the corneal stroma with breaks in the Bowman layer. In contrast, the endothelium is usually normal. Bullous keratopathy results from damage to the endothelium by a number of causes, leading to stromal edema and the formation of subepithelial bullae. Chronic actinic keratopathy is the accumulation of protein globules in the superficial stroma of the cornea and results from chronic exposure to ultraviolet light. Herpes simplex type 1 is the most common cause of chronic keratitis. Histologically, the cornea shows epithelium of irregular thickness, disrupted Bowman layer, pannus formation (collagenous tissue between epithelium and Bowman layer), and chronic inflammation of the stroma.

**3. Correct choice: A.**

Corneal dystrophies (CDs) are a group of hereditary bilateral corneal disorders. CDs can be divided into three groups: anterior CD, involving the epithelium, Bowman layer, and superficial corneal stroma; stromal CD, involving the corneal stroma; and posterior CD, involving the Descemet membrane and endothelium. Fuchs endothelial dystrophy is the most commonly submitted corneal specimen for pathologic examination. Fuchs endothelial dystrophy is characterized by wartlike excrescences (guttae) of the Descemet membrane associated with loss of endothelial lining. It is associated with *COL8A2* alterations. Granular dystrophy is characterized by subepithelial stromal deposits of an abnormal protein derived from mutation of the *TGFBI* gene. The corneal deposits appear bright red on Masson trichrome and are immunoreactive for transforming growth factor-β (TGF-β)–induced protein. Macular dystrophy is caused by a mutation in the *CHST6* gene and is characterized by the accumulation of keratan sulfate–related glycosaminoglycans within the stroma and endothelium. CDs with amyloid deposition are characterized by irregular linear opacities resulting from stromal amyloid deposition. The amyloid in this dystrophy reacts with antibodies to the TGF-β–induced protein.

**4. Correct choice: C.**

The eyes are involved in up to 38% of patients with sarcoidosis. The conjunctiva and uvea are the most frequently involved sites, and thus, a conjunctival biopsy is often used to confirm a diagnosis. Granulomatous inflammation is not associated with necrosis. Fungal and mycobacterial infections are ruled out by special stains. Tularemia and cat scratch fever are associated with necrosis.

**5. Correct choice: E.**

Lymphoma in the conjunctiva presents as salmon-colored masses. Since the lymphoid tissue in the conjunctiva and probably the whole orbit is of mucosa-associated lymphoid tissue (MALT) type, most lymphomas arising in this region are marginal zone B-cell lymphomas. They consist of well-differentiated small lymphocytes and remain localized for a long time. Follicular lymphoma, diffuse large B-cell lymphoma, and mantle cell lymphoma may be seen in the conjunctiva and orbit. Hodgkin disease rarely involves the orbit. Burkitt lymphoma of the orbit is common in Africa but not in the United States.

**6. Correct choice: C.**

Sebaceous carcinoma represents 1% to 3% of eyelid malignancies, but this potentially lethal neoplasm is often misdiagnosed by both clinicians and pathologists. The tumor most often originates in the upper eyelid and is clinically indistinguishable from chalazion or blepharoconjunctivitis. Histologically, it may have a lobular, comedocarcinoma, or papillary pattern. Tumor cells with obvious sebaceous differentiation (abundant foamy cytoplasm and well-defined cell borders) are found in the center of lobules. Poorly differentiated sebaceous carcinoma may be difficult to distinguish from squamous cell carcinoma or basal cell carcinoma, so immunohistochemical analysis may be necessary. More than 90% of sebaceous neoplasms are immunoreactive for adipophilin, a newly identified marker of sebaceous differentiation. Recurrence after excision is observed in one-third of cases, while 20% of patients die of metastases.

**7. Correct choice: B.**

Retinoblastoma (RB) is the most common malignant tumor of the eye in childhood, caused by biallelic inactive of the *RB1* gene. Histologically, the appearance of RB varies with the degree of differentiation. Small, undifferentiated cells with scant cytoplasm and hyperchromatic nuclei make up the bulk of many RBs. Flexner-Wintersteiner rosettes consist of neoplastic cells arranged around a central lumen and represent important diagnostic features. Retinoblastomas have a tendency to spread along the optic nerves, and the extent of optic nerve invasion should be carefully recorded because it is directly related to prognosis. Necrosis and calcification are common in retinoblastomas but do not have prognostic significance. Other histologic features of prognostic significance include tumor size, seeding of vitreous, degree of differentiation, involvement of anterior segment, growth pattern, and involvement of the sclera.

**8. Correct choice: D.**

Uveal melanoma (UM) is the most frequent of adult intraocular tumors and develops from melanocytes of the uveal tract (iris, ciliary body, and choroid). Histologically, UMs can be divided into spindle cell, epithelioid cell, or mixed types. The spindle cell type grows in a cohesive manner, and mitotic activity is rarely, if ever, seen, while prominent in the epithelioid cell type. In contrast to retinoblastoma, UM rarely extends into the optic nerve and spreads through scleral emissaria canals. The prognosis of UM is related to several factors. Histopathologic prognosis factors include tumor size, tumor site (ciliary body UM has a worse prognosis than choroidal UM; iris UM usually has the best prognosis among them), extrascleral extension, cell type, mitotic activity, and lymphocytic infiltration. Genetic analyses have shown that in UM, loss of a copy of chromosome 3 (monosomy 3) is the most prognostically significant chromosomal marker. These tumors have a high metastatic rate, and mortality is also high.

# 25 Nonneoplastic Pulmonary Disease

1. A 65-year-old man presents with slowly progressive respiratory insufficiency. Chest x-rays show a diffuse infiltrative process most prominent at the lung base. An open lung biopsy shows extensive fibrosis of the interalveolar septa, dilatation of alveolar ducts, and chronic inflammatory infiltration of the septa. Histopathologic changes are patchy, with areas of new and advanced fibrosis with scattered foci of immature fibrosis. These findings are most consistent with

   A. desquamative interstitial pneumonia.
   B. giant-cell interstitial pneumonia.
   C. lymphocytic interstitial pneumonia.
   D. nonspecific interstitial pneumonia.
   E. usual interstitial pneumonia.

2. A 38-year-old woman with a history of heavy smoking presents with slowly progressive respiratory insufficiency. Chest x-rays show a bilateral ground-glass interstitial infiltrate involving the lung base. An open lung biopsy reveals the following histopathologic changes: alveolar spaces filled with histiocytes, hyperplasia of alveolar type II cells, and a mixed lymphocytic, plasma cell, and neutrophilic interstitial infiltrate. These changes are relatively homogeneous. The most likely diagnosis is

   A. centriacinar emphysema with chronic bronchitis.
   B. desquamative interstitial pneumonia.
   C. nonspecific interstitial pneumonia.
   D. respiratory bronchiolitis.
   E. usual interstitial pneumonia.

3. Hypersensitivity pneumonitis is a reaction to long-term exposure to various antigens of animal or plant origin. The inflammatory infiltrate present in the lung is predominantly composed of

   A. cytotoxic T lymphocytes and plasma cells.
   B. eosinophils and neutrophils.
   C. helper T lymphocytes and plasma cells.
   D. histiocytes and multinucleated giant cells.
   E. plasma cells and histiocytes.

4. A 23-year-old female with a heavy smoking history presents with progressive shortness of breath. Chest computed tomography (CT) scan shows multiple small centrilobular nodules. The lesional cells are characterized by distinctive, longitudinal nuclei with coffee-bean grooves and an undulating or indented nuclear membrane, and have pentalaminar, rod-shaped intracytoplasmic inclusion bodies on electron microscopy. Which of the following immunohistochemical stains, if positive, would be most diagnostic of this entity?

   A. CD1a and S100
   B. CD163 and CD1a
   C. CD68 and CD21
   D. Cyclin D1 and CD68
   E. S100 and CD163

All figures in this chapter are from Longacre TA, Greenson JK, Hornick JL, Reuter VE, eds. *Mills and Sternberg's Diagnostic Surgical Pathology*. 7th ed. Wolters Kluwer; 2022 except for those noted at the end of this book.

5. A 38-year-old female office worker presents with computed tomography (CT) findings of mediastinal and hilar opacities as well as micronodularity of perilymphatic and bronchocentric distribution. Figure 1 shows microscopic findings from a lung wedge biopsy with nonnecrotizing granulomas. What is the most likely diagnosis and which stains should be performed on the biopsy before sign out?

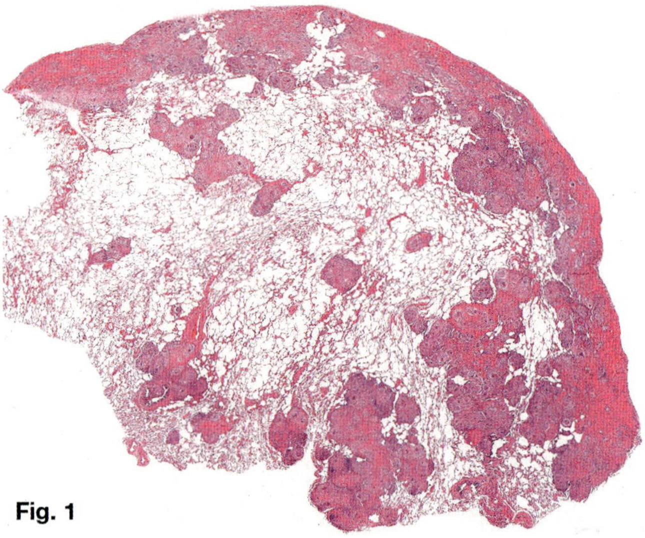

Fig. 1

A. Asbestosis; stains: Trichrome, Prussian blue
B. Berylliosis; stains: acid-fast bacilli (AFB), Gomori methenamine silver (GMS)
C. Hypersensitivity pneumonitis; stains: CD4 and CD8
D. Infectious process; stains: AFB and GMS
E. Sarcoidosis; stains: AFB, GMS

6. Which of the following histopathologic findings is considered the most characteristic of organizing pneumonia?

A. Hyaline membranes
B. Interstitial fibrosis
C. Intra-alveolar fibroblastic plugs
D. Macrophages within alveolar spaces
E. Peribronchial granulomas

7. A lymphoma originating from BALT (bronchial-associated lymphoid tissue) is usually

A. an aggressive high-grade lymphoma.
B. associated with lymphatic tracking.
C. composed of T lymphocytes, similar to lymphocytic interstitial pneumonia (LIP).
D. not associated with lymphoepithelial lesions.
E. seen in young patients.

8. The entity known as lymphomatoid granulomatosis is a/an

A. infectious condition due to mycobacteria.
B. leukemic infiltration.
C. malignant lymphoid proliferation.
D. process akin to mycobacterial pseudotumor.
E. reactive lymphoid process.

9. Figures 1 and 2 are characteristic findings in which of the following conditions?

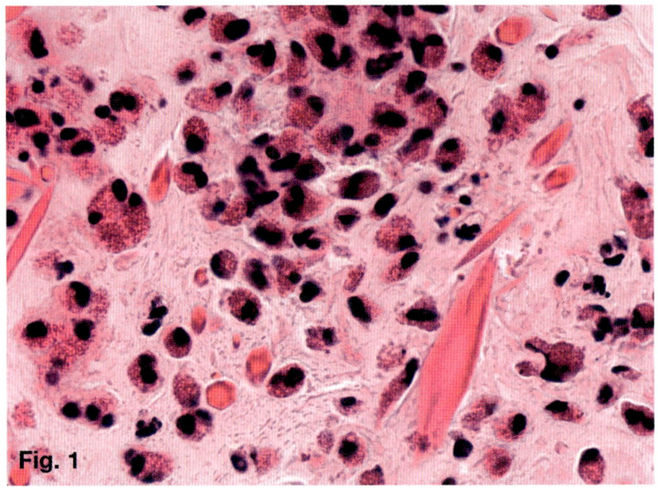

Fig. 1

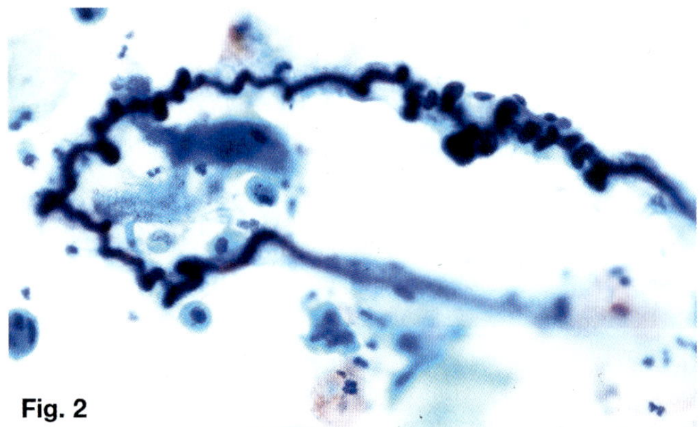

Fig. 2

A. Aspiration pneumonia
B. Asthma
C. Bronchiectasis
D. Bronchiolitis
E. Parasitic infection

10. Which of the following pulmonary conditions is due to the accumulation of surfactant apoprotein within alveoli?

A. Alveolar proteinosis
B. Amyloidosis
C. Goodpasture syndrome
D. Idiopathic hemosiderosis
E. Pulmonary alveolar microlithiasis

11. A 45-year-old patient with a lung nodule and glomerulonephritis undergoes a lung wedge resection. Figure 1 shows the findings from the lung wedge resection. The patient is c-ANCA (cytoplasmic antineutrophil cytoplasmic antibodies) positive. Which of the following is the most likely diagnosis?

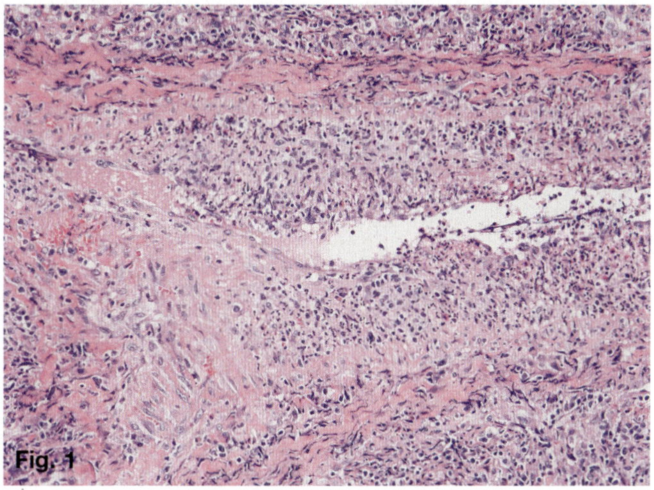


A. Eosinophilic granulomatosis with polyangiitis
B. Granulomatosis with polyangiitis
C. Infectious etiology
D. Lymphomatoid granulomatosis
E. Microscopic polyangiitis

12. Which of the following is true regarding pulmonary hypertensive vasculopathy?

A. Limited to changes in small pulmonary artery and veins
B. Mean pulmonary arterial pressure equal to or greater than 20 mm Hg at rest
C. No known associated genetic abnormalities
D. Pathologic evaluation required for diagnosis
E. Pulmonary arteriopathy has the worst prognosis and requires lung transplantation

13. Which of the following is the characteristic finding in pulmonary immunoglobulin G subclass 4 (IgG4)-related disease?

A. Dense lymphoplasmacytic infiltrate, fibrosis, and obliterative phlebitis
B. Electron microscopy demonstrates coarsely granular electron-dense deposits
C. Patchy deposition of amorphous eosinophilic material that is negative on Congo red stain
D. Plasma cells usually present and reveal light-chain restriction
E. Xanthogranulomatous lesions characterized by clonal foamy CD68($^{+}$)/CD1a($^{-}$) histiocytes

14. The lesion in Figure 1 is most likely

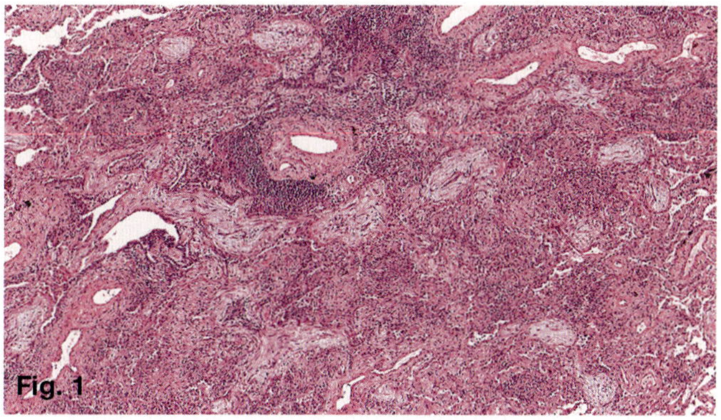


A. cryptogenic organizing pneumonia (COP).
B. desquamative interstitial pneumonia (DIP).
C. diffuse alveolar damage (DAD).
D. respiratory bronchiolitis (RB).
E. usual interstitial pneumonitis (UIP).

15. The lesion in Figure 1 is most likely

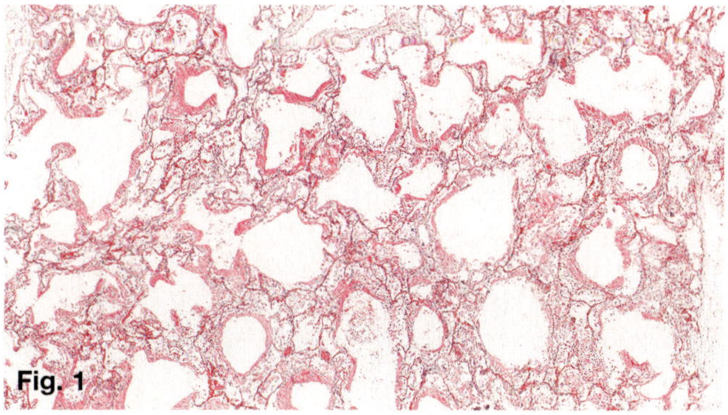


A. bronchocentric granulomatosis.
B. bronchopneumonia.
C. desquamative interstitial pneumonitis.
D. diffuse alveolar damage.
E. extrinsic allergic alveolitis.

16. The lesion in Figure 1 is most likely

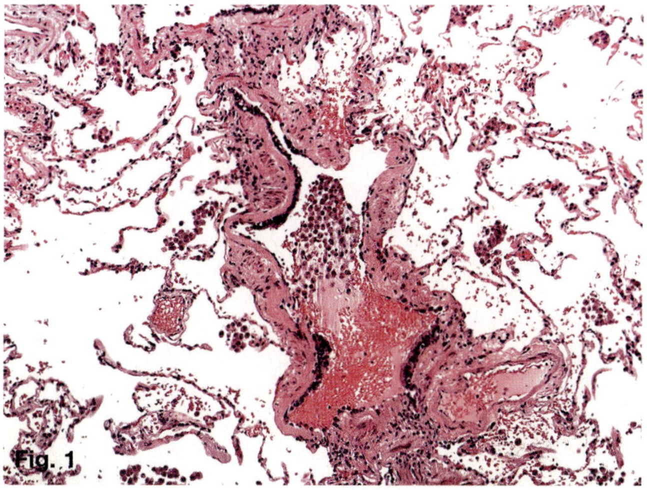


A. bronchiocentric granulomatosis.
B. desquamative interstitial pneumonia.
C. immunoglobulin G subclass 4 (IgG4)-related disease.
D. lymphangioleiomyomatosis.
E. respiratory bronchiolitis.

17. The lesion in Figure 1 is most likely

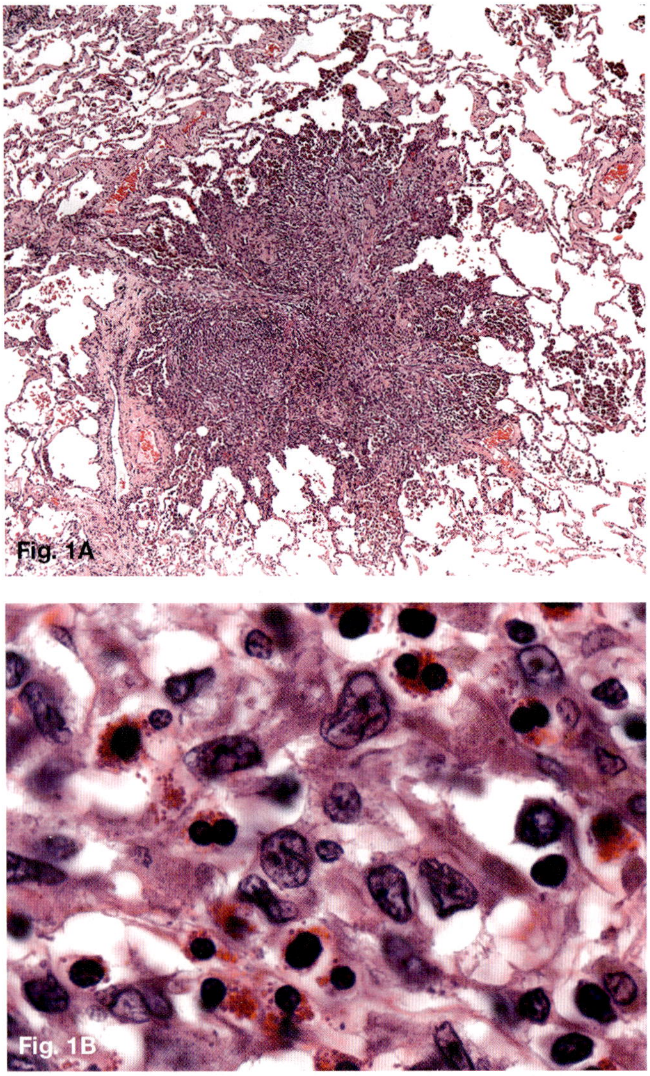


A. giant-cell pneumonia.
B. immunoglobulin G subclass 4 (IgG4)-related disease.
C. nonspecific interstitial pneumonia.
D. pulmonary Langerhans histiocytosis.
E. usual interstitial pneumonia.

18. The lesion in Figure 1 is most likely

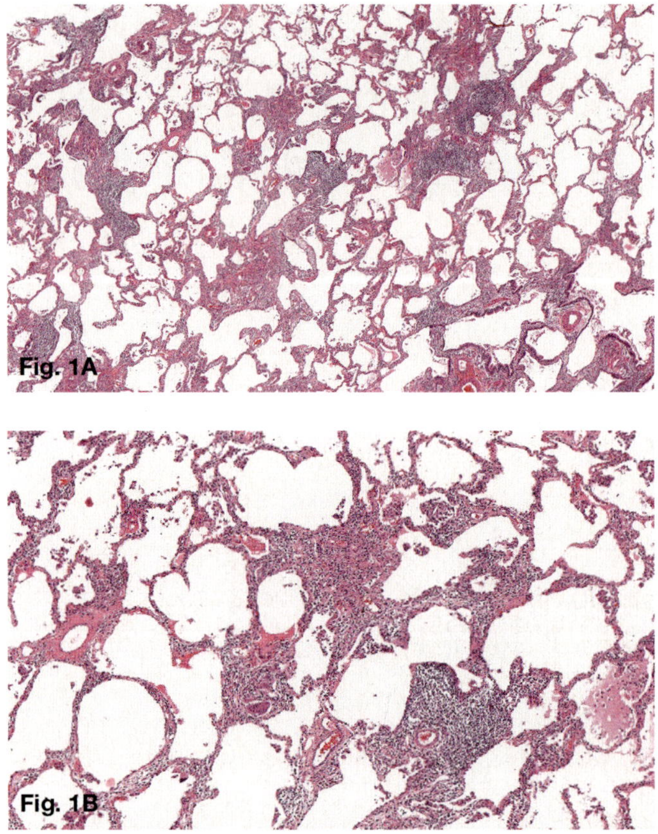


A. bronchocentric granulomatosis.
B. cryptogenic organizing pneumonia.
C. hypersensitivity pneumonitis.
D. immunoglobulin G subclass 4 (IgG4)-related disease.
E. nonspecific interstitial pneumonitis.

19. The illustrated lesion, shown in Figure 1, is most likely

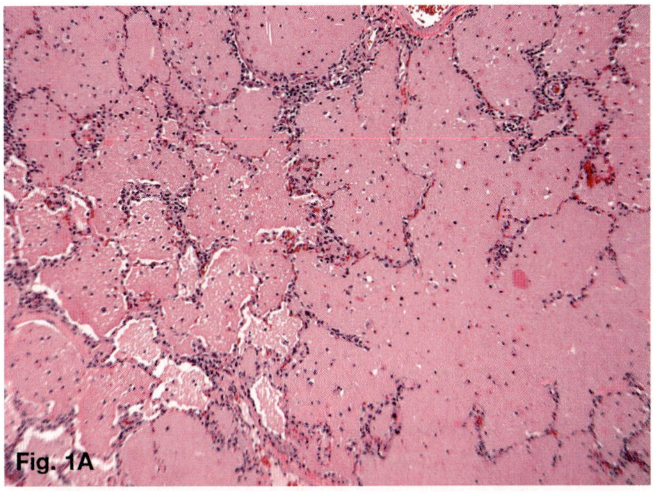
Fig. 1A

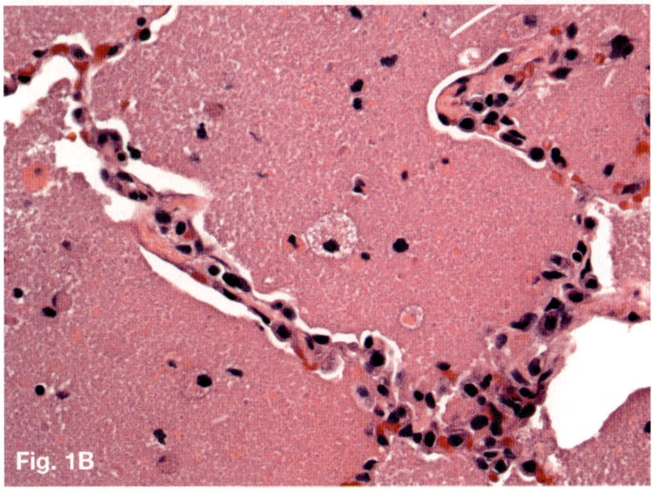
Fig. 1B

A. diffuse alveolar damage.
B. eosinophilic pneumonia.
C. exogenous lipid pneumonia.
D. pulmonary alveolar proteinosis.
E. pulmonary edema.

20. The illustrated lesion, shown in Figure 1, is most likely

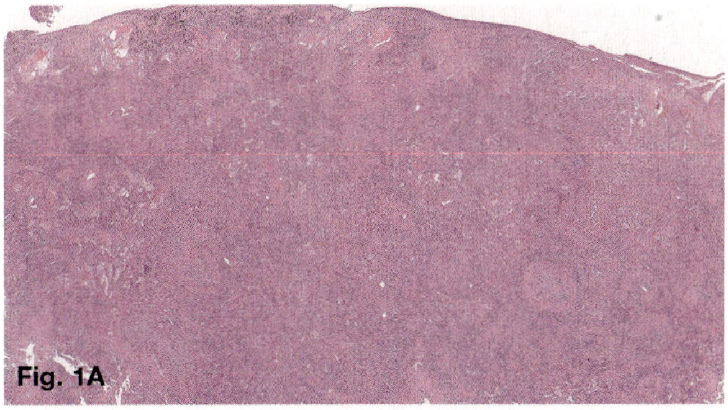
Fig. 1A

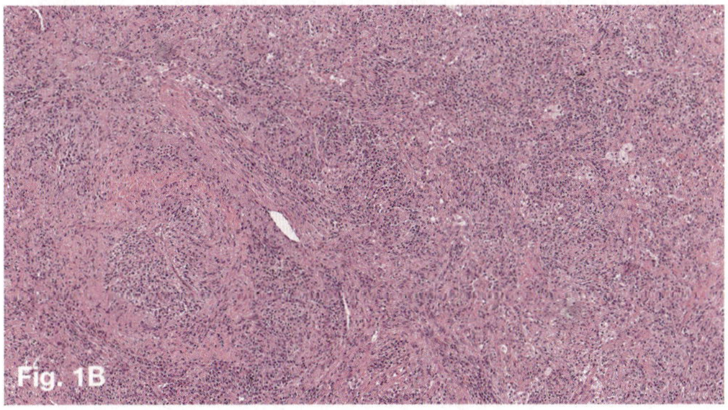
Fig. 1B

A. cryptogenic organizing pneumonia.
B. immunoglobulin G subclass 4 (IgG4)-related lung disease.
C. lymphoid interstitial pneumonia.
D. pulmonary Langerhans histiocytosis.
E. usual interstitial pneumonia.

21. The illustrated lesion, shown in Figure 1, is most likely

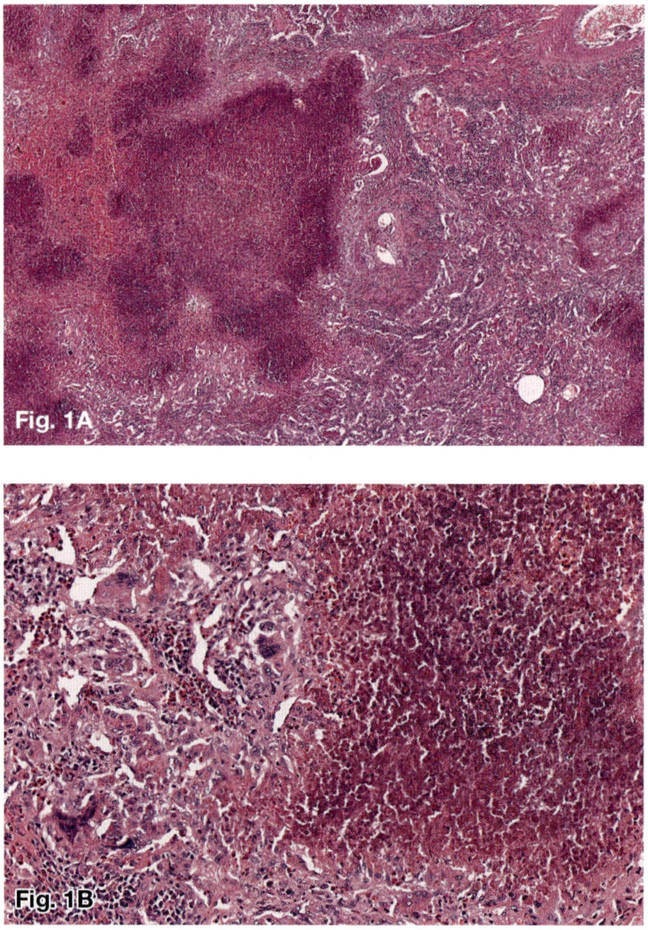


A. eosinophilic granulomatosis with polyangiitis.
B. granulomatosis with polyangiitis.
C. lymphomatoid granulomatosis.
D. periarteritis nodosa.
E. tuberculosis.

22. The illustrated lesion, shown in Figure 1, is most likely

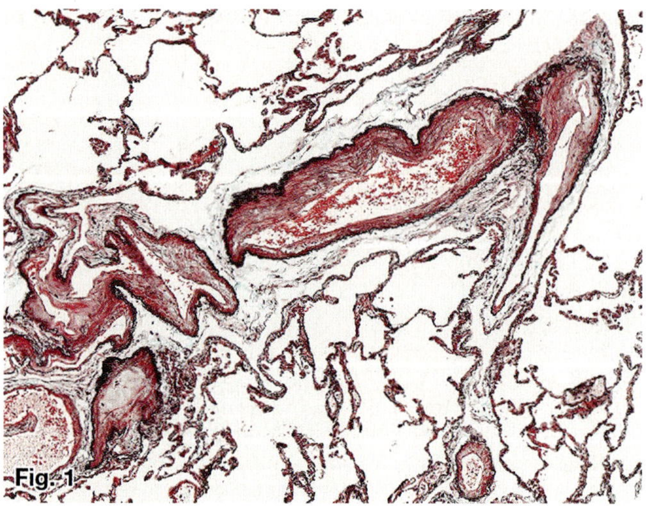


A. granulomatous pulmonary arteritis.
B. plexogenic arteriopathy.
C. pulmonary hypertension.
D. usual interstitial pneumonia.
E. venoocclusive disease.

23. Which of the following is the characteristic finding in measles pneumonia?

A. Basophilic inclusion that completely replaces the nuclei
B. Diffuse alveolar damage with well-formed hyaline membranes
C. Eosinophilic intranuclear inclusion and clear halo
D. Intranuclear and basophilic intracytoplasmic inclusions
E. Multinucleated giant cells with more than 20 nuclei per cell

24. What is the causative agent of the finding in Figure 1?

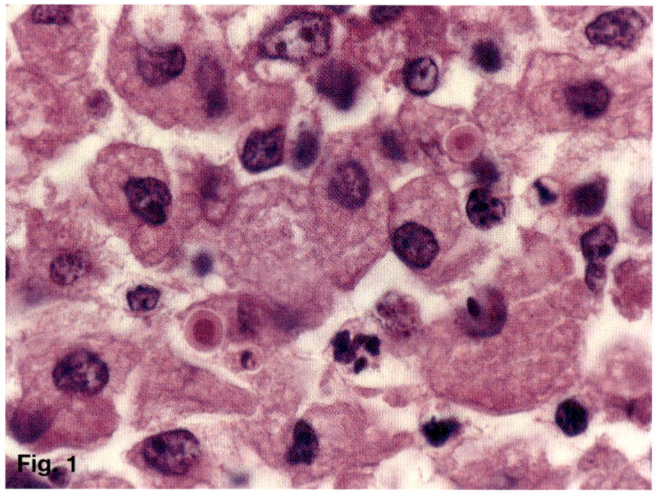


A. *Blastomyces dermatitidis*
B. *Escherichia coli*
C. *Histoplasma capsulatum*
D. *Legionella pneumophila*
E. *Rhodococcus equi*

# ANSWERS AND EXPLANATIONS

**1. Correct choice: E.**

Usual interstitial pneumonia (UIP) is commonly associated with the clinical term idiopathic pulmonary fibrosis. Patients with UIP usually present in the fifth to seventh decade of life; it is twice as common in men as in women. There may be an association with autoimmune diseases such as rheumatoid arthritis or scleroderma, but most cases are idiopathic. UIP shows interstitial fibrosis with an uneven distribution of recent and old fibrotic changes, leading to honeycombing in the late stage. This pattern is also referred to as temporal heterogeneity. Dense collagen deposition in these areas is accompanied by scattered foci of immature fibrosis, otherwise known as fibroblastic foci, which are composed of loose myxoid stroma with spindle cells that align in a roughly parallel manner underneath regenerating surface pneumocytes. The prognosis of UIP is poor, with a median survival of 3 to 5 years.

**2. Correct choice: B.**

Desquamative interstitial pneumonia (DIP) type of smoking-related interstitial pneumonia characterized by a marked accumulation of alveolar macrophages with pronounced inflammatory features. DIP usually affects male smokers in the fourth to fifth decade of life. The histopathologic hallmark is an intra-alveolar accumulation of pigmented macrophages, with hyperplasia of type II pneumocytes. Alveolar septa are thickened by mild fibrosis and chronic inflammation with plasma cells, eosinophils, and scattered lymphoid follicles. DIP may progress to end-stage (honeycomb) lung but usually responds to steroid treatment, hence the importance of differentiating DIP in lung biopsies from other forms of interstitial lung disease. Respiratory bronchiolitis may mimic DIP, affects smokers preferentially, but is associated with a predominantly peribronchiolar pattern of inflammatory changes.

**3. Correct choice: A.**

Hypersensitivity pneumonitis (HP) fibrosing lung disease, representing 15% of all interstitial lung diseases, is caused by repeated inhalation exposure to occupational, recreational, or domestic environmental antigens. Histologic changes are composed of a triad of (a) cellular bronchiolitis, (b) cellular interstitial pneumonia centered around the airways, and (c) small, poorly formed nonnecrotizing granulomas and/or single multinucleated histiocytic giant cells. The inflammatory process has a bronchiolocentric distribution and is composed predominantly of small lymphocytes.

Cytotoxic T cells and plasma cells are the predominant inflammatory elements, but scattered histiocytes and multinucleated giant cells are present. Eosinophils and neutrophils are infrequent, whereas granulomas may be found in terminal airways.

**4. Correct choice: A.**

Langerhans cell histiocytosis (LCH) is a relatively rare interstitial lung disease and usually affects adults, aged 20 to 40 years, with a strong association with cigarette smoking. Chest imaging usually shows diffuse bilateral upper and middle lung interstitial or reticulonodular infiltrates that are more pronounced in the peripheral lung fields. Microscopically, LCH is characterized by bronchiocentric stellate fibrotic nodules that extend into the surrounding interstitium. Langerhans cells have distinctive longitudinal nuclei with a coffee-bean shape and longitudinal grooves with an undulating or indented nuclear membrane. Eosinophils are present in the surrounding cellular infiltrate. Electron microscopy shows a pentalaminar, rod-shaped intracytoplasmic inclusion body in the Langerhans cell called a "Birbeck granule." Immunohistochemically, the nucleus and cytoplasm stain positively with antibodies to CD1a, S100 protein, Langerin, and cyclin-D1, and are negative for CD168 and CD21. There is variable CD68 expression. Background alveolar macrophages are negative for S100 and CD1a. Although positive expression for cyclin D1 and CD68 can be seen in LCH, it is not diagnostic as this combination is also found in extranodal Rosai-Dorfman disease. In about 50% of cases, there are *BRAF* V600E gene mutations.

**5. Correct choice: E.**

The image shows well-formed, nonnecrotizing granulomas in the subpleural and interlobular septa, and around the bronchovascular areas in the wedge biopsy. These findings are characteristic of sarcoidosis, which is a diagnosis of exclusion and which requires special stains and cultures for infectious agents in all cases. The granulomas of sarcoidosis are composed of epithelioid histiocytes and multinucleated giant cells that sometimes contain nonspecific birefringent crystalline, asteroid, or Schaumann bodies. The CD4/CD8 T-cell ratio is usually greater than 3-5:1 and can be a useful diagnostic test in active sarcoidosis. Infectious processes present with necrotizing granulomas. Hypersensitivity pneumonitis presents with ill-formed granulomas and is associated with interstitial chronic inflammation/pneumonitis. Berylliosis is histologically indistinguishable from sarcoidosis, requiring a history of occupational exposure. Asbestos causes interstitial fibrosis that starts from bronchiolar walls. Multinucleated giant cells can be seen but not granulomas.

**6. Correct choice: C.**

Organizing pneumonia (OP) is considered a clinicopathologic airspace-predominant disease of acute and organizing lung injury and is associated with a number of conditions, including infections, drugs, connective tissue diseases, and inhalation injury. The idiopathic variant is called cryptogenic organizing pneumonia (COP), which is a diagnosis of exclusion. Clinical presentation may be acute (dyspnea, cough, fever) or insidious. Histologically, the main feature is the formation of fibrous plugs (Masson plugs) filling alveolar spaces. Other features include interstitial inflammatory infiltration and endoluminal macrophages leading to consolidation of pulmonary parenchyma. Masson plugs have a characteristic serpiginous shape.

**7. Correct choice: B.**

Bronchial-associated lymphoid tissue (BALT) lymphoma is a low-grade lymphoma that is usually discovered in asymptomatic middle-aged or older patients. It is sometimes difficult to differentiate a pulmonary lymphoma from benign lymphoid infiltrates such as lymphocytic interstitial pneumonia (LIP) or pulmonary pseudolymphoma (PL), and pulmonary lymphoma probably arises from progressive degrees of BALT hyperplasia. Features favoring BALT lymphoma include sheets or confluent nodules of uniform small lymphocytes, B-cell composition (in contrast to LIP), characteristic lymphoepithelial lesions (similar to mucosa-associated lymphoid tissue [MALT] lymphoma of the gastrointestinal [GI] tract), and spread along lymphatics and blood vessels. The latter feature is referred to as lymphatic tracking. The prognosis is excellent.

**8. Correct choice: C.**

Lymphomatoid granulomatosis is a lymphoproliferative disorder characterized by an angiocentric/angiodestructive proliferation of a polymorphic cell population. It can be thought of as a T-cell–rich B-cell lymphoma. Infiltrates consist of mixtures of atypical lymphocytes, histiocytes, and plasma cells, but B lymphocytes are the true neoplastic element. T lymphocytes and other inflammatory cells are reactive. The angioinvasive nature of this process leads to large areas of coagulation necrosis. Lymphomatoid granulomatosis eventually evolves into aggressive lymphoma with a poor prognosis. The Epstein-Barr virus (EBV) genome has been found in up to 70% of cases. Lungs, skin, and the central nervous system are the most commonly involved sites.

**9. Correct choice: B.**

Asthma is a very common lung disease, with a clinical course characterized by acute, episodic paroxysmal, and usually reversible airway narrowing. The lungs are overexpanded with alternating areas of atelectasis, bronchiectasis, and mucus plugs. Bronchial and bronchiolar lumens contain mucin mixed with sloughed bronchial epithelium (creola bodies), inflammatory cells, and elongated bipyramidal needle-shaped (Charcot-Leyden) crystals (Figure 1). Eosinophils are scattered throughout the mucin, and small airways may contain mucous casts known as Curschmann spirals (Figure 2). Airway walls, especially the subepithelial compartment, are expanded by eosinophils, plasma cells, lymphocytes (particularly $CD8^+$ T cells), mast cells, occasional neutrophils, and dilated blood vessels.

**10. Correct choice: A.**

Pulmonary alveolar proteinosis (PAP) is defined by the abnormal accumulation of surfactant in the alveoli due to macrophage dysfunction that results in hypoxemia and, eventually, respiratory failure. Microscopically, alveoli are filled with homogeneous, eosinophilic, periodic acid-Schiff (PAS)-positive, granular material with cholesterol clefts as well as degenerated macrophages while alveolar septa remain unremarkable. PAP is classified into primary and secondary diseases based on the etiology of the macrophage dysfunction:

- Primary PAP: Disruption of signaling by granulocyte-macrophage colony-stimulating factor (GM-CSF) in lung alveolar macrophages. This category can be divided into autoimmune and hereditary PAP. Autoimmune PAP accounts for 90% of primary PAP cases and is due to circulating, neutralizing antibodies against GM-CSF that decrease or block GM-CSF signaling in the alveolar macrophages.
- Secondary PAP: Result of environmental exposure or pharmaceutical agents that reduce the number or function of alveolar macrophages. Environmental factors implicated include cigarette smoke, welding fumes, organic and inorganic dusts, aluminum, cellulose fibers, and titanium dioxide.

**11. Correct choice: B.**

Granulomatosis with polyangiitis (GPA) is characterized by a clinical and pathologic triad of necrotizing granulomatous inflammation, angiitis, and necrotizing glomerulonephritis. Upper and lower respiratory tracts and the kidney are most commonly affected, but it can also target peripheral nerves and the central nervous system, orbit, skin, ear, breast, and other sites. Lung involvement is documented in 65% to 85% of patients, and necrotizing glomerulonephritis affects as many as 80% of patients over the course of the disease. Ninety percent of patients with active GPA are ANCA (antineutrophil cytoplasmic antibodies) positive. Microscopically, GPA usually first manifests as lung parenchyma necrosis with granulomatous microabscesses. As the disease progresses, the necrotic zones expand and coalesce to form areas of geographic necrosis. Vasculitis in GPA is considered the defining feature, which presents as edema of the vessel wall and transmural infiltration by neutrophils, eosinophils, and plasma cells (as seen in the image).

**12. Correct choice: B.**

Pulmonary hypertensive vasculopathy is defined as sustained mean pulmonary arterial pressure equal to or greater than 20 mm Hg at rest, as measured by right heart catheterization. Mutations in *PAH, BMPR2,* and *EIF2AK4* genes have been identified in multiple forms of pulmonary hypertensive vasculopathies with the associated familial presentation. There are major categories based on the pathologic patterns present:

- Pulmonary arteriopathy (PA): Characterized by medial hypertrophy, concentric intimal thickening, eccentric, nonlaminar thickening, plexiform, and/or dilatation lesions and arteritis. Therapies are mainly composed of vasodilator drugs, anticoagulants, and supportive measures.
- Pulmonary veno-occlusive disease (PVOD): Changes in predominantly postcapillary pulmonary vasculature, such as venous intimal fibrosis and medial hypertrophy, venous intraluminal recanalization, interlobular septal thickening, and capillary congestion. Lung transplantation remains the treatment of choice.
- Pulmonary capillary hemangiomatosis (PCH): Characterized patchy distribution of orange-tan nodules throughout the lung, composed of atypical proliferations of capillaries. Lung transplantation remains the treatment of choice.

Tissue is not commonly needed for a diagnosis and is usually obtained to rule out other possible pathologies.

**13. Correct choice: A.**

Immunoglobulin G subclass 4 (IgG4)-related disease is a fibroinflammatory condition with diverse organ manifestations linked by similar histologic findings. In general, diagnosis requires an appropriate histologic appearance along with increased numbers of $IgG4^+$ plasma cells, an elevated $IgG4^+/IgG^+$ cell ratio in the tissue sample, and elevation of serum IgG4. The three major histopathologic features of the lung are (a) dense lymphoplasmacytic infiltrate; (b) fibrosis, at least focally in a storiform pattern; and (c) obliterative phlebitis. Lung lesions manifest as a nodule or mass with lymphangitic extension, interstitial disease, or a bronchocentric distribution. Options B and C characterize light-chain deposition disease. Option E characterizes Erdheim-Chester disease (ECD).

**14. Correct choice: A.**

Cryptogenic organizing pneumonia (COP) is characterized by fibromyxoid plugs filling the air spaces (see the answer for question 6 for additional information). Usual interstitial pneumonitis (UIP) is also characterized by acute and chronic scarring, but the scarring process is in different phases and is also characterized by the presence of fibroblastic foci. Desquamative interstitial pneumonia (DIP) is characterized by the presence of clumps of alveolar macrophages, which are generally without scarring of the interstitium, although in later changes, they may be associated with some scarring. Diffuse alveolar damage is characterized by an exudative process in the presence of inflammatory cells, which include lymphocytes as well as some neutrophils. The pathognomonic feature is the presence of hyaline fibrinous membranes surrounding the alveolar spaces and applied to the alveolar surfaces. Respiratory bronchiolitis is characterized by filling of the alveolar spaces with alveolar macrophages containing brown and black pigment and peribronchiolar chronic inflammation. The interstitium may become scarred, at which time the lesion is considered respiratory bronchiolitis with interstitial lung disease.

**15. Correct choice: D.**

Diffuse alveolar damage (DAD) is an exudative process with inflammatory cells and the characteristic hyaline membrane identifies the lesion as alveolar damage. The diffuseness of the process has to be confirmed from the biopsy or from its radiographic appearance. As noted earlier, DAD may clear entirely or it may result in interstitial fibrosis. Bronchiocentric granulomatosis is also bronchiocentric or bronchiolocentric, but it is characterized by extensive well-formed granulomas, which efface the bronchi, but generally spare the adjacent arteries. Bronchopneumonia is characterized by an exudative process, but the air spaces are filled with inflammatory cells, and a hyaline membrane is not present. The hyaline membrane of DAD can be thought of as the result of capillary damage with leakage of fibrin, which elicits the intense inflammatory response. Desquamative interstitial pneumonitis is characterized by the filling of the alveolar spaces with clumps of alveolar macrophages usually with little to no damage to the interstitium and without the presence of lymphocytes or neutrophils. The macrophages may assume an epithelioid appearance. Extrinsic allergic alveolitis is a bronchiolocentric lesion, which is characterized by the presence of poorly formed granulomas and alveolar inflammation, which is sometimes granulomatous but more often chronic inflammatory.

**16. Correct choice: E.**

The image shows the presence of peribronchiolar inflammation and alveolar macrophages containing brown pigment scattered throughout the air spaces, which is consistent with respiratory bronchiolitis. Interstitial fibrosis may or may not accompany this lesion. Bronchocentric granulomatosis is characterized by the presence of extensive granulomas, which are well formed and affect the peribronchiolar or peribronchial area and efface the bronchus, but spare the arteries. Desquamative interstitial pneumonitis is characterized by the filling of air spaces with macrophages. Immunoglobulin G subclass 4 (IgG4)-related disease is characterized by compression of the airspaces, which are filled with foamy macrophages. It is associated with scarring and a lymphoplasmacytic infiltrate in the interstitium. Lymphangioleiomyomatosis is characterized by bronchiolar cysts surrounded by smooth muscle and containing hemosiderin-laden macrophages. The smooth muscles surrounding these dilated bronchial-based spaces stain positively for HMB45.

**17. Correct choice: D.**

The stellate interstitial lesion is the result of fibrosis associated with the presence of Langerhans cells, which are characterized by large and grooved nuclei. Eosinophils are often present but are not required for the diagnosis of pulmonary Langerhans histiocytosis or eosinophilic granuloma. In later stages, there may be a paucity or even absence of the atypical histiocytes, which are replaced by fibrosis. However, a stellate bronchiolocentric interstitial scar is suggestive of the presence of "burned-out" pulmonary Langerhans histiocytosis. Giant-cell pneumonia is characterized by the presence of an intense interstitial pulmonary fibrosis with inflammation and the presence of multinucleated giant cells. Immunoglobulin G subclass 4 (IgG4)-related disease is characterized by compressed airspaces filled with foamy macrophages, interstitial fibrosis, and a lymphoplasmacytic infiltration staining for IgG4. Nonspecific interstitial pulmonary fibrosis is similar in many ways to usual interstitial pneumonia, but it lacks the variation in the stage of the inflammatory process and fibrosis, and it also lacks the fibroblastic foci. Usual interstitial pneumonia is characterized by the presence of interstitial fibrosis of varying ages and areas of interstitial inflammation with fibroblastic foci.

**18. Correct choice: C.**

Extrinsic allergic alveolitis is bronchiolocentric and is characterized by interstitial inflammation, organizing pneumonia, and the presence of poorly defined granulomas, which usually contain one or a few multinucleated histiocytes. Bronchocentric granulomatosis is characterized by well-formed granulomas compressing and effacing the bronchi. Cryptogenic organizing pneumonia is characterized by fibromyxoid plugs in the alveolar spaces but does not contain granulomas. Immunoglobulin G subclass 4 (IgG4)-related disease is characterized by compressed air spaces with foamy macrophage scarring and a lymphoplasmacytic infiltrate. Nonspecific interstitial pneumonitis is characterized by interstitial fibrosis but without variation in the stage of the fibrosis across the lesion. Interstitial inflammation may be a small or fairly prominent part of the process.

**19. Correct choice: D.**

Pulmonary alveolar proteinosis is a rare disease characterized by the accumulation of acellular surfactant presumably due to impaired clearance, likely due to dysfunction of alveolar macrophages. There are primary (idiopathic) and secondary forms. Congenital cases are usually due to mutation in surfactant protein or granulocyte-macrophage colony-stimulating factor (GM-CSF) receptor genes. Secondary (most common) pulmonary alveolar proteinosis is associated with silica dust, aluminum, fiberglass, chemicals, immunosuppression, and hematologic malignancies. Infection with *Nocardia*, mycobacteria, and *Aspergillosis* may complicate the clinical course. The intra-alveolar exudate in *Pneumocystis jirovecii* may closely resemble pulmonary alveolar proteinosis; special stains are often helpful in excluding Pneumocystis pneumonia.

**20. Correct choice: B.**

Immunoglobulin G subclass 4 (IgG4)-related disease is characterized by the presence of an intense lymphoplasmacytic infiltrate, which is associated with fibrosis and compression of the air spaces. Identification of the lesion requires documentation of the presence of IgG4-producing cells by immunohistochemistry. However, the histology is relatively nonspecific in appearance, and the constellation requires clinical pathologic correlation. Cryptogenic organizing pneumonia is characterized by the fibromyxoid lesions, which are usually confined to the air spaces and rarely involve the interstitium. A lymphoplasmacytic infiltrate is not a characteristic. Lymphocytic interstitial pneumonia is characterized by the presence of large amounts of lymphoid cells, which are usually without plasma cell differentiation. They tend to track along the septa of the lung and are not associated with extensive fibrosis. Pulmonary Langerhans histiocytosis is associated with interstitial fibrosis and the presence of large mononuclear cells, which are histiocytic in type, S100 positive by immunohistochemistry, and characterized by the presence of nuclear grooves. Usual interstitial pneumonia is characterized by temporal differences in the fibrosis as well as the presence of fibroblastic foci.

**21. Correct choice: A.**

Eosinophilic granulomatosis with polyangiitis is characterized by the presence of an eosinophilic infiltrate with preservation of the architecture of the arteries. Granulomatosis with polyangiitis is characterized by a lymphoplasmacytic infiltrate of the arterial wall, frequently with compression and obstruction of the wall and association with geographic necrosis in the surrounding lung. Lymphomatoid granulomatosis is characterized by the presence of atypical lymphocytes, which are angiocentric and angiodestructive. The characterization of the atypical cells by immunohistochemistry reveals that they are a T-cell–rich B-cell lymphoma. Periarteritis nodosa is characterized by a lymphoplasmacytic infiltrate frequently with fibrinoid necrosis of the arteries. Tuberculosis may mimic all of the lesions noted above. The arteritis may be intense, and the destruction of the lung may be similar to that seen in granulomatous pulmonary arteritis. The diagnostic feature is the presence of the tubercle bacilli.

**22. Correct choice: E.**

The location indicates that the vessels involved are veins. There is fibrosis and scarring of the veins without necrosis. In granulomatous pulmonary arteritis (Wegener granulomatosis [WG]), the lesions are angiocentric and usually involve arteries. Geographic necrosis is a common accompaniment of this lesion. Plexogenic arteriopathy is characterized by the presence of sievelike vascular channels in muscular arteries and does not usually involve veins. Pulmonary hypertension is usually restricted to the arterial component, which is normally found in conjunction with the bronchial or bronchiolar structures. Usual interstitial pneumonia is characterized by variation in the temporal stage of interstitial fibrosis and fibroplastic foci. Arterial involvement is usually not intense.

**23. Correct choice: E.**

Measles pneumonia is an uncommon complication of measles infection but may occur, especially in infants and children, in unvaccinated populations. Characteristic multinucleated giant cells, usually with more than 20 nuclei per cell, set within a background of interstitial pneumonia and/or diffuse alveolar damage (DAD). Options A, B, C, and D are characteristic findings in adenovirus, SARS-CoV2, herpes simplex virus (HSV), and cytomegalovirus (CMV) infections, respectively.

**24. Correct choice: E.**

Malakoplakia can involve the lung, and contrary to the urinary bladder or kidney where the common causative organism is *Escherichia coli*, the causative pathogen in 70% of pulmonary infections is *Rhodococcus equi*. Microscopically, malakoplakia is composed of intra-alveolar collections of pink or foamy histiocytes that often contain intracellular periodic acid-Schiff (PAS)-positive bacteria mixed with lymphocytes, plasma cells, and neutrophils. The pathognomonic Michaelis-Gutmann bodies are deeply staining round or oval structures that measure between 5 and 20 μm in diameter and have a laminated or targetoid appearance.

# 26 Pulmonary Neoplasms

1. Which of the following clinical *or* pathologic features is most commonly associated with squamous cell carcinoma of the lung?

   A. Development in close proximity to lung scars
   B. Diffuse pneumonia-like infiltrate on chest x-rays
   C. Lambert-Eaton syndrome
   D. Origin from a major bronchus
   E. Presence of human papillomavirus (HPV) in close to 100% of cases

2. The benign entity in Figure 1 is associated with which of the following?

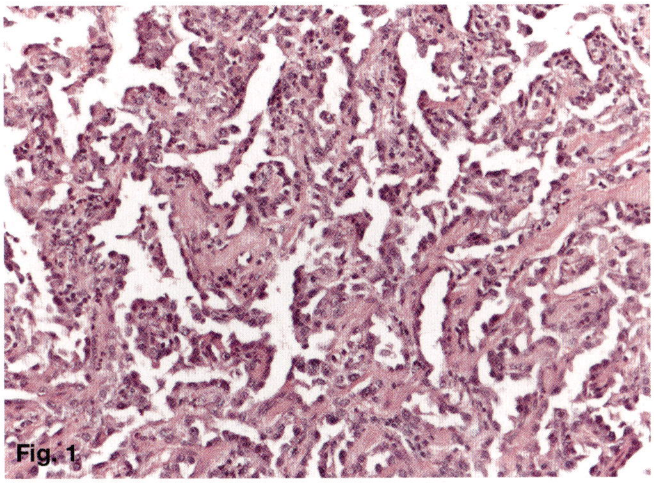

Fig. 1

   A. Cigarette smoking
   B. DICER1 syndrome
   C. High-risk human papillomavirus (HPV) serotypes
   D. Lambert-Eaton syndrome
   E. Tuberous sclerosis complex (TSC)

3. Figure 1 is of a 2.5-cm lung lesion. The alveolar spaces are lined by frankly atypical pneumocytes. Which of the following is the most appropriate diagnosis?

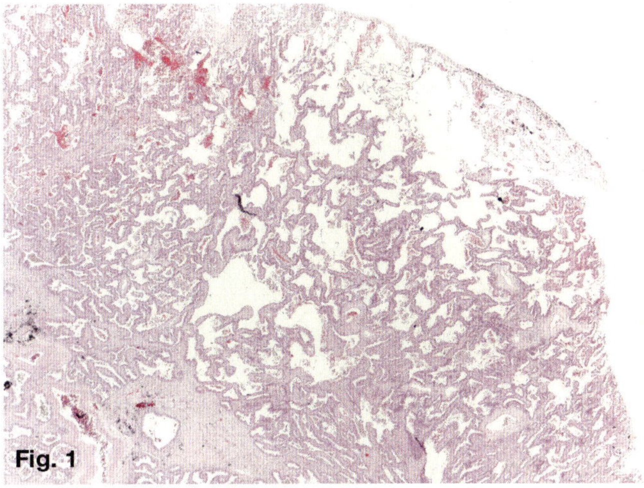

Fig. 1

   A. Adenocarcinoma in situ
   B. Alveolar adenoma
   C. Atypical adenomatous hyperplasia
   D. Invasive adenocarcinoma
   E. Minimally invasive adenocarcinoma

4. Which of the following is true regarding typical carcinoid tumors of the lung?

   A. Bizarre pleomorphism that does not affect prognosis
   B. Frequent areas of punctuate, comedo-like necrosis
   C. Ki-67 index of 5% to 20%
   D. Poor prognosis when regional lymph node metastasis is present
   E. Strong association with cigarette smoking

5. A lung nodule shows tumor cells with a Ki-67 index of 25%. Which of the following combination of immunohistochemical stains and results is most useful to distinguish the diagnosis of neuroendocrine carcinoma from an atypical carcinoid tumor?

   A. Pan-cytokeratin (pan-CK) negative; Rb loss
   B. Pan-CK positive; PAX5 negative
   C. Pan-CK positive; PAX5 positive
   D. Rb intact; p53 wild type
   E. Rb loss; p53 null type

All figures in this chapter are from Longacre TA, Greenson JK, Hornick JL, Reuter VE, eds. *Mills and Sternberg's Diagnostic Surgical Pathology.* 7th ed. Wolters Kluwer; 2022 except for those noted at the end of this book.

6. Which of the following lung adenocarcinomas has the worst prognosis?

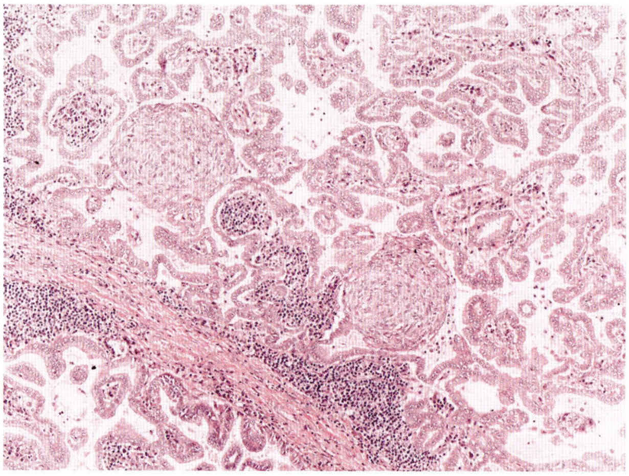
A.

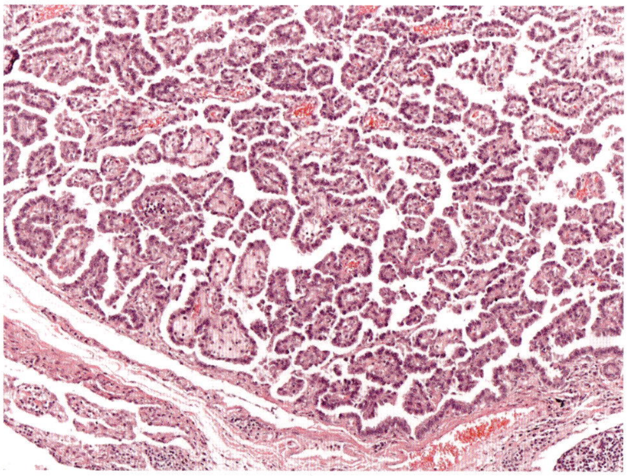
B.

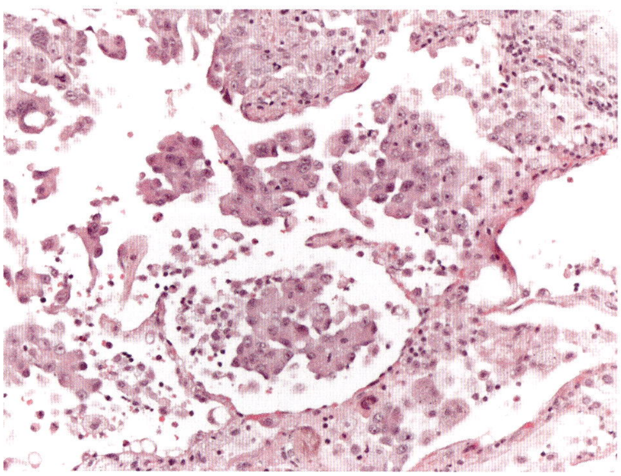
C.

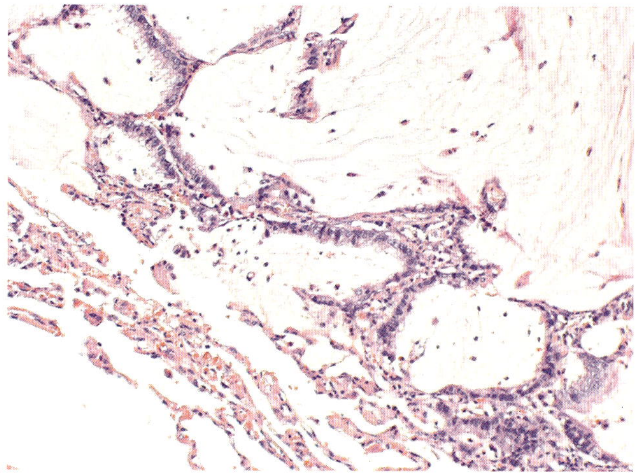
D.

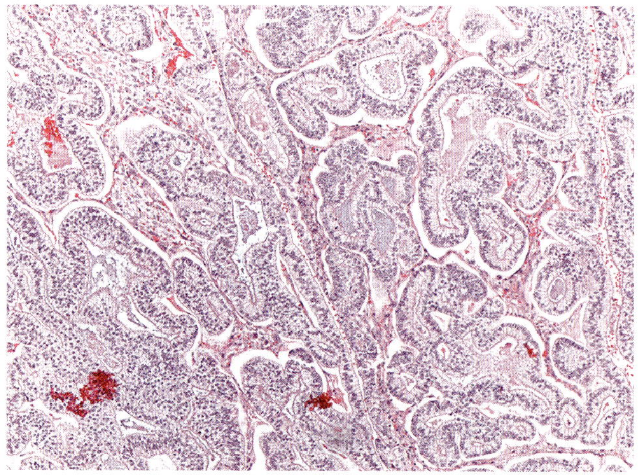
E.

7. The most common salivary gland–like tumor arising in the lungs is

   A. acinic cell carcinoma.
   B. adenoid cystic carcinoma.
   C. mucoepidermoid carcinoma.
   D. oncocytoma.
   E. pleomorphic adenoma.

8. The most common lymphoma of the lungs is characterized by which of the following molecular alterations?

   A. *BCL10::IGH* fusion
   B. *BIRC3::MALT1* fusion
   C. *CCND1::IGH* fusion
   D. *FOXP1::IGH* fusion
   E. *IGH::MALT* fusion

9. A lobectomy is submitted for intraoperative consultation. It contains a well-circumscribed tumor with a tan, bulging cut surface. It can be easily shelled out. A specimen taken from the periphery shows papillary structures with minimal cellular atypia and angiomatous features. What is the most likely diagnosis?

   A. Adenocarcinoma
   B. Bronchioloalveolar carcinoma
   C. Perivascular epithelioid cell tumor (PEComa)
   D. Pulmonary blastoma
   E. Sclerosing pneumocytoma

10. A 3-cm, round, subpleural nodule is found on computed tomography (CT) scan in the left lung of a 14-year-old boy. Grossly, the nodule has a yellow-whitish cut surface with a round-to-lobulated shape. Histologically, it consists of a proliferation of bland spindle mesenchymal cells arranged in irregular fascicles and a dense inflammatory infiltrate. Expression of which of the following is most helpful for the diagnosis?

A. ALK1
B. CD117
C. Desmin
D. Immunoglobulin G subclass 4 (IgG4)
E. Smooth muscle actin

11. A 3-cm coin lesion with a "popcorn" pattern of calcification on a chest x-ray is excised. Histologically, it consists of islands of cartilage mixed with adipose and smooth muscle tissue with occasional epithelium-lined clefts. Which of the following is the most likely pathogenesis of this lesion?

A. Acquired lesion resulting from overgrowth of mesenchymal tissue
B. Congenital lesion caused by developmental anomalies
C. Congenital lesion caused by separation of lung parenchyma from the bronchial tree
D. Inflammatory proliferation of mesenchymal elements
E. Neoplastic transformation of bronchial cartilage

12. A vascular tumor from a 32-year-old female is shown in Figure 1. The diagnostic immunohistochemical stain is

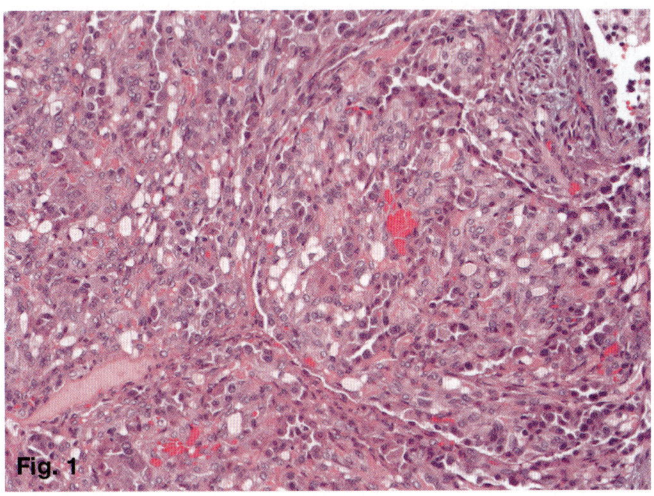

Fig. 1

A. CAMTA-1.
B. FL1-1.
C. GLUT-1.
D. HHV8.
E. vimentin.

13. Which of the following is the molecular abnormality in pleuropulmonary blastoma?

A. *BRAF* mutation
B. *DICER1* mutation
C. *EWSR1-CREB1* fusion
D. *MECT1-MAML2* fusion
E. *MYC* amplification

14. The illustrated lesion, shown in Figure 1, is most likely

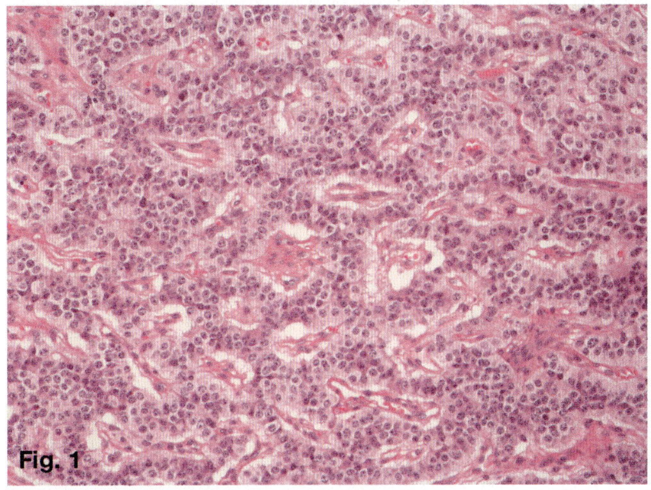

Fig. 1

A. atypical adenomatous hyperplasia.
B. granular cell tumor.
C. paraganglioma.
D. peripheral carcinoid.
E. typical carcinoid.

15. The illustrated lesion, shown in Figure 1, is most likely

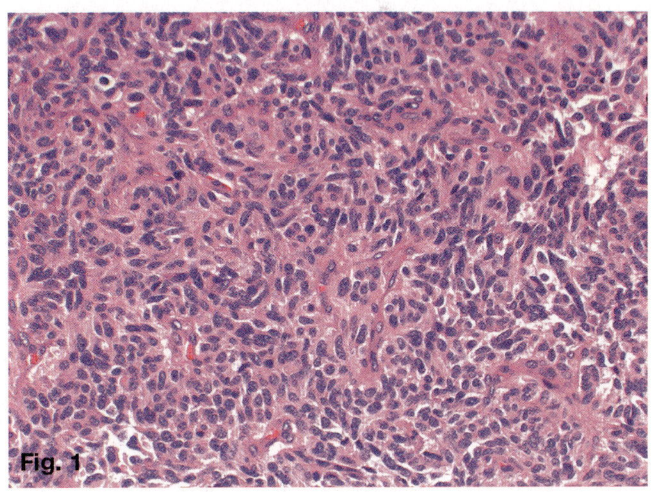

Fig. 1

A. atypical adenomatous hyperplasia.
B. granular cell tumor.
C. paraganglioma.
D. peripheral carcinoid.
E. typical carcinoid.

16. The illustrated lesion, shown in Figure 1, is most likely

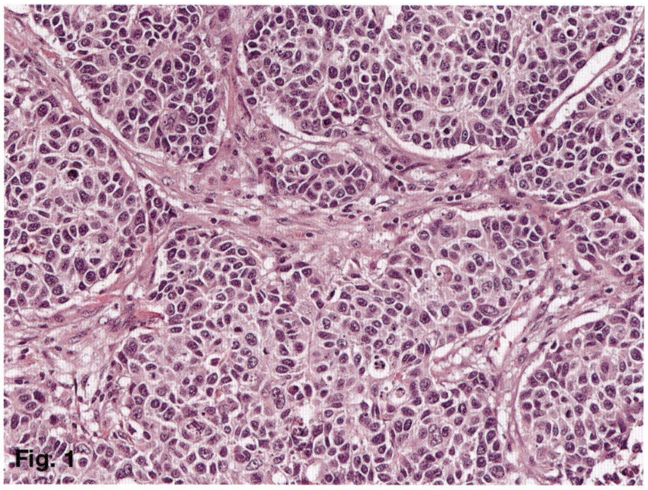


A. large cell carcinoma.
B. large cell neuroendocrine carcinoma.
C. peripheral carcinoid.
D. poorly differentiated adenocarcinoma.
E. poorly differentiated squamous cell carcinoma.

17. The illustrated lesion, shown in Figure 1, is most likely

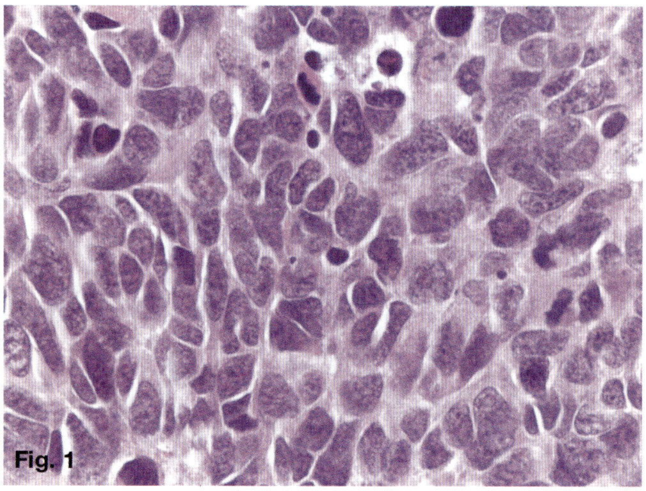


A. B-cell lymphoma.
B. large cell neuroendocrine carcinoma.
C. mantle cell lymphoma.
D. poorly differentiated squamous cell carcinoma.
E. small cell lung carcinoma.

18. The illustrated lesion, seen in Figure 1, shows positive nuclear expression of β-catenin and is most likely

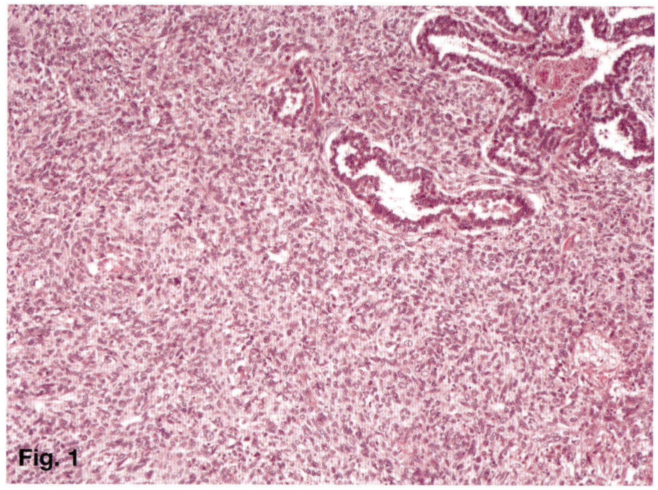


A. inflammatory myofibroblastic tumor.
B. melanoma.
C. mesothelioma.
D. pulmonary blastoma.
E. spindle cell carcinoma.

19. The illustrated lesion, shown in Figure 1, is most likely

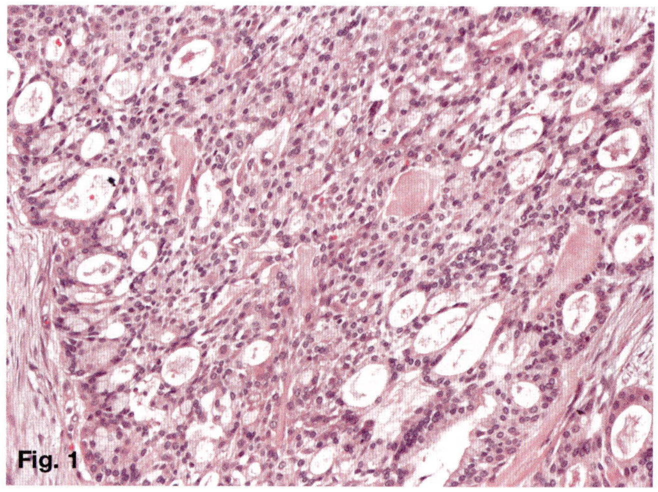


A. acinic cell tumor.
B. adenosquamous carcinoma.
C. alveolar adenoma.
D. mucoepidermoid carcinoma.
E. mucous gland adenoma.

20. The illustrated lesion, shown in Figure 1, is most likely

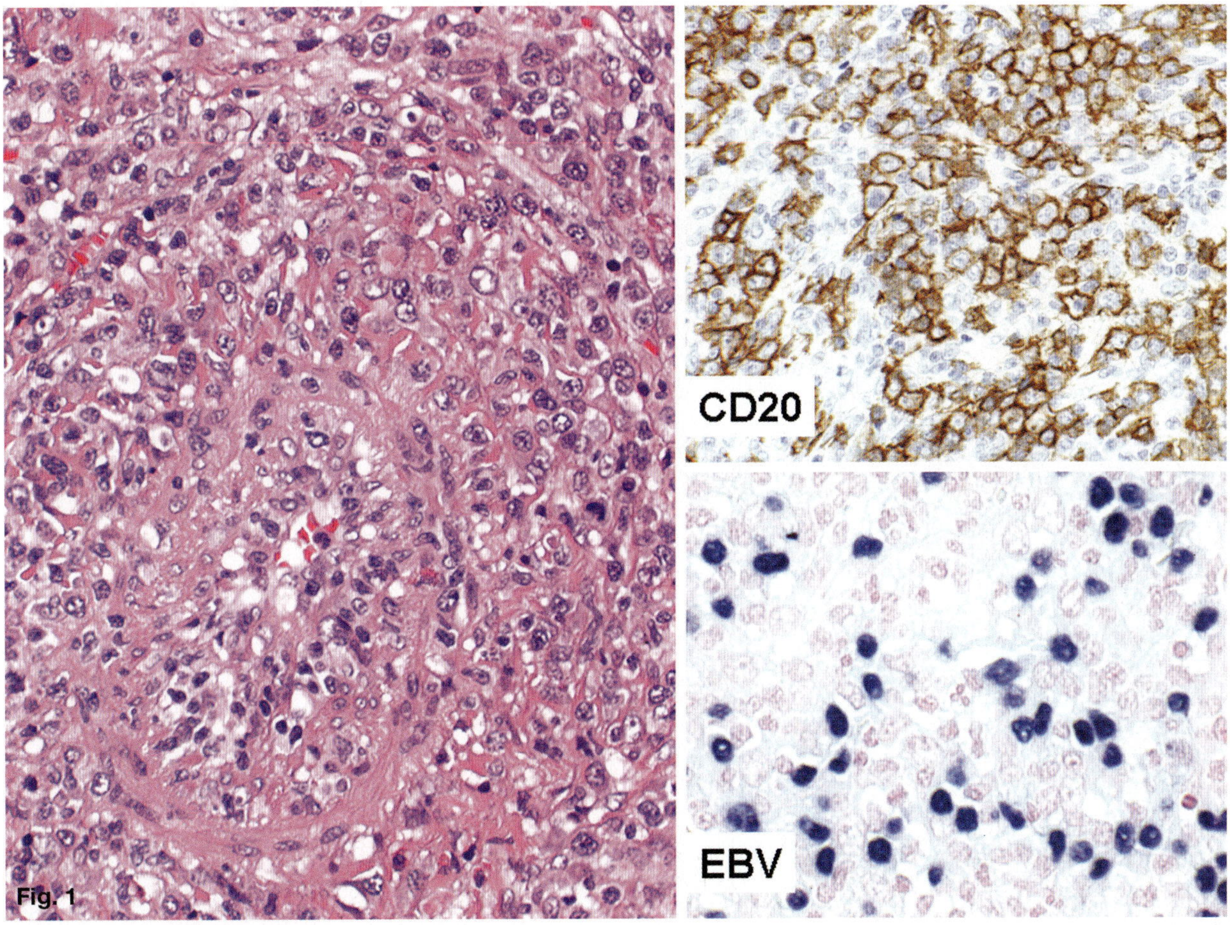


Fig. 1

A. diffuse large B-cell lymphoma.
B. eosinophilic granulomatosis with polyangiitis.
C. granulomatosis with polyangiitis.
D. lymphomatoid granulomatosis.
E. T-cell lymphoma.

21. The illustrated lesion, shown in Figure 1, is most likely positive for which of the following?

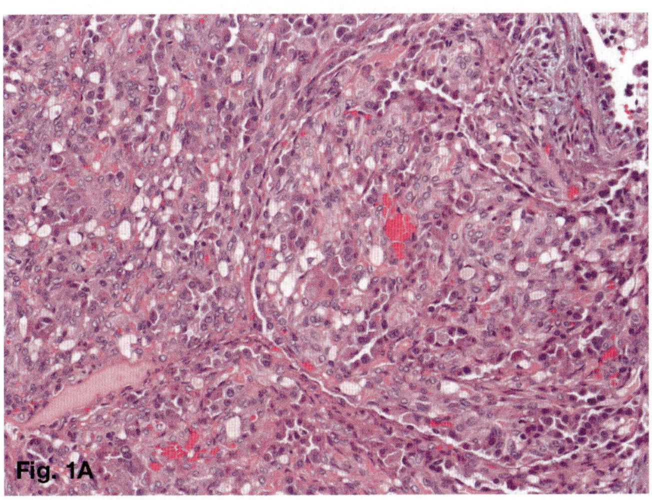

Fig. 1A

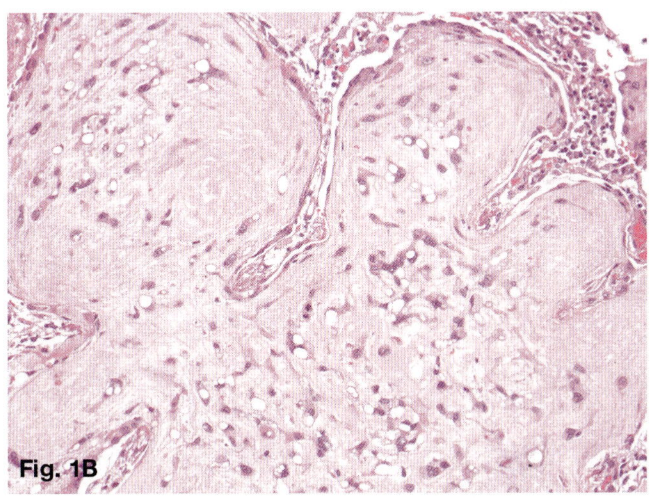

Fig. 1B

A. BEREP4 positive
B. CD31 positive
C. CK5/CK6 positive
D. CK7 positive
E. TTF-1

22. The illustrated lesion, shown in Figure 1, is most likely due to

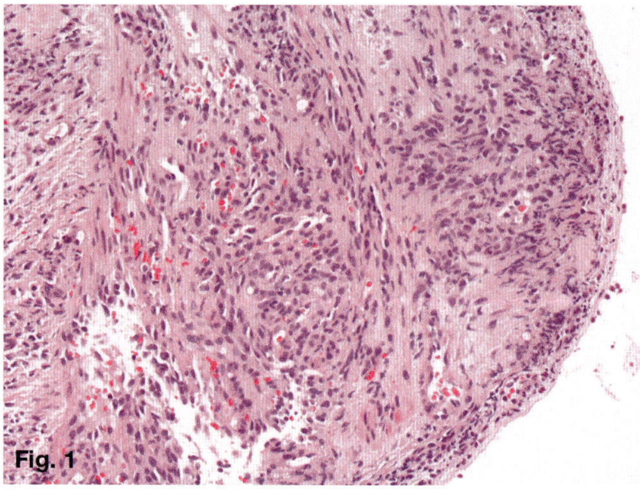
Fig. 1

A. *Aspergillus*.
B. atypical mycobacterium.
C. Epstein-Barr virus.
D. herpes virus type 8.
E. human papillomavirus.

23. The illustrated lesion, shown in Figure 1, is most likely

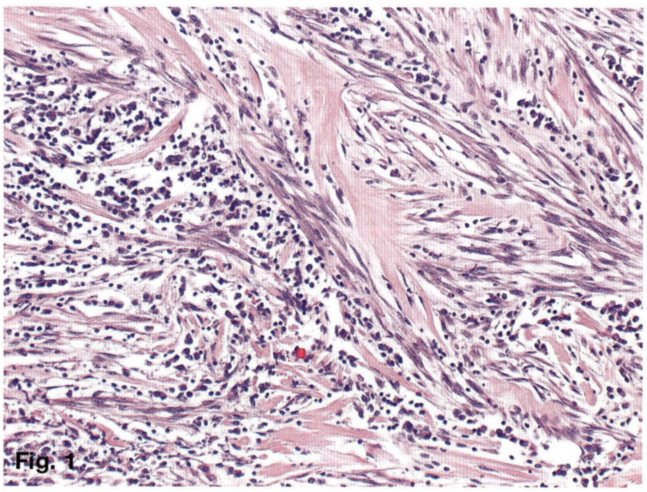
Fig. 1

A. inflammatory myofibroblastic tumor.
B. metastatic leiomyosarcoma.
C. metastatic liposarcoma.
D. nodular sclerosis classical Hodgkin lymphoma.
E. pulmonary artery sarcoma.

24. Which of the following is true of the illustrated lesion, shown in Figure 1?

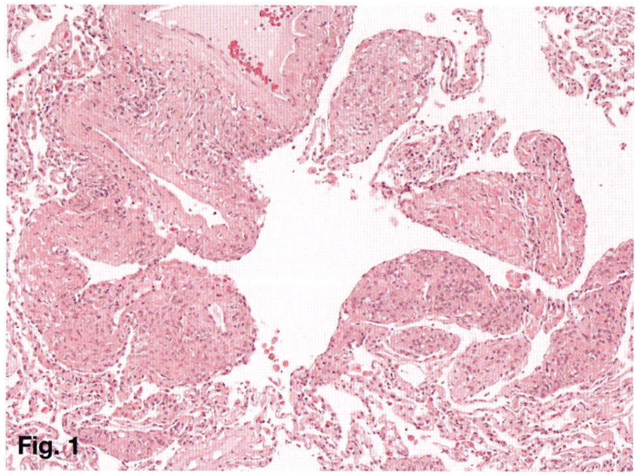
Fig. 1

A. Congenital abnormality
B. Does not recur after lung transplant
C. Found in older men and women
D. HMB45 positive lesional cells
E. Perivascular epithelial cell origin

25. What is the most likely positive immunohistochemical stain for the lesion seen in Figure 1?

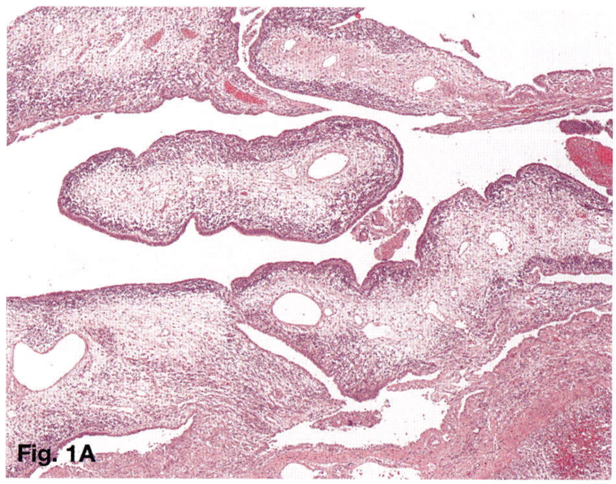
Fig. 1A

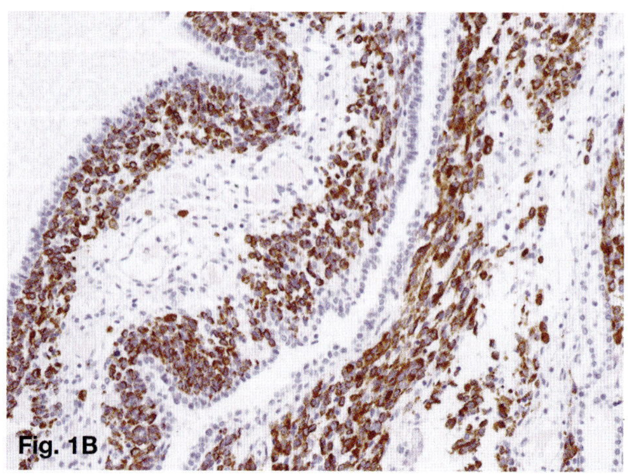
Fig. 1B

A. Desmin
B. HMB45
C. INSM1
D. Pan-CKs
E. S100 protein

26. The illustrated lesion, shown in Figure 1, is most likely

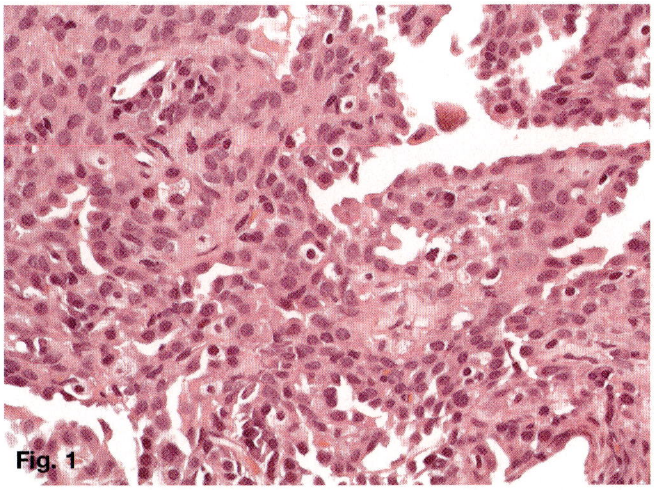


A. adenocarcinoma in situ.
B. adenocarcinoma, invasive with lepidic pattern.
C. epithelioid hemangioendothelioma.
D. metastatic breast carcinoma.
E. sclerosing pneumocytoma.

27. The illustrated lesion, shown in Figure 1, is most likely positive for which of the following?

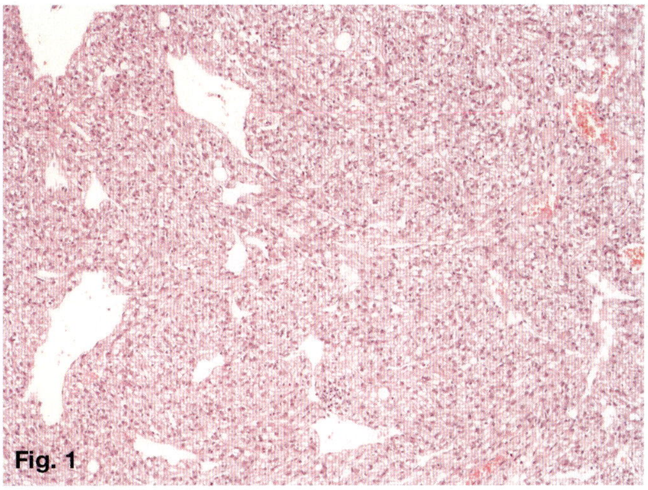


A. Atypical carcinoid
B. Clear cell variant of large cell carcinoma
C. Metastatic renal cell carcinoma
D. Paraganglioma
E. Perivascular epithelioid cell tumor (PEComa)

# ANSWERS AND EXPLANATIONS

**1. Correct choice: D.**

Squamous cell carcinoma of the lung usually arises from segmental bronchi (thus perihilar), undergoes central cavitation, is associated with human papillomavirus (HPV) in up to 20% of cases, and does not arise in proximity to pulmonary scars. Most cases of lung cancer associated with peripheral scars are adenocarcinomas. Lambert-Eaton (myasthenic) syndrome is most commonly associated with small cell carcinoma. Hyperparathyroidism is the most common paraneoplastic syndrome associated with squamous cell carcinoma.

**2. Correct choice: E.**

Micronodular pneumocyte hyperplasia consists of multiple small nodules, frequently arising in patients with tuberous sclerosis complex (TSC) and composed of bland pneumocytes with mild interstitial thickening. The lack of cellular atypia and lepidic growth distinguishes micronodular pneumocyte hyperplasia from atypical adenomatous hyperplasia (AAH).

**3. Correct choice: E.**

The image shows adenocarcinoma with lepidic pattern with focal invasion seen on the bottom left corner, consisting of small acini embedded in a desmoplastic stroma. This is characteristic of minimally invasive adenocarcinoma, which is defined as a single lesion, 3 cm or less, with a predominant lepidic pattern and with foci of invasion 5 mm or less. If multiple foci of invasion are present, only the size of the largest invasive area should be measured. Vascular and pleural invasion and tumor necrosis must be absent. Adenocarcinoma in situ is 3 cm or less without invasion. Atypical adenomatous hyperplasia is less than 5 mm. Invasive adenocarcinoma has invasive foci greater than 5 mm.

**4. Correct choice: A.**

Typical carcinoid tumors of the lung arise in the fourth to fifth decades, with an equal sex distribution. The majority of patients are nonsmokers. Overall, 5- and 10-year survival of typical carcinoids ranges from 90% to 100% and from 80% to 90%, respectively. Regional lymph node metastasis and lymphovascular invasion does not change staging. Typical carcinoids show finely dispersed nuclear chromatin with absence of extensive necrosis and high mitotic activity. Several histologic changes without clinical significance have been described in carcinoids: papillary, oncocytic, melanocytic type, psammoma rich, signet ring, acinic like, mucin producing, and clear cell. Even cellular pleomorphism does not have diagnostic or prognostic value. The proliferative activity assessed by Ki-67/MIB-1 index is generally low (<5%) in typical and significantly higher in atypical forms (ranging from 5% to 20%).

**5. Correct choice: E.**

Distinguishing between atypical carcinoid tumor, large cell neuroendocrine carcinoma, and small cell lung carcinoma may be difficult by histology alone. All three entities show expression for pan-CKs, CK7, and PAX5. A proliferative index exceeding 25% by Ki-67/MIB-1 generally favors neuroendocrine carcinoma over carcinoids. Loss of Rb and abnormal p53 expression is associated with neuroendocrine carcinoma.

**6. Correct choice: C.**

Micropapillary-predominant adenocarcinoma is composed of papillary tufts with the absence of fibrovascular cores. Micropapillae may be connected to alveolar lumina or may "float" within alveoli and, sometimes, infiltrate the stroma as small clusters reminiscent of the "budding" of colonic adenocarcinoma. It is associated with poor prognosis and even 1% of tumors with micropapillary foci demonstrate an adverse prognostic effect.

**7. Correct choice: C.**

Salivary gland–type carcinomas of the lung usually present in young (third to fourth decade of life) nonsmoking patients. Mucoepidermoid carcinoma represents about 1% of all primary lung tumors. A low-grade and a high-grade type are recognized. Low-grade mucoepidermoid carcinoma is more common and has an excellent prognosis after complete excision. It is characterized by cystic changes and a mixture of nonkeratinizing squamoid elements closely admixed with bland-looking, mucin-producing columnar cells arranged in tubuloglandular formations. The high-grade form is very rare and has an aggressive behavior. The presence of numerous mitoses, necrosis, and pleomorphism distinguishes high-grade from low-grade mucoepidermoid carcinoma. Adenoid cystic carcinoma is the second most common salivary gland–type tumor of the lung.

**8. Correct choice: B.**

Pulmonary extranodal marginal zone lymphoma (MZL) is the most common primary lymphoma of the lung, accounting for approximately 70% to 90% of cases. MZL commonly occurs in the fifth to seventh decades, with a slight male predilection. MZL is a low-grade B-cell lymphoma, but transformation to a high-grade diffuse large B-cell lymphoma (DLBCL) may rarely occur. Lymphoma cells express CD20, CD19, CD79a, bcl-2, and PAX5 but are negative for CD5, CD10, cyclin D1, and bcl6. Lung MZL is commonly associated with BIRC3::MALT1 t(11;18). Answers A and C are most associated with MZL of the stomach and thyroid, respectively. DLBCL is the second most common type of primary pulmonary lymphoma.

**9. Correct choice: E.**

Sclerosing pneumocytoma is a benign slow-growing lesion that is usually discovered incidentally in young women. It is a well-demarcated, solid, tan mass composed of polygonal cells arranged in a nesting or papillary pattern. The cells have eosinophilic cytoplasm. Characteristic is a sort of zonal pattern: Peripheral regions show a papillary architecture and increased cellular atypia (which may lead to an erroneous diagnosis of adenocarcinoma), whereas central areas have an angiomatous appearance. Features favoring an origin from type II pneumocytes include immunoreactivity for Napsin A, as well as lamellated bodies and short microvilli on electron microscopy (EM; all features of normal type II pneumocytes). Thus, this lesion is not a hemangioma.

**10. Correct choice: A.**

Inflammatory myofibroblastic tumor (IMT, also known as inflammatory pseudotumor) is a neoplasm encompassing several conditions ranging from reactive lesions to true sarcomas. It is most often found in children or young adults. Histologically, a proliferation of bland spindle mesenchymal cells arranged in irregular fascicles into a cellular stroma with inflammatory infiltrate. The tumor may invade the blood vessels or the pleura. At immunohistochemistry, it expresses the markers of myofibroblastic differentiation (smooth muscle actin and, rarely, desmin) but lacks myogenin, CD117, and S100. A weak staining for cytokeratins (CKs) is observed in one-third of cases, whereas about 40% to 50% of IMT express ALK1.

**11. Correct choice: A.**

Pulmonary hamartoma is a benign lesion that is usually discovered as an incidental finding on chest x-rays. An admixture of cartilage, smooth muscle, epithelium-lined clefts, and adipose tissue is characteristic. In contrast to previous hypotheses, lung hamartoma is an acquired lesion. It probably arises from overgrowth of mesenchymal components of the bronchial walls, with secondary entrapment of bronchial epithelium.

**12. Correct choice: A.**

Epithelioid hemangioendothelioma (EHE) is an intermediate-grade malignant vascular tumor that mainly affects young adult females and often presents as an asymptomatic indolent disease. EHE generally presents as multiple, bilateral nodules of a few centimeters. Microscopically, the neoplastic cells have an eosinophilic cytoplasm, with intracytoplasmic vacuoles sometimes containing erythrocytes, and, frequently, intranuclear inclusions. They are typically arranged in cords within a chondromyxoid or hyaline stroma. Tumor cells stain with at least one vascular marker, and CAMTA-1 expression is quite specific to EHE.

**13. Correct choice: B.**

Pleuropulmonary blastoma (PPB) is a rare pediatric mesenchymal tumor occurring before 4 years of life without gender predilection. Type 1 PPB (cystic variant) consists of multiloculated cysts lined by respiratory epithelium and surrounded by a blastematous proliferation of small primitive malignant cells with rhabdomyoblastic differentiation. From type II (mixed cystic/solid) to type III (pure solid) form, there is an overgrowth of the blastematous component in the septal stroma, with nodules of chondrosarcoma, fibrosarcoma, or pleomorphic sarcoma. PPB is part of an inherited cancer syndrome due to germline *DICER1* mutations.

**14. Correct choice: E.**

The lesion is a typical carcinoid characterized by the presence of pseudorosettes. It is characterized by the absence of anaplastic nuclei, mitotic figures, and necrosis. Peripheral carcinoids are frequently spindled, but are still classified as typical carcinoids if they lack anaplasia, mitoses, and necrosis; they may have the appearance of this epithelioid carcinoid. Atypical adenomatous hyperplasia is a proliferation of type II pneumocytes on alveolar walls. Paraganglioma is characterized by neuroendocrine and sustentacular cells. Granular cell tumors are characterized by large granular cells without pattern and without neuroendocrine markers.

**15. Correct choice: D.**

The spindle cell lesion is a peripheral carcinoid. It is without mitotic figures and necrosis and therefore falls under the classification of typical carcinoid for prognostic purposes. Atypical adenomatous hyperplasia is a proliferation of type II pneumocytes on the alveolar structure. Paraganglioma is characterized by neuroendocrine and sustentacular cells. Granular cell tumor is characterized by large epithelioid cells without pattern and not by spindle cells.

**16. Correct choice: B.**

Large cell neuroendocrine carcinoma is characterized by anaplastic large nuclei with prominent nucleoli and numerous mitotic figures. It is the only neuroendocrine tumor with anaplastic nuclei and prominent nucleoli. In this way, it is distinct from the spindle cell peripheral carcinoid. Large cell carcinoma lacks neuroendocrine differentiation both histologically and by immunohistochemistry. Poorly differentiated adenocarcinoma is characterized by acini and not pseudorosettes and lacks neuroendocrine markers. Squamous cell carcinoma is characterized by hyalinized cytoplasm, intercellular bridges, and stains for p63 and p40.

**17. Correct choice: E.**

Small cell lung carcinoma (SCLC) is characterized by small epithelial cells, which are distinguished by the molding of nuclei by nuclei of adjacent cells. The nuclei are two-and-a-half times the size of normal lymphocytes and are characterized by an even common distribution and a high mitotic rate, which can be documented by Ki-67 staining (usually >50%). B-cell lymphoma and mantle cell lymphoma lack the molding seen in small cell carcinoma and express lymphocytic markers. Large cell neuroendocrine carcinoma has neuroendocrine features and a high mitotic rate but is characterized by anaplastic open nuclei with prominent nucleoli. Poorly differentiated squamous cell carcinoma lacks neuroendocrine differentiation and has squamous features. However, the distinction between poorly differentiated squamous cell carcinoma and small cell carcinoma may be difficult, especially on small biopsies. Small cell carcinoma is distinguished from squamous cell carcinoma by the presence of neuroendocrine features and markers.

**18. Correct choice: D.**

The lesion is a biphasic tumor consistent with a pulmonary blastoma, in which a fetal-type adenocarcinoma is associated with primitive malignant mesenchymal tissue. The mesenchymal component has a blastema-like appearance and may differentiate toward striated muscle, smooth muscle, cartilage, or a combination of these. Both glandular and blastematous components of pulmonary blastoma have a nuclear expression of β-catenin.

**19. Correct choice: D.**

The lesion is mucoepidermoid carcinoma characterized by the presence of intermediate cells. Mucous gland adenoma, alveolar adenoma, acinic cell tumor, and adenosquamous cell carcinoma do not contain intermediate cells. Mucous gland adenoma may give a very bland appearance but lacks intermediate cells. Alveolar adenoma is characterized by a stromal component. Acinic cell tumor is characterized by the presence of periodic acid-Schiff (PAS)-positive, diastase-resistant granules, and adenosquamous carcinoma lacks intermediate cells. Mucoepidermoid carcinomas show a range from low grade, which may be difficult to distinguish from mucous gland adenoma, to high grade, which may be difficult to distinguish from adenosquamous carcinoma.

**20. Correct choice: D.**

The illustrated lesion is lymphomatoid granulomatosis (LYG). It is an angiocentric and angiodestructive process characterized by the infiltration of vascular structures by CD20-positive lymphocytes. LYG and granulomatosis with polyangiitis share a low-magnification appearance of necrosis due to the vascular compromise of the affected arteries. Granulomatosis with polyangiitis has vasculitis that is not characterized by CD20-positive lymphocytes. LYG prevails in males in the fifth to sixth decades, frequently in a setting of immunodeficiency. Grading of LYG depends on the proportion of Epstein-Barr virus (EBV)-positive large B cells.

**21. Correct choice: B.**

This lesion is an epithelioid hemangioendothelioma with prominent myxoid stroma. Because it is an endothelial neoplasm, it is positive for CD31. It is found in the lung and frequently in associated organs such as the liver. Although it may assume an epithelioid appearance, stains for BEREP4, TTF-1, CK5/CK6, and CK7 and other epithelial markers are not positive.

**22. Correct choice: D.**

The lesion is a Kaposi sarcoma, and these have been found to be associated with herpesvirus type 8 infection. They are not associated with human papillomavirus or Epstein-Barr virus (EBV), although it is associated with HIV infection. Because Kaposi is found in immunocompromised hosts, mycobacterial infection and *Aspergillus* may be secondary invaders but are not part of the genesis of Kaposi sarcoma.

**23. Correct choice: A.**

The lesion is an inflammatory myofibroblastic tumor. It is characterized by the florid proliferation of fibroblasts but is also associated with a lymphocytic or plasma cell infiltrate, which may be predominant. Pulmonary artery sarcoma, metastatic leiomyosarcoma, and liposarcoma may also contain proliferating and mitotically active spindle cells, but they usually lack the inflammatory component and are characterized by cells differentiating toward either smooth muscle or adipose tissue. Nodular sclerosis classical Hodgkin lymphoma is associated with a lymphocytic infiltrate but is characterized by the presence of Reed-Sternberg cells with their bilobed nuclei and prominent nucleoli.

**24. Correct choice: D.**

The lesion is lymphangioleiomyomatosis (LAM), a low-grade progressive neoplasm consisting of short spindle cells with myoid differentiation infiltrating the interstitium and remodeling the lung parenchyma, leading to micronodules and cysts of variable size involving both lungs without any site predilection. LAM is usually seen in women in their childbearing years. The LAM cells express smooth muscle actin, desmin, HMB45, hormonal receptors, and cathepsin K. LAM occurs in about 40% of women with tuberous sclerosis complex (TSC) and is associated with *TSC1* and *TSC2* mutations. LAM cells may migrate through the lymphatic system, and recurrent LAM lesions in the allograft of lung transplants seem to derive from the recipient.

**25. Correct choice: A.**

The illustrated lesion is a pleuropulmonary blastoma, which is found in children younger than age 4 without gender predilection. It is distinguished from congenital cystic adenomatoid malformation by the presence of a primitive stromal component, which may be found in a "cambium" layer distribution with myogenic differentiation (desmin).

**26. Correct choice: E.**

The lesion is a sclerosing pneumocytoma, which may be confused with all four of the malignant lesions listed. At low magnification, the tumor is well circumscribed and has a variable combination of four patterns: solid, hemorrhagic, papillary, and sclerotic. Two cell types occur: round interstitial cells and surface cells. It is an epithelial lesion expressing TTF-1 and keratin.

**27. Correct choice: E.**

The lesion is perivascular epithelioid cell tumor (PEComa; also known as a clear cell "sugar" tumor) characterized by well-circumscribed nodules composed of round-to-oval cells with abundant clear cytoplasm. Mitoses and necrosis are usually absent. PEComas are immunoreactivity for melanocytic markers such as HMB45. Virtually, all PEComas in the lung have a benign clinical behavior.

# 27 Pleura

1. Subserosal fibroblast-like cells are responsible for regeneration of the mesothelial lining in response to injury. Immunohistochemically, such cells are characterized by expression of vimentin and

   A. Cam 5.2.
   B. CD34.
   C. CD99.
   D. Carcinoembryonic antigen (CEA).
   E. S100 protein.

2. Which of the following is true?

   A. Localized mesothelioma has the same prognosis as a diffuse counterpart.
   B. Long and narrow microvilli cover the surface of tumor cells on electron microscopy.
   C. Sarcomatoid mesothelioma rarely shows a storiform growth pattern.
   D. There is a strong association with asbestos and tobacco smoke.
   E. Well-differentiated papillary mesothelial tumor is most common on the pleura.

3. A 65-year-old man presents with persistent chest pain and unexplained weight loss. On initial examination, he is found to have a hemorrhagic pleural effusion, which is evacuated. A computed tomography (CT) scan reveals irregular pleural thickening. A biopsy of the pleural lesions demonstrates an epithelioid tubulopapillary tumor, which has diffuse expression of pan-cytokeratin. Which of the following markers, if positive, would support a diagnosis of mesothelioma and rule out adenocarcinoma?

   A. Calretinin
   B. CK7
   C. Claudin-4
   D. D2-40
   E. WT-1

4. Which of the following mesothelial markers show both nuclear and cytoplasmic expression?

   A. Calretinin
   B. CK5/6
   C. Mesothelin
   D. Thrombomodulin
   E. WT-1

5. Which of the following immunohistochemical stains is most useful to distinguish mesothelioma from a benign mesothelial proliferation?

   A. BAP1
   B. Glucose transporter protein 1 (GLUT-1)
   C. IMP3
   D. P16
   E. P53

6. A well-circumscribed 5-cm nodule is excised from the visceral pleura of a 40-year-old presenting with chest pain and hypoglycemia. The histologic appearance of the lesion is shown in Figure 1. *NAB2::STAT6* fusion is detected. Which of the following is the most likely diagnosis?

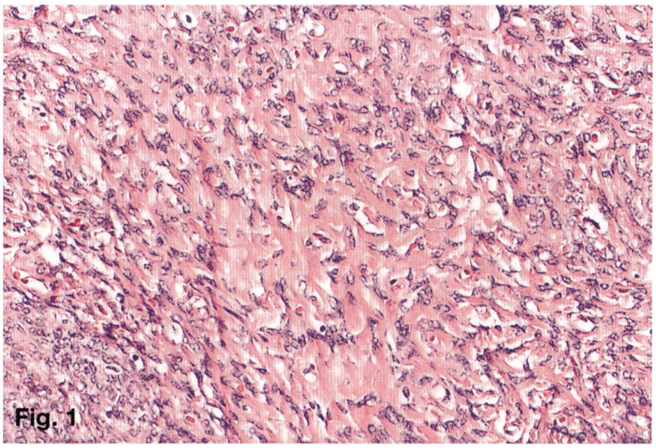

Fig. 1

   A. Epithelioid hemangioendothelioma
   B. Fibrosarcoma
   C. Mesothelioma
   D. Schwannoma
   E. Solitary fibrous tumor

---

All figures in this chapter are from Longacre TA, Greenson JK, Hornick JL, Reuter VE, eds. *Mills and Sternberg's Diagnostic Surgical Pathology*. 7th ed. Wolters Kluwer; 2022 except for those noted at the end of this book.

# ANSWERS AND EXPLANATIONS

**1. Correct choice: A.**

Regenerating mesothelium has been shown to derive from subserosal fibroblast-like cells that migrate toward the surface and acquire an epithelial/mesothelial phenotype. Originally, such cells express only vimentin, but they retain the ability to express low-molecular-weight keratin and actin in response to noxious stimuli. This phenotypical change has been observed in other serosal sites. A common problem in the differential diagnosis of serosal lesions is distinguishing reactive from neoplastic cells. Keratin-positive reactive cells do not show infiltrative behavior and are arranged in a bandlike manner parallel to the serosal surface.

**2. Correct choice: B.**

Mesothelioma has a strong association with asbestos fibers; however, contributions of other factors (including heredity and exposure to other carcinogens such as tobacco smoke) to the pathogenesis of mesothelioma are not clear in most cases. Three major histologic types of diffuse mesothelioma are described: epithelioid, sarcomatoid, and biphasic. Localized mesothelioma is histologically and immunophenotypically indistinguishable from diffuse mesothelioma but exhibits a different biologic behavior, with many patients having a long survival after surgical resection. A well-differentiated papillary mesothelial tumor is most commonly seen in the peritoneal cavity of women. It is typically identified incidentally during surgery. Well-differentiated papillary mesothelial tumors of the peritoneum and pleura have an indolent clinical course. Diffuse sarcomatoid mesothelioma is made up predominantly of malignant-appearing spindle cells arranged in a storiform pattern with fibrous stroma. Electron micrographs of mesothelioma cells show the presence of abundant long and narrow microvilli over much of the free surfaces of the tumor cells.

**3. Correct choice: A.**

Immunohistochemistry for mesothelioma is similar to reactive and resting mesothelial cells. Both mesotheliomas and adenocarcinomas have a strong and diffuse expression of pan-cytokeratin. Immunostains for cytokeratins 7 and 20 are useful in localizing the site of origin of metastatic adenocarcinoma but not in distinguishing adenocarcinoma from epithelioid mesothelioma. Calretinin, D2-40, and WT-1 are mesothelial markers; however, D2-40 and WT-1 are also expressed in carcinoma. Calretinin expression is seen in both normal mesothelial cells and mesothelioma, but rarely in adenocarcinoma.

**4. Correct choice: A.**

All answer choices are mesothelial markers. Only calretinin has both nuclear and cytoplasmic expression. WT-1 has nuclear expression. CK5/6 has cytoplasmic expression. Mesothelin and thrombomodulin have membranous expressions.

**5. Correct choice: A.**

BAP1 immunohistochemistry has been shown to be most helpful for distinguishing between benign and malignant mesothelial proliferations because nuclear expression is lost in the majority of epithelioid mesotheliomas and a subset of sarcomatoid mesotheliomas, whereas it is always expressed in benign mesothelial lesions. Positive glucose transporter protein 1 (GLUT-1), p53 overexpression, and loss of p16 have also been reported to have potential for distinguishing benign reactive mesothelium from mesothelioma but are not as useful as BAP1.

**6. Correct choice: E.**

The clinical and histologic features are consistent with solitary fibrous tumor (SFT) of the pleura. Histologically, SFT is composed of a mixture of spindle-shaped, fibroblast-like cells lying within a variable amount of collagenous stroma. Cytologic atypia and mitoses are uncommon. *NAB2::STAT6* fusion genes are identified in the majority of SFTs, and almost 100% of cases will show nuclear expression of STAT6 by immunohistochemistry. A keloid-like fibrous stroma is a frequent feature of SFT. Recurrence of SFT after excision is approximately 16%, and malignant transformation is rare.

# 28 Mediastinum

1. Which of the following is true regarding the most common congenital cyst of the mediastinum?

   A. Associated with myasthenia gravis or Sjögren syndrome
   B. Contains chylous fluid that grossly appears milky
   C. Limited to the mediastinum
   D. Lined by respiratory-type pseudostratified columnar epithelium
   E. Often communicates with large airways

2. Which of the following is true of thymic cysts?

   A. Multilocular cysts lack significant inflammation and cholesterol granulomas.
   B. Pseudoepitheliomatous hyperplasia can be seen in acquired cysts.
   C. The cysts usually do not grow bigger than 5 cm.
   D. There is no association with autoimmune diseases.
   E. Unilocular cysts are usually congenital.

3. A mediastinal cyst is incidentally discovered in a 45-year-old man at the right cardiophrenic angle. The microscopic appearance of the cyst wall is shown in Figure 1. The cyst is lined by cells that are positive WT-1 (Figure 2). Which of the following is the most likely diagnosis?

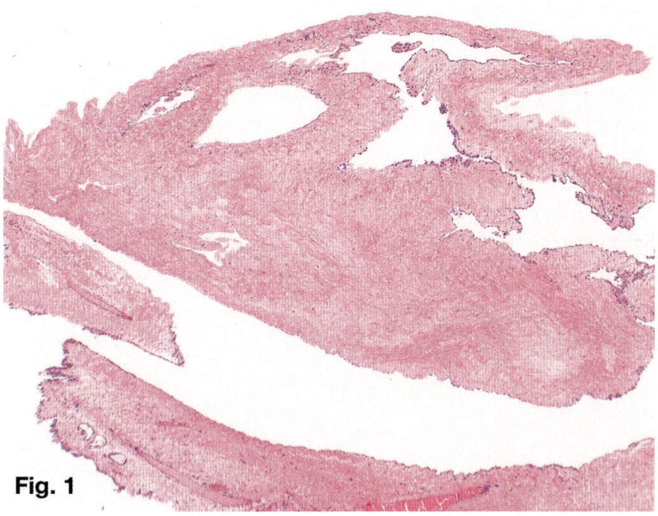
Fig. 1

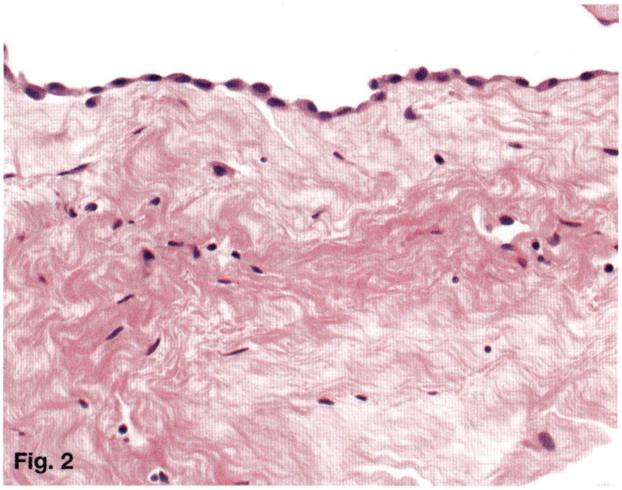
Fig. 2

   A. Bronchogenic cyst
   B. Cystic hygroma
   C. Müllerian cyst
   D. Pericardial cyst
   E. Unilocular thymic cyst

4. Figure 1 shows the histopathologic features of a cystic mass in the mediastinum of a 20-year-old man who presented with chest pain and dyspnea. Which of the following is the most likely diagnosis?

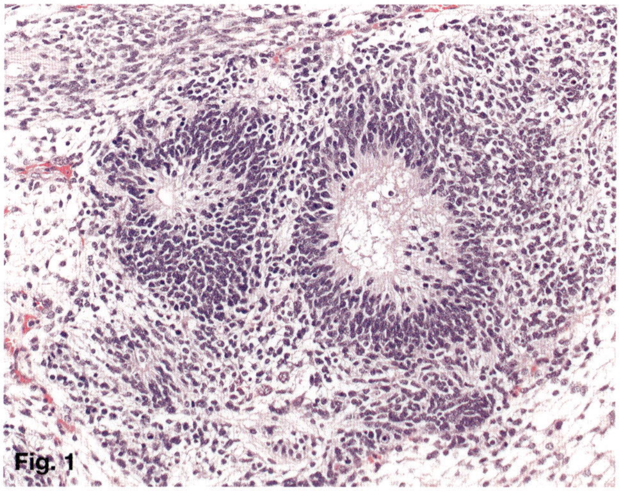
Fig. 1

   A. Ganglioneuroma
   B. Immature teratoma
   C. Malignant mixed germ cell tumor
   D. Mature teratoma
   E. Thymic carcinoma

All figures in this chapter are from Longacre TA, Greenson JK, Hornick JL, Reuter VE, eds. *Mills and Sternberg's Diagnostic Surgical Pathology.* 7th ed. Wolters Kluwer; 2022 except for those noted at the end of this book.

Questions 5-10: Match the following histologic features to the appropriate World Health Organization (WHO) classification for thymomas.

5. Type A

6. Type B1

7. Type B2

8. Type B3

9. Metaplastic thymomas

10. Micronodular thymoma

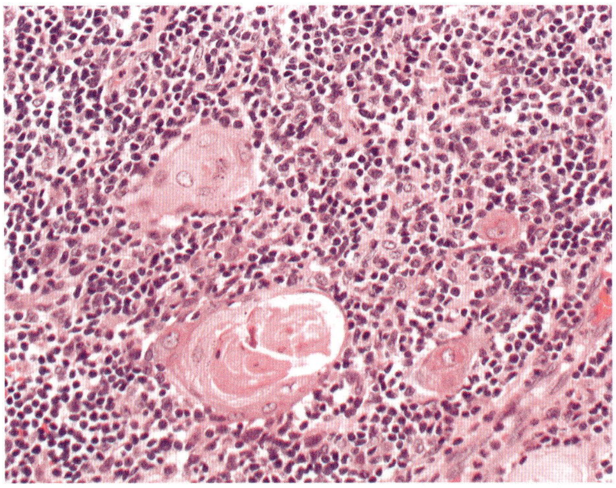

A.

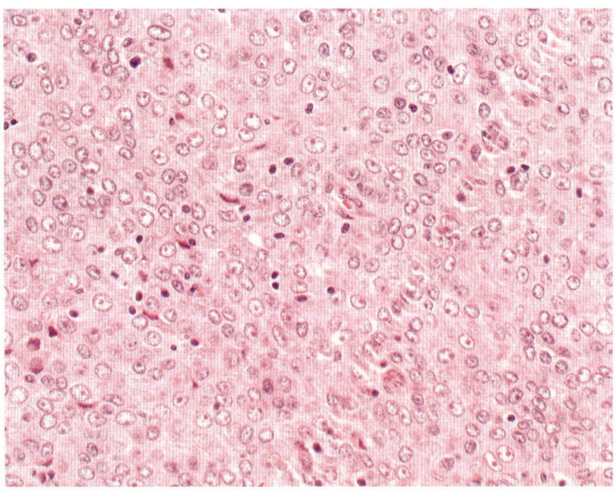

B.

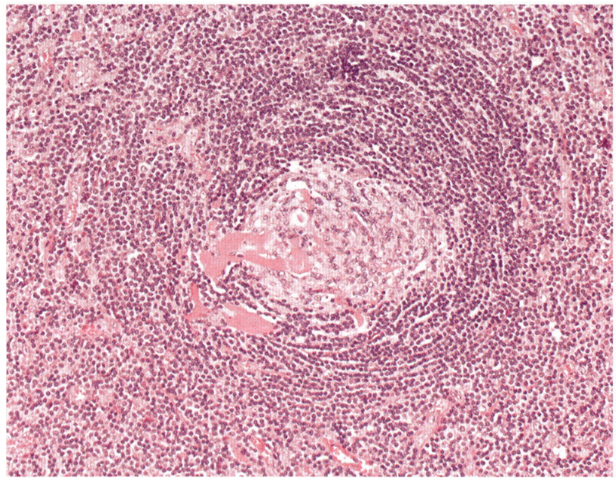

C.

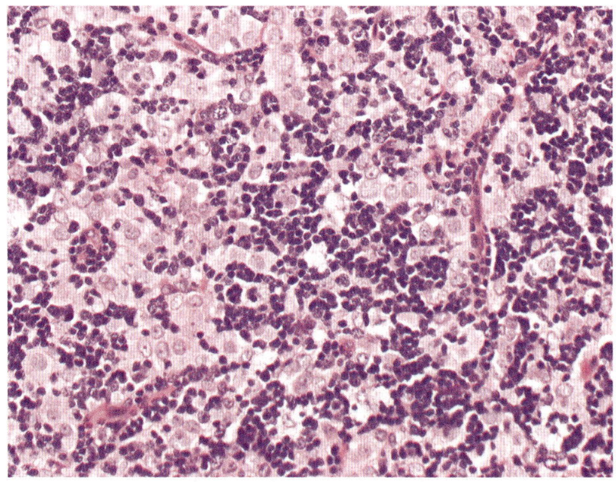

D.

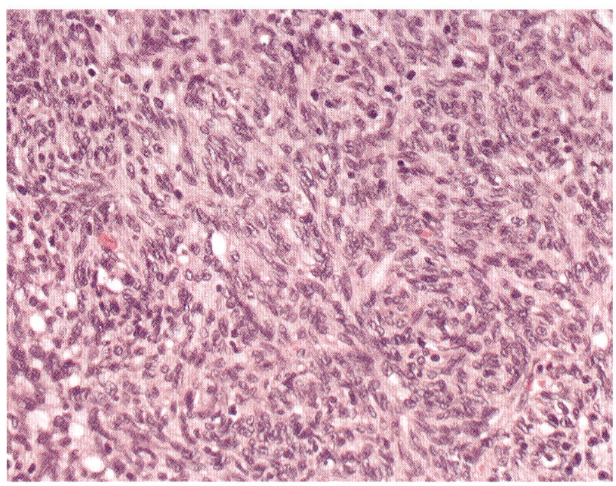

E.

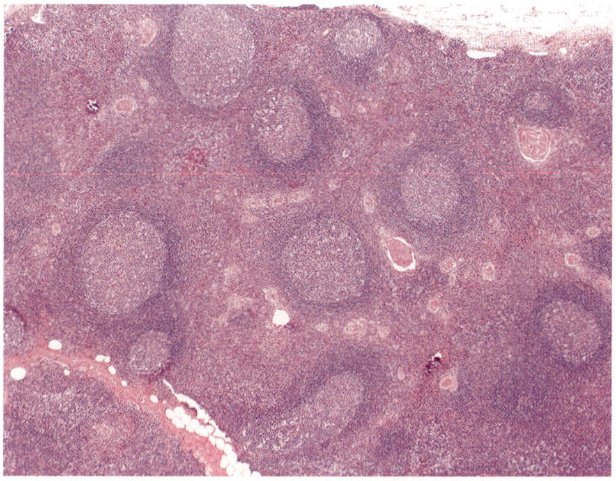

F.

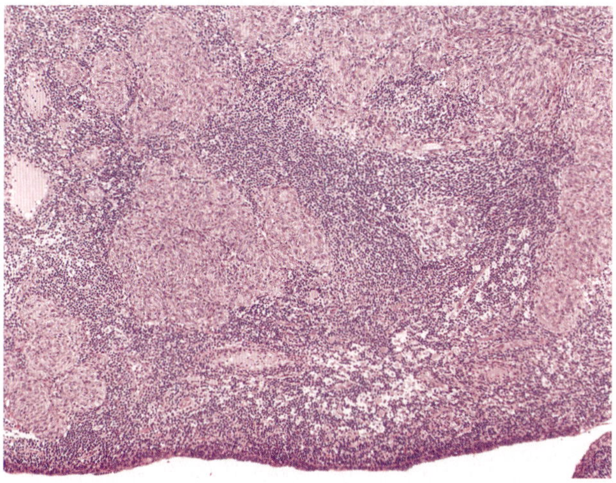

G.

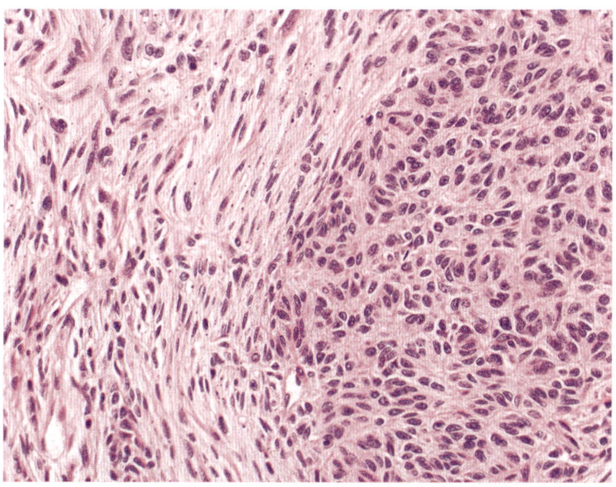

H.

11. A 33-year-old woman with myasthenia gravis undergoes resection of an enlarged thymus. Which of the following features favors lymphocyte-predominant thymoma over thymic hyperplasia?

    A. Effacement of thymic architecture
    B. Fibrous bands separating cellular lobules
    C. Keratin immunoreactivity in an arborizing pattern
    D. Rare lymphoid follicles
    E. All of the above

12. Which of the following is true of "true thymic hyperplasia"?

    A. Associated with myasthenia gravis
    B. Can occur after chemotherapy
    C. Diagnosis by biopsies alone
    D. Follicles encircled by "onionskin" layers of lymphocytes
    E. Weighs the same as the normal thymic gland based on age

13. A mediastinal lesion comes to the pathologist's attention. The patient has fever, anemia, weight loss, and hypergammaglobulinemia. Histologically, the specimen displays the features shown in Figure 1. Which of the following is true regarding this entity?

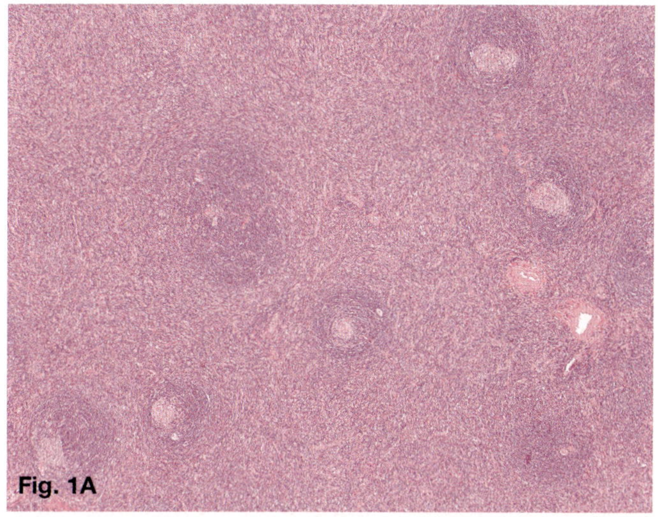

Fig. 1A

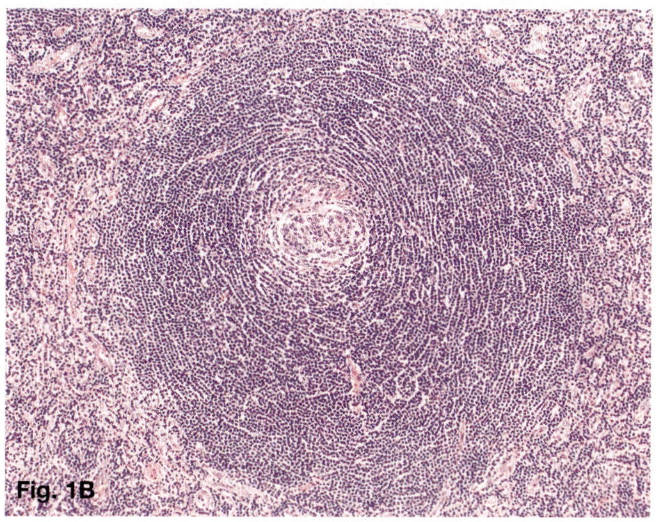

Fig. 1B

    A. It affects both the thymus and lymph nodes.
    B. Lymphocytes are CD5(+), CD20(+), and cyclin-D1(+).
    C. There is prominent interfollicular vascular proliferation.
    D. t(11;14) is the most commonly molecular abnormality.
    E. All of the above are correct.

14. A 33-year-old man presents with a thymic mass and an elevated white blood cell count. A thymic resection shows histologic features highly suggestive of lymphocyte-predominant thymoma, but lymphoblastic lymphoma cannot be ruled out. Which of the following immunostains is most helpful in this differential diagnosis?

A. CD3
B. CD43
C. CD99 (MIC-2)
D. Cytokeratin
E. Terminal deoxynucleotidyl transferase

15. The histologic type of thymoma shown in Figure 1 has a strong resemblance to

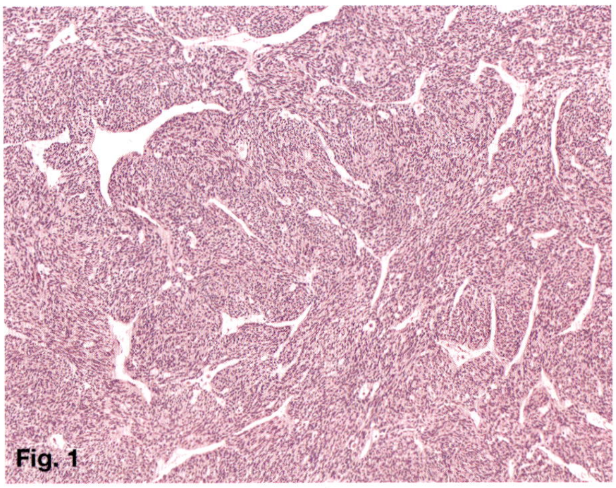
Fig. 1

A. atypical carcinoid.
B. Castleman disease.
C. neurofibroma.
D. schwannoma.
E. solitary fibrous tumor.

16. A 32-year-old male has a cystic mediastinal mass. Figure 1 shows its microscopic appearance. The lesional cells are positive for CD117 and show focal dot-like positivity for AE1/AE3. What is the most likely diagnosis?

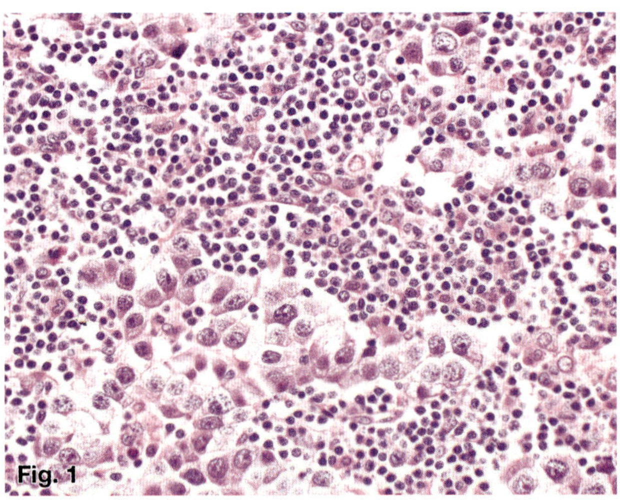
Fig. 1

A. Mature teratoma
B. Micronodular thymoma
C. Seminoma
D. Thymic carcinoma
E. Thymoma, type B1

17. The mediastinal neoplasm depicted in Figure 1 is characterized by

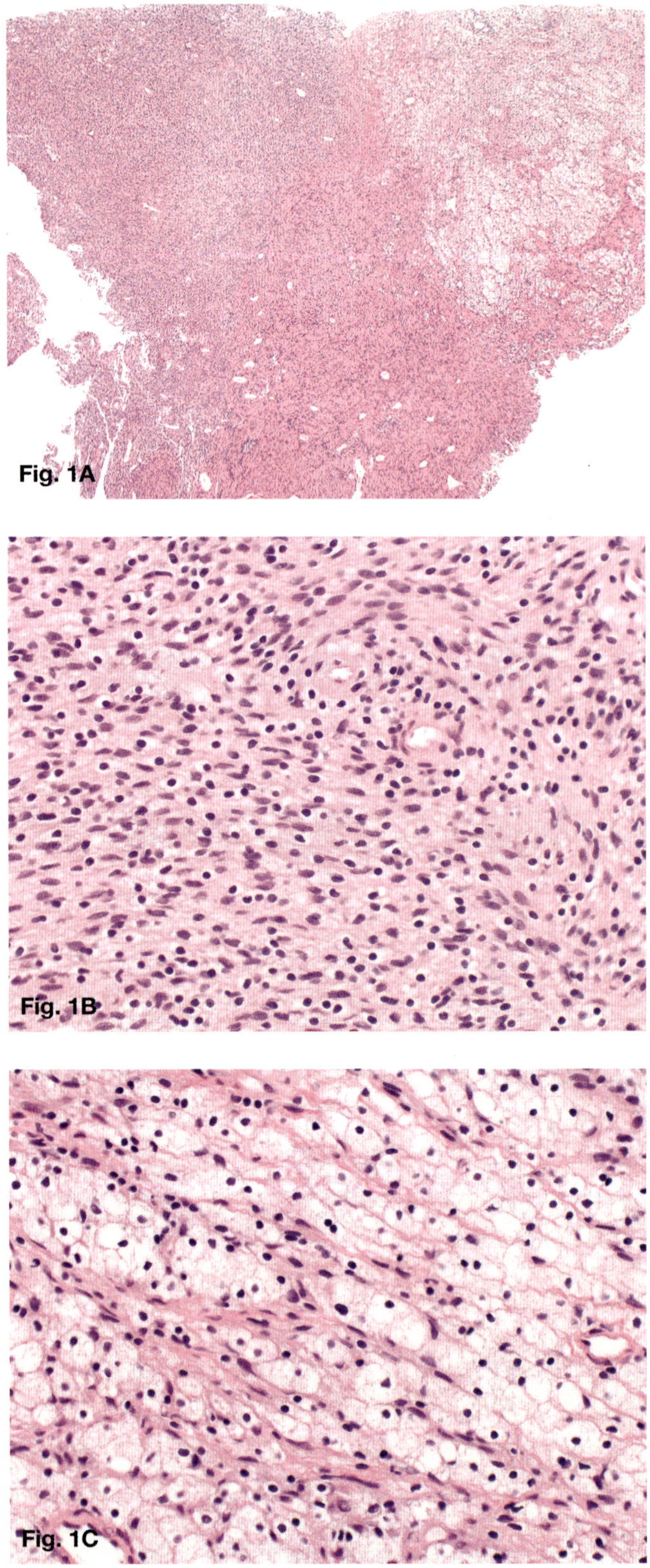
Fig. 1A
Fig. 1B
Fig. 1C

A. early clinical manifestations.
B. lack of a well-defined capsule.
C. large size and prominent regressive changes.
D. poorer prognosis compared to retroperitoneal location.
E. presence of clusters of well-differentiated ganglion cells.

18. A 36-year-old male presents with superior vena cava syndrome. A poorly demarcated mediastinal mass is identified. Histologically, the specimen displays the features shown in Figure 1. The tumor cells are elongated, slender, spindled cells of uniform appearance without cytologic atypia or mitotic activity. What is the molecular abnormality associated with this entity?

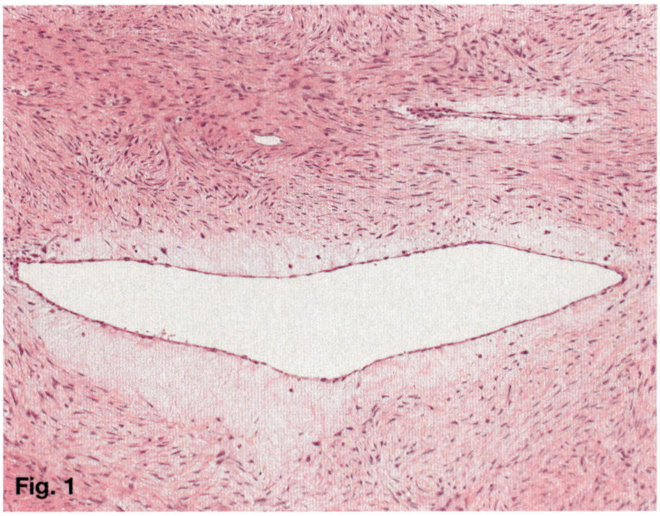
Fig. 1

A. *CTNNB1* mutation
B. *EML4::ALK* fusion
C. *NF1* mutation
D. *STAT6* mutation
E. *YAP1::MAML2* fusion

19. Which of the following is true of mediastinal small cell carcinoma?

A. Commonly present as Cushing syndrome
B. Majority metastatic in nature
C. Most commonly located in the prevascular mediastinum
D. Positive for CAM 5.2 with distinct speckled nuclear expression
E. Primary mediastinal small cell carcinoma negative for TTF-1

20. The microscopic appearance of a posterior mediastinal mass in a 5-year-old child is demonstrated in Figure 1. The differential diagnosis includes neuroblastoma, Ewing sarcoma, and rhabdomyosarcoma. Which of the following would support the diagnosis of Ewing sarcoma and rule out the other tumors?

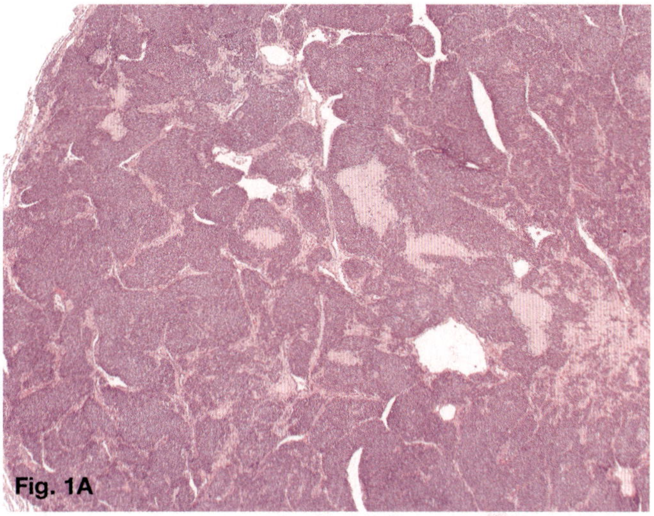
Fig. 1A

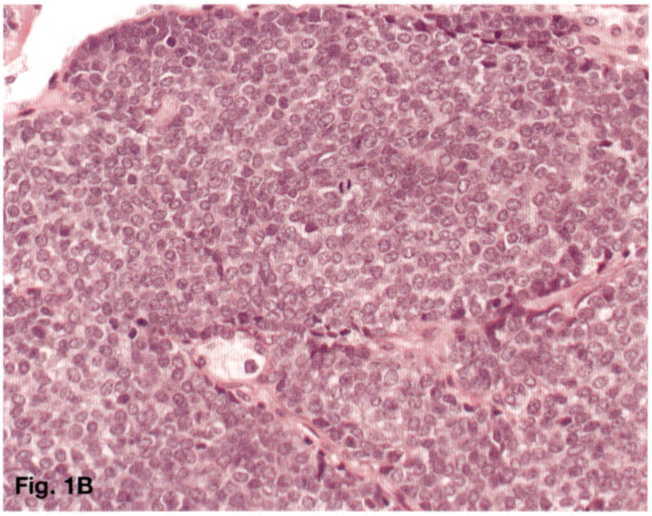
Fig. 1B

A. Cytogenetic evidence of t(11;22)(q24;q12)
B. Immunoreactivity for desmin
C. Immunoreactivity for neuroendocrine markers
D. Ultrastructural demonstration of elongated cell processes
E. Ultrastructural demonstration of intermediate filament skeins

21. A 45-year-old woman undergoes resection of an anterior mediastinal neoplasm located in proximity to the aorticopulmonary roots. Figure 1 shows its microscopic appearance. Which of the following is the most likely diagnosis?

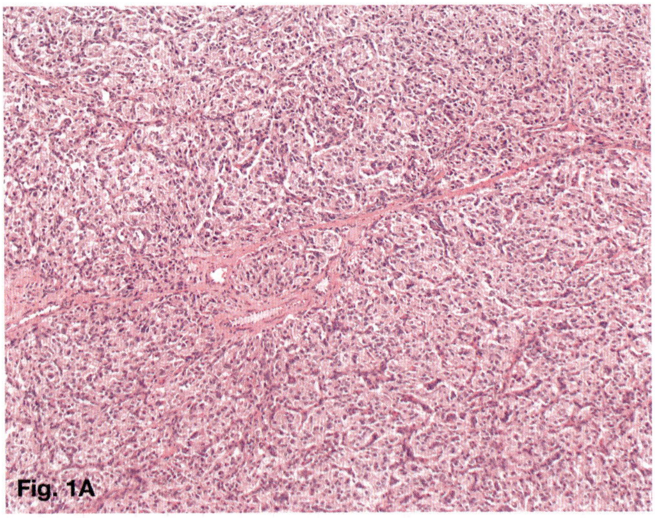


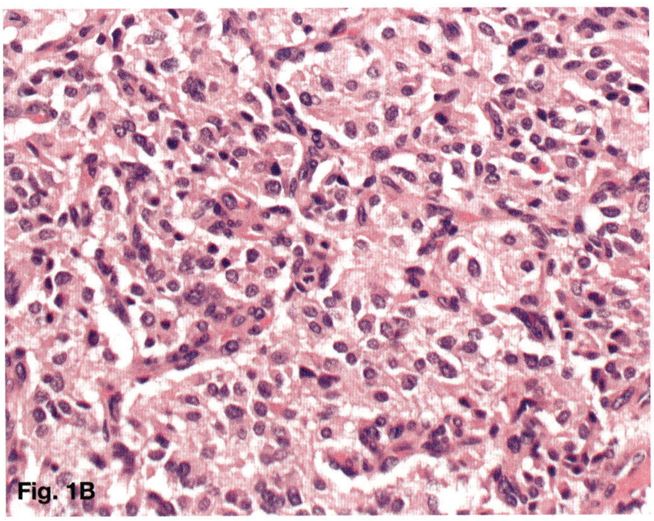


A. Carcinoid
B. Large cell non-Hodgkin lymphoma
C. Paraganglioma
D. Parathyroid carcinoma
E. Seminoma

22. Which of the following is the most important factor to distinguish thymic carcinoma from thymoma?

A. Distorted architecture and desmoplastic stromal reaction
B. Lack of clusters of terminal deoxynucleotidyl transferase (TdT)-positive thymocytes
C. Positive expression of CD5 and CD117
D. Presence of cytologic atypia

23. An adolescent male presents with a cervical tumor around the thyroid. Histologic examination of the tumor reveals a biphasic pattern similar to synovial sarcoma, with a mesenchymal spindle cell component containing scattered mucin-secreting glandular structures as seen in Figure 1. The tumor cells are positive for pan-keratins, CK7 and CD99. Which of the following is the most likely diagnosis?

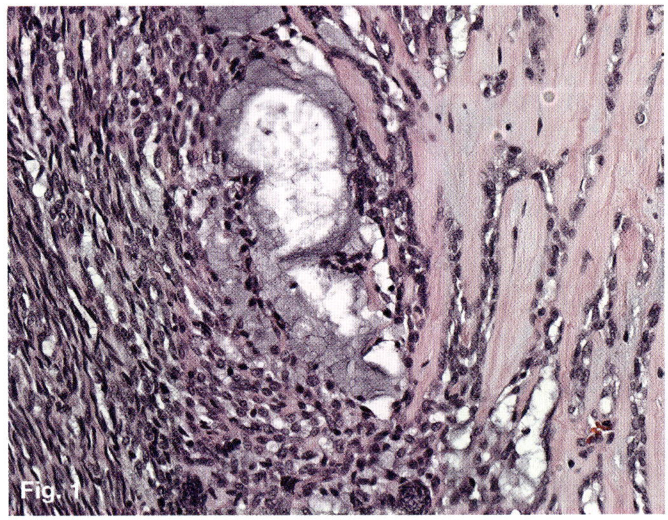


(Courtesy of Dr Todd M. Stevens, University of Alabama at Birmingham, AL.)

A. Carcinoma showing thymus-like differentiation (CASTLE)
B. Ectopic cervical thymoma
C. Ectopic hamartomatous thymoma
D. Spindle epithelial tumor with thymus-like differentiation (SETTLE)
E. Synovial sarcoma

# ANSWERS AND EXPLANATIONS

**1. Correct choice: D.**

Bronchogenic cysts are the most common congenital cysts in the mediastinum and can also be seen in the lung and the pericardium. Whereas intrapulmonary cysts of this type often communicate with large airways, mediastinal bronchogenic cysts are not associated with airways and are often asymptomatic. Histologically, the key feature of bronchogenic cysts is the presence of a respiratory-type (ciliated) pseudostratified columnar epithelium. In addition, the wall usually contains elements of a benign bronchial wall, such as cartilage, seromucinous glands, smooth muscle, and/or nerve.

**2. Correct choice: E.**

Thymic cysts are generally located in the prevascular mediastinum and are often asymptomatic. Thymic cysts might occur in patients with autoimmune disease, such as myasthenia gravis or Sjögren syndrome. Congenital cysts are usually unilocular, while acquired cysts are often multilocular and of inflammatory/postinflammatory nature. Thymic cysts can become very large and have been reported up to 30 cm. Microscopically, thymic cysts characteristically contain thymic gland parenchyma in their walls. In unilocular cysts, the epithelial lining of the cyst cavity is only a few layers in thickness and lacks significant inflammation, hemorrhage, or cholesterol granulomas. Multilocular thymic cysts are often more proliferative in nature and are characterized by multiple layers of simple or multilayered squamous, cuboidal, columnar, ciliated, or glandular epithelium. Abundant lymphocytes, granulation tissue, hemorrhage, clusters of histiocytes, and cholesterol granulomas are often present in the fibrous walls. Multilocular thymic cysts might show pseudoepitheliomatous hyperplasia.

**3. Correct choice: D.**

Pericardial cysts are usually congenital but can be acquired. They are typically located in the right cardiophrenic angle. The gross appearance is that of thin fibrous-walled cyst with smooth internal surfaces. The cyst fluid is serous. Microscopically, pericardial cysts are characterized by thin fibrous tissue that is usually mantled by a single layer of bland mesothelium. Smooth muscle, cartilage, and cholesterol granulomas are lacking.

**4. Correct choice: B.**

Cystic teratoma is the most common primary germ cell tumor of the mediastinum, comprising 43% to 75% of these lesions. Teratomas are neoplasms that contain tissue usually from at least two of the three germinal cell layers, endoderm, ectoderm, and mesoderm. These germ cell tumors can consist of mature tissue only (mature teratoma, 63% of all mediastinal teratomas), immature tissue with or without mature tissue (immature teratomas, 4%), or harbor other malignant components such as other germ cell tumors (mixed germ cell tumor), carcinoma, sarcoma, or hematologic malignancy (33%). The presence of immature neuroepithelium (eg, with rosette-like structures mimicking primitive neural tubules, as seen in the image) justifies a diagnosis of *immature teratoma.*

**5-10. Correct choices: 5 E; 6 A; 7 D; 8 B; 9 H; 10 G.**

Thymoma World Health Organization (WHO) classification is based on the cytologic features of the neoplastic cells: bland elongated to spindled tumor cells in type A, and polygonal tumor cells in type B (Table 1). Type B thymomas are further subtyped depending on the ratio of thymocytes and tumor cells (highest in type B1, lowest in type B3). Thymomas can be morphologically heterogeneous and may be composed of various subtypes. Both combinations of types A and B1 or types A and B2 will result in a designation of type AB thymoma. Rare subtypes of thymomas include micronodular thymoma with lymphoid stroma and metaplastic thymoma. Micronodular thymoma with lymphoid stroma is characterized by nodules and strands of bland-appearing oval to slightly spindled neoplastic cells. Lymphocytes focally form germinal centers and are in between the epithelial cell nodules. Metaplastic thymoma is biphasic composed of a darker component of nests and sheets of neoplastic cells and a paler component of spindled cells.

**11. Correct choice: E.**

Of all patients with myasthenia gravis (MG), 65% will have thymic follicular hyperplasia, 10% a thymoma, and 25% no thymic changes. The listed features help in distinguishing lymphocyte-predominant thymoma (type B1) from thymic follicular hyperplasia. Type B1 thymoma results in effacement of the thymic architecture and has a thick capsule and intersecting fibrous bands within the mass. Diagnostic features of thymic follicular hyperplasia include preserved microscopic cortical and medullary glandular distinction with Hassall corpuscles, together with the presence of multiple well-formed intrathymic lymphoid follicles, which often contain germinal centers, complete with tingible body macrophages. Keratin stain will be helpful as it will highlight a diffuse meshwork of keratin-positive neoplastic cells

**TABLE 1 Morphologic Features of Thymic Epithelial Tumors Based on WHO Classification**

| WHO Subtype | Morphologic Features |
|---|---|
| A | Bland spindled cells, no or only scattered thymocytes |
| A/B | A + B1 or B2 |
| B1 | Scattered neoplastic polygonal epithelial cells in background of thymocytes<br>Medullary islands |
| B2 | **Mixture of neoplastic polygonal epithelial cells and thymocytes;** epithelial cells forming small clusters<br>Medullary islands—rare |
| B3 | Polygonal epithelial cells, no or only scattered thymocytes |

WHO, World Health Organization.

in thymomas, whereas in benign thymic glands, keratin-positive epithelial cells are rather focal and/or scattered single cells.

**12. Correct choice: B.**

True thymic hyperplasia is an enlarged thymic gland of normal morphology that weighs more than the normal weight of the thymic gland based on age or an increased volume. True thymic hyperplasia can occur after chemotherapy as a rebound thymic gland or because of the failure to involute. This diagnosis cannot be established on biopsies because the weight or volume of the entire thymic gland is necessary to establish the diagnosis.

**13. Correct choice: C.**

Castleman disease (CD) in the mediastinum affects lymph nodes and not the thymus itself. Hyaline-vascular type is the most common type encountered in the mediastinum. The main differential diagnosis in the mediastinum is with lymphocyte-predominant thymoma (type B1). CD leads to architectural distortion by aggregates of small, mature lymphoid cells. The most typical microscopic features are (a) proliferation of small blood vessels embedded in a fibrohyaline eosinophilic matrix and (b) follicles encircled by "onionskin" layers of lymphocytes that mimic mantle zones surrounding small atrophic germinal centers.

**14. Correct choice: D.**

Although lymphoblastic lymphoma (LBL) occurs at a younger age than thymoma type B1, radiologic and clinical features overlap to such an extent that morphologic diagnosis is of crucial importance. CD1, CD2, CD3, CD99, *bcl-2*, and terminal deoxynucleotidyl transferase are expressed by lymphocytes in both tumors. Immunohistochemistry for p63 (an intranuclear transcription factor expressed in squamous and transitional epithelium) and cytokeratin immunohistochemistry will highlight a fine meshwork of interconnecting epithelial cells in thymoma, but not in LBL. Immunohistochemical studies are crucial in the differential diagnosis between thymoma and LBL.

**15. Correct choice: E.**

Type A thymomas composed of plump or elongated fusiform cells may be difficult to distinguish from fibrous histiocytomas or solitary fibrous tumors on purely histologic grounds. The image shows a hemangiopericytoma-like pattern. Solitary fibrous tumors and fibrous histiocytomas usually do not have a thick fibrous capsule. Immunohistochemistry is helpful: Type A thymoma will be positive for keratin, whereas solitary fibrous tumor expresses STAT6 and CD34, and benign fibrous histiocytoma may be highlighted by CD34 and/or smooth muscle actin (SMA) stains, which are negative in thymoma.

**16. Correct choice: C.**

Seminomas (termed dysgerminoma in women) are malignant germ cell tumors and are the second most common primary mediastinal germ cell tumors after teratomas. Although mediastinal seminomas immunophenotypically and genetically resemble their gonadal counterparts, there are a few histopathologic features that appear to be unique to the mediastinal location, including induction of thymic epithelial cell hyperplasia and cyst formation. The tumor cells are composed of epithelioid tumor cells characterized by mostly clear or eosinophilic cytoplasm, large round to slightly oval nuclei with a prominent nucleolus, and well-defined cell borders. A high level of suspicion and low threshold for use of immunostains such as OCT4 and CD117 to highlight the seminoma cells is necessary to identify these tumors in a cystic and/or lymphocyte-rich lesion of the thymus.

**17. Correct choice: C.**

Mediastinal schwannomas usually grow to a large size before manifesting clinically. The presence of a capsule is a unique feature compared to schwannomas developing in other sites. The tumor often grows from a large nerve trunk hanging from the nerve "like a pod on a tree branch." Schwannomas have a characteristic *biphasic* arrangement (Antoni A areas, highly cellular, alternating with Antoni B areas, paucicellular and myxoid) and contain eye-catching *Verocay bodies*, as seen in the first picture. Regressive changes are common and include hemorrhage, cystic degeneration, hemosiderin deposition, and vascular wall hyalinization. By the time the tumor is discovered and removed, regressive changes may be so pronounced as to make histologic diagnosis rather difficult (*ancient schwannoma*). The prognosis is excellent.

**18. Correct choice: A.**

Desmoid-type fibromatosis is a poorly demarcated tumefactive proliferation of spindle cells that is centered in the soft tissue and usually invades into surrounding soft tissue. Microscopically, desmoid-type fibromatosis is composed of elongated, slender, spindled cells of uniform appearance growing in long sweeping bundles. There is no nuclear hyperchromasia or cytologic atypia. Mitotic activity is variable but usually low or nonexistent. One of the most characteristic histologic attributes of desmoid-type fibromatosis is numerous venule-sized vessels with thick walls interspersed regularly throughout the mass (as seen in the image). Nuclear β-catenin expression is seen in 70% to 75% of tumors, and 85% of tumors harbor a *CTNNB1* mutation.

**19. Correct choice: B.**

The overwhelming majority of small cell carcinomas that present as mediastinal masses are metastatic in nature, most commonly from the lung. A minority of individuals have paraneoplastic syndrome, such as Cushing syndrome. There is no immunostain specific for thymic origin of small cell carcinomas, and TTF-1 expression can be seen in small cell carcinomas of any origin. Small cell carcinomas show at least dotlike to diffuse staining patterns with keratins such as AE1/AE3 and CAM5.2. Therefore, clinicoradiologic correlation is necessary.

**20. Correct choice: A.**

Neuroblastoma, Ewing sarcoma, and rhabdomyosarcoma may develop in the same mediastinal location, and all occur in children/young adults. H&E (hematoxylin and eosin) morphology alone is usually not specific enough to allow distinguishing between these entities without ancillary tests. Ewing sarcoma and neuroblastoma share immunoreactivity for neuroendocrine markers (synaptophysin, neurofilaments, CD57). Desmin expression and ultrastructural evidence of cytoplasmic masses of actin and myosin intermediate filaments (sometimes forming rudimentary sarcomeres) are found in rhabdomyosarcoma. Elongated filaments can be demonstrated by ultrastructural analysis of neuroblastoma. Demonstration of the characteristic t(11;22) translocation by cytogenetic analysis is the ultimate test supporting a diagnosis of Ewing sarcoma.

**21. Correct choice: C.**

Paraganglioma is rare in the mediastinum (<0.5%), where it includes aorticopulmonary and paravertebral forms. The aorticopulmonary form occurs at an average age of 49 years and more frequently in women, while the paravertebral form is more frequent in men at an average age of 29 years. On low-power examination, one can appreciate the typical nesting arrangement (often referred to as "zellballen"), in which round nests of neoplastic cells are surrounded by delicate fibrovascular septa. Immunohistochemistry confirms the diagnosis: Neoplastic cells within zellballen are immunoreactive for synaptophysin and similar neural markers, whereas sustentacular cells around the zellballen are positive for S100 protein. *Thymic carcinoids* display organoid arrangements and frequent rosettes; artifactual detachment of necrotic "balls" is typical. *Large cell non-Hodgkin lymphoma* is the most frequent lymphoid malignancy in the mediastinum. It is composed of a uniform population of large lymphoid cells with slightly irregular nuclear contours. Interdigitating bands of sclerosis may compartmentalize the tumor in an epithelial-like manner. *Parathyroid carcinoma* may arise in the thymus and manifests with hyperparathyroidism. It consists of polygonal cells arranged in a trabecular or nesting pattern, with uniform round nuclei. The constituent cells are immunoreactive for parathyroid hormone (PTH) and GATA-3, and occasionally for synaptophysin. *Seminoma* is composed of clusters of polygonal cells with clear cytoplasm, open nuclei, and prominent nucleoli, separated by lymphocyte-rich stroma. Tumor cells express CD117 and podoplanin (D2-40).

**22. Correct choice: A.**

The distinction between thymic carcinoma and thymoma can be problematic, particularly on small biopsies. Morphology is most helpful as thymomas show a lobulated architecture with fibrous bands, while thymic carcinomas are characterized by a distorted architecture and desmoplastic stromal reaction. Cytologic atypia can be seen in both. Thymic carcinomas lack clusters of terminal deoxynucleotidyl transferase (TdT)-positive thymocytes; however, the lack of thymocytes is not unique to carcinomas because it also can occur in type A and B3 thymomas. Therefore, the absence of thymocytes is not specific to thymic carcinoma, but their presence is indicative of thymoma. Some studies have suggested that the expression of CD5 and/or CD117 might aid in the distinction of thymic carcinomas from thymomas. Studies comparing B3 thymomas with thymic carcinomas show that CD5, CD117, and monoclonal carcinoembryonic antigen (CEA) are most specific for thymic squamous cell carcinomas, with sensitivities of 67% to 84%, 77% to 90%, and 75%, respectively. Rare B3 thymomas have been reported to express CD5 or CD117. Currently, no immunostain is specific for thymic carcinoma.

**23. Correct choice: D.**

Spindle epithelial tumor with thymus-like differentiation (SETTLE) is a low-grade thyroid neoplasm that affects adolescents and young adults (mostly males). Morphologically, these neoplasms are infiltrative and have a vaguely lobulated architecture with cellular lobules composed of compact bland-appearing spindle cells intersected by thick fibrous bands. The spindle cells are plump and monotonous, with elongated nuclei with fine chromatin. The spindle cells grow in streaming or storiform fascicles that blend in with cuboidal or ciliated respiratory epithelial cells. Immunohistochemistry shows expression of keratin, specifically high-molecular-weight keratins and CK7, and the cells are often also positive for CD99 and CD117. Carcinoma showing thymus-like differentiation (CASTLE) is a thymic carcinoma commonly found in the thyroid gland. Ectopic cervical thymoma occurs almost exclusively in females around the thyroid and is histologically indistinguishable from its thymic counterpart. *Ectopic hamartomatous thymoma* is a benign tumor developing in the supraclavicular/suprasternal regions composed of a spindle cell epithelial component amid anastomosing squamous cell strands.

# 29 Heart

1. Figure 1 shows the explanted heart of a 20-year-old man undergoing orthotopic heart transplantation. With respect to its cause, this cardiac disorder is most frequently

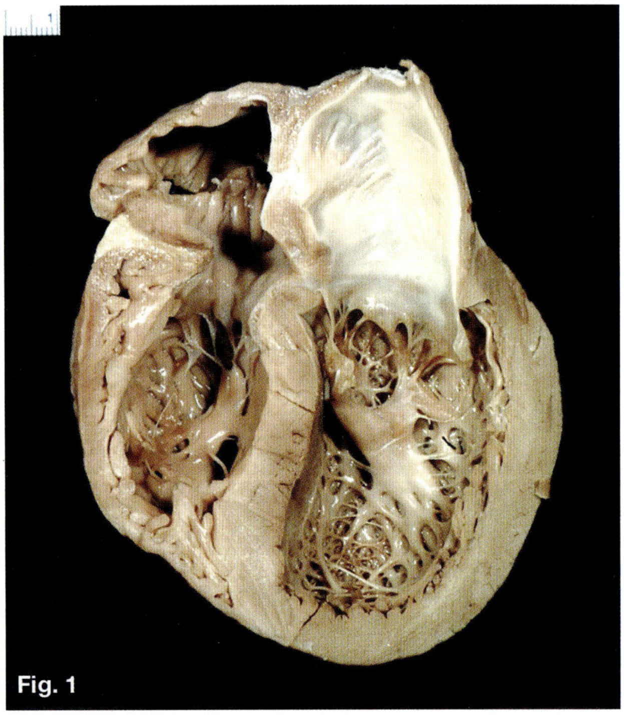

Fig. 1

A. hereditary.
B. idiopathic.
C. infectious.
D. metabolic.
E. toxic.

2. A 24-year-old male suffers from congestive heart failure. He has no history of therapeutic or illicit drug use, valvular disease, or systemic disorder. A myocardial biopsy shows myofibers arranged as seen in Figure 1. Occasional fibers contain basophilic granules. These morphologic features are most consistent with

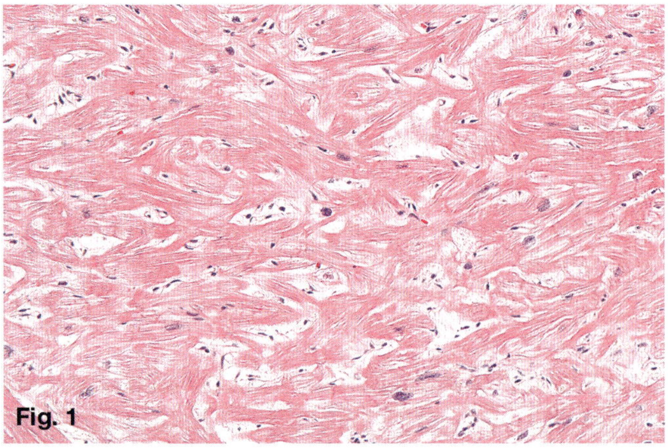

Fig. 1

A. amyloidosis.
B. dilated cardiomyopathy.
C. hypertrophic cardiomyopathy.
D. infiltrative cardiomyopathy.
E. myocarditis.

All figures in this chapter are from Longacre TA, Greenson JK, Hornick JL, Reuter VE, eds. *Mills and Sternberg's Diagnostic Surgical Pathology*. 7th ed. Wolters Kluwer; 2022 except for those noted at the end of this book.

3. A 30-year-old woman presents with skin rash and signs and symptoms of congestive heart failure. Investigations reveal impaired diastolic function with preserved systolic function. An endomyocardial biopsy shows thickened endocardium covered with thrombus, as seen in Figure 1. A mononuclear and eosinophilic infiltrate is seen in the endocardium. Which of the following is the most likely diagnosis?

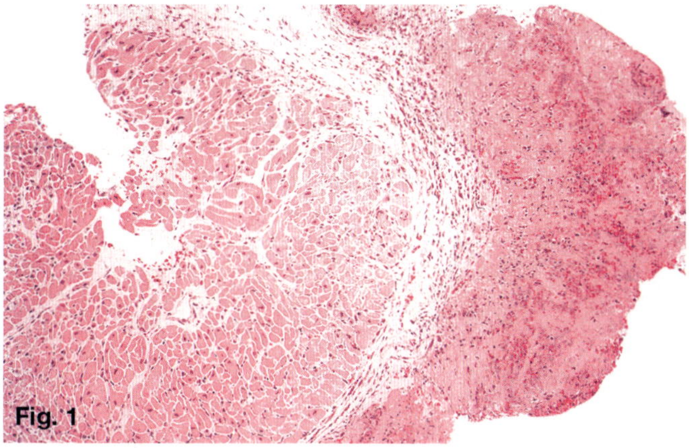


A. Acute rheumatic fever
B. Arrhythmogenic right ventricular cardiomyopathy/dysplasia
C. Endocardial fibroelastosis
D. Idiopathic restrictive cardiomyopathy
E. Loeffler endocarditis

4. An endomyocardial biopsy reveals expansion of the myocardial interstitium by an amorphous pale eosinophilic substance. Congo red staining is positive. Deposition of which of the following is the most frequent cause of this condition?

A. AA type (inflammatory)
B. AL type (immunoglobulin associated)
C. Atrial natriuretic factor
D. β2 Microglobulin
E. Transthyretin protein

5. A patient treated with chemotherapy for a lymphoid malignancy undergoes an endomyocardial biopsy, which is fixed in glutaraldehyde for ultrastructural analysis. The light microscopic appearance of toluidine-stained thick sections and the changes detected by electron microscopy (EM) are shown in Figure 1. Which of the following is the most likely cause of these findings?

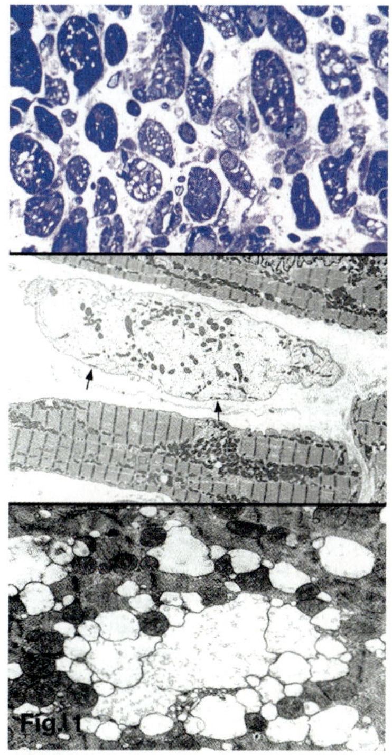


A. Anthracycline toxicity
B. Busulfan toxicity
C. Chloroquine toxicity
D. Cyclophosphamide toxicity
E. Fabry disease

6. In order to make a morphologic diagnosis of definite myocarditis, which of the following changes is required?

A. Eosinophilic infiltration
B. Giant cells
C. Inflammatory infiltration
D. Inflammatory infiltration and fibrosis
E. Inflammatory infiltration and myocyte necrosis

7. A 27-year-old man presents with rapid onset of heart failure and ventricular arrhythmias. An endomyocardial biopsy reveals the changes shown in Figure 1. Which of the following is the most likely diagnosis?

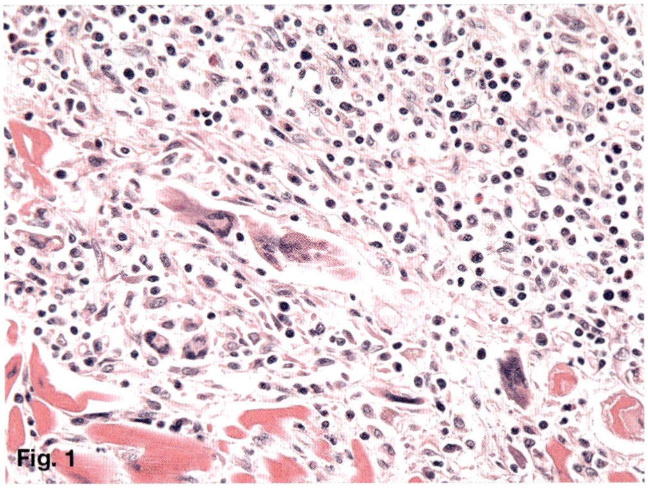

Fig. 1

A. Giant cell myocarditis
B. Hypersensitivity myocarditis
C. Lymphocytic myocarditis
D. Sarcoidosis
E. Trypanosomiasis

8. According to the 2004 revised grading system of the International Society for Heart and Lung Transplantation (ISHLT), an endomyocardial biopsy with a single infiltrate of mononuclear infiltrates distorting the myocardial architecture and associated with myocyte damage is graded as

A. 0 R.
B. 1 R.
C. 2 R.
D. 3 R.

9. Two weeks after cardiac transplantation, an endomyocardial biopsy demonstrates a single well-demarcated, mononuclear infiltrate in a subendocardial location, as shown in Figure 1. Numerous plasma cells are found within the aggregate. Immunostains reveal CD20-positive B lymphocytes and CD21-positive dendritic cells in the core of the lesion, surrounded by a rim of CD3-positive T cells. Which of the following is the most likely morphologic diagnosis?

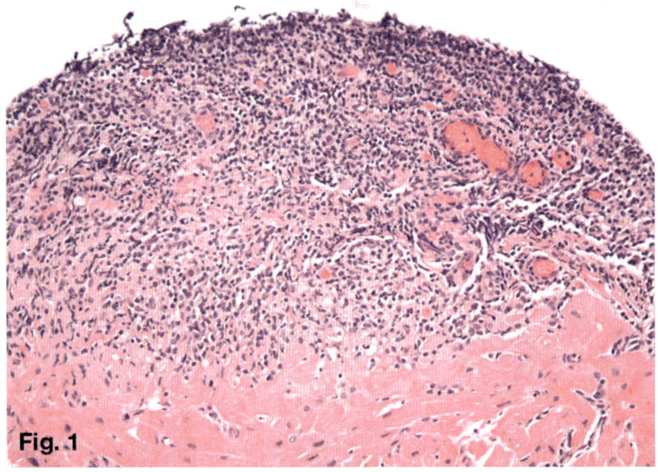

Fig. 1

A. Acute rejection, grade 2
B. Cyclosporin A toxicity
C. Nodular endocardial infiltrate (Quilty effect)
D. Posttransplantation lymphoproliferative disorder
E. Prior biopsy site changes

10. An endomyocardial biopsy of a heart allograft reveals interstitial edema, sparse lymphohistiocytic infiltrates, and swelling of capillary endothelium. The key findings of immunohistochemistry for CD68 and complement component C4d are shown in Figure 1. These findings are typically associated with

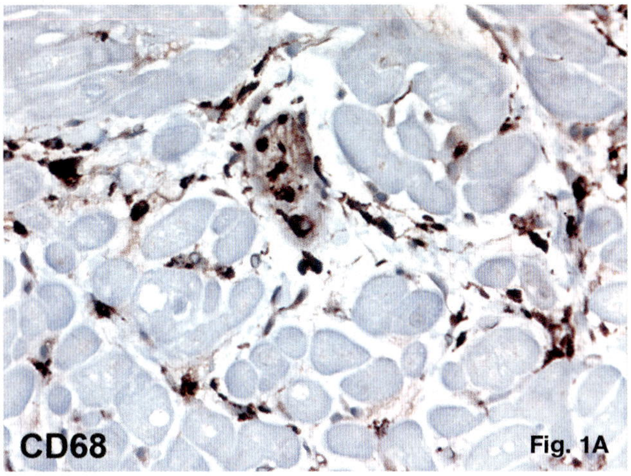


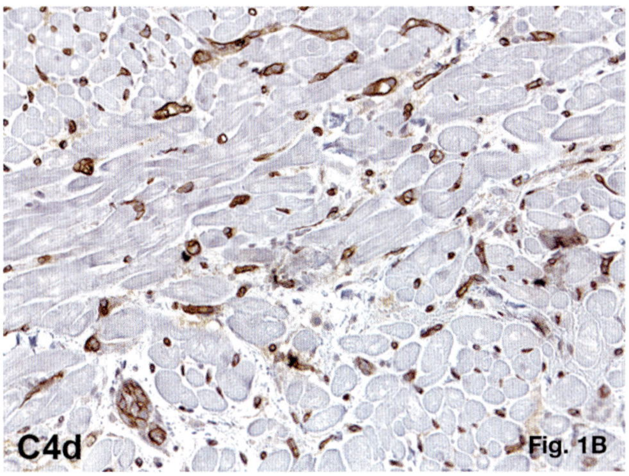


A. acute antibody-mediated rejection.
B. acute cellular rejection.
C. cardiac allograft vasculopathy.
D. posttransplantation lymphoproliferative disorder.
E. transplantation coronary artery disease.

11. Echocardiography reveals a solid mass filling the left atrium in a 44-year-old female with signs and symptoms of mitral valve obstruction. The histologic appearance of the lesion is shown in Figure 1. Which of the following is the most likely diagnosis?

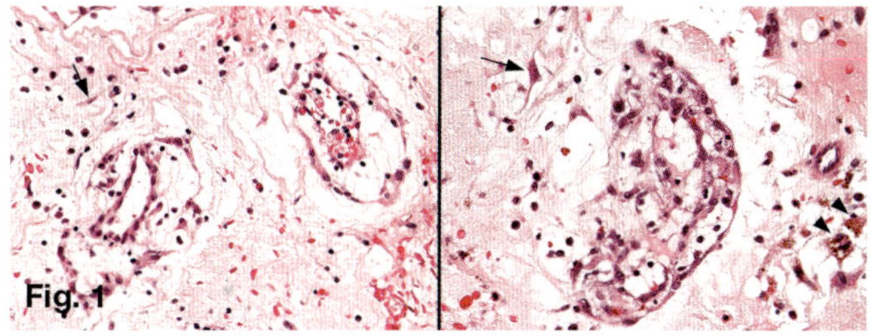


A. Angiosarcoma
B. Fibroma
C. Myxoma
D. Papillary fibroelastoma
E. Rhabdomyoma

12. A surgically resected mitral valve is shown in Figure 1. These changes are most likely the result of

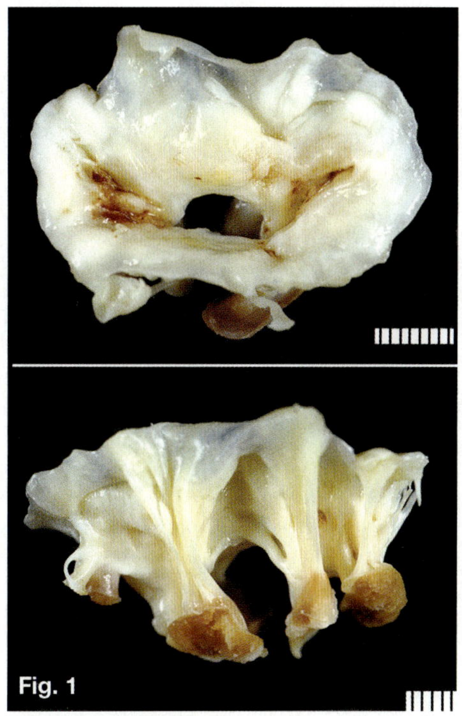


A. infective endocarditis.
B. left ventricular enlargement.
C. myxomatous degeneration.
D. papillary muscle rupture.
E. rheumatic heart disease.

# ANSWERS AND EXPLANATIONS

**1. Correct choice: B.**

Dilated cardiomyopathy (DCM) is the most frequent form of cardiomyopathy and a common indication for heart transplantation. It consists of progressive four-chamber dilatation resulting in thinning of ventricular walls, systolic dysfunction, and reduced ejection fraction. The heart acquires a characteristic globular shape. Mural thrombi and endocardial fibrosis are frequent. Microscopic changes are nonspecific: attenuated and hypertrophic myocytes and interstitial fibrosis. About 50% of cases are idiopathic, while the remaining cases are genetically determined or due to alcohol or metal toxicity or peripartum factors. Approximately 50 different mutations may cause DCM, which involve genes coding for sarcomeric, cytoskeletal, and nuclear proteins or proteins regulating calcium metabolism. The role of endomyocardial biopsy is to rule out conditions that may mimic DCM, including lymphocytic myocarditis, sarcoidosis, hemochromatosis, anthracycline toxicity, and others.

**2. Correct choice: C.**

Hypertrophic cardiomyopathy (HCM) is characterized by asymmetric left ventricular hypertrophy, which results in abnormal thickening of the interventricular septum, decreased compliance, and stenosis of the outflow aortic segment. Histologically, HCM is characterized by disarray of myofibers, myofiber hypertrophy, basophilic degeneration, and interstitial fibrosis. Most cases are due to autosomal dominant mutations of genes coding for sarcomeric proteins with β-myosin heavy chain (*MYH7*) and myosin-binding protein C (*MYBPC3*) accounting for the majority. The cardiomyopathy associated with metabolic and storage disorders (glycogen storage diseases, carnitine deficiency, Fabry disease, etc), mitochondrial disorders (Friedreich ataxia), and syndromic forms of HCM (Noonan and LEOPARD syndromes) is phenotypically identical to the sarcomeric form. Right ventricular endomyocardial biopsies cannot confirm a diagnosis of HCM because myofiber disarray is normally present in the apex and trabecular muscles of the right ventricle, but they are useful to rule out amyloidosis or hemochromatosis, which may manifest similarly.

**3. Correct choice: E.**

Restrictive cardiomyopathies (RCMs) are a heterogeneous group characterized by diastolic dysfunction as a result of thickened or "stiff" ventricles. Two forms of the primary disorder have been described:

- Primary idiopathic RCM: sporadic disorder usually affecting children and occasionally associated with myopathy. There is progression from diastolic dysfunction to systolic heart failure requiring transplantation. Microscopic sections display variable degrees of myocyte hypertrophy and interstitial fibrosis in both distributions.
- Obliterative cardiomyopathy: characterized by endomyocardial abnormalities and consists of an acute form (Loffler endocarditis) and a chronic form (endomyocardial fibrosis). The endocardium of the inflow tracts and apices are covered by thrombus. Eosinophils are admixed with the thrombus and may extend into the underlying myocardium. In the later stages, the number of eosinophils diminishes and the endocardial plaques are thick and fibrotic.

*Arrhythmogenic right ventricular cardiomyopathy/dysplasia* (ARVC/D) is an uncommon disorder characterized by replacement of the right ventricular wall with fibroadipose tissue and manifesting in adolescents and young adults with exercise-induced ventricular arrhythmias and sudden death. The disease is inherited as an autosomal dominant trait and is due to mutations in genes encoding desmosomal proteins such as plakoglobin.

**4. Correct choice: B.**

Cardiac amyloidosis clinically presents with restrictive ventricular dysfunction, congestive heart failure refractory to therapy, low voltage on electrocardiogram (ECG) in spite of myocardial hypertrophy, or cardiac dysfunction in association with plasma cell dyscrasia or chronic inflammatory conditions. The most frequent amyloid depositing in the heart is the *AL* type, derived from immunoglobulin (Ig) light chains and caused by *multiple myeloma* or other plasma cell dyscrasias. AA type of amyloid involves the heart infrequently and causes minor dysfunction. Atrial natriuretic factor is found in *senile atrial amyloidosis*, which is usually an incidental autopsy finding. Amyloid consisting of transthyretin (TTR) is found in two forms: (a) *familial*, an autosomal dominant disease caused by mutations of the gene encoding TTR, which leads to deposition of mutated TTR in peripheral nerves and heart, and (b) *acquired*, in which wild-type TTR accumulates in the heart of middle-aged and older men. β2 microglobulin accumulates in association with *chronic dialysis*.

**5. Correct choice: A.**

The changes seen in the images are typical (although not pathognomonic) of anthracycline (doxorubicin, daunorubicin) toxicity. Evaluation of a posttransplant rejection and the assessment of adriamycin toxicity are the two most common reasons for performing an endomyocardial biopsy (EMB). Anthracycline toxicity may have an early or a late onset. The late-onset form manifests years after administration, with congestive heart failure or arrhythmias. The entire EMB specimen should be fixed in glutaraldehyde for electron microscopy (EM) analysis. Grading anthracycline toxicity by the Billingham criteria requires 10 1-μm plastic-embedded sections stained with toluidine blue. Ultrastructurally, myofibrillar loss with partial or complete loss of fibrils and retention of Z-band remnants (**as noted by arrows**) along the cytoplasmic membrane are more common than the swelling and coalescence of vacuolar change to form sarcotubular distension. *Chloroquine* toxicity produces changes similar to Fabry disease, with vacuolization of the cytoplasm on light microscopy and lamellar myelin bodies (*zebra bodies*) on EM. The *alkylating agents* busulfan and cyclophosphamide cause endomyocardial fibrosis and, respectively, pericarditis/myocarditis.

**6. Correct choice: E.**

Myocarditis was defined as a myocardial process characterized by the presence of both an inflammatory infiltrate and myocyte damage or necrosis not typical of the myocardial damage of ischemic heart disease. In active myocarditis, both inflammation and myocyte damage are present. The composition of the cellular infiltrate delineates the specific type of myocarditis (eg, lymphocytic, eosinophilic, neutrophilic, giant cell, granulomatous, or mixed cell types). Any form of inflammatory infiltrate alone is considered consistent with *borderline* myocarditis.

**7. Correct choice: A.**

The image shows a mixed chronic inflammatory infiltrate characterized by many multinucleated giant cells, which is the histologic hallmark of *idiopathic giant cell myocarditis*, a disorder of unknown etiology that seems to be mediated by abnormal T-cell reactivity. This condition affects young people and carries a dismal prognosis. Death occurs within weeks or months of onset of symptoms, unless aggressive immunosuppression and cardiac transplantation are implemented. The microscopic features consist of regions of diffuse, serpiginous necrosis containing multinucleated giant cells, lymphocytes, histiocytes, and eosinophils in the absence of sarcoid-like granulomas. *Hypersensitivity myocarditis* is usually the result of allergic reactions to medications. *Lymphocytic myocarditis* is caused by viruses, most commonly Coxsackie B virus, echovirus, and adenovirus. Cardiac *sarcoidosis* is characterized by nonnecrotizing granulomas. *Trypanosomiasis* (*Chagas disease*) leads to dilatation of the heart with formation of ventricular aneurysms; endomyocardial biopsy (EMB) is rarely performed in this case.

**8. Correct choice: B.**

Grading of acute cardiac allograft rejection follows the revised International Society for Heart and Lung Transplantation (ISHLT) system. The morphologic changes associated with increasing grades of acute rejection are depicted in the accompanying image.

- Grade 0 R: no mononuclear infiltration or myocyte damage
- Grade 1 R: focal infiltrate without necrosis; diffuse sparse infiltrate with no necrosis; single focus of infiltrate distorting the normal architecture with or without myocyte damage
- 2 R: two or more foci of mononuclear infiltration with myocyte damage
- 3 R: diffuse chronic inflammation and multifocal myocyte damage or diffuse infiltrates including neutrophils and eosinophils associated with myocyte necrosis and, in the most severe cases, edema, hemorrhage, and vasculitis

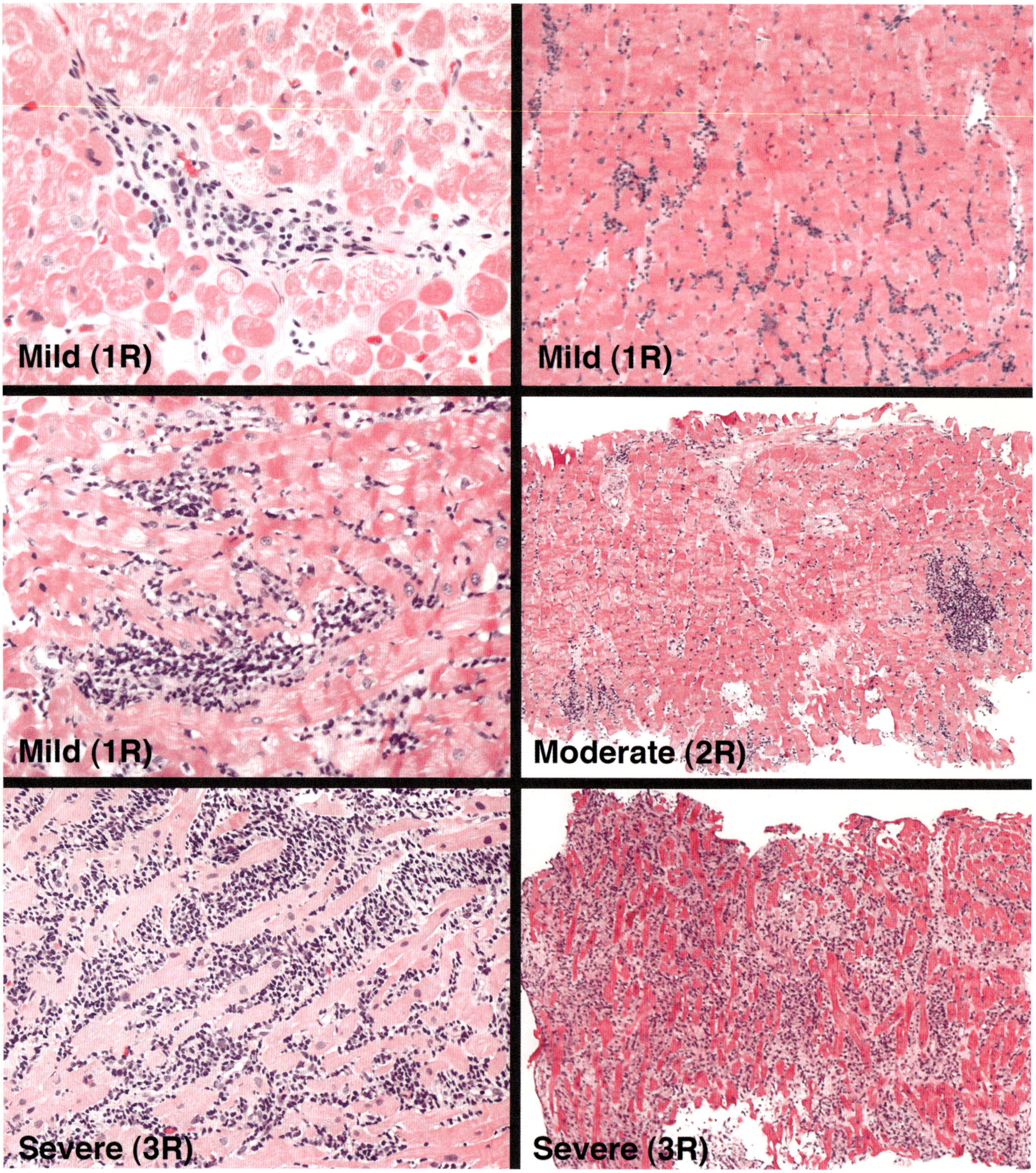
Mild (1R)
Mild (1R)
Mild (1R)
Moderate (2R)
Severe (3R)
Severe (3R)

**9. Correct choice: C.**

Nodular endocardial infiltrate (Quilty effect) is observed in 39% to 74% of endomyocardial biopsies (EMBs) following transplantation. It does not imply rejection and is not due to drug toxicity. Quilty lesions may be confined to the endocardial surface or extend to the adjacent subendocardial myocardium. Myocardial extension can be misinterpreted as acute rejection. Quilty lesions extending into the myocardium is a mimic of grade 2 rejection. Posttransplantation lymphoproliferative disorder is characterized by a lymphoid infiltrate showing prominent atypia and mitotic activity. Prior biopsies lead to healing foci of ischemic injury, which should not be confused with acute rejection.

**10. Correct choice: A.**

Antibody-mediated rejection (AMR; humoral rejection) is characterized by interstitial capillary injury with swollen endothelial cells and intravascular accumulations of macrophages. Vascular thrombi, edema, hemorrhage, and capillary and myocyte necrosis are seen in severe cases. The confirmation requires the demonstration of complement deposition in the tissues. Immunohistochemical evidence of C4d in more than 50% of small vessels is considered diagnostic of AMR. Immunohistochemical demonstration of CD68-positive macrophages within the lumina of at least 10% of the microvasculature is an alternative diagnostic confirmation. *Hyperacute rejection* is a rare but fulminant form of AMR. It is caused by preformed immunoglobulin G (IgG) or IgM, which binds to endothelial cells, leading to complement activation, vascular damage, thrombosis, and myocardial necrosis. Graft failure is extremely rapid and can be appreciated during surgery as the allograft heart becomes edematous and hemorrhagic.

**11. Correct choice: C.**

Cardiac myxoma, the most common primary cardiac tumor, is defined as a benign neoplasm characterized by an abundant mucopolysaccharide matrix and stellate "myxoma" cells. These tumors arise on the endocardial surface of the left atrium adjacent to the foramen ovale in 80% of cases. Grossly, these gelatinous tumors attach by either a broad base or delicate stalk to the endocardium and protrude into the cardiac cavity. Microscopically, the myxoma is composed of spindled or stellate cells with eosinophilic cytoplasm and uniform, round nuclei with inconspicuous nucleoli.

The cellularity can be variable, including foci of increased cellularity, but marked pleomorphism, increased mitotic activity, and abnormal division forms are absent. The degree of myxoid stroma is also variable, and collections of pigment-laden macrophages, calcification or ossification, and extramedullary hematopoietic elements have been reported. The familial form of myxoma is associated with extracardiac anomalies in *Carney syndrome.*

**12. Correct choice: E.**

The image shows commissural fusion, which is highly characteristic of rheumatic heart disease, giving rise to a "fish mouth" appearance (upper panel of the picture), usually associated with fused and shortened chordae tendineae (lower panel). *Myxomatous degeneration* is associated with the ballooning of leaflets and stretching of chordae tendineae. Left ventricular enlargement leads to widening of the annulus and mitral valve insufficiency. Defects in valve leaflets and rupture of chordae tendineae are often the results of infective endocarditis.

# 30 Blood Vessels

1. A Movat-stained section of the thoracic aorta of a 33-year-old man who died in a motor vehicle accident is shown in Figure 1. Which of the following conditions is frequently associated with these microscopic changes?

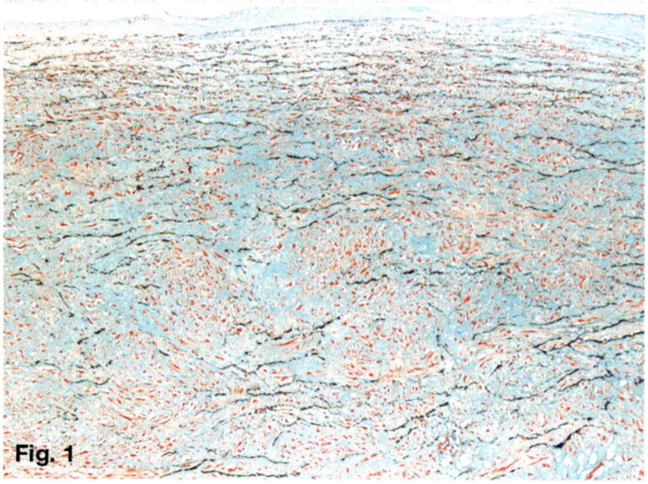

Fig. 1

A. Giant cell arteritis
B. Marfan syndrome
C. Rheumatoid arthritis
D. Syphilis
E. Takayasu disease

2. Which of the following aneurysms is caused by atherosclerotic weakening of the arterial wall?

A. Abdominal aortic aneurysm
B. Aneurysm associated with fibromuscular dysplasia
C. Berry aneurysm
D. Pseudoaneurysm
E. Syphilitic infection

3. A 42-year-old man with a 35 pack-year history presents with sudden low back pain. A computed tomography (CT) scan of the abdomen reveals a fusiform dilatation of the infrarenal aortic segment, with prominent nodular thickening of its wall and adherence of the adjacent structures. Figure 1 demonstrates the typical histologic features of this type of aortic aneurysm. Which of the following is the most likely condition associated with this aortic lesion?

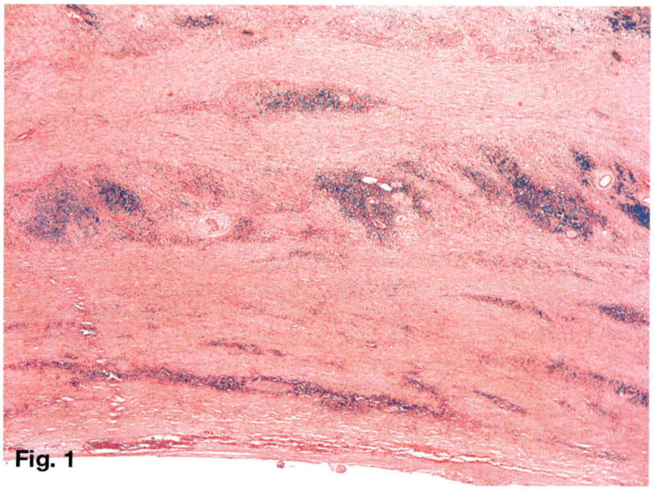

Fig. 1

A. Giant cell arteritis
B. Immunoglobulin G subclass 4 (IgG4)–related disease
C. Kawasaki disease
D. Polyarteritis nodosa
E. Takayasu disease

4. Which of the following forms of vasculitis affects elastic arteries?

A. Eosinophilic granulomatosis with polyangiitis
B. Immunoglobulin A (IgA) vasculitis
C. Kawasaki disease
D. Polyarteritis nodosa
E. Takayasu disease

All figures in this chapter are from Longacre TA, Greenson JK, Hornick JL, Reuter VE, eds. *Mills and Sternberg's Diagnostic Surgical Pathology*. 7th ed. Wolters Kluwer; 2022 except for those noted at the end of this book.

5. A 70-year-old patient presents with temporal headache of acute onset, fever of unknown origin, and a high erythrocyte sedimentation rate. A temporal artery biopsy reveals the changes shown in Figure 1. Elastic stain shows near-total destruction of the internal elastic lamina. Which of the following is true of this entity?

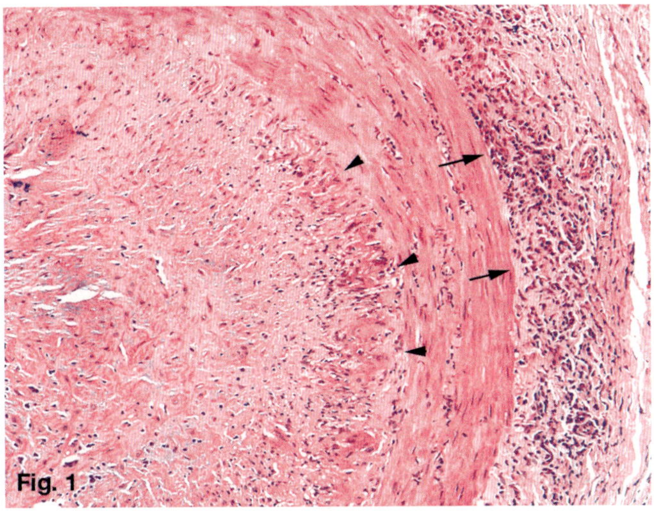


A. Human leukocyte antigen (HLA) polymorphisms is a critical risk factor.
B. It is limited to the temporal and ophthalmic arteries.
C. It predominantly involves the intima.
D. Negative biopsy does rule out the disease.
E. Presence of giant cells is not required for diagnosis.

6. A renal biopsy reveals the histopathologic changes shown in Figure 1, affecting medium-sized arteries. Vascular lesions appear at different stages of evolution. Laboratory tests indicate a recent hepatitis B infection; antineutrophil cytoplasmic antibodies (ANCAs) are negative. These features are most consistent with

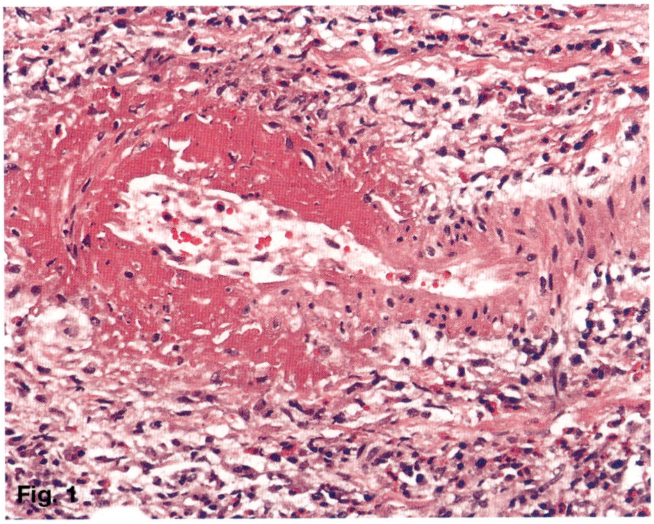


A. eosinophilic granulomatosis with polyangiitis.
B. giant cell arteritis.
C. granulomatosis with polyangiitis.
D. leukocytoclastic cutaneous arteritis.
E. polyarteritis nodosa.

7. A 3-year-old boy is brought to the family physician because of a 7-day history of fever unresponsive to over-the-counter medications, bilateral conjunctivitis, strawberry tongue, palmar and plantar erythema with skin peeling, and swollen cervical lymph nodes. This condition is most likely due to

A. eosinophilic granulomatosis with polyangiitis.
B. granulomatosis with polyangiitis.
C. Kawasaki disease.
D. leukocytoclastic cutaneous arteritis.
E. polyarteritis nodosa.

8. A lung biopsy reveals the lesions shown in Figure 1. The patient has similar lesions in the sinonasal mucosa and kidneys. Laboratory test results are positive for circulating antineutrophil cytoplasmic antibodies (c-ANCA). Which of the following is the most likely diagnosis?

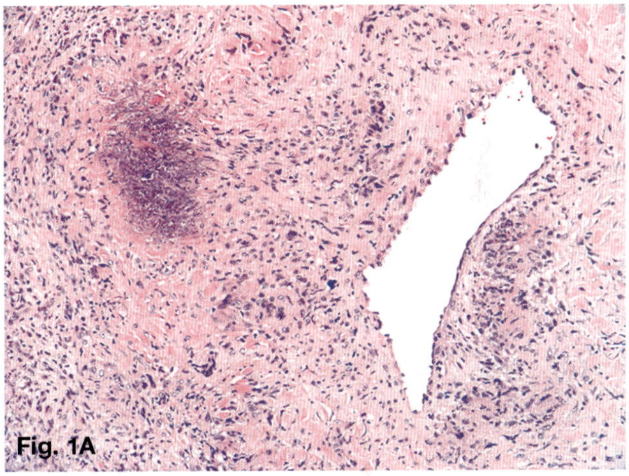


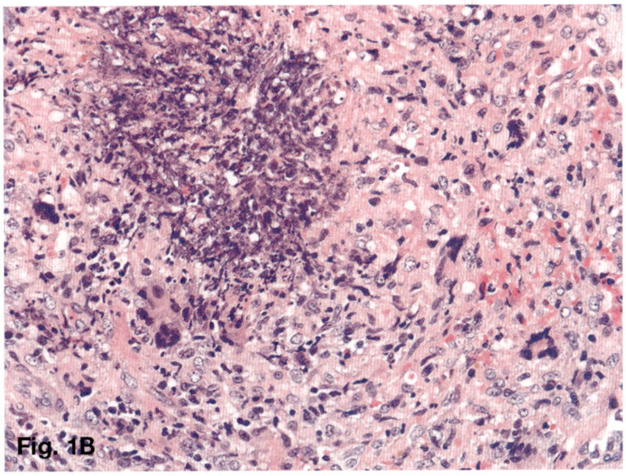


A. Eosinophilic granulomatosis with polyangiitis
B. Granulomatosis with polyangiitis
C. Immune complex vasculitis
D. Immunoglobulin A (IgA) vasculitis
E. Polyarteritis nodosa

9. A 35-year-old woman with a 10-year-history of asthma is evaluated for weight loss, fatigue, gastrointestinal pain, and hemoptysis. Chest x-rays reveal pulmonary infiltrates. The patient is positive for perinuclear antineutrophil cytoplasmic antibodies (p-ANCA). A biopsy of the pulmonary lesions reveals a necrotizing vasculitis associated with the lesion, shown in Figure 1. Which of the following is the most likely diagnosis?

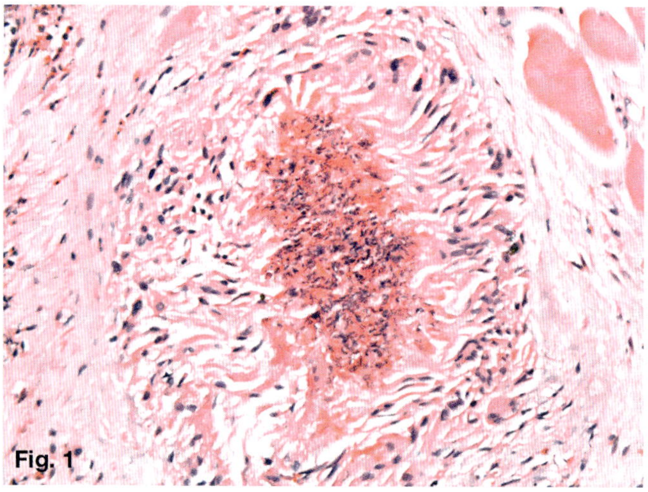


A. Eosinophilic granulomatosis with polyangiitis
B. Granulomatosis with polyangiitis
C. Immunoglobulin A (IgA) vasculitis
D. Microscopic polyangiitis
E. Polyarteritis nodosa

10. A 36-year-old patient with joint hypermobility presents with severe back pain. Computed tomography (CT) imaging shows thoracic aorta dissection as well as aneurysms of the renal and hepatic arteries. On microscopic examination, media is histologically normal without loss of elastic layers and smooth muscle cells. What is the molecular abnormality is associated with this diagnosis?

A. *COL3A1*
B. *FBN1*
C. *JAG1*
D. *NOTCH1*
E. *TSC2*

11. A 50-year-old woman came to the emergency room (ER) with chest pain and breathlessness. Computed tomography (CT) scan showed a left pulmonary artery mass. On microscopy, there is a malignant spindle cell tumor arising from the intimal layer of the pulmonary artery. Immunostains showed that the tumor cells were positive for smooth muscle actin (SMA) and CD31 and negative for AE1/AE3. What is the most common molecular alteration seen in this entity?

A. *EGFR* amplification
B. *ETV6::NTRK3* fusion
C. *EWSR1::FLI1* fusion
D. *MDM2* amplification
E. *MYH11* mutation

# ANSWERS AND EXPLANATIONS

**1. Correct choice: B.**

Marfan syndrome is an autosomal dominant condition caused by mutations in the fibrillin gene. Cardiovascular manifestations include proximal aortic aneurysms, which may lead to aortic dissections and rupture, aortic incompetence; mitral valve prolapse; and peripheral artery aneurysms. The characteristic histologic finding is cystic medial degeneration (CMD), as shown in the image, which is characterized by the loss of elastic lamellae and smooth muscle cells, with replacement by pools of proteoglycan matrix. Keep in mind that only 3% to 5% of patients with aortic aneurysm/dissection have Marfan syndrome. Takayasu disease, giant cell arteritis, and rheumatoid arthritis cause a necrotizing arteritis with macrophage or giant cell reaction. Syphilitic aortitis is due to inflammation of the vasa vasorum with a plasma cell–rich infiltrate.

**2. Correct choice: A.**

The list of choices includes different conditions associated with different types of aneurysms. Abdominal aortic aneurysm (AAA) usually develops in the infrarenal portion of the descending aorta and is caused by severe calcific atherosclerosis leading to disruption of the arterial elastic laminae. Atherosclerosis alone is probably not sufficient to explain the pathogenesis of AAA; genetic factors, smoking, White population, hypertension, and elevated circulating matrix metalloproteinases are suspected predisposing conditions. A similar process occurs in the aneurysm developing in the basilar artery in the brain (*fusiform aneurysm*). *Pseudoaneurysms* (also called *traumatic aneurysms*) are due to trauma and result from development of a false arterial wall around a hematoma. *Berry aneurysms* presumably result from congenital defects in the internal elastic lamina and involve arteries in the circle of Willis at the point of bifurcation. *Syphilitic* infection of the ascending aorta causes inflammation of the vasa vasorum, with subsequent necrosis of the aortic media and development of a usually very large aneurysm.

**3. Correct choice: B.**

Inflammatory aortic aneurysm is a variant of abdominal aortic aneurysm (AAA) (~10%). The purported etiologies include autoimmune disease, and immunoglobulin G subclass 4 (IgG4)–related disease. Grossly, there is marked thickening of the aneurysm wall, fibrosis of the adjacent retroperitoneum, and adherence of the adjacent structures to the anterior aneurysm wall. Histologically, there is expansion of the adventitia with fibrosis, lymphocytes, and plasma cells infiltration.

**4. Correct choice: E.**

Takayasu disease (TD) is a necrotizing vasculitis that involves the aorta and branch vessels and usually resulting in aortic root dilatation and valvular insufficiency. TD ranges in age from 20 to more than 80 years, has no gender predilection, while in a subset of patients (women <50 of age), the vasculitis extends to peripheral arteries in a diffuse manner, leading to stenosis. Grossly, the intima looks wrinkled (*tree-barking* appearance similar to syphilitic aortitis) and the wall thickened. Histologically, there is medial necrosis surrounded by multinucleated giant cells. TD comes to the pathologist's attention when aortic root biopsies are taken during aortic aneurysm repair.

**5. Correct choice: B.**

Giant cell arteritis (GCA) is a granulomatous inflammation (**as noted by arrows and arrowheads**) of medium- to large-sized vessels and manifests with fever of unknown origin in older patients. Advanced age (patients ≥50 years) is a critical risk factor. GCA classically involves cranial arteries such as the temporal artery and the ophthalmic artery but can also involve arteries outside the head, most commonly the aorta but also the carotid, subclavian, axillary, iliac, and femoral arteries. Histologic features include intimal thickening and granulomatous inflammation, including lymphocytes and giant cells, often in close proximity to a fragmented elastic lamina. Giant cells are frequently absent and not required for diagnosis. The pathologic changes may be patchy, and, therefore, biopsy segments of the temporal artery should be as large as possible. Furthermore, multiple levels should be examined histologically. Large vessel involvement may result in complications of aortic dissection, aortic aneurysm, and large artery stenosis.

Life-threatening complications such as acute dissection, rupture, and congestive heart failure may present as late features.

**6. Correct choice: E.**

Polyarteritis nodosa (PAN) is a primary systemic necrotizing vasculitis predominantly targeting medium-sized muscular arteries. The skin, kidneys, heart, gastrointestinal (GI) tract, and joints are most frequently involved, but renal pathology is the most important source of morbidity and mortality. Transmural inflammation, fibrinoid necrosis, thrombosis, and scarring are found at different stages in different vessels or within the same vessel. PAN derives its name from the nodularity imparted by alternating dilatations and stenotic segments (fibrinoid necrosis with pseudoaneurysm formation as shown in the image). Antineutrophil cytoplasmic antibodies (ANCAs) are not present in classic PAN.

**7. Correct choice: C.**

Kawasaki disease (KD) is a necrotizing vasculitis affecting muscular arteries at various sites, including coronary arteries. It affects children younger than 5 years. The diagnosis is made clinically. KD is suspected when a child presents with fever lasting longer than 4 days plus four of the following features: bilateral conjunctivitis, red and swollen tongue (strawberry tongue), erythema of palms and soles, skin peeling, and enlarged lymph nodes (usually cervical). TD needs urgent treatment to prevent cardiac complications (infarct and arrhythmias).

**8. Correct choice: B.**

Granulomatosis with polyangiitis (GPA) is a necrotizing vasculitis that involves small arteries, arterioles, capillaries, and venules. Necrotizing granulomas are also found in the parenchyma of affected organs, as seen in the image. It is strongly associated with circulating *antineutrophil cytoplasmic antibodies* (ANCA), which usually are of the *cytoplasmic* type (c-ANCA). These are autoantibodies directed to *proteinase 3*, an enzyme present in cytoplasmic granules. Histologically, GPA vasculitis is indistinguishable from that of PAN, but the triad of organ involvement (lungs, sinonasal region, and kidneys) is highly characteristic of GOA.

**9. Correct choice: A.**

Eosinophilic granulomatosis with polyangiitis (EGPA) is defined as necrotizing granulomatous inflammation that is rich in eosinophils, often with involvement of the respiratory tract. EGPA is diagnosed if at least four of the following features are demonstrated: (1) asthma, (2) blood eosinophilia (at least 10% of white blood cells [WBCs]), (3) paranasal sinusitis, (4) nonfixed (transient) pulmonary infiltrates, (5) histologic evidence of vasculitis with extravascular eosinophils, and (6) mononeuritis multiplex or polyneuropathy. The image shows eosinophilic granuloma, which is the histopathologic hallmark of EGPA. Approximately 40% of patients have circulating antineutrophil cytoplasmic antibodies (ANCA), usually perinuclear antineutrophil cytoplasmic antibodies (p-ANCA).

**10. Correct choice: A.**

Elhers-Danlos syndrome (EDS) type IV, the vascular type, results from mutations in the gene for type III procollagen (*COL3A1*). It is characterized by generalized joint hypermobility and related osteoarticular complications, dermal dysplasia, and vascular fragility. Affected patients are at risk for arterial, bowel, and uterine rupture. Most lesions occur in the thoracic or abdominal aorta, and/or its proximal branches such as the renal, hepatic, splenic, and iliac arteries, and especially prone to aneurysms, dissections, and rupture. In many cases of EDS, the media is histologically normal and rupture and pseudoaneurysm formation are in an otherwise apparently normal vessel.

**11. Correct choice: D.**

Sarcomas of the pulmonary artery are usually divided into mural and intimal sarcomas. The mural sarcomas are typically leiomyosarcomas that develop from the smooth muscle cells of large veins. Intimal sarcomas are generally intraluminal tumors that cause symptoms that mimic those of pulmonary embolism. The histologic examination usually shows a poorly differentiated malignant spindle or epithelioid cell tumor with varying degrees of atypia. Routine immunohistochemical staining shows expression of vimentin, desmin, and smooth muscle actin, and an endothelial cell marker such as CD31 might be expressed. *MDM2* gene amplification is most important for diagnosis.

# 31 Esophagus

1. A patient undergoes endoscopic examination for the evaluation of gastroesophageal reflux disease (GERD). The distal esophagus was biopsied for histologic evaluation. Which of the following is the most sensitive histologic feature for the diagnosis of reflux esophagitis?

   A. Epithelial hyperplasia
   B. Intercellular edema
   C. Intraepithelial eosinophils
   D. Intraepithelial neutrophils
   E. Mucosal ulceration

2. A patient undergoes endoscopic examination for the evaluation of generalized abdominal pain. The mucosa of the distal esophagus is hyperemic with erosions and irregular Z-line. Biopsies from this area reveal a few scattered intraepithelial eosinophils and lymphocytes, basal layer hyperplasia, and lamina propria papillae elongation. What is the most likely diagnosis?

   A. Barrett esophagus
   B. Candida esophagitis
   C. Eosinophilic esophagitis
   D. Lymphocytic esophagitis
   E. Reflux esophagitis

3. A patient with a recent heart transplant presents with odynophagia. On endoscopic examination, scattered erosions are seen in the distal esophagus. A biopsy from the distal esophagus is performed (see Figure 1). What is the diagnosis?

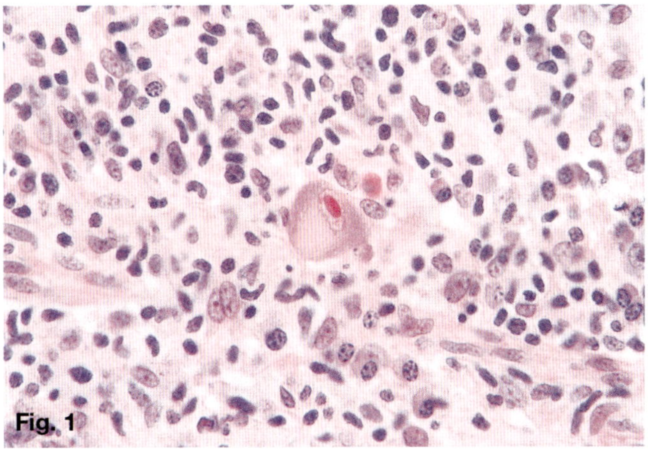

Fig. 1

   A. Cytomegalovirus (CMV) esophagitis
   B. Fungal esophagitis
   C. Herpes simplex virus (HSV) esophagitis
   D. No significant abnormality
   E. Reflux esophagitis

4. A patient with long-standing gastroesophageal reflux disease (GERD) undergoes surveillance endoscopy. On endoscopy, the distal esophagus shows an irregular Z-line and a 2.0-cm pink salmon-colored mucosal tongue. The histology on the biopsy of the distal esophagus shows fragments of squamous and columnar mucosa. The squamous mucosa shows a few scattered intraepithelial lymphocytes. The columnar mucosa shows increased lamina propria plasma cells and lymphocytes and pancreatic acinar metaplasia. What is the most likely diagnosis?

   A. Barrett esophagus
   B. Chronic gastritis
   C. Lymphocytic esophagitis
   D. No significant abnormality
   E. Reflux esophagitis

All figures in this chapter are from Longacre TA, Greenson JK, Hornick JL, Reuter VE, eds. *Mills and Sternberg's Diagnostic Surgical Pathology.* 7th ed. Wolters Kluwer; 2022 except for those noted at the end of this book.

5. Along with the endoscopic finding of a "salmon-colored" tongue in the distal esophagus, which of the following histologic changes is needed to diagnose Barrett esophagus?

   A. Antral-type glands
   B. Cardia-type glands
   C. Goblet cells
   D. Oxyntic glands
   E. Pancreatic acinar metaplasia

6. A histologic section from the mid esophagus of a 45-year-old female with dysphagia shows basal layer hyperplasia, hyperkeratosis, and intraepithelial eosinophils numbering up to 35 in a single high-power field. What is the diagnosis and the most common endoscopic finding?

   A. Eosinophilic esophagitis; "feline" rings and furrows
   B. Eosinophilic esophagitis; salmon-colored patches
   C. Fungal esophagitis; large white plaques
   D. Reflux esophagitis; longitudinal mucosal tears
   E. Reflux esophagitis; mucosa erythema and small ulcers

7. A 55-year-old male with a long-standing history of Barrett esophagus undergoes surveillance endoscopy. Figure 1 is the histologic section of a biopsy taken at 40 cm from the incisors. What is the appropriate diagnosis?

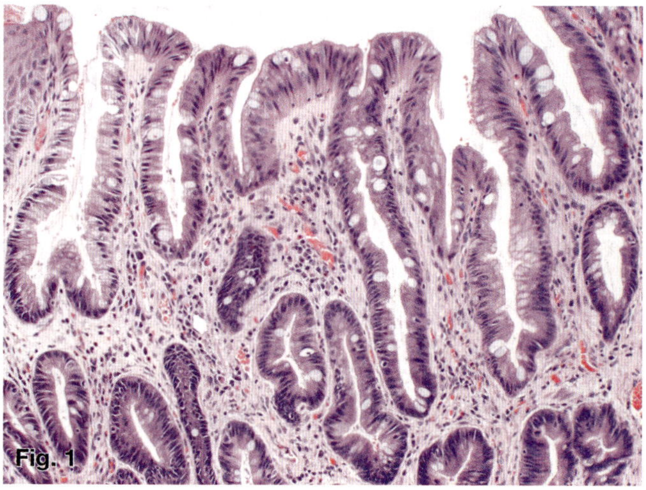

Fig. 1

   A. High-grade dysplasia
   B. Indefinite for dysplasia
   C. Intramucosal adenocarcinoma
   D. Low-grade dysplasia
   E. Negative for dysplasia

8. A 55-year-old male with a long-standing history of Barrett esophagus undergoes surveillance endoscopy. Figure 1 is the histologic section of a biopsy taken at 38 cm from the incisors. What is the appropriate diagnosis?

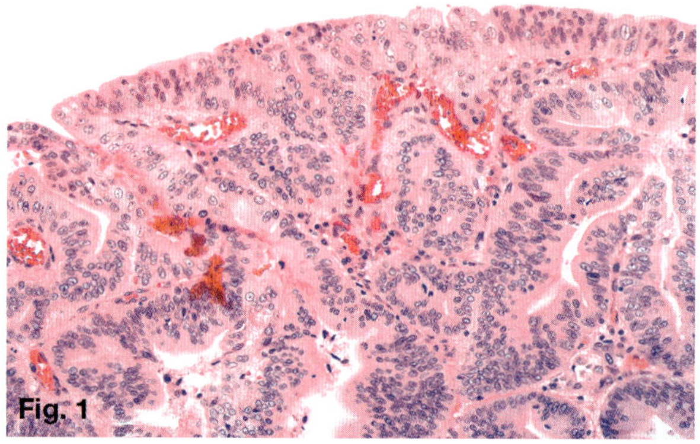

Fig. 1

   A. High-grade dysplasia
   B. Indefinite for dysplasia
   C. Intramucosal adenocarcinoma
   D. Low-grade dysplasia
   E. Negative for dysplasia

9. A 0.5-cm nodule is found in the esophagus of a 45-year-old female with gastroesophageal reflux disease (GERD). Figure 1 is the histologic section of the lesion. What is the diagnosis?

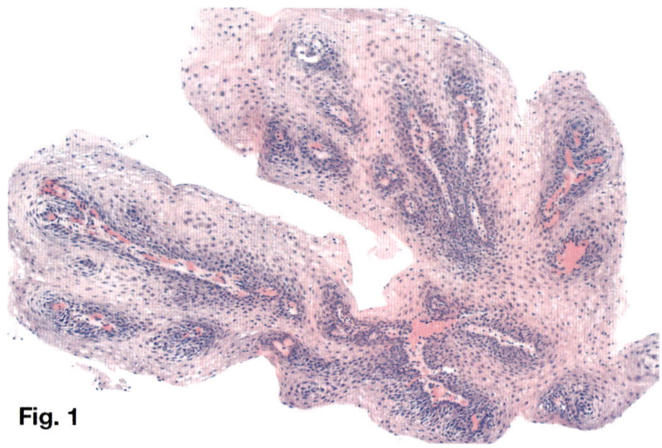

Fig. 1

   A. Condyloma
   B. Fibrovascular polyp
   C. Inflammatory fibroid polyp
   D. Squamous papilloma
   E. Verrucous carcinoma

10. Which of the following is the greatest risk factor for esophageal squamous cell carcinoma in the US population?

    A. Gastroesophageal reflux disease
    B. Human papillomavirus
    C. Ingestion of hot beverages
    D. Nitrosamines rich foods
    E. Tobacco

11. A 60-year-old male undergoes an endoscopy procedure. A 1.5-cm submucosal nodule is identified in the esophagus. Figure 1 is the histologic section of the lesion. What is the diagnosis?

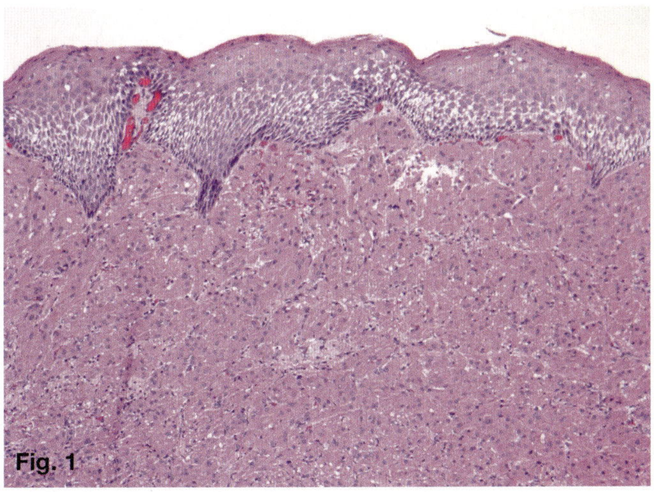

Fig. 1

    A. Glomus tumor
    B. Granular cell tumor
    C. Leiomyoma
    D. Low-grade squamous dysplasia
    E. Squamous cell carcinoma

12. A 62-year-old woman presents with dysphagia. Endoscopy shows narrowing of the distal esophageal lumen. A segmental esophagectomy is performed. Histologic sections show extensive ganglion cell loss in the myenteric plexus, which is additionally infiltrated by inflammatory infiltrate composed predominantly of cytotoxic T cells. What is the diagnosis?

    A. Achalasia
    B. Idiopathic muscular hypertrophy
    C. Neurofibroma
    D. Schwannoma
    E. Systemic sclerosis

13. A 62-year-old female presents with dysphagia. On endoscopy, the distal esophagus was erythematous and friable. Biopsy from this area was taken and histologic features shown in Figure 1. What is the diagnosis?

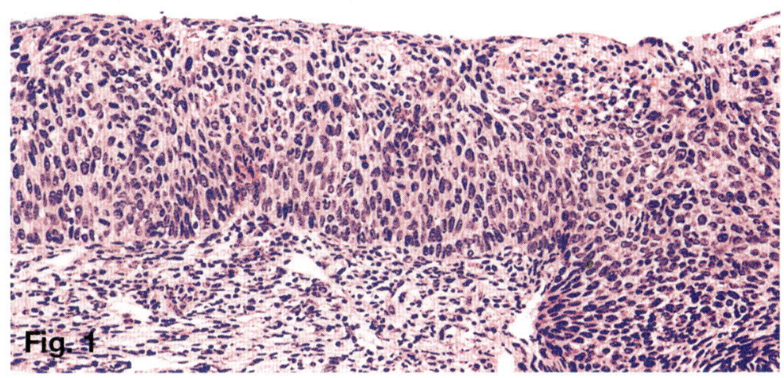

Fig. 1

    A. High-grade squamous dysplasia
    B. Lichen planus
    C. Low-grade squamous dysplasia
    D. Lymphocytic esophagitis
    E. Squamous cell carcinoma

# ANSWERS AND EXPLANATIONS

**1. Correct choice: A.**

Epithelial hyperplasia is the most sensitive diagnostic feature for reflux esophagitis. It is composed of two elements. The first is basal zone hyperplasia, which is characterized as a basal zone exceeding 15% of the total epithelial thickness. The second is elongation of the lamina propria papillae, which is defined as papillae lengthening greater than two-thirds of the epithelial thickness (see Table 1).

**TABLE 1 Histologic Features in Gastroesophageal Reflux Disease**

| Feature | Diagnostic Sensitivity (%) | Comments and Differential Considerations |
|---|---|---|
| Epithelial mucosal injury<br>Basal zone hyperplasia, >15%<br>Elongation of papillae, >67% | 60-90 | Associated with capillary congestion and ultimately mucosal erosion<br>Normally one to four cells thick<br>Exclude tangential cut |
| Dilated intercellular spaces, intercellular edema (spongiosis) | | Exclude artifactual cell separation at edges of biopsy; less prominent with PPI use |
| Intraepithelial eosinophils | 20-40 | Other causes of low-grade epithelial insult including infectious esophagitis, pill-induced esophagitis, eosinophilic esophagitis |
| Intraepithelial neutrophils | 10-30 | |
| Intraepithelial lymphocytes | | "Squiggle cells"; exclude lymphocytic esophagitis |
| Mucosal erosion/ulceration | 10-40 | Infectious esophagitis, pill-induced esophagitis |
| Inflammation of cardiac-type mucosa | | Often mild with eosinophils and few neutrophils, exclude *Helicobacter pylori* gastritis |

PPI, proton pump inhibitor.

**2. Correct choice: E.**

The diagnosis of gastroesophageal reflux disease (GERD) rests on clinicopathologic correlation. The most common findings in reflux esophagitis are epithelial hyperplasia as defined as basal layer hyperplasia (basal layer >15% of the total epithelial thickness) and elongation of the lamina propria papillae (>2/3 into the total epithelial thickness), and intraepithelial eosinophilic infiltration. In addition, other reactive changes can be seen, such as parakeratosis, ballooned squamous cells, and spongiosis. The differential diagnosis includes infectious esophagitis and pill esophagitis. Infectious esophagitis, especially fungal esophagitis, presents with significant intraepithelial neutrophils with superficial neutrophilic microabscesses. Eosinophilic esophagitis is usually found to affect the upper esophagus, and histologically, requires 15 or more intraepithelial lymphocytes in a single high-power field.

**3. Correct choice: A.**

In the bottom right quadrant, the picture shows enlarged endothelial cells with nucleomegaly and cytoplasmic amphophilic inclusions that contain eosinophilic granules, characteristic of cytomegalovirus (CMV) infection. CMV infects endothelial cells and glandular epithelium but not squamous cells. The main pathogens that cause infectious esophagitis are fungal, CMV, and herpes simplex virus (HSV). These infections are more frequent in patients who are immunocompromised. In patients who are immunocompromised, there may not always be an associated inflammatory infiltrate.

**4. Correct choice: D.**

This is a normal variant histology in the gastroesophageal junction (GEJ). Foci of pancreatic acinar cells are a common finding at the GEJ in approximately 20% of unselected individuals. This represents an incidental, likely congenital, occurrence without clinical significance or association with reflux disease. Many adult patients have metaplastic cardiac-type mucosa in the distal esophagus (up to 2-3 cm proximal to the GEJ), which can also appear as pink patches on endoscopy. This finding alone does not provide histologic support for gastroesophageal reflux disease (GERD). Distal esophageal biopsies often show inflamed cardia-type mucosa. Without the presence of intestinal metaplasia, this is also not diagnostic of Barrett esophagus.

**5. Correct choice: C.**

For the definitive diagnosis of Barrett esophagus, both endoscopic and histologic findings must be met. On endoscopy, there must be findings in support of glandular metaplasia, which is present as pink patches or "salmon-colored" tongues of velvety glandular mucosa in the distal esophagus, extending 1 cm or more from the gastroesophageal junction (GEJ). On histology, there must be goblet cells, which are also known as intestinal metaplasia, present in a background of columnar metaplasia.

**6. Correct choice: A.**

Eosinophilic esophagitis is commonly associated with the pediatric population; however, it also affects patients in third to fifth decades of life. Frequent endoscopic findings are esophageal rings. These may be fixed (trachealization) or transient (felinization). The histologic hallmark of this condition is marked eosinophilic infiltration of the squamous epithelium. The diagnostic requirement is that more than 15 intraepithelial eosinophils should be found and usually affects the proximal and mid esophagus. Another diagnostic feature is the presence of superficial eosinophilic microabscesses, defined as a cluster of at least four eosinophils. Other changes include superficial layering of eosinophils, eosinophil degranulation, spongiosis, basal zone expansion, and elongation of papillae. Reflux esophagitis is the main differential diagnostic consideration. Even though 15 or more intraepithelial eosinophils are the cutoff for eosinophilic esophagitis, this amount can also be seen in reflux esophagitis as well, thus clinicopathologic correlation is required.

**7. Correct choice: E.**

The histologic section shows columnar mucosa within the distal esophagus with scattered goblet cells, consistent with Barrett esophagus, negative for dysplasia. Low-grade dysplasia is defined by minimal crypt architectural distortion and cytologically overlapping, elongated, variably hyperchromatic basally located nuclei. High-grade dysplasia has marked architectural distortion, such as fused and cribriform glands, and cytologically shows loss of nuclear polarity and enlarged rounded pleomorphic nuclei with irregular nuclear contours. Intramucosal adenocarcinoma occurs when neoplastic cells penetrate the crypt's basement membrane and invade into the lamina propria or muscularis mucosae.

**8. Correct choice: A.**

Barrett esophagus, high-grade dysplasia—see earlier explanation for high-grade dysplasia.

**9. Correct choice: D.**

Squamous papilloma is the most common benign esophageal neoplasm, although overall incidence is low. Most squamous papillomas are small (<0.5 cm) lesions, usually solitary, composed of mature acanthotic squamous epithelium arranged along branching fibrovascular stalks. They are most commonly located in the distal esophagus in association with reflux. On occasion, features such as koilocytosis, parakeratosis, hypergranulosis, and binucleated cells can be seen; however, no squamous dysplasia is present. Treatment is endoscopic removal.

**10. Correct choice: E.**

Tobacco is the most common cause of esophageal cancer in Western countries, although all of the answer choices are considered to be risk factors for esophageal squamous cell carcinoma. Squamous cell carcinoma is rare in the United States and has the highest incidence in Eastern Asia.

**11. Correct choice: B.**

Esophagus is a favored site for granular cell tumors. They are slow-growing, benign lesions. They appear as poorly circumscribed intramural nodules that are usually less than 2 cm in size. Histologically, they resemble granular cell tumors from other sites and are composed of sheets of uniform cells with small nuclei and abundant granular PAS (periodic acid-Schiff)-positive cytoplasm. The tumor cells will show expression for S100, CD68, and SOX10 by immunohistochemistry. The overlying squamous epithelium can undergo pseudoepitheliomatous hyperplasia that may be so profound as to be mistaken for squamous cell carcinoma.

**12. Correct choice: A.**

Achalasia is an esophageal motor disorder characterized by failure of relaxation of the lower esophageal sphincter and lack of progressive peristalsis in the esophageal body. Most cases are idiopathic. The cardinal morphologic feature is the decreased or complete absence of myenteric ganglion cells associated with an inflammatory infiltrate composed predominantly of cytotoxic T cells. Patients with achalasia have a significantly increased risk of esophageal squamous cell carcinoma.

**13. Correct choice: A.**

Squamous dysplasia is characterized by nuclear enlargement, hyperchromasia, and pleomorphism with abnormal mitoses and varying degrees of altered maturation. Squamous dysplasia is categorized as low grade (mild-to-moderate dysplasia) when the abnormal cells are limited to the basal half of the mucosa and as high grade (severe dysplasia to carcinoma in situ) when they extend to the upper half. There is no invasion into the lamina propria. Dysplastic epithelium may spread to involve submucosal gland ducts and can be a mimic of invasion.

# 32 Stomach

1. A 68-year-old female with dyspepsia undergoes an endoscopic examination. The gastric antrum shows erythema, and the histologic section of the antral biopsy is shown in Figure 1. What is the appropriate classification of this finding?

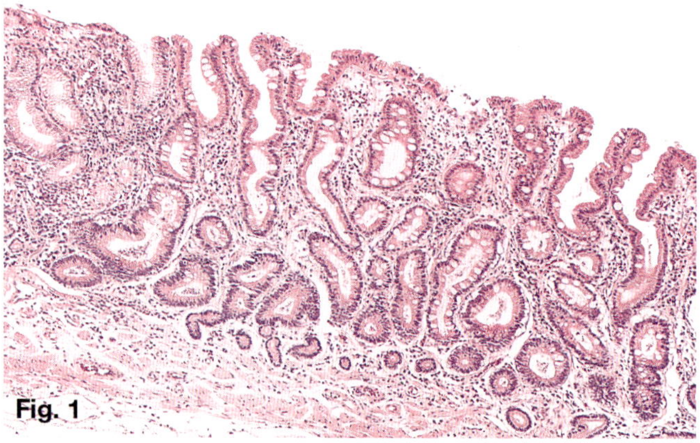

Fig. 1

A. Duodenal mucosa with foveolar metaplasia
B. Gastric adenoma, intestinal type
C. Gastric intestinal metaplasia, complete type
D. Gastric intestinal metaplasia, incomplete type
E. Reactive gastropathy

2. A 55-year-old male with a history of gastric intestinal metaplasia undergoes an endoscopic examination. Five biopsies were taken: two from the antrum, two from the fundus, and one from the incisura. The pathologist grades the histologic findings by the degree of inflammation, intestinal metaplasia, atrophy, dysplasia, and *Helicobacter pylori* density. Which of the following describes the above protocol?

A. Bethesda system
B. Nancy system
C. Nottingham score
D. Sydney system
E. Weiss score

3. A 63-year-old male with melena undergoes endoscopic examination. Figure 1 is best described as

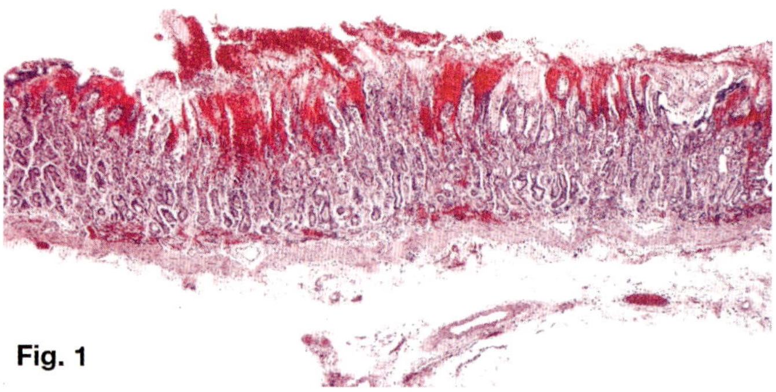

Fig. 1

A. autoimmune gastritis.
B. chronic gastritis.
C. erosive gastritis.
D. pill gastritis.
E. reactive gastropathy.

All figures in this chapter are from Longacre TA, Greenson JK, Hornick JL, Reuter VE, eds. *Mills and Sternberg's Diagnostic Surgical Pathology*. 7th ed. Wolters Kluwer; 2022 except for those noted at the end of this book.

4. Which of the following forms of gastritis is typically associated with the mucosal changes seen in the antrum as shown in Figure 1?

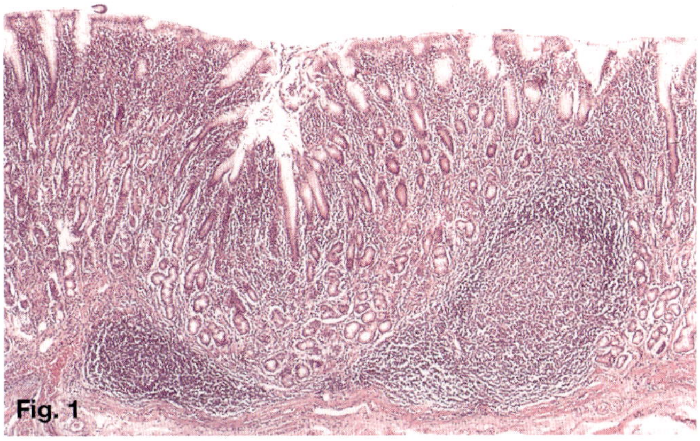

Fig. 1

A. Autoimmune gastritis
B. Focal enhancing gastritis
C. Granulomatous gastritis
D. *Helicobacter*-associated gastritis
E. Lymphocytic gastritis

5. A 64-year-old female presents with a 6-month history of progressive fatigue and megaloblastic anemia identified on complete blood count (CBC). Endoscopic examination reveals diffuse erythema. Histologic sections of a biopsy from the body show severe chronic atrophic gastritis with intestinal metaplasia, and the antrum shows mild chronic gastritis. Which of the following pathogenetic mechanisms is most likely associated with this form of gastritis?

A. Autoimmune process
B. Chronic *Helicobacter pylori* infection
C. Combined tobacco and alcohol use
D. Increased gastric acid production
E. Zollinger-Ellison syndrome

6. Figure 1 shows a representative section of a random gastric biopsy. What is the best diagnosis?

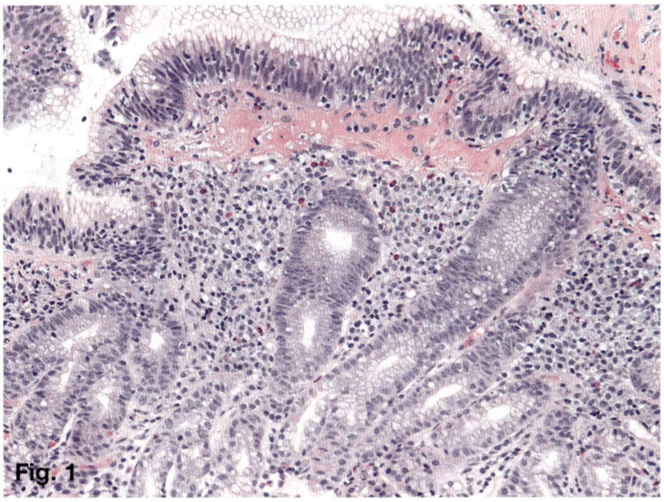

Fig. 1

A. Autoimmune gastritis
B. Collagenous gastritis
C. *Helicobacter*-associated gastritis
D. Infectious gastritis
E. Lymphocytic gastritis

7. A 24-year-old male status post allograft bone marrow transplant 6 months ago presents with altered bowel habits. A biopsy from the stomach is represented in Figure 1. What is the most likely etiology of these findings?

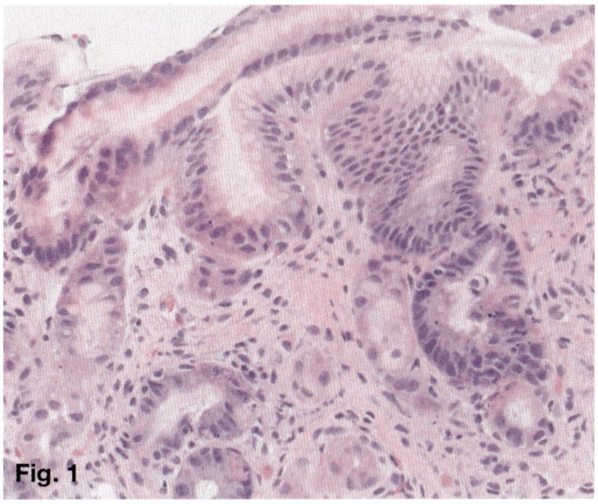

Fig. 1

A. Adenovirus infection
B. Chemotherapy-induced injury
C. Cytomegalovirus infection
D. Graft versus host disease
E. Human papillomavirus infection

8. Gastric polyps are discovered in approximately 6% of individuals undergoing endoscopic examination. Figure 1 shows the characteristic morphology of which type of gastric polyp?

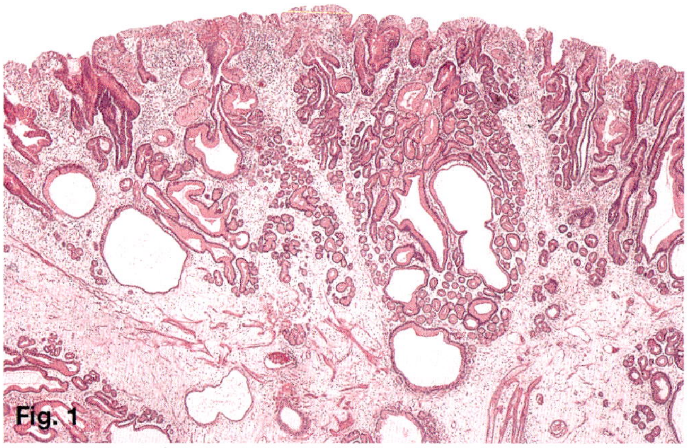


A. Adenomatous polyp
B. Fundic gland polyp
C. Hamartomatous polyp
D. Hyperplastic polyp
E. Mucosal prolapse type polyp

9. A 35-year-old male has numerous gastric polyps on screening endoscopy. On histology, multiple fundic gland polyps with low-grade dysplasia and gastric adenomas are seen. Which of the following germline genetic alterations does this patient most likely have?

A. *APC*
B. *MLH1*
C. *MSH2*
D. *P53*
E. *WT1*

10. Figure 1 is a representative histologic section of a gastric polyp. Which of the following is the most accurate diagnosis?

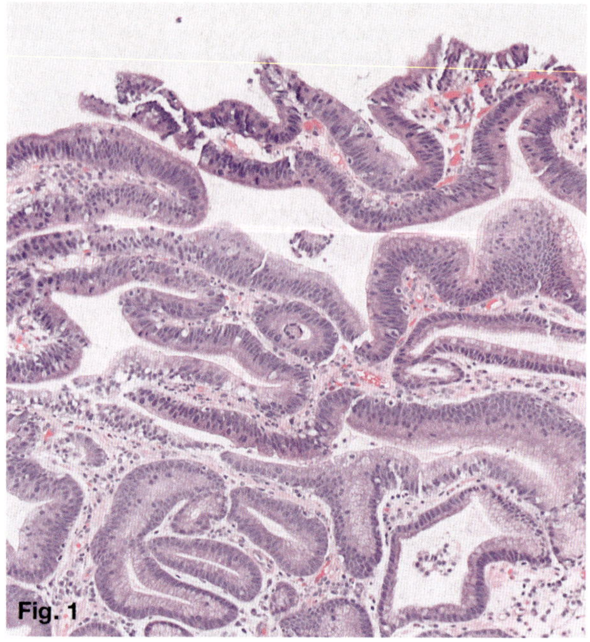


A. Fundic gland polyp
B. Gastric adenoma, foveolar type
C. Gastric adenoma, intestinal type
D. Hyperplastic polyp
E. Pyloric gland adenoma

11. A 56-year-old female presents with hypochlorhydria and weight loss. Endoscopic examination shows the gastric body has prominent rugal folds. A biopsy of the affected region is shown in Figure 1. The patient most likely has which of the following conditions?

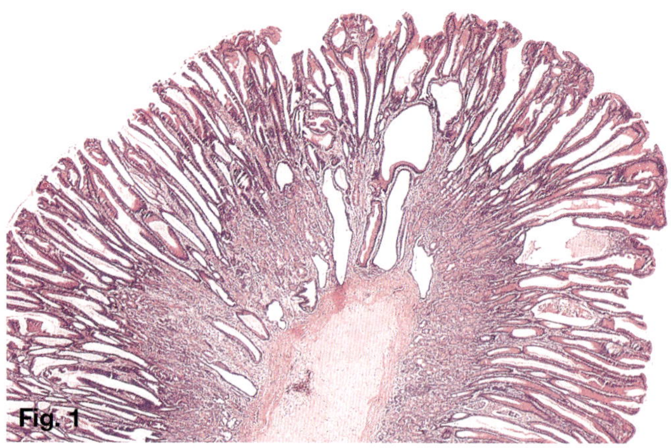


A. Autoimmune gastritis
B. Cowden syndrome
C. Gastric adenocarcinoma and proximal polyposis syndrome
D. Menetrier disease
E. Peutz-Jeghers syndrome

12. A 38-year-old female with a history of breast cancer undergoes screening endoscopy. On endoscopy, no lesions are seen in the entire stomach. Multiple random biopsies are taken. Figure 1 is a histologic section from one of the biopsies. Which of the following germline genetic alterations does this patient most likely have?

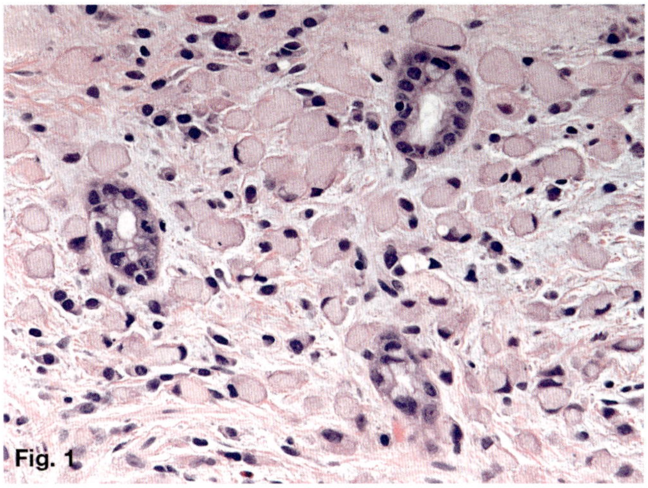

Fig. 1

A. *APC*
B. *BRCA1*
C. *BRCA2*
D. *CDH1*
E. *SMAD4*

13. Chronic *Helicobacter pylori* infections increase a person's risk for which of the following?

A. Adenocarcinoma
B. Autoimmune gastritis
C. Mantle cell lymphoma
D. Neuroendocrine carcinoma
E. Well-differentiated neuroendocrine tumors

14. Which of the following statements regarding gastric carcinoma is correct?

A. Early onset gastric cancers are defined by gastric carcinoma in patients less than 30 years old.
B. Lauren intestinal type is synonymous with well differentiated by World Health Organization (WHO) classification.
C. Matched stage for stage, there is no prognostic difference between papillary adenocarcinoma and micropapillary carcinoma.
D. Splenic involvement by gastric carcinoma is not always considered to be a metastasis.
E. WHO classification has three histologic types: intestinal, diffuse, and mixed.

15. A patient with a gastric mass undergoes endoscopic biopsy. The tumor cells are positive for AE1/AE3 and synaptophysin by immunohistochemistry. The tumor cells are hyperchromatic with scant cytoplasm and nuclear molding. Tumor necrosis is present. Ki-67 index shows nuclear expression in 45% of the tumor cells. Which of the following is the proper classification of this neoplasm?

A. Neuroendocrine carcinoma, large cell type
B. Neuroendocrine carcinoma, small cell type
C. Poorly cohesive adenocarcinoma
D. Poorly differentiated squamous cell carcinoma
E. Well-differentiated neuroendocrine tumor, WHO (World Health Organization) grade 3

16. A 55-year-old man with a history of refractory *Helicobacter pylori* infection has prominent accentuation of mucosal rugae of the stomach on endoscopy. Biopsies show a diffuse infiltrate by sheets of tumor cells, which are negative for CK7 and positive for CD20 by immunohistochemistry as seen on the H&E (hematoxylin and eosin) image in Figure 1. Which of the following is the most likely diagnosis?

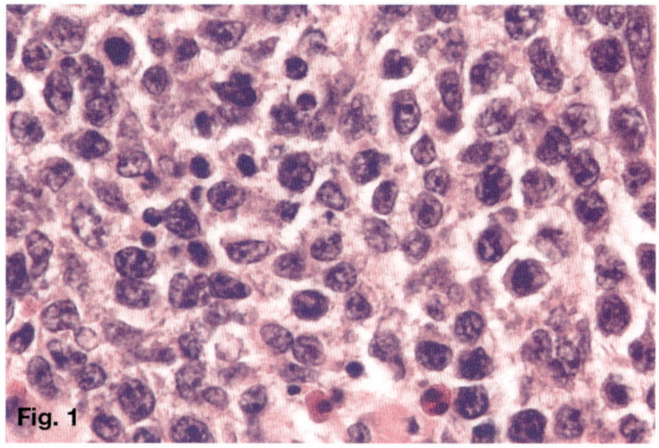

Fig. 1

A. Diffuse large B-cell lymphoma
B. Gastric carcinoma with lymphoid stroma
C. Mucosa-associated lymphoid tissue lymphoma
D. Neuroendocrine carcinoma
E. Poorly cohesive adenocarcinoma

17. A patient undergoes partial gastrectomy for a neoplasm with the histologic appearance as shown in Figure 1. This class of tumor is presumably derived from

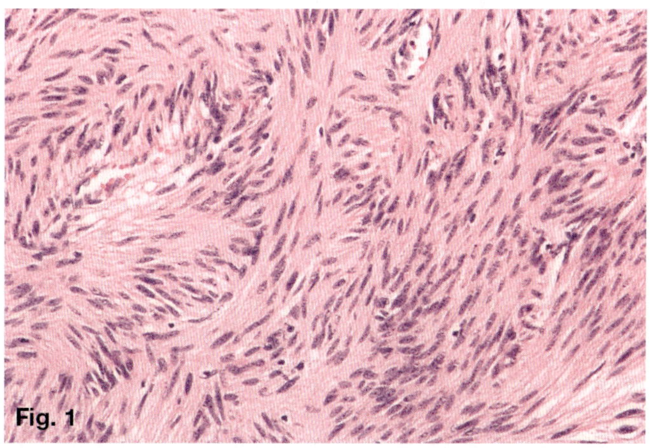

Fig. 1

A. interstitial cells of Cajal.
B. myofibroblasts.
C. Schwann cells.
D. smooth muscle cells.
E. undifferentiated mesenchymal cells.

18. A 33-year-old female with a history of abdominal paraganglioma now has a 3.2-cm gastric submucosal lesion. Histologically, the tumor cells have round nuclei with clear to lightly eosinophilic cytoplasm and cytoplasmic vacuoles. The tumor is negative for mixed cytokeratins and positive for DOG-1 by immunohistochemistry. A succinate dehydrogenase (SDH) immunohistochemical stain was performed and the results are seen in Figure 1. Which of the following syndromes does the patient most likely have?

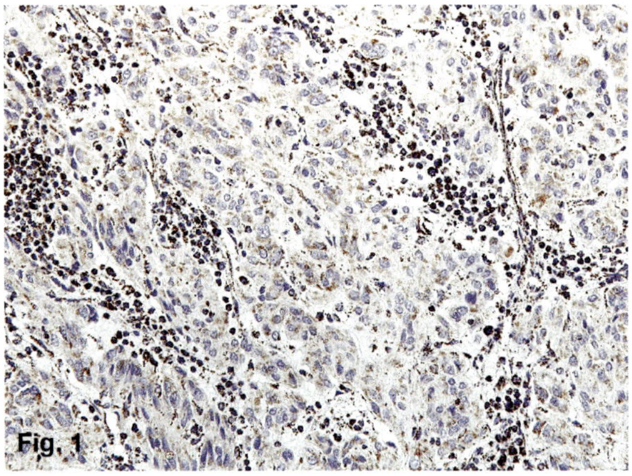
Fig. 1

A. Carney complex
B. Carney-Stratakis syndrome
C. Carney triad
D. Gardner syndrome
E. Maffucci syndrome

19. A 62-year-old male with a 1.7-cm submucosal lesion in the gastric antrum undergoes surgical resection. The histologic appearance of the lesion is shown in Figure 1. What is the most likely diagnosis?

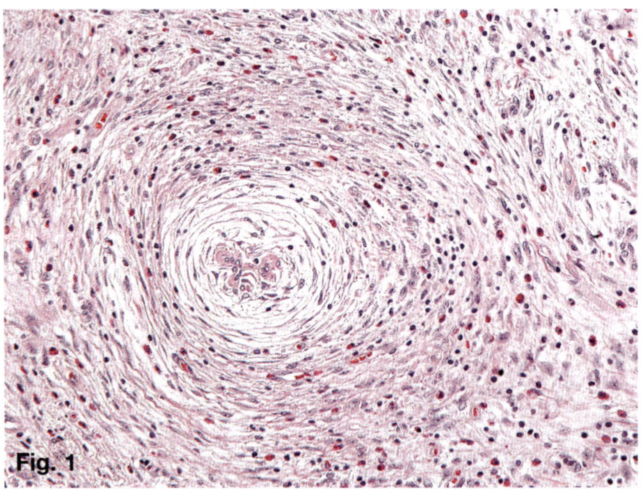
Fig. 1

A. Gastrointestinal stromal tumor
B. Inflammatory fibroid polyp
C. Neurofibroma
D. Plexiform fibromyxoma
E. Schwannoma

20. An 82-year-old female with anemia undergoes endoscopy. Endoscopic findings show mucosal red stripes that radiate from the gastric pylorus. A biopsy was taken from the gastric antrum and a representative histologic section is shown in Figure 1. What is the correct diagnosis?

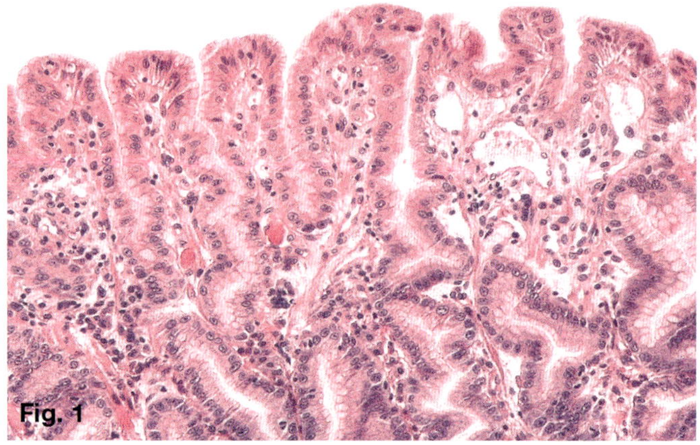
Fig. 1

A. Arteriovenous malformations
B. Autoimmune gastritis
C. Chronic gastritis
D. Gastric antral vascular ectasia
E. No significant abnormality

21. Which of the following statements is true of pyloric gland adenomas?

A. Almost no risk of progressing to high-grade dysplasia or adenocarcinoma
B. Background gastric mucosa usually without significant abnormality
C. Dilated glands lined by columnar cells with basally located nuclei and apical mucin cap
D. No association with polyposis syndromes
E. Tightly packed glands lined by cuboidal cells with basally located nuclei and pale ground-glass cytoplasm

# ANSWERS AND EXPLANATIONS

**1. Correct choice: D.**

In intestinal metaplasia (IM), areas of gastric foveolar epithelium are replaced by intestinal-type epithelium, as defined as the presence of goblet cells. This can be split into three categories: complete, incomplete, or mixed type. Complete type IM recapitulates small intestinal epithelium with the presence of goblet cells and absorptive enterocytes with a brush border and may also contain Paneth and enteroendocrine cells. In contrast, incomplete IM is characterized by goblet cells and goblet-like columnar cells, which contain variably sized pale-blue cytoplasmic mucin intermixed with intervening foveolar epithelium. Mixed type shows features of both complete and incomplete types.

**2. Correct choice: D.**

The Sydney system is a system for the classification and description of gastritis. Full application of the system requires that a minimum of five biopsies be taken: two from antral mucosa, two from fundic mucosa, and one from the incisura. Biopsies from each area are graded based on the degree of inflammation, intestinal metaplasia, atrophy, dysplasia, and *Helicobacter pylori* density. The Nancy system is used to grade ulcerative colitis. The Bethesda system is used in cytology. Weiss score is used for adrenal cortical carcinoma. Nottingham score is used for breast carcinoma.

**3. Correct choice: C.**

Erosive gastritis is characterized by a gastric erosion, an ulcer-like process that does not extend beyond the muscularis mucosae, whereas an ulcer extends beyond the muscularis mucosae. Common etiologies for both gastric erosions and ulcers are medications (especially nonsteroidal anti-inflammatory drugs [NSAIDs]), ischemia, cardiogenic shock, alcohol, increased acid production, and *Helicobacter pylori* infection.

**4. Correct choice: D.**

*Helicobacter*-associated gastritis usually presents as superficial gastritis and can be seen with or without active inflammation. Neutrophilic infiltration of the epithelium is a sign of active gastritis, which may even result in pit abscesses. Formation of lymphoid follicles with active germinal centers within the deep mucosa (the so-called follicular gastritis) is almost always associated with *Helicobacter pylori*. As such, chronic *H. pylori* infection increases the risk of developing mucosa-associated lymphoid tissue (MALT) lymphomas. This gram-negative organism can be identified on goodwill-stained H&E (hematoxylin and eosin) sections; on immunohistochemistry; or on sections stained with modified Steiner, Giemsa, or Leung stains.

**5. Correct choice: A.**

Autoimmune gastritis accounts for less than 5% of cases of chronic gastritis. Typically, this affects the gastric fundus and body, while sparing the antrum; however, rare cases of atrophic autoimmune pan-gastritis have been identified. Microscopically, it is characterized by chronic inflammation with loss of parietal cells and pyloric metaplasia. The mechanism of this disease is caused by autoantibodies against parietal cells and/or intrinsic factors, which causes elevated blood gastrin levels and pernicious (megaloblastic) anemia. This results in increased gastrin production due to hypochlorhydria. Enterochromaffin-like (ECL) cells within oxyntic mucosa are stimulated and may develop into well-differentiated neuroendocrine tumors.

**6. Correct choice: B.**

Collagenous gastritis is characterized by a prominent subepithelial collagen band (often 30-40 µm in thickness) that entraps capillaries but does not extend down along the neck glands. In adults, it is commonly associated with microscopic colitis or celiac disease. In the pediatric population, it presents as anemia and is not associated with microscopic colitis or celiac disease.

**7. Correct choice: D.**

Gastrointestinal graft versus host disease (GVHD) may be encountered after allograft bone marrow transplantation. Early changes consist of increased epithelial cell apoptosis with associated karyorrhectic debris. In severe disease, mucosal denudation will occur. The bottom right of the image shows a crypt with numerous apoptotic bodies. There are no viral cytopathic changes seen.

**8. Correct choice: D.**

Hyperplastic polyps can occur in adults and children and account for 17% of gastric polyps. They are thought to develop as a florid regenerative reaction to any kind of mucosal injury. They can be solitary or multiple with variable size (0.5-2.5 cm). They are usually found at the junction between pyloric and corpus mucosa. Histologically, hyperplastic polyps consist of cystically dilated and tortuous foveolae in a chronically inflamed and edematous stroma. Intestinal metaplasia and dysplasia are rarely seen but can occur in gastric hyperplastic polyps; however, they rarely undergo malignant change.

**9. Correct choice: A.**

Fundic gland polyps (FGPs) account for almost 80% of all gastric polyps. Histologically, FGPs show cystically dilated fundic glands, lined by a flattened layer of chief cells, parietal cells, and mucous neck cells. Sporadic forms are most frequent but may also occur (1) after treatment for gastric acid suppression and (2) in polyposis syndromes. Patients with FAP (familial adenomatous polyposis) and GAPPS (gastric adenocarcinoma and proximal polyposis syndrome) both commonly present with numerous polyps with a 25% to 50% prevalence of dysplasia in the foveolar epithelium. Both of these syndromes frequently show mutations in the *APC* gene. *CDH1*, *MLH1*, *TP53*, and *WT1* alterations are associated with hereditary diffuse gastric cancer (HDGC) syndrome, Lynch syndrome, Li-Fraumeni syndrome, and Wilms tumor, respectively.

**10. Correct choice: B.**

This figure depicts a gastric adenoma, foveolar type. Adenomas account for just 1% of all gastric polyps. They develop from foveolar epithelium and may present as polypoid or flat lesions. The two most common types of gastric adenomas are (1) **intestinal type**, which resembles features seen in colorectal adenomas with hyperchromatic, elongated, pseudostratified nuclei and variable amounts of goblet and Paneth cells and (2) **foveolar type**, which arises in mucosa that either is normal or shows minor inflammatory features, and is lined by columnar cells with elongated, hyperchromatic nuclei, and an apical mucin cap. Intestinal-type gastric adenoma is more likely to progress to gastric cancer as compared to foveolar-type gastric adenoma.

**11. Correct choice: D.**

Menetrier disease is a condition that most commonly manifests as prominent gastric folds and low acid production even after stimulation, for which no other primary cause can be identified. The mucosal folds most commonly occur in the gastric body, but rarely, can affect the antrum. Histologically, the gastric mucosa shows elongated foveolae with deep cystically dilated glands and fundic gland atrophy. Gastric adenocarcinoma and proximal polyposis syndrome (GAPPS) presents at a young age with numerous fundic gland polyps, with or without dysplasia. Peutz-Jeghers syndrome presents at a young age with hamartomatous polyps that have arborizing branches of smooth muscle. Cowden syndrome is associated with mucocutaneous lesions and polyps in the gastrointestinal (GI) tract.

**12. Correct choice: D.**

Hereditary diffuse gastric cancer (HDGC) syndrome is commonly associated with a germline mutation in the E-cadherin gene *CDH1*. In the early stages, it presents as multiple discontinuous foci of in situ signet-ring cells in the neck glands or as intramucosal signet-ring carcinoma. Patients usually undergo prophylactic total gastrectomy at a young age (30-40s). A subset of these patients are also at risk for lobular breast cancer.

**13. Correct choice: A.**

Gastric adenocarcinomas are strongly associated with *Helicobacter pylori* infection. The pathway to adenocarcinoma starts with chronic *H. pylori* infection leading to complete or incomplete intestinal metaplasia, which has an increased risk of dysplasia and carcinoma. Chronic *H. pylori* infection is also associated with the development of gastric mucosa-associated lymphoid tissue (MALT) lymphoma. Autoimmune gastritis increases the risk of developing well-differentiated neuroendocrine tumors (type 1).

**14. Correct choice: D.**

The classification of gastric cancer as intestinal, diffuse, and mixed histologic types is based on the Lauren classification. When matched stage for stage, there is no difference in survival between the tumor types, except gastric carcinoma with an invasive micropapillary pattern, which has been reported to have a poor prognosis and rapid progression. The World Health Organization (WHO) classifies adenocarcinomas as papillary carcinoma, tubular carcinoma, mucinous carcinoma, poorly cohesive carcinoma, and signet-ring cell carcinoma among other variants. The grading is based on the percentage of glandular formation. Intestinal-type carcinoma tends to be well demarcated and is characterized predominantly by a glandular pattern; however, the glandular pattern can range from well to poorly differentiated. Splenic involvement can occur via the transperitoneal route, and these tumors would be staged as pT4b, M0. A patient with gastric carcinoma is considered to have "early onset gastric cancer" if less than 50 years of age.

**15. Correct choice: B.**

This photomicrograph depicts a neuroendocrine carcinoma, a small cell type. The World Health Organization (WHO) grades well-differentiated neuroendocrine tumors (WDNET) and poorly differentiated (neuroendocrine carcinoma) based on morphology and Ki-67 and/or mitotic index (Table 1). For this case, based on the Ki-67 index, this neoplasm can either be WDNET, grade 3, or neuroendocrine carcinoma. Based on the morphologic description, it would be the neuroendocrine carcinoma, a small cell type.

**TABLE 1 World Health Organization Classification of Gastrointestinal Neuroendocrine Tumors**

| | Ki-67[a] Index (%) | Mitotic Index/10 HPF[b] |
|---|---|---|
| **Well-Differentiated Neuroendocrine Neoplasms (NENS)** | | |
| NET grade 1 (G1) | <3 | <2 |
| NET grade 2 (G2) | 3-20 | 2-20 |
| NET grade 3 (G3) | >20 | >20 |
| **Poorly Differentiated Neuroendocrine Neoplasms (NENS)** | | |
| Neuroendocrine carcinoma | >20 | >20 |
| Small cell | | |
| Large cell | | |
| **Mixed Neuroendocrine-Nonneuroendocrine Neoplasms (MINEN)** | | |
| Mixed adenocarcinoma NET | 0-20 | 0-20 |
| Mixed adenocarcinoma NEC (mixed adenoneuroendocrine carcinoma) | >20 | >20 |

HPF, high-power field; NEC, neuroendocrine carcinoma; NET, neuroendocrine tumor.

[a]MIB1 antibody % positive of 500 to 2,000 tumor cells in the area of highest labeling.

[b]10 HPF = 2 $mm^2$. At least 50 HPF (at 40×) must be evaluated in the area of highest mitotic index.

Adapted from La Rosa S, Rindi G, Solcia E, et al. Gastric neuroendocrine neoplasms. In: WHO Classification of Tumours Editorial Board, ed. *Digestive System Tumours*, WHO Classification of Tumours Series. 5th ed. Vol 1. International Agency for Research on Cancer; 2019:104-109. With permission.

**16. Correct choice: A.**

This is an example of diffuse large B-cell lymphoma. The majority of primary gastric lymphomas are thought to arise from the extranodal marginal zone of follicles comprising mucosa-associated lymphoid tissue (MALT). They arise in a background of chronic gastritis, typically caused by infection with *Helicobacter pylori*. Approximately 75% of MALT lymphomas respond to antibiotic therapy directed against *H. pylori* and, following treatment, may become reduced in size or regress entirely. MALT lymphoma is a low-grade B-cell lymphoma, but it may transform into a high-grade lymphoma, namely, diffuse large B-cell lymphoma (DLBCL). The cells become more epithelioid and the nuclei are characteristically vesicular, with prominent nucleoli and nuclear membranes. A major diagnostic challenge with biopsy material from suspected DLBCL is to separate lymphoma from a poorly differentiated carcinoma.

**17. Correct choice: A.**

Gastrointestinal stromal tumor (GIST) has a highly variable morphology, although many subtypes fall into two categories: spindle and epithelioid cell types. The spindle cell type is the most common and consists of fascicles and whorls of elongated cells. Cells have ovoid vesicular nuclei and eosinophilic cytoplasm. Epithelioid cell types are composed of round cells with artifactual clearing of their cytoplasm. Immunohistochemical and ultrastructural evidence show that GIST is derived from gastrointestinal (GI) pacemaker cells, also known as the interstitial cells of Cajal. Both tumor cells of GIST and interstitial cells of Cajal are immunoreactive for CD117, the protein encoded by the *KIT* protooncogene. Most gastric GISTs (95%) have gain-of-function mutations of the *KIT* gene and express CD117. Most of the remaining 5% of gastric GISTs have mutations in the *PDGFRA* gene. Such mutations result in constitutive activation of the KIT tyrosine kinase receptor. The development of specific tyrosine kinase inhibitors, such as imatinib, has radically changed the treatment of advanced GIST. *PDGFRA* D842V-mutant GISTs may respond to platelet-derived growth factor receptor-α (PDGFRA)-targeted therapy.

**18. Correct choice: B.**

Carney-Stratakis syndrome is an autosomal dominant disorder that usually affects young adults who have germline mutations in one of the succinate dehydrogenase genes (*SDHB, SDHC,* or *SDHD*). It is characterized by gastrointestinal stromal tumor (GIST), commonly epithelioid, and paraganglioma. The image shows the loss of SDHB by immunohistochemistry. Tumors in this setting also demonstrate relatively indolent behavior.

**19. Correct choice: B.**

Inflammatory fibroid polyps may develop in any segment of the gastrointestinal (GI) tract, but 35% of them are found in the stomach, usually in the antral region. These are mesenchymal neoplasms caused by mutations in the gene coding for the platelet-derived growth factor receptor-α or *PDGFRA*. They result from the growth of a loose connective tissue expanding the submucosa, partly replacing the muscularis mucosae and resulting in mucosal ulceration. Numerous small vessels surrounded by hypocellular stroma represent a characteristic feature. The accompanying chronic inflammatory infiltrate is mild but rich in eosinophils. All polyps are positive for vimentin and the majority are positive for CD34.

**20. Correct choice: D.**

Gastric antral vascular ectasia (GAVE) is also commonly known as "watermelon stomach" due to the endoscopic presence of red patches, spots, or mucosal red stripes that radiate from the gastric pylorus. Biopsy of the reddened area shows dilated capillaries in the superficial lamina propria immediately below the surface epithelium. These capillaries may contain fibrin thrombi and may be surrounded by eosinophilic homogeneous material (fibrohyalinosis).

**21. Correct choice: E.**

Pyloric gland adenoma consists of tightly packed pyloric glands lined by a monolayer of cuboidal to low columnar epithelium. The cytoplasm is lightly eosinophilic with a pale ground-glass appearance. Nuclei are round to oval in shape and basally oriented. Pyloric gland adenomas lack an apical mucin cap and goblet cells. Sporadic pyloric gland adenomas are associated with background atrophic gastritis and intestinal metaplasia. Pyloric gland adenomas can be seen in familial adenomatous polyposis (FAP) and gastric adenocarcinoma and proximal polyposis of the stomach (GAPPS), Lynch syndrome, juvenile polyposis syndrome, and McCune-Albright syndrome. Approximately 40% to 50% of pyloric gland adenomas exhibit high-grade dysplasia, and 12% to 46% are associated with intramucosal or more deeply invasive adenocarcinoma.

# 33 Nonneoplastic Intestinal Diseases

1. Which of the following histologic features constitutes an abnormal finding if seen in a duodenal biopsy?

   A. Brown-black pigment in macrophages of the lamina propria
   B. Lamina propria inflammation composed of only lymphocytes, eosinophils, and mast cells
   C. One intraepithelial lymphocyte per four to five enterocyte
   D. Ratio of villus-to-crypt length of 3:1 to 5:1
   E. Shortened, distorted villi overlying lymphoid aggregates

2. A 33-year-old female presents with abdominal pain, diarrhea, and weight loss. Lab tests show that the patient is positive for HLA-DQ2. A duodenal biopsy shows the changes seen in Figure 1. What is the most likely diagnosis?

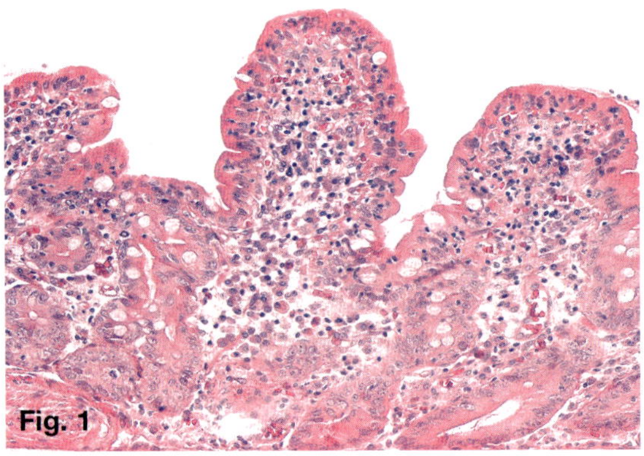

Fig. 1

   A. Autoimmune enteropathy
   B. Celiac disease
   C. Common variable immunodeficiency
   D. Systemic mastocytosis
   E. Tropical sprue

3. A 33-year-old female presents with abdominal pain, diarrhea, and weight loss. She has recently returned from her temporary position in Mexico. A duodenal biopsy shows the changes seen in Figure 1. Her symptoms quickly responded to the administration of folate, vitamin B12, and broad-spectrum antibiotics. Which of the following is the most likely diagnosis?

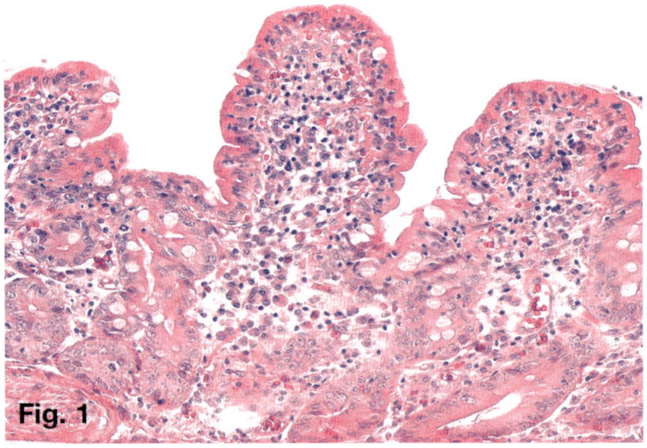

Fig. 1

   A. Autoimmune enteropathy
   B. Celiac disease
   C. Common variable immunodeficiency
   D. Systemic mastocytosis
   E. Tropical sprue

All figures in this chapter are from Longacre TA, Greenson JK, Hornick JL, Reuter VE, eds. *Mills and Sternberg's Diagnostic Surgical Pathology.* 7th ed. Wolters Kluwer; 2022 except for those noted at the end of this book.

4. A 33-year-old female presents with abdominal pain, diarrhea, and weight loss. A duodenal biopsy shows the changes seen in Figure 1. Immunohistochemical testing highlights clusters of cells (>15 cells) that are positive for CD117 and CD25. Which of the following is the most likely diagnosis?

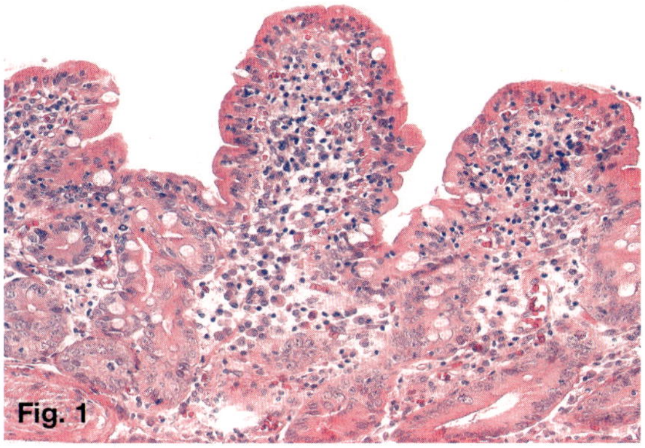
Fig. 1

A. Autoimmune enteropathy
B. Celiac disease
C. Common variable immunodeficiency
D. Systemic mastocytosis
E. Tropical sprue

5. A 26-year-old male presents with diarrhea, malabsorption, and recurrent Giardia infections. A small bowel biopsy shows mild villous blunting, increased intraepithelial lymphocytes, prominent lymphoid aggregates, and rare lamina propria plasma cells. Which of the following is the most likely diagnosis?

A. Autoimmune enteropathy
B. Celiac disease
C. Common variable immunodeficiency
D. Systemic mastocytosis
E. Tropical sprue

6. A newborn infant has intractable diarrhea. The clinical team suspects microvillus inclusion disease. A small intestine biopsy is performed. Which of the following findings is seen in this disease?

A. Enlarged enterocytes with eosinophilic cytoplasmic inclusions
B. Foveolar metaplasia and active duodenitis
C. Loss of lamina propria plasma cells
D. Retained enterocyte microvilli on electron microscopy
E. Severe villous blunting with crypt hypoplasia

7. A duodenal biopsy from a patient suffering from explosive, foul-smell diarrhea is shown in the representative histologic section in Figure 1. Which of the following is the most appropriate diagnosis?

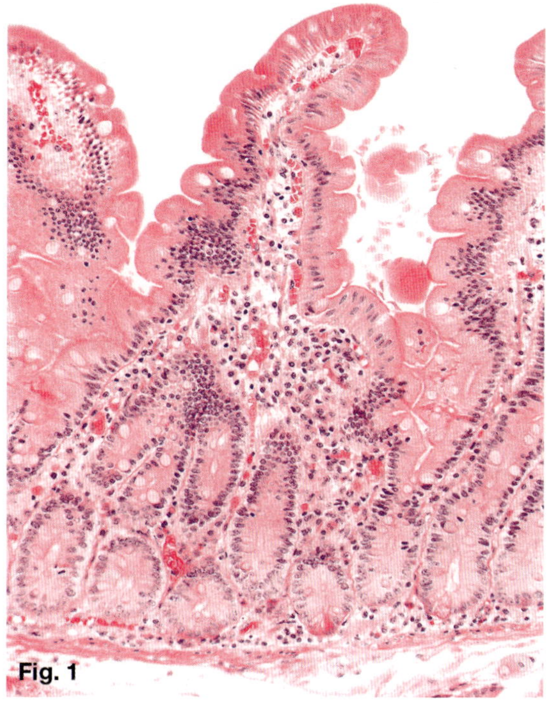
Fig. 1

A. Cryptosporidiosis
B. Eosinophilic duodenitis
C. Giardiasis
D. Inflammatory bowel disease
E. No significant abnormality

8. A 72-year-old male was recently discharged from the hospital after treatment of aspiration-induced bacterial pneumonia. Now he presents to the emergency room with watery foul-smelling diarrhea, abdominal pain, nausea, and bloating. On colonoscopy, numerous elevated yellow-white plaques are identified. A colon biopsy from the areas with the plaques is obtained, shown in Figure 1. What is the most likely etiology?

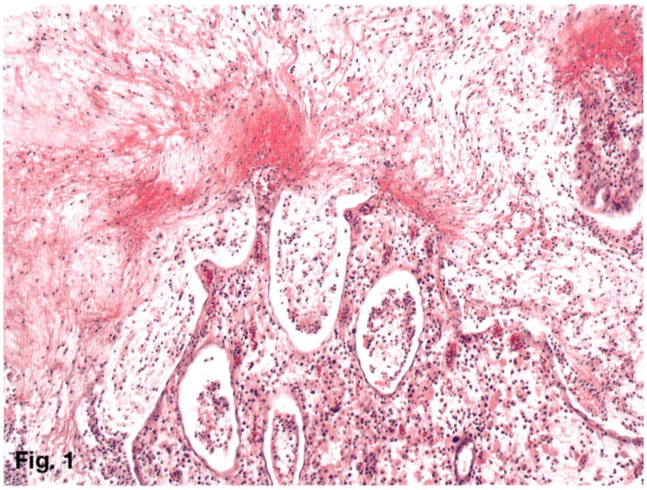
Fig. 1

A. Amebiasis
B. *Clostridium difficile* colitis
C. Cryptosporidiosis
D. Enterohemorrhagic *Escherichia coli*
E. Inflammatory bowel disease

9. A 72-year-old female presents with chronic watery diarrhea and weight loss. On colonoscopy, random colon biopsies are obtained showing features depicted in Figure 1. What is the most likely diagnosis?

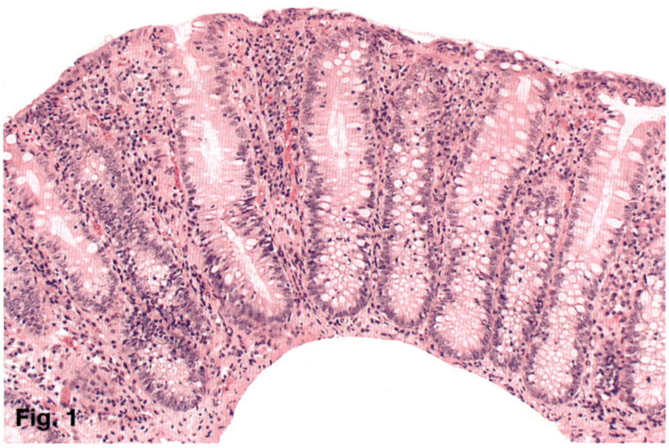
Fig. 1

A. Collagenous colitis
B. Inflammatory bowel disease
C. Lymphocytic colitis
D. Mucosal prolapse
E. No significant abnormality

10. A 32-year-old male with chronic back pain presents with bright red blood per rectum and constipation. On colonoscopy, several ulcers and polypoid erythematous mucosa are identified in the rectum. Figure 1 is a representative histologic section of the erythematous mucosa adjacent to an ulcer. What is the most likely diagnosis?

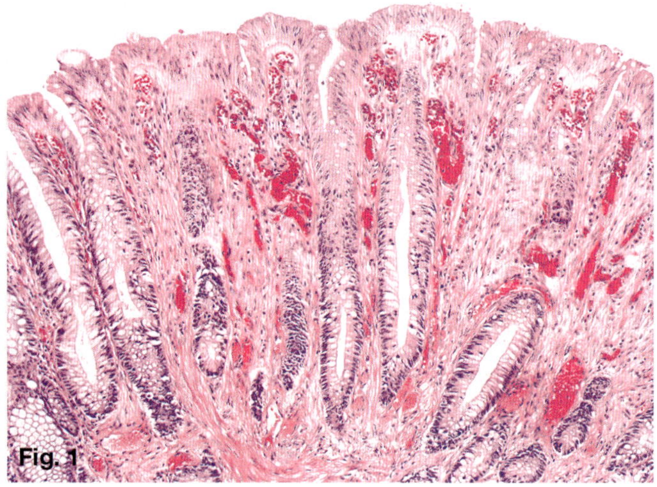
Fig. 1

A. Acute ischemic injury
B. Crohn disease
C. Medication-induced colitis
D. Solitary rectal ulcer syndrome
E. Ulcerative colitis

11. In the gross room, you receive an ileal resection specimen removed from a 42-year-old patient with small bowel obstruction. You notice that the distal ileum is tortuous and involved by abundant adhesions. Once opened, the affected small bowel has multiple fistulas connecting separate loops of bowel and linear ulcerations. The bowel wall is variably thickened. The mesentery shows fat wrapping and contains easily identifiable enlarged lymph nodes. Based on this gross description, what is the most likely clinical history for this patient?

A. Chronic parasitic infection
B. *Clostridium difficile* infection
C. Crohn disease
D. Ischemic enteritis
E. Ulcerative colitis

12. A 45-year-old male is a recent immigrant from China. He presents with bloody diarrhea, abdominal pain, and weight loss. On colonoscopy, skip lesions are identified in the ileum and cecum. In the affected areas, the mucosa shows erythema, friability, and delineated ulcers. There are multiple areas of luminal narrowing, suggestive of strictures. Biopsies taken from the affected areas show chronic active enteritis and colitis with numerous scattered and coalescing granulomas, of which some are necrotizing. Based on this information, what is the most likely diagnosis?

A. Chronic strongyloidiasis
B. Chronic tuberculosis
C. Crohn disease
D. Ischemic colitis
E. Ulcerative colitis

13. A patient with severe Crohn disease undergoes an ileocolectomy with ileostomy placement and creation of a Hartmann pouch. A couple of months after the surgery, the patient undergoes pouchoscopy for bloody anal discharge, which shows erythematous, friable, and nodular mucosa. A representative histologic section of the biopsy is shown in Figure 1. What is the most likely diagnosis?

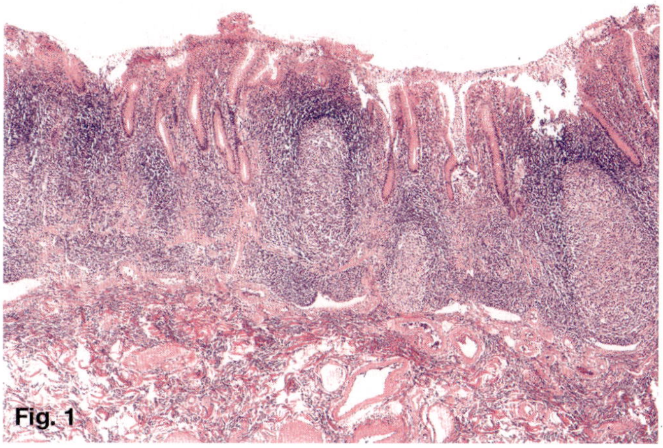

Fig. 1

A. Diversion colitis
B. Follicular lymphoma
C. Ischemic colitis
D. New diagnosis of ulcerative colitis
E. Reemergence of Crohn disease

14. A previously healthy 70-year-old woman presents with recurrent melena and undergoes a colonoscopy. Multiple sources of bleeding are identified in the cecum and ascending colon. Which of the following is the most likely cause of this patient's bleeding?

A. Angioectasia
B. Diverticular disease
C. Hemangioma
D. Inflammatory bowel disease
E. Varices

15. Which of the following is a feature of Hirschsprung disease?

A. Aganglionosis affecting only the myenteric plexus
B. Associated with germline *PTEN* mutation
C. Histologic diagnosis made on resection specimen
D. Suction biopsy showing anal canal mucosa considered inadequate
E. Suction biopsy showing any amount of submucosa considered adequate

16. A patient with familial adenomatous polyposis is undergoing total colectomy. During the surgery, a firm mesenteric mass is identified and resected. Histologic sections of the mesenteric mass show a pale spindle cell lesion with areas of increased cellularity, arranged in interlacing bundles with infiltration into adjacent adipose tissue. There is a paucity of inflammatory and foam cells. Which of the following immunohistochemical stains would be most helpful?

A. β-Catenin
B. CD117
C. Desmin
D. S100 protein
E. Smooth muscle actin (SMA)

17. Which of the following is true regarding inflammatory bowel disease (IBD) associated dysplasia and carcinoma?

A. Colitis-associated carcinomas are usually visualized by standard endoscopic techniques.
B. Crohn disease carcinoma does not occur in bypassed or out-of-circuit segments of small bowel.
C. IBD dysplasia is distinguished from reactive changes by the presence of nuclear enlargement and hyperchromasia, increased mitotic activity, and decreased intracellular mucin.
D. Patients with IBD with visible dysplasia that is completely removed endoscopically can continue with surveillance colonoscopy, rather than colectomy.
E. Visible dysplasia does not include sporadic colonic adenomas that occur in patients with IBD.

18. A 42-year-old female develops altered bowel habits and gastrointestinal (GI) bleeding 1 week after allogeneic stem cell transplant following induction chemotherapy for acute lymphocytic leukemia. The colonoscopy shows patchy colitis with scattered small ulcers. Histologic examination shows the following finding in Figure 1. What is the likely etiology?

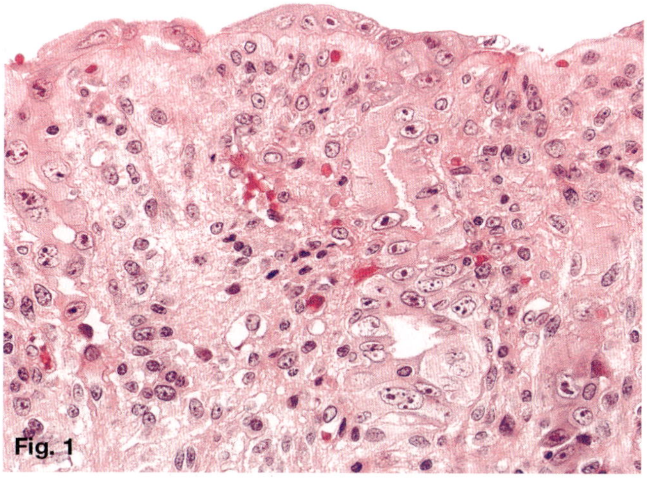

Fig. 1

A. Chemotherapy effect
B. Graft versus host disease (GVHD)
C. High-grade dysplasia
D. Inflammatory bowel disease
E. Viral infection

# ANSWERS AND EXPLANATIONS

**1. Correct choice: B.**

A loss of lamina propria plasma cells is associated with common variable immunodeficiency and immunoglobulin A (IgA) immunodeficiency. Normal features of duodenal biopsies include (1) villus-to-crypt length of 3:1 to 5:1, (2) villi can appear shorter and distorted in areas overlying lymphoid aggregates or Brunner glands, (3) brown-black pigment that may be found in the lamina propria macrophages (pseudomelanosis duodeni), (4) lymphocytes are scattered among the individual epithelial cells in the ratio of one lymphocyte for every four or five cells in the proximal small intestine or in macrophages of Peyer patches, and (5) inflammatory cells in the lamina propria, including lymphocytes, plasma cells, and occasional eosinophils. In general, identifying four villi in a row indicates that the villous architecture of the whole biopsy specimen is *probably* normal.

**2. Correct choice: B.**

Celiac sprue, also known as gluten-induced enteropathy, is in the end a clinical diagnosis. The pathogenesis involves immunologic injury to the enterocyte associated with the ingestion of gluten found in wheat, rye, and barley. It is associated with specific major histocompatibility complex (MHC) class II alleles: 90% of patients have HLA-DQ2, and the remaining have HLA-DQ8. The principal histologic features are crypt hyperplasia, loss of villous height, chronic inflammatory cell infiltration, and surface intraepithelial lymphocytosis (>40 per 100 enterocytes). The histologic abnormalities are most severe in the proximal intestinal mucosa, gradually lessening distally. With gluten withdrawal, the abnormalities recede from distal to proximal. The list of choices includes the most common conditions presenting with a pattern of nonspecific variable villous abnormality, characterized by variable villous shortening and increased intraepithelial lymphocytes.

**3. Correct choice: E.**

Tropical sprue is endemic in tropical regions of Asia, West Africa, Mexico, Puerto Rico, the Caribbean, and Central and South America, but it may be seen in patients who traveled to those regions. These patients have no response to gluten withdrawal trials. Patients most often respond dramatically to the administration of folate, vitamin B12, and tetracycline or other broad-spectrum antibiotics, implying that an infectious agent may be important in the etiology.

**4. Correct choice: D.**

Systemic mastocytosis is a rare, clonal myeloproliferative disorder characterized by infiltration of mast cells in tissues. The major criterion for diagnosis is the finding of mast cell infiltrates, consisting of at least 15 cells in aggregate, in the bone marrow or extracutaneous sites. Minor diagnostic criteria include (1) atypical or spindle-shaped morphology affecting more than 25% of the mast cells, (2) detection of the D816V *KIT* mutation, (3) aberrant expression of CD2 and/or CD25 on mast cells, and (4) a serum tryptase level greater than 20 ng/mL. Diagnosis requires the major and one minor criteria or three minor criteria. Gastrointestinal involvement is common and may result in abdominal pain, diarrhea, and/or malabsorption. Rare patients have had histologic and clinical features of celiac sprue but usually present with mucosal nodules, erosions, and friability on endoscopy.

**5. Correct choice: C.**

Common variable immunodeficiency disease (CVID) is characterized by chronic diarrhea, malabsorption, and recurrent gastrointestinal giardiasis and can often be misdiagnosed as celiac sprue. Although histologic findings are variable, the most frequent findings are intraepithelial lymphocytosis, reduction in or absence of plasma cells, and lymphoid hyperplasia. There is usually mild or no villous blunting. In contrast to celiac sprue, where they are increased, plasma cells in CVID are usually markedly decreased and immunoglobulin A (IgA)-containing plasma cells are typically absent.

**6. Correct choice: E.**

Microvillus inclusion disease is an autosomal recessive disease characterized by severe secretory diarrhea, typically within the first week of life. Small intestine biopsy specimens exhibit a severe villous abnormality with crypt hypoplasia. On electron microscopy, enterocytes have an absence of membranous microvilli, with an accumulation of "inclusions" of microvilli within the cytoplasm. These intracytoplasmic aggregates are apparent on periodic acid-Schiff stain with diastase (PAS-D) and CD10, which also highlight an absent brush border.

**7. Correct choice: C.**

Giardiasis is the most common protozoal disease in the United States. The first signs of infection usually appear after 6 to 15 days of infection and include explosive, foul-smelling watery diarrhea, nausea, epigastric pain, and malabsorption. Most biopsies in patients with giardiasis are essentially unremarkable apart from the presence of the organisms; however, they can occasionally have mild villous blunting with inflammatory expansion of the lamina propria. Morphologically, the trophozoite has a "pear-shaped" appearance with two prominent nuclei. They often appear as if they are "falling off" the mucosa-like leaves and, for this reason, may be overlooked under the assumption that they are simply mucus from the goblet cells on the villi.

**8. Correct choice: B.**

*Clostridium difficile* colitis, caused by a toxin-producing gram-positive, anaerobic bacterium, is the leading cause of healthcare-associated infection in the United States. Patients at highest risk are hospitalized patients older than 65 years with recent antibiotic exposure. Typical symptoms include watery diarrhea, anorexia, nausea, abdominal pain, and leukocytosis with a neutrophilic predominance. Diagnosis is based on the presence of *C. difficile* organisms/toxins in stool or pseudomembranous colitis on colonoscopy, which is characterized by an elevated yellow-white plaque on the mucosal surface of the colon. Microscopically, an inflammatory pseudomembrane, which consists of karyorrhectic debris and neutrophils, exudes from dilated and degenerating crypts in an eruptive fashion.

**9. Correct choice: C.**

Lymphocytic colitis is a form of microscopic colitis. Microscopic colitis consists of two major histologic subtypes: collagenous colitis and lymphocytic colitis. Mean age at diagnosis is 60 to 65 years, and there is a female predominance. Patients typically present with chronic watery, nonbloody diarrhea. Endoscopically, the mucosa is unremarkable. Histologically, lymphocytic colitis is characterized by increased intraepithelial lymphocytes and evidence of surface epithelial injury. At least 20 lymphocytes should be present per 100 epithelial cells to meet the criteria for this diagnosis. Collagenous colitis is characterized by a thickened subepithelial collagen band measuring greater than 10 μm with irregular collagen tendrils creeping down into the lamina propria and entrapping capillaries.

**10. Correct choice: D.**

Solitary rectal ulcer syndrome is a misnomer because multiple ulcers have been reported in 30% of cases and can occur at the end of stomas, hemorrhoids, and adjacent to mass lesions. The characteristic histopathologic changes of mucosal prolapse consist of fibromuscular obliteration of the lamina propria associated with mucosal architectural distortion, often with a hyperplastic or villiform appearance. Basal crypts can appear characteristically "pinched" or pointed owing to the bundles of smooth muscle from the muscularis mucosae extending upward and surrounding them. Inflammation is typically mild or absent. The histology of specimens obtained from ulcerated areas is usually nonspecific, consisting of fibrinopurulent debris and granulation tissue.

**11. Correct choice: C.**

This is a classic gross description of Crohn disease (CD). The gross specimen received from patients with CD and ulcerative colitis (UC) can be distinguished by a variety of gross features. See Table 1.

**TABLE 1 Distinguishing Gross Features of Crohn Disease and Ulcerative Colitis**

| Feature | Crohn Enteritis | Crohn Colitis | Ulcerative Colitis |
|---|---|---|---|
| Serositis | Yes | Yes | No, except in fulminant colitis |
| Thick bowel wall | Yes | Yes | No, except when complicated by carcinoma |
| Stricture | Often | Sometimes | No, except when complicated by carcinoma |
| Mucosal edema | Yes | Yes | Usually, no |
| Discrete mucosal ulcers | Yes | Yes | Usually no, except in fulminant colitis |
| Fat wrapping | Often present | Often present | Usually, no |
| Fistula | Common | Sometimes | No |
| Distribution | Focal or patchy | Focal or patchy | Diffuse |
| Rectal involvement | No | Sometimes | Yes |
| Inflammatory polyps | Rare | Sometimes | Sometimes |

**12. Correct choice: B.**

Tuberculosis infection is one of the multiple mimics of Crohn disease, which also include ischemic colitis and other infectious conditions (eg, Yersinia). See Table 1.

**TABLE 1 Differential Diagnosis of Crohn Disease**

| Feature | Crohn Disease | Ischemic Bowel Disease | Tuberculosis |
|---|---|---|---|
| Discrete ulcers | Yes | Yes | Yes |
| Longitudinally running ulcers | Yes | Yes | Usually, no |
| Stricture | Yes | Yes | Yes |
| Lymphoid aggregates | Yes | No | Usually, no |
| Hemorrhage and necrosis | No | Yes (acute) | No |
| Granulation tissue and fibrosis | No | Yes (late) | Sometimes |
| Hemosiderin deposition | Usually, no | Often | Usually, no |
| Preferred location | Ileum and cecum | Watershed zones (eg, splenic flexure) | Ileum and cecum |
| Granulomas | Often | No | Yes |
| Confluence of granulomas | No | Not applicable | Sometimes |
| Necrotizing granulomas | No | Not applicable | Sometimes |
| Fibrosis of muscularis propria | Usually, no | Yes | Yes |

**13. Correct choice: A.**

Diversion colitis develops when a segment of colon, most commonly the rectum, is bypassed from the fecal stream either surgically or by another means such as a fistula. Patients are usually asymptomatic but can present with tenesmus and blood discharge; the mucosa of the diverted segment is erythematous, granular, and friable. Histologically, there is nodular lymphoid hyperplasia with germinal centers, accompanied by chronic lamina propria inflammation, cryptitis, and crypt abscesses.

These changes may be indistinguishable from inflammatory bowel disease (IBD), but the history of diversion is a critical component of the diagnosis.

**14. Correct choice: A.**

Angioectasia, also known as vascular ectasia, angiodysplasia, and arteriovenous malformation, typically affects older adults who have episodes of recurrent low-grade lower gastrointestinal bleeding. The lesions, which are generally confined to the cecum or ascending colon and are often multiple, may be endoscopically inconspicuous. Once identified, these lesions are usually treated by endoscopic methods. On histology, abnormal, thin-walled, ectatic veins, venules, and capillaries can be seen extending into the mucosa from the submucosa.

**15. Correct choice: D.**

Hirschsprung disease (HD) is caused by the absence of ganglion cells in both the submucosal and myenteric plexuses, which is usually accompanied by hypertrophy of the muscularis mucosae and of the nerves of both plexuses. HD has been linked to inactivating mutations of the *RET* proto-oncogene. HD has a predilection for males, and 90% of patients are first seen in the neonatal period, usually with constipation, abdominal distention, vomiting, and delay of meconium stool. Diarrhea may also occur, and some patients develop life-threatening enterocolitis. The abnormalities in the submucosal and myenteric plexuses parallel each other. Suction biopsy of the mucosa and submucosa is now considered the standard method for evaluation for patients suspected to have HD. If the amount of submucosa occupies less than half the thickness of the biopsy or anal canal epithelium, these biopsies are considered inadequate.

**16. Correct choice: A.**

Mesenteric fibromatosis affects the mesentery or retroperitoneum and can be associated with the Gardner syndrome variant of familial adenomatous polyposis. Key histologic features include uniform fibroblastic proliferation with areas of increased cellularity, an arrangement of spindle cells in interlacing bundles, an infiltrative character of the spindle cell population as it interacts with the muscularis propria of the intestines and adjacent adipose tissue, and a paucity of inflammatory and foam cells. There is typically nuclear positivity for β-catenin in fibromatosis.

**17. Correct choice: D.**

Patients with inflammatory bowel disease (IBD) with visible dysplasia that is completely removed on endoscopy can continue with surveillance colonoscopy, rather than colectomy. Colitis-associated carcinomas are often morphologically atypical and difficult to visualize by standard radiographic techniques. The cytologic criteria for dysplasia are well established, although the diagnosis, separation from reactive or reparative changes in association with inflammation or other injury, and grading are not always so straightforward. Dysplasia and repair both have nuclear enlargement and hyperchromasia, increased mitotic activity, and decreased intracellular mucin. Visible dysplasia can be seen endoscopically and is, therefore, potentially amenable to endoscopic removal. This category includes both colitis-associated dysplasia that creates visible lesions and sporadic colonic adenomas that occur in patients who also have IBD.

**18. Correct choice: A.**

Chemotherapeutic-associated injury, characterized by necrosis, ulcers, and acute and chronic inflammation of the mucosa, usually occurs within 1 or 2 weeks after cessation of chemotherapy. Typically, the abnormalities subside in 1 to 2 months. Features include marked cellular enlargement of the crypt epithelium with large, extremely atypical nuclei and mucin depletion. The epithelial atypia associated with radiation and chemotherapy may be significant enough to simulate the appearance of carcinoma. Features that favor therapy effect rather than neoplasia include a general preservation of mucosal architecture, preservation of a relatively normal nuclear-to-cytoplasmic ratio despite the presence of atypia, a lack of mitotic activity, similar atypical changes in fibroblasts and endothelium, and the lack of an infiltrative pattern or a desmoplastic stromal reaction.

# 34 Intestinal Neoplasms

1. A histologic section of a colon polyp is shown in Figure 1. What is the proper diagnosis?

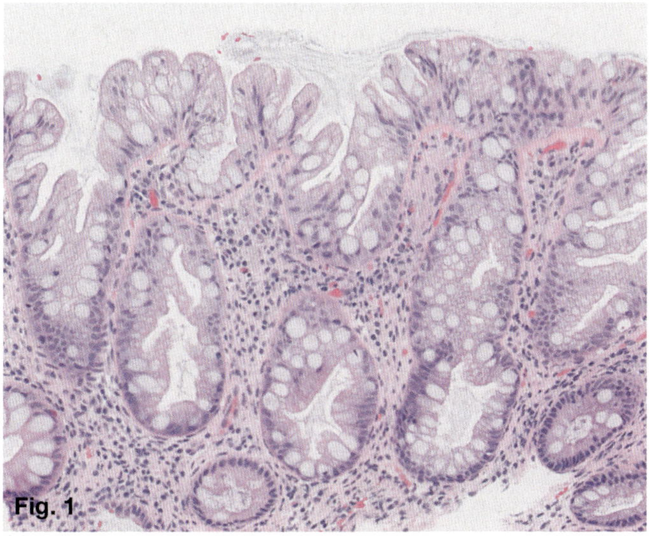

Fig. 1

A. Hyperplastic polyp, goblet cell rich
B. Hyperplastic polyp, microvesicular
C. Sessile serrated polyp
D. Traditional serrated adenoma
E. Tubular adenoma

2. A histologic section of a colon polyp is shown in Figure 1. What is the proper diagnosis?

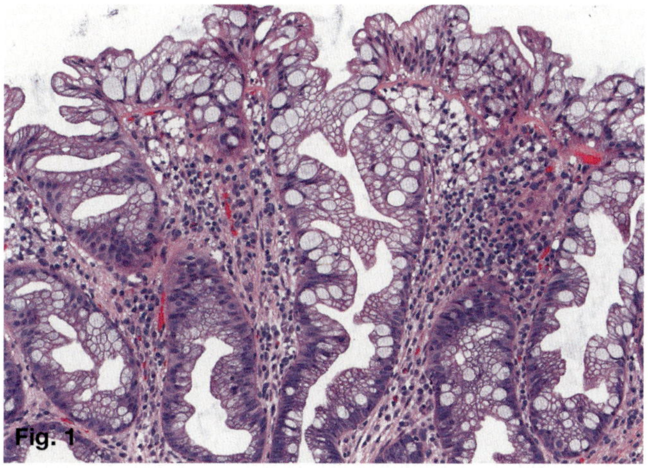

Fig. 1

A. Hyperplastic polyp, goblet cell rich
B. Hyperplastic polyp, microvesicular
C. Sessile serrated polyp
D. Traditional serrated adenoma
E. Tubular adenoma

3. Which of the following polyps are thought to be precursor lesions of adenocarcinomas characterized by CpG island methylator phenotype and often show loss of MLH1 expression?

A. Conventional adenomas
B. Hamartomatous polyps
C. Hyperplastic polyps
D. Juvenile polyps
E. Sessile serrated polyps with dysplasia

4. Which of the following is true about traditional serrated adenomas?

A. Crypts show slit-like serrations with basal dilation and horizontal growth.
B. Greater than 90% of traditional serrated adenomas show *BRAF* mutation.
C. Most traditional serrated adenomas are found in patients with familial adenomatous polyposis.
D. They can be found in both the small bowel and proximal colon.
E. They are lined by goblet cell–rich epithelium with eosinophilic cytoplasm with pencillate nuclei.

---

All figures in this chapter are from Longacre TA, Greenson JK, Hornick JL, Reuter VE, eds. *Mills and Sternberg's Diagnostic Surgical Pathology.* 7th ed. Wolters Kluwer; 2022 except for those noted at the end of this book.

5. A pedunculated polyp is excised from the descending colon. Histologically, it is composed of crypts with pseudostratified, elongated, and hyperchromatic nuclei with smooth nuclear contours and inconspicuous nucleoli aligned along the basal layer. There is little cytoplasm and rare goblet cells. Some of the dysplastic crypts have luminal serration and 20% of the lesional polyp has a villous component. There is prominent epithelial apoptosis. What is the diagnosis?

   A. Sessile serrated polyp with dysplasia
   B. Traditional serrated adenoma
   C. Tubular adenoma
   D. Tubulovillous adenoma
   E. Villous adenoma

6. A pedunculated polyp is excised from the rectum. Histologically, it is mostly composed of a cytologically low-grade epithelium that shows a 75% villous component. There is an area near the surface of the polyp that shows high-grade morphology. Focally, some adenomatous crypts that are surrounded by mixed inflammation are identified in the submucosa of the polyp near the junction with the stalk. Within the submucosa directly adjacent to these crypts, there are extensive hemosiderin deposition, extravasated red blood cells, and distortion of the muscularis mucosa. What is the most likely diagnosis?

   A. Intramucosal adenocarcinoma
   B. Invasive adenocarcinoma
   C. Tubular adenoma with high-grade dysplasia
   D. Tubulovillous adenoma with high-grade dysplasia
   E. Villous adenoma with high-grade dysplasia

7. A 56-year-old male patient with a long-standing history of left-sided ulcerative colitis that has been medically managed undergoes a surveillance colonoscopy, which shows scattered erythema without discrete lesions or masses. Random biopsies are taken from all parts of the colon. Figure 1 is of a representative histologic section from the sigmoid colon. What is the most appropriate diagnosis?

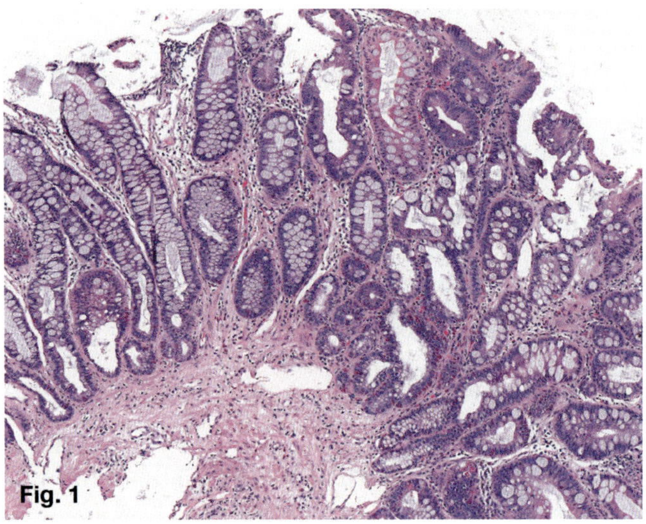

Fig. 1

   A. Chronic active colitis
   B. Flat low-grade dysplasia
   C. Polypoid low-grade dysplasia
   D. Quiescent colitis
   E. Tubular adenoma

8. A pedunculated polyp is resected from the proximal portion of the jejunum. Histologically, it consists of nondysplastic intestinal-type epithelium. There are arborizing bundles of smooth muscle that emanate from the muscularis mucosae that gives the polyp a "branching" appearance. Which of the following additional features is most likely to be observed in this patient?

   A. Cranial and cardiac abnormalities
   B. Gastrointestinal tumors
   C. Innumerable adenomatous polyps
   D. Mucocutaneous hyperpigmentation
   E. Osteomas of the mandible and long bones

9. A 34-year-old patient with a history of multiple trichilemmomas underwent an esophagogastroduodenoscopy (EGD) and colonoscopy, which showed multifocal esophageal glycogenic acanthosis and multiple sessile polyps in the colon. The colon polyps are identified as ganglioneuromas and intramucosal lipomas. This patient then undergoes genetic testing. Which of the following germline mutations would most likely be found in this patient?

   A. *APC*
   B. *MUTYH*
   C. *PTEN*
   D. *SMAD4*
   E. *STK11*

10. A 66-year-old female patient with recurrent pancreatitis undergoes an esophagogastroduodenoscopy (EGD). A nodule is resected from the first third of the duodenum. Histologic sections of this nodule show frond-like mucinous epithelium composed of cuboidal-to-columnar cells with low-grade dysplasia arranged in a tubulopapillary architecture. Immunohistochemical stains show that the tumor cells show expression for epithelial membrane antigen (EMA), MUC5AC, CK7, and CK20. Adjacent to the lesion is benign duodenal mucosa. What is the likely diagnosis?

   A. Ampullary adenoma
   B. Duodenal adenoma
   C. Intra-ampullary papillary-tubular neoplasm
   D. Intraductal papillary mucinous neoplasm
   E. Peutz-Jeghers hamartomatous polyp

11. Which of the following most accurately reflects intramucosal carcinoma in the tubular gastrointestinal tract?

   A. Defined as submucosal lymphoglandular complexes with low-grade cytology
   B. Invasion beyond the muscularis mucosae
   C. Invasion into the lamina propria
   D. No malignant potential
   E. Synonymous with high-grade dysplasia

12. A 3.4-cm malignant polyp of the sigmoid colon is removed in one piece by endoscopic mucosal resection. Which of the following statements is true?

    A. Histologic subtype and a synoptic report need to be reported.
    B. Representative sampling of the polyp (1 section/cm) is considered adequate.
    C. Submucosal lymphoglandular complexes with high-grade cytology are staged as pTis.
    D. Submucosal mucin pools with strips of atypical epithelium reflect misplaced epithelium.
    E. There is no need to evaluate for tumor bedding in malignant polyps.

13. Which of the following is true about a carcinoma identified in the small bowel?

    A. If it is a small bowel primary, it is most likely to arise in the duodenum.
    B. Most tumors present with symptoms of small bowel obstruction.
    C. Periampullary adenocarcinomas are almost always of pancreatobiliary type.
    D. Small bowel adenocarcinomas are usually low stage and good prognosis.
    E. There is a low frequency of *KRAS* mutation, similar to carcinoma of the colon.

14. A resected colon carcinoma shows the following histologic feature seen in Figure 1, which accounts for 40% of total tumor volume. The rest of the tumor volume consists of cribriform and angulated glandular architecture. Which of the following is the proper histologic classification of this carcinoma?

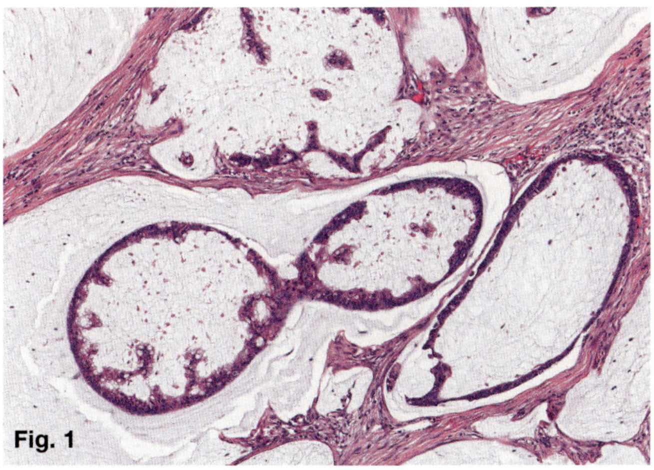
Fig. 1

    A. Adenocarcinoma, conventional
    B. Medullary carcinoma
    C. Micropapillary adenocarcinoma
    D. Mucinous adenocarcinoma
    E. Signet-ring cell carcinoma

15. A 70-year-old woman undergoes resection of a bulky, well-circumscribed mass in the proximal colon. Figure 1 shows the histologic appearance of the tumor, which is diffusely infiltrated by lymphocytes. The tumor was found to be high microsatellite instability (MSI-H) and lacks expression of CK20, CDX-2, synaptophysin, and INSM1. Which of the following is the most likely diagnosis?

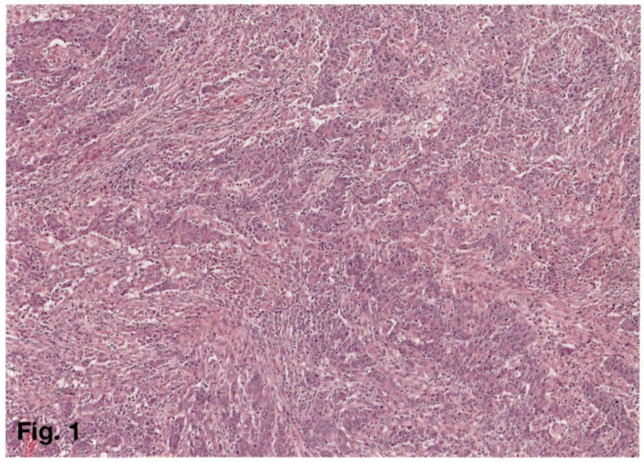
Fig. 1

    A. Adenocarcinoma, conventional
    B. Enteroblastoma
    C. Medullary carcinoma
    D. Neuroendocrine carcinoma
    E. Undifferentiated carcinoma

16. Which of the following is true about tumor budding?

    A. A tumor bud is a cluster of up to five tumor cells intimately associated with invasive glands.
    B. High-tumor budding score is associated with increased risk for regional lymph node metastases.
    C. High-tumor budding score is indicative of an adenocarcinoma with poor differentiation.
    D. It is an important independent prognostic feature in neoadjuvant-treated adenocarcinomas.
    E. It is more commonly seen in mismatch repair–deficient neoplasms.

17. A full-thickness section of a colon cancer is shown in Figure 1. What is the appropriate pathologic stage?

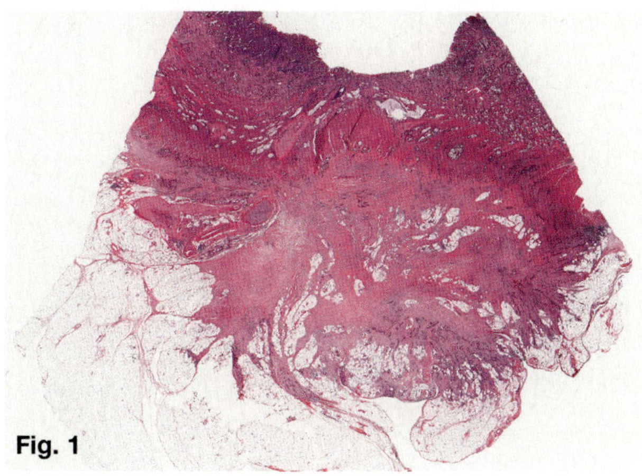
Fig. 1

    A. pT1
    B. pT2
    C. pT3
    D. pT4a
    E. pT4b

18. DNA mismatch repair protein testing by immunohistochemistry is performed on a moderately differentiated adenocarcinoma in the colon. The immunostain for MLH1 is shown in Figure 1. Which of the following is a correct statement about the result of this testing?

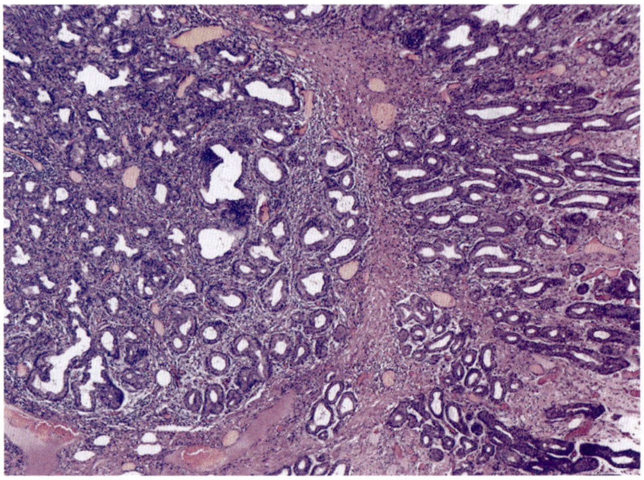

A. Intact MLH1 expression
B. Patient has Lynch syndrome
C. Predicts loss of MSH2
D. Send for DNA methylation testing
E. Test for BRAF by immunohistochemistry

19. Figure 1 is a histologic section of a colectomy specimen from a 35-year-old patient with a history of osteomas and innumerable small intestinal and gastric polyps. In addition, multiple desmoid tumors were identified in the mesentery. The patient most likely has which of the following syndromes and germline mutations?

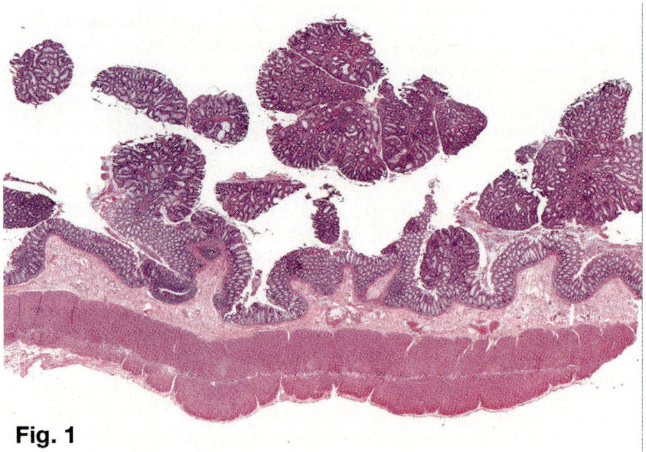

Fig. 1

A. Cowden syndrome; *PTEN*
B. Familial adenomatous polyposis; *KRAS*
C. Gardner syndrome; *APC*
D. Hereditary mixed polyposis syndrome; *GERM1*
E. Lynch syndrome; *MSH6*

20. According to the World Health Organization (WHO), the tumor shown in Figure 1 is graded by which of the following parameters?

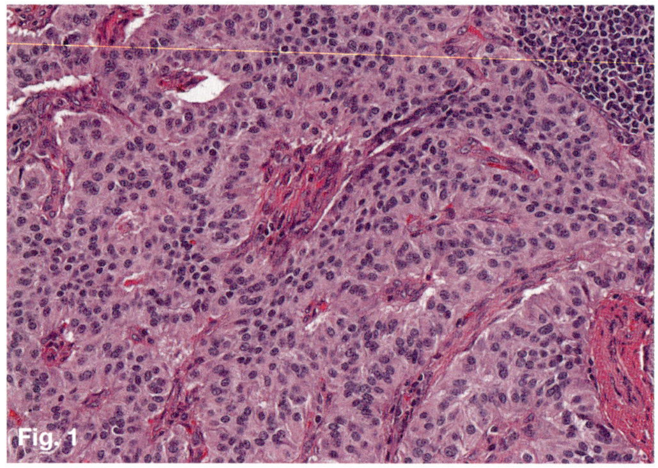

Fig. 1

A. Amount of tumor necrosis
B. Degree of cytologic atypia
C. Mitotic count
D. Status of MLH1 by immunohistochemistry
E. Tumor architectural features

21. A 0.8-cm submucosal nodule was excised from the colon. Figure 1 is a representative histologic section of the nodule. Which of the following immunostains would be most helpful to confirm the diagnosis?

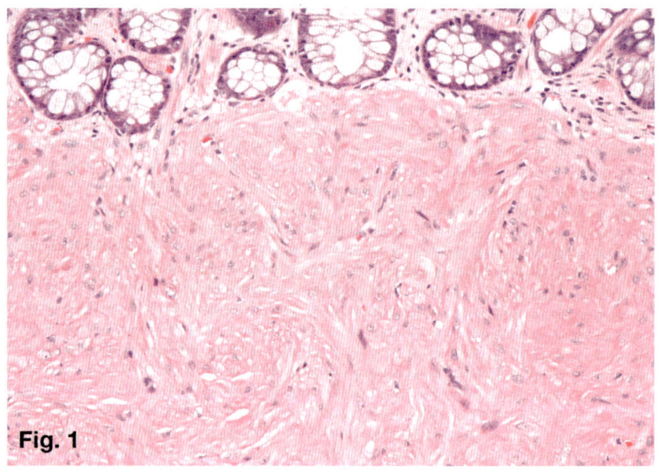

Fig. 1

A. CD117
B. Desmin
C. Epithelial membrane antigen (EMA)
D. S100
E. SOX10

22. You received a segmental colectomy with large purple submucosal nodules and spongy appearance in the gross room. Figure 1 is a histologic section of the lesion. What is the most likely diagnosis?

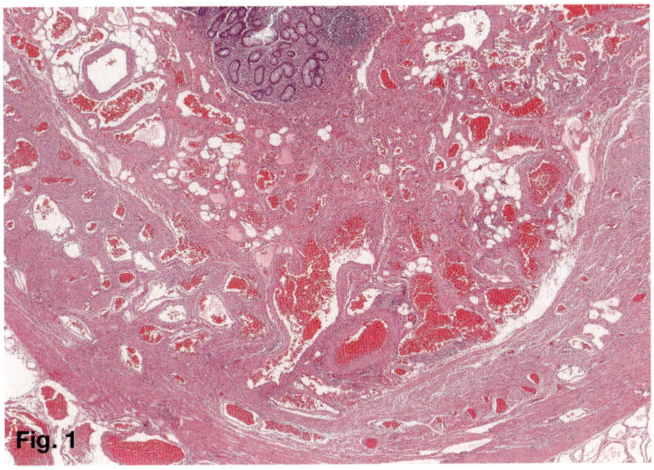

Fig. 1

A. Angiodysplasia
B. Arteriovenous malformation
C. Cavernous hemangioma
D. Lobular capillary hemangioma
E. Telangiectasia

23. A 36-year-old female with a history of severe dysmenorrhea and medically intractable left-sided ulcerative colitis undergoes a proctocolectomy. On gross examination, there is severe colitis involving the rectum and extending into the proximal left colon. In addition, there is a nodular, ulcerated, and circumferential lesion in the sigmoid colon with associated luminal narrowing and transmural thickening. Figure 1 shows a section of the involved muscularis propria. What is the most likely diagnosis?

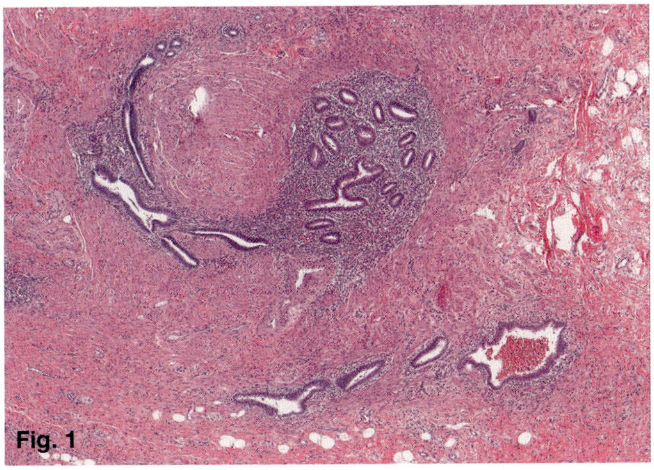

Fig. 1

A. Crohn disease
B. Diverticulosis
C. Endometriosis
D. Invasive adenocarcinoma
E. Lymphoglandular complexes

24. A patient with celiac sprue (gluten-sensitive enteropathy) is prone to developing which of the following types of small intestinal lymphomas?

A. Histiocytic lymphoma
B. Hodgkin disease
C. Immunoproliferative small intestinal disease
D. Mucosa-associated lymphoid tissue (MALT)-associated lymphoma
E. T-cell lymphoma

25. A 36-year-old male with a history of celiac disease undergoes an upper gastrointestinal (GI) endoscopy, which reveals nodular mucosa in the duodenum. Histologic section of a biopsied duodenal polyp is shown in Figure 1. The small lymphocytes show expression for CD20, CD10, BCL6, and BCL2. What is the diagnosis?

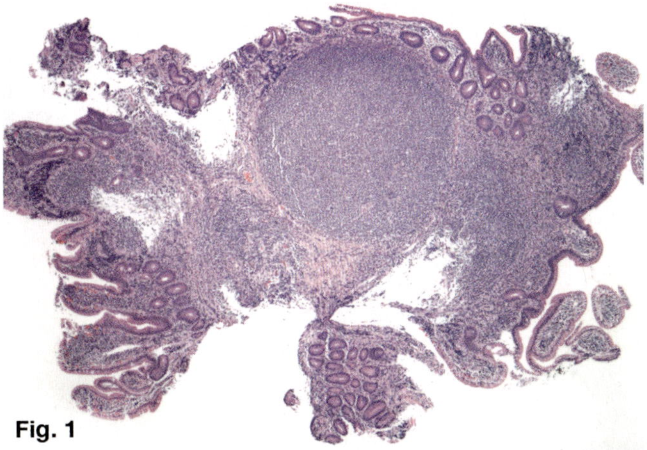

Fig. 1

A. Burkitt lymphoma
B. Enteropathy-associated T-cell lymphomas
C. Follicular lymphoma
D. Mantle cell lymphoma
E. Marginal zone lymphoma

26. Which of the following is true of posttransplant lymphoproliferative disorder?

A. Cannot be detected on endoscopy
B. Caused by acute rejection
C. Caused by new infection or reactivation of Epstein-Barr virus (EBV)
D. Comprises atypical T-cell population
E. Treat by increasing immunosuppression

27. A patient undergoes appendectomy for acute appendicitis. The appendix is enlarged and distended. When sectioned, the lumen is filled with mucinous material and diffuse wall thinning. A representative histologic section of the mucosal surface is shown in Figure 1. What is the most likely diagnosis?

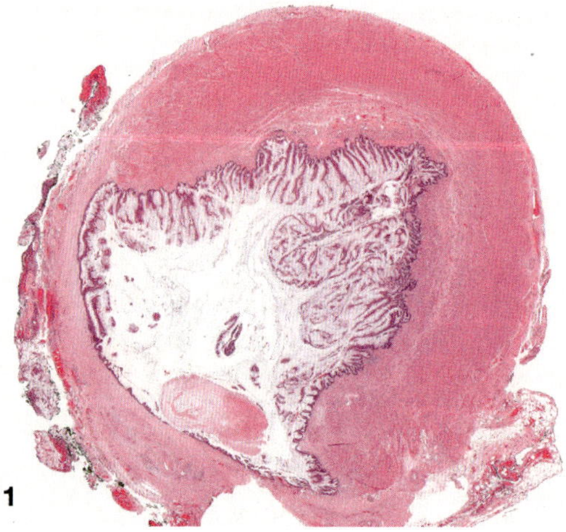

Fig. 1

A. Conventional adenoma
B. Hyperplastic polyp
C. Invasive low-grade adenocarcinoma
D. Low-grade appendiceal mucinous neoplasm
E. Mucinous adenoma

# ANSWERS AND EXPLANATIONS

**1. Correct choice: B.**

Hyperplastic polyps (HP) are the most common colorectal polyps and have a predilection for the distal colon/rectum. Two variants are recognized based on morphologic and molecular differences: microvesicular HP and goblet cell–rich HP. Microvesicular HPs are the most common. Histologically, they show evenly spaced, funnel-shaped crypts that show prominent infoldings of the epithelium composed of a mixed population of goblet cells and non–goblet mucinous cells, particularly in the upper crypt region. Goblet cell–rich HPs are easily overlooked in biopsy samples because they resemble normal mucosa. Subclassifying HPs in clinical practice is currently not warranted.

**2. Correct choice: C.**

Sessile serrated polyps (SSP) are nondysplastic serrated colorectal polyps with predilection for proximal colon/cecum. SSPs are precursors to a subset of sporadic mismatch repair–deficient colonic adenocarcinomas. Even though the epithelium is nondysplastic, it has a comparable biologic risk to that of conventional adenomas. Histologically, SSPs have lesional crypts that have horizontal growth with branching or budding above the muscularis mucosae. The crypts contain a dual population of goblet cells and non–goblet columnar cells with microvesicular mucin. Distinction of SSP from hyperplastic polyp (HP) is subject to a high degree of interobserver variability.

**3. Correct choice: E.**

Sessile serrated polyp (SSP) with cytologic dysplasia is associated with *BRAF* mutations with DNA methylation (CpG island methylator phenotype). Thus, it is commonly associated with sporadic loss of MLH1 expression and high microsatellite instability (MSI-H) via *MLH1* promoter methylation. Conventional adenomas and traditional serrated adenomas usually show preserved MLH1 staining and are mismatch repair proficient.

**4. Correct choice: D.**

Traditional serrated adenomas (TSA) are uncommon dysplastic polyps that account for 1% to 2% of endoscopically removed colorectal adenomas. Most TSAs are sporadic, but they have been described in patients with familial adenomatous polyposis and serrated polyposis. TSAs show predilection for the sigmoid colon and rectum but can be found in the right colon and rarely in the proximal small bowel. TSAs are composed of crypts with slit-like serrations and villi with small invaginations in the lateral aspect of the epithelium, which have been termed aberrant crypt foci. Crypts and villous projections are lined by non–goblet epithelial cells with abundant eosinophilic cytoplasm and indistinct cell borders. Most show low-grade cytologic features with elongated, pencillate nuclei that are slightly lifted from the basal aspect and usually have less mitotic activity and apoptosis compared to conventional adenomas. Some contain foci of nondysplastic serrated crypts similar to that of a sessile serrated polyp, and others acquire different types of dysplasia, often with high-grade cytologic features. Unlike hyperplastic and sessile serrated polyps, *BRAF* mutation is not the predominant molecular feature of TSA (40% *BRAF* mutation vs 50% *KRAS* mutation).

**5. Correct choice: C.**

Tubular adenomas account for nearly 50% of all endoscopically removed colorectal polyps. The likelihood of malignant adenoma is directly related to size: invasive carcinoma is detected in 0.5% of adenomas less than 1.0 cm and 10% of adenomas greater than 2.0 cm. Adenomas are further categorized as tubular adenoma, tubulovillous adenoma, and villous adenoma. Tubular adenomas have 75% or more volume composed of straight tubular or branched crypts, whereas villous adenomas contain slender fronds of dysplastic epithelium that account for 75% or more of the polyp volume. Anything in between is considered tubulovillous. Villous adenomas carry a worse prognosis as invasive carcinoma is more likely to be present when compared to a tubular adenoma. By convention, the term "adenoma" is cytologically low grade, and a distinction must be made when there is a component of high-grade dysplasia.

**6. Correct choice: D.**

Epithelial misplacement can be seen in large pedunculated adenomas of the distal colon/rectum secondary to intermittent ischemic injury and increased luminal pressure. These forces lead to the herniation of adenomatous crypts and surrounding lamina propria into the submucosa. This "pseudoinvasion" is associated with hemorrhage, hemosiderin deposition, and fibrosis. Epithelial misplacement can also occur when adenomatous crypts involve lymphoid aggregates located immediately adjacent to the muscularis mucosae, which is commonly seen in the proximal colon. The epithelium in these lymphoglandular complexes is usually cytologically similar to the rest of the adenoma.

**7. Correct choice: B.**

Inflammatory bowel disease (IBD)-associated dysplasia most often occurs in the setting of long-standing ulcerative colitis (UC), increasing the risk of developing colorectal adenocarcinoma. IBD-associated dysplasia, both low and high, is divided into categories of visible and invisible dysplasia. Visible dysplasia can be seen endoscopically with white light and/or augmented techniques and is therefore potentially amenable to endoscopic removal. This category includes both colitis-associated dysplasia that creates visible lesions and sporadic colonic adenomas. Invisible dysplasia is identified only on biopsies taken randomly and cannot be targeted for endoscopic therapeutic techniques.

**8. Correct choice: D.**

Peutz-Jeghers syndrome (PJS) is caused by mutations of the *STK11* tumor-suppressor gene. This syndrome is characterized by hamartomatous polyps of the gastrointestinal (GI) tract, mucocutaneous hyperpigmentation (ie, around the mouth), and increased risk for cancers of the breast, testis, gynecologic tract, colon, pancreas, and stomach. The PJS polyps are hamartomatous polyps that are lined by absorptive cells, goblet cells, endocrine cells, and Paneth cells, showing a branching pattern and bundles of arborizing smooth muscle extending from the muscularis propria. These classical features are usually seen in polyps of the small bowel, as PJS polyps in the colon may present as an inflamed mucosal prolapse-type polyp. Despite the risk for carcinoma, foci of dysplasia and/or invasive carcinoma are rarely present in PJS polyps.

**9. Correct choice: C.**

Cowden syndrome is an autosomal dominant disorder caused by germline *PTEN* mutations. Affected patients can develop gastrointestinal (GI) tract, oral, and cutaneous hamartomatous lesions. See Table 1 for criteria for diagnosis of Cowden syndrome.

**TABLE 1 Diagnostic Criteria for Cowden Syndrome**

| Organ System | Major Criteria | Minor Criteria |
|---|---|---|
| Gastrointestinal | Three or more hamartomas | Esophageal glycogenic acanthosis<br>Colon carcinoma |
| Genitourinary/Gynecologic | Endometrial carcinoma | Testicular lipomatosis<br>Renal cell carcinoma |
| Neurologic | Dysplastic gangliocytoma of the cerebellum (Lhermitte-Duclos disease)<br>Macrocephaly | Intracranial venous anomalies and other vascular anomalies<br>Autism spectrum disorder<br>IQ ≤ 75 |
| Endocrine | Follicular thyroid carcinoma | Papillary thyroid carcinoma<br>Thyroid follicular adenoma<br>Multinodular goiter |
| Mucocutaneous | Three or more trichilemmomas<br>Three or more acral keratosis<br>Three or more neuromas<br>Three or more oral papillomas | Lipomas |
| Breast | Carcinoma | |

From Pilarski R, Burt R, Kohlman W, et al. Cowden syndrome and the PTEN hamartoma tumor syndrome: systematic review and revised diagnostic criteria. *J Natl Cancer Inst.* 2013;105(21):1607-1616. Copyright © 2013 The Author. Reproduced by permission of Oxford University Press.

**10. Correct choice: C.**

Adenomas that develop within the intra-ampullary channel are classified as intra-ampullary papillary-tubular neoplasms (IPTNs), which typically have a frond-like appearance with tubulopapillary architecture reminiscent of pancreatic intraductal papillary mucinous neoplasms. Ampullary adenomas can also occur in the ampullary/periampullary duodenal mucosa. Small adenomas are usually seen incidentally during esophagogastroduodenoscopy (EGD). Large adenomas cause biliary symptoms such as pancreatitis or cholangitis. Adenomas of the ampullary and/or periampullary duodenal mucosa are usually of intestinal type similar to duodenal adenomas and can extend into ampullary ducts and glands. By immunohistochemistry, intestinal-type ampullary adenomas are positive for CDX2, CK7, CK20 and negative for epithelial membrane antigen (EMA). Intra-ampullary papillary-tubular neoplasms (IPTNs) are positive for EMA, MUC5AC, CK7 and CK20.

**11. Correct choice: C.**

Intramucosal adenocarcinoma is defined as adenocarcinoma that invades the lamina propria but is confined to the muscularis mucosae. There is no associated desmoplastic tissue reaction. It is essential to distinguish such lesions from those with malignant growth extending into the submucosa. Intramucosal carcinoma of the colorectum has a negligible risk for metastasis due to the paucity of lymphatic vessels within the lamina propria and is categorized as in situ neoplasm (pTis). However, intramucosal carcinomas of the esophagus and stomach are associated with a more significant metastatic potential. In these sites, there are lymphatic vessels in the lamina propria and these are categorized as malignant (pT1).

**12. Correct choice: A.**

Endoscopically resected malignant polyps have invasive adenocarcinoma, thus should be histologically subtyped and a synoptic report needs to be reported. Regardless of the nature of the specimen, endoscopically removed material should be entirely submitted for histologic evaluation. The most important features that should be reported include depth of invasion, distance from resection margins, status of resection margins, tumor budding score, angiolymphatic invasion, perineural invasion, and pathologic stage (pT). Submucosal mucin pool with peripheral strips of atypical epithelium is considered invasive adenocarcinoma, as well as submucosal lymphoglandular complexes with high-grade cytology.

**13. Correct choice: A.**

Nonampullary carcinomas of the small intestine can arise sporadically or in association with hereditary cancer syndromes or chronic inflammatory conditions, such as Crohn disease and celiac disease. Small bowel primary adenocarcinomas are very rare gastrointestinal (GI) malignancies (0.3%) and primary duodenal adenocarcinomas account for greater than 50%. Periampullary duodenal adenocarcinomas usually show intestinal-type differentiation with intestinal-type dysplasia in the adjacent mucosa. Most tumors are asymptomatic until locally advanced and, thus, the overall prognosis is poor. Unlike their colorectal counterparts, *KRAS* mutations are the most common molecular alteration and are present in greater than two-thirds of small bowel adenocarcinomas.

**14. Correct choice: A.**

Multiple variants of adenocarcinoma have been identified, of which the most are mucinous adenocarcinoma, signet-ring cell carcinoma, medullary carcinoma, and micropapillary adenocarcinoma. The carcinoma described in the question stem is an adenocarcinoma with mucinous features. Mucinous adenocarcinoma is defined by greater than 50% mucinous tumor volume. Carcinomas that show at least 50% signet-ring cell differentiation are classified as signet-ring cell carcinomas. Medullary carcinomas are solid tumors with broad-front, pushing invasion and minimal gland formation. Micropapillary carcinomas feature clusters or balls of tumor cells within lacunar spaces that are unaccompanied by supportive stroma. This variant is associated with a worse prognosis than that of stage-matched advanced adenocarcinomas.

**15. Correct choice: C.**

Medullary carcinoma tends to develop as bulky masses with an expansile growth with a predilection for older female patients. Tumor cells are arranged in trabeculae or solid nests embedded in a lymphocyte-rich stroma with prominent intraepithelial lymphocytes. The architectural growth pattern mimics that of neuroendocrine tumors, but there is no significant expression of neuroendocrine markers. In contrast to conventional adenocarcinoma, medullary carcinomas do not express CDX-2 and often lack CK20 as well. In addition, they are microsatellite instability-high (MSI-H). Medullary carcinoma has a better prognosis than the conventional type.

**16. Correct choice: B.**

Tumor budding is defined as the presence of single infiltrating cells or groups of up to four neoplastic cells intimately associated with larger invasive glands. It is classified as low (0-4 buds), intermediate (5-9 buds), and high grade (≥10 buds) by assessing the number of tumor buds per 0.785 $mm^2$ in the area of maximal budding. High-tumor budding is associated with increased risk for regional lymph node metastases when evaluated in non–treated colorectal adenocarcinoma. Tumor budding is more common among mismatch repair proficient tumors than mismatch repair–deficient neoplasms but predicts aggressive behavior in both types of tumors.

**17. Correct choice: D.**

The tumor, node, metastasis (TNM) staging system of the American Joint Committee on Cancer (AJCC) and the Union for International Cancer Control (UICC) provide standardized criteria for cancer reporting. The T category denotes the pathologic tumor stage and describes the deepest point of penetration in the intestinal wall, surrounding fat, or adjacent structures. pTis is reserved for intramucosal adenocarcinomas. pT1 tumors are confined to the submucosal. pT2 tumors are confined to muscularis propria, and pT3 tumors extend into the subserosal soft tissue. pT4 is divided into serosal involvement (pT4a) or invasion into non-adjacent structures (pT4b). Distinguishing between pT3 and pT4a is important, as the latter will receive adjuvant chemotherapy.

**18. Correct choice: D.**

*MLH1* promoter methylation should be performed on any non–colorectal gastrointestinal (GI) cancer with loss of MLH1 and PMS2 expression. It is common practice to use immunohistochemical testing for DNA repair proteins MLH1, MSH2, MSH6, and PMS2 as a surrogate for evaluating microsatellite instability (MSI) status. MLH1 and PMS2 are paired proteins where loss of MLH1 will cause loss of PMS2, while loss of PMS2 does not necessarily mean loss of MLH1. The sample principle applies to MSH2 and MSH6. Patients with germline mutations in the genes which encode either four of the proteins have Lynch syndrome; however, just because there is loss of expression by immunohistochemistry, this is not definitive for Lynch syndrome, especially with the loss of both MLH1 and PMS2 by immunohistochemistry. Sporadic mutations may occur in all four, but *MLH1* can be silenced by methylation of the promoter region, which can be tested for by *MLH1* promoter methylation assay. In colorectal adenocarcinomas with MLH1 loss, *BRAF* molecular testing can be performed as a surrogate marker for DNA methylation.

**19. Correct choice: C.**

Gardner syndrome is an autosomal dominant condition due to germline *APC* mutations on chromosome 5q21. It is characterized by the development of hundreds to thousands of colorectal adenomatous polyps and a colorectal cancer risk of nearly 100% by age 40. Patients with Gardner syndrome develop gastrointestinal polyposis, osteomas, and intraabdominal fibromatosis (ie, desmoid tumors), etc.

**20. Correct choice: C.**

Well-differentiated neuroendocrine tumors (WDNETs) may arise along the entire gastrointestinal (GI) tract. They are characterized by uniform tumor cells arranged in nests, trabeculae, acini, or ribbon-like cords embedded in the hyalinized stroma. The cells are polygonal with pale cytoplasm and round or slightly ovoid nuclei containing coarse, granular chromatin and inconspicuous nuclei. They are graded by mitotic rate and/or Ki-67 index. See Table 1.

**TABLE 1** World Health Organization Classification of Gastrointestinal Neuroendocrine Tumors

| | Ki-67[a] Index (%) | Mitotic Index/10 HPF[b] |
|---|---|---|
| **Well-Differentiated Neuroendocrine Neoplasms (NENS)** | | |
| NET grade 1 (G1) | <3 | <2 |
| NET grade 2 (G2) | 3-20 | 2-20 |
| NET grade 3 (G3) | >20 | >20 |
| **Poorly Differentiated Neuroendocrine Neoplasms (NENS)** | | |
| Neuroendocrine carcinoma | >20 | >20 |
| Small cell | | |
| Large cell | | |

HPF, high-power field; NET, neuroendocrine tumor.
[a]MIB1 antibody percentage positive of 500 to 2,000 tumor cells in the area of highest labeling.
[b]10 HPF = 2 $mm^2$. At least 50 HPF (at 40 times) must be evaluated in the area of highest mitotic index.

Adapted from La Rosa S, Rindi G, Solcia E, et al. Gastric neuroendocrine neoplasms. In: WHO Classification of Tumours Editorial Board, ed. *Digestive System Tumours, WHO Classification of Tumours Series.* 5th ed. Vol 1. International Agency for Research on Cancer; 2019:104-109. With permission.

**21. Correct choice: B.**

Leiomyomas generally arise from the muscularis mucosae of the colon and present as well-circumscribed, unencapsulated nodules. They are composed of paucicellular proliferations of smooth muscle cells arranged in short intersecting fascicles. They generally lack mitotic activity and cytologic atypia. The tumor cells would stain positive for desmin, smooth muscle actin, and caldesmon.

**22. Correct choice: B.**

Arteriovenous malformations (AVMs) are congenital abnormalities that result from aberrant communications between arteries and veins. AVMs can affect all layers of the bowel wall, producing large purple nodules that protrude into the lumen and a spongy appearance on cross section. Histologic sections show disorganized aggregates of tortuous arteries and veins with thick muscular walls surrounded by ectatic, thin-walled vessels. Solitary lesions are usually sporadic, but multiple AVMs are seen in patients with Maffucci syndrome, Klippel-Trénaunay syndrome, and Osler-Weber-Rendu syndrome.

**23. Correct choice: C.**

Endometriosis has a predilection for the rectosigmoid or ileocecal region. Histologically, it is characterized by aggregates of endometrial glands that are intimately associated with stromal cells and adjacent hemosiderin. Extensive mural disease can cause gastrointestinal bleeding or bowel obstruction, whereas appendiceal endometriosis may mimic acute appendicitis. When present in the muscularis propria, it induces smooth muscle cell hypertrophy that distorts and expands the muscularis propria, causing strictures that simulate malignancy.

**24. Correct choice: E.**

Enteropathy-Associated T-Cell Lymphoma (EATCL)—Patients with malabsorption, and especially those with celiac disease, are at increased risk of developing small intestinal lymphomas. Such lymphomas are usually of T-cell origin. Clinically, these lymphomas manifest after a long latency period (20 or more years) with recurrence of malabsorption (despite a gluten-free diet), bowel ulcerations and strictures, and elevated serum immunoglobulin A (IgA) levels. Because of the presence of multinucleated RS (Reed-Sternberg)-like cells, EATCL may lead to a mistaken diagnosis of Hodgkin disease. Hodgkin disease is rare in the small bowel.

**25. Correct choice: C.**

Duodenal-type follicular lymphoma accounts for 4% of gastrointestinal lymphomas and shows a predilection for the second part of the duodenum. Tumors are generally discovered incidentally during endoscopic examinations performed for other reasons. Most patients are older adults with an equal gender distribution, but approximately 10% of patients are young adults. Morphologically, they resemble follicular lymphomas in other parts of the gastrointestinal (GI) tract with nodular proliferations of neoplastic "follicles" containing follicular dendritic cells as well as small B-cells and larger centroblast-like cells. Tumor cells express B-cell markers in addition to CD10, BCL6, and BLC2. They harbor t(14;18) translocations that result in *BCL2-IGH* fusions.

**26. Correct choice: C.**

Posttransplant lymphoproliferative disorder occurs in patients who undergo bone marrow or solid-organ transplants. Chronic immunosuppression leads to impaired T-cell function and facilitates the proliferation of Epstein-Barr virus (EBV)-positive B-cell populations. Symptoms include a mononucleosis-like syndrome, diarrhea, abdominal pain, and declining graft function. On endoscopy, small lesions may appear as ulcers or polyps, and larger lesions appear as fungating masses. The World Health Organization classifies posttransplant lymphoproliferative disorders according to morphologic and molecular features. Treatment consists of decreased immunosuppression in conjunction with chemotherapy, surgery, and/or radiation.

**27. Correct choice: D.**

Low-grade appendiceal mucinous neoplasm (LAMN) confers uncertain biologic risk. The appendix is dilated and contains thick, tenacious mucin. The low-grade dysplastic epithelium, obliteration of muscularis mucosa, and atrophy of lymphoid tissue are characteristic of this entity. Dissecting acellular mucin can be seen deep in the hyalinized muscularis propria. When cellular mucin is present on the serosal surface, this commonly leads to pseudomyxoma peritonei.

# 35 Pancreas

1. Which of the following statements defines the condition nesidioblastosis?

   A. Diffuse or focal acinar ectasia with acinar cell dysplasia
   B. Enlarged islets with large β cells with enlarged hyperchromatic nuclei
   C. Failure of the dorsal and ventral pancreatic duct system to fuse
   D. Malformation of the pancreas causing duodenal obstruction
   E. Multiple sites of ectopic pancreatic tissue involving upper gastrointestinal (GI) tract

2. An endoscopic ultrasound-guided fine needle aspiration (FNA) of a pancreatic mass yields the cellular population shown in Figure 1. What kind of cells are these?

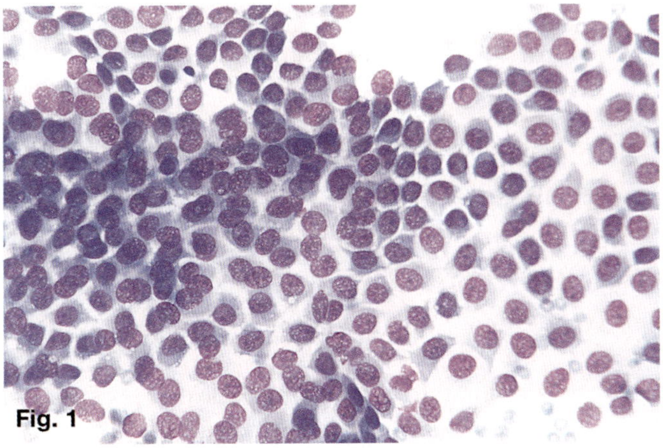

Fig. 1

   A. Acinar cells
   B. Ductal cells
   C. Hepatocytes
   D. Islet cells
   E. Mesothelial cells

3. Which of the following is true regarding acute pancreatitis?

   A. Cytopathologists commonly see these samples.
   B. Fine needle aspiration (FNA) will always show high cellularity and abundant neutrophils.
   C. Grayish-yellow plaques and nodules can be seen in the extrapancreatic adipose tissue.
   D. In the setting of severe acute pancreatitis, the plasma cells frequently express immunoglobulin G subclass 4 (IgG4).
   E. Zonal necrosis of acinar tissue is commonly seen.

4. A 69-year-old man presents with chronic diarrhea, steatorrhea, weight loss, and painless jaundice. A computed tomography (CT) scan reveals diffuse, sausage-shaped enlargement of the pancreas with narrowing of the main duct. His serum immunoglobulin G subclass 4 (IgG4) level is elevated. Out of concern for possible cancer, a biopsy of the pancreas is performed, revealing the histologic changes shown in Figure 1. Also, the inflammatory reaction is noted to involve veins with inflammatory cells undermining the endothelium. Which of the following is the most appropriate diagnosis?

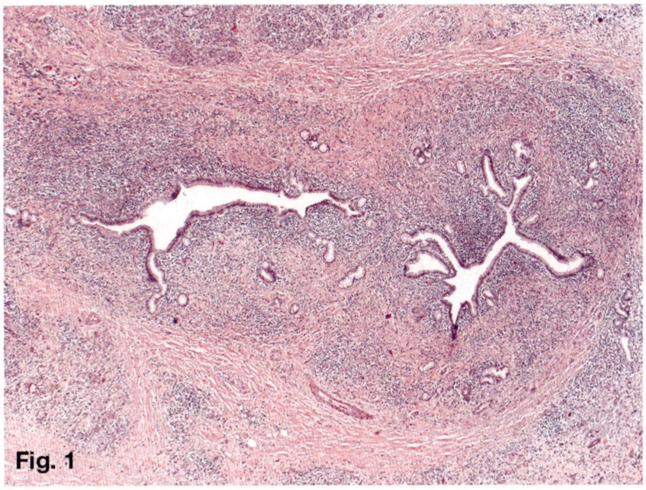

Fig. 1

   A. Alcoholic pancreatitis
   B. Autoimmune pancreatitis, type 1
   C. Autoimmune pancreatitis, type 2
   D. Chronic pancreatitis
   E. Hereditary pancreatitis

All figures in this chapter are from Longacre TA, Greenson JK, Hornick JL, Reuter VE, eds. *Mills and Sternberg's Diagnostic Surgical Pathology.* 7th ed. Wolters Kluwer; 2022 except for those noted at the end of this book.

5. A previously healthy 68-year-old male presents with jaundice and abdominal pain. He undergoes a computed tomography (CT) scan, which reveals lymphadenopathy, a mass in the head of the pancreas, and multiple lesions in the liver. An endoscopic retrograde cholangiopancreatography (ERCP) shows segmental attenuation of the main pancreatic duct. A core biopsy of the mass is shown in Figure 1. Which of the following is the most logical next step?

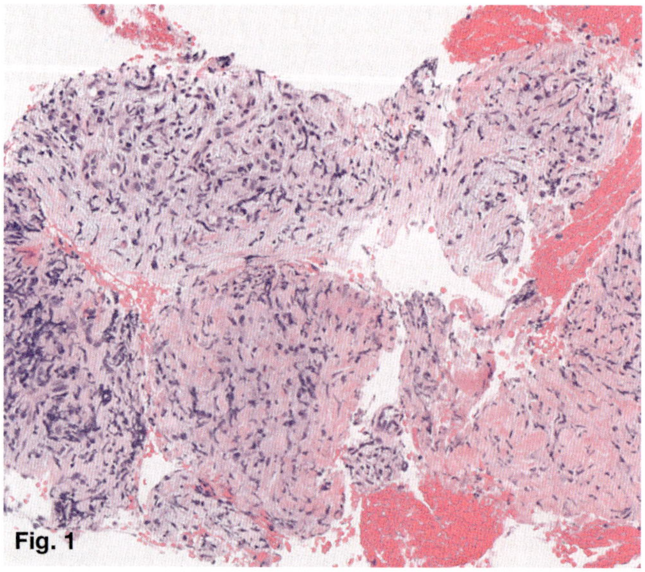
Fig. 1

A. Consult hematopathology for a lymphoma workup.
B. Give a diagnosis of pancreatic ductal adenocarcinoma.
C. Perform immunoglobulin G (IgG), IgG4, and CD138 testing by immunohistochemistry.
D. Report chronic pancreatitis, negative for tumor.
E. Report that the biopsy sample was inadequate for evaluation.

6. While looking through slides for a distal pancreatectomy for a well-differentiated neuroendocrine tumor, you see some cystically dilated ducts with the following epithelium, seen in Figure 1. What is the appropriate diagnosis?

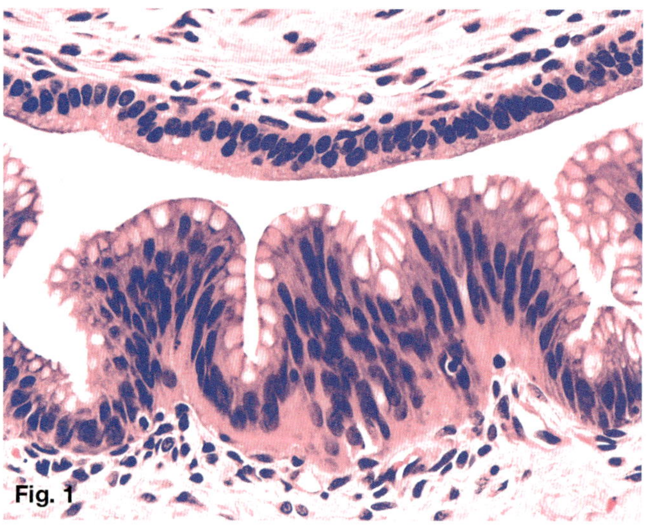
Fig. 1

A. High-grade intraductal mucinous neoplasm
B. High-grade pancreatic intraepithelial neoplasia
C. Low-grade intraductal mucinous neoplasm
D. Low-grade pancreatic intraepithelial neoplasia
E. Reactive atypia

7. A 56-year-old male undergoes a distal pancreatomy for a 4.5-cm cystic mass. The cystic mass is multiloculated. The cyst lining is mostly smooth with multiple excrescences. Figure 1 shows a representative section of the cyst lining. What is the appropriate diagnosis?

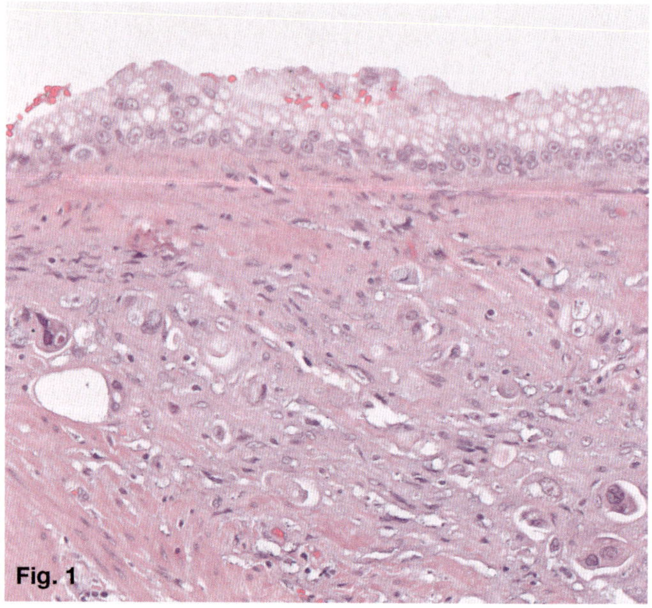
Fig. 1

A. High-grade intraductal papillary mucinous neoplasm
B. High-grade pancreatic intraepithelial neoplasia
C. Low-grade intraductal papillary mucinous neoplasm
D. Low-grade pancreatic intraepithelial neoplasia
E. Pancreatic ductal adenocarcinoma

8. An ultrasound-guided fine needle aspiration (FNA) of a pancreatic lesion reveals the cell clusters shown in Figure 1. Which of the following is the most likely diagnosis?

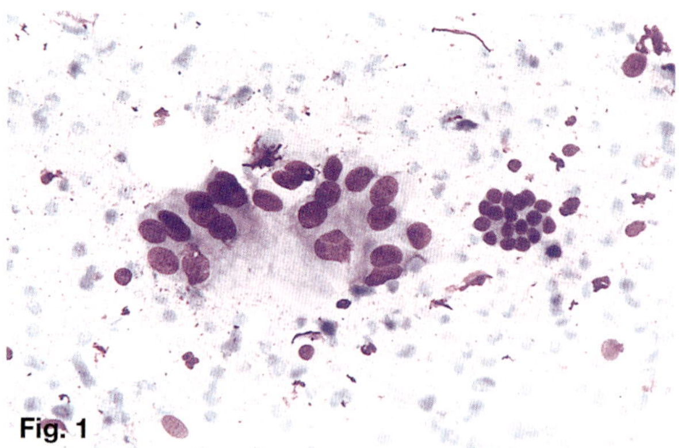
Fig. 1

A. Acinar cells
B. Ductal cells
C. Hepatocytes
D. Mesothelial cells
E. Pancreatic ductal adenocarcinoma

9. Figure 1 shows the fine needle aspiration (FNA) of a pancreatic mass. Which of the following is the most likely diagnosis?

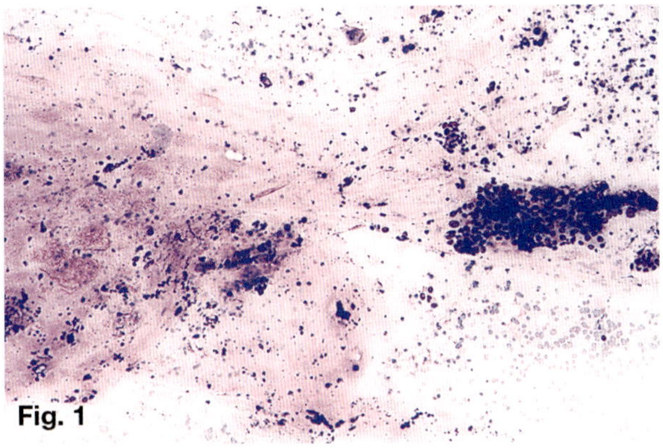

Fig. 1

A. Adenosquamous carcinoma
B. Colloid carcinoma
C. Ductal carcinoma
D. Medullary carcinoma
E. Undifferentiated carcinoma

10. Figure 1 is a representative section from a Whipple specimen of a 3.5-cm pancreatic head mass. Which of the following is the most likely diagnosis?

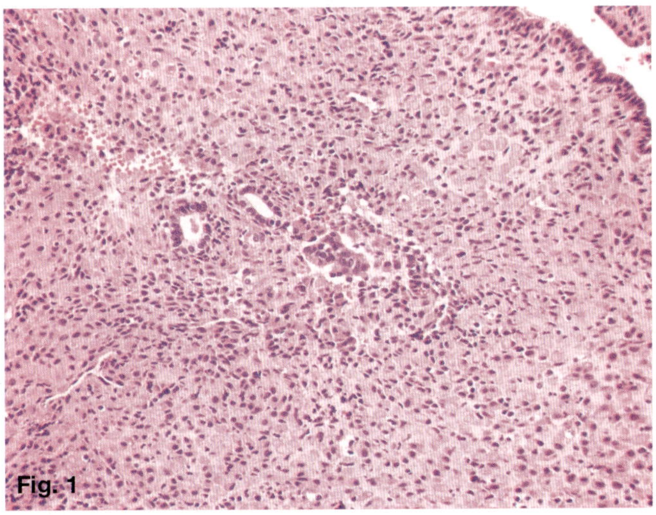

Fig. 1

A. High-grade intraductal papillary neoplasm
B. Low-grade intraductal papillary neoplasm
C. Pancreatic ductal adenocarcinoma, foamy gland variant
D. Pancreatic ductal adenocarcinoma, large duct variant
E. Pancreatic ductal adenocarcinoma, poorly cohesive variant

11. Which of the following immunohistochemical stains, if negative, would be most helpful to differentiate pancreatic ductal carcinoma from reactive (nonneoplastic) ducts?

A. CK7
B. CK20
C. SATB2
D. SMAD4
E. Vimentin

12. Figure 1 is a representative section from a pancreatic mass. Which of the following is true regarding this entity?

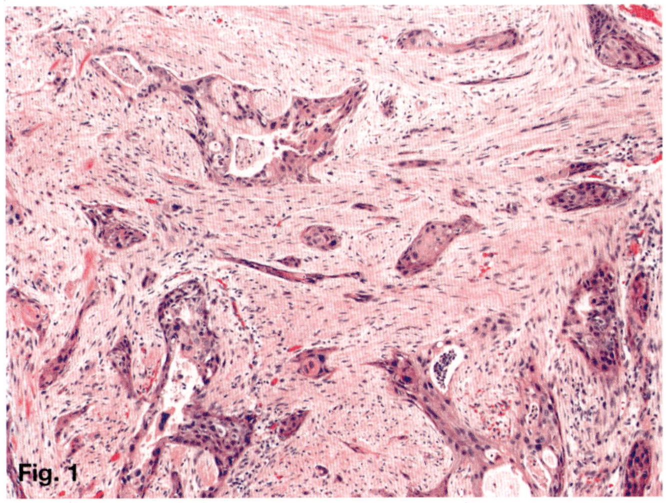

Fig. 1

A. Any amount of squamous differentiation is sufficient for the diagnosis.
B. Metastasis is most commonly composed of the squamous component.
C. It is more aggressive than conventional pancreatic ductal adenocarcinoma.
D. It is most commonly found in the pancreatic head.
E. It is usually found in the distal pancreas of young women.

13. Which of the following histologic types of pancreatic carcinoma is associated with microsatellite instability (MSI)?

A. Adenosquamous carcinoma
B. Colloid carcinoma
C. Medullary carcinoma
D. Undifferentiated carcinoma
E. Undifferentiated carcinoma with osteoclast-like giant cells

14. Figure 1 is a representative section from a Whipple specimen. Which of the following is the most likely diagnosis?

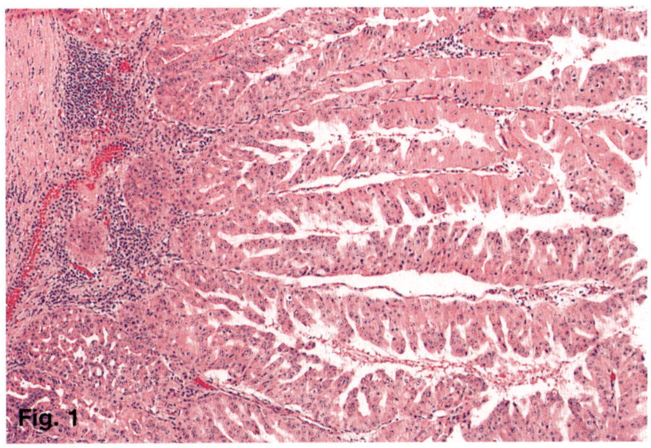

Fig. 1

A. Intraductal mucinous neoplasm
B. Intraductal oncocytic papillary neoplasm
C. Intraductal tubulopapillary neoplasm
D. Mucinous cystic neoplasm
E. Serous cystadenoma

15. Figure 1 is a representative section from a distal pancreatectomy specimen from a 57-year-old female. Which of the following is the most likely diagnosis?

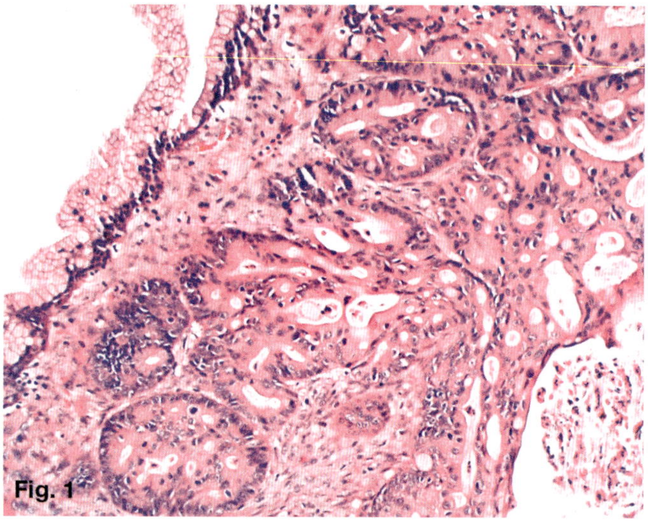

Fig. 1

A. Intraductal mucinous neoplasm
B. Intraductal oncocytic papillary neoplasm
C. Intraductal tubulopapillary neoplasm
D. Mucinous cystic neoplasm
E. Serous cystadenoma

16. A pancreatic tumor is found at the autopsy of a 75-year-old woman who died of a myocardial infarction. On the cut surface, the tumor shows small cysts filled with serous fluid. Histologically, the septa between cysts are lined by cuboidal cells with clear cytoplasm and contain scattered islets of Langerhans. Which of the following is the most likely diagnosis?

A. Acinar cell carcinoma
B. Chronic pancreatitis
C. Microcystic serous cystadenoma
D. Mucinous cystadenoma
E. Polycystic disease

17. The most frequent pancreatic neuroendocrine tumor is also the most commonly benign. Which one is it?

A. Gastrinoma
B. Glucagonoma
C. Insulinoma
D. Somatostatinoma
E. VIPoma

18. Figure 1 is a representative section from a distal pancreatectomy specimen. The neoplasm contains 15 mitoses per 10 HPF (high-power field) and shows the expression for CK18/8 and synaptophysin. Which of the following is the most likely diagnosis?

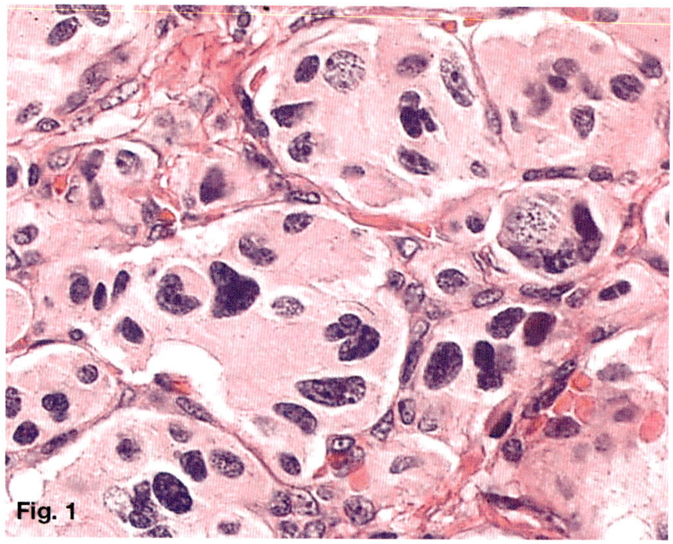

Fig. 1

A. Acinar cell carcinoma
B. Metastatic hepatocellular carcinoma
C. Neuroendocrine carcinoma, large cell type
D. Pancreatic ductal adenocarcinoma
E. Pancreatic neuroendocrine tumor

19. A pancreatic neoplasm resected from an 18-year-old woman is characterized by a pseudopapillary architecture and shows the histologic features demonstrated in Figure 1. Which of the following additional features are characteristic of this tumor?

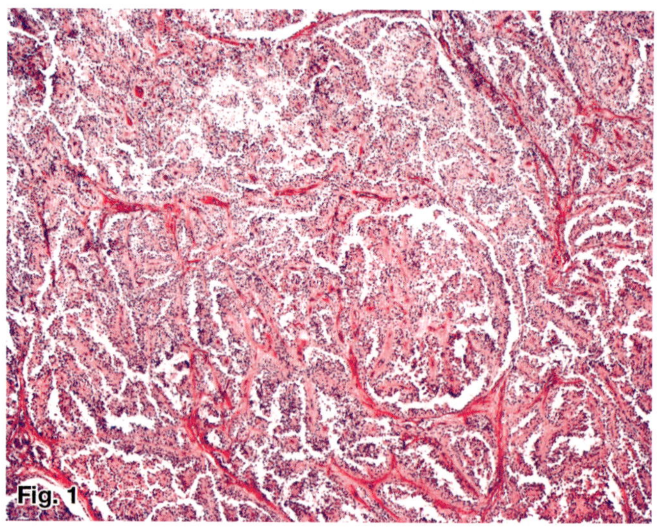

Fig. 1

A. Butyrate esterase positivity
B. Innumerable mitochondria
C. Osteoclast-like giant cells
D. $\alpha$1-Antitrypsin immunoreactive globules
E. Squamoid corpuscles

# ANSWERS AND EXPLANATIONS

**1. Correct choice: B.**

Nesidioblastosis is an abnormality that was originally defined as enlarged islets seen in newborns of mothers with hyperglycemia, which leads to in utero suppression and postpartum compensatory hyperactivity of the islets of Langerhans. On histology, large, hypertrophic collections of islet cells displace acinar tissue in close association with ducts (ductuloinsular complexes). Currently, it is thought that this condition can also be seen in adults with hyperinsulinemic hypoglycemia. Answer choice A defines pancreas divisum and B defines annular pancreas.

**2. Correct choice: E.**

Fine needle aspiration (FNA) is currently the preferred method for the histologic diagnosis of pancreatic lesions. Pathologists need to know the appearance of the following normal cells can be a contaminant in pancreatic FNAs: acinar cells, ductal cells, gastrointestinal (GI) epithelium (gastric or duodenal), mesothelial cells, and hepatocytes, depending on which organs are transected to reach the targeted pancreatic mass.

**3. Correct choice: C.**

Acute pancreatitis is fundamentally a clinical diagnosis. Pathologists rarely receive tissue, but occasionally, a pancreatic biopsy or partial resection of damaged tissue is performed. The gross appearance ranges from a slightly swollen, wet, firm, fibrotic organ to hemorrhagic and/or necrotic tissue. Due to severity, it should be kept in mind that neutrophils may be limited in acute pancreatitis. Fat necrosis is manifested as grayish-yellow plaques and nodules in extrapancreatic and intrapancreatic adipose tissue. The pancreatic acini will show a variable degree of autodigestive tissue necrosis. However, zonal necrosis of acinar tissue is very uncommon in conventional acute pancreatitis. A small portion of acute pancreatitis can be attributed to autoimmune pancreatitis where plasma cells express immunoglobulin G subclass 4 (IgG4).

**4. Correct choice: B.**

Autoimmune Pancreatitis (AIP)—AIP is separated into AIP, type 1 and AIP, type 2, which are entirely different conditions. AIP-1 is a manifestation of systemic *immunoglobulin G subclass 4 (IgG4)-related disease*. Elevated serum levels of IgG4 are found in more than 60% of patients. Histologically, the disease is characterized by a dense lymphoplasmacellular infiltrate surrounding ducts and vascular structures, with associated fibrosis and obliterative phlebitis. The latter feature is unique to AIP-1 and not found in the other type AIP-2. Immunohistochemistry shows that the majority of infiltrating plasma cells are positive for IgG4. Fibrosis is florid and exhibits a storiform pattern.

**5. Correct choice: C.**

Immunoglobulin G subclass 4 (IgG4)-related disease can involve many organs as well as lymph nodes. In the pancreas, it is called autoimmune pancreatitis (AIP), type 1. The patients exhibit symptoms of chronic pancreatitis and painless obstructive jaundice. The serum IgG4 concentration is elevated (>135 mg/dL) in many patients. Diffuse pancreatic involvement on computed tomography (CT) shows sausage-shaped enlargement with homogeneous attenuation. Focal disease can mimic pancreatic carcinoma. Endoscopic retrograde cholangiopancreatography (ERCP) shows focal, diffuse, or segmental attenuation of the main pancreatic duct with loss of branches. The three characteristic histopathologic features are (1) dense lymphoplasmacytic infiltrate with ductitis, (2) venulitis, and (3) fibrosis of the pancreatic parenchyma. By immunohistochemistry, the majority of plasma cells are positive for IgG4 with more than 50 IgG4+ plasma cells per HPF.

**6. Correct choice: D.**

Pancreatic intraepithelial neoplasia (PanIN) is composed of a spectrum of intraductal precursor lesions of the pancreas often seen as an incidental microscopic finding in contrast to intraductal mucinous neoplasm, which is a grossly visible lesion. PanIN can be subdivided into PanIN 1-3; however, in clinical practice, PanIN is graded based on the cytologic morphology. Low-grade PanIN encompasses both PanIN 1-2 and is believed to be clinically inconsequential, whereas high-grade PanIN is equivalent to PanIN 3 (carcinoma in situ). If PanIN 3 is identified, a thorough investigation of the pancreas is warranted because there is a very high likelihood of an invasive carcinoma.

**7. Correct choice: E.**

The image depicts intraductal papillary mucinous neoplasm (IPMN) with invasive pancreatic ductal adenocarcinoma (PDAC). IPMN of the pancreas is a grossly visible (typically >5 mm) intraductal epithelial neoplasm of mucin-producing cells. Clinically, it is subdivided into three groups based on the location within the pancreatic ductal system: (1) branch duct type, (2) main duct type, and (3) mixed duct type. PDAC is reported in 1% to 36% of branch duct IPMNs, 11% to 80% of main duct IPMNs, and 20% to 65% mixed duct IPMNs. Histologically, IPMNs are characterized by an intraductal proliferation of columnar mucin-producing cells that can be flat to papillary in appearance. IPMNs can be subclassified into histologic subtypes: gastric, intestinal, and pancreatobiliary. Based on the degree of cytoarchitectural atypia, the noninvasive component of an IPMN is subclassified as low grade or high grade.

**8. Correct choice: D.**

Differential Diagnosis in Pancreatic Ductal Adenocarcinoma (PDAC)—The primary differential diagnosis of PDAC is with benign noninvasive ducts. Pancreatic ducts lack a basal or myoepithelial cell layer, as in prostate or breast, so immunohistochemistry for those markers is not applicable. Malignant duct proliferation is associated with the following features: (1) abnormal "angulated" configuration of ducts; (2) partial rupture of ducts, with intraluminal debris/neutrophils; (3) abnormal location of ducts, around nerves or vessels, within adipose tissue, in the duodenal wall, etc; (4) myxoid reaction in the stroma; and (5) nuclear changes as seen in cytologic in fine needle aspiration (FNA). Benign processes are associated with (1) preserved lobular architecture, as mentioned previously; (2) lack of ductal irregularities; and (3) corpora amylacea–like secretions.

**9. Correct choice: B.**

Colloid Carcinoma—Colloid carcinoma of the pancreas is morphologically similar to colloid carcinoma in the skin and breast. The tumor contains abundant mucin, in which malignant cells seem to be floating. Fine needle aspirations (FNAs) of colloid carcinomas are difficult to smear because of the mucus. Infiltration of the surrounding stroma is minimal, perhaps because the mucin itself acts as a barrier to neoplastic spread. Many cases arise in association with *intraductal papillary mucinous neoplasms* (IPMNs), which are known to express "intestinal" markers, such as MUC-2 and CDX-2. Colloid carcinoma also expresses MUC-2 and CDX-2, which are not present in normal pancreatic cells. Colloid carcinomas have a better prognosis than pancreatic ductal adenocarcinoma (PDAC).

**10. Correct choice: C.**

Pancreatic ductal adenocarcinomas (PDACs) can exhibit a variety of morphologic variants that may be helpful in their accurate diagnosis. The foamy gland variant is characterized by abundant very pale foamy/microvesicular cytoplasm and well-formed glands; thus, the overall pattern is deceptively benign in appearance. In addition, foamy cell change is also fairly common in cases after neoadjuvant treatment. Large duct variant presents as large and well-defined infiltrating glands that mimic preinvasive neoplasia, such as pancreatic intraepithelial neoplasia (PanIN) or intraductal papillary mucinous neoplasms (IPMNs). The poorly cohesive variant can exhibit cordlike and even individual cell infiltration that is closely admixed with a conventional tubular pattern.

**11. Correct choice: D.**

*SMAD4* alterations are reported to be inactivating (SMAD4 loss) and present in approximately 50% of pancreatic ductal adenocarcinomas (PDACs), and usually occur as a late finding in the pathogenesis of PDAC. SMAD4 loss by immunohistochemistry (IHC) can be used to establish a diagnosis of PDAC in the pancreas in scenarios where the differential diagnosis is between PDAC and reactive (nonneoplastic) ducts such as those associated with chronic pancreatitis. The neoplastic cells in PDAC also show immunohistochemical reactivity for CK7, CK19, CAM5.2, CA19-9, CA125, and CEA(m) (carcinoembryonic antigen [modified]), whereas they are negative with vimentin and β-catenin. CK20, if present, is usually focal.

**12. Correct choice: C.**

Adenosquamous carcinoma is more common in older men than in women and affects the pancreatic body and tail more often than the pancreatic head. Histologically, it shows dual differentiation toward adenocarcinoma and squamous cell carcinoma. An arbitrary squamous component of 30% has been proposed for a carcinoma to be regarded as adenosquamous carcinoma. Although the squamous elements may be extensive in the primary neoplasm, the adenocarcinomatous element may predominate or may be the only pattern in metastatic foci. P40 and p63 expression by immunohistochemistry is present only in the squamous component and is a useful tool to assess the amount of squamous component. Immunohistochemically, these neoplasms show loss of SMAD4 protein expression and strong nuclear p53 immunoreactivity.

**13. Correct choice: C.**

Medullary Carcinoma—Medullary carcinoma in the pancreas is morphologically similar to that occurring in the colon or breast. It is characterized by a pushing pattern of growth and contains chronic inflammatory infiltrates. Medullary carcinoma of the pancreas has an even stronger association with microsatellite instability (MSI) than the colonic form. Its prognosis seems to be better than that of ordinary pancreatic ductal adenocarcinoma (PDAC).

**14. Correct choice: B.**

Intraductal oncocytic papillary neoplasms (IOPNs), similar to intraductal papillary mucinous neoplasms (IPMNs), are grossly cystic epithelial neoplasms that grow within the pancreatic ducts and are composed of architecturally complex papillary masses with oncocytic cells. Grossly, IOPNs are usually unilocular or multilocular intraductal papillary masses with a mean size of 6.0 cm; most do not involve the main pancreatic duct. Microscopically, IOPNs are composed of neoplastic oncocytic cells arranged in arborizing and cribriforming papillae, and solid nests that grow within dilated ducts. Invasive carcinomas are found in approximately 30% of IOPNs and may retain the oncocytic cytology. IOPNs stain strongly for HepPar-1; alterations in *TP53* and *SMAD4* are absent.

**15. Correct choice: D.**

Mucinous cystic neoplasms (MCNs) are seen almost exclusively in perimenopausal women. MCNs typically form a thick-walled multilocular, encapsulated cyst in the body or the tail of the pancreas. Histologically, they are composed of columnar epithelium similar to that of the large pancreatic ducts (and colon) and have the requisite ovarian-type stroma composed of spindle cells, which shows expression for progesterone receptor (PR) on immunohistochemistry. The ovarian-type stroma can vary from cellular to slightly more hyalinized. The grade of the lesion is associated with the clinical outcome, and the cases classified as low-grade dysplasia are typically cured by complete removal. There are also mesenchymal neoplasms that presumably derive from the ovarian stroma of these tumors.

**16. Correct choice: C.**

Serous Cystadenoma, Microcystic Type—Most pancreatic serous neoplasms are *serous cystadenomas*. They are usually discovered in older individuals, often located in the pancreatic body or tail. One may see two patterns, with cysts that may be minute and regular (the *microcystic* type) or large and irregular. The cut surface is highly characteristic, resembling the spongy appearance of the infantile form of polycystic kidney disease. Whether diagnosed incidentally or manifesting with clinical symptoms, the tumor is associated with a good prognosis.

**17. Correct choice: C.**

Pancreatic Neuroendocrine Tumors (PanNETs)—Insulinoma is the most common PanNET. Fewer than 10% of insulinomas are malignant tumors, showing infiltrative and metastatic behavior. In contrast to insulinomas, most of the other islet cell tumors have a malignant behavior. The World Health Organization (WHO) grading system of PanNETs is based on mitotic count and Ki-67 labeling index and recognizes three grades: grade I (well differentiated), grade II (atypical), and grade III (neuroendocrine carcinoma, NEC). The WHO system gives the false impression that NEC is part of the spectrum of well-differentiated PanNETs, whereas NEC is in fact a highly aggressive neoplasm and a separate entity.

**18. Correct choice: E.**

Pancreatic neuroendocrine tumors (PanNETs) may exhibit a variety of morphologies such as clear cell, lipid-rich, oncocytic, and pleomorphic variants, that are peculiar and diagnostically challenging. PanNETs, similar to those seen in other endocrine organs, may show the so-called endocrine atypia, which is characterized by large cells, sometimes irregular in shape, with large or even giant nuclei. Fundamentally, this is a degenerative atypia. PanNETs are graded essentially like neuroendocrine tumors elsewhere in the gastrointestinal (GI) tract. Thus, based on the mitotic count, the diagnosis is a well-differentiated neuroendocrine tumor, grade 2.

**19. Correct choice: D.**

Solid pseudopapillary neoplasm occurs almost exclusively in young adolescent girls and young women of all races. Histologically, the neoplasm appears to begin as solid masses in which there are many poorly supported tiny vessels. A pseudopapillary pattern emerges as the cells farthest from the small vessels undergo swelling and degenerative changes, whereas the cells next to the vessels remain. The cells are small to medium sized and polygonal to elongated, with ovoid nuclei that often are grooved or indented. Periodic acid-Schiff with diastase (PAS-D) positive eosinophilic globules composed of $\alpha$1-antitrypsin might also be seen. Clusters of lipid crystals surrounded by foreign body macrophages are often present.

# 36 Nonneoplastic Liver Disease

1. Which of the following immunohistochemical stains would produce the pattern seen in Figure 1?

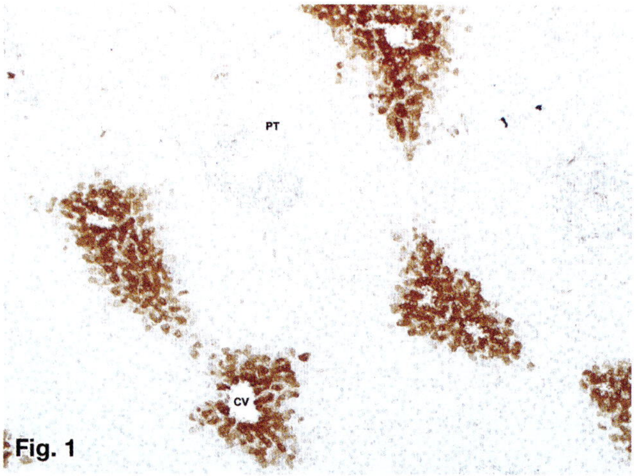


Fig. 1

A. CD34
B. CK7
C. CK8
D. Glial fibrillary acidic protein
E. Glutamine synthetase

2. Figure 1 shows a cellular change resulting from damage to

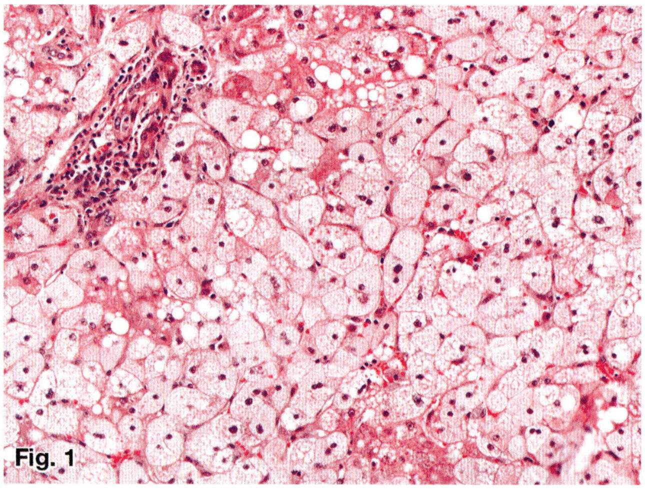

Fig. 1

A. Golgi complex.
B. lysosomes.
C. mitochondria.
D. nucleus.
E. smooth endoplasmic reticulum.

3. According to the Batts-Ludwig system, the extent of hepatic inflammation and injury shown in Figure 1 should be graded as

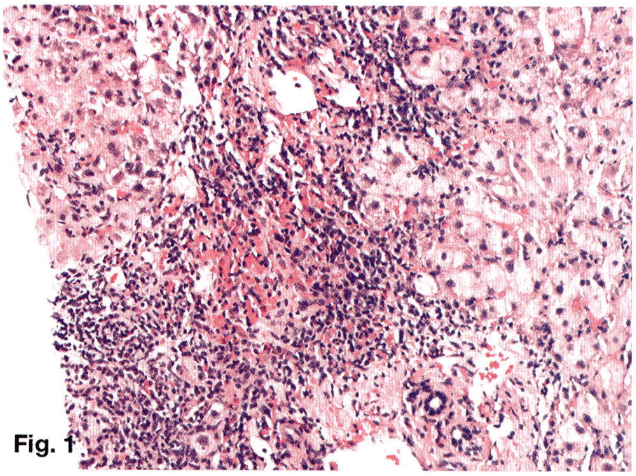

Fig. 1

A. grade 0.
B. grade 1.
C. grade 2.
D. grade 3.
E. grade 4.

4. According to the Batts-Ludwig system, the stage of liver fibrosis seen in Figure 1 is

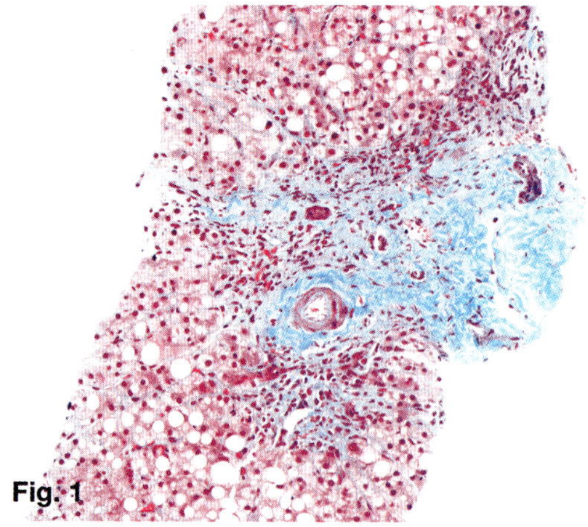

Fig. 1

A. stage 0.
B. stage 1.
C. stage 2.
D. stage 3.
E. stage 4.

All figures in this chapter are from Longacre TA, Greenson JK, Hornick JL, Reuter VE, eds. *Mills and Sternberg's Diagnostic Surgical Pathology*. 7th ed. Wolters Kluwer; 2022 except for those noted at the end of this book.

5. Figure 1 shows a section of liver immunostained with an antibody to CD34. Which of the following pathologic reactions is demonstrated by this immunostain?

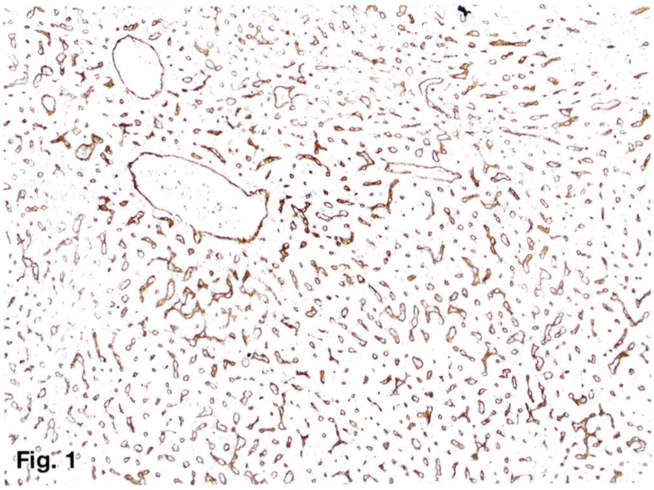

Fig. 1

A. Activation of Kupffer cells
B. Activation of stellate cells (Ito cells)
C. Cholestasis
D. Deposition of elastin in the space of Disse
E. Sinusoidal capillarization

6. A 30-year-old woman is found to have laboratory evidence of acute hepatitis. A liver biopsy shows the changes seen in Figure 1. Which of the following is the most likely diagnosis?

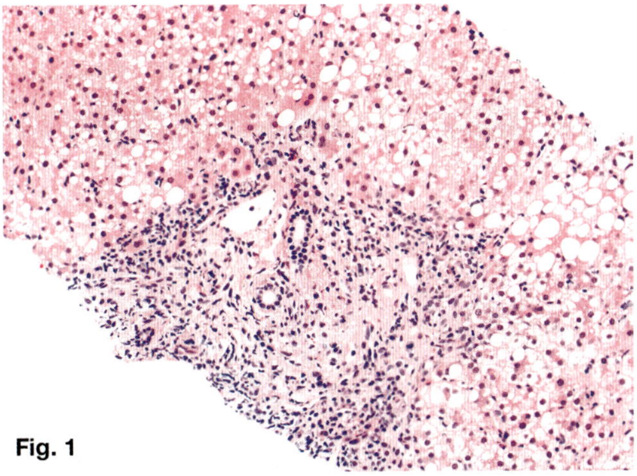

Fig. 1

A. Acute viral hepatitis
B. Autoimmune hepatitis
C. Celiac disease
D. Drug-induced liver injury
E. Wilson disease

7. A patient with laboratory evidence of liver dysfunction has a history of chronic intake of anabolic steroids. Which of the following patterns of liver injury would be expected?

A. Cholestasis
B. Granulomatous inflammation
C. Hepatocyte necrosis
D. Macrovesicular steatosis
E. Microvesicular steatosis

8. Which of the following histopathologic features is usually absent or minimal in the so-called *toxic* pattern of acute hepatitis?

A. Cholestasis
B. Granulomas
C. Inflammation
D. Necrosis
E. Steatosis

9. Which of the following patterns of acute hepatitis would be favored by the finding of sinusoidal pigmented macrophages clustered around central veins?

A. Cholestatic
B. Giant cell
C. Inflammatory
D. Resolving
E. Toxic

10. A 55-year-old male immigrant from Africa undergoes a liver biopsy for evaluation of chronic hepatitis. A key histologic finding is demonstrated in Figure 1. Which of the following is the most likely etiologic agent?

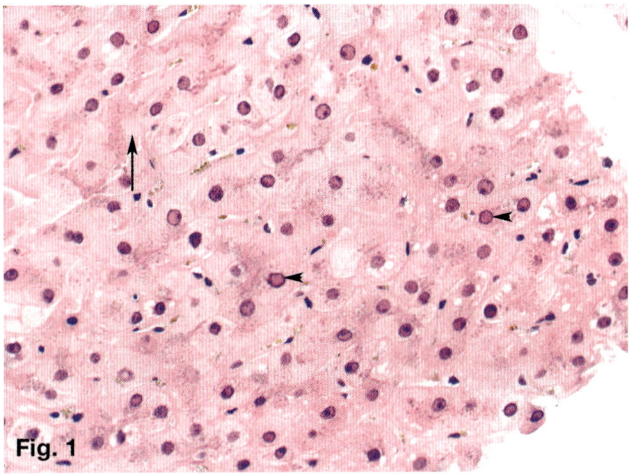

Fig. 1

A. Adenovirus
B. Cytomegalovirus
C. Epstein-Barr virus
D. Hepatitis B
E. Hepatitis C

11. A patient undergoes serum testing for hepatitis B virus (HBV), which is positive for immunoglobulin G (IgG) anti–hepatitis B surface antigen (HBsAg) and anti–hepatitis B core (HBc). A liver biopsy is performed and immunohistochemical studies for HBV are performed, which show positive cytoplasmic staining for hepatitis HBsAg and negative staining for HBcAg. Which of the following best describes the patient's current HBV status?

A. Acutely infected
B. Chronically infected
C. Immune due to hepatitis B vaccination
D. Immune due to natural infection
E. Serum and immunohistochemical testing not congruent

12. A 55-year-old male undergoes a liver biopsy for evaluation of chronic hepatitis. Along with marked macrovesicular steatosis, another key histologic finding is demonstrated in Figure 1. Which of the following is the most likely etiologic agent?

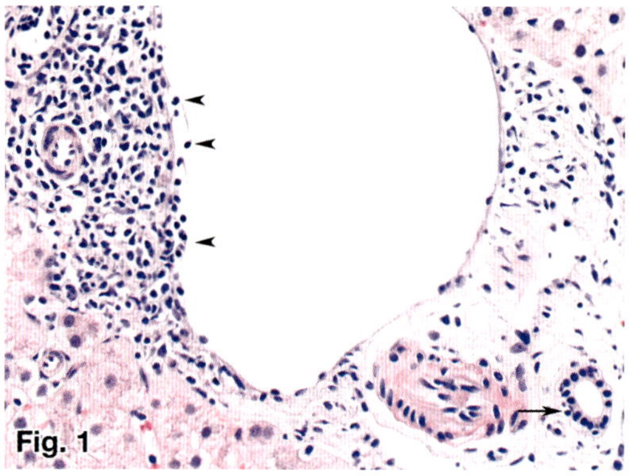

Fig. 1

A. Adenovirus
B. Cytomegalovirus
C. Epstein-Barr virus
D. Hepatitis B
E. Hepatitis C

13. A liver biopsy from a 50-year-old man with type 2 diabetes reveals the following changes: extensive macrovesicular steatosis involving approximately 50% of the tissue, more pronounced in the centrilobular region; mild chronic inflammation within the lobule; ballooning change of hepatocytes; and pericellular fibrosis in the centrilobular region. Occasional Mallory bodies are found. There are small clusters of neutrophils surrounding ballooned hepatocytes. There is no evidence of cholestasis. This histopathologic picture is most consistent with

A. autoimmune hepatitis.
B. chronic viral hepatitis.
C. drug-induced liver injury.
D. nonalcoholic fatty liver.
E. nonalcoholic steatohepatitis.

14. Figure 1 is a representative histologic section of a liver biopsy. What is the appropriate breakdown of the nonalcoholic steatohepatitis (NASH) activity score?

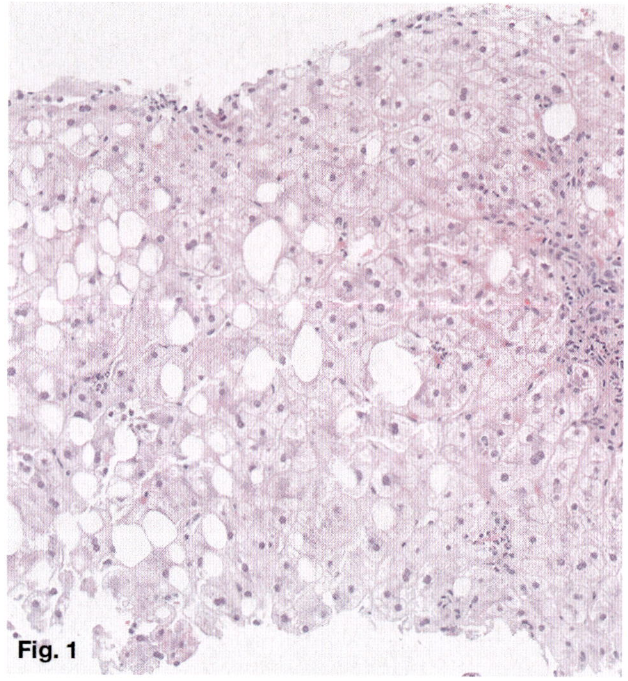

Fig. 1

A. Steatosis 1, Lobular inflammation 1, Ballooning 1
B. Steatosis 1, Lobular inflammation 2, Ballooning 2
C. Steatosis 2, Lobular inflammation 2, Ballooning 1
D. Steatosis 2, Lobular inflammation 3, Ballooning 2
E. Steatosis 3, Lobular inflammation 3, Ballooning 2

15. Figure 1 is a trichrome stain performed on a liver biopsy showing nonalcoholic steatohepatitis (NASH). What is the most appropriate stage?

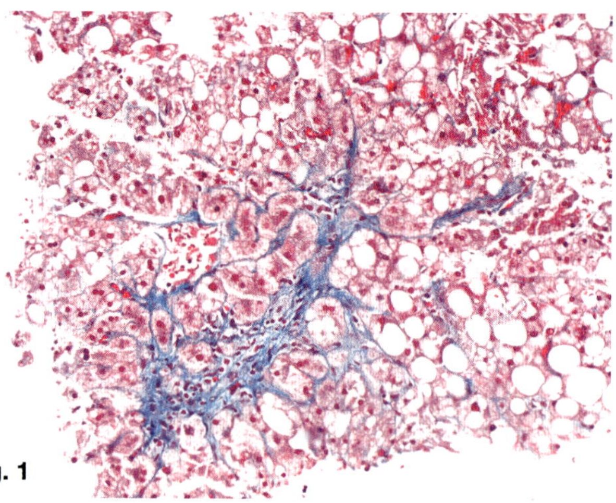

Fig. 1

Figure 1 Reproduced from Gill RM, Kakar S. Nonalcoholic steatohepatitis. *Surg Pathol Clin*. 2013;6(2):227-257. Copyright © 2013 Elsevier. With permission.

A. Stage 1A
B. Stage 1B
C. Stage 1C
D. Stage 2
E. Stage 3

16. Figure 1 shows a characteristic histologic feature of which of the following?

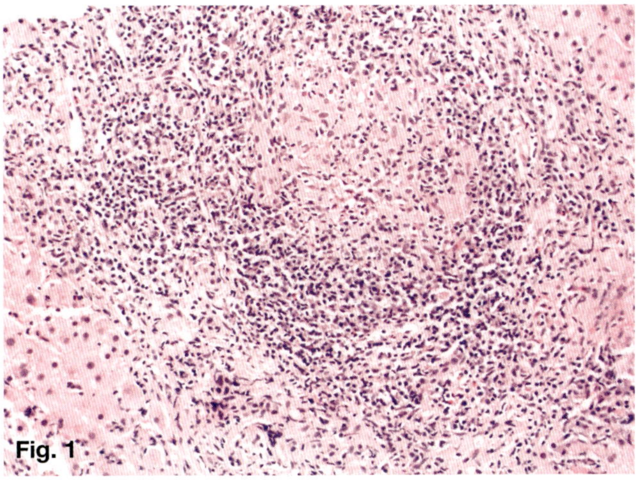

Fig. 1

A. Anabolic steroids
B. Autoimmune hepatitis
C. Large bile duct obstruction
D. Primary biliary cirrhosis
E. Viral infection

17. Which of the following ancillary studies is most useful in support of a chronic cholestasis pattern of injury?

A. CD34 and periodic acid-Schiff (PAS) with diastase stain
B. CD34 and reticulin stain
C. CD34 and rhodanine stain
D. CK7 and PAS with diastase stain
E. CK7 and rhodanine stain

18. Figure 1 shows a characteristic histologic feature of which of the following?

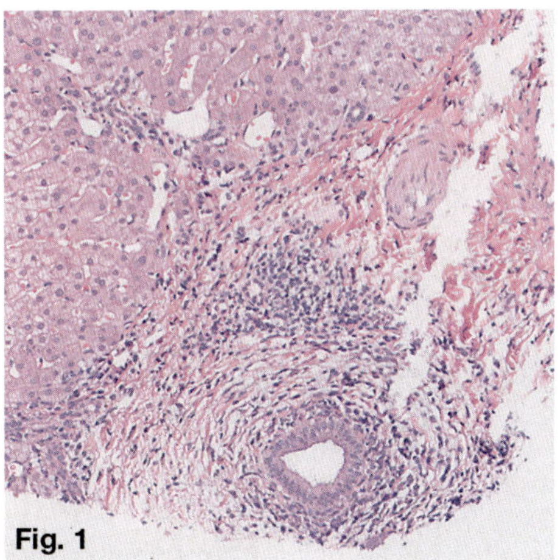

Fig. 1

A. Autoimmune hepatitis
B. IgG4 (immunoglobulin G subclass 4)-related sclerosing cholangitis
C. Large bile duct obstruction
D. Primary biliary cirrhosis
E. Primary sclerosing cholangitis

19. A liver biopsy from a 2-month-old infant with cholestatic jaundice reveals prominent small bile duct proliferation, bile plugs, portal edema, and scattered hepatic giant cells. The lobular architecture is preserved. Which of the following is the most likely cause of these changes?

A. α-1-Antitrypsin deficiency
B. Extrahepatic biliary atresia
C. Galactosemia
D. Hereditary fructose intolerance
E. Infection

20. A 26-year-old female with jaundice undergoes liver biopsy that shows cholestasis and ductular reaction pattern of injury. Figure 1 is stained with periodic acid–Schiff with diastase stain. Pathogenic mutation in which of the following genes is associated with this disorder?

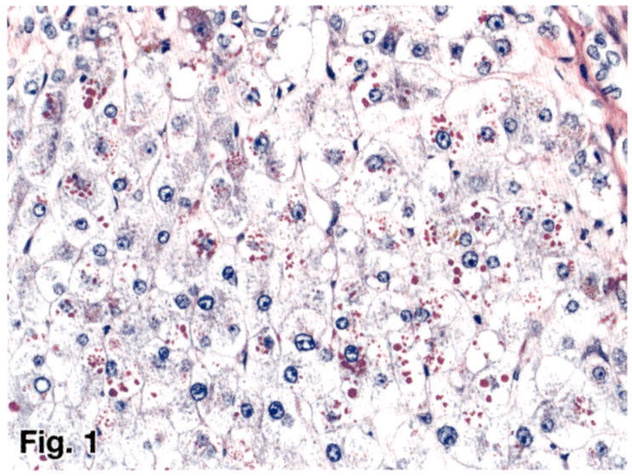

Fig. 1

A. *BSEP*
B. *FIC1*
C. *HFE*
D. *NOTCH2*
E. *SERPINA1*

21. A 3-week-old neonate with jaundice undergoes liver biopsy that shows paucity of bile ducts. Genetic testing identifies a mutation in the *JAG1* gene. Which of the following abnormalities is most likely also present in this neonate?

A. Cleft palate
B. Ductal plate malformation
C. Hepatosplenomegaly
D. Hypopituitarism
E. Tetralogy of Fallot

22. A 32-year-old pregnant female with a history of sickle cell anemia undergoes a liver biopsy, which shows some steatosis and increased iron deposition in a mixed hepatocellular-Kupffer cell distribution. Which of the following is the most likely cause of this increase in iron deposition?

A. Cirrhosis
B. Hemochromatosis
C. Juvenile hemochromatosis
D. Prenatal vitamins
E. Recurrent blood transfusions

23. The liver disorder known as *nodular regenerative hyperplasia* (NRH) is most likely due to

A. drug-mediated injury to hepatocytes.
B. hormonal contraception.
C. obliteration of small portal veins.
D. thrombosis of large hepatic veins or inferior vena cava.
E. viral infection.

24. Figure 1 shows the main histologic changes of a liver biopsy obtained 14 days after orthotopic liver transplantation. This histologic picture is most consistent with

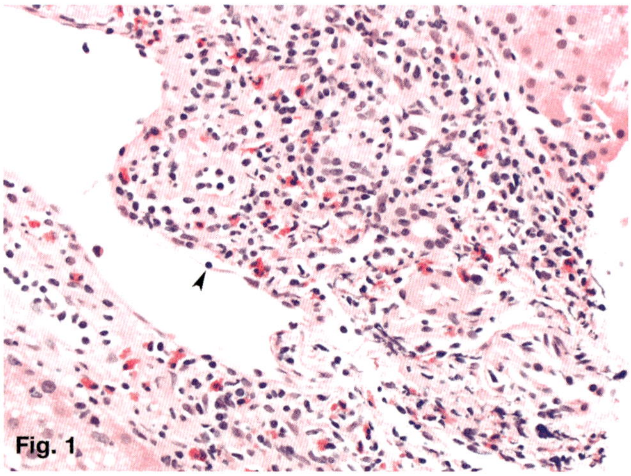
Fig. 1

A. acute cellular rejection.
B. acute parenchymal rejection.
C. chronic ductopenic rejection.
D. chronic vascular rejection.
E. preservation injury.

# ANSWERS AND EXPLANATIONS

**1. Correct choice: E.**

The complex architecture of the liver lobule leads to functional heterogeneity, such as central ammonium metabolism with associated zone 3 (area around the central venule) glutamine synthetase expression.

**2. Correct choice: C.**

Fat droplets, or steatosis, is a diagnostic feature of fatty liver disease. Steatosis may be separated into microvesicular and macrovesicular forms. Microvesicular steatosis is defined by very small/fine fat globules and is a result of mitochondrial injury. Diffuse microvesicular steatosis can be seen in Reye syndrome as well as in congenital metabolic disorders, such as in fatty acid metabolism defects, and lysosomal acid lipase deficiency. Macrovesicular steatosis may show multiple fat droplets that do not displace the nucleus (small droplet steatosis) or coalescent fat vacuoles that displace the nucleus (large droplet steatosis).

**3. Correct choice: D.**

The Batts-Ludwig system (see Table 1) is one of the most widely recognized systems for grading liver injury. The image shows portal inflammation with moderate interface hepatitis, grade 3.

**4. Correct choice: C.**

The image shows periportal septal fibrosis, stage 2 (also see Table 1).

**TABLE 1 Staging of Liver Fibrosis**

| Stage | Scheuer | Batts-Ludwig |
|---|---|---|
| 0 | No fibrosis | Normal connective tissue |
| 1 | Enlarged fibrotic portal areas[a] | Fibrous portal expansion[a] |
| 2 | Periportal septa or portal-portal septa but intact architecture | Periportal, or rare portal-portal, septa |
| 3 | Fibrosis with architectural distortion but no obvious cirrhosis | Fibrous septa with architectural distortion, no obvious cirrhosis |
| 4 | Probable or definite cirrhosis | Cirrhosis |

[a]Small, thin periportal extensions are considered part of stage 1.
Adapted by permission from *Nature*: Theise ND. Liver biopsy assessment in chronic viral hepatitis: a personal, practical approach. *Mod Pathol.* 2007;20(suppl 1):S3-S14.

**TABLE 1 Grading Inflammation/Liver Injury**

| | Batts-Ludwig | | |
|---|---|---|---|
| **Grade** | **Classifier of Activity** | **Interface Hepatitis (Piecemeal Necrosis)** | **Lobular Activity** |
| 0 | None | No significant inflammation | None |
| 1 | Minimal | Minimal to no interface hepatitis | Rare spotty necrosis |
| 2 | Mild | Portal inflammation with mild (1-3 foci) interface hepatitis | Spotty necrosis |
| 3 | Moderate | Portal inflammation with moderate interface hepatitis (~3 or more foci) in multiple portal tracts | Confluent necrosis |
| 4 | Severe | Severe interface hepatitis (diffuse/continuous along interface) | Bridging or extensive necrosis |

Adapted with permission from Batts KP, Ludwig J. Chronic hepatitis: an update on terminology and reporting. *Am J Surg Pathol.* 1995;19(12):1409-1417.

**5. Correct choice: E.**

Chronic injury leads to fibrosis, which affects blood flow and leads to sinusoidal capillarization (which can be highlighted on CD34 immunohistochemical staining). Normal hepatic sinusoids do not express CD34.

**6. Correct choice: B.**

Acute hepatitis can be divided into six morphologic subpatterns (Table 1), each with its distinct morphologic features and differential diagnoses. The inflammation-predominant pattern is the most common and shows hepatocellular injury accompanied by a prominent inflammatory infiltrate. The differential diagnosis includes acute viral hepatitis, drug-induced liver injury, autoimmune hepatitis, Wilson disease, and celiac disease. Acute hepatitis with abundant portal plasma cells is a common feature of autoimmune hepatitis, which can present as acute hepatitis, including a fulminant form, chronic hepatitis, and cirrhosis.

**TABLE 1 Patterns of Acute Hepatitis**

1. Inflammation-predominant pattern (with variable necrosis) → acute viral hepatitis, idiosyncratic drug reaction, autoimmune hepatitis, Wilson disease, or celiac disease
2. Cholestatic pattern → nonspecific, most commonly with acute hepatitis due to drug, hepatitis A, or hepatitis E
3. Toxic pattern → direct hepatocellular injury (halothane, acetaminophen, cocaine, MDMA, organic solvents, toxic mushrooms, some herbal medications, HSV, and adenovirus) or acute vascular injury/ischemia
4. Resolving pattern → nonspecific but common in idiosyncratic drug reaction and in systemic autoimmune and inflammatory disorders
5. Giant cell pattern → nonspecific in adults, most common in autoimmune hepatitis
6. Mild nonspecific pattern → raises consideration for early acute hepatitis vs early biliary injury, requires clinical and laboratory correlation

HSV, herpes simplex virus; MDMA, 3,4-methylenedioxy-*N*-methylamphetamine.

**7. Correct choice: A.**

A great number of substances may injure the liver. Morphologic changes related to drugs or toxins are nonspecific. The classification is based on two parameters: (i) intrinsic reactions (predictable, dose related) versus idiosyncratic reactions (unpredictable, dose unrelated) and (ii) histopathologic changes. The pattern of morphologic changes may suggest the underlying cause. Pure bland cholestasis, which appears as hepatocanalicular bile plugs without significant bile ductular reaction, inflammation, or hepatocellular injury, is nearly always associated with drugs (such as anabolic steroids). Additional examples are provided below.

| Pattern of Liver Injury | Causes |
|---|---|
| Macrovesicular steatosis | Ethanol, amiodarone |
| Microvesicular steatosis | Tetracyclines, valproate |
| Centrilobular necrosis | Acetaminophen |
| Massive necrosis | Acetaminophen, halothane, *Amanita phalloides* |
| Hepatitis | Isoniazid, methyldopa |
| Granulomatous inflammation | Sulfonamides, methyldopa |
| Cholestasis | Anabolic steroids, oral contraceptives, chlorpromazine |

**8. Correct choice: D.**

Toxic hepatitis is caused by agents that are direct liver toxins (ie, not immune mediated). Thus, liver damage will manifest as hepatocellular necrosis without significant inflammation. Causes of toxic hepatitis include halothane, acetaminophen, cocaine, 3,4-methylenedioxy-*N*-methylamphetamine (MDMA), organic solvents, poison mushrooms, some herbal medications, herpes simplex virus (HSV), and adenovirus. This pattern can also be seen in ischemic injury and acute vascular outflow obstruction (Budd-Chiari syndrome).

**9. Correct choice: D.**

The resolving hepatitis pattern of injury is characterized by mild portal and lobular inflammation with scattered pigmented macrophages (also called ceroid-laden macrophages) in sinusoids, often clustered around central veins. There is usually only mild hepatocellular necrosis manifested by rare/spotty acidophil bodies.

**10. Correct choice: D.**

Typical histologic findings of hepatitis B virus (HBV) infection show ground glass cytoplasmic inclusions (due to hepatitis B surface antigen [HBsAg]) and sanded nuclear change (due to hepatitis B core antigen [HBcAg]). Only HBV produces inclusions among the hepatotropic viruses. A majority of the patients (~65%) remain asymptomatic after acquisition of HBV infection. Chronic disease develops in less than 5% of infected individuals.

**11. Correct choice: B.**

This combination of serum and immunohistologic testing is consistent with chronic hepatitis B virus (HBV) hepatitis without active viral replication. If serum testing for immunoglobulin M (IgM) anti–hepatitis B core (anti-HBc) was performed, it would be negative. In this setting, if additional testing shows positive immunoglobulin M (IgM) anti-HBc and positive HBc by immunohistochemistry (IHC), this will represent an episode of acute on chronic HBV hepatitis.

**12. Correct choice: E.**

Among hepatotropic viruses, hepatitis C is the most commonly encountered etiology of chronic hepatitis in the United States, with the majority of infections progressing to a chronic stage. Histologically, it presents with severe large and small droplet macrovesicular steatosis and portal venule endotheliitis (arrowheads), and bile duct damage (arrow) may also be present.

**13. Correct choice: E.**

Nonalcoholic steatohepatitis (NASH) encompasses nonalcoholic fatty liver (NAFL) and NASH. NAFL consists of macrovesicular steatosis without accompanying inflammation or liver damage, whereas NASH consists of macrovesicular steatosis with accompanying inflammation and liver damage. Risk factors for NASH include diabetes mellitus type 2, Wilson disease, amiodarone, and lipodystrophy. See Table 1 for histologic features of NASH.

**TABLE 1 Histologic Features of Nonalcoholic Steatohepatitis**

| | |
|---|---|
| **Essential features** | **Often present, not essential for diagnosis** |
| 1. Steatosis, predominantly macrovesicular, concentrated in zone 3 | 1. Glycogenated nuclei in zone 1 |
| 2. Mild mixed acinar inflammation | 2. Lipogranulomas in the lobular parenchyma or portal tracts |
| 3. Hepatocellular injury in the form of: Hepatocellular ballooning, often most prominent in zone 3, and/or pericellular fibrosis | 3. Occasional acidophil bodies |
| **May be present, not essential for diagnosis** | **Unusual features** |
| 1. Mallory hyaline in zone 3, typically inconspicuous | 1. Predominantly microvesicular steatosis |
| 2. Mild iron deposits in hepatocytes or sinusoidal cells | 2. Prominent portal and/or acinar inflammation, numerous plasma cells |
| 3. Megamitochondria | 3. Prominent bile ductular reaction, cholestasis |
| | 4. Perivenular fibrosis, hyaline sclerosis |
| | 5. Marked lobular inflammation |

From Neuschwander-Tetri BA, Caldwell SH. Nonalcoholic steatohepatitis: summary of an AASLD single topic conference. *Hepatology*. 2003;37(5):1202-1219. Copyright © 2003 by the American Association for the Study of Liver Diseases. Adapted by permission of John Wiley & Sons, Inc.

**14. Correct choice: B.**

Steatosis ~30%, Lobular inflammation 4 foci, Ballooning prominent. Although hepatologists are often interested in the grade of steatosis, there is no need to present a formal evaluation of the NASH activity score, which is primarily a research tool (see Table 1).

**TABLE 1 Nonalcoholic Steatohepatitis Activity Score**

| Histologic Feature | Definition | Score |
|---|---|---|
| Steatosis | <5% | 0 |
| | 5%-33% | 1 |
| | 33%-66% | 2 |
| | >66% | 3 |
| Lobular inflammation[a] | None | 0 |
| | <2 foci | 1 |
| | 2-4 foci | 2 |
| | >4 foci | 3 |
| Ballooning[b] | None | 0 |
| | Few cells | 1 |
| | Prominent | 2 |

[a]The number of foci was counted per ×200 field for lobular inflammation.

[b]Few ballooned cells indicate rare but definite ballooned hepatocytes as well as cases that are diagnostically borderline.

From Kleiner DE, Brunt EM, Van Natta M, et al. Design and validation of a histological scoring system for nonalcoholic fatty liver disease. *Hepatology*. 2005;41(6):1313-1321. Copyright © 2005 American Association for the Study of Liver Diseases. Reprinted by permission of John Wiley & Sons, Inc.

**15. Correct choice: A.**

Evaluation of the stage of fibrosis is important in nonalcoholic steatohepatitis (NASH) and can influence treatment decisions. Advanced fibrosis (stages 3 and 4) will prompt consideration of future transplantation. Steatohepatitis fibrosis usually starts around the central vein and thus should not be staged using the Batts-Ludwig methodology. The Brunt methodology is provided in Table 1.

**TABLE 1 Staging of Steatohepatitis**

| | |
|---|---|
| Stage 0 | No fibrosis |
| Stage 1 | Perisinusoidal or periportal fibrosis<br>1A. Mild zone 3 pericellular fibrosis, requires trichrome for identification<br>1B. Moderate zone 3 pericellular fibrosis, often apparent on H&E stain<br>1C. Portal/periportal fibrosis only |
| Stage 2 | As in stage 1 plus portal/periportal fibrosis, focal or extensive |
| Stage 3 | Bridging fibrosis, focal or extensive |
| Stage 4 | Cirrhosis (and/or residual pericellular fibrosis) |

H&E, hematoxylin and eosin.

**16. Correct choice: D.**

Primary biliary cirrhosis (PBC) commonly affects middle-aged women and manifests with cholestatic jaundice. PBC is characterized by lymphocytic infiltration of the bile duct with epithelial injury and duct-centric inflammation composed of lymphoplasmacytic cells, eosinophils, and epithelioid macrophages in ill-defined clusters. The image is of a florid duct lesion, which is defined as lymphocytic cholangitis in a background of a dense lymphoplasmacytic infiltrate and granulomatous inflammation. Florid duct lesions are a characteristic feature of PBC.

**17. Correct choice: E.**

In the setting of chronic cholestasis, periportal hepatocytes often acquire a biliary phenotype, which can be highlighted by CK7 immunohistochemical stain, and have periportal hepatocyte copper deposition, which can be highlighted by a rhodanine stain. Copper accumulation can occur in a nonspecific manner in advanced fibrosis of any etiology; thus, in this setting, a copper stain is not useful. The absence of periportal copper and/or CK7-positive hepatocytes does not exclude chronic cholestasis.

**18. Correct choice: E.**

Primary sclerosing cholangitis (PSC) is a chronic cholestatic disease characterized by inflammation and fibrosis of intrahepatic and extrahepatic bile ducts. Inflammatory bowel disease, especially ulcerative colitis, is present in 60% to 80% of cases. Histologically, sections show ductular reaction with or without bile duct injury. The image shows concentric periductal fibrosis ("onion-skin" fibrosis), which is a characteristic finding of PSC.

**19. Correct choice: B.**

Extrahepatic Biliary Atresia (EBA) is an idiopathic biliary disease presenting in the first few months of life. Ductular reaction develops around 4 to 6 weeks with variable portal inflammation and periportal/portal-portal fibrosis, which can quickly progress to cirrhosis. It is the most common reason for pediatric liver transplantation and may manifest with atresia of common bile duct or of the more proximal structures, possibly with a hypoplastic gallbladder.

**20. Correct choice: E.**

Alpha-1-antitrypsin (AAT) deficiency is an autosomal recessive condition due to inheritance of biallelic pathogenic variants in the *SERPINA1* gene, which results in abnormally low levels of AAT. The genotype, protease inhibitor (Pi) typing, PiZZ leads to levels of AAT that are 10% of normal values, whereas PiMM is normal phenotype. This biochemical defect results in (i) progressive accumulation of AAT within hepatocytes, identifiable as diastase-resistant periodic acid-Schiff (PAS)-positive intracytoplasmic globules, or by immunohistochemistry (IHC), with subsequent chronic hepatitis and cirrhosis, and (ii) panacinar emphysema. Liver biopsy is intended to assess liver disease and its stage. Since the PAS-positive globules are not specific for AAT deficiency (it may be seen in acute inflammation and alcoholic liver disease), the diagnosis must be confirmed by Pi typing.

**21. Correct choice: E.**

Alagille syndrome is a cause of paucity of bile ducts and is recognized clinically by facial irregularity (triangular facies) and abnormalities in the kidney, eyes, spine, and/or heart (eg, tetralogy of Fallot). Histologically, a liver biopsy will show a cholestatic pattern of injury with loss of interlobular bile ducts. The diagnosis is confirmed by genetic testing and demonstration of *NOTCH2* or *JAG1* mutations.

**22. Correct choice: E.**

Iron deposition is Kupffer cell dominant or demonstrates a mixed hepatocellular-Kupffer cell distribution and is seen in secondary iron overload, unlike in hemochromatosis, where iron deposition is limited to periportal hepatocytes. Common causes of secondary iron overload include hemolytic anemia, excess iron intake, chronic inflammatory conditions, fatty liver disease, metabolic syndrome, frequent blood transfusions, and cirrhosis of any etiology. Liver involvement in sickle cell anemia is frequently caused by acute sickle hepatic crisis (ischemic injury), iron overload, and viral hepatitis from frequent blood transfusions.

**23. Correct choice: C.**

Nodular Regenerative Hyperplasia (NRH) is a rare disorder in which the normal liver architecture is replaced by small regenerative nodules without fibrosis. NRH manifests with portal hypertension. NRH is a diffuse process that involves the whole hepatic parenchyma. It is found in association with different types of conditions and is caused by obliteration of small portal vein radicles. Nodular regeneration is probably a reaction to alterations in blood flow. Nodules measure 1 to 3 mm and are devoid of fibrous septa. The appearance in liver biopsies is characteristic, as the regenerative nodules are demarcated by darker, congested rims of atrophic parenchyma.

**24. Correct choice: A.**

Acute cellular rejection can manifest as early as 5 to 30 days and can occur years after transplantation, especially if the patient goes off immunosuppressants. The reaction has two main epithelial cell targets: bile ducts and endothelial cells. The defining morphologic features are (i) mixed portal inflammation, with lymphocytes, eosinophils, neutrophils, and plasma cells; (ii) bile duct damage; and (iii) endotheliitis affecting central or portal veins (arrowhead in the picture), where lymphocytes insinuate themselves into the subendothelial space. Vascular damage may lead to hepatocyte necrosis. Rejection is graded as mild, moderate, or severe according to the Banff classification.

# 37 Masses of the Liver

1. Aspiration of a cystic lesion in the right hepatic lobe yields odorless, orange, pasty material. Microscopic examination of this material shows necrotic debris, with no neutrophils. Occasional histiocyte-like round cells with a small, round nucleus with a karyosome are identified. Which of the following is the most likely diagnosis?

   A. Amebiasis
   B. Biliary cystadenoma
   C. Echinococcosis
   D. Pyogenic abscess
   E. Solitary unilocular cyst

2. A 45-year-old female presents with abdominal pain and distension, and a computed tomography (CT) scan reveals a multilocular cystic tumor in the right lobe of the liver. Blood tests show elevated carbohydrate antigen 19-9 (CA19-9) levels. The tumor is excised, and its histologic appearance is shown in Figure 1. Which of the following is the most likely diagnosis?

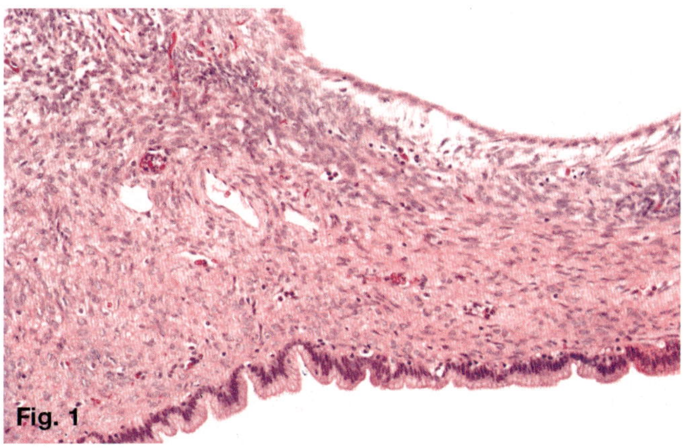


   A. Mesenchymal hamartoma
   B. Mucinous cystic neoplasm
   C. Polycystic liver disease
   D. Serous cystadenoma
   E. Simple biliary cyst

3. A well-demarcated subcapsular nodule is identified by magnetic resonance imaging (MRI) in the right hepatic lobe of a 35-year-old woman with abdominal discomfort. The lesion is removed. Its cut section is shown in the macroscopic photograph in Figure 1. Microscopic examination shows liver lobules with fatty changes separated by thick fibrous bands. The central scar contains thick-walled arteries. These gross and microscopic features are consistent with

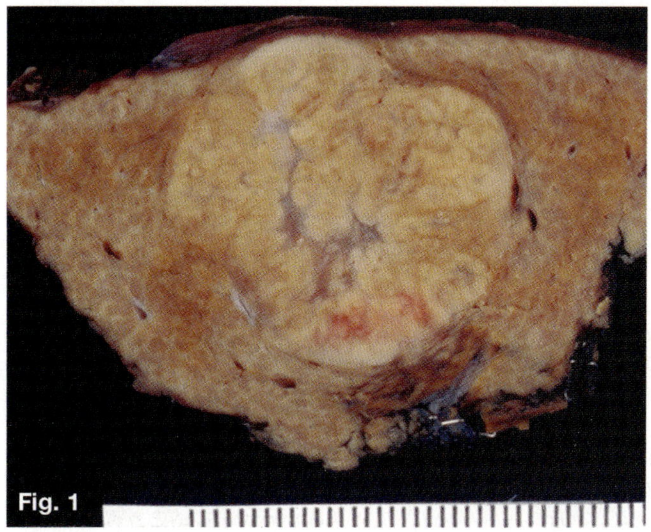


Di Patre PL, Carter D. Sternberg's Diagnostic Surgical Pathology Review. 2nd ed. Wolters Kluwer; 2015.

   A. early cirrhosis.
   B. focal nodular hyperplasia.
   C. hepatoblastoma.
   D. liver adenoma.
   E. nodular regenerative hyperplasia.

All figures in this chapter are from Longacre TA, Greenson JK, Hornick JL, Reuter VE, eds. *Mills and Sternberg's Diagnostic Surgical Pathology*. 7th ed. Wolters Kluwer; 2022 except for those noted at the end of this book.

4. Figure 1 shows the histologic appearance of a subcapsular nodular liver lesion. Which of the following stains is most helpful in making a diagnosis?

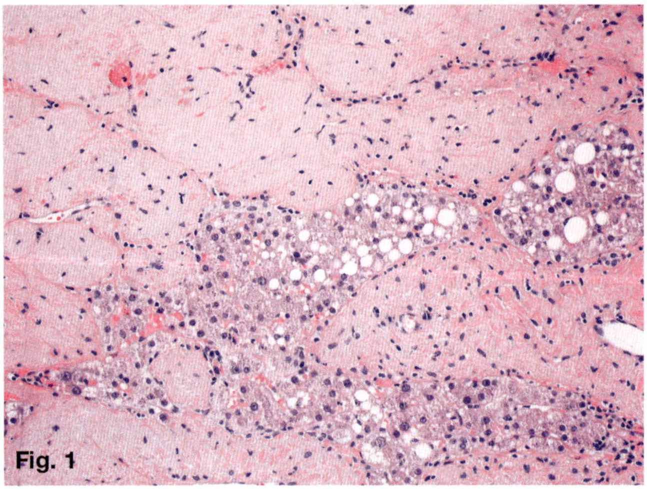

Fig. 1

A. CD34
B. Congo red
C. Elastin Van Gieson
D. Glutamine synthetase
E. Reticulin

5. A 2.3-cm solitary liver mass was resected. The background liver shows no significant fibrosis. Figure 1 shows the result of liver fatty acid–binding protein (LFABP) immunohistochemical testing. What is the appropriate diagnosis?

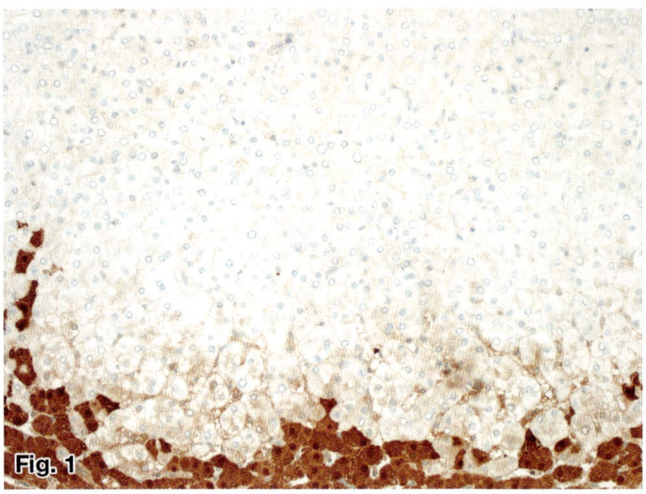

Fig. 1

A. Focal nodular hyperplasia
B. Hepatocellular adenoma, β-catenin–activated subtype
C. Hepatocellular adenoma, hepatocyte nuclear factor 1-α (HNF1α)–inactivated subtype
D. Hepatocellular adenoma, inflammatory subtype
E. Hepatocellular carcinoma

6. Several small nodules measuring 1.0 to 1.8 cm in greatest dimension are seen in a liver explant for cirrhosis. Figure 1 shows a representative histologic section of one of the nodules. Reticulin stain shows hepatocyte cords that are one to two cells thick, and the hepatocytes are cytologically bland. The proliferation index by Ki-67 is 0.6%. What is the appropriate diagnosis?

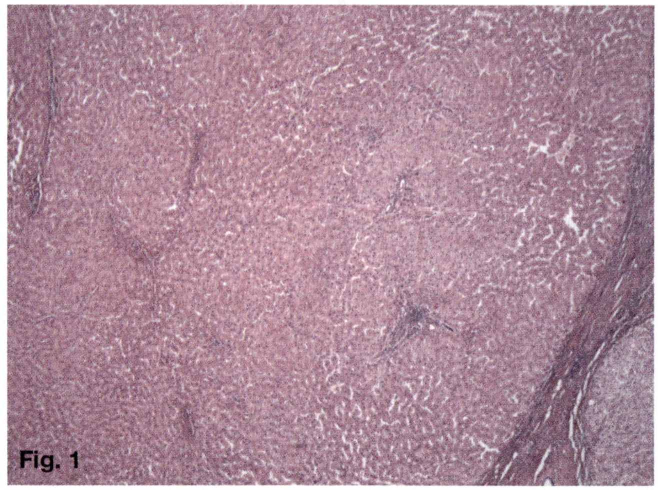

Fig. 1

A. Dysplastic nodule
B. Focal nodular hyperplasia
C. Hepatocellular adenoma
D. Hepatocellular carcinoma
E. Macroregenerative nodule

7. The following is a list of factors or conditions that predispose to the development of hepatocellular carcinoma (HCC). In which of them does HCC occur constantly in noncirrhotic livers?

A. Alcohol use
B. Hepatitis B virus
C. Hepatitis C virus
D. Hereditary hemochromatosis
E. Hypercitrullinemia

8. Which of the following morphologic patterns of hepatocellular carcinoma (HCC) is represented in Figure 1?

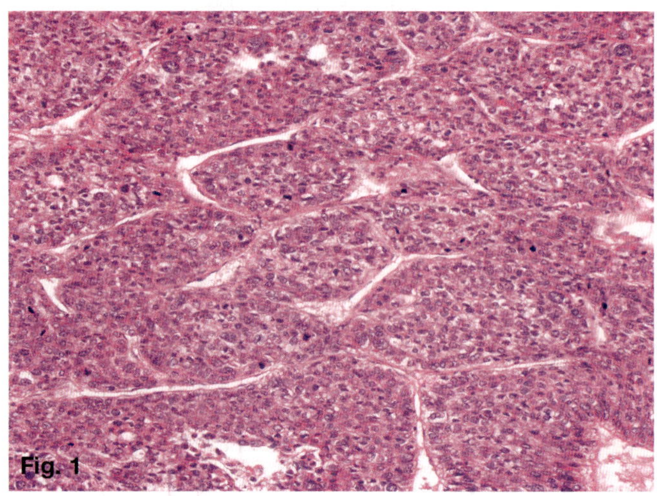

Fig. 1

A. Macrotrabecular
B. Pseudoglandular
C. Scirrhous
D. Solid
E. Trabecular

9. Which of the following subtypes of hepatocellular carcinoma converse a worse prognosis compared to conventional hepatocellular carcinoma?

   A. Clear cell
   B. Fibrolamellar
   C. Lymphocyte rich
   D. Macrotrabecular
   E. Steatohepatitic

10. A patient undergoes partial hepatectomy for a solitary liver mass. A representative histologic section of the mass is shown in Figure 1. Which of the following is the most likely clinical setting associated with this tumor?

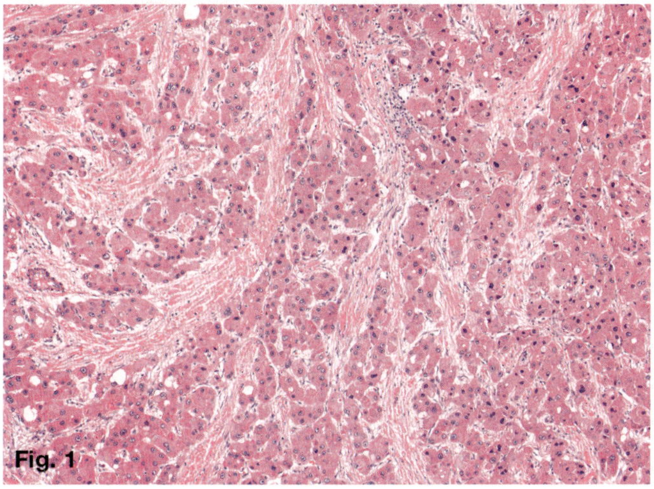

Fig. 1

   A. 20-year-old with chronic hepatitis B
   B. 30-year-old with background noncirrhotic liver
   C. 50-year-old with alcoholic cirrhosis
   D. Markedly elevated serum α-fetoprotein
   E. Older patients with hemochromatosis

11. Figure 1 is a representative section of a liver mass. Which of the following statements is true regarding this tumor?

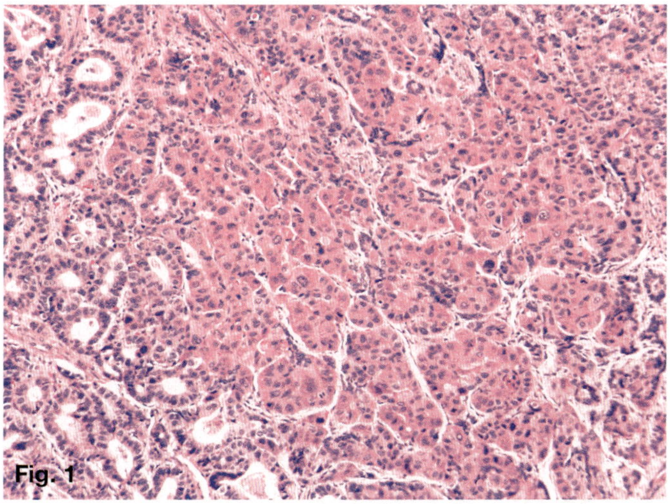

Fig. 1

   A. Diffusely expresses Arginase-1 by immunohistochemistry
   B. Has unique and distinguishing macroscopic features
   C. Has a similar prognosis relative to conventional hepatocellular carcinoma
   D. Exhibits a glandular component that can be positive for albumin by in situ hybridization
   E. Is the most common primary liver carcinoma

12. A 56-year-old patient has a solitary liver mass. Which of the following immunostains, if positive, would be most helpful to differentiate between a benign hepatocellular proliferation from a hepatocellular carcinoma?

   A. Albumin in situ hybridization (ISH)
   B. Arginase-1
   C. Glypican-3
   D. HepPar-1
   E. Monoclonal carcinoembryonic antigen (mCEA)

13. A 16-month-old baby is diagnosed with a liver tumor. On histologic examination, the tumor is characterized by a "light/dark" biphasic pattern, as shown in the low-power photomicrograph in Figure 1. This tumor is most likely a

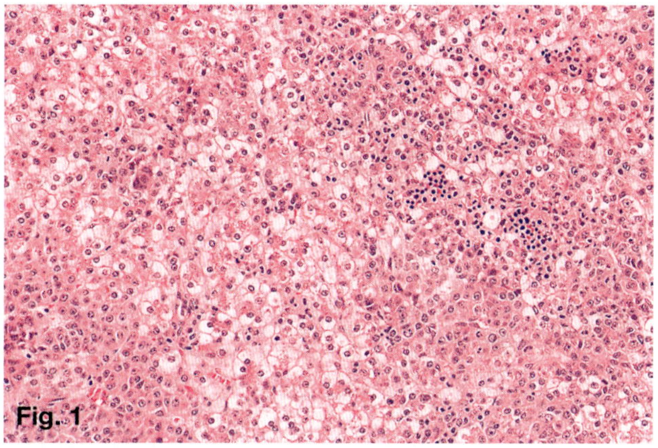

Fig. 1

   A. bile duct hamartoma.
   B. hemangioblastoma.
   C. hepatoblastoma.
   D. malignant mesenchymoma.
   E. mesenchymal hamartoma.

14. A 56-year-old patient with pancreatic ductal adenocarcinoma is undergoing a Whipple procedure. Intraoperatively, a 0.8-cm lesion is seen in the subcapsular liver, which was sent to pathology for intraoperative diagnosis. Figure 1 shows a representative hematoxylin and eosin (H&E) section of the frozen remnant. What is the diagnosis?

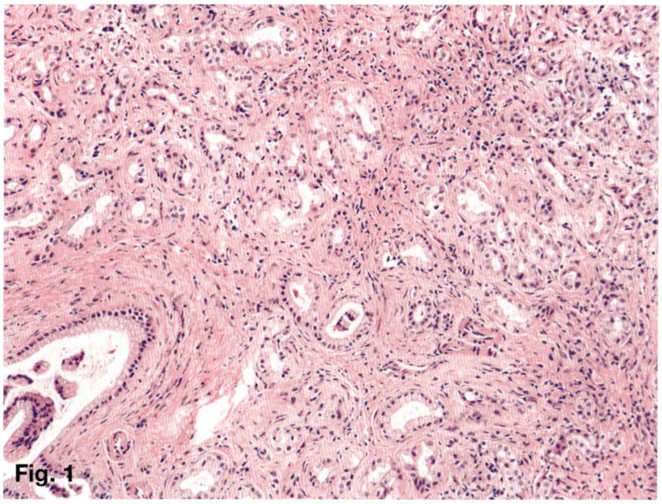

Fig. 1

   A. Bile duct adenoma
   B. Bile duct hamartoma
   C. Biliary adenofibroma
   D. Intrahepatic cholangiocarcinoma
   E. Metastatic adenocarcinoma

15. Multiple tan-white masses are found in the liver of a 65-year-old man at autopsy. Premortem blood tests show elevated serum carcinoembryonic antigen (CEA) and carbohydrate antigen 19-9 (CA19-9) levels. Figure 1 is a representative hematoxylin and eosin (H&E) section of one of the masses. The tumor cells are positive for CK7, monoclonal CEA (mCEA), and albumin in situ hybridization. Which of the following is the most likely diagnosis for the liver masses described?

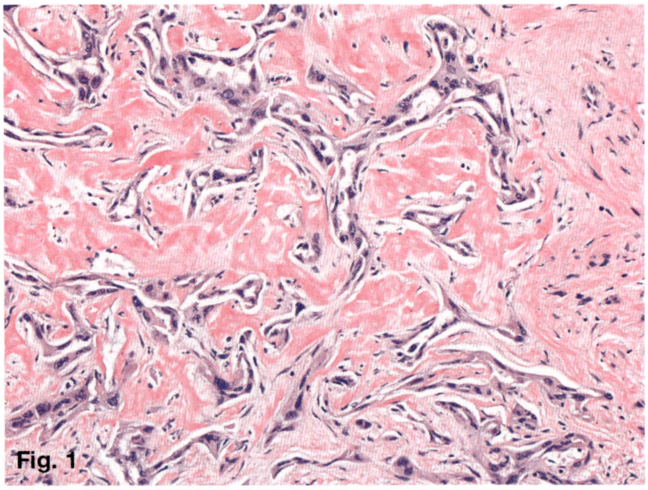

Fig. 1

A. Angiosarcoma
B. Bile duct adenoma
C. Hepatocellular carcinoma
D. Intrahepatic cholangiocarcinoma
E. Metastatic carcinoma

16. A 6-month-old baby girl undergoes resection of a 3-cm mass in the left lobe of the liver. Figure 1 shows its histologic appearance. Which of the following is the most likely diagnosis?

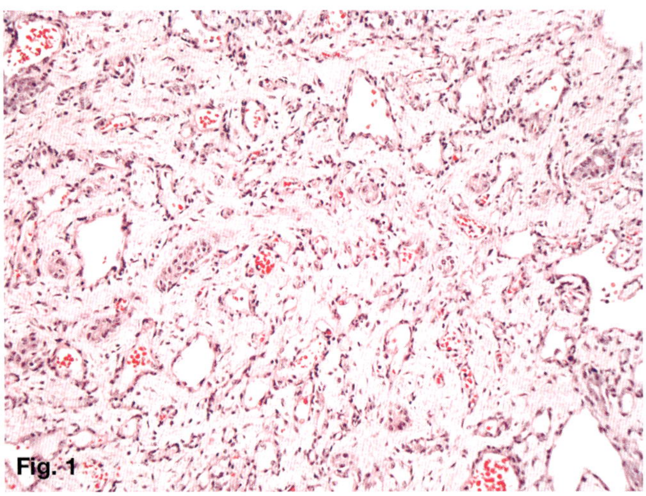

Fig. 1

A. Angiosarcoma
B. Arteriovascular malformation
C. Cavernous hemangioma
D. Infantile hemangioma
E. Mesenchymal hamartoma

17. Which of the following factors is known to increase the risk of developing angiosarcoma of the liver but not that of cholangiocarcinoma or hepatocellular carcinoma?

A. Anabolic steroid treatment
B. Cirrhosis of any etiology
C. Clonorchis parasite infestation
D. Occupational exposure to vinyl chloride
E. Thorotrast exposure

18. A 34-year-old woman who takes oral contraceptives undergoes surgery for resection of multiple intrahepatic tumors. Histologically, the lesions consist of plump cells with acidophilic and vacuolated cytoplasm. Neoplastic cells infiltrate vascular channels. Immunoreactivity for factor VIII–related antigen and CD34 is detected. Ultrastructural studies reveal Weibel-Palade bodies. Which of the following is the most likely diagnosis?

A. Angiosarcoma
B. Epithelioid hemangioendothelioma
C. Focal nodular hyperplasia
D. Hemangioma
E. Liver cell adenoma

19. What is the most common molecular abnormality associated with the entity in Question 18?

A. *DNAJB1-PRKACA* fusion
B. *NAB2-STAT6* fusion
C. *WWTR1-CAMTA1* fusion
D. *YAP1-TFE3* fusion
E. *ZFP36-FOSB* fusion

20. Which of the following is true of inflammatory myofibroblastic tumors of the liver?

A. Anaplastic lymphoma kinase (ALK)–positive neoplastic proliferations
B. Exhibit phlebitis and storiform fibrosis as defining characteristics
C. Sequelae to bacterial liver infections
D. Synonymous to immunoglobulin G4 (IgG4) disease of the liver
E. Will shrink in size or disappear with antibiotic therapy

# ANSWERS AND EXPLANATIONS

**1. Correct choice: A.**

Hepatic "abscesses" are observed in up to 9% of amebic infections. The term "abscess" is incorrect because no neutrophils are seen in the cystic fluid. *Entamoeba histolytica* trophozoites are similar to histiocytes but have a small, round nucleus with a distinct karyosome. Trophozoites are recovered in greater numbers from the periphery of the cyst, but they are rare in the central region. Biliary cystadenoma is a cystic tumor, usually multilocular and of mucinous type, and with a distinctive ovarian stroma, 85% of which occur in women. *Echinococcus* cysts contain typical protoscolices. Pyogenic abscesses contain foul-smelling neutrophil-rich fluid; *Escherichia coli* is the most frequent agent.

**2. Correct choice: B.**

Mucinous cyst neoplasms (MCNs) account for approximately 5% of solitary hepatic cysts and are commonly mistaken for simple biliary cysts. Most MCNs are intrahepatic (84%), although they can rarely arise within the common bile duct, hepatic ducts, cystic duct, or gallbladder. Elevated levels of carbohydrate antigen 19-9 (CA19-9) and carcinoembryonic antigen (CEA) in cyst fluid may be helpful in distinguishing MCN from simple biliary cysts. MCNs are lined by a single layer of mucinous epithelium that is usually columnar but may be focally flattened, denuded, or pseudostratified. The defining feature is the presence of dense subepithelial mesenchymal stroma that resembles normal ovarian stroma, which can be focal and quite inconspicuous in some cases, requiring stains for its confident identification.

**3. Correct choice: B.**

Focal nodular hyperplasia (FNH) is asymptomatic in 80% of cases and found incidentally during surgery or at autopsy. It may manifest with pain or abdominal discomfort. Arteriographic examination yields a typical centrifugal pattern. The characteristic gross appearance is that of a nonencapsulated but well-circumscribed nodule containing a central scar with radiating fibrous septa. All the normal histologic components of the liver are present in FNH, so that on biopsy the morphologic features may resemble focal cirrhosis. Hepatocytes may show fatty change, glycogen accumulation, and/or α-1-antitrypsin globules. Morphologic variations include cases where bile ductule proliferation is pronounced or dilated vessels are particularly abundant. The latter variant, called telangiectatic, is now believed to correspond to the inflammatory type of hepatocellular adenoma.

**4. Correct choice: C.**

Segmental atrophy/nodular elastosis shows the following progressive histologic changes: (1) parenchymal collapse with bile ductular proliferation and mixed neutrophilic and lymphocytic inflammation; (2) reduction and eventual loss of the bile ductular proliferation, inflammation, and increasing deposition of elastosis; (3) nodular lesion composed of elastosis with occasional islands of hepatocytes; and (4) replacement of elastosis by fibrosis, leading to a nodular scar of dense collagen, often with still a few islands of hepatocytes. Nodular elastosis is secondary to thrombosis of blood vessels feeding a small subsegment of the liver, usually in a subcapsular location. The elastin Van Gieson stain will highlight the elastosis.

**5. Correct choice: C.**

Hepatic adenomas are benign hepatocellular neoplasms that arise in normal or nearly, normal livers. The four most common subtypes, based on molecular and immunohistochemical findings, are hepatocyte nuclear factor 1-α (HNF1α)-inactivated, β-catenin–activated, inflammatory, and unclassified adenomas. The image shows loss of liver fatty acid–binding protein (LFABP) expression in the tumor cells, which is consistent with the HNF1α-inactivated hepatocellular adenoma (see Table 1).

**TABLE 1 Common Subtypes of Hepatic Adenoma**

| Subtype | Molecular Features | Microscopic Features | Clinical Associations | Immunohistochemistry |
|---|---|---|---|---|
| HNF1α-inactivated | Biallelic inactivation of HNF1α | Fatty change in many; not specific | Most cases sporadic, but rare cases in patient with MODY3 | LFABP negative |
| β-Catenin activated | Mutation in *CTNNB1* | No specific features | Higher rate of malignant transformation and hemorrhage | Nuclear β-catenin positive<br>Strong diffuse glutamine synthetase staining |
| Inflammatory | Activation of IL6/JAK/STAT pathway | Sinusoidal dilation; patchy inflammation; variable number of faux portal tracts | Obesity, alcohol<br>Higher rate of hemorrhage<br>More frequently develops secondary β-catenin mutations, compared to HNF1α | Cytoplasmic positivity for serum amyloid A–associated protein (SAA) for C-reactive protein (CRP)<br>There can be nonspecific patchy staining in FNH, so staining should be strong and diffuse. |
| Unclassified | No specific genetic abnormalities | No specific features | No specific features | |

FNH, focal nodular hyperplasia; HNF1α, hepatocyte nuclear factor 1α; JAK, Janus kinase; LFABP, liver fatty acid–binding protein; MODY3, maturity-onset diabetes of the young type 3; NF1α, hepatocyte nuclear factor 1α; STAT, signal transducer and activator of transcription.

**6. Correct choice: E.**

Macroregenerative nodules (MRNs) are nonneoplastic and stand out from the background cirrhotic nodules based on their noticeably larger size. MRNs are usually multiple and most measure less than 1.5 cm in diameter. They are found in about 15% of cirrhotic livers. Hepatocytes within MRNs are identical to those in the surrounding liver and are cytologically bland. The hepatocellular plates are one or two cells thick and the reticulin framework is intact. Portal tracts are scattered throughout the nodule, but are frequently fewer in number compared with the background liver. Macroscopically, MRNs cannot be distinguished grossly from dysplastic nodules. Dysplastic nodules show cytologic and/or architectural atypia and are further subdivided into low-grade and high-grade, depending on the degree of atypia.

**7. Correct choice: E.**

The great majority of cases of hepatocellular carcinoma develop in cirrhotic livers. Alcohol, hepatitis B virus, and hepatitis C virus are the most important etiologic factors worldwide. Several conditions may lead to hepatocellular carcinoma without causing cirrhosis. Among these are hypercitrullinemia (a high rate of association with hepatocellular carcinoma), glycogen storage disease (an intermediate rate), and several others with a low rate of association with hepatocellular carcinoma (eg, oral contraceptive use, hereditary fructose intolerance).

**8. Correct choice: A.**

Histologic growth patterns seen within hepatocellular carcinoma (HCC) do not have prognostic significance, and multiple histologic growth patterns are often found in the same tumor. Most of these patterns are helpful for pathologists in recognizing HCC but do not need to be included in pathology reports.

- Trabecular: This is the most common pattern (~70%) and resembles normal hepatic architecture with tumor cells growing in cords or plates that are separated by vascular channels lined by endothelial cells. The trabeculae can have varying thickness.
- Macrotrabecular: Defined by trabeculae that are at least 10 cells thick.
- Solid: Seen in about 20% of HCC and is composed of sheets of cells without well-defined trabeculae at low power. This pattern is typically mixed with the conventional trabecular pattern.
- Pseudoglandular: Seen in about 10% to 20% of HCC and shows pseudogland (acinar) formation that ranges from focal to diffuse. The pseudoglands are secondary to dilated bile canaliculi and are lined by a single layer of tumor cells.

**9. Correct choice: D.**

The macrotrabecular subtype is defined by a macrotrabecular growth pattern in at least 50% of tumor and has a worse prognosis compared to conventional hepatocellular carcinoma. The steatohepatitic subtype is defined by steatohepatitis in at least 50% of the tumor and has a similar prognosis to conventional hepatocellular carcinoma. Clear cell, fibrolamellar, and lymphocyte rich subtypes have a better prognosis compared to conventional hepatocellular carcinoma.

**10. Correct choice: B.**

Although the most important risk factors for the conventional histologic type of hepatocellular carcinoma include hepatitis B virus infection and cirrhosis, the fibrolamellar variant develops in young patients (between 20 and 40 years of age) with an otherwise normal liver. This type is associated with a far better prognosis than classic hepatocellular carcinoma. The characteristic histologic findings are sheets, nests, and trabeculae of large polygonal cells with prominent nucleoli, with intervening hyalinized, relatively acellular, bands of fibrosis. The eosinophilic tumor cells have well-defined cell borders and coarsely granular cytoplasm due to the accumulation of large numbers of mitochondria and lysosomes. Mild nuclear pleomorphism may be seen. α-Fetoprotein (AFP) levels are markedly elevated in patients with hepatocellular carcinoma but not in those with fibrolamellar hepatocellular carcinoma.

**11. Correct choice: D.**

Combined hepatocellular carcinoma-cholangiocarcinoma (HCC-CC) is a rare tumor that requires the presence of distinct and separate HCC and CC elements within the same tumor. The interface between the two cell types can be sharply defined or more admixed. The CC component can display glandular formation that is positive for CK7 and negative for hepatocellular markers, such as Arginase-1. It is essential to distinguish this tumor from conventional HCC with pseudoglandular formation. The pseudogland formation may be recognized by the similarity of the lining cells to hepatocytes and the presence of bile rather than mucin. Macroscopically, many combined HCC-CC cannot be distinguished from HCC. The prognosis of HCC-CC has been reported to be worse relative to conventional HCC. The overall 5-year survival rate reported in one series was 23.1% for combined HCC-CC, as compared to 66.2% for HCC. Albumin in situ hybridization has greater than 99% sensitivity for HCC and can also be positive in cholangiocarcinomas.

**12. Correct choice: C.**

Immunohistochemistry may be necessary in distinguishing hepatocellular carcinoma (HCC) from hepatic benign or dysplastic lesions. Albumin in situ hybridization (ISH), Arginase-1, and HepPar-1 are all markers of hepatic differentiation; however, it does not distinguish between HCC and benign hepatocellular proliferations. Although Glypican-3 is a marker of hepatocellular differentiation, it is generally negative in benign hepatic lesions. Thus, when positive, it is useful in the diagnosis of well-differentiated HCC. HCCs, unlike adenocarcinomas, rarely show strong or diffuse cytoplasmic immunoreactivity with monoclonal carcinoembryonic antigen (mCEA).

**13. Correct choice: C.**

Hepatoblastoma is a malignant tumor that may be considered the hepatic counterpart of Wilms tumor. It probably arises from a precursor that differentiates along epithelial and mesenchymal lines. Variably immature (small) hepatocytes represent the main epithelial component, but this may be associated with a mesenchymal component containing bone or muscle tissue. Six histologic variants are recognized. The most frequent fetal variant is characterized by an alternating light/dark pattern on low power (as seen in the picture) due to the uneven distribution of glycogen-rich and glycogen-depleted areas. The prognosis depends on the stage and degree of differentiation of the epithelial component. Malignant mesenchymoma is an infantile hepatic sarcoma with giant cells and PAS (periodic acid-Schiff)-positive globules.

**14. Correct choice: A.**

Bile duct adenomas are small, well-circumscribed, wedge-shaped nodules commonly found incidentally during surgery or autopsy. Bile duct adenomas are composed of compact, well-differentiated small tubules with absent to inconspicuous lumens, embedded in variable amounts of fibrous stroma. Bile duct hamartomas are characterized by small, often multiple nodules (<5 mm) associated with portal tracts. They are composed of angulated, dilated ductal structures, often containing bile, within a hyalinized stroma that may contain sparse chronic inflammation. Unlike bile duct adenomas, the lumens do not contain bile. Biliary adenofibromas are larger than most bile duct adenomas or Von Meyenburg complexes, ranging in size from 2 to 20 cm. They are characterized by dilated tubulocystic structures that show areas of inter-anastomosing growth. It is important to distinguish benign bile duct lesions from metastatic adenocarcinoma in the intraoperative setting.

**15. Correct choice: D.**

Intrahepatic cholangiocarcinoma (ICC) is a carcinoma arising from any portion of the intrahepatic bile ducts. Grossly, ICC appears as large, very firm, tan-white, and nodular masses often with satellite nodules. Microscopically, ICC arising in the hilar or larger branches of the biliary tree often shows large, well-defined glands lined by columnar tumor cells that are typically periodic acid-Schiff (PAS) positive and show mucin production; this morphology is called the large duct pattern. ICC arising from peripheral smaller bile ducts often contains smaller sized glands or grows as branching cords of tumor cells without well-formed glands; this morphology is called the small duct pattern. The morphology seen in the image is of the small duct pattern. Architecture showing anastomosing cords or tumor cells reminiscent of a bile ductular proliferation is called the cholangiolocellular pattern. ICC tumor cells will be positive for CK7 and CK19, and negative for HepPar-1 and Arginase-1. Approximately 80% of ICCs are positive for albumin in situ hybridization (ISH).

**16. Correct choice: D.**

Infantile hemangioma is the second most common liver tumor of childhood. It manifests in the first year of life with nonspecific gastrointestinal symptoms, high-output congestive heart failure (due to extensive shunting within the tumor), or liver failure, rarely with Kasabach-Merritt syndrome (bleeding diathesis due to platelet sequestration). It can be solitary or multiple. The main differential diagnosis is with angiosarcoma (irregular vascular spaces lined by atypical endothelial cells with hyperchromatic nuclei and mitotic figures), mesenchymal hamartoma (loose, myxoid stroma arranged in a concentric manner around bile ducts), and vascular malformations such as cavernous hemangioma (large, thin-walled vascular spaces) and arteriovenous malformation (disorganized cluster of arterial, venous channels, and arterialized veins).

**17. Correct choice: D.**

Angiosarcoma is a rare malignant vasogenic neoplasm in the liver, but it is inordinately more common in workers with chronic exposure to vinyl chloride used in the polyvinyl chloride (PVC) industry. Vinyl chloride exposure does not increase the risk of hepatocellular carcinoma (HCC) or intrahepatic cholangiocarcinoma (ICC). Anabolic steroid treatment is known to increase the risk of a variety of liver neoplasms, including ICC (but not angiosarcoma). Cirrhosis is associated with an increased risk of both HCC and angiosarcoma, but not ICC. *Clonorchis* infestation may lead to ICC. Thorotrast exposure is associated with increased prevalence of both ICC and angiosarcoma.

**18. Correct choice: B.**

Epithelioid hemangioendothelioma is a malignant vascular tumor that develops in noncirrhotic liver, usually in women. The tumor is often multifocal. Tumor cells infiltrate the liver parenchyma in short cords or as single cells with myxoid to fibrotic stroma. Neoplastic cells resemble epithelial cells with intracytoplasmic vacuoles. Tumor cells may infiltrate veins to produce intravascular tufts. The endothelial origin of this neoplasm is supported by immunohistochemistry and ultrastructural studies. Epithelioid hemangioendothelioma has a better prognosis than angiosarcoma. The latter is characterized by more pronounced cellular atypia.

**19. Correct choice: C.**

Molecular studies of epithelioid hemangioendothelioma have shown translocations leading to a *WWTR1-CAMTA1* fusion gene in most cases. Other fusions in *YAP1-TFE3* and *ZFP36-FOSB* have been seen. Fluorescence in situ hybridization (FISH) or polymerase chain reaction (PCR) for detection of these arrangements can help confirm the diagnosis in difficult cases. Confirmatory immunostaining for calmodulin-binding transcription activator 1 (CAMTA1) can also be performed.

**20. Correct choice: A.**

Inflammatory myofibroblastic tumor (IMT) is composed of neoplastic spindled to epithelioid myofibroblasts mixed with lymphocytes, plasma cells, and eosinophils. IMT is now reserved for anaplastic lymphoma kinase (ALK)–positive neoplastic proliferations and is not a synonym for inflammatory pseudotumor, which is a benign reactive process. Inflammatory myofibroblastic tumors (IMTs) are solitary in the majority of cases and are well circumscribed and firm. Phlebitis and storiform fibrosis are more characteristic of immunoglobulin G4 (IgG4) disease.

# 38 Gallbladder, Extrahepatic Biliary Tree, and Ampulla

1. Which of the following types of gallstones is commonly found in infected bile?

   A. Black stones
   B. Brown stones
   C. Cholesterol stones
   D. Disappearing stones
   E. Intramural stones

2. Which of the following is true regarding acute cholecystitis?

   A. Acute acalculous cholecystitis is associated with exceptionally low mortality rate.
   B. Acute cholecystitis is defined by the presence of intraepithelial neutrophils.
   C. Acute gangrenous cholecystitis is defined by the presence of mural infarction.
   D. Perimuscular myofibroblastic proliferation peaks within 24 hours of onset of acute injury.
   E. Recurrence after nonsurgical management is rare and presents as less severe disease.

3. Which of the following variants of chronic cholecystitis is associated with the highest risk of cancer?

   A. Eosinophilic
   B. Follicular
   C. Hyalinizing
   D. Immunoglobulin G subclass 4 (IgG4) related
   E. Lymphoplasmacytic

4. Most cases of carcinoma of the gallbladder are associated with

   A. cholelithiasis.
   B. Gardner syndrome.
   C. porcelain gallbladder.
   D. sclerosing cholangitis.
   E. ulcerative colitis.

5. A 65-year-old female with acute cholecystitis undergoes cholecystectomy. On sectioning of the gallbladder, a white, firm, nodular lesion with sievelike cystic areas is seen in the fundus. Representative section is shown in Figure 1. What is the diagnosis?

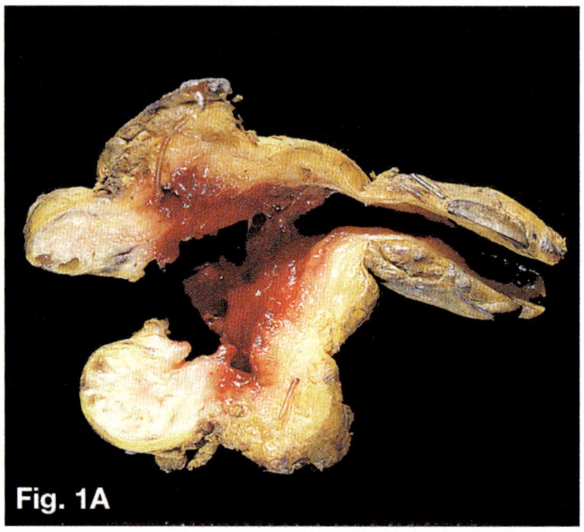

Fig. 1A

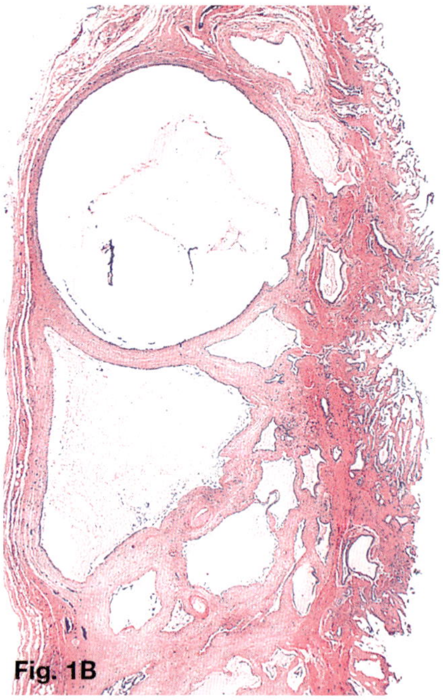

Fig. 1B

   A. Adenomyomatous hyperplasia
   B. Fibromyoglandular polyp
   C. Invasive adenocarcinoma
   D. Primary papillary hyperplasia
   E. Pyloric gland adenoma

All figures in this chapter are from Longacre TA, Greenson JK, Hornick JL, Reuter VE, eds. *Mills and Sternberg's Diagnostic Surgical Pathology*. 7th ed. Wolters Kluwer; 2022 except for those noted at the end of this book.

6. Abnormalities in which of the following genes is most commonly seen in gallbladder carcinomas?

   A. *GNAS*
   B. *HER2*
   C. *KRAS*
   D. *SMAD4*
   E. *TP53*

7. A 10-year-old female presents with signs and symptoms of cholestatic jaundice. A lesion involving the common bile duct is resected. The surgical specimen is shown in the gross photograph in Figure 1. The diagnosis is

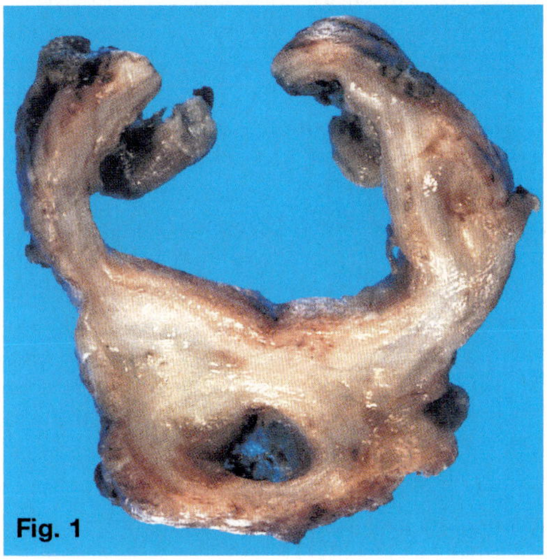

Fig. 1

   A. biliary atresia.
   B. Caroli disease.
   C. choledochal cyst.
   D. Phrygian cap.
   E. sclerosing cholangitis.

8. An incidental small polypoid lesion is seen on a routine cholecystectomy specimen. Representative section is shown in Figure 1. What is the diagnosis?

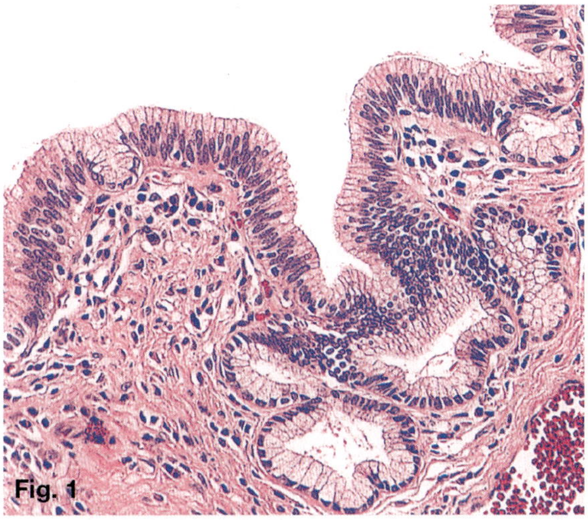

Fig. 1

   A. Adenocarcinoma
   B. High-grade dysplasia
   C. Low-grade dysplasia
   D. No dysplasia

9. Which of the following is the most common malignant tumor of extrahepatic bile ducts in children?

   A. Cholangiocarcinoma
   B. Embryonal rhabdomyosarcoma
   C. Leiomyosarcoma
   D. Malignant peripheral nerve sheath tumor
   E. Neuroendocrine carcinoma

10. Which of the following is true of intra-ampullary papillary tubular neoplasm (IAPN)?

   A. Approximately 80% of the cases have a concurrent focus of invasive carcinoma.
   B. Invasive carcinoma arising from IAPNs has a poorer prognosis compared to conventional invasive carcinoma.
   C. It is defined by the presence of more than 50% of the tumor localized within the ampullary channel.
   D. The term is used when intraductal tubulopapillary neoplasm of the pancreas extends into the lumen of the ampulla.
   E. Virtually all have an intestinal-type morphology with tubular, villous, or tubulovillous growth patterns.

# ANSWERS AND EXPLANATIONS

**1. Correct choice: B.**

There are two types of pigment stones: (i) black stones form in sterile bile from excess bilirubin in the context of hemolytic anemia, cirrhosis, or sclerosing cholangitis; while (ii) brown stones form in infected bile. *Escherichia coli* and parasites (*Ascaris lumbricoides* and *Opisthorchis sinensis*) are the most common infectious agents found in bile. The organisms produce phospholipases and glucuronidases, with formation of free fatty acids and unconjugated bilirubin, leading to formation of calcium salts. Pure cholesterol stones develop in bile supersaturated with cholesterol. Disappearing stones are those that spontaneously dissolve or pass through the common bile duct or a cholecystoenteric fistula. Intramural stones have become embedded in the gallbladder wall.

**2. Correct choice: C.**

Acute cholecystitis is clinically defined as acute injury of the gallbladder. Up to 95% of cases of acute cholecystitis are associated with gallstones, while acute acalculous cholecystitis accounts for about 5% of all cases and is typically seen in the context of severe debilitating conditions such as major trauma, burns, and multisystem organ failure. Acute cholecystitis does not necessarily contain neutrophils, which is usually secondary to infection. Microscopic findings of early-acute cholecystitis are prominent edema, congestion, hemorrhage, and fibrin deposition. Widespread myofibroblastic proliferation begins by the fifth day and peaks around the 10th day. Acute gangrenous cholecystitis is defined by true necrosis of the gallbladder wall of the gallbladder. The treatment of acute cholecystitis is cholecystectomy. In untreated patients, the attack subsides in 7 to 10 days and often within 24 hours; however, recurrences are common. The overall mortality rate for acute calculous cholecystitis is about 1%, while acute acalculous cholecystitis has a more fulminant clinical course with a mortality rate approaching 40%.

**3. Correct choice: C.**

Features of chronic cholecystitis include chronic inflammation, fibrosis, epithelial changes (atrophy, hyperplasia, metaplasia), and Aschoff-Rokitansky sinuses. Hyalinizing cholecystitis, better known as porcelain gallbladder, results from long-standing injury and refers to the development of a diffuse, hyaline type of fibrosis, associated with calcium deposition and complete effacement of the wall structures. Carcinomas developing in this setting are difficult to diagnose and stage.

**4. Correct choice: A.**

All of the named conditions predispose to this cancer, but cholelithiasis has the strongest association. Up to 90% of gallbladders removed, due to carcinoma, contain stones; however, 1% to 3% of patients with gallstones develop gallbladder carcinoma. Older people are most commonly affected. Histologically, this tumor is usually an adenocarcinoma. Typically, it appears well differentiated on low power (with well-developed glandular structures), but poorly differentiated cytologically (with anaplastic cuboidal cells in a single or double row). Concentric desmoplastic reactions around neoplastic glands are frequent. Intestinal metaplasia is commonly found in areas adjacent to the tumor. The prognosis is poor, with a 5-year survival of 5%, but tumors limited to mucosa and muscularis can be cured by simple cholecystectomy.

**5. Correct choice: A.**

Adenomyomatous hyperplasia (aka, adenomyoma) is technically not a hyperplasia but an exaggerated form of diverticular changes, or a malformation, and does not involve epithelial hyperplasia. Macroscopically, it presents as a firm, white, nodular lesion with sievelike cystic areas. Microscopically, it consists of an intramural conglomerate of cystic glands with intervening fibrotic stroma. Although it is called adenomyoma, the participation of muscle is often minimal. It is a nonneoplastic process, although dysplasia and carcinoma can occasionally evolve from adenomyomatous hyperplasia. Primary papillary hyperplasia is characterized by a thickened gallbladder mucosa, which exhibits villous-like folds that are taller than normal and closer together, without any distinct nodule formation. The epithelium appears normal, and no Paneth cells, endocrine cells, or metaplastic goblet cells are seen. The process may be focal, segmental, or diffuse.

**6. Correct choice: E.**

Molecular and genetic studies have revealed that mutations and loss of heterozygosity in the *TP53* gene are very common in gallbladder carcinomas. Immunohistochemical testing with p53 may aid in distinguishing it from benign mimics. Loss of heterozygosity of 8p, 9p, and 18q and amplification of HER2 are detected in close to half of the tumors. Although gallbladder carcinoma is regarded as a biliary-type adenocarcinoma by morphology, mutations in *KRAS*, which is present in the vast majority of pancreatic ductal adenocarcinomas and extrahepatic cholangiocarcinomas, is very rare in gallbladder carcinoma. Similarly, loss of *SMAD4* is also much less common. Microsatellite instability is reported in 10% of the cases.

**7. Correct choice: C.**

Choledochal cyst consists of a fusiform dilatation of the common bile duct, whose wall undergoes calcification. It is the most common cause of cholestatic jaundice in children after the first year of life. Choledochal cysts predispose to the development of gallstones and carcinoma. Caroli disease refers to multiple cysts of the intrahepatic ducts. Phrygian cap is a clinically silent deformity of the fundus of the gallbladder.

**8. Correct choice: D.**

Some parts of the biliary tract tend to form more stratified epithelium without being dysplastic. Even though pseudostratification of thin, columnar cells may be regarded as low-grade dysplasia elsewhere in the gastrointestinal (GI) tract or pancreas, in the gallbladder and in the surface epithelium of extrahepatic bile ducts with mucous glands these changes can be seen as a part of a reactive/regenerative process. Unlike the cells in low-grade dysplasia, these remain slender and parallel with no significant nuclear enlargement. Basal polarity of the nuclei is maintained; the cells do not extend to the surface of the epithelium.

**9. Correct choice: B.**

Embryonal rhabdomyosarcoma (botryoid subtype) is the most common malignant tumor of extrahepatic bile ducts in children, with patients typically presenting at the ages of 3 to 4 years. It can also involve the gallbladder. The most common site is the common bile duct. Macroscopically, the tumor usually consists of a conglomerate of soft, mucosa-covered polyps that may fill the lumen. The polypoid fragments are usually covered by a layer of flattened biliary epithelium overlying a dense zone of primitive spindle cells representing the cambium layer. Metastases occur in about 40% of cases.

**10. Correct choice: A.**

Intra-ampullary papillary tubular neoplasms (IAPNs) are classified as adenoma or "noninvasive papillary neoplasm" and occur predominantly (>75%) within the ampulla. IAPNs should be distinguished from histologically analogous neoplasms that occur in neighboring sites such as intraductal tubulopapillary neoplasms of the pancreas or intraductal tubulopapillary neoplasms of the distal common bile duct. While adenomas of the ampullary duodenum are virtually all intestinal type, IAPNs often have gastric and pancreatobiliary features, and most are of mixed type. Most IAPNs tend to have substantial cytologic atypia and architectural complexity that warrants the diagnosis of high-grade dysplasia. Invasive carcinomas are identified in 80% of the cases and often exhibit mixed pancreatobiliary and intestinal patterns. Noninvasive IAPNs have a very good prognosis, and cases with invasive carcinoma have a better prognosis than conventional invasive carcinomas (unaccompanied by IAPN).

# 39 Anus and Perianal Area

1. Which of the following is true about anal squamous cell carcinoma?

   A. It is commonly discovered in the anal canal on endoscopy.
   B. Patients with human immunodeficiency virus (HIV) have a better prognosis.
   C. The basaloid variant has the worst prognosis.
   D. The first line therapy is surgical resection.
   E. There is no difference in human papillomavirus (HPV) associations based on tumor morphology.

2. An anal biopsy from a 32-year-old female with human papillomavirus (HPV) is seen in Figure 1. What is the best diagnosis?

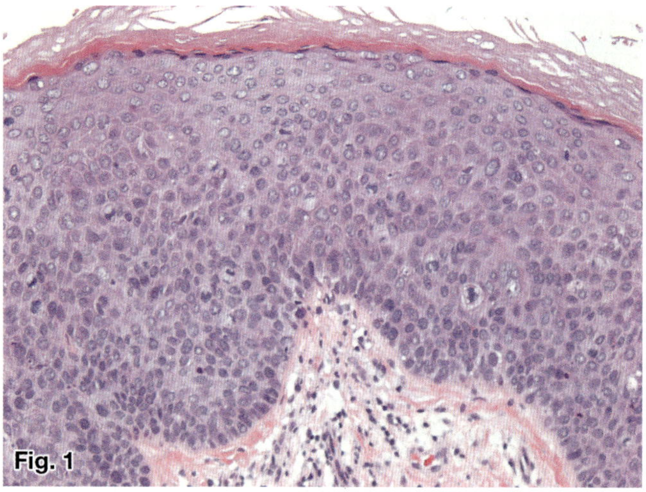


   A. Condyloma acuminatum
   B. Epidermoid metaplasia
   C. High-grade squamous intraepithelial neoplasia
   D. Low-grade squamous intraepithelial neoplasia
   E. Reactive epithelial changes

3. Which of the following human papillomavirus (HPV) serotypes is most commonly associated with anal invasive squamous cell carcinoma?

   A. 6
   B. 11
   C. 16
   D. 18
   E. 31

4. Which of the following is true about primary adenocarcinomas of the anal canal?

   A. All cases are due to extension from rectal tumors.
   B. They are associated with long-standing perianal disease.
   C. They are commonly associated with human papillomavirus (HPV) infection.
   D. They are histologically similar to conventional-type colorectal adenocarcinoma.
   E. They are usually poorly differentiated and rapidly growing.

5. Figure 1 is from a biopsy from the anal canal of a patient with a history of rectal adenocarcinoma that was resected 1 years ago. What is the expected immunoprofile of this lesion?

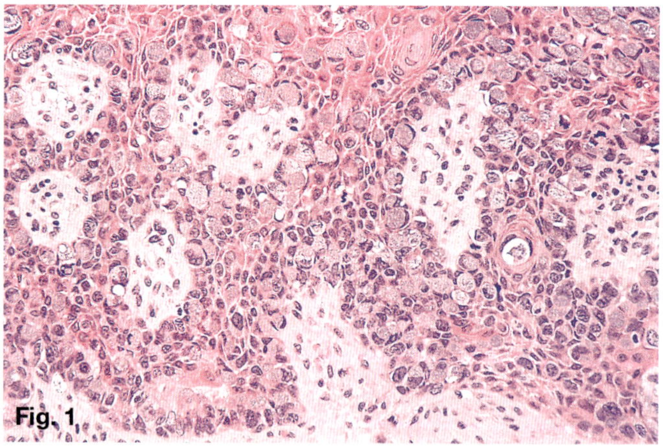


   A. CK7(+), GCDFP-15(+), CK20(−), CDX2(−)
   B. CK7(−), GCDFP-15(−), CK20(+), CDX2(+)
   C. CK7(+), GCDFP-15(−), CK20(−), CDX2(+)
   D. CK7(−), GCDFP-15(+), CK20(−), SOX10(+)
   E. CK7(−), GCDFP-15(−), CK20(−), SOX10(+)

All figures in this chapter are from Longacre TA, Greenson JK, Hornick JL, Reuter VE, eds. *Mills and Sternberg's Diagnostic Surgical Pathology*. 7th ed. Wolters Kluwer; 2022 except for those noted at the end of this book.

# ANSWERS AND EXPLANATIONS

**1. Correct choice: E.**

Most carcinomas of the anal canal are variants of squamous cell carcinomas, many of which have mixed histologic features: keratinizing squamous cell, carcinomas that resemble urothelial carcinoma, carcinomas with a basaloid appearance, and carcinomas with mucin-containing cells. Although there is a wide range of morphologic features, there is no clinical significance to subtyping, and all the carcinoma subtypes share a common association with human papillomavirus (HPV). Squamous cell carcinomas of the anal canal are often discovered on biopsies of the distal rectum due to difficulty associated with examining the anus endoscopically and the tendency of these carcinomas to undermine the mucosa above it and invade proximally. Squamous cell carcinomas of the anal canal used to be treated surgically but are now treated with radiation, so tumor stages are defined by imaging modalities. Poor prognostic factors in anal squamous cell carcinoma include older age, male sex, and human immunodeficiency virus (HIV) positivity.

**2. Correct choice: C.**

Precursor lesions for anal squamous cell carcinomas (SCCs) used based on a three-grade classification of anal intraepithelial neoplasia (AIN1-3); but recently, a two-tier system of low-grade squamous intraepithelial neoplasia (LSIL/AIN1) and high-grade squamous intraepithelial neoplasia (HSIL/AIN2-3) has been used. The histologic features are similar to those of cervical intraepithelial neoplasia. The image shows nearly full thickness dysplasia (HSIL/AIN3). Blocklike p16-positive immunostaining will additionally support HSIL.

**3. Correct choice: C.**

Human papillomavirus (HPV) serotypes 6 and 11 are associated with low-grade squamous intraepithelial neoplasia (LSIL/anal intraepithelial neoplasia 1 [AIN1]). Serotypes 16, 18, 31, 33, and 35 are associated with high-grade squamous intraepithelial neoplasia (HSIL/AIN2-3), with 16 being most prevalent.

**4. Correct choicer: B.**

Most (not all) adenocarcinomas involving the anal canal are downward extensions of rectal cancer, but a primary adenocarcinoma of the anal canal does exist and has the following features: (1) associated with long-standing perianal disease, that is, fissures and abscesses; (2) mucinous type; (3) indolent growth, with better prognosis than conventional colorectal carcinoma, although most cases are diagnosed at advanced stages; and (4) rarely associated with human papillomavirus (HPV) infection, in contrast to anal squamous cell carcinoma.

**5. Correct choice: B.**

Anal and perianal Paget disease is often associated with an underlying carcinoma of the rectum (secondary Paget disease), which is either concurrent with the discovery of the Paget disease or develops later. Paget disease associated with a rectal carcinoma is likely to be CK20 and CDX2 positive, and CK7 and GCDFP-15 negative. Primary Paget disease is thought to arise from perianal skin sweat glands and show negative CK20 and CDX2, and positive CK7 and GCDFP-15. Top differential diagnosis includes anal melanoma, which will be SOX10 positive.

# 40 Developmental Abnormalities of the Kidney

1. These images show a kidney biopsy from a 10-year-old boy with abnormally small kidneys (Figure 1) and from an age-matched normal kidney (Figure 2). Which of the following developmental conditions is most consistent with the microscopic abnormalities seen in (A)?

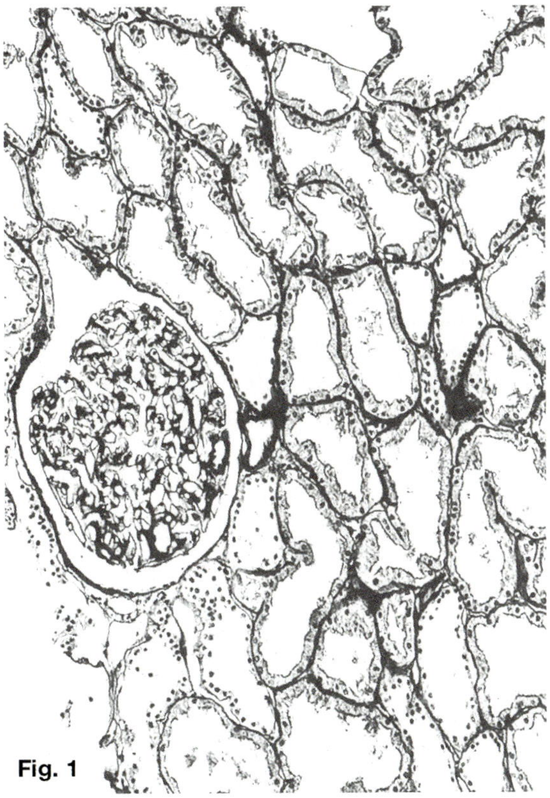

Fig. 1

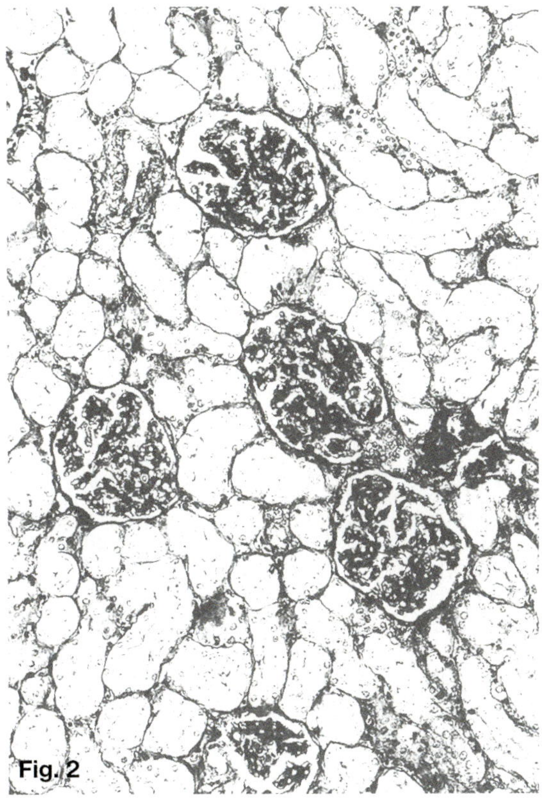

Fig. 2

A. Congenital nephromegaly
B. Oligonephronic hypoplasia
C. Renal dysplasia
D. Renal segmental atrophy
E. Renal tubular dysgenesis

All figures in this chapter are from Longacre TA, Greenson JK, Hornick JL, Reuter VE, eds. *Mills and Sternberg's Diagnostic Surgical Pathology*. 7th ed. Wolters Kluwer; 2022 except for those noted at the end of this book.

2. Figure 1 depicts a condition found in the left kidney of a 7-year-old girl. The changes seen in the kidney are most likely due to

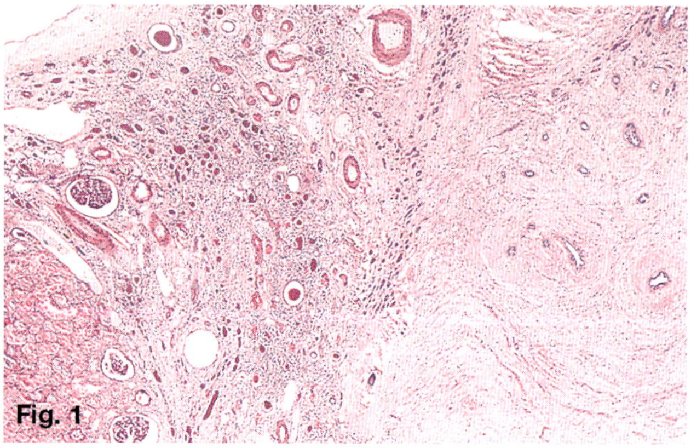

Fig. 1

A. autosomal dominant genetic defect.
B. autosomal recessive genetic defect.
C. congenital anomaly of ureteral muscle.
D. segmental hypoplasia.
E. vesicoureteral reflux.

3. Figure 1 shows the histopathologic appearance of an enlarged, cystic kidney removed from a 2-day-old girl. Which of the following is true about this congenital renal condition?

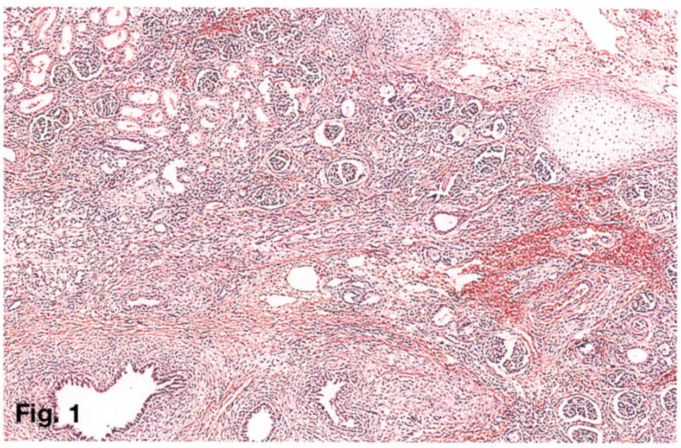

Fig. 1

A. Affected kidneys retain their function.
B. Calices, pelvis, and ureter are usually patent.
C. It is inherited as an autosomal recessive disorder.
D. Malformations in other systems are common.
E. They are most often bilateral.

4. Figure 1 demonstrates the developmental anomaly that has been linked to maternal use of angiotensin-converting enzyme (ACE) inhibitors and maternal cocaine abuse. Which of the following is it?

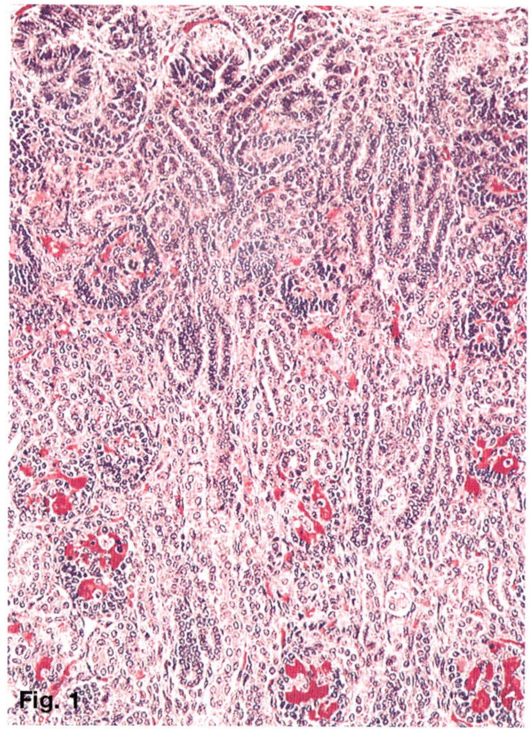

Fig. 1

A. Congenital hydronephrosis
B. Renal dysplasia
C. Renal hypoplasia
D. Renal segmental atrophy
E. Renal tubular dysgenesis

5. A 9-month-old infant comes to clinical attention because of renal insufficiency and enlarged kidneys. Radiologic and sonographic studies show large hyperechoic kidneys. A renal biopsy shows the changes depicted in Figure 1. Which of the following pathologic lesions is most likely to be associated with this kidney condition?

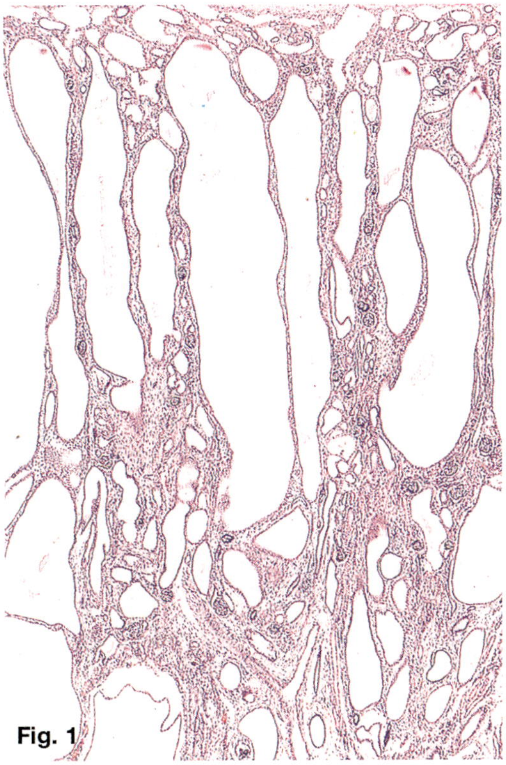

Fig. 1

A. Angiomas in the retina and cerebellum
B. Angiomyolipoma
C. Cardiac rhabdomyoma
D. Hepatic fibrosis
E. Pancreatic cysts

6. Which of the following features is not characteristic of the renal pathology in autosomal dominant polycystic kidney disease?

A. Lithiasis and infection are frequent in renal cysts.
B. Renal cysts are lined by hyperplastic epithelium with papillary formations.
C. Renal parenchyma between cysts is dysplastic.
D. Renal pathology is usually associated with pyelocalyceal occlusion.
E. Virtually all nephrons are affected by cystic dilatation.

7. Figure 1 demonstrates the histologic features of the kidney cysts in an 18-month-old infant with hypertension who was found to have enlarged kidneys with diffuse cystic changes. What is the most likely diagnosis?

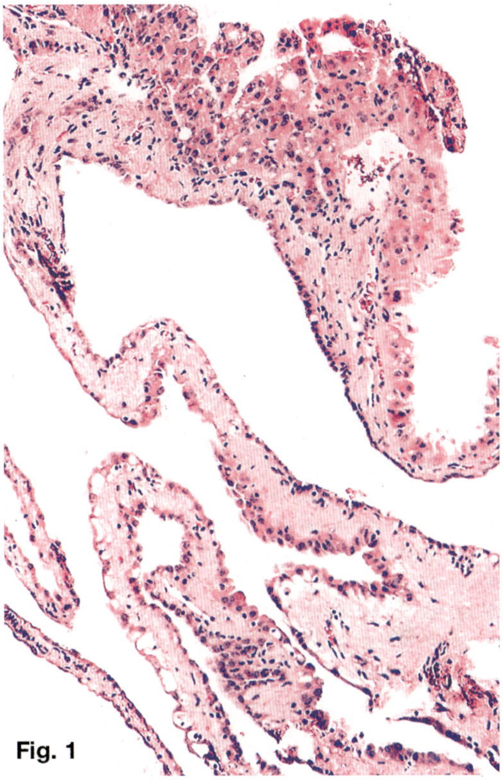

Fig. 1

A. Autosomal recessive polycystic kidney disease
B. Congenital hydronephrosis
C. Congenital nephromegaly
D. Renal dysplasia
E. Tuberous sclerosis

8. Which of the following is true of von Hippel-Lindau (VHL) disease?

A. Associated with pheochromocytomas in a subset of patients
B. Autosomal dominant inheritance
C. Characterized by retinal angiomatosis, cerebellar angiomas, and cysts
D. Clear cell renal cell carcinoma developing in about one-third of patients
E. All of the above

9. An infant with no obvious malformations and no significant family history is found to have renal insufficiency with large kidneys. Figure 1 shows the histologic findings of the kidney with a large number of glomerular cysts. What is the most likely diagnosis?

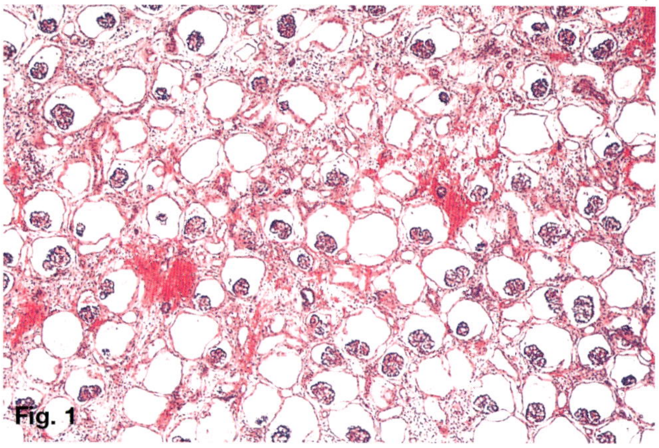
Fig. 1

A. Autosomal recessive polycystic kidney disease
B. Congenital hydronephrosis
C. Congenital nephromegaly
D. Glomerulocystic kidney
E. Tuberous sclerosis

# ANSWERS AND EXPLANATIONS

**1. Correct choice: B.**

Hypoplastic kidneys are pathologically small but normally differentiated. Renal hypoplasia is probably caused by aberrant interaction between metanephric blastema and ureteric bud, leading to the formation of insufficient renal parenchyma. Oligonephronic hypoplasia is the most common form of renal hypoplasia, which is due to a reduced number of glomeruli. Microscopically, the condition is characterized by markedly enlarged glomeruli and large dilated tubules, as seen in the image. Oligonephronic hypoplasia progresses to chronic renal failure within 10 to 12 years.

**2. Correct choice: E.**

Segmental or lobar atrophy is an acquired condition due to vesicoureteral and intrarenal reflux. Vesicoureteral reflux, however, is not always demonstrable in all cases. The salient macroscopic feature is a shrunken lobe with effacement of the cortex and medullary pyramid. In affected lobes, the cortex is virtually devoid of glomeruli: it contains dilated tubules with intraluminal casts, and the medulla contains few ducts. The remaining renal parenchyma undergoes hypertrophy and often develops focal segmental glomerulosclerosis. Hypertension is the most frequent initial sign.

**3. Correct choice: D.**

Renal dysplasia is a sporadic disorder that is usually diagnosed by ultrasound in utero. The condition affects only one kidney in the majority of cases and is associated with ureteral atresia and pyelocalyceal occlusion on the involved side. The aplastic kidney is not functional and is often surgically removed for fear of malignant transformation, although a more conservative approach is gaining favor. Renal dysplasia is caused by disturbances of metanephric differentiation manifesting microscopically as a persistence of abnormal structures, including cartilage, immature collecting ducts, and undifferentiated mesenchyme, along with architectural disorganization. Abnormal ducts become cystic. Depending on the extent of cystic transformation, two variants are recognized: multicystic kidney dysplasia (MCKD, the most common, with numerous cysts) and aplastic dysplasia (few or no cysts). Renal dysplasia is usually associated with other malformations of the urinary tract and of other systems.

**4. Correct choice: E.**

Renal tubular dysgenesis is an uncommon cause of neonatal oliguria that is due to aberrant development of renal tubules. It is inherited as an autosomal recessive condition or in association with prenatal exposure to several drugs, notably, angiotensin-converting enzyme (ACE) inhibitors and cocaine; a similar renal abnormality has been linked to in utero exposure to nonsteroidal anti-inflammatory drugs (NSAIDs). Congenital hydronephrosis is due to congenital obstruction at the ureteropelvic junction. In renal dysplasia, there is an abnormal organization of metaphrenic elements, usually associated with other congenital anomalies of the urinary tract. Renal hypoplasia may be sporadic, due to chromosomal deletion syndromes, or associated with Down syndrome (15% of cases).

**5. Correct choice: D.**

Autosomal recessive polycystic kidney disease (AR-PKD) is a hereditary condition characterized by congenital cystic anomalies of the kidneys and liver. The mutated gene, located on the short arm of chromosome 6, encodes fibrocystin. Renal cysts derive from dilated collecting ducts, whereas hepatic cysts develop from abnormal bile ducts. In the liver, cystically dilated bile ducts are associated with portal fibrosis, which progresses to a picture mimicking micronodular cirrhosis and leading to portal hypertension. Hepatic abnormalities become increasingly severe with age. Cerebellar/retinal angiomas and pancreatic cysts are seen in von Hippel-Lindau syndrome; angiomyolipomas and cardiac rhabdomyomas are seen in tuberous sclerosis.

**6. Correct choice: E.**

About 90% of adult (autosomal dominant) polycystic kidney disease (AD-PKD) cases are due to mutations of a gene on chromosome 16 that encodes polycystin-1, involved in cell-matrix interactions or another one on chromosome 4 coding for polycystin-2. A third gene has not yet been mapped. The disease manifests in the fourth or fifth decade with hypertension, microhematuria, and/or enlarged kidneys. Renal cysts derive from virtually all segments of the nephron. Their wall is lined by a hyperplastic micropapillary epithelium. Papillary formations cause luminal obstruction and cause or facilitate cyst development. Only 20% of the nephrons are affected. The remaining ones suffer from cyst compression but are structurally normal. Lithiasis and infections are common in AD-PKD. Pyelocalyceal occlusion and ureteral agenesis are usually associated with renal dysplasia.

**7. Correct choice: E.**

Severe cystic disease of tuberous sclerosis occurs more often in infancy/childhood and causes renal enlargement, moderate renal insufficiency, and severe hypertension. The renal manifestations sometimes precede the obvious development of other stigmata. Cystic disease may present as unilateral renal enlargement. The cysts are lined with a distinctive, hyperplastic epithelium seemingly unique to this syndrome, and cellular hyperplasia is probably responsible for both cyst formation and an increased risk of neoplasia. The cysts occasionally predominate in glomeruli. Cysts and angiomyolipomas often coexist, and large angiomyolipomas may rupture and cause life-threatening hemorrhage. Deletion of the *TSC2* and *PKD1* genes is associated with severe infantile polycystic kidney disease—a contiguous gene syndrome.

**8. Correct choice: E.**

Von Hippel-Lindau (VHL) disease is a condition inherited as an autosomal dominant trait characterized by a variable combination of retinal angiomatosis, cerebellar angiomas, and cysts as well as tumors of abdominal organs, particularly the pancreas and kidneys. The VHL disease tumor suppressor cyclin D1 gene maps to chromosome 3p25-26. Germline mutations in the VHL tumor suppressor gene predispose to renal cell carcinoma, hemangioblastoma of the central nervous system, and pheochromocytoma. Renal cysts are found in two-thirds of patients with VHL disease. Cysts are usually multiple and bilateral and are often lined with hyperplastic, atypical cells that form mural nodules of intracystic carcinoma. Renal cell carcinoma develops in about one-third of the patients, and in 15%, it is bilateral. Diagnosis of renal cell carcinoma is made an average of 15 years earlier than in sporadic cases. The carcinomas are usually clear cell type, low grade, with a relatively good prognosis. In a small subset of patients, pheochromocytomas occur as a manifestation of VHL disease.

**9. Correct choice: D.**

Glomerular cysts have long been recognized in infants' kidneys, occurring in a variety of primary and secondary disorders. It can be classified into etiologic categories as follows: familial nonsyndromic, associated with inheritable malformation syndromes, syndromic (non-Mendelian, sporadic, or acquired). In particular, it is part of a clinical spectrum of the renal cysts and diabetes syndrome that is associated with mutations in hepatocyte nuclear factor-1β (HNF-1β). Acquired form can also be seen as a component of renal dysplasia and has developed following hemolytic uremic syndrome. After prolonged peritoneal dialysis, severe hypertension and normal-sized kidneys without the development of macroscopic cysts are common features.

# 41 Adult Renal Diseases

1. Which of the following statements on glomerular diseases is true?

   A. Different renal morphologic patterns can cause the same clinical syndrome.
   B. One renal disease may be associated with different morphologic patterns.
   C. One specific morphologic pattern may be associated with different diseases.
   D. Renal biopsy alone is diagnostic of only few conditions.
   E. All of the above.

2. Electron microscopy on a renal biopsy from a 9-year-old boy with nephritic syndrome and elevated antistreptococcal antibody titers reveals the glomerular changes shown in Figure 1. Which of the following is the morphologic pattern most probably present with light microscopic examination?

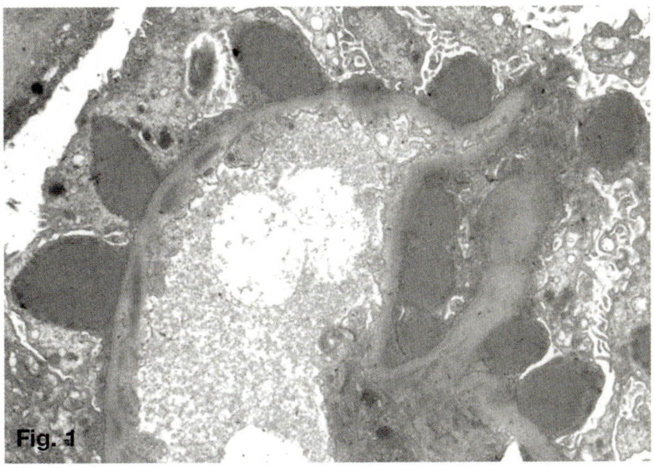

Fig. 1

   A. Diffuse extracapillary proliferative glomerulonephritis
   B. Diffuse intracapillary proliferative glomerulonephritis
   C. Focal glomerulonephritis
   D. Membranous glomerulopathy
   E. Normal glomerular morphology

3. A renal biopsy from a patient with a severe infection reveals a diffuse intracapillary proliferation with leukocytic infiltration and obliteration of capillary lumina. Subepithelial electron-dense "humps" are found on electron microscopy (EM). Which of the following immunofluorescence (IF) findings would be consistent with an infection caused by *Staphylococcus aureus*?

   A. Diffuse capillary loop deposits of C3
   B. Diffuse mesangial immunoglobulin M (IgM) deposits
   C. Granular mesangial and glomerular capillary IgA deposits
   D. Granular mesangial and glomerular capillary IgG and C3 deposits
   E. Linear deposition of IgG and C3 along glioblastoma multiforme (GBM)

4. Which of the following morphologic or immunofluorescence (IF) features favor a diagnosis of C3 glomerulopathy over that of classic membranoproliferative glomerulonephritis (MPGN)?

   A. Mesangial and intramembranous deposits of C3 alone
   B. Mesangial and subendothelial deposits of C3 and immunoglobulin G (IgG)
   C. Mesangial interposition with glioblastoma multiforme (GBM) duplication
   D. Mesangial proliferation
   E. Mesangial, subendothelial, and intramembranous deposits of C3 and IgG

All figures in this chapter are from Longacre TA, Greenson JK, Hornick JL, Reuter VE, eds. *Mills and Sternberg's Diagnostic Surgical Pathology*. 7th ed. Wolters Kluwer; 2022 except for those noted at the end of this book.

5. A 12-year-old boy has nephrotic syndrome and low complement levels. The most significant findings on renal biopsy are demonstrated in the periodic acid-Schiff (PAS) (Figure 1) and methenamine silver–stained (Figure 2) sections. Mesangial and glomerular capillary deposition of C3 and immunoglobulin G (IgG) was detected by immunofluorescence (IF). Electron microscopy (EM) showed large subendothelial electron-dense deposits with mesangial interposition. Which of the following is the most likely diagnosis?

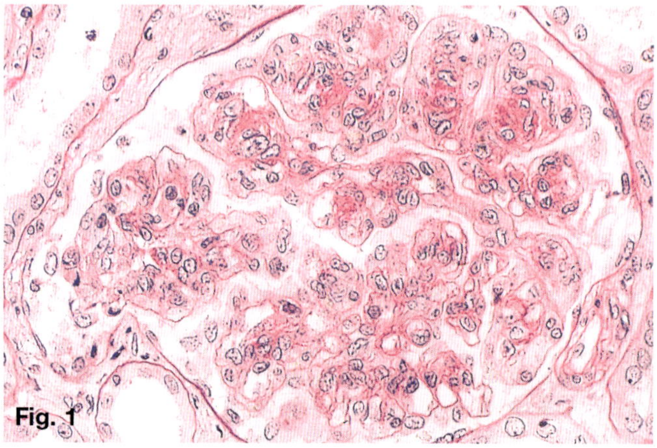


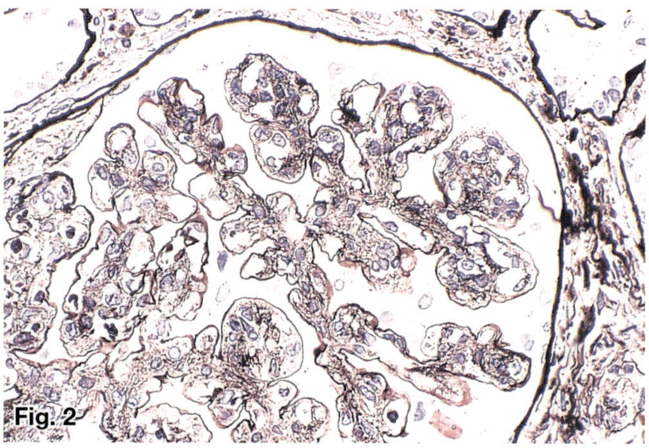


A. Dense deposit disease (membranoproliferative glomerulonephritis [MPGN], type II)
B. Membranous glomerulopathy
C. Minimal change glomerulopathy
D. MPGN, type I
E. Postinfectious glomerulonephritis

6. The ultrastructural changes seen in the electron microscopy (EM) picture, shown in Figure 1, are pathognomonic of

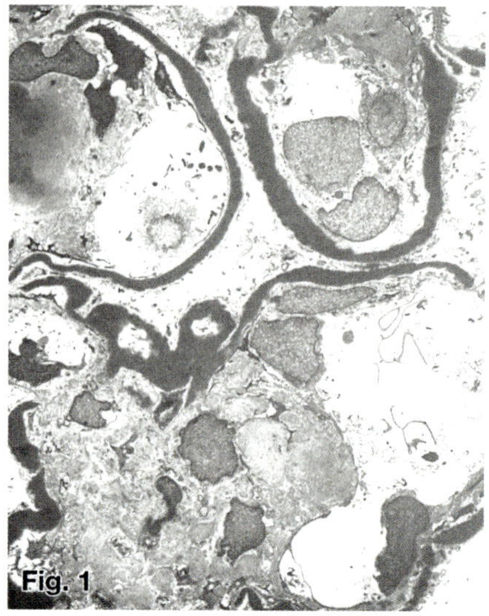


A. dense deposit disease.
B. light-chain disease.
C. membranoproliferative (mesangiocapillary) glomerulonephritis, type I.
D. membranous glomerulopathy.
E. minimal change glomerulopathy.

7. Which of the following is true about crescentic glomerulonephritis?

A. Crescents consist exclusively of parietal cells of the Bowman capsule.
B. Finding 20% of glomeruli with crescents supports the diagnosis.
C. Most cases are associated with a known underlying condition.
D. Most cases are associated with linear deposition of anti-glioblastoma multiforme (GBM) immunoglobulin G (IgG).
E. Prognosis depends on the extent of crescent formation and immunofluorescence (IF) pattern.

8. Which of the following glomerular lesions is shown in Figure 1 of a periodic acid-Schiff (PAS)-stained section?

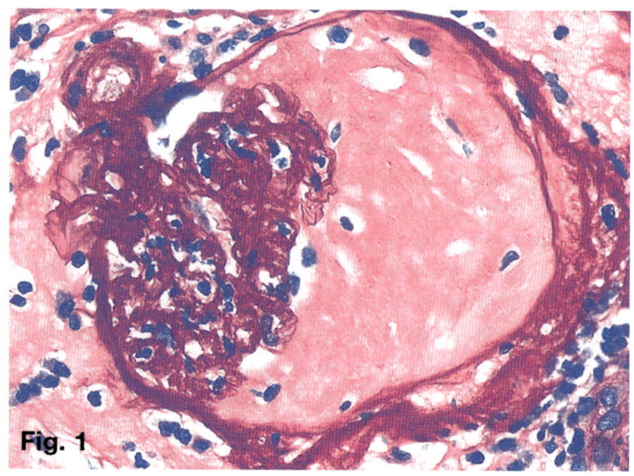


A. Cellular crescent
B. Fibrocellular crescent
C. Fibrous crescent
D. Obsolescent glomerulus
E. Segmental scarring

9. A 4-year-old child presents with nephrotic syndrome, and a renal biopsy shows no light microscopic changes. Ultrastructural changes are shown in Figure 1. Which of the following immunofluorescence findings would be most likely present?

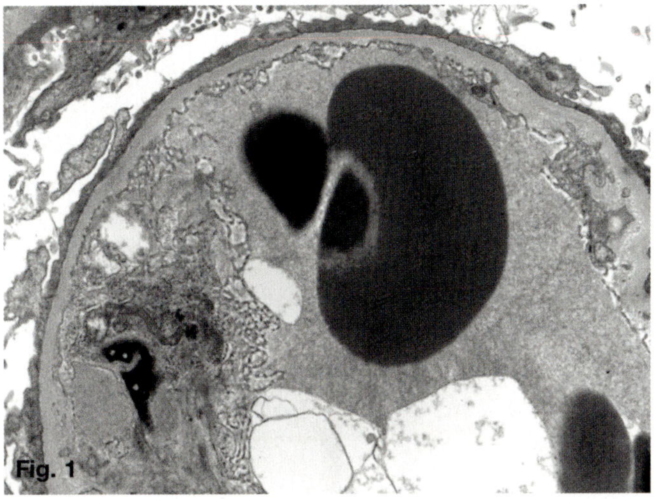

Fig. 1

A. Absence of C3 and immunoglobulin (Ig) deposits
B. Continuous granular C3 deposition along the capillary wall
C. Granular IgG/C3 deposits along glioblastoma multiforme (GBM)
D. Linear IgG deposition along GBM
E. Mesangial IgA deposits

10. A clinical evaluation of a young adult with generalized edema shows heavy proteinuria (4.5 g/d). The past medical history is unremarkable. In the United States, which of the following is the most common glomerular disease accounting for this presentation?

A. Diabetic nephropathy
B. Focal segmental glomerulosclerosis
C. Immunoglobulin A (IgA) nephropathy (Berger disease)
D. Membranous glomerulonephritis
E. Minimal change disease

11. An adult patient presents with nephrotic syndrome, and a renal biopsy reveals the glomerular changes shown in Figure 1. Which of the following ultrastructural alterations is most likely found in the glomeruli that appear normal on light microscopy?

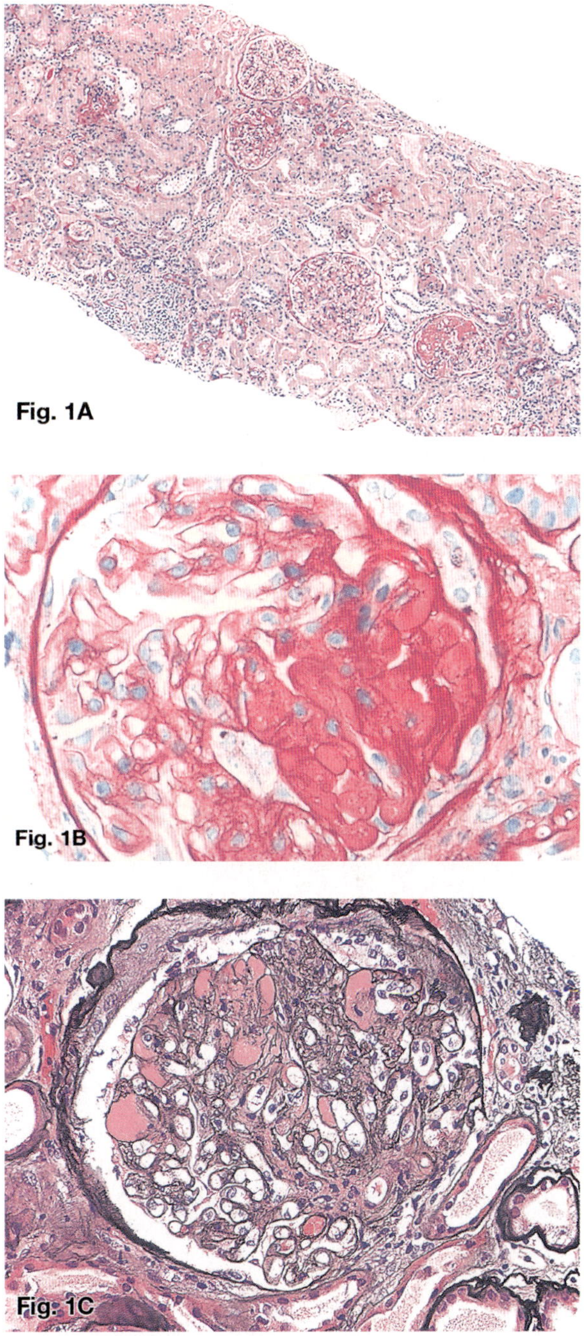

Fig. 1A

Fig. 1B

Fig. 1C

A. Effacement of epithelial cell foot processes
B. Mesangial interposition
C. Subendothelial deposits
D. Subepithelial deposits with spikes of glioblastoma multiforme (GBM) material
E. Subepithelial humps

12. Focal segmental glomerulosclerosis (FSGS) is the usual morphologic pattern of HIV-associated nephropathy (HIVAN). Which of the following light microscopic changes is most characteristic of HIVAN?

    A. Argyrophilic spikes on the basement membrane
    B. Crescent formation
    C. Glomerular collapse and tubular interstitial fibrosis
    D. Obsolescent glomeruli
    E. None of the above

13. A renal biopsy is performed on a 34-year-old man for the evaluation of proteinuria in the nephrotic range. A representative silver-stained section is shown in Figure 1. Immunofluorescence (IF) demonstrates finely granular deposits of immunoglobulin G (IgG) and C3 along the capillary wall. Electron microscopy (EM) shows effacement of foot processes, associated with numerous subepithelial electron-dense deposits, which are separated from each other by extensions of the basement membrane. Which of the following is the most likely diagnosis?

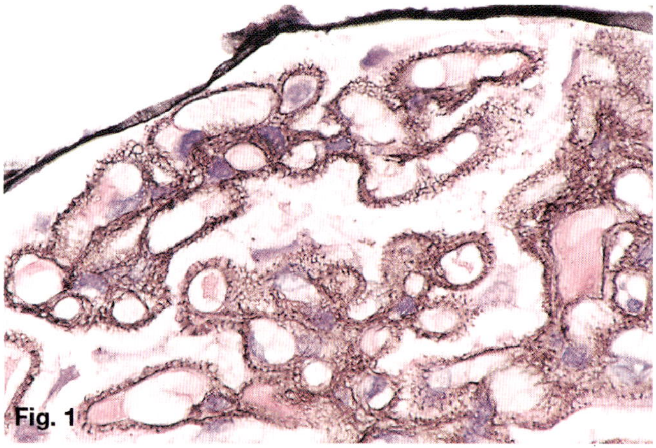


    A. Dense deposit disease
    B. Focal segmental glomerulosclerosis
    C. Membranoproliferative glomerulonephritis
    D. Membranous glomerulonephritis
    E. Minimal change glomerulopathy

14. A previously healthy 35-year-old woman presents with nephrotic syndrome. She has no other known significant condition. Laboratory tests reveal circulating immunoglobulin G subclass 4 (IgG4) directed against the phospholipase A2 receptor (PLA2R). Which of the following is the most likely glomerular disease?

    A. Dense deposit disease
    B. Focal segmental glomerulosclerosis
    C. Membranoproliferative glomerulonephritis
    D. Membranous glomerulonephritis
    E. Minimal change nephrotic syndrome

15. A 55-year-old woman with a 15-year history of type 2 diabetes mellitus is found to have microalbuminuria. All other renal function tests are normal. At this early stage, what is the most likely glomerular change of diabetic nephropathy?

    A. Expansion of the mesangial matrix
    B. Fibroepithelial crescents
    C. Insudative lesions such as fibrin caps and capsular drops
    D. Mesangial intercapillary nodules (of Kimmelstiel-Wilson)
    E. Thickening of the basement membrane

16. The glomerular lesion seen in Figure 1 was found in a renal biopsy from a patient with long-standing diabetes mellitus. What is this glomerular change called?

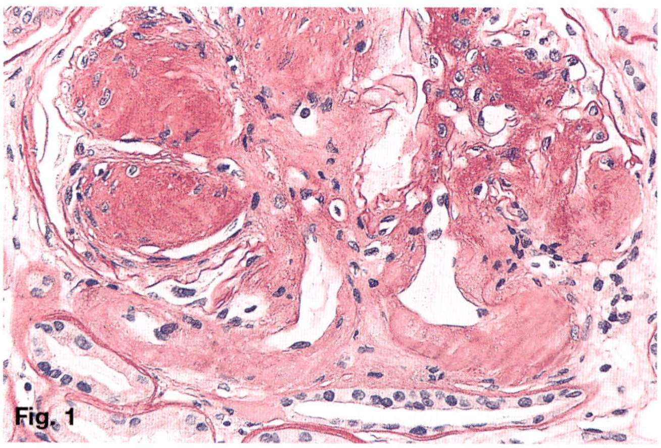


    A. Capsular drop
    B. Diffuse diabetic glomerulosclerosis
    C. Fibrin cap
    D. Microaneurysm
    E. Nodular diabetic glomerulosclerosis

17. Which of the following is the most common form of glomerulonephritis worldwide and manifests with recurrent gross or microhematuria?

    A. Alport syndrome
    B. Immunoglobulin A (IgA) nephropathy (Berger disease)
    C. Pauci-immune crescentic glomerulonephritis
    D. Postinfectious glomerulonephritis
    E. Thin membrane disease

18. Microscopic hematuria is discovered in an otherwise healthy 20-year-old man. There is a family history of similar abnormality. A renal biopsy appears normal on light microscopy, but the glomerular basement membrane is less than 200 nm thick on electron microscopy (EM). Which of the following extrarenal abnormalities is most likely associated with this condition?

    A. Deafness
    B. Hypoplasia of patella
    C. Lens dislocation
    D. Nail dysplasia
    E. None of the above

19. A hereditary form of glomerulopathy caused by defective collagen synthesis and associated with sensorineural deafness and ocular abnormalities is

A. Alport syndrome.
B. Berger disease.
C. Fabry disease.
D. onycho-osteodysplasia.
E. thin membrane disease.

20. Which of the following conditions is most likely to be associated with the type of "bloodless" glomerulus, as depicted in Figure 1?

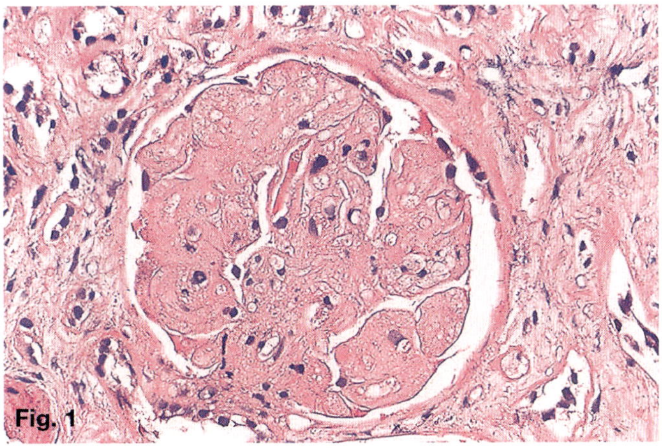

Fig. 1

A. Cryoglobulinemia
B. Hemolytic-uremic syndrome
C. Multiple myeloma
D. Streptococcal infection
E. Systemic lupus erythematosus

21. A 35-year-old man presents with nephritic syndrome. Several years prior to this, he suffered from an episode of generalized purpura due to cryoglobulinemia. Which of the following ultrastructural changes is most characteristic of glomerular disease secondary to cryoglobulinemia?

A. Diffuse vacuolization of glomerular endothelial cells
B. Laminated intraepithelial inclusions called "zebra bodies"
C. Subendothelial deposits with a fingerprint-like pattern
D. Subepithelial electron-dense "humps"
E. Tubulovesicular inclusions in endothelial cells

22. A 60-year-old woman with a long history of rheumatoid arthritis comes to medical attention because of heavy proteinuria. Which of the following alterations is most likely to be identified on a renal biopsy?

A. Amyloid deposition
B. Immune complex deposition
C. Immunoglobulin A (IgA) mesangial deposition
D. Light-chain mesangial deposition
E. Urate crystal deposition within tubules

23. A 40-year-old man presents with proteinuria in the nephrotic range, microhematuria, and hypertension. The patient does not have monoclonal gammopathy, lymphoproliferative disorders, or cryoglobulinemia. A renal biopsy reveals expansion of the mesangium and thickening of the glomerular capillary wall. Immunofluorescence (IF) staining with antibodies to immunoglobulin A (IgG) is shown in Figure 1. Congo red stain is negative. Which of the following types of glomerular deposits would be most likely found by electron microscope (EM)?

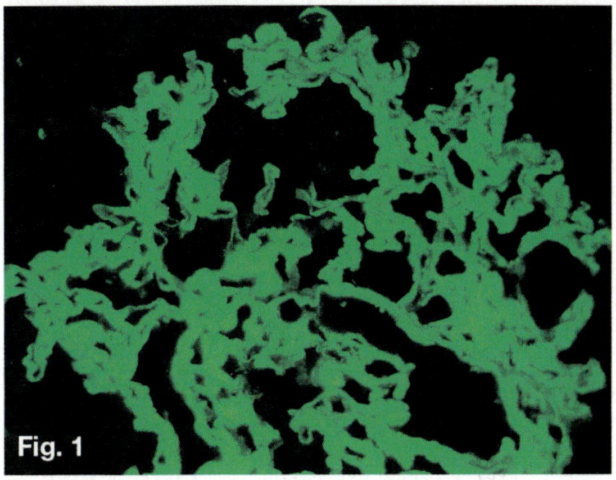

Fig. 1

A. Microtubular structures with a 20 to 50 nm diameter
B. Randomly arranged, rigid 8- to 10-nm fibrils
C. Randomly arranged, rigid 18- to 24-nm fibrils

24. A 30-year-old woman with systemic lupus erythematosus (SLE) undergoes a renal biopsy because of proteinuria and microhematuria. The biopsy shows glomerular changes consistent with class IV lupus nephritis according to the new classification by the International Society of Nephrology and the Renal Pathology Society (ISN/RPS). Which of the following glomerular changes is present in this renal biopsy?

A. Diffuse lupus nephritis
B. Focal lupus nephritis
C. Membranous lupus nephritis
D. Mesangial proliferative lupus nephritis
E. Minimal mesangial lupus nephritis

25. Which of the following morphologic parameters is used in the evaluation of the activity of lupus nephritis?

A. Cellular crescents
B. Fibrous crescents
C. Glomerulosclerosis
D. Interstitial fibrosis
E. Tubular atrophy

26. A 65-year-old man with heavy proteinuria and hypertension undergoes a renal biopsy. The main biopsy finding consists of diffuse and nodular mesangial accumulation of periodic acid-Schiff (PAS)-positive material. Immunofluorescence (IF) reveals deposition of κ light-chain throughout the mesangium and along the glioblastoma multiforme (GBM), as shown in Figure 1. On light microscopy, the glomerular changes of this condition may be very similar to

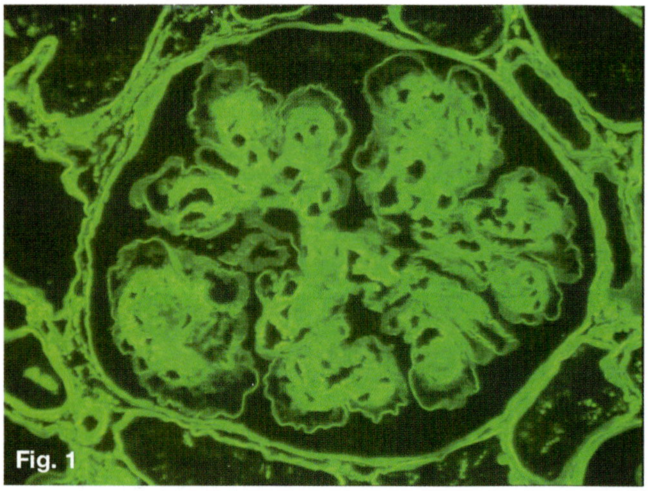
Fig. 1

A. amyloidosis.
B. diabetic nephropathy.
C. fibrillary glomerulonephritis.
D. focal segmental glomerulosclerosis.
E. immunoglobulin A (IgA) nephropathy.

27. Which of the following morphologic changes is not commonly found in acute tubular necrosis (ATN)?

A. Frank necrosis of tubular epithelium
B. Granular casts in distal tubules and collecting ducts
C. Loss of brush border in proximal tubules
D. Mononuclear cells in the vasa recta
E. Regenerative changes of tubular epithelium

28. A 55-year-old man presents with slowly progressive renal insufficiency. Imaging studies reveal abnormal renal morphology, more pronounced on the left. A left renal biopsy reveals extensive interstitial changes with chronic inflammatory infiltration alternating with paucicellular areas of fibrosis. The inflammatory infiltrate is rich in plasma cells. Immunohistochemistry should be performed for which of the following markers?

A. Complement C3
B. Immunoglobulin G (IgG)
C. IgG4
D. κ and λ light chains
E. Phospholipase A2 receptor

29. Figure 1 shows the gross findings of the kidney of a young child with chronic renal failure. The following microscopic changes are observed: periglomerular fibrosis, atrophic and dilated tubules, and interstitial fibrosis. These histopathologic findings are most likely due to

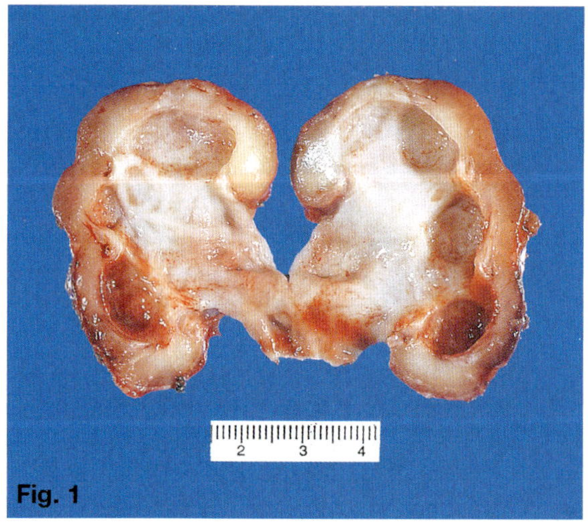

Fig. 1

A. acute pyelonephritis.
B. allergic tubulointerstitial nephritis.
C. chronic pyelonephritis.
D. malakoplakia.
E. xanthogranulomatous pyelonephritis.

30. The kidney shown in Figure 1 was removed from a patient with moderate renal insufficiency, microhematuria, mild proteinuria, and hypertension. Which of the following is the most likely diagnosis?

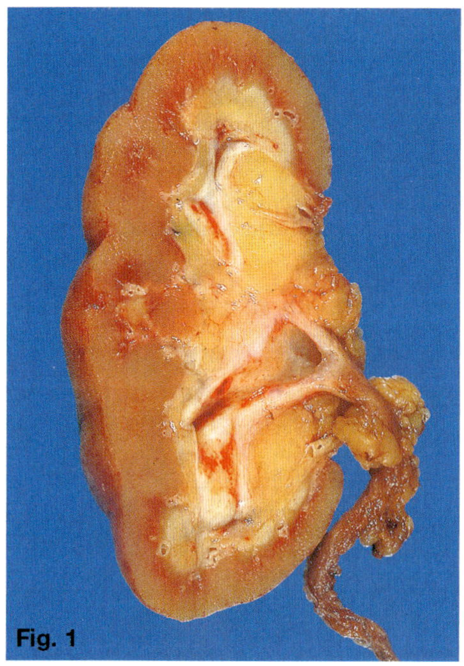
Fig. 1

A. Analgesic nephropathy
B. Arteriolar nephrosclerosis
C. Chronic pyelonephritis
D. End-stage renal disease
E. Xanthogranulomatous pyelonephritis

31. In the United States, the most common cause of end-stage renal disease (ESRD) among Caucasians is diabetic nephropathy. What is the most common cause in African Americans?

A. Autosomal dominant polycystic kidney disease (AD-PKD)
B. Chronic interstitial nephritis
C. Diabetic nephropathy
D. Glomerulonephritides
E. Hypertension

32. Hyperacute rejection of renal allograft is

A. characterized by emperipolesis of tubular epithelium.
B. characterized by swelling and detachment of endothelium.
C. mediated principally by cytotoxic lymphocyte.
D. preventable by cyclosporine treatment.
E. preventable by routine pretransplant cross-matching.

33. Figure 1 shows a biopsy of a transplanted kidney 2 weeks after surgery. Based on these findings, acute antibody-mediated rejection is suspected. Immunohistochemistry for which of the following markers can confirm this diagnosis?

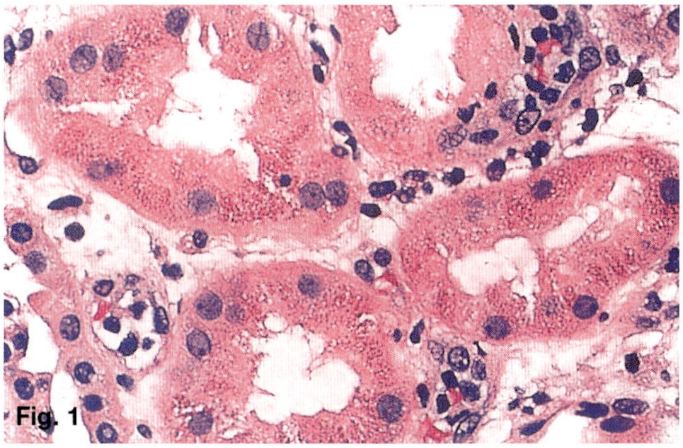
Fig. 1

A. C3
B. C4d
C. CD4
D. CD8
E. CD45

34. Figure 1 shows the most significant microscopic change identified in a biopsy of a transplanted kidney. This change is most consistent with

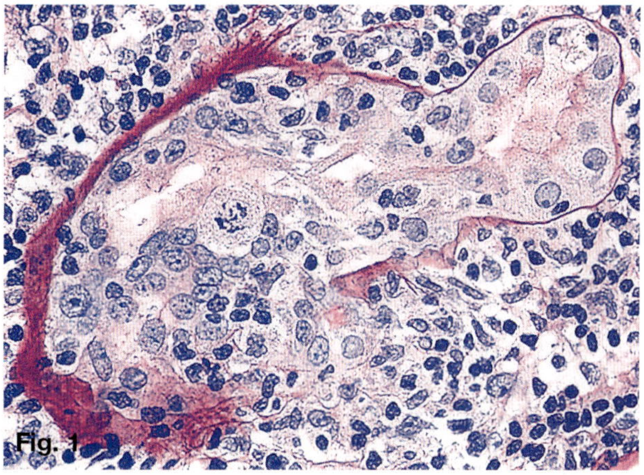
Fig. 1

A. acute antibody-mediated rejection.
B. acute cellular rejection.
C. chronic graft injury.
D. humoral rejection.
E. hyperacute rejection.

35. A patient presents with progressive decline in renal function and hypertension 4 years after receiving allograft renal transplantation. Which of the following changes is the most likely underlying cause of this presentation?

A. Destruction of tubules
B. Endothelial swelling
C. Fibrointimal thickening of vessels
D. Interstitial lymphomonocytic infiltration
E. Mesangial prominence with "tram-tracking" of glioblastoma multiforme (GBM)

36. Which of the following toxic effects of cyclosporine closely mimics hemolytic-uremic syndrome and is reversible upon drug withdrawal?

A. Functional toxicity
B. Tubular toxicity
C. Vascular interstitial toxicity, acute
D. Vascular interstitial toxicity, chronic
E. None of the above

37. Figure 1 shows a microscopic change detected in a biopsy of a transplanted kidney. Which of the following is the most likely diagnosis?

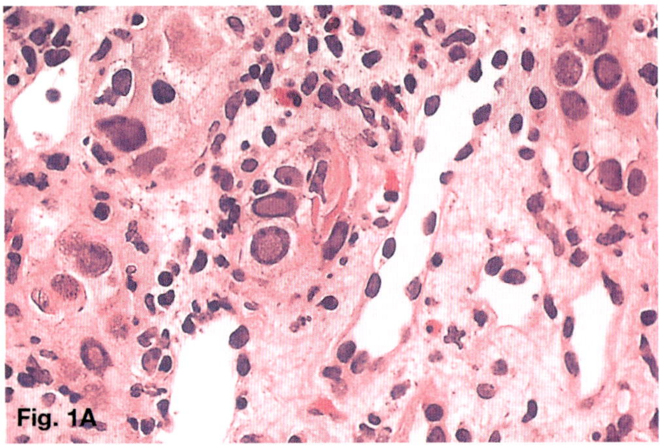

Fig. 1A

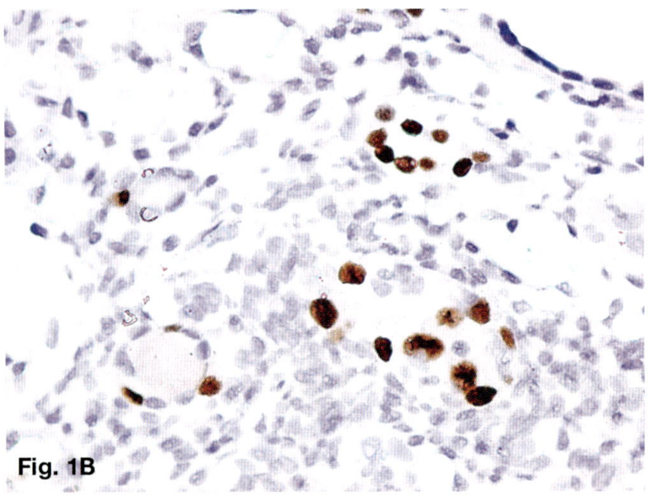

Fig. 1B

A. Acute cellular rejection
B. Cytomegalovirus (CMV) infection
C. Polyomavirus infection
D. Regenerative changes of acute tubular necrosis (ATN)
E. Tacrolimus toxicity

# ANSWERS AND EXPLANATIONS

**1. Correct choice: E.**

To the list of considerations concerning the relationship between patterns of glomerular injury and renal diseases/syndromes, one must add that a renal syndrome may be associated with different renal diseases but have the same pathogenetic mechanism. Example of the latter is crescentic glomerulonephritis (GN), which may be seen in vasculitides, systemic lupus erythematosus (SLE), and acute GN, but the underlying mechanism is the same, that is, exudation of fibrinogen-related antigens (FRAs) and other plasma proteins into the Bowman space through gaps in the glioblastoma multiforme (GBM). This complex interrelationship between morphologic patterns of glomerular injury and clinical/laboratory manifestations makes the diagnosis of these disorders an exercise in correlation of morphologic findings in renal biopsies (by light microscopy [LM], electron microscopy [EM], and immunofluorescence [IF]) with clinical and laboratory findings.

**2. Correct choice: B.**

The history suggests a nephritic syndrome secondary to streptococcal infection. Subepithelial electron-dense deposits, called humps, are characteristic of diffuse intracapillary proliferative GN. On light microscopy, this condition is characterized by hypercellular glomeruli due to increased mesangial and intracapillary cells and acute inflammatory cell infiltration, leading to obliteration of capillary lumina. The disease resolves spontaneously with supportive treatment. Increased glomerular cellularity is usually consistent with GN. Intracapillary hypercellularity with obliteration of the capillary lumina, if diffuse, suggests postinfectious GN or membranoproliferative GN. Extracapillary hypercellularity is diagnostic of crescentic GN.

**3. Correct choice: C.**

Acute proliferative glomerulonephritis (GN) morphologically similar to poststreptococcal GN can be rarely seen in other bacterial infections, especially endocarditis, deep-seated abscesses, and infected cardiac shunts. Granular mesangial and glomerular capillary deposition of immunoglobulin G (IgG) and C3 is similar to that found in poststreptococcal GN, but the form associated with staphylococcal infection is characterized by additional deposits of IgA in the mesangium and glomerular capillaries.

**4. Correct choice: A.**

Advances in understanding glomerulonephritis (GN) associated with prominent C3 deposition have led to reclassification of membranoproliferative glomerulonephritis (MPGN) and identification of a new form of glomerular disease, C3 glomerulopathy. A significant number of MPGN cases were recognized to be associated with predominant C3 deposition without Ig deposition. Such cases turned out to be diagnosed in patients who had genetic or acquired anomalies in factors regulating the alternate complement pathway. C3G includes glomerular lesions with C3-dominant immune complex deposits with little or no immunoglobulin (Ig) deposition and in the presence of detectable gene mutations or acquired nephritic factors causing dysregulation of the alternate complement pathway. C3G encompasses the following:

1. C3GN, a proliferative GN resembling MPGN type I with little or no Ig deposits
2. Dense deposit disease (formerly known as type II MPGN) where elongated (ribbon-like, highly osmiophilic) dense glomerular intramembranous deposits are present in the glomerular capillary loops, which stain for C3 only by immunofluorescence (IF)

**5. Correct choice: D.**

Clinical presentation (nephritic syndrome with or without nephrotic syndrome) and progression are similar for all types of membranoproliferative glomerulonephritis (MPGN). MPGN may manifest at all ages. Most cases are idiopathic, but some occur in association with certain systemic conditions (eg, hepatitis B, lupus erythematosus, sickle cell disease). The microscopic features outlined in the question stem are characteristic of MPGN type I, especially the tram-track appearance of glioblastoma multiforme (GBM), which is due to the interposition of mesangial cells between the GBM and the endothelium. Pronounced lobularity may mimic diabetic nodular glomerulosclerosis. immunofluorescence (IF) usually shows mesangial deposits of both C3 and immunoglobulin G (IgG). Large subendothelial electron-dense deposits are highly characteristic of MPGN type I.

**6. Correct choice: A.**

Dense deposit disease is classified as C3 glomerulopathy, since virtually all cases are associated with defects in the alternate complement pathway. The diagnostic feature is the presence of highly electron-dense deposits within the glioblastoma multiforme (GBM). Such deposits produce a ribbon-like thickening of the glomerular basement membrane, which can be appreciated on silver/periodic acid-Schiff (PAS) stains. immunofluorescence (IF) shows continuous staining for C3 and properdin along the capillary membrane and around the GBM deposits.

**7. Correct choice: E.**

At least 50% of glomeruli must show crescents for a diagnosis of crescentic glomerulonephritis (GN). Crescents are masses of cells and fibrin accumulating into and obliterating the urinary space of the Bowman capsule. They originate from breaks of the glioblastoma multiforme (GBM), resulting in extravasation of proteins (fibrinogen-related antigens [FRAs]) and inflammatory cells (monocytes and neutrophils) and subsequent hyperplasia of visceral and parietal cells. Most cases are idiopathic. The immunofluorescence (IF) pattern recognizes three different forms:

- Pauci-immune: Minimal or no immune deposits, often associated with circulating antineutrophil cytoplasmic autoantibodies (ANCAs). Idiopathic or associated with granulomatosis with polyangiitis, microscopic polyangiitis, and others. Most common form of crescentic GN.

- Anti-GBM disease: Linear deposition of anti-GBM immunoglobulin G (IgG) and C3. Idiopathic or associated with Goodpasture syndrome. Least common form.
- Primary immune complex: Granular deposition of immune complex. Idiopathic or associated with postinfectious glomerulonephritis, Henoch-Schönlein syndrome, systemic lupus erythematosus (SLE), IgA nephropathy, and others.

**8. Correct choice: D.**

Crescents undergo a morphologic evolution. Cellular crescents consist of cells derived from glomerular parietal epithelial cells and inflammatory cells, admixed with fibrin. Cellular crescents become fibrocellular crescents, with myofibroblasts and deposition of extracellular matrix, including collagen. Fibrous crescents develop as collagen accumulates, and the lesion becomes progressively less cellular. Fibrous crescent must be distinguished from obsolescent glomeruli (shown in the image), which results from chronic ischemia or arteriolonephrosclerosis. Crescents are associated with disruption of the Bowman capsular basement membrane, identifiable by periodic acid-Schiff (PAS) staining, which is associated with old crescents, but not with obsolescent glomeruli.

**9. Correct choice: A.**

Minimal change nephrotic syndrome is the most common cause of nephrotic syndrome in children, usually presenting before 6 years of age. On light microscopy, glomeruli look virtually normal, but electron microscopy (EM) reveals diffuse effacement (detachment and fusion) of epithelial foot processes. Immunofluorescence is usually negative. The disease commonly resolves with steroid treatment. Relapses may occur, but only infrequently does the disease progress to chronic renal failure. Continuous granular C3 deposition along the capillary wall is seen in dense deposit disease, now reclassified as C3 glomerulopathy. Granular immunoglobulin G (IgG)/C3 deposits along glioblastoma multiforme (GBM) are found in various glomerular diseases, for example, membranous glomerulonephritis and postinfectious glomerulonephritis. Linear IgG deposition along GBM is pathognomonic of Goodpasture syndrome. Mesangial IgA deposits are associated with Berger disease (IgA nephropathy).

**10. Correct choice: B.**

Focal segmental glomerulosclerosis (FSGS) is currently the most common glomerular pattern seen in adults with idiopathic nephrotic syndrome. It is characterized by the collapse of glomerular basement membrane with the deposition of hyaline material (sclerosis) in a segmental and focal distribution. Lipid droplets and foam cells are characteristic. FSGS is a pattern of glomerular injury, which may occur as a primary disorder (idiopathic FSGS) or (1) with other known conditions, such as AIDS, heroin abuse, sickle cell disease, and morbid obesity; (2) secondary to scarring due to focal glomerulonephritides, such as immunoglobulin A (IgA) nephropathy; (3) as a compensatory phenomenon due to the loss of renal tissue, as with renal ablation, unilateral renal agenesis, and advanced renal disorders; and (4) in uncommon familial disorders.

**11. Correct choice: A.**

All glomeruli in focal segmental glomerulosclerosis (FSGS) display the same ultrastructural changes seen in minimal change nephrotic syndrome (MCNS), that is, visceral epithelial cell foot process effacement. The sclerotic glomerular portions have increased mesangial matrix and capillary obliteration. Vacuolation and focal detachment of the visceral epithelial cells from the glioblastoma multiforme (GBM) are also noted. Because of the focal nature of FSGS, and since the changes of FSGS begin in the juxtamedullary region, a superficial biopsy or a biopsy with few glomeruli may not contain the diagnostic segmentally sclerosed glomeruli. Thus, the electron microscopy (EM) finding of podocyte effacement may lead to an erroneous diagnosis of MCNS.

**12. Correct choice: C.**

HIV-associated nephropathy (HIVAN) is an AIDS-associated complication that is particularly prevalent in African American males. Although focal segmental glomerulosclerosis (FSGS) is the predominant pattern of glomerular involvement, there are specific clinical and morphologic features suggesting that HIVAN may be a unique entity. The morphologic changes characteristic of HIVAN include the collapse of glomerular loops, interstitial fibrosis with chronic inflammation, and tubuloreticular inclusions in endothelial cells (identifiable by electron microscopy [EM]). Furthermore, podocytes become conspicuously hypertrophic, resulting in crescent-like formations. Resorption droplets are particularly abundant. HIVAN causes rapidly progressive renal failure.

**13. Correct choice: D.**

The subepithelial deposits detected on electron microscopy (EM) between the basement membrane and visceral epithelium consist of antigen-antibody complexes, which are highlighted by immunofluorescence (IF), consistent with membranous glomerulonephritis. In most cases, they result from in situ production. The basement membrane extensions between such deposits (but not the deposits themselves) are stained by silver methods, resulting in the characteristic spiked appearance, as shown in the image. Most cases are idiopathic, but some are associated with infections (hepatitis B and syphilis), systemic lupus erythematosus (SLE), drugs/toxins (mercury exposure), or cancer (eg, renal cell carcinoma). About one-third of idiopathic cases progress to chronic renal failure, whereas the secondary forms usually abate on elimination of the inciting factors. Staging does not have prognostic significance.

**14. Correct choice: D.**

The majority of Membranous glomerulonephritis (MG) cases are idiopathic, not associated with any known disease, while secondary MG accounts for 20% to 50% of cases. Morphologically, primary and secondary MG are indistinguishable. Recently, most patients with primary MG have been found to have circulating anti-phospholipase A2 receptor (anti-PLA2R) antibodies, which are present in the glomerular deposits.

**15. Correct choice: E.**

Diabetic nephropathy is the most common cause of end-stage renal disease (ESRD) in the United States. Thickening of the glomerular and tubular basement membranes has been observed as early as 1 to 2 years following the onset of diabetes. It appears before the second most frequent glomerular change, that is, the expansion of the mesangial matrix (diffuse glomerulosclerosis). Nodular glomerulosclerosis (Kimmelstiel-Wilson disease) is less commonly associated with, but more specific of, diabetic nephropathy and consists of spherical deposits of periodic acid-Schiff (PAS)-positive material within the peripheral mesangium. Insudative lesions, including fibrin caps and capsular drops, are less specific and result from accumulation of plasma proteins and lipids.

**16. Correct choice: E.**

Kimmelstiel-Wilson nodule in nodular diabetic glomerulosclerosis is a sclerotic acellular nodule located in intercapillary or mesangial regions and consists of mesangial matrix-like and glioblastoma multiforme (GBM)-like material. Kimmelstiel-Wilson nodules are often surrounded by microaneurysms (dilated capillary loops). Kimmelstiel-Wilson nodules are usually associated with diffuse diabetic glomerulosclerosis (mesangial expansion) and increase with time. Insudative lesions derive from the extravasation of plasma fluid. Plasma proteins accumulate between the endothelial wall and the GBM in the fibrin cap, whereas they accumulate between the parietal epithelial cells and the Bowman capsule in the capsular drop. Insudative lesions are common but not pathognomonic of diabetic nephropathy. Both afferent and efferent arterioles are affected by the accumulation of plasma proteins (hyalinosis) as occurs in the glomeruli, a feature called arteriolar hyalinosis. Involvement of the efferent arteriole is thought to be more specific of diabetic nephropathy.

**17. Correct choice: B.**

Immunoglobulin A (IgA) nephropathy/Berger disease is related to the mesangial deposition of IgA. It is probably the most common form of glomerulonephritis worldwide. Recurrent hematuria, often discovered incidentally, is the most frequent presentation, sometimes associated with mild proteinuria. The only way to diagnose the disease is to demonstrate IgA deposits in the mesangium by immunofluorescence (IF). Overproduction of IgA in response to infectious agents is the most likely underlying mechanism. Episodes of hematuria manifest transiently following respiratory or gastrointestinal infections. Light microscopic alterations are highly variable, but mesangial expansion and hypercellularity without interstitial changes represent the earliest and most common features. Most cases tend to have a remission/relapsing course, but approximately 30% will eventually progress to renal failure over a 20-year period. Glomerular changes of Henoch-Schönlein purpura are indistinguishable from those of Berger disease.

**18. Correct choice: E.**

Clinical symptomatology and ultrastructural findings are consistent with thin basement membrane disease. Note that glioblastoma multiforme (GBM) thickness varies with age and sex: a value of 300 to 480 nm is considered normal in adults. Some authors suggest using a value of 264 nm as a low cutoff for the diagnosis of thin basement membrane disease. This condition is benign and does not progress to renal failure. No associated extrarenal abnormalities have been reported. Recent finding indicates that abnormalities of α4 or α3 chains of type IV may play a pathogenetic role. Alport syndrome initially manifests with ultrastructural features of thin basement membrane disease.

**19. Correct choice: A.**

This syndrome includes several hereditary conditions, the most frequent of which (the classic form) is inherited as an X-linked dominant disorder (thus, females may manifest the disease). The most characteristic glomerular alterations are visualized by electron microscopy (EM): splitting and variable thickening of the glioblastoma multiforme (GBM). GBM changes lead to recurrent hematuria (similar to thin basement membrane disease). The classic (X-linked) form is due to mutations of the genes encoding α3, α4, and α5 chains of type IV collagen, which are present in the GBM, Bowman capsule, and basement membrane of the distal tubules. Immunostaining with antibodies to these collagen chains is absent in Alport syndrome. Ocular defects, leiomyomatosis, and blood cell anomalies occasionally coexist. All men with Alport syndrome and 10% of women with the X-linked variant will eventually progress to renal failure.

**20. Correct choice: B.**

Thrombotic microangiopathy (TMA) is most commonly associated with hemolytic-uremic syndrome (HUS) and thrombotic thrombocytopenic purpura (TTP) and less frequently with postpartum renal failure, severe preeclampsia and eclampsia, malignant hypertension, antiphospholipid syndrome, systemic lupus erythematosus (SLE), and malignancy. Clinical presentation depends on the underlying condition. Light microscopic changes include swelling of endothelial cells and subendothelial deposition of amorphous material, leading to narrowing of the glomerular capillary lumina, which produces the bloodless appearance. Glomerular capillary thrombi may develop. Characteristic changes also affect arteries and arterioles, including intimal myxoid fibroplasia and fibrinoid necrosis.

**21. Correct choice: C.**

Cryoglobulinemic glomerulonephritis (GN) is a condition is due to the formation of cryoglobulins, which precipitate at 4 °C and become soluble at 30 °C. One-third of cases are idiopathic, whereas the remaining cases are associated with various conditions (eg, collagen vascular diseases, liver disease, lymphomas). The acute manifestation consists of purpura, joint inflammation, hepatosplenomegaly, and lymphadenopathy. Intracapillary proliferative GN may develop in the acute phase or years thereafter. Cryoglobulin thrombi are evident within the capillary lumen on periodic acid-Schiff (PAS) staining. Electron microscopy (EM) demonstrates subendothelial or intracapillary accumulation of material showing a microtubular substructure often described as a fingerprint-like pattern.

**22. Correct choice: A.**

Renal amyloidosis always affects the glomeruli and may develop in various forms of systemic amyloidosis, particularly as a result of chronic inflammatory conditions such as rheumatoid arthritis, collagen vascular diseases, and bronchiectasis. This form is due to the accumulation of AA (amyloid-associated) protein, which can be demonstrated by Congo red staining or immunohistochemistry (IHC) for AA. Glomerular disease due to amyloidosis usually manifests with nephrotic syndrome.

**23. Correct choice: C.**

Fibrillary glomerulonephritis is a rare form of glomerulopathy that manifests in adults with nephrotic syndrome and microhematuria. On light microscopy, the changes are variable, but mesangial expansion and thickening of the capillary walls are common findings. immunofluorescence (IF) for immunoglobulin G (IgG) shows a characteristic intense, diffuse, and smudgy staining of both mesangium and capillary walls. Electron microscopy (EM) shows deposits of rigid, nonbranching fibrils that measure 18 to 24 nm in diameter (amyloid fibrils are 8-10 nm thick). Fibrils with a microtubular structure measuring 20 to 50 nm in diameter are found in the very rare immunotactoid glomerulonephritis, which is often associated with lymphoproliferative disorders, cryoglobulinemia, or monoclonal gammopathy.

**24. Correct choice: A.**

Glomerular pathology is extremely common and morphologically diverse in systemic lupus erythematosus (SLE). The recent International Society of Nephrology and the Renal Pathology Society (ISN/RPS) classification of lupus nephritis has replaced the World Health Organization (WHO) classification but has retained the stratification of SLE-associated glomerular disease into six classes (I-VI). The answer choices reflect the diagnostic features of those six classes. Here are the main pathologic changes associated with each of the ISN/RPS classes.

Class I: Minimal mesangial lupus nephritis. Normal glomeruli by light microscopy (LM). Immunofluorescence (IF) and electron microscopy (EM) show mesangial immune complex deposits.

Class II: Mesangial proliferative lupus nephritis. Mesangial hypercellularity with patent capillaries and mesangial immune complex deposits

Class III: Focal lupus nephritis. Focal and segmental lesions involving fewer than 50% of glomeruli. The lesions can be proliferative (intracapillary or extracapillary), necrotizing, or sclerosing.

Class IV: Diffuse lupus nephritis. Lesions are the same type as class III, but more severe and involve more than 50% of the glomeruli. Characteristics of this stage are thick, glassy glomerular capillary walls having a "wire loop" appearance due to subendothelial deposits.

Class V: Membranous lupus nephritis. Membranous glomerulonephritis (GN) with associated mesangial hypercellularity

Class VI: Advanced sclerosing lupus nephritis. Advanced disease, with more than 90% glomerular sclerosis

**25. Correct choice: A.**

Renal biopsies in lupus nephritis are carried out in order to determine the type of renal injury and assess its severity for therapeutic purposes. Active disease requires more aggressive immune suppression. On the other hand, more aggressive treatment is not likely to produce benefits if the renal pathology is limited to mesangial involvement or consists of chronic, irreversible changes, such as glomerulosclerosis and interstitial fibrosis. Thus, a widely used scoring system is based on evaluating and comparing parameters of activity and chronicity.

A. The activity index includes cellular crescents, fibrinoid necrosis/karyorrhexis, endocapillary hypercellularity, leukocyte infiltration, large subendothelial deposits (wire loops), and interstitial inflammation.
B. The chronicity index includes glomerulosclerosis, fibrous crescents, tubular atrophy, and interstitial fibrosis.

**26. Correct choice: B.**

Light-chain deposition disease (LCDD) is a condition that may produce light microscopic changes extremely similar to those associated with diabetes mellitus (diffuse and nodular glomerulosclerosis). LCDD is caused by the accumulation of light chains in a nonamyloidotic, nonfibrillary form. Deposition of κ chain is present in the great majority of cases, whereas λ chain is preferentially deposited in amyloidotic form. Electron-dense subendothelial deposits are seen on electron microscopy (EM). In two-thirds of cases, multiple myeloma or analogous lymphoplasmacellular proliferation occurs concomitantly with LCDD or develops later. Sometimes, there is no evidence of plasma cell dyscrasia. It is not known why κ light chains give rise to nonamyloidotic/granular deposits, while λ light chains result in amyloidotic/fibrillary deposits. Other factors, such as amyloid P component and apolipoprotein E, may play a role.

**27. Correct choice: A.**

Light microscopic changes of ATN detectable in renal biopsies can be subtle. Frank necrosis of tubular epithelium is uncommon and found only in the most severe injury. Detachment of tubular cells from the basement membrane leaves denuded segments of tubules, but the detached cells are still viable. Common findings include loss of brush border in proximal tubules, granular casts in distal tubules and collecting ducts, interstitial edema, mononuclear cells filling the vasa recta, regenerative changes such as flattening of epithelial cells, and large nuclei with visible nucleoli. Specific causes of ATN produce distinctive changes: (1) coarse vacuolization and oxalate crystal in the tubular lumen; (2) myoglobin or hemoglobin casts in myoglobinuric or hemoglobinuric ATN; (3) fine vacuolation of proximal tubular cells after infusion of macromolecules (mannitol) or administration of immunoglobulin, contrast media, or calcineurin inhibitors; and (4) bile casts in hepatic failure with jaundice.

**28. Correct choice: C.**

Acute and chronic interstitial nephritis may result from a number of causes: drugs, infections, systemic disease (IgG4 [immunoglobulin G subclass 4]-related systemic disease, Sjögren syndrome, sarcoidosis), and other rare conditions. IgG4-related nephritis is part of the systemic IgG4-related disease and should be suspected when the chronic inflammatory infiltrate contains numerous plasma cells. Immunohistochemistry for IgG4 should reveal at least 10 IgG4-positive plasma cells per high-power field. The diagnosis, however, rests on correlating renal biopsy findings with clinical and laboratory data (high circulating serum IgG4 levels, low complement). IgG4-related nephritis responds to steroid treatment.

**29. Correct choice: C.**

Chronic pyelonephritis is caused by recurrent insults to the pelvicalyceal system secondary to causes that can be obstructive (ie, urolithiasis) or nonobstructive (ie, vesicoureteral reflux with recurrent infection). Grossly, the kidneys show irregular scarring, blunted papillae, and dilated calyces. Histologically, there is interstitial chronic inflammation and fibrosis, tubular atrophy or dilatation, accumulation of inspissated protein within tubular lumina, interstitial deposits of Tamm-Horsfall protein, and periglomerular fibrosis. Widespread dilatation of the tubules containing eosinophilic material may mimic thyroid tissue (thyroidization). A diagnosis of chronic pyelonephritis cannot be made solely on microscopic examination.

**30. Correct choice: A.**

The incidence of analgesic nephropathy, a tubulointerstitial kidney disease, is declining, but it continues to be seen in association with long-standing abuse of nonphenacetin analgesic medications (salicylates, acetaminophen). Papillary necrosis is the most characteristic gross change of analgesic nephropathy. The cortex has a bumpy appearance due to atrophic areas (overlying necrotic papillae) alternating with areas of compensatory hypertrophy. Papillary necrosis can also be caused by diabetes mellitus and sickle cell anemia. The mechanism of action seems to be related to glutathione depletion, with accumulation of toxic lipid peroxides and vascular damage leading to ischemic necrosis of the renal papillae.

**31. Correct choice: E.**

The three most common underlying causes of end-stage renal disease (ESRD) in the United States include diabetes (46%), hypertension (29%), and glomerulonephritis (7%). Diabetes is the prevalent cause among Whites and hypertension among Blacks. Chronic interstitial nephritis and autosomal dominant polycystic kidney disease (AD-PKD) are important but less frequent causes of ESRD. Grossly, end-stage kidneys are very small, with markedly thinned cortex and a blurred corticomedullary junction. The surface is granular with an adherent capsule. Scars, hydronephrosis, and various other abnormalities can be seen depending on the original etiology. Microscopic changes are often nonspecific.

**32. Correct choice: E.**

Hyperacute renal rejection is a rare complication because cross-matching techniques have become routine before renal transplantation. It is due to preformed circulating antibodies against allograft antigens. Such antibodies develop in the recipient because of prior immunologic exposure, which may result from past pregnancies, blood transfusions, or transplantation. A few minutes or hours following transplantation, the patient develops a sudden decrease in urine output. The recipient's antibodies react with endothelial cells, triggering thrombosis and rapid failure of the graft. Infarction of renal parenchyma, fibrin thrombi, and extensive leukocytic infiltration are seen histologically.

**33. Correct choice: B.**

Acute antibody-mediated (humoral) rejection is a type of rejection that usually manifests 2 weeks after transplantation, but it may also occur anytime thereafter. The humoral form is mediated by the recipient's antidonor antibodies targeting endothelial cells. Margination of leukocytes in peritubular capillaries (as seen in the picture) is the most common and specific change. Severe forms lead to vasculitis with fibrinoid necrosis and thrombosis. Immunohistochemistry for C4d (a complement degradation product) is now used routinely in the diagnosis of acute rejection. Diffuse immunostaining of peritubular capillaries for C4d is considered the hallmark of acute humoral rejection. Acute humoral rejection is less responsive to immunosuppressive therapy than acute cellular rejection.

**34. Correct choice: B.**

Acute cellular rejection is the most frequent form of rejection and develops typically days to weeks after transplantation (rarely after months). It is mediated by T lymphocytes and characterized by interstitial mononuclear inflammatory infiltrate. Lymphocytes permeate through the tubular epithelium, resulting in tubulitis, the morphologic hallmark (shown in the image). Features of acute cellular rejection are usually combined with those of acute humoral rejection (endothelial damage). The reports on renal biopsies for follow-up of transplant patients should quantify the relative degrees of both acute humoral and cellular rejection patterns. Acute cellular rejection is highly responsive to appropriate treatment.

**35. Correct choice: C.**

Chronic rejection is the most common cause of long-term failure of renal allografts. It manifests clinically with progressive renal insufficiency, often associated with proteinuria and hypertension. The most distinctive histopathologic change consists of fibrointimal sclerosis of arteries and arterioles, mimicking arteriolosclerosis. This complication may arise from recurrent episodes of acute rejection and is not per se a unique immunologic pattern of rejection. It always progresses to irreversible renal failure. Mesangial prominence with glioblastoma multiforme (GBM) "tram-tracking" refers to transplant glomerulopathy, a glomerular change mimicking membranoproliferative glomerulonephritis (GN) and occurring in 25% of long-term renal transplants.

**36. Correct choice: C.**

Effects of calcineurin inhibitors such as cyclosporine and FK506 (tacrolimus) include:

- Acute functional: manifests with a rapid decline in renal function; no morphologic changes
- Acute tubular: dose related but infrequent since the adoption of lower dosages; epithelial cells of the proximal convoluted tubules develop isometric vacuolation and inclusion bodies (the latter are giant mitochondria).
- Chronic vascular interstitial: the most important form, which manifests with progressive interstitial fibrosis, arteriolosclerosis, and tubular atrophy.

**37. Correct choice: D.**

The picture shows the typical nuclear inclusions caused by polyomavirus in tubular cells. Polyomavirus interstitial nephritis is reported in 1% to 10% of kidney transplants and can lead to rapid graft failure. BK virus is the specific type involved. Detection of BK virus in the blood by polymerase chain reaction (PCR) is the screening method for polyomavirus infection of the graft. Worsening of renal function in spite of adequate immune suppression is the typical presentation. In biopsies, the most important differential diagnosis is with acute cellular rejection, since the two conditions require opposite therapeutic adjustments. Cytomegalovirus (CMV) inclusions and nuclear regenerative changes may mimic polyomavirus inclusions, and immunohistochemistry for virus-specific antigens can be used to solve this diagnostic problem.

# 42 Adult Renal Tumors

1. Papillary renal cell carcinomas develop in patients with a hereditary renal tumor syndrome caused by

   A. activating mutations of the proto-oncogene c-MET on chromosome 7.
   B. inactivation of the von Hippel-Lindau tumor suppressor gene.
   C. mutations in the gene coding for folliculin.
   D. mutations in the gene coding for fumarate hydratase.
   E. mutations in the gene coding for succinate dehydrogenase.

2. Cytogenetic studies performed on a renal tumor demonstrate the presence of terminal deletion of the short arm of chromosome 3. Which of the following is the most likely neoplasm?

   A. Collecting duct carcinoma
   B. Oncocytoma
   C. Renal cell carcinoma, chromophobe type
   D. Renal cell carcinoma, clear cell type
   E. Renal cell carcinoma, papillary type

3. In addition to nucleoli, which of the following elements should be assessed according to the Fuhrman system in grading renal cell carcinoma (RCC)?

   A. Cytoplasmic features (clear vs granular)
   B. Growth pattern (solid vs acinar)
   C. Mitotic figures
   D. Nuclear size
   E. Nucleocytoplasmic ratio

4. A biopsy of a renal mass shows an epithelial tumor composed predominantly of cells with abundant granular cytoplasm. This feature can be found in

   A. chromophobe carcinoma.
   B. conventional (clear cell) carcinoma.
   C. oncocytoma.
   D. papillary carcinoma.
   E. all of the above.

5. The morphologic type of renal cell carcinoma (RCC) shown in Figure 1 is characterized by expression of a marker that is not found in other RCC types. Which marker is it?

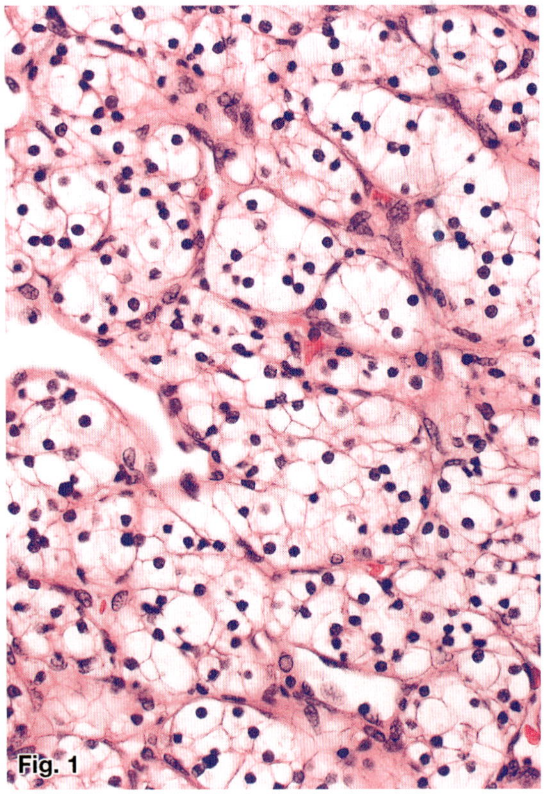

Fig. 1

   A. Carbonic anhydrase IX
   B. CD10
   C. CK7
   D. EMA (epithelial membrane antigen)
   E. Pax2

All figures in this chapter are from Longacre TA, Greenson JK, Hornick JL, Reuter VE, eds. *Mills and Sternberg's Diagnostic Surgical Pathology*. 7th ed. Wolters Kluwer; 2022 except for those noted at the end of this book.

6. A 50-year-old man undergoes resection of a renal neoplasm, which grossly appears as a well-circumscribed, multilocular cystic mass. Microscopically, the tumor is composed of thin-walled cysts lined by one or several layers of clear cells, as shown in Figure 1. In which of the following features does this variant differ from the clear cell (conventional) renal cell carcinoma (RCC)?

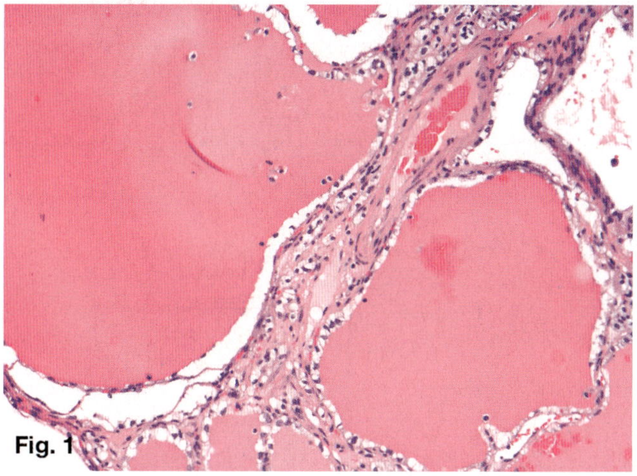

Fig. 1

A. Cytologic characteristics
B. Immunoreactivity for carbonic anhydrase IX (CAIX)
C. Indolent growth and lack of invasion
D. Underlying genetic alterations
E. None of the above

7. A partially cystic, encapsulated renal neoplasm displays the histologic appearance shown in Figure 1. Neoplastic cells are immunoreactive for carbonic anhydrase IX (CAIX) in a "cup-like" manner, where the luminal border is not stained. The tumor is also positive for CK7 and PAX2, but negative for CD10. Cytogenetic and molecular studies show no 3p losses, *VHL* gene mutations, or promoter hypermethylation, nor trisomy of chromosomes 7/17. Which of the following is this type of renal tumor?

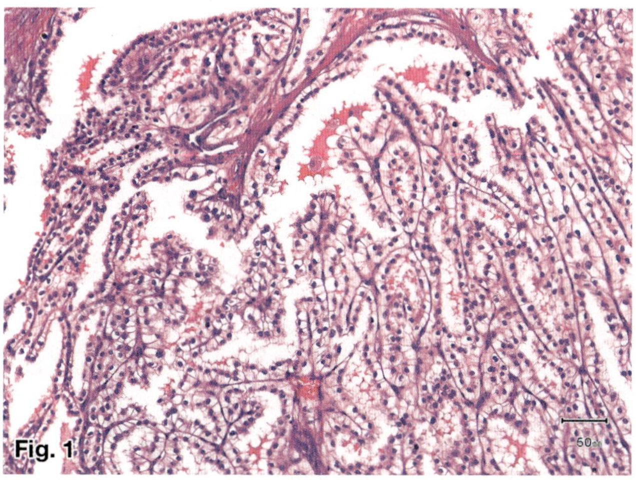

Fig. 1

A. Clear cell (conventional) renal cell carcinoma (RCC)
B. Clear cell papillary RCC
C. Cystic nephroma/mixed epithelial stromal tumor
D. Multilocular cystic RCC
E. Papillary RCC

8. The microscopic features of a 5-cm cortical renal tumor are shown in Figure 1. Tumor cells express Pax2, CD10, CK7, and α-methyl CoA racemase (AMACR), but not carbonic anhydrase IX (CAIX) or CD117. Cytogenetic studies reveal various chromosomal abnormalities, including trisomies 7 and 17 and loss of chromosome Y. Which of the following histologic features can be found in this tumor?

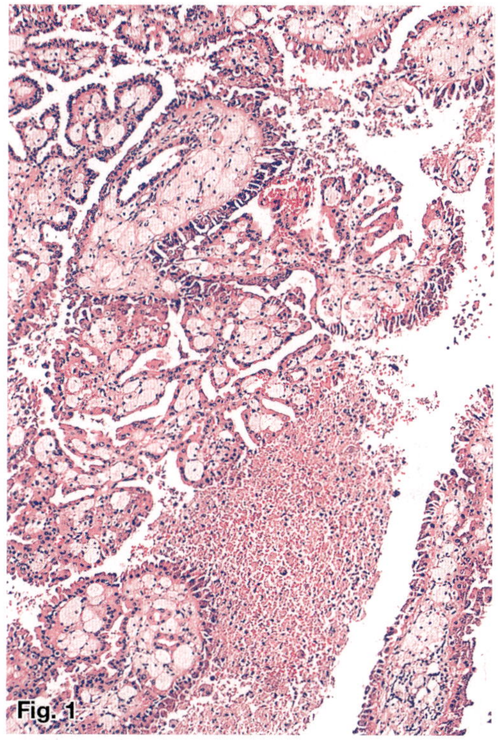

Fig. 1

A. Foamy macrophages in fibrovascular stalks
B. Geographic necrosis
C. Hemosiderin within tumor cells
D. Psammoma bodies in fibrovascular stalks
E. All of the above

9. A 51-year-old woman undergoes resection of a well-circumscribed 8-cm renal tumor. On gross examination, the tumor has tan brown cut surfaces, and microscopically, it has the features shown in Figure 1. This type of renal cell tumor arises from

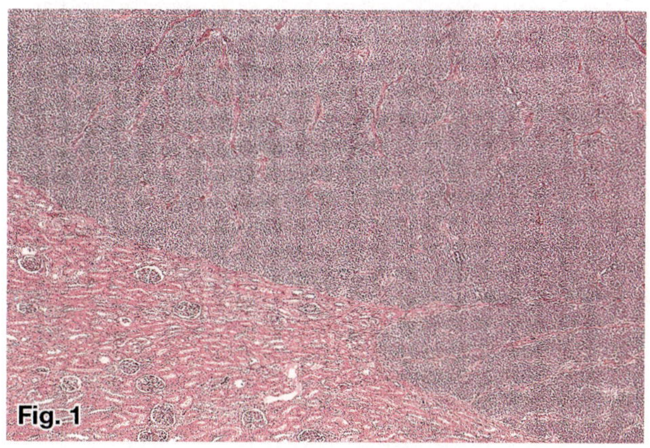

Fig. 1

A. cells from the distal convoluted tubule.
B. cells of the proximal convoluted tubule.
C. collecting ducts of the renal medulla.
D. intercalated cells of the renal cortex.
E. urothelial cells of the pelvis.

10. On gross examination, a renal tumor displays the features shown in Figure 1. Which of the following microscopic features will be most likely associated with such gross appearance?

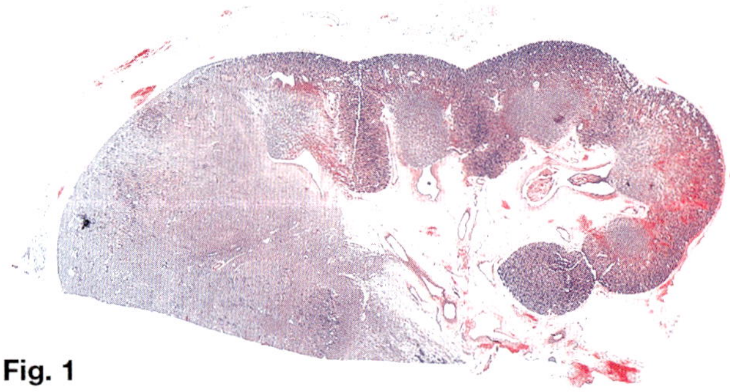

Fig. 1

A. Neoplastic ducts and tubules in a desmoplastic stroma
B. Nests and tubules of malignant cells with prominent nucleoli
C. Oncocytic cells with eosinophilic cytoplasm and round nuclei
D. Papillary architecture lined by hemosiderin-laden epithelial cells
E. Solid sheets of cells with sharp borders and perinuclear clearing

11. Figure 1 shows the morphology of a type of renal cell carcinoma (RCC) typically located in the renal medulla. This tumor may have light microscopic features and immunohistochemical profile indistinguishable from

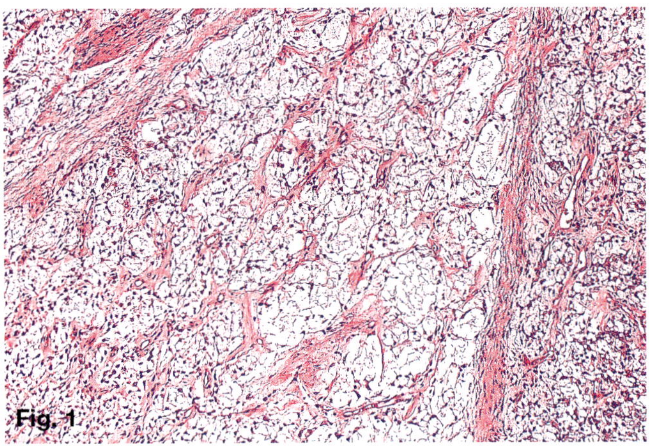

Fig. 1

A. clear cell RCC.
B. mixed epithelial and stromal tumor.
C. papillary renal cell carcinoma (PRCC).
D. renal medullary carcinoma.
E. urothelial carcinoma.

12. A 20-year-old African American male with sickle cell trait undergoes removal of a renal tumor, which has the histologic features shown in Figure 1. What is this tumor most likely be?

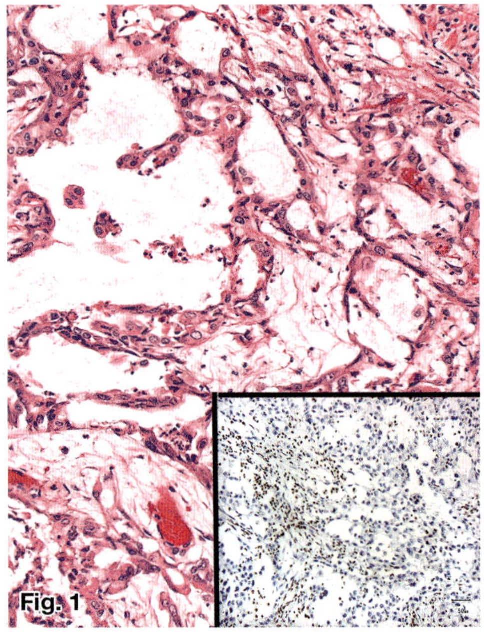

Fig. 1

A. Chromophobe cell carcinoma
B. Clear cell (classic) renal cell carcinoma
C. Collecting duct carcinoma
D. Medullary carcinoma
E. Oncocytoma

13. Figure 1 taken under partially polarized light shows scattered deposits of oxalate crystals in this type of renal cell carcinoma (RCC). Which type is it?

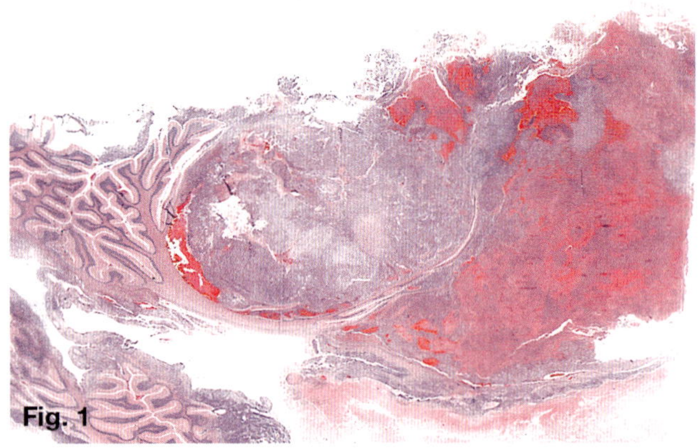

Fig. 1

A. Acquired cystic disease of kidney-associated RCC
B. Clear cell (conventional) RCC
C. Clear cell papillary RCC
D. Mucinous tubular and spindle cell carcinoma
E. Papillary RCC

14. The renal neoplasms known as mixed epithelial and stromal tumors affect preferentially

A. African American men with sickle cell disease.
B. patients with end-stage renal disease.
C. patients with tuberous sclerosis.
D. patients with von Hippel-Lindau syndrome.
E. women of perimenopausal age.

15. Ultrastructural analysis of a tumor from a patient presenting with hypertension and hypokalemia reveals the cytoplasmic crystals shown in Figure 1. Which of the following is the most likely diagnosis?

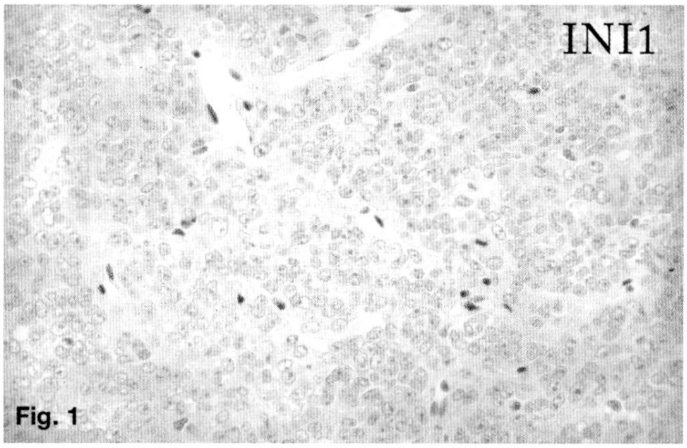


Fig. 1

A. Angiomyolipoma
B. Carcinoid tumor
C. Juxtaglomerular cell tumor
D. Metanephric neoplasm
E. Oncocytoma

16. Metanephric adenomas are frequent tumors found in approximately 15% to 20% of adult autopsies. They are characterized by which of the following features?

A. Associated more frequently with tuberous sclerosis
B. Contain foamy histiocytes
C. Histologically similar to papillary carcinoma
D. Located most frequently in the medulla
E. Presence of deletion of short arm of chromosome 3

17. A renal tumor composed of a mixture of adipose tissue, vessels, and HMB45—reactive smooth muscle cells is frequently associated with

A. Beckwith-Wiedemann syndrome.
B. neurofibromatosis.
C. sickle cell trait.
D. tuberous sclerosis.
E. von Hippel-Lindau syndrome.

# ANSWERS AND EXPLANATIONS

**1. Correct choice: A.**

Activating mutations of the proto-oncogene c-MET on chromosome 7 have been found in a hereditary syndrome, leading to the development of numerous bilateral papillary renal cell carcinoma (RCC). Activation of the gene results in activation of a MET tyrosine kinase, which is a receptor for hepatocyte growth factor/scatter factor. Of note, this is the only syndrome whose underlying genetic abnormality does not involve upregulation of hypoxia-inducible factor 1-α (HIF1α), which is the common mechanisms found in all other hereditary syndromes as well as most of sporadic renal cancers. Inactivation of von Hippel-Lindau tumor suppressor gene on chromosome 3p is the cause of von Hippel-Lindau disease as well as the underlying genetic abnormalities of sporadic clear cell RCC. Mutations in the gene coding for folliculin have been found to be the cause of Birt-Hogg-Dubé (BHD) syndrome, which manifests with oncocytomas or chromophobe RCC as well as a host of other lesions. Mutations in the gene coding for fumarate hydratase are the cause of hereditary leiomyomatosis RCC (HLRCC), characterized by cutaneous and uterine leiomyomas and clear cell RCC. Mutations in the gene coding for succinate dehydrogenase have been recently described as the cause of hereditary RCC, predominantly of the oncocytic type.

**2. Correct choice: D.**

The majority of cases of the conventional type of renal cell carcinoma show abnormalities of the short arm of chromosome 3. These anomalies result in loss of the region containing the *VHL* (von Hippel-Lindau) gene. In the majority of cases, the nondeleted allele of the *VHL* gene is found to be inactivated by mutations or hypermethylation. Thus, the *VHL* gene is thought to act as a tumor suppressor gene. This genetic abnormality occurs in both familial and sporadic forms of the clear cell type of renal carcinoma, but not in the papillary type or the chromophobe type. The normal product of the *VHL* gene, pVHL, degrades hydroxylated hypoxia-inducible factor 1-α (HIF1-α) in normoxemic states. If pVHL is absent or abnormal, HIF1-α escapes degradation and activates downstream molecules such as vascular endothelial growth factor (VEGF), glucose transporter 1 (GLUT1), carbonic anhydrase IX (CAIX), and epidermal- and platelet-derived growth factors (EDGF and PDGF), leading to carcinogenesis.

**3. Correct choice: D.**

The Fuhrman system is based entirely on nuclear and nucleolar features. Nuclear size should be evaluated. In practice, grading can be performed as follows:

Grade 1: Nucleoli are inconspicuous (examined at 400 times).
Grade 2: Nucleoli are visible (examined at 400 times).
Grade 3: Nucleoli are large (visible at 100 times).
Grade 4: Nucleoli are large (visible at 100 times), and nuclei measure greater than 20 μm.

**4. Correct choice: E.**

Conventional (clear cell) renal cell carcinoma (RCC) is often composed of a mixture of clear and granular cells. A granular cell pattern is a nonspecific feature that can also be found in chromophobe RCC, papillary RCC, RCC unclassified, collecting duct carcinoma, epithelioid angiomyolipoma, and oncocytoma. Thus, a renal tumor should never be diagnosed as a "granular cell" tumor. Similarly, a sarcomatoid pattern can be seen in conventional (clear cell) RCC, chromophobe RCC, and collecting duct carcinoma.

**5. Correct choice: A.**

An increasing number of immunohistochemical markers are becoming available to help in the differential diagnosis of renal cell carcinoma (RCC) versus tumors from other sites and of different histologic types of RCC. Clear cell RCC displays a diffuse and strong membranous reactivity for carbonic anhydrase IX (CAIX), whereas all other common subtypes of renal cell tumors are negative for CAIX. CK7 is expressed by papillary RCC, but not by clear cell RCC. Virtually all cases and subtypes of RCC are immunoreactive for PAX2 and PAX8. CD10 is positive in both clear cell and papillary RCC, but negative in some other subtypes.

**6. Correct choice: C.**

Multilocular cystic renal cell carcinoma (RCC) is a variant that represents approximately 5% of clear cell RCC. Tumor cells express epithelial membrane antigen (EMA), pan-keratin, and carbonic anhydrase IX (CAIX), like clear cell RCC. In contrast to clear cell RCC, multilocular cystic RCC often shows focal or diffuse positivity for CK7. As with conventional RCC, this variant has been found to harbor 3p deletions and inactivation of the *VHL* gene. Most importantly, multilocular cystic RCC does not recur or metastasize.

**7. Correct choice: B.**

Clear cell papillary renal cell carcinoma (RCC) is a subtype of RCC that was first described in patients with end-stage renal disease (ESRD), but it has been found in normal kidneys as well. This partially cystic tumor consists of clear cells arranged in tubular structures, which may show branching simulating a papillary architecture. The linear arrangement of the nuclei far from the basement membrane is highly characteristic of this tumor. Clear cell papillary RCC has the genetic abnormalities typical of clear cell RCC (3p−) and papillary carcinoma (trisomy of chromosomes 7 and 17). Its immunohistochemical profile is also quite characteristic, showing membranous expression of carbonic anhydrase IX (CAIX) in a cup-like manner, diffuse expression of CK7, but lack of CD10. Clear cell papillary RCC has a good prognosis.

**8. Correct choice: E.**

Papillary renal cell carcinoma (PRCC) accounts for approximately 15% of RCC. It is composed of a predominantly papillary

**TABLE 1 Distinguishing Features of Renal Oncocytoma and Chromophobe Renal Cell Carcinoma**

| Features | Oncocytoma | Chromophobe RCC |
|---|---|---|
| **GROSS** | | |
| Color | Brown red | Brown red (eosinophilic variant) or yellow- tan (classic) |
| Central scar | Common | Less common |
| **CELLULAR** | | |
| Architecture | Nested and tubular | Solid sheets with incomplete septations; nested and tubular |
| Necrosis | Absent | Not uncommon |
| Cytoplasm | Densely granular | Reticular; densely granular in eosinophilic variant |
| Perinuclear halo | Absent | Always present, at least focally |
| **NUCLEAR** | | |
| Shape | Round | Irregular, raisinoid |
| Hyperchromatic, smudgy atypical pleomorphic foci | Common | Less common |
| Nucleoli | Common | Usually small or absent; may be present |
| Binucleate | Common | Almost always |
| **Ultrastructural** | Mitochondria with long lamellae | Microvesicles; mitochondria with tubulocystic lamellae |
| **Hale colloidal iron** | Negative or luminal | Diffuse, granular, or reticular |

RCC, renal cell carcinoma.
Modified from Perez-Ordonez B, Hamed G, Campbell S, et al. Renal oncocytoma: a clinicopathologic study of 70 cases. *Am J Surg Pathol.* 1997;21(8):871-883.

or papillary-solid architecture. Other morphologic features that are frequently seen in PRCC include those listed in the answers. The most common genetic abnormalities include trisomies 7 and 17 and loss of chromosome Y. The prognosis is better than that of conventional (clear cell) carcinoma. The immunohistochemical profile allows distinguishing PRCC from other RCC types in ambiguous cases. The designation of papillary adenoma refers to papillary lesions less than 0.5 cm in diameter, which, although morphologically identical to PRCC, has no metastatic potential.

**9. Correct choice: C.**

Chromophobe renal cell carcinoma (CRCC) constitutes approximately 5% to 10% of RCCs and is characterized by an excellent prognosis compared to the more frequent clear cell and papillary RCCs. Histologically, it consists of sheets of cells with sharp cytoplasmic borders, pale cytoplasm, and frequent perinuclear halos. Characteristically, large cells are clustered around vessels. Neoplastic cells contain acid mucin, which accounts for the characteristic positivity for colloidal iron. Electron microscopy (EM) reveals innumerable cytoplasmic vesicles. CRCC is thought to arise from intercalated cells of the collecting ducts. CRCC should be distinguished from oncocytoma (see Table 1). Tumor cells are positive for epithelial membrane antigen (EMA), pan-cytokeratin, CK7, and CD117. Hypodiploidy and multiple monosomies, with loss of 1, 2, 6, 10, 13, 17, 21, or Y, are detectable in these tumors. CRCC has a very good prognosis.

**10. Correct choice: C.**

Oncocytoma is a benign tumor that accounts for 3% to 7% of all resected renal neoplasms. It is derived from the intercalated duct and composed of uniform cells with intensely eosinophilic granular cytoplasm. The nuclei are monotonous and have a central nucleolus. Mitotic activity is inconspicuous. Architectural patterns are variable, including tubular-acinar, solid sheets, and biphasic. The gross appearance is highly characteristic because the tumor shows a mahogany brown color and, when large, a central stellate scar. The latter feature is infrequent in tumors measuring less than 5 cm in main diameter. Choice A is characteristic of collecting duct carcinoma, choice B of medullary carcinoma, choice D of papillary carcinoma, and choice E of chromophobe cell carcinoma.

**11. Correct choice: E.**

Collecting duct carcinoma (CDC) is a highly aggressive renal cell carcinoma (RCC) that accounts for less than 1% of renal tumors. It originates from the ducts of Bellini, which explains its medullary location. They tend to occur in patients younger than those with conventional RCC. Histologically, CDC is composed of complex tubular, ductal, and papillary formations embedded in a dense desmoplastic stroma. Tumor cells have high-grade nuclei with prominent nucleoli. papillary renal cell carcinoma (PRCC) and urothelial carcinoma are to be considered in the differential diagnosis. Negative immunostains for α-methyl CoA racemase (AMACR), CD10, and RCC favor PRCC. Unfortunately, immunohistochemical profiles and many microscopic features of CDC overlap with those of urothelial carcinoma, so the best approach to the differential diagnosis in challenging cases is to sample the renal pelvis extensively to find or rule out in situ lesions.

**12. Correct choice: D.**

Renal medullary carcinoma is a rare type of renal carcinoma with a striking propensity to affect young people with sickle cell trait, whether of African American or Mediterranean descent. It is probably a variant of collecting duct carcinoma, with which it shares histologic and histogenetic features. Often, the tumor consists of anastomosing tubules and cords with microcystic spaces that impart a vague resemblance to yolk sac tumors. Unique to renal medullary carcinoma is the loss of nuclear expression of the transcriptional regulator INI1, whereas all other markers are similar to collecting duct carcinoma (CDC). This is a very aggressive tumor.

**13. Correct choice: A.**

Various types of renal cell carcinoma (RCC) can develop in end-stage kidneys with acquired cystic disease (ACD), but ACD-associated RCC is the most common. It is a high-grade RCC characterized by variable architecture, including tubular, papillary, and cribriform. Tumor cells have high-grade nuclei with prominent nucleoli and brightly eosinophilic cytoplasm. Intratumoral deposition of oxalate crystals is the most characteristic feature. The tumor is strongly and diffusely positive for α-methyl CoA racemase (AMACR) and negative for CK7.

**14. Correct choice: E.**

These rare tumors are biphasic and consist of an epithelial and a mesenchymal component. The latter is similar to ovarian stroma and displays expression of estrogen and progesterone receptors. These tumors affect almost exclusively women, usually with obesity or receiving exogenous hormones. They are benign. Cystic nephroma is classified within the spectrum of mixed epithelial and stromal tumors.

**15. Correct choice: C.**

Juxtaglomerular cell tumor (JCT) is a very rare, benign, renin-secreting tumor occurring in young individuals with a prevalence of women. It manifests with severe hypertension associated with hyperreninism and hypokalemia. The tumor is solid and well demarcated and consists of sheets of round to spindly cells with well-defined borders and eosinophilic cytoplasm. JCT shows diffuse immunoreactivity for renin, vimentin, CD34, and CD117. Membrane-bound rhomboid crystals are highly characteristic ultrastructural features.

**16. Correct choice: C.**

Metanephric adenoma is a tumor that is invariably located in the cortex and represents a frequent incidental finding. Histologically, it consists of uniform bland cells arranged in papillary or tubular formations. Cells have eosinophilic (not clear) cytoplasm and lack 3p deletions. A papillary architecture may pose a diagnostic challenge in distinguishing metanephric adenoma from papillary carcinoma. Metanephric adenofibroma is closely related to metanephric adenoma: it is composed of an epithelial component (like that of metanephric adenoma) and a mesenchymal, fibroblast-like component. Recently, BRAF (v-raf murine sarcoma viral oncogene homolog B1) mutations (V600E) have been demonstrated in 90% of metanephric adenomas.

**17. Correct choice: D.**

Angiomyolipoma is a neoplasm of probable hamartomatous (developmental) genesis, seen in approximately 40% of patients with tuberous sclerosis (TS). TS causes various developmental anomalies, including cortical tubers (consisting of a disorganized neocortex), skin angiofibromas, and cardiac rhabdomyomas. HMB45 immunoreactivity is also found in similar hamartomatous TS-related lesions, such as lymphangiomyomatosis. Beckwith-Wiedemann syndrome is associated with omphalocele, macroglossia, and Wilms tumor. Renal medullary carcinoma is associated with sickle cell trait. von Hippel-Lindau syndrome is associated with conventional (clear cell) renal cell carcinoma (RCC).

# 43 Renal Neoplasms of Childhood

1. A nephrectomy specimen is received for staging of a previously diagnosed Wilms tumor. The tumor appears confined within the kidney and completely resected. In distinguishing between stage I and stage II, which of the following anatomic structures should be examined?

   A. Hilar plane
   B. Lymph nodes
   C. Peritoneum
   D. Renal sinus
   E. Renal vein

2. A 3-year-old child undergoes surgery for resection of a large abdominal mass centered in the right kidney. The tumor is composed of various histologic elements, as shown in Figure 1. Areas of skeletal muscle differentiation are seen in the stromal component. Which of the following morphologic patterns of this tumor is considered "favorable histology"?

   A. Diffuse blastemal
   B. Mixed
   C. Nested blastemal
   D. Tubular
   E. All of the above

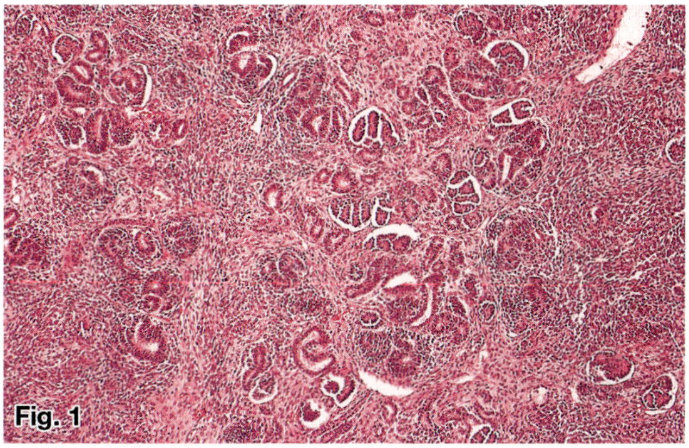

Fig. 1

3. A Wilms tumor with the morphologic changes shown in Figure 1 will most likely have which of the following genetic alterations?

   A. Inactivation of the *INI1* gene
   B. *TP53* mutations
   C. Translocation t(10;17)
   D. Translocation t(12;15)
   E. Translocation t(X;18)

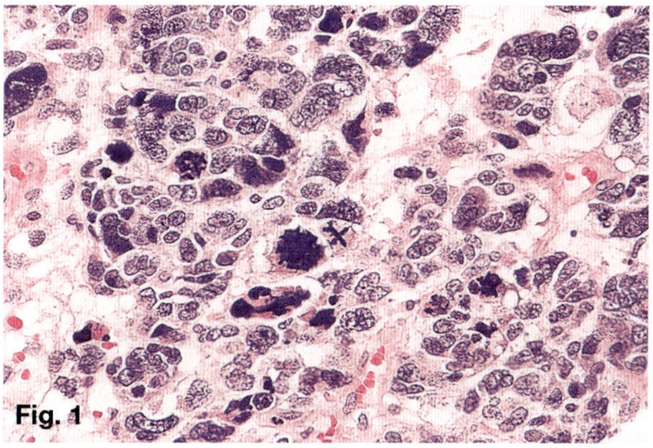

Fig. 1

4. The renal tumor known as mesoblastic nephroma is characterized by

   A. development in fetal life.
   B. highly aggressive behavior.
   C. mesenchymal and epithelial elements.
   D. multiple cysts lined by tubular epithelium.
   E. small round cell morphology.

---

All figures in this chapter are from Longacre TA, Greenson JK, Hornick JL, Reuter VE, eds. *Mills and Sternberg's Diagnostic Surgical Pathology*. 7th ed. Wolters Kluwer; 2022 except for those noted at the end of this book.

5. A nephrectomy specimen from a 2-year-old boy shows a well-circumscribed homogeneous tumor in the medullary region. Its histologic features are shown in Figure 1. Mitoses are frequent. Only vimentin immunoreactivity is demonstrated in tumor cells. The child has metastases in the skull and the brain. Which of the following is the most likely diagnosis?

   A. Clear cell sarcoma
   B. Medullary fibroma
   C. Mesoblastic nephroma
   D. Multicystic nephroma
   E. Wilms tumor

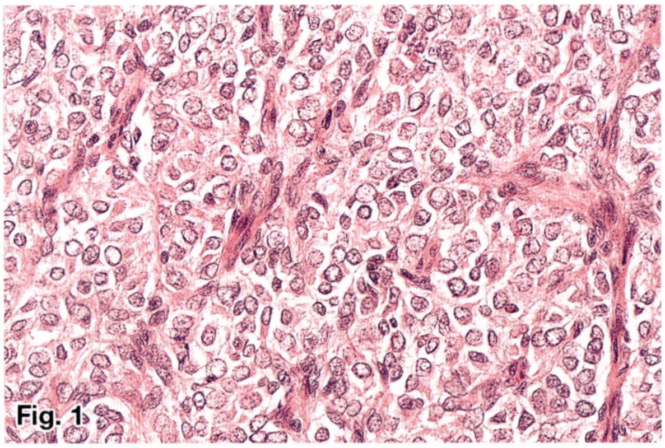

Fig. 1

6. Figure 1 shows the histologic appearance of a renal tumor from a 1-year-old boy. Tumor cells express vimentin, keratin, and epithelial membrane antigen (EMA) and are negative for INI1. Which of the following is the diagnosis?

   A. Clear cell sarcoma
   B. Primitive neuroectodermal tumor
   C. Renal cell carcinoma
   D. Rhabdoid tumor
   E. Synovial sarcoma

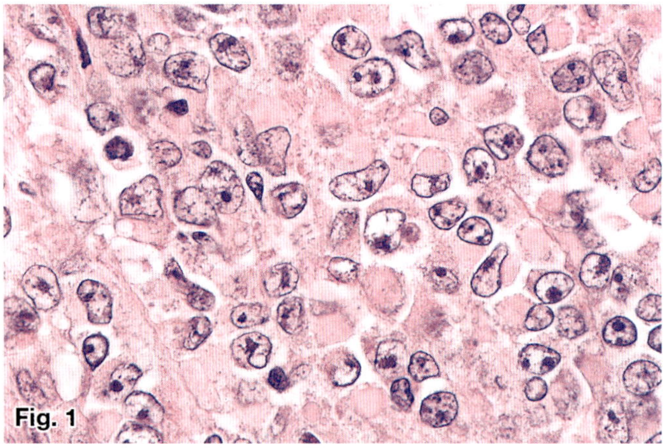

Fig. 1

# ANSWERS AND EXPLANATIONS

**1. Correct choice: D.**

The renal sinus is the concave region of the kidney containing major vascular and pelvicalyceal structures, where tumor invasion may gain access to blood and lymphatic vessels and spread to distant sites. Vascular invasion within the renal sinus is a primary discriminant between stage I and stage II. If resection margins are involved or there is peritoneal spread, but the tumor is still confined within the abdomen, the tumor is in stage III. Hematogenous spread corresponds to stage IV, and bilateral tumors to stage V.

**2. Correct choice: E.**

Ninety percent of Wilms tumors (WTs) occur before the age of 6 years. Histologically, they consist of variable mixtures of three cellular lineages: blastemal, stromal, and epithelial. WTs show a tremendous morphologic variability because each of the three components may present with varying degrees of differentiation and patterns. Most tumors are triphasic, but biphasic and monophasic tumors are not rare. Blastemal cells are small, undifferentiated cells with a high nuclear-to-cytoplasmic ratio. Blastema may be diffuse or nested. The epithelial component most often presents with a tubular pattern. The stromal component consists of spindly mesenchymal cells in a myxoid matrix; heterologous differentiation may produce skeletal muscle. Tubular-dominant pattern is usually diagnosed at stage I, reflecting a slow growth, while the diffuse blastemal pattern is usually seen at stages II and IV. However, tumors with the diffuse blastemal pattern respond well to current therapeutic protocols and are still classified in the favorable histology category. Staging is the most important prognostic factor.

**3. Correct choice: B.**

Anaplastic nuclear change is detected in 5% of Wilms tumors (WTs) and is the only morphologic indicator of "unfavorable histology." It is associated with extreme polyploidy. It is defined by prominent nuclear enlargement, hyperchromasia, and atypical mitotic figures (multipolar or polyploidy). Absolute neutrophil count (ANC) imparts increased resistance to chemotherapy. The majority of anaplastic WTs have been shown to harbor mutations of p53, which is never present in WTs with favorable histology. This molecular change accounts for increased resistance to chemotherapy, since chemotherapy-induced apoptosis requires an intact p53 protein. Choice A: Rhabdoid tumor. Choice C: Clear cell sarcoma. Choice D: Mesoblastic nephroma. Choice E: Synovial sarcoma.

**4. Correct choice: A.**

Mesoblastic nephroma is a congenital neoplasm that represents 3% of childhood renal tumors and usually becomes apparent in the first 3 months of life. It is a well-circumscribed mass often located near the renal sinus. It consists of a monotonous mesenchymal growth of fibroblast-like spindly cells; this is referred to as the classic pattern. The cellular pattern is more common and is similar to fibrosarcoma, with high cellularity and numerous mitoses. The tumor often shows focal myofibroblastic smooth muscle or cartilage differentiation. It is a benign tumor, which infrequently displays local infiltrative behavior or metastatic spread. Cystic nephroma, a rare variant of Wilms tumor (WT), is characterized by multiple cysts lined by tubular epithelium.

**5. Correct choice: A.**

This highly malignant renal tumor has a controversial histogenesis, which is distinct from that of Wilms tumor (WT). Despite its name, the clear cell appearance is seen in a minority of cases. The classic pattern consists of uniform cells arranged in nests and cords separated by a chicken wire network of thin intersecting vascular septa. Other morphologic patterns are epithelioid, spindled, and myxoid. Helpful diagnostic features include extreme uniformity of gross and microscopic features, a scalloped border, negative immunostains except for vimentin, and the propensity of this tumor to metastasize to bones and the brain (utterly unusual for other childhood renal tumors). The prognosis is poor, but it has recently improved due to the use of doxorubicin. Metastases often manifest a long time after the initial diagnosis.

**6. Correct choice: D.**

Rhabdoid tumor of the kidney (RTK) is one of the most aggressive neoplasms of childhood. It accounts for 2% of renal neoplasms in children. Peak age at presentation is 13 months. Most patients present with metastatic disease. Inactivation of the *hSNF5/INI1* gene on chromosome 22 is the pathognomonic molecular feature of RTK. Immunohistochemical demonstration of lack of INI1 expression in tumor cells is diagnostic of RTK. Extrarenal rhabdoid tumors occur in the brain and soft tissues and have the same morphology and genetic alteration as RTK.

# 44 Urothelial Tract: Renal Pelvis, Ureter, Urinary Bladder, and Urethra

1. Histologic examination of a bladder specimen reveals glandular structures and cystic spaces within the bladder wall, as shown in Figure 1. This finding is most consistent with

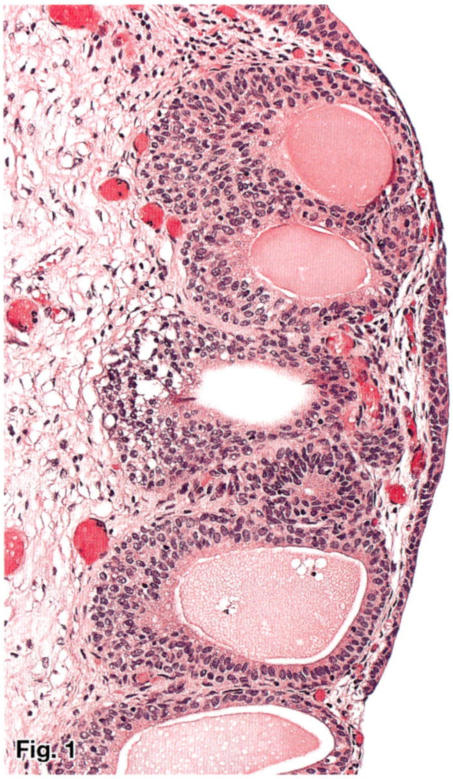

Fig. 1

A. Bacillus Calmette-Guerin (BCG) treatment.
B. follicular cystitis.
C. invasive adenocarcinoma.
D. mesonephroid metaplasia.
E. reactive change.

2. A middle-aged woman presents with a 3-month history of suprapubic discomfort, dysuria, and frequency. Urine cultures are negative. The finding of mucosal fissures on cystoscopy and mucosal/submucosal chronic inflammation with mast cells on biopsy is most consistent with

A. cystitis glandularis.
B. follicular cystitis.
C. interstitial cystitis.
D. malakoplakia.
E. ulcerative cystitis.

3. A 68-year-old woman undergoes excision of an easily bleeding polypoid mass protruding through the urethral meatus. Histologically, it is composed of vascular tissue with chronic inflammatory cells and islands of squamous epithelium. What is the most likely diagnosis?

A. Crohn disease
B. Fibroepithelial polyp
C. Mesonephric adenoma
D. Urethral carcinoma
E. Urethral caruncle

4. A plaque of the urinary bladder mucosa is biopsied. The biopsy shows a mixed inflammatory infiltrate predominantly located within the lamina propria, consisting of nodules of histiocytes surrounded by lymphoid aggregates. Figure 1 shows round laminated inclusions. Which of the following mechanisms is related to this lesion?

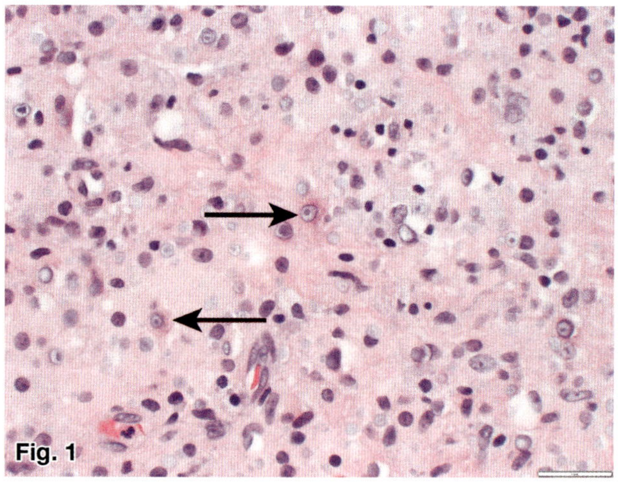

Fig. 1

A. Autoimmune response
B. Defects in phagocytic function
C. Drug toxicity
D. Metaplastic change
E. Response to radiation

5. Which of the following is the most important predisposing condition for the development of bladder cancer in the United States?

A. Arylamine exposure
B. Cigarette smoking
C. Cyclophosphamide treatment
D. Human papillomavirus infection
E. *Schistosoma haematobium* infection

All figures in this chapter are from Longacre TA, Greenson JK, Hornick JL, Reuter VE, eds. *Mills and Sternberg's Diagnostic Surgical Pathology.* 7th ed. Wolters Kluwer; 2022 except for those noted at the end of this book.

6. Pathologic staging of urothelial carcinoma (UC) of the bladder shows the poorest interobserver reliability in evaluating the depth of invasion into the

A. lamina propria.
B. muscularis propria.
C. pelvic wall.
D. perivesical fat.
E. prostate.

7. Biopsies of a 2.0-cm exophytic tumor in the bladder trigone of a 57-year-old man show papillary structures lined by more than 10 layers of epithelial cells. Nuclear atypia is moderate, mitoses are rare, and there are foci of necrosis. The neoplasm infiltrates the underlying muscularis propria. Which of the following is the most important parameter influencing the prognosis?

A. Cell layers
B. Infiltration of the muscularis
C. Mitoses
D. Necrosis
E. Nuclear atypia

8. A 60-year-old woman without prior history of cancer presents with newly onset right hemiparesis. A magnetic resonance imaging (MRI) shows a ring-enhancing mass in the left frontal lobe. A biopsy reveals a carcinoma immunoreactive for CK7, CK20, and GATA3. Which of the following is the most likely source of this metastasis?

A. Kidney
B. Lungs
C. Prostate
D. Skin
E. Urinary bladder

9. Figure 1 depicts a papillary urothelial lesion. What is the most likely diagnosis?

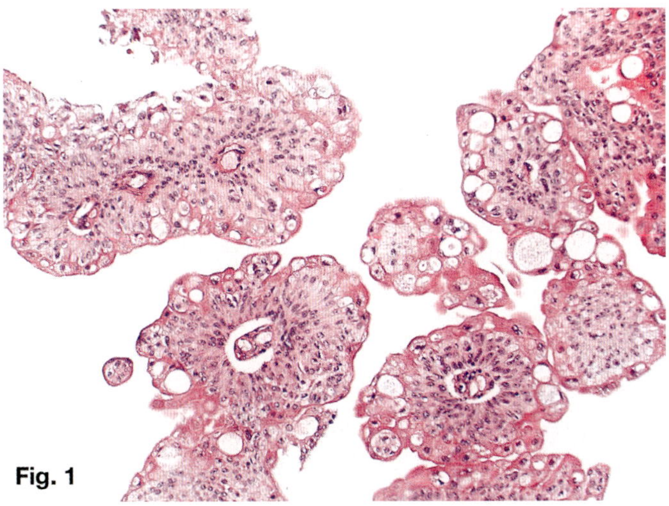

Fig. 1

A. High-grade noninvasive urothelial carcinoma
B. Inverted urothelial papilloma
C. Low-grade noninvasive urothelial carcinoma
D. Papillary hyperplasia
E. Urothelial papilloma

10. The degree of cytologic and architectural atypia present in the urothelial lesion in Figure 1 is most compatible with

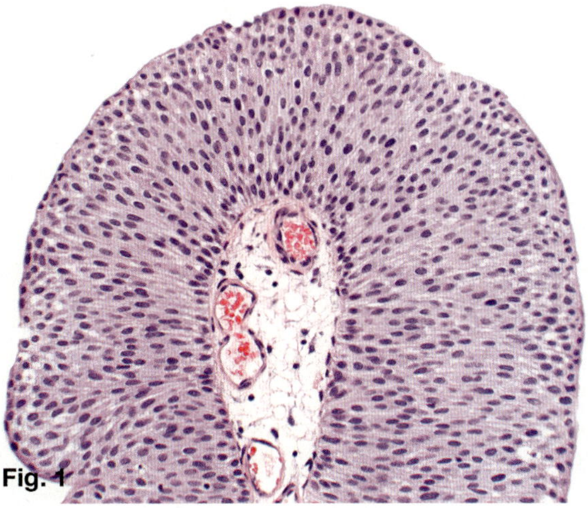

Fig. 1

A. carcinoma in situ.
B. high-grade noninvasive urothelial carcinoma.
C. low-grade noninvasive urothelial carcinoma.
D. papillary urothelial neoplasm of low malignant potential.
E. urothelial papilloma.

11. A papillary tumor of the bladder exhibits the cytologic and architectural features shown in Figure 1. Which of the following is urothelial lesion?

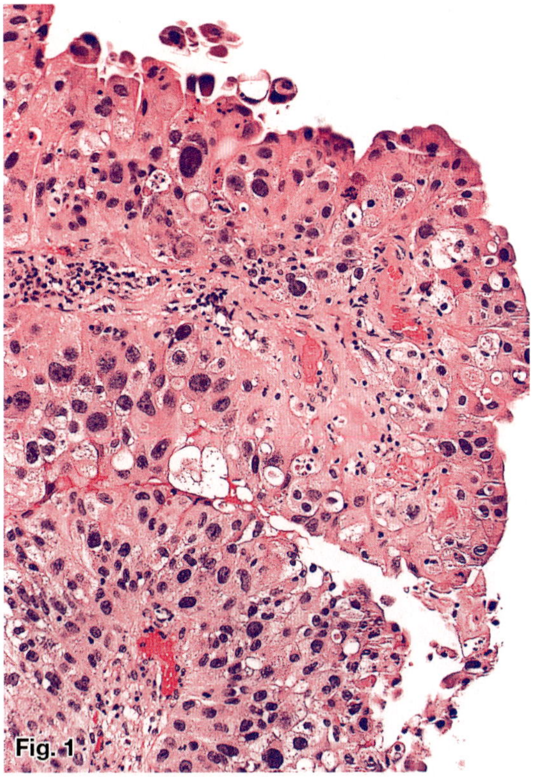

Fig. 1

A. Carcinoma in situ
B. High-grade noninvasive urothelial carcinoma
C. Low-grade noninvasive urothelial carcinoma
D. Papillary urothelial neoplasm of low malignant potential
E. Urothelial papilloma

12. A 66-year-old man presents with dysuria, urgency, and microscopic hematuria. Following cytologic studies and cystoscopy, biopsies reveal the presence of the lesion shown in Figure 1. Which of the following is true about this lesion?

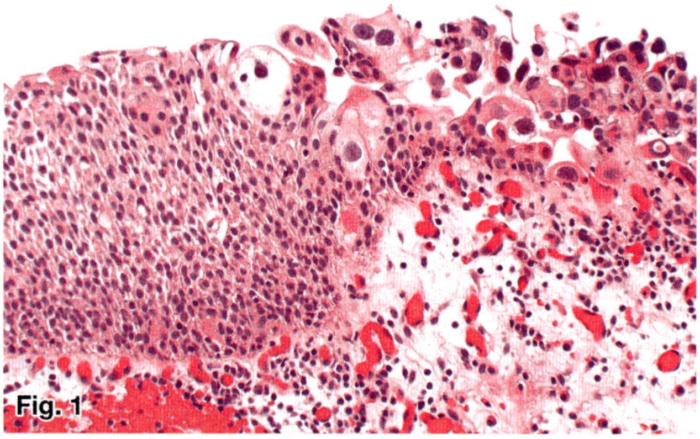
Fig. 1

A. Characterized by full-thickness cellular atypia
B. Detected usually in association with papillary or invasive tumors
C. High nuclear-to-cytoplasmic ratio always present
D. Manifests usually with dysuria and hematuria
E. Umbrella cells always absent

13. Of the following types of urothelial carcinoma (UC) with divergent differentiation, which one is the most common?

A. Glandular
B. Mucinous
C. Sarcomatoid
D. Squamous
E. Trophoblastic

14. In the United States, the histologic type of urinary bladder cancer shown in Figure 1 is most frequently associated with

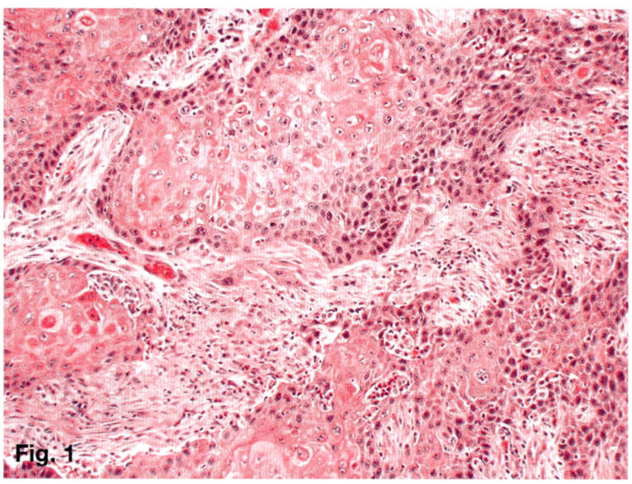
Fig. 1

A. bladder diverticula.
B. neurogenic bladder.
C. renal transplantation.
D. smoking.
E. vesicolithiasis.

15. A biopsy of a mass in the trigone area of the urinary bladder shows a malignant tumor with microscopic features similar to those in Figure 1. This type of urinary bladder cancer is most frequently associated with

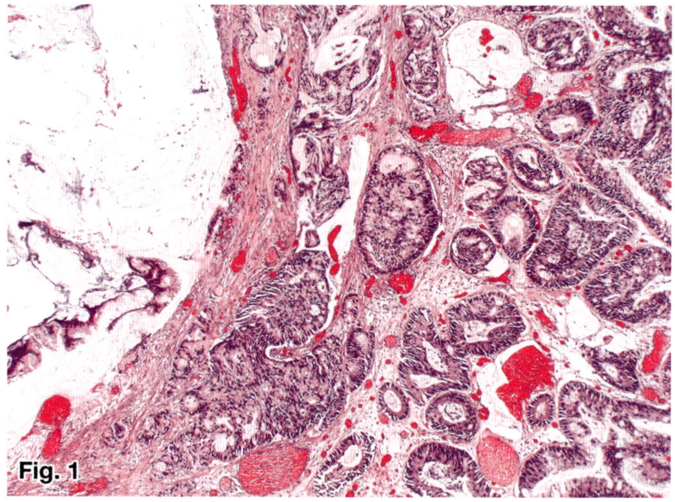
Fig. 1

A. bladder exstrophy.
B. cigarette smoking.
C. cystitis glandularis/cystica.
D. mesonephric rests in the bladder mucosa.
E. *Schistosoma haematobium* infection.

16. Which of the following is the most common type of cancer arising from urachal remnants?

A. Adenocarcinoma
B. Anaplastic carcinoma
C. Small cell/neuroendocrine carcinoma
D. Squamous cell carcinoma
E. Urothelial carcinoma, usual type

17. Which of the following variants of urothelial carcinoma (UC) is characterized by amplification of the *HER2* gene?

A. Lymphoepithelioma like
B. Micropapillary
C. Nested
D. Sarcomatoid
E. Small cell/neuroendocrine

18. Cystoscopic studies reveal a large polypoid mass in the urinary bladder of a 6-year-old child. Histologically, the tumor is composed of a mucinous matrix with sheets of small blue cells. It exhibits a conspicuous "cambium layer," consisting of an accumulation of neoplastic cells beneath the mucosa. Which of the following is the most likely diagnosis?

A. Adenocarcinoma
B. Leiomyosarcoma
C. Lymphoma
D. Rhabdomyosarcoma
E. Sarcomatoid carcinoma

19. Four weeks following transurethral resection of the prostate, a 60-year-old man undergoes a follow-up cystoscopic examination, which reveals a small nodule in the bladder neck. A biopsy of this lesion shows a cellular infiltrate such as that shown in Figure 1. The cells display immunoreactivity for cytokeratin and actin. What is the most likely diagnosis?

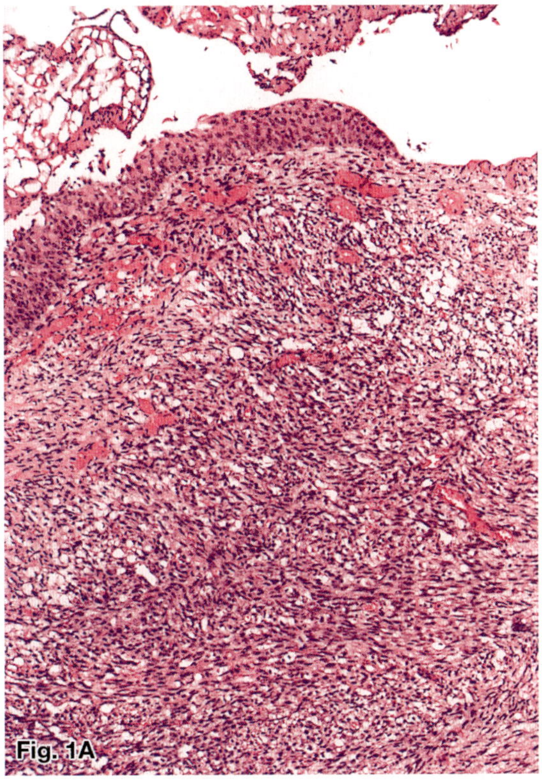
Fig. 1A

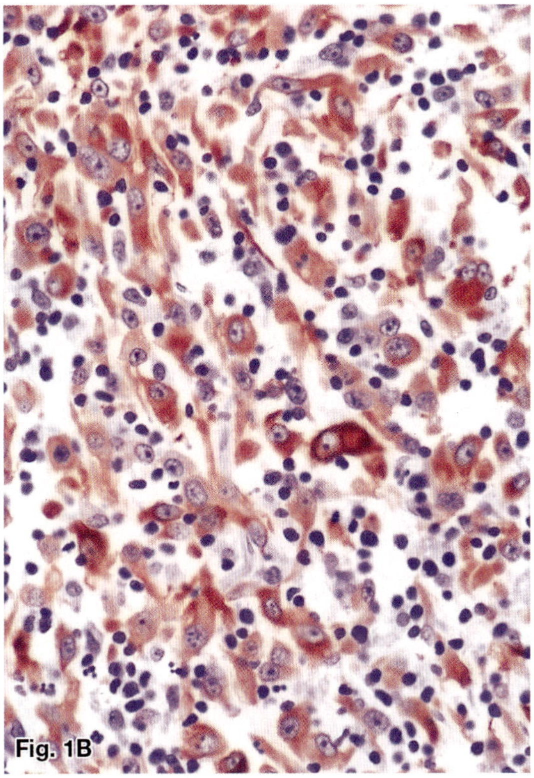
Fig. 1B

A. Inflammatory pseudotumor
B. Leiomyosarcoma
C. Mesonephroid metaplasia
D. Postoperative granuloma
E. Postoperative spindle cell nodule

# ANSWERS AND EXPLANATIONS

**1. Correct choice: E.**

Cystitis glandularis/cystica is a pattern of reaction that may be due to a number of chronic stimuli, such as recurrent cystitis, neurogenic bladder, and bladder exstrophy. Nests of urothelium (Brunn nests) grow inward and undergo metaplastic changes (cystitis glandularis) and/or cystic dilatation (cystitis cystica). There is no evidence that this change predisposes to carcinoma. Mesonephroid metaplasia also occurs in response to various irritative stimuli: It consists of papillary or sessile masses composed of tubules lined by cuboidal cells. Follicular cystitis refers to chronic cystitis associated with the formation of lymphoid follicles.

**2. Correct choice: C.**

Interstitial cystitis is a form of cystitis that is probably of autoimmune nature. Cultures are usually negative. The condition is most commonly seen in women with systemic lupus erythematosus or other autoimmune disorders. A chronic inflammatory infiltrate of mucosa and submucosa with numerous mast cells is the typical morphologic substrate. Mucosal fissures are frequent.

**3. Correct choice: E.**

Urethral caruncle is a benign lesion that manifests characteristically as a small, friable, raspberry-like mass that protrudes from the meatus. It occurs exclusively in older women and is probably reactive. It is composed of highly vascular and chronically inflamed granulation tissue with accompanying islands of metaplastic squamous epithelium. The latter may mimic a malignant growth. Urethral carcinoma develops in the region of the meatus, is associated with human papillomavirus (HPV) infection, and has a predilection for older women. Mesonephric adenoma (also called nephrogenic adenoma) is a reactive lesion morphologically similar to the homonymous lesion in the bladder.

**4. Correct choice: B.**

Malakoplakia is a reaction characterized by multiple yellow nodules and plaques in the trigone region that may be mistaken for cancer on cystoscopy. Microscopically, the lesion consists of histiocytic collections. Michaelis-Guttmann bodies are frequently identified in the cytoplasm of macrophages and in the interstitium. They consist of concentrically layered corpuscles that contain iron and calcium. Malakoplakia probably results from the deficient phagocytic function of macrophages and is more common in patients who are immunosuppressed. *Escherichia coli* and less frequently *Proteus* are frequently involved. It may also develop in the kidneys, colon, lung, prostate, and other sites.

**5. Correct choice: B.**

Cigarette smoking is the most important risk factor in transitional cell carcinoma in industrialized countries. Increased risk of bladder cancer was first reported in dye industry employees at the end of the 19th century. Aromatic amines (naphthylamines, benzidine, and biphenyls) are the chemicals that cause bladder cancer. Exposure to such chemicals occurs in various occupations, for example, dyestuff, rubber, paint, textile, leather, and printing industries. Cyclophosphamide causes hemorrhagic cystitis and increased risk for urinary bladder cancer following long-term administration. The association between human papillomavirus (HPV) and bladder cancer is at best controversial. *Schistosoma haematobium* is an important risk factor for squamous cell (less frequently transitional) carcinoma of the urinary bladder in regions where this infection is endemic.

**6. Correct choice: A.**

Staging is the most important prognostic factor in urothelial carcinoma of the bladder. Clinical staging is highly inaccurate, and thus, pathologic staging acquires a great importance. Crushing and cautery artifact, biopsy orientation, and distortion due to prior biopsy all account for difficulty in evaluating invasion of the lamina propria. Important parameters in assessing lamina propria invasion include pattern of infiltrating cells, continuity of basement membrane, stromal reaction, retraction artifact around tumor cells, and paradoxical differentiation of infiltrating cells, which shows better differentiation compared to the primary focus.

**7. Correct choice: B.**

Urothelial carcinoma (UC) accounts for 90% of urothelial neoplasms of the bladder. Pathologic staging is the most powerful determinant of metastatic potential and survival in UCs. The 5-year survival rate is 75% for tumors infiltrating no deeper than the lamina propria, 50% for those infiltrating the muscularis propria, and 20% for those invading perivesical fat. Other prognostic factors include (a) gross tumor morphology (papillary tumors are less aggressive than nonpapillary/sessile tumors), (b) small vessel invasion, and (c) tumor type and grade.

**8. Correct choice: E.**

Immunostains positive in urothelial carcinoma include CK7, CK20, high-molecular-weight keratin identified by the 34βE12 antibody, uroplakin, thrombomodulin, and GATA3. Immunohistochemical (IHC) is usually not necessary in the diagnosis of primary urothelial carcinoma (UC) in the bladder, but it becomes a useful tool in the identification of metastatic UC, especially when the primary is not known. Metastatic UC tends to be poorly differentiated and mimics other poorly differentiated tumors, such as nonkeratinizing squamous cell carcinoma.

**9. Correct choice: E.**

Urothelial papilloma is a rare but entirely benign papillary lesion consisting of fibrovascular stalk lined by urothelium that is cytologically and architecturally normal. It has no malignant potential.

**10. Correct choice: D.**

The image shows urothelium of increased thickness, but with minimal architectural and cytologic atypias, which are the defining features of papillary urothelial neoplasm of low malignant potential (PUNLMP). Mitotic figures are rare and limited to the basal layers.

**11. Correct choice: B.**

High-grade noninvasive urothelial carcinoma displays marked architectural and cytologic atypia, as shown in the image. There is moderate-to-severe cellular pleomorphism, mitotic activity, atypical mitotic figures, and apoptotic bodies. These features often involve the full thickness of the urothelium. These high-grade lesions are usually invasive by the time of detection. As mentioned previously, malignant progression rate is 15% to 40%. If a papillary urothelial tumor has both low-grade and high-grade areas, it should be diagnosed as high grade.

**12. Correct choice: B.**

Urothelial carcinoma in situ (CIS) refers to areas of bladder mucosa where the normal urothelium has been replaced by neoplastic epithelium that does not invade through the basement membrane. CIS is a recognized precancerous lesion but is usually asymptomatic. It is frequently detected (90% of cases) in association with other urothelial neoplasms or in patients with a history of prior bladder tumors, whereas the presentation described in the question stem is rare (on the other hand, microscopic hematuria is common with CIS). Most cases of CIS progress to invasive cancer if not appropriately treated. To make a diagnosis of urothelial CIS, one should remember that cytologic atypia need not be full thickness, CIS cells may have a pagetoid spread, a high nuclear-to-cytoplasmic ratio is not a constant feature of CIS, umbrella cells may still be present, and the degree of cytologic atypia is variable.

**13. Correct choice: D.**

Urothelial carcinoma (UC), especially if high grade, shows marked morphologic heterogeneity. Up to 27% of UCs contain areas of divergent differentiation, in which the tumor may mimic histologically diverse neoplasms. The most frequent of these cases is UC with squamous differentiation, which seems to impart a worse response to conventional treatments. Squamous differentiation is detected in 20% of invasive UC. The other types are rare. Sarcomatoid UC is a biphasic tumor with a malignant epithelial (usually urothelial) and mesenchymal component (usually undifferentiated sarcoma).

**14. Correct choice: B.**

The image shows squamous cell carcinoma (SCC), which is the most common urinary bladder tumor in regions of the world where schistosomiasis is endemic (eg, Middle East and parts of Africa). In contrast, it represents only 5% of urinary bladder tumors in Western countries. Chronic inflammation of the urinary bladder due to any condition (lithiasis, indwelling catheters, diverticula) is a common predisposing factor, but nonfunctioning neurogenic bladders are the most common risk factor in the United States. Often, SCC arising in neurogenic bladders has a basaloid appearance and is associated with human papillomavirus (HPV) infection. Urinary bladder SCC presents as invasive cancer and has a worse prognosis than urothelial carcinoma. Squamous metaplasia and in situ carcinoma are commonly found in areas adjacent to invasive SCC, supporting the notion that SCC in the bladder arises through the usual metaplasia-dysplasia sequence.

**15. Correct choice: A.**

Adenocarcinoma of the bladder represents 2% of all bladder cancers, but it constitutes the great majority of those associated with bladder exstrophy. It usually grows as a polypoid mass in the trigone. Sometimes, it behaves like a signet-ring carcinoma, with diffuse infiltration of the bladder wall. Urachal remnants and bladder diverticula are other anatomic abnormalities that predispose to the development of adenocarcinoma of the bladder. Cigarette smoking is associated with an increased risk of urothelial and squamous cell carcinoma, not adenocarcinoma. Mesonephric rests may be related to some cases of the mesonephric type of adenocarcinoma (clear cell type). *Schistosoma haematobium* infection predisposes to squamous cell carcinoma. The coexistence of cystitis glandularis/cystica and adenocarcinoma is frequent but coincidental.

**16. Correct choice: A.**

The urachus is the conduit connecting the urinary bladder to the umbilicus. It regresses after birth, becoming the median umbilical ligament. Urachal remnants, consisting of allantoid endoderm, are found in one-third of bladders analyzed postmortem. They are usually located on the dome. Such remnants may give rise, rarely, to carcinomas, of which mucinous adenocarcinoma, enteric type, is the most frequent. Squamous cell, small cell/neuroendocrine, urothelial, and anaplastic have also been reported. Since urachal carcinoma involves the free surface of the bladder (dome) and urachal remnants in the median umbilical ligaments can give rise to other neoplasms, the treatment of choice is partial cystectomy with en bloc resection of the entire median umbilical ligament, including the umbilicus. Staging entails documenting neoplastic spread in the urachus and adjacent structures.

**17. Correct choice: B.**

All variants of urothelial carcinoma are aggressive neoplasms associated with a much worse prognosis than the usual type of urothelial carcinoma (UC), and the micropapillary variant is no exception. However, the majority of micropapillary carcinomas of the bladder have been recently found to harbor HER2 amplification, which may be exploited for therapeutic purposes by using monoclonal antibodies (such as trastuzumab) that disrupt HER2 receptors.

**18. Correct choice: D.**

Rhabdomyosarcoma of the bladder is a mesenchymal neoplasm that is the most common bladder malignancy in pediatric age. Most cases are exophytic embryonal rhabdomyosarcomas that may or may not contain a botryoid component. The tumor presents as a large polypoid mass protruding into the vesicle lumen in the trigone area, covered by atrophic mucosa. Diffuse infiltration of the bladder wall without an exophytic component is a less frequent growth pattern. Neoplastic cells tend to form a condensation underneath the mucosa, which is a highly characteristic microscopic feature known as cambium layer. Cross-striations and immunohistochemical markers of skeletal muscle differentiation (desmin, myogenin, myoglobin) are identifiable in better-differentiated neoplastic cells. Leiomyosarcoma is the most common bladder sarcoma in adults.

**19. Correct choice: E.**

Postoperative spindle cell nodule is a small nodular lesion that may develop after transurethral surgical interventions and has been reported in the vagina as well. It may generate confusion with sarcoma because of its high proliferative rate and immunoreactivity for actin. Delicate vascular network with scattered inflammatory cells and a myxoid matrix favor a benign lesion. An inflammatory pseudotumor, also of a reactive nature, develops most commonly in children and is composed of spindle cells within a myxoid background and a chronic inflammatory infiltrate. Postoperative granuloma may develop as a result of surgery.

# 45 Prostate and Seminal Vesicles

1. Which of the following is true about prostatic infarcts in surgically resected specimens?

    A. Clinically silent
    B. Found in fewer than 2% of specimens
    C. Frequently associated with areas of squamous metaplasia
    D. Frequently associated with foci of carcinoma
    E. Occur in small glands as often as in enlarged glands

2. A needle biopsy reveals the lesion shown in Figure 1. Which of the following is the cause of this prostatic lesion?

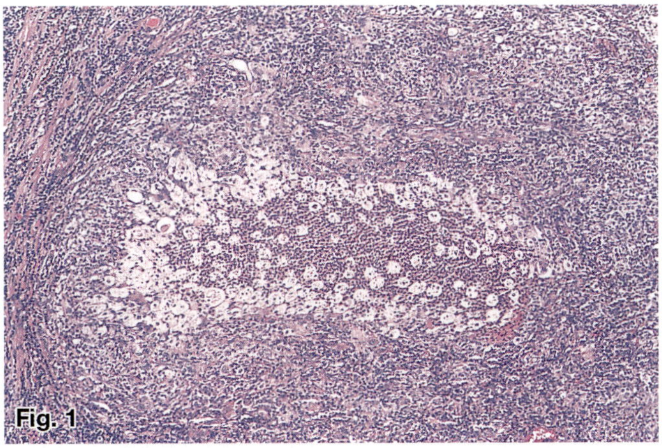

Fig. 1

    A. Allergic reaction
    B. Infarct
    C. Mycobacterial infection
    D. Previous biopsy
    E. Rupture of ducts and acini

3. Besides age, which of the following is a well-recognized factor that influences the incidence of prostatic carcinoma?

    A. Exposure to environmental toxins
    B. Fat consumption
    C. Nodular hyperplasia
    D. Race
    E. Vitamin A intake

4. Which of the following is true of prostate cancer screening?

    A. Complex form of prostate-specific antigen (PSA) is released predominantly by hyperplastic prostate.
    B. False-negative rate of core biopsies is approximately 25%.
    C. Free form of PSA is released predominantly by prostate cancer.
    D. Transrectal ultrasonography (TRUS) has a 95% sensitivity.
    E. Tumor seeding after transrectal needle biopsy is not uncommon.

5. A prostatic carcinoma is detected by needle biopsy. The tumor has only one pattern, which is illustrated in Figure 1. Which of the following is the corresponding Gleason score?

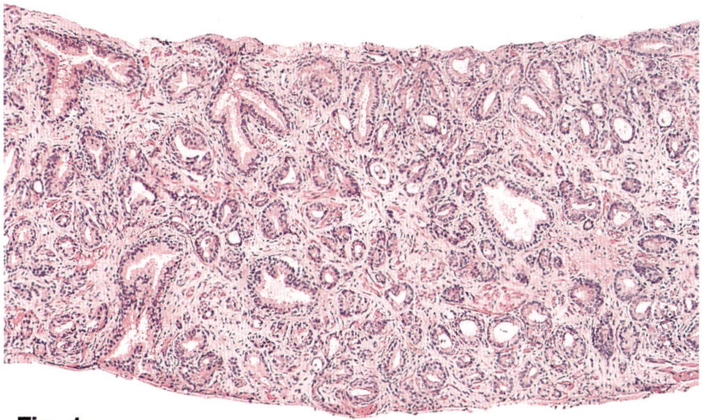

Fig. 1

    A. 2
    B. 3
    C. 6
    D. 9
    E. 10

All figures in this chapter are from Longacre TA, Greenson JK, Hornick JL, Reuter VE, eds. *Mills and Sternberg's Diagnostic Surgical Pathology*. 7th ed. Wolters Kluwer; 2022 except for those noted at the end of this book.

6. A prostatic carcinoma is detected by needle biopsy. Figure 1 shows the tumor's dominant pattern (on the lower right) and secondary pattern (on the upper left). Which of the following is the corresponding Gleason score?

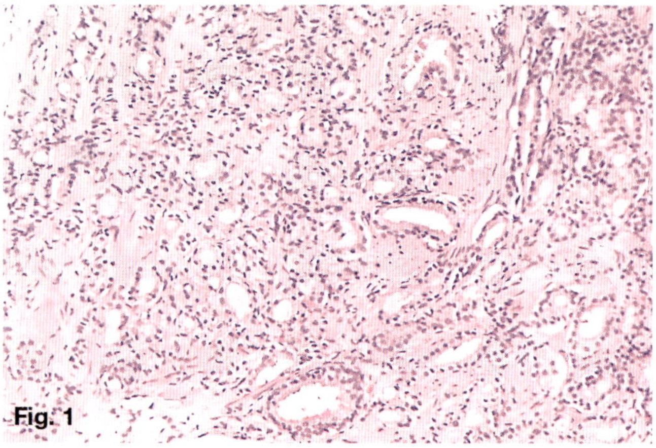

Fig. 1

A. 3
B. 5
C. 7
D. 9
E. 10

7. Gleason score assessed in needle biopsies is a powerful predictor of the pathologic findings in prostatectomy specimens, prognosis after radical prostatectomy, and prognosis following radiotherapy. Which of the following Gleason scores represents the major divide between low-risk and medium-risk prostate cancer?

A. 2 to 3
B. 4 to 5
C. 5 to 6
D. 6 to 7
E. 7 to 8

8. Which of the following histopathologic features in a prostatic biopsy favors a diagnosis of adenocarcinoma over that of prostatic hyperplasia?

A. Atrophic glands
B. Conspicuous nucleoli
C. Corpora amylacea
D. Inflammatory infiltrate
E. Large glands with papillary infoldings

9. A prostatic needle biopsy from a patient with an elevated serum prostate-specific antigen (PSA) is submitted for histopathologic evaluation. Most of the tissue in the biopsy consists of normal glands and stroma, but there is a small focus of crowded small glands suspicious for malignancy. In this context, which of the following parameters is most helpful in making a diagnosis of cancer?

A. Intraluminal crystalloids
B. Mitoses
C. Nuclear hyperchromasia/enlargement
D. Prominent nucleoli
E. All of the above

10. A prostatic needle biopsy reveals the lesion shown in Figure 1. What is the most likely diagnosis?

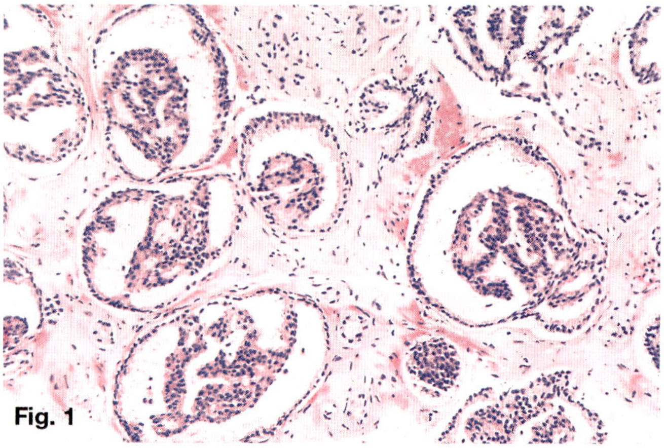

Fig. 1

A. Adenocarcinoma
B. Atrophic gland
C. Atypical adenomatous hyperplasia (adenosis)
D. Benign prostatic hyperplasia
E. Mucous gland metaplasia

11. A section of a prostatic needle biopsy is immunohistochemically stained for α-methyl acyl-CoA racemase (AMACR). The result is shown in Figure 1. What is the most likely diagnosis?

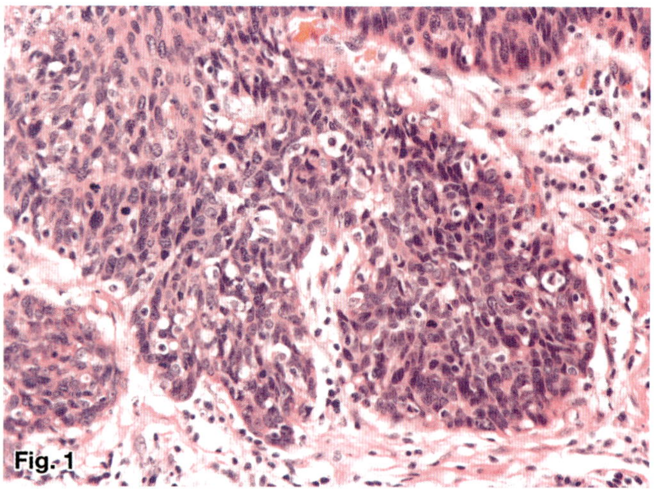

Fig. 1

A. Adenocarcinoma
B. Atrophic gland
C. Atypical adenomatous hyperplasia (adenosis)
D. Benign prostatic hyperplasia
E. Mucous gland metaplasia

12. In transurethral prostate resection (TUPR) specimens, which of the following parameters is most helpful in the differential diagnosis between prostatic atypical adenomatous hyperplasia (adenosis) and low-grade adenocarcinoma?

A. Architectural features
B. Back-to-back glands
C. Intraluminal crystalloids
D. Medium-sized nucleoli
E. Minimal infiltrative behavior

13. Figure 1 shows the most significant finding in a prostatic needle biopsy of a 60-year-old man with a slightly elevated serum prostate-specific antigen (PSA). What is the most likely diagnosis?

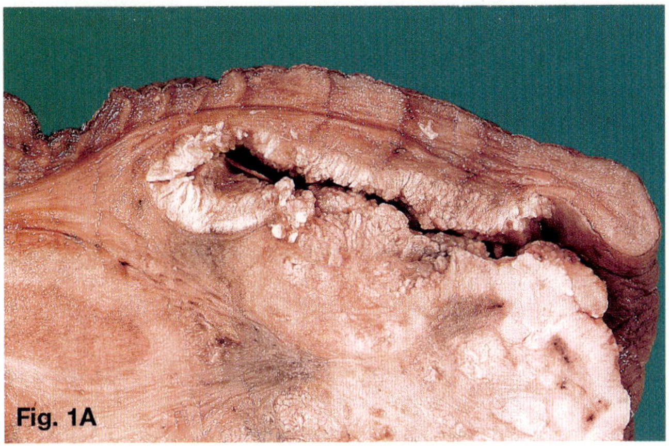
Fig. 1A

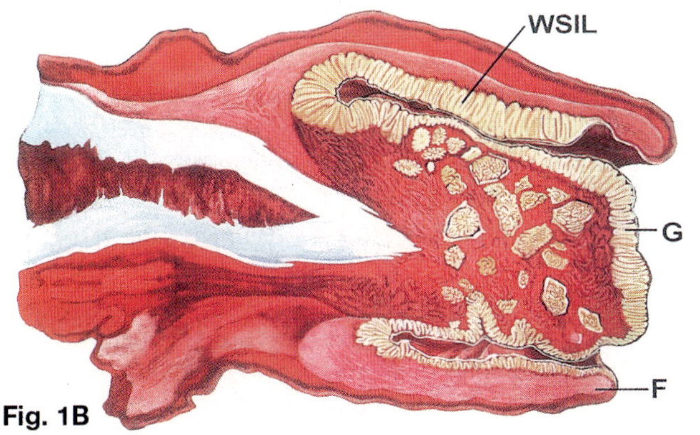

Fig. 1B

A. Atrophic glands
B. Colonic mucosa
C. Cowper glands
D. Seminal vesicles
E. Verumontanum hyperplasia

14. Which of the following features will differentiate low-grade from high-grade prostatic intraepithelial neoplasia (PIN)?

A. Absence of immunolabeling for basal cell–specific markers
B. Architectural features
C. Macronucleoli
D. Mitotic figures
E. Nuclear enlargement

15. A patient undergoes radical prostatectomy because of a palpable (stage II) carcinoma. Which of the following is correct regarding the pathologic staging of this cancer?

A. Capsular invasion is seldom detected.
B. Extracapsular extension usually occurs anteriorly.
C. Microscopic extraprostatic extension is found in 50% of cases.
D. Perineural infiltration has prognostic significance.
E. Tumor is usually difficult to detect on gross examination.

16. A poorly differentiated carcinoma is detected in a transurethral prostate resection (TUPR) specimen, raising the differential diagnosis between prostatic adenocarcinoma and urothelial carcinoma infiltrating from the urinary bladder. Which of the following is the most sensitive and specific marker of urothelial cancer that does not stain prostatic carcinoma?

A. CK7
B. CK20
C. GATA3
D. NKX3.1
E. p501S (prostein)

17. A prostatic biopsy reveals the lesion shown in Figure 1. What is the most likely diagnosis?

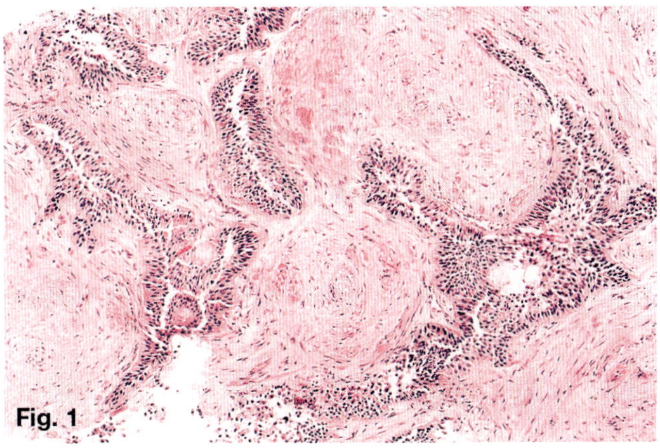
Fig. 1

A. Adenocarcinoma
B. Atypical adenomatous hyperplasia
C. Basal cell carcinoma
D. Basal cell hyperplasia (BCH)
E. High-grade prostatic intraepithelial neoplasia (PIN)

# ANSWERS AND EXPLANATIONS

**1. Correct choice: C.**

Prostatic infarcts are common, involving up to 25% of surgical specimens (much less often in needle biopsies). They are usually found in enlarged glands and are accompanied by acute urinary retention and hematuria. The symptoms, however, are probably due to the gland enlargement rather than the infarct itself. Acute infarcts are areas of coagulative necrosis, which later heal by scarring. Areas of squamous metaplasia are commonly found around infarcts and may be confused for cancer because of the presence of pleomorphism and atypical mitotic figures. There is no association between infarcts and carcinoma.

**2. Correct choice: E.**

The image shows the typical appearance of nonspecific granulomatous prostatitis, a common condition thought to result from an inflammatory reaction to prostatic secretions released into the stroma by ruptured ducts and acini. It consists of a lobular infiltrate of lymphocytes, plasma cells, foamy histiocytes, and small numbers of neutrophils. In early stages, a dilated duct is seen at the center of the lesion (as evident in the picture). The condition manifests with symptoms of urinary obstruction or lower urinary tract infection. Nodularity on palpation accompanied by elevated prostate-specific antigen (PSA) clinically mimics carcinoma. Mycobacterial prostatitis produces caseating granulomas. Allergic prostatitis is a very rare condition associated with other allergic manifestations, such as asthma. Postbiopsy granulomas consist of a central region of fibrinoid necrosis surrounded by palisading histiocytes.

**3. Correct choice: D.**

Of the mentioned factors, only age and race seem to affect the risk of developing prostatic carcinoma. By the age of 50, up to 34% of men will have occult foci of prostatic carcinoma, a rate that increases to 70% by the age of 70. The age-adjusted incidence (cases/100,000) rate varies dramatically among different ethnic groups: 3 to 4 for Japanese men, 50 for American White men, and higher rates for Blacks. Environmental influences are suspected of playing a role in the development of this cancer, but no specific toxin has been identified. The role played by fat consumption and vitamin A intake is currently under investigation. Benign prostatic hyperplasia (BPH), although often associated with cancer, does not predispose to cancer according to most studies.

**4. Correct choice: B.**

Prostate-specific antigen (PSA) levels with or without transrectal ultrasonography (TRUS) are the mainstay of most screening programs. TRUS alone has a low sensitivity and low specificity. Methods to increase the sensitivity and specificity of PSA measurement include determination of the PSA index (PSA/gram of tissue determined by TRUS), age-specific reference ranges, and percentage of free PSA. Free PSA is released predominantly by hyperplastic tissue, whereas the complex form of PSA is released mainly by cancer. Core needle biopsies may be performed by transrectal or, seldom, transperineal route. Tumor seeding along needle track does not occur with transrectal biopsies, while occasionally, it does occur with transperineal biopsies. Overall, the false-negative rate of core needle biopsies by the transrectal route is 25%.

**5. Correct choice: C.**

Gleason grading is a widely used grading system that is based on architectural features evaluated on low power. Two main patterns are identified, the dominant pattern (to which a score from 1 to 5 is assigned) and a subdominant pattern (to which another score of 1-5 is applied). The Gleason score is determined by adding the two scores. If only one pattern is identifiable, its score is doubled. The image shows a pattern 3; thus, in this example, the Gleason score is 6.

**6. Correct choice: C.**

In the lower right, the tumor is composed of well-formed glands, which is consistent with a Gleason pattern 3. In the upper right, the glands are fused and have infiltrating edges, consistent with Gleason pattern 4. Since the former is the dominant pattern, and the latter is the secondary pattern, the Gleason score is $3 + 4 = 7$.

**7. Correct choice: D.**

Most prostatic adenocarcinomas detected by needle biopsies are given Gleason scores of 6 and 7. Carcinoma with a Gleason score of 6 or less is considered low risk and usually followed with watchful waiting, without further treatment. Carcinoma with a Gleason score of 7 or higher needs treatment.

**8. Correct choice: B.**

The features listed in choices A, C, D, and E are variably present in prostatic hyperplasia, but nucleoli of epithelial cells remain inconspicuous. Prostatic adenocarcinoma, on the contrary, is composed of cells that usually show prominent nucleoli (larger than 1 μm).

**9. Correct choice: E.**

One of the most difficult problems is diagnosing prostatic cancer in biopsies where the amount of neoplastic tissue is scanty. This problem is obviously more frequent in needle biopsies than in transurethral resection (TUR) material. In these cases, one should not rely on a single parameter (eg, nuclear enlargement or macronucleoli) but rather on the full spectrum of cytologic changes. Cytologic features are more important than architectural ones in needle biopsy specimens. Atrophic glands and seminal vesicles are two of the most common sources of diagnostic difficulties in needle biopsies.

**10. Correct choice: A.**

There are three morphologic features that are characteristic of prostatic adenocarcinoma and never found in benign prostatic tissue: glomerulations (shown in the image), perineural invasion, and mucinous fibroplasia (collagenous nodules).

**11. Correct choice: A.**

α-Methyl acyl-CoA racemase (AMACR) is a marker of prostatic malignancy that can be very helpful in difficult cases when a limited amount of tumor is present in biopsies. Benign glands are negative for this marker, whereas about 80% of prostatic adenocarcinomas are positive. Furthermore, many cases of prostatic intraepithelial neoplasia (PIN) and some cases of adenosis and atrophic glands are positive for the marker. Basal cell layer can be immunostained with antibodies to high-molecular-weight cytokeratin and p63. Lack of a basal cell layer favors cancer.

**12. Correct choice: A.**

Distinguishing between adenosis and low-grade adenocarcinoma of the prostate is particularly challenging with transurethral resection (TUR) specimens. Adenosis may show atypical features, such as minimal infiltration at the periphery, occasionally prominent nucleoli, and back-to-back crowding of glands. Adenosis, however, is composed of glands with a lobular configuration, whereas in adenocarcinoma, the glands are arranged haphazardly. Furthermore, in adenosis, there is a gradual transition with adjacent normal-appearing glands. Immunolabeling with basal cell–specific antibodies to high-molecular-weight cytokeratin or p63 may help in the differential diagnosis.

**13. Correct choice: D.**

In needle biopsies, seminal vesicles may result in overdiagnosis of prostatic adenocarcinoma. Seminal vesicles are often seen at the edge of the tissue sample and appear as glands arranged around a central lumen. Their lipofuscin pigment is a helpful diagnostic feature. Atrophic glands may produce a seemingly infiltrative pattern, but they appear more basophilic than carcinoma. Cowper glands consist of ducts surrounded by mucinous glands. Verumontanum glands are located beneath the urethra and contain pale red concretions and corpora amylacea.

**14. Correct choice: C.**

PIN refers to the presence of cytologically atypical cells lining architecturally normal acini or ducts. It can be low or high grade, and the distinction between the two grades relies on the presence of prominent nucleoli (eg, visible at 20 times magnification). High-grade prostatic intraepithelial neoplasia (PIN) is found in approximately 5% of prostate needle biopsies. When high-grade PIN is diagnosed on biopsy, there is a 23% to 35% probability of finding prostate cancer on a subsequent biopsy. Glands in PIN are architecturally similar to benign glands, but more basophilic owing to hyperplasia, nuclear enlargement and hyperchromasia, and amphophilic cytoplasm. The tufting pattern is the most common type of high-grade PIN, with papillary tufts lined by atypical cells.

**15. Correct choice: C.**

Clinically, stage II cancer is palpable, but it does not spread outside the prostate. Histologic evaluation shows that 50% of these cases have microscopic extracapsular extension, thus becoming stage III. Extracapsular extension occurs in the posterolateral region. The tumor is grossly evident in up to 85% of specimens. Capsular invasion is frequent, but it should not be confused with extracapsular extension, that is, infiltration of extraprostatic tissues. Perineural infiltration is a common finding in prostatic adenocarcinoma and correlates with the likelihood of extracapsular extension; however, it is not an independent prognostic factor.

**16. Correct choice: C.**

The distinction between poorly differentiated prostatic and urothelial carcinomas can be challenging or impossible based on hematoxylin and eosin (H&E) morphology alone. About 95% of poorly differentiated prostatic cancer is immunoreactive for prostate-specific antigen (PSA), and those tumors negative for PSA may be positive for the newer prostate-specific markers, NKX3.1 and p501S (prostein). GATA3 is the most specific and sensitive immunohistochemical marker for urothelial carcinoma.

**17. Correct choice: D.**

The image shows the classic appearance of basal cell hyperplasia (BCH), which consists of solid nests of uniform cells resembling normal basal cells. The nests display characteristic peripheral palisading, occasionally with a small central lumen. Lamellar calcifications and intracytoplasmic eosinophilic globules are features characteristic of BCH, but not of carcinoma. However, cells in BCH may have prominent nucleoli, enlarged hyperchromatic nuclei, mitotic figures, and blue-tinged mucinous secretions. Table 1 lists the features allowing a differential diagnosis between BCH and high-grade prostatic intraepithelial neoplasia (PIN). There is no association between BCH and acinar adenocarcinoma or basal cell carcinoma.

**TABLE 1 Differential Diagnosis: High-Grade Prostatic Intraepithelial Neoplasia and Basal Cell Hyperplasia With Nucleoli**

| Basal Cell Hyperplasia | HGPIN |
|---|---|
| Often small, crowded glands | Large glands without crowding |
| Occasional solid nests | Glands with well-formed lumina |
| Basal cells with atypical nuclei (blue) undermine secretory cells with benign nuclei (red/violet) | No two distinct cell populations |
| Basal cell nuclei stream parallel to basement membrane | Atypical cells oriented perpendicular to basement membrane |
| Atypical nuclei positive for basal cell markers | Atypical nuclei negative for basal cell markers; underlying flattened, benign-appearing cells positive |

HGPIN, high-grade intraepithelial neoplasia.

# 46 Nonneoplastic Diseases of the Testis

1. Persons undergoing vasectomy are particularly prone to developing which of the following conditions?

   A. Fibrosarcoma
   B. Lipoma
   C. Proliferative funiculitis
   D. Testicular infarction
   E. Vasitis nodosa

2. A 55-year-old man presents with unilateral painless enlargement of the testis. A biopsy discloses granulomatous inflammation within the stroma without evidence of neoplasm. Numerous neutrophils and plasma cells are also present. Special stains for fungi or acid-fast bacilli are negative. Michaelis-Gutmann bodies are not seen. Which of the following is the prevalent etiologic/pathogenetic factor in this condition?

   A. Autoimmune
   B. Genetic
   C. Infectious
   D. Sarcoidosis
   E. Treponema

3. A diagnosis of "normal spermatogenesis" is made on a testicular biopsy from a patient with azoospermia. Which of the following causes is compatible with this diagnosis?

   A. Excurrent duct obstruction
   B. Exposure to excess heat
   C. Hypothyroidism
   D. Klinefelter syndrome
   E. Radiation effect

All figures in this chapter are from Longacre TA, Greenson JK, Hornick JL, Reuter VE, eds. *Mills and Sternberg's Diagnostic Surgical Pathology*. 7th ed. Wolters Kluwer; 2022 except for those noted at the end of this book.

# ANSWERS AND EXPLANATIONS

**1. Correct choice: E.**

Vasitis nodosa is a benign granulomatous reaction around the vas deferens, which most commonly arises following vasectomy or herniorrhaphy. Proliferative funiculitis is a peculiar entity histologically identical to proliferative fasciitis. It constitutes a frequent incidental finding in hernia sacs. Lipomas are the most common neoplasms of the spermatic cord.

**2. Correct choice: A.**

Nonspecific granulomatous orchitis is thought to result from an autoimmune reaction against testicular antigens, perhaps unmasked by traumatic injury. Indeed, a history of trauma can be elicited in a significant number of cases. It usually presents in middle-aged or older men in a manner simulating carcinoma. Histologically, it may be confused with malakoplakia.

**3. Correct choice: A.**

Excurrent duct obstruction is caused by obstruction of the excurrent duct system distal to the rete testis. It can be congenital (atresia of components of the excurrent duct system) or acquired (as in cystic fibrosis, infection, sterilization). The typical presentation is a triad of azoospermia, normal-sized testes, and active spermatogenesis. Active spermatogenesis can continue for years after the obstruction. On the other hand, all of the other conditions listed present with diminished or absent spermatogenesis.

# 47 Testicular and Paratesticular Tumors

1. Which of the following is the risk factor with the strongest correlation with testicular germ cell tumors?

   A. Cryptorchidism
   B. Disorders of sex development (intersex syndromes)
   C. Family history of testicular germ cell tumor
   D. Oligospermic infertility
   E. Prior testicular germ cell tumor

2. The testicular lesion shown in Figure 1 is not considered a precursor for which germ cell tumor?

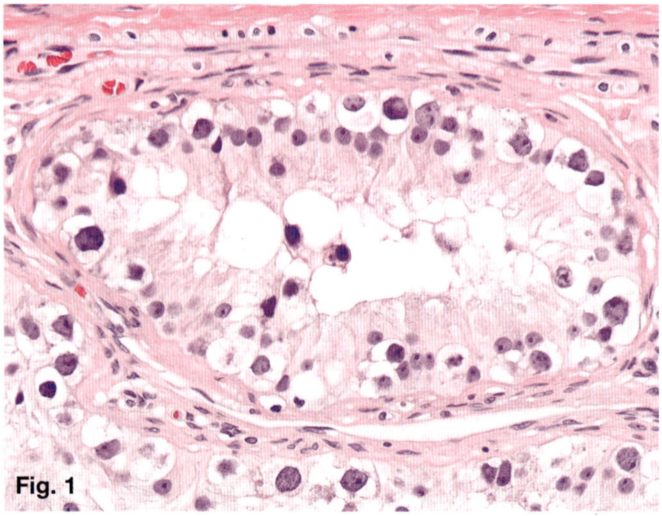

Fig. 1

   A. Choriocarcinoma
   B. Classic seminoma
   C. Embryonal carcinoma
   D. Spermatocytic seminoma
   E. Teratoma

3. A testicular biopsy in a 40-year-old patient shows a neoplasm consisting of cells with conspicuous nucleoli and clear cytoplasm arranged in a nesting pattern, as shown in Figure 1. Fibrous septae between neoplastic nests contain numerous lymphocytes. Mitotic figures are rare. Tumor cells are immunoreactive for placental alkaline phosphatase (PLAP). Which of the following is the most likely diagnosis?

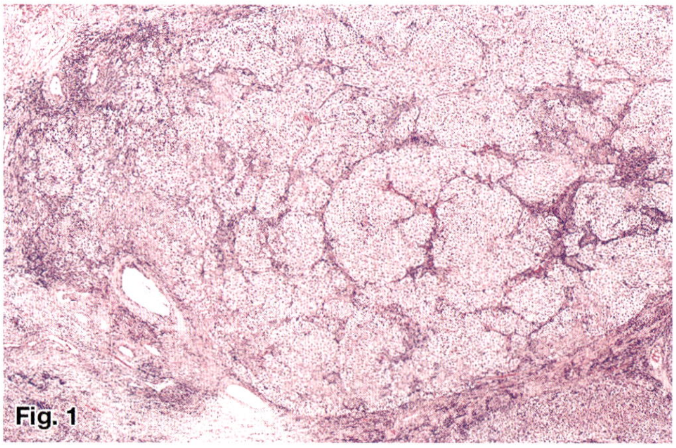

Fig. 1

   A. Anaplastic seminoma
   B. Embryonal cell carcinoma
   C. Lymphoma
   D. Seminoma
   E. Spermatocytic seminoma

---

All figures in this chapter are from Longacre TA, Greenson JK, Hornick JL, Reuter VE, eds. *Mills and Sternberg's Diagnostic Surgical Pathology*. 7th ed. Wolters Kluwer; 2022, except for those noted at the end of this book.

4. A 70-year-old man undergoes an orchiectomy for a testicular tumor. Histologically, the tumor consists of a polymorphic population of small, intermediate, and giant cells, as seen in Figure 1. Mitotic activity is present. Which of the following features is typical of this tumor?

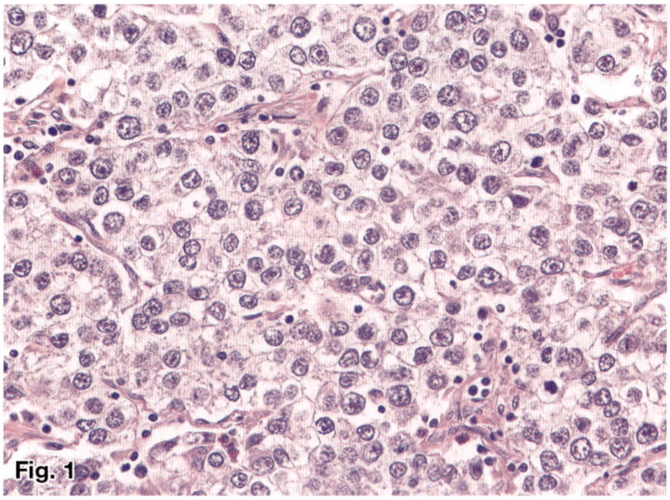
Fig. 1

A. It is associated with cryptorchidism.
B. It may occur in extratesticular sites.
C. Metastatic spread is rare.
D. Orchiectomy and radiation are the recommended treatments.
E. Placental alkaline phosphatase (PLAP) immunoreactivity is usually detected.

5. A testicular tumor from a 30-year-old man consists of highly anaplastic epithelial cells with poorly defined borders arranged in papillary structures, as seen in Figure 1. Multifocal coagulative necrosis is noted. Neoplastic cells express CK8, CK18, and CD30. Which of the following is true about this tumor?

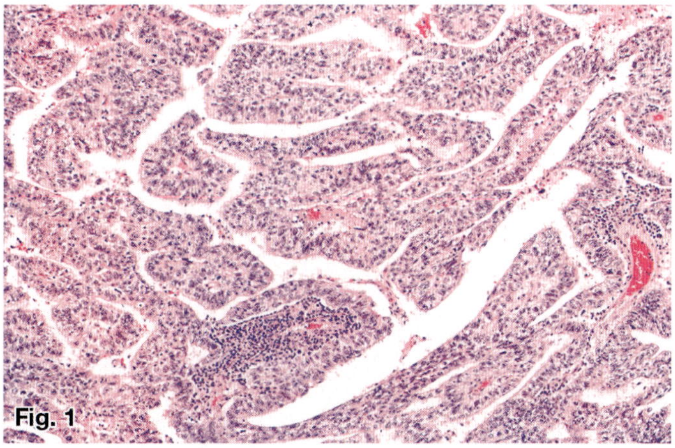
Fig. 1

A. In its pure form it accounts for 30% of testicular neoplasms.
B. It is most commonly associated with yolk sac or trophoblastic components.
C. It is most frequent in children under 3 years.
D. It is uniformly positive for placental alkaline phosphatase (PLAP).
E. Mitotic activity is low or absent.

6. The most common testicular neoplasm in children less than 3 years of age is characterized by a spongy texture on the surface. Microscopically, its most typical pattern is characterized by fibrovascular cores "festooned" by tumor cells, as shown in Figure 1. Which of the following is it?

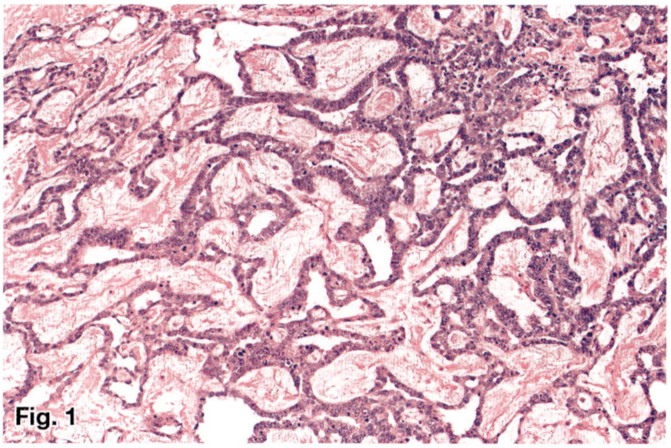
Fig. 1

A. Choriocarcinoma
B. Embryonal carcinoma
C. Seminoma
D. Teratoma
E. Yolk sac tumor

7. A testicular teratoma

A. behaves as a malignant tumor in children and as a benign tumor in adults.
B. consists of a cyst filled with keratin and hair.
C. is usually associated with other germ cell tumors in adults.
D. is usually immature in prepubertal age.
E. occurs more frequently in pure form in adult patients.

8. Which of the following testicular tumors is a specialized form of teratoma?

A. Carcinoid tumor
B. Dermoid cyst
C. Epidermoid cyst
D. Primitive neuroectodermal tumor (PNET)
E. All of the above

9. An 18-year-old male is evaluated for the acute onset of right hemiplegia. A computed tomography (CT) scan shows a well-demarcated hemorrhagic mass in the left frontal lobe. The mass is removed and reveals the neoplasm shown in Figure 1. Further investigations lead to the discovery of a testicular tumor. Which of the following is the most likely diagnosis?

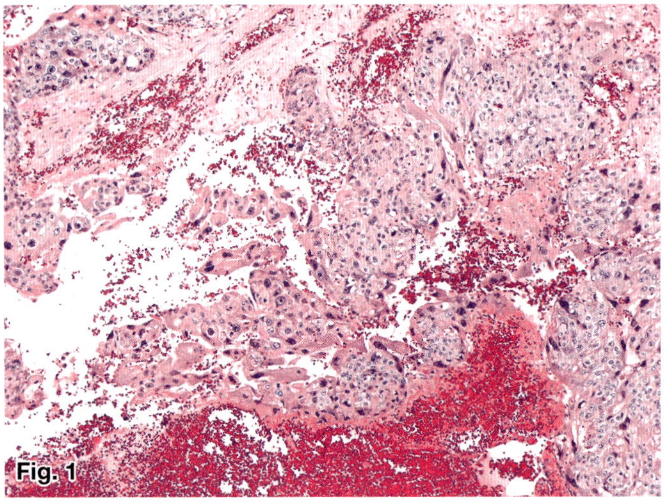

Fig. 1

A. Choriocarcinoma
B. Embryonal carcinoma
C. Seminoma
D. Teratoma
E. Yolk sac tumor

10. Histologic analysis of an orchiectomy specimen reveals a neoplasm whose microscopic appearance is shown in Figure 1. Which of the following is the diagnosis?

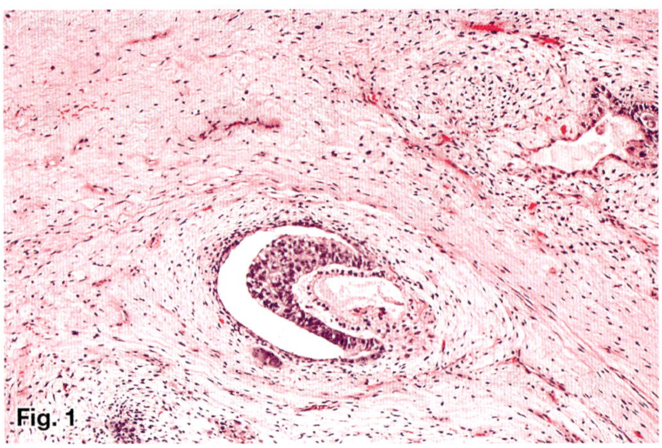

Fig. 1

A. Burned-out germ cell tumor
B. Diffuse embryoma
C. Placental site trophoblastic tumor
D. Polyembryoma
E. Yolk sac tumor

11. Histologic examination of a 2-cm testicular tumor from a 40-year-old man with gynecomastia shows sheets of polygonal cells with eosinophilic cytoplasm. Many rod-shaped intracytoplasmic crystals are identified, as shown in Figure 1. Electron microscopy reveals abundant smooth endoplasmic reticulum, mitochondria with tubular cristae, lipid droplets, and cytoplasmic elongated crystalloids. Which of the following is the most likely diagnosis?

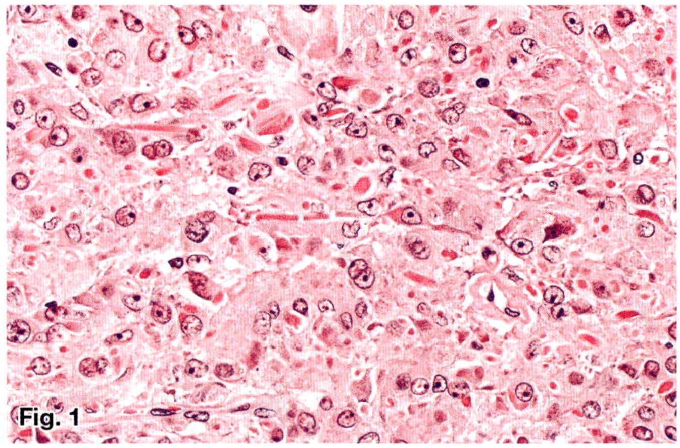

Fig. 1

A. Adrenogenital syndrome
B. Choriocarcinoma
C. Leydig cell hyperplasia
D. Leydig cell tumor
E. Sertoli cell tumor

12. Which of the following histologic patterns is most characteristic of Sertoli cell tumors?

A. Glandular arrangement
B. Mixture of cytotrophoblast and syncytiotrophoblast
C. Round nests between lymphocyte-rich septa
D. Stromal fibrovascular core surrounded by double-cell layer
E. Structures reminiscent of immature seminiferous tubules

13. Which of the following is a mixed germ cell-sex cord-stromal tumor that develops in patients with gonadal dysgenesis?

A. Diffuse embryoma
B. Gonadoblastoma
C. Granulosa cell tumor
D. Polyembryoma
E. Sertoli-Leydig cell tumor

14. Which of the following is the most common testicular neoplasm in patients over the age of 60 years?

A. Classic seminoma
B. Embryonal carcinoma
C. Lymphoma
D. Mixed germ cell tumor
E. Spermatocytic seminoma

15. Which of the following is the most common source of metastatic neoplasm to the testis in adults?

A. Colon
B. Kidney
C. Lungs
D. Melanoma
E. Prostate

16. A tumor attached to the epididymis is resected. Its histologic appearance is shown in Figure 1. Which of the following is the most likely diagnosis?

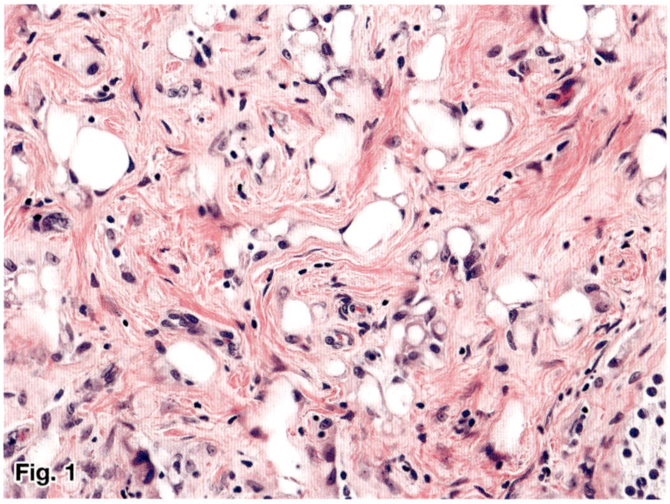
Fig. 1

A. Adenomatoid tumor
B. Lipoma
C. Melanotic neuroectodermal tumor
D. Papillary cystadenoma
E. Rhabdomyosarcoma

17. A 30-year-old man presents with bilateral tumors of the epididymal head. Surgically removed, both tumors present the histologic appearance depicted in Figure 1. Which of the following genetic conditions is associated with this type of tumor?

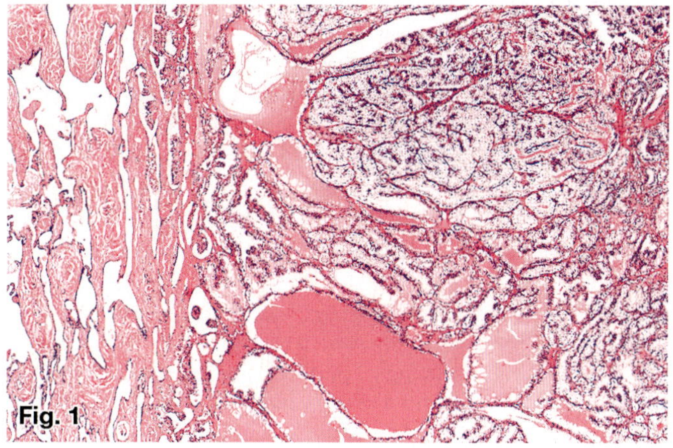
Fig. 1

A. Androgen insensitivity syndrome
B. Intersex syndromes
C. Klinefelter syndrome
D. Turner syndrome
E. von Hippel-Lindau syndrome

18. Which of the following is true about rhabdomyosarcoma of the spermatic cord?

A. It affects adults more frequently than children.
B. It is extremely rare in this location.
C. It is usually of the embryonal type.
D. Spindle cell subtype has the worst prognosis.
E. Tumor size and age have no prognostic impact.

# ANSWERS AND EXPLANATIONS

**1. Correct choice: A.**

Of all those factors, cryptorchidism is the most common, with 10% of germ cell tumors (GCTs) associated with history of corrected or uncorrected cryptorchidism. Intratubular germ cell neoplasia, unclassified (IGCNU), the precursor lesion of GCTs, is present in 2% to 4% of cryptorchid testes; 50% of patients who have IGCNU on biopsy will develop a GCT within 5 years. All other conditions listed are associated with variably increased risk of GCTs.

**2. Correct choice: D.**

Intratubular germ cell neoplasia, unclassified (IGCNU) is analogous to carcinoma in situ. It describes an intratubular precursor lesion consisting of germ cells with enlarged nuclei, prominent nucleoli, and periodic acid-Schiff (PAS)-positive/diastase-sensitive clear cytoplasm. Cells of IGCNU can be identified, thanks to their immunoreactivity for placental alkaline phosphatase (PLAP). Other positive markers in IGCNU include D2-40 (podoplanin), OCT3/OCT4, and CD117. Patients with a diagnosis of IGCNU eventually develop germ cell tumors in 50% of cases at 5 years. IGCNU is most commonly found in patients with cryptorchidism, patients with infertility, and in the testis contralateral to a testis affected by a germ cell tumor. IGCNU may be seen in association with virtually all germ cell tumors except spermatocytic seminoma. Conversely, spermatocytic seminoma is the only germ cell neoplasm reported not to occur in an undescended testis. The association of IGCNU with prepubertal yolk sac tumor is controversial.

**3. Correct choice: D.**

In its pure form, seminoma represents 50% of germ cell tumors (GCTs). It is composed of two cell types, neoplastic germ cells with central conspicuous nucleoli and reactive lymphocytes within the stroma. The architectural features may vary from the classic multinodular pattern, to sheetlike, a cord-like, tubular, or pseudomicrocystic pattern. It is important to differentiate these neoplasms from embryonal carcinoma and spermatocytic carcinoma. Embryonal carcinoma displays more severe pleomorphism and high mitotic activity and retains an epithelial-like appearance even in the most anaplastic types. Several immunohistochemical markers have become available to aid in the differential diagnosis. Seminomas are positive for placental alkaline phosphatase (PLAP), CD117, podoplanin (D2-40), and OCT3/OCT4 and negative for pan-keratin, epithelial membrane antigen (EMA), and CD30. Also, seminomas express SOX17 but not SOX2. Embryonal carcinoma is positive for pan-keratin, CD30, and SOX2 and negative for CD117, podoplanin (D2-40), and SOX17.

**4. Correct choice: C.**

Spermatocytic seminoma occurs in patients over 50 years of age. Variability in cell size is a peculiarity of this neoplasm, which consists of round small (lymphocyte-like) and medium-sized cells with scattered multinucleated giant cells. The cytoplasm is scanty and eosinophilic without glycogen vacuoles. Tumor cells are usually negative for placental alkaline phosphatase (PLAP), OCT3/OCT4, carcinoembryonic antigen (CEA), α-fetoprotein (AFP), leukocyte common antigen (LCA), human chorionic gonadotropin (hCG), and keratin. Studies support an origin from the primary spermatocyte. This slowly growing tumor rarely metastasizes and is thus associated with a good prognosis. Orchiectomy alone is usually curative.

**5. Correct choice: B.**

Embryonal carcinoma is a malignant tumor composed of pleomorphic epithelial-like cells that consistently express keratin but less often placental alkaline phosphatase (PLAP). Mitotic activity is brisk, and tumor giant cells are frequent. Neoplastic cells are arranged in glandular, papillary, or solid patterns. Tumor cells express CK8, CK18, CD30, OCT3/OCT4, and SOX2. In its pure form, it is rare (<5% of all testicular neoplasms), but embryonal carcinomas mixed with either choriocarcinoma or yolk sac tumor are common. Note that patients with embryonal carcinoma are on average 10 years younger than those with seminoma. In contrast to seminoma, embryonal carcinoma is treated with orchiectomy and chemotherapy. The overall survival rate is about 80%.

**6. Correct choice: E.**

Yolk sac tumor is the most common, whereas teratoma is the second most common testicular tumor in children less than 3 years old. The cut surface of a yolk sac tumor has a spongy appearance due to numerous microcysts. Eleven microscopic patterns have been described, but several of these patterns are commonly present in various combinations within the same tumor. Typically, yolk sac tumor has an organoid architecture characterized by cuboidal cells arranged in glandular, alveolar, and papillary formations, mixed with mesenchymal components. Schiller-Duval bodies consist of a central vessel within a core of mesenchymal tissue, surrounded by cuboidal to columnar malignant cells within a cystic space. Schiller-Duval bodies are characteristic of the endodermal sinus pattern. Hyaline globules are also a common diagnostic feature of yolk sac tumors: They are round, eosinophilic, periodic acid-Schiff (PAS)-positive, diastase-resistant globules from 1 to 50 μm in diameter. Tumor cells express α-fetoprotein (AFP) and pan-keratin and are aneuploid. In adults, yolk sac components are most often seen in mixed germ cell tumors (GCTs). The hepatoid pattern (more common in ovarian tumors) has a striking resemblance to hepatocellular carcinoma. Almost all patients with GCTs containing a yolk sac component have high serum levels of AFP.

**7. Correct choice: C.**

Teratoma is the second most common testicular tumor in children (after yolk sac tumor). The pure form is usually found in children but is distinctly rare in adults, in whom it is usually associated with other forms of germ cell neoplasms. Paradoxically, mature teratomas are more frequent in children than in adults. Childhood teratomas behave as benign tumors treatable with simple orchiectomy, whereas adult teratomas have a higher propensity for metastatic spread. Association with intratubular germ cell neoplasia, unclassified (IGCNU) is another important feature present in adult cases but absent in prepubertal cases. Dermoid cysts are a rare form of testicular mature teratoma. The distinction between "mature" and "immature" teratomas is no longer present in the most recent World Health Organization (WHO) classification since this feature has been found to have no prognostic significance.

**8. Correct choice: E.**

All of these lesions are rare in the testis. Epidermoid cysts are composed of keratinized squamous epithelium without adnexal structures. Dermoid cysts contain adnexal structures. Both lesions should be considered as specialized forms of teratoma. Testicular carcinoid and primitive neuroectodermal tumor (PNET) are considered monodermal variants of teratoma. Twenty percent of testicular carcinoids are associated with teratoma-like components. PNET results from overgrowth of primitive neural elements in teratoma.

**9. Correct choice: A.**

In its pure form, choriocarcinoma is found in 1 of 300 testicular neoplasms, but it is present in 15% of mixed germ cell tumors. Its hemorrhagic appearance and propensity for cerebral metastatic spread are highly characteristic. The classic histologic pattern of this tumor is that of a combination of cytotrophoblastic cells with pale cytoplasm capped by multinucleated syncytiotrophoblastic cells with dark cytoplasm. Neoplastic cells express human chorionic gonadotropin (hCG, whose plasma levels are usually elevated as well), keratin, epithelial membrane antigen (EMA), and sometimes placental alkaline phosphatase (PLAP). The most important differentials in orchiectomy specimens include testicular torsion and infarction.

**10. Correct choice: D.**

Polyembryoma is a mixed germ cell tumor, whose histologic hallmark, the embryoid body, is shown in the image. This is an embryo-like body with a central core of embryonal carcinoma cells within an amniotic-like cavity, associated with a yolk sac tumor component resembling the embryonic yolk sac. Diffuse embryoma, instead, consists of a haphazard admixture of embryonal and yolk sac tumor elements in equal proportion. Placental site trophoblastic tumor is composed of an admixture of intermediate trophoblast with Leydig cells. Regression of the primary testicular tumor is observed in about 10% of patients dying of metastatic disease. Microscopically, burned-out tumors consist of scars with small blood vessels, lymphoplasmacytic infiltrates, hemosiderin-laden macrophages, ghost tubules, and intratubular calcifications.

**11. Correct choice: D.**

Although the so-called crystals of Reinke are found in only 40% of Leydig cell tumors, they constitute a pathognomonic feature. Neoplastic cells produce androgens and estrogens and have ultrastructural features of steroid hormone–producing cells. These tumors occur in children as well as in adults. Children usually manifest sexual precocity, whereas adults present with a testicular mass and, occasionally, gynecomastia. Histologically, they are composed of sheets of polygonal cells with sharp borders and eosinophilic cytoplasm. The differential diagnosis is with Leydig cell hyperplasia (interstitial growth pattern), malakoplakia (Michaelis-Gutmann bodies), and nodules associated with adrenogenital syndrome (multifocal, without crystals of Reinke). Leydig cell tumor is positive for inhibin-α, melan-A, and calretinin.

**12. Correct choice: E.**

Sertoli cell tumor is a rare testicular neoplasm that is composed of neoplastic Sertoli cells that form solid cords resembling primitive seminiferous tubules. Each cord is surrounded by an artifactual, but diagnostically significant, separation from the adjacent stroma. These tumors may produce estrogens and manifest with gynecomastia without associated virilism (in contrast to Leydig cell tumors). Approximately 10% are malignant.

**13. Correct choice: B.**

Gonadoblastoma is a rare benign tumor composed of a mixture of gonadal elements, including large primordial germ cells, sex cord elements (immature Sertoli cells or granulosa cells), and gonadal stromal cells. There are three histologic patterns, the most common of which consists of clusters of immature Sertoli cells and germ cells surrounded by a rim of basement membrane. They occur in patients with intersex syndromes, of whom 80% are phenotypically females and 20% phenotypically males. Syndromes that impart increased risk for gonadoblastomas are Denys-Drash, Frasier, Sawyer, and partial androgen insensitivity. Deficient development of Sertoli cells appears to be the common underlying condition that allows delayed germ cell maturation and subsequent evolution to germ cell neoplasia.

**14. Correct choice: C.**

Testicular lymphoma represents approximately 5% of all testicular tumors, but at least 50% of testicular neoplasms over the age of 60. Not uncommonly, testicular involvement is the first manifestation of disease, but in most cases, lymphoma is widely disseminated when the testicular tumor becomes clinically apparent. Testicular biopsies are thus used for staging purposes. Most cases are high-grade, usually diffuse large B-cell lymphomas. An interstitial growth pattern with relative sparing of tubules is the most important low-power clue to diagnosis of testicular lymphoma. Primary lymphoma of the testis has a 60% 5-year survival.

**15. Correct choice: E.**

The most common testicular metastases come from (in decreasing frequency) (a) adults: prostate, lungs, melanoma, colon, and kidney; (b) children: neuroblastoma, rhabdomyosarcoma, and Wilms tumor. Metastases to the testis may be the presenting manifestation in the absence of a known primary. Microscopically, metastases are characterized by an intertubular pattern associated with lymphatic and vascular invasion.

**16. Correct choice: A.**

Adenomatoid tumor is the most common tumor of the epididymis and is also commonly seen in the spermatic cord, fallopian tube, and uterus. It is thought to be of mesothelial origin and usually presents with a painless testicular mass. Histologically, it is composed of tubular structures lined by cuboidal cells with large cytoplasmic vacuoles. Long, slender apical microvilli of the mesothelial type are detected on ultrastructural examination. Lipoma is the most common tumor of the spermatic cord. Melanotic neuroectodermal tumor is similar to the homonymous tumor of the jaw. Papillary cystadenoma is characterized by papillary structures lined by clear cells within cystic spaces, often associated with von Hippel-Lindau syndrome. Rhabdomyosarcoma is the most common malignant tumor of the spermatic cord.

**17. Correct choice: E.**

The image shows the typical appearance of papillary cystadenoma, with papillary formations lined by a single or double layer of cuboidal-columnar epithelium that projects into cystic spaces containing a colloid-like secretion. The tumor is bilateral in 40% of cases, most of which are associated with von Hippel-Lindau syndrome. Both sporadic and syndromic cases have mutations in the *VHL* gene. Lesions associated with von Hippel-Lindau include hemangioblastomas of retina, cerebellum, and spinal cord, renal cell carcinoma, pheochromocytoma, pancreatic cysts, endolymphatic sac tumor, and bilateral papillary cystadenoma of the epididymis or broad ligament.

**18. Correct choice: C.**

Rhabdomyosarcoma is the most common malignant tumor of the spermatic cord, and 20% of all rhabdomyosarcomas indeed occur at this location. The mean age at presentation is 7 years. Most tumors are of the embryonal type, and most of these have a spindle cell morphology. The spindle cell subtype of embryonal rhabdomyosarcoma is associated with a better prognosis. Few cases are alveolar or pleomorphic types. Immunostains to confirm the diagnosis include MyoD1, myogenin, desmin, and muscle-specific actin. After orchiectomy and chemotherapy or radiotherapy, the overall survival rate is 80%. Poor prognostic factors are alveolar subtype, tumor size greater than 5 cm, and age older than 10 years.

# 48 Penis

1. Which of the following is the cause of Fournier gangrene?

   A. Excessive sexual activity
   B. Implantation of foreign material
   C. Penile torsion
   D. Staphylococci and streptococci
   E. Syphilis

2. A 25-year-old male presents with an ulcerated painless perianal mass, clinically diagnosed as carcinoma. Biopsy of the lesion shows extensive lymphohistiocytic and plasmacellular infiltration. Scrapings of the lesions stained with Wright stain demonstrate large histiocytic cells containing microcysts filled with deeply stained bodies. Which of the following is the etiologic agent?

   A. *Bartonella henselae*
   B. *Calymmatobacterium granulomatis*
   C. *Chlamydia trachomatis*
   D. *Haemophilus ducreyi*
   E. *Treponema pallidum*

3. Figure 1 shows the histologic appearance of a gray-white, atrophic area involving the inner aspect of the foreskin and the glans. Which of the following is the diagnosis?

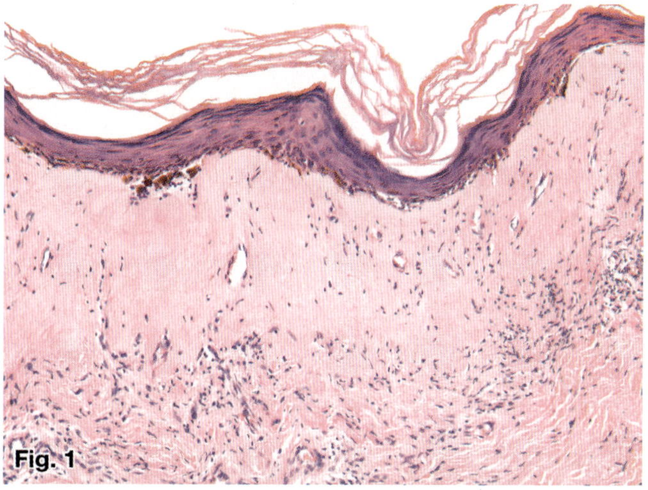


   A. Balanitis circumscripta plasmacellularis
   B. Lichen sclerosus
   C. Penile melanosis
   D. Peyronie disease
   E. Sclerosing lymphangitis of the penis

4. Erythroplasia of Queyrat and Bowen disease refer to conditions histologically characterized by

   A. acanthosis with spotty proliferation of atypical cells.
   B. carcinoma in situ.
   C. prominent koilocytic atypia.
   D. squamous hyperplasia with papillomatosis.
   E. superficial spreading squamous cell carcinoma.

All figures in this chapter are from Longacre TA, Greenson JK, Hornick JL, Reuter VE, eds. *Mills and Sternberg's Diagnostic Surgical Pathology*. 7th ed. Wolters Kluwer; 2022 except for those noted at the end of this book.

5. Figure 1 to Figure 3 show three squamous lesions associated with increased risk of penile squamous cell carcinoma (SCC). Which one of them is most often associated with human papillomavirus (HPV) infection?

A. Figure 1
B. Figure 2
C. Figure 3

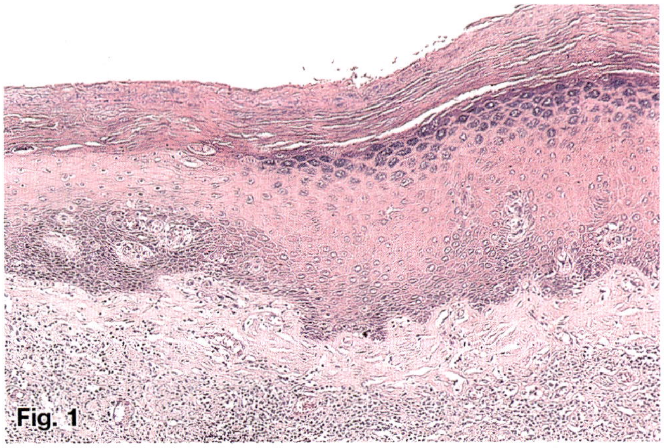


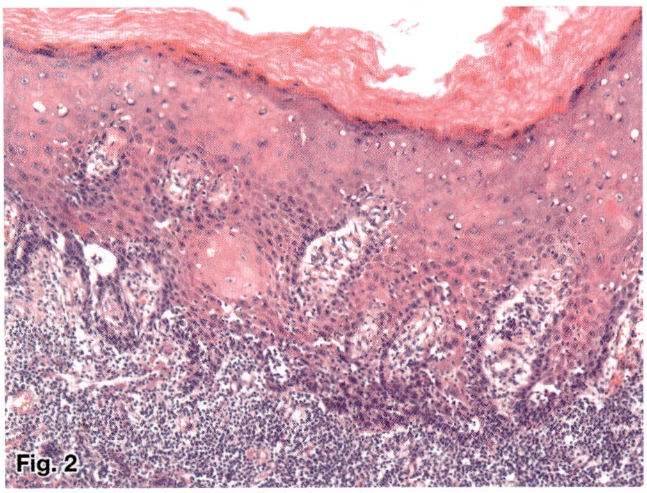


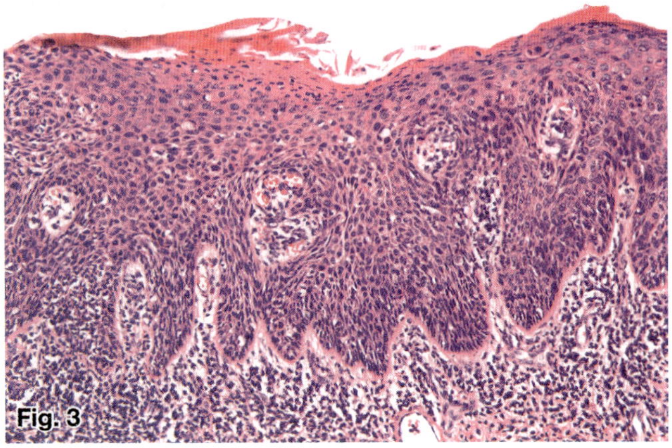


6. The variant of penile squamous cell carcinoma (SCC) shown in Figure 1 is

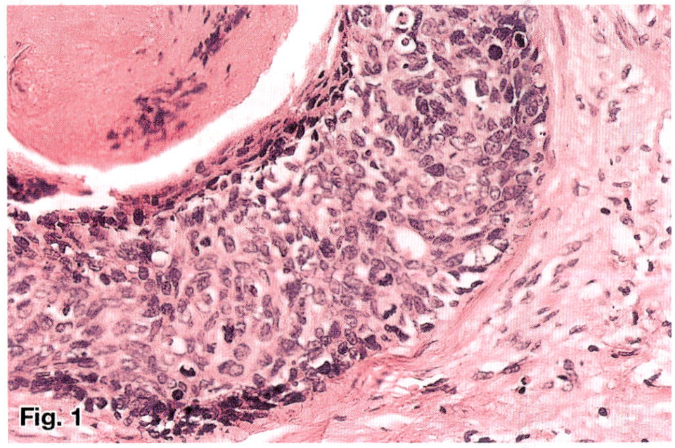


A. basaloid.
B. papillary.
C. sarcomatoid.
D. usual.
E. warty.

# ANSWERS AND EXPLANATIONS

**1. Correct choice: D.**

Fournier gangrene is a life-threatening necrotizing fasciitis of the genitalia. Dartos and penile fascia are preferred sites of involvement. Predisposing factors are local or perineal trauma, burns, or anorectal disease added to debilitating conditions such as diabetes, leukemia, and alcoholic cirrhosis. Streptococci and staphylococci are the most common causative agents in children, as gram-negative bacilli and anaerobic bacteria are in adults. Fournier gangrene is akin to necrotizing balanitis (Corbus disease).

**2. Correct choice: B.**

Granuloma inguinale is an infection that manifests with slowly enlarging painless perianal nodules that become ulcerated. The etiologic agent is *Calymmatobacterium granulomatis* (*donovani*), now renamed *Klebsiella granulomatis.* On tissue sections or scrapings, the bacteria are identified as Donovan bodies by Giemsa or Wright staining. These are intracytoplasmic deeply staining bodies contained within a cystic structure in large histiocytes. The incidence of this sexually transmitted disease has been increasing. Clinically, the lesions are often interpreted as carcinoma. *Bartonella henselae* is the etiologic agent of cat scratch disease, *Chlamydia trachomatis* of lymphogranuloma venereum and nongonococcal urethritis, *Haemophilus ducreyi* of chancroid, and *Treponema pallidum* of syphilis.

**3. Correct choice: B.**

Lichen sclerosus (aka balanitis xerotica obliterans) is a condition that affects men in their 50s and 60s and appears grossly as patchy gray-white atrophic areas involving the inner foreskin and glans. Histologically, the epithelium is atrophic but frequently associated with hyperplastic foci and vacuolar alteration of the basal layer. The lamina propria is thickened and sclerotic, and a band-like lymphocytic infiltration is present underneath. This lesion is clinically important because it predisposes to squamous cell carcinoma (SCC), with about 9% of SCC arising in association with long-standing lichen sclerosus. Lichen sclerosus tends to be associated with the differentiated/non–human papillomavirus (HPV)-related type of penile intraepithelial neoplasia (PeIN). Balanitis circumscripta plasmacellularis (Zoon balanitis) is an inflammatory condition that clinically mimics erythroplasia of Queyrat. Penile melanosis refers to multiple pigmented macules involving the foreskin and glans. Peyronie disease consists of dense fibrosis of the penile fascia that results in penile deformity. Sclerosing lymphangitis of the penis is a self-limited condition manifesting with cord-like induration on the dorsal aspect of the penile shaft.

**4. Correct choice: B.**

Erythroplasia of Queyrat and Bowen disease refer to in situ carcinoma: Erythroplasia of Queyrat involves the glans, whereas Bowen disease involves the skin of the shaft. Acanthosis with spotty proliferation of atypical cells is seen in bowenoid papulosis. Koilocytic atypia is commonly associated with human papillomavirus (HPV)-related lesions such as the warty type of penile carcinoma. Superficial spreading is the most frequent pattern of squamous cell carcinoma of the penis, analogous to the horizontal growth phase of melanoma.

**5. Correct choice: C.**

The images show squamous hyperplasia, differentiated penile intraepithelial neoplasia (PeIN), and basaloid PeIN, respectively. Squamous hyperplasia is not per se a precursor of cancer, but it is often found in close proximity to differentiated PeIN and invasive squamous cell carcinoma (SCC). Development of SCC follows two distinct pathways, which morphologically correspond to differentiated PeIN and basaloid PeIN.

**6. Correct choice: A.**

Penile squamous cell carcinoma (SCC) is rare in the United States (incidence, 0.3/100,000), but frequent in some parts of Asia, Africa, and South America. Circumcision protects against penile cancer, if performed before age 10. It is more common in lower socioeconomic populations, Hispanic and Black men. Risk factors include phimosis, paraphimosis, long foreskin, smoking, and chronic balanitis. Human papillomavirus (HPV) is present in up to 50% of cases, usually types 16 and 18. HPV-related variants are basaloid, warty, and warty-basaloid. Penile SCC has great morphologic variability, with many recognized histologic types (the ones in the list of choices are the most frequent). The usual type is the most common, accounts for 50% to 60% of cases, and is a conventional SCC. The basaloid type is the second most frequent: it consists of monotonous small basaloid cells with high mitotic activity, comedo-like necrosis, and artifactual clefts separating tumor lobules from surrounding stroma. Prognosis depends on tumor type, grade, depth of infiltration, angiolymphatic invasion, perineural invasion, and of course presence of node involvement.

# 49 Gestational Trophoblastic Disease

1. Which of the following histologic features are characteristic of a complete hydatidiform molar pregnancy?

   A. Absence of fetal parts or nonvillous placental structures
   B. Diffuse villous hydrops with cistern formation
   C. Marked trophoblastic hyperplasia that is nonpolar, multifocal, and circumferential
   D. Significant increase in villous size
   E. All of the above

2. Upon gross examination, the abortus from a 14-week gestation consists of a mass of vesicles that vary in size from 0.1 to 3.0 cm. Microscopically, all trophoblastic villi are swollen and devoid of central vessels, as shown in Figure 1. The lining trophoblastic cells are variably hyperplastic circumferentially. No fetal parts or nucleated red blood cells are identified. This condition is characterized by

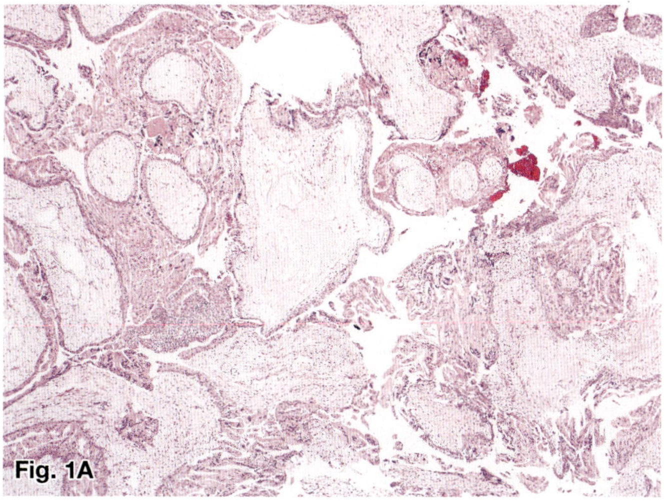
Fig. 1A

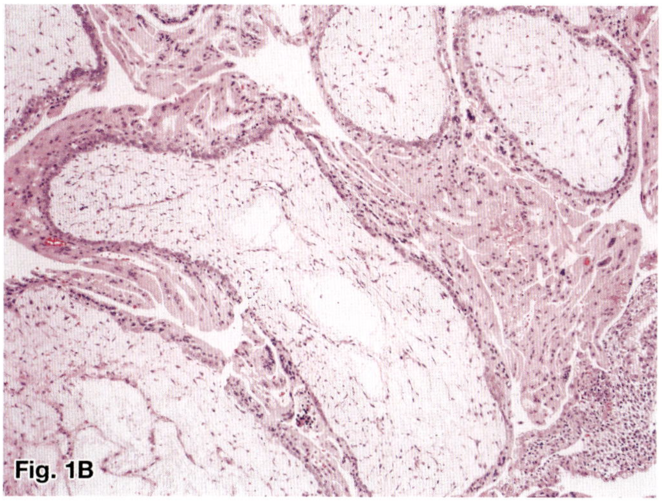
Fig. 1B

   A. diploidy (46,XX or 46,XY).
   B. no significant risk of choriocarcinoma.
   C. normal volume of uterus.
   D. parthenogenetic origin.
   E. triploidy (69,XXX or 69,XXY).

3. The products of conception from a 20-week gestation are analyzed by p57 immunohistochemistry. Expression of p57 is detected in villous trophoblast and stromal cells. Subsequently, genotyping demonstrates biparental diploidy, with one chromosomal complement from the father and one from the mother. These findings are consistent with

   A. complete hydatidiform mole.
   B. incomplete mole.
   C. nonmolar pregnancy.
   D. partial hydatidiform mole.
   E. very early complete hydatidiform mole.

All figures in this chapter are from Longacre TA, Greenson JK, Hornick JL, Reuter VE, eds. *Mills and Sternberg's Diagnostic Surgical Pathology.* 7th ed. Wolters Kluwer; 2022 except for those noted at the end of this book.

4. Which of the following are true regarding complete hydatidiform molar pregnancies?

   A. All patients must undergo the molar surveillance serum β-human chorionic gonadotropin (β-hCG) monitoring program.
   B. Heterozygous/dispermic complete moles are clinically more aggressive.
   C. There is a 2% to 3% risk of gestational choriocarcinoma.
   D. There is a 15% to 20% risk of developing postmolar gestational trophoblastic disease.
   E. All of the above.

5. Which of the following clinical presentations favors a partial molar pregnancy over a complete molar gestation?

   A. Maternal preeclampsia
   B. Presence of a fetus
   C. Significantly elevated serum β-human chorionic gonadotropin (β-hCG) level
   D. Ultrasound with "snowstorm" appearance due to well-developed molar vesicles
   E. Uterine size that is large for gestational age

6. Which of the following histologic features are seen in partial hydatidiform molar pregnancy?

   A. Admixture of two villous populations
   B. Cistern formation
   C. Round or oval trophoblastic pseudoinclusions
   D. Villous hydrops
   E. All of the above

7. Figure 1 demonstrates the histologic features of a missed abortion in a 38-year-old woman. Without knowing the short tandem repeat (STR) genotyping or p57 immunolabeling results, the differential diagnosis includes

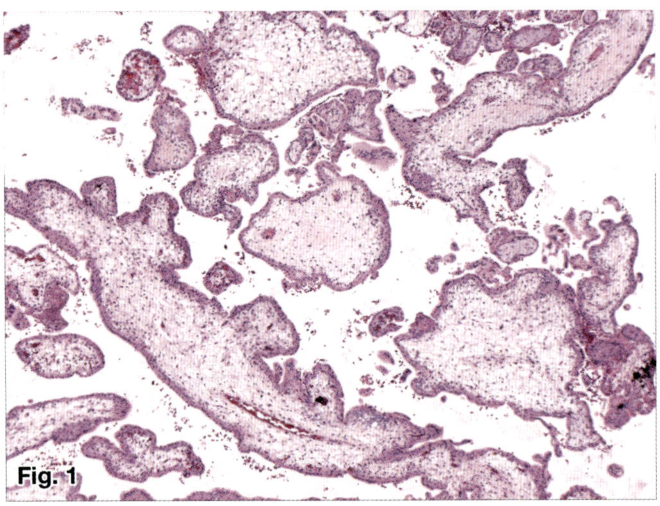


   A. complete hydatidiform mole.
   B. partial hydatidiform mole.
   C. triploid digynic monoandric gestation.
   D. trisomy 21 gestation.
   E. all of the above.

8. Figure 1 shows a non–mass-forming lesion in the endometrial curettage specimen in a 32-year-old woman who had a missed abortion. There is no increase in necrosis, cellularity, or mitotic activity noted. p63 immunostain is negative in the lesional cells. This lesion is characterized by an increased number of

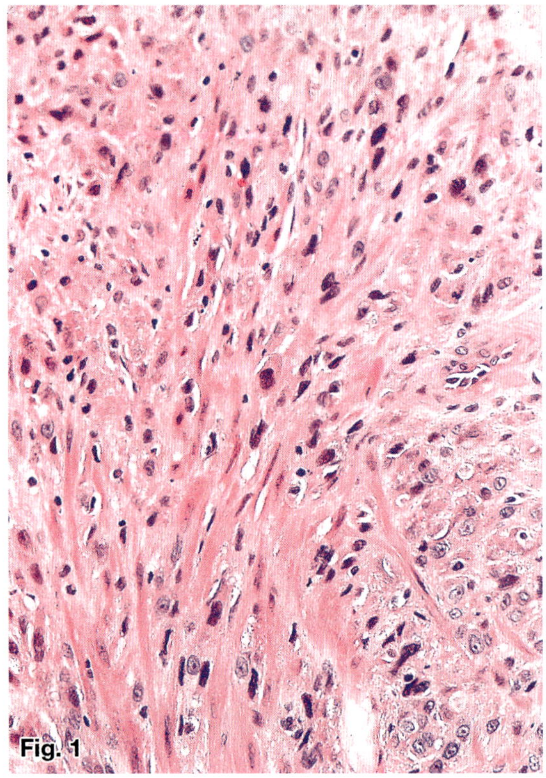


   A. cytotrophoblastic cells.
   B. intermediate trophoblastic cells.
   C. smooth muscle cells.
   D. syncytiotrophoblastic cells.
   E. all of the above.

9. The histologic features of a well-circumscribed hyalinized lesion that was incidentally found in an endometrial biopsy from a 35-year-old G2P2 woman are shown in Figure 1. There is no significant cytologic atypia, necrosis, or hypercellularity noted. Ki-67 expression is highlighted in scattered lesional cells, which are positive for p63, focally positive for human placental lactogen (hPL), and negative for β-human chorionic gonadotropin (β-hCG). What is the most likely diagnosis?

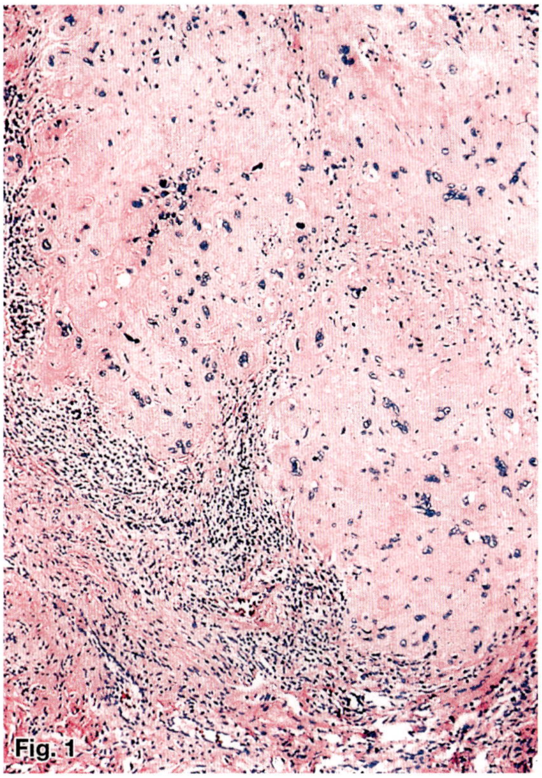
Fig. 1

A. Choriocarcinoma
B. Epithelioid trophoblastic tumor
C. Exaggerated placental site
D. Placental site nodule
E. Placental site trophoblastic tumor

10. Which of the following statements is true about the gestational trophoblastic disease shown in Figure 1?

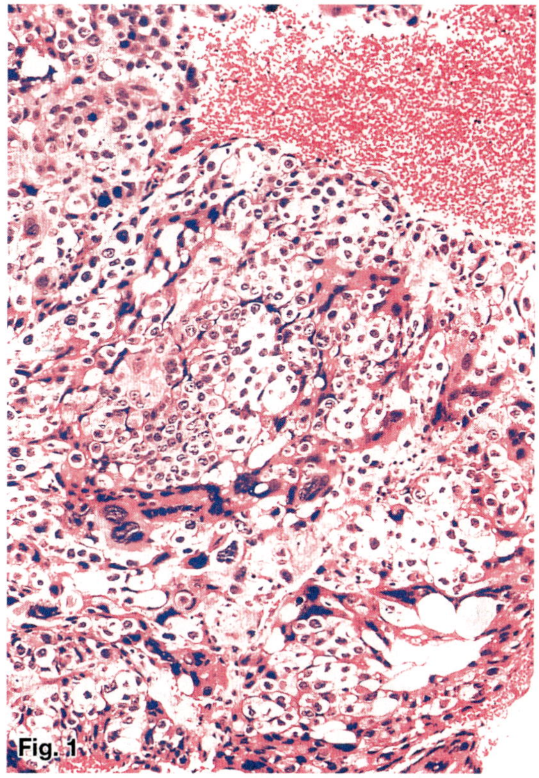
Fig. 1

A. It develops most frequently from ectopic pregnancy.
B. It is poorly responsive to chemotherapy.
C. It rarely metastasizes to the brain.
D. Most cases arise from a partial hydatidiform molar gestation.
E. Risk is influenced by blood group.

11. One year after a term pregnancy, a 40-year-old woman undergoes hysterectomy because of a neoplasm infiltrating the uterine fundus to the serosa. Its histologic appearance is shown in Figure 1. Cells are immunoreactive for cytokeratin and human placental lactogen (hPL), but negative for p63. The Ki-67 labeling index is approximately 15%. What is the diagnosis?

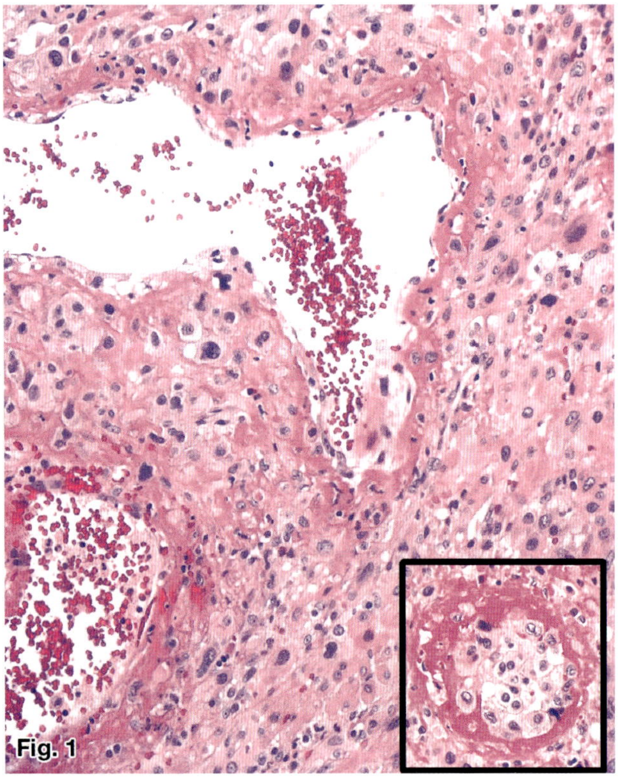

Fig. 1

A. Choriocarcinoma
B. Epithelioid trophoblastic tumor
C. Exaggerated placental site
D. Placental site nodule
E. Placental site trophoblastic tumor

12. A 40-year-old woman, gravida 3, para 2, spontaneous abortion 1, presents with vaginal bleeding. Her last pregnancy was a molar pregnancy treated with dilatation and curettage 5 years earlier. Her serum human chorionic gonadotropin (hCG) is 115 IU/L (normal <2 IU/L). A computed tomography (CT) scan shows a 6-cm solid cystic mass in the lower uterine segment. The patient undergoes a total abdominal hysterectomy with bilateral salpingo-oophorectomy. Microscopically, the tumor shows extensive necrosis. The microscopic appearance of a viable area is shown in Figure 1. Tumor cells are immunoreactive for cytokeratin and p63. Ki-67 labeling index is 20%. The most likely diagnosis is

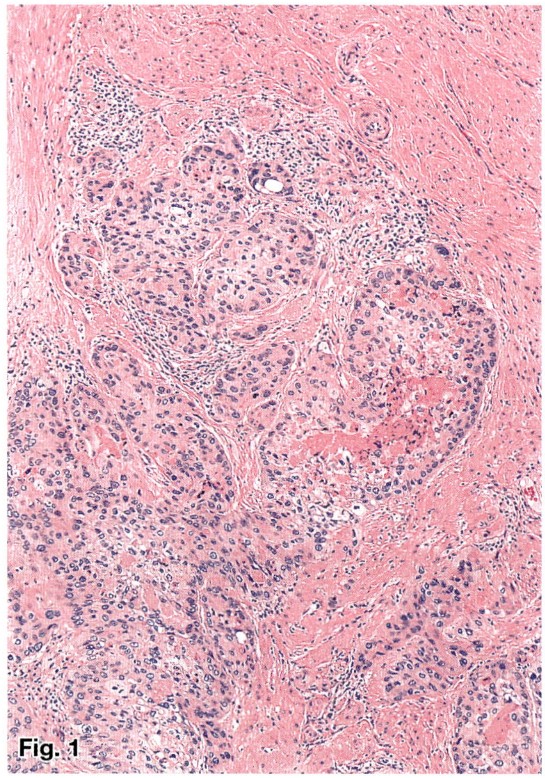

Fig. 1

A. choriocarcinoma.
B. epithelioid trophoblastic tumor.
C. exaggerated placental site.
D. placental site nodule.
E. placental site trophoblastic tumor.

# ANSWERS AND EXPLANATIONS

**1. Correct choice: E.**

Microscopically, diffuse villous hydrops and marked trophoblastic hyperplasia are hallmarks of a well-developed complete hydatidiform mole (CHM). The villous hydropic changes involve all chorionic villi with extensive edematous stroma and cistern formation. Cistern formation is defined as central cystic spaces that are completely devoid of cellular components occupying at least 50% of the villous stromal area. There is a significant increase in the villous size, and the shapes of the chorionic villi are round, oval, or irregular. Trophoblastic hyperplasia is characterized by irregular to diffuse trophoblastic proliferation involving a significant portion of chorionic villi. In contrast to a polarized distribution of trophoblasts in a nonmolar gestation, the trophoblastic hyperplasia in complete mole is nonpolar, multifocal, and frequently circumferential. Fetal parts or nonvillous placental structures, including amnion, yolk sac, and chorionic membrane, are essentially absent. Of note, fetal nucleated red blood cells are not observed in a fully developed complete mole but can be rarely seen in very early complete mole, and so their utility for the diagnosis for CHM depends greatly on gestational age.

**2. Correct choice: A.**

Complete moles arise from (a) androgenesis due to fertilization of an empty ovum (ie, lacking functional maternal chromosomes) by one X-sperm that undergoes duplication, thus resulting in a 46,XX karyotype (90% of cases); or (b) dispermy, which is due to fertilization of an empty ovum by two spermatozoa, resulting in a 46,XY phenotype (10% of cases). Microscopically, diffuse villous hydrops and marked abnormal circumferential trophoblastic hyperplasia, consisting of sheets or confluent aggregates of villous intermediate trophoblast admixed with cytotrophoblast and syncytiotrophoblast, are hallmarks of a well-developed complete mole. Histologically, all villi undergo hydropic degeneration and cistern formation, defined as central cystic spaces that are completely devoid of cellular components occupying at least 50% of the villous stromal area, and contain few or no blood vessels. The uterus becomes enlarged, and levels of human chorionic gonadotropin (hCG) rise above normal limits by the third month of pregnancy. This form is associated with a 2% risk of choriocarcinoma. In contrast, partial moles are triploid with two sets of chromosomes of paternal origin and a haploid maternal set. The triploid set is XXY (58%), XXX (40%), or XYY (2%). The differential diagnosis between complete and partial moles is presented in Table 1.

**3. Correct choice: C.**

The differential diagnosis between nonmolar products of conception (POC) and complete and incomplete moles is now aided by immunohistochemistry for p57 and short tandem repeat genotyping. p57 is a paternally imprinted maternally expressed gene. Therefore, its expression is lacking in trophoblasts and stromal cells of complete moles, which do not have maternal genes. On the other hand, incomplete and nonmolar POCs show p57 expression. Immunohistochemistry for p57 is therefore the first test to distinguish between complete mole and nonmolar specimens or incomplete moles. Genotyping is then used to identify the parental source of polymorphic alleles as well as ploidy. Complete hydatidiform mole is associated with androgenetic diploidy, partial hydatidiform mole with diandric triploidy, and nonmolar placenta with biparental diploidy.

**4. Correct choice: E.**

Complete moles have a 15% to 20% risk of developing postmolar gestational trophoblastic disease (GTD) and a 2% to 3% risk of gestational choriocarcinoma, regardless of the gestational age at the initial evacuation. All patients with a diagnosis of complete mole will undergo the molar surveillance serum β-human chorionic gonadotropin (β-hCG) monitoring program. Recent investigations have confirmed that heterozygous/dispermic complete moles are clinically more aggressive with a significantly higher risk for the development of postmolar GTD than homozygous/monospermic complete moles. Genotyping classification of complete moles into precise subtypes based on their genetic zygosity is therefore important for risk assessment of postmolar GTD and subsequent patient management.

**5. Correct choice: B.**

Most cases of partial hydatidiform molar pregnancies are not suspected clinically prior to evacuation. The uterine size is small or appropriate for the gestational age. Vaginal bleeding is less common than with complete mole. Serum β-human chorionic gonadotropin (β-hCG) is normal or only mildly elevated. Ultrasound may show focal placental cystic changes, and a fetus may be detectable. In contrast, patients with well-developed complete hydatidiform mole evacuated at late first trimester or early second trimester present classic symptoms including vaginal bleeding, enlarged uterus, hyperemesis, hyperthyroidism, and preeclampsia as result of markedly elevated serum β-hCG. Ultrasound shows no evidence of fetal development or fetal heartbeat; instead, the typical "snowstorm" or mixed echogenic appearance is seen due to well-developed molar vesicles admixed with blood.

**6. Correct choice: E.**

Partial hydatidiform moles (PHMs) typically demonstrate an admixture of two villous populations: a small, fibrotic villi and enlarged, irregularly shaped villi with scalloped contours, a variable degree of hydrops, and mild to moderate circumferential trophoblastic proliferation. Cistern formation and trophoblastic pseudoinclusions are common. Cistern formation with a maze-like acellular pattern is usually seen in advanced cases. Round to oval trophoblastic pseudoinclusions due to invaginations of villous surface trophoblast are frequent findings. Mild to moderate circumferential nonpolar trophoblastic hyperplasia is usually present, generally without significant cytologic atypia. Focally prominent syncytiotrophoblast "knuckles" (or "sprouts") with intracytoplasmic lacunae are also a characteristic finding in partial mole. Fetal blood vessels and nucleated red blood cells are often present as well. The following morphologic parameters are important for the initial screening for PHM: villi size enlargement, presence of two villous populations, round or oval trophoblastic pseudoinclusions, at least moderate villous hydrops, cistern formation, and abnormal trophoblastic hyperplasia.

**TABLE 1 Comparison of Complete and Partial Mole**

| | Complete Mole | Partial Mole |
|---|---|---|
| Preoperative diagnosis of hydatidiform mole | +++ | +/− |
| Spontaneous abortion | ++ | ++ |
| Missed abortion | +/− | +++ |
| Heavy bleeding | +++ | + |
| Toxemia | ++ | +/− |
| Uterus large for dates | ++ | +/− |
| Uterus small for dates | +/− | ++ |
| Fetal tissue present | − | + |
| Serum hCG level | +++ | +/++ |
| Cytogenetics | Androgenetic diploid; XX or XY (all paternal) | Diandric triploid; XXY or XXX (paternal:maternal, 2:1) |
| p57 staining | − | + |
| Percentage to develop persistent GTD | 10-30 | 0-5.6[a] |

GTD, gestational trophoblastic disease; hCG, human chorionic gonadotropin.
[a]The percentage may be overestimated due to possible misclassification of complete moles for partial moles.

**7. Correct choice: E.**

The image is of a trisomy 21 gestation, which will also demonstrate irregular villous shapes, hydropic changes, and trophoblastic pseudoinclusions. The differential diagnoses of partial hydatidiform moles (PHMs), in addition to complete moles, also include a variety of nonmolar gestations that exhibit overlapping morphologic features. Trisomy gestations can be microscopically indistinguishable from PHM, as they often show abnormal villous configurations with trophoblastic pseudoinclusions and villous hydrops. Triploid digynic monoandric gestations may mimic partial moles at both the morphologic level and DNA ploidy level. Although most cases are without abnormal villous morphology, in rare cases, digynic triploidy may simulate a PHM mainly due to the presence of hydropic villi and, less commonly, cistern formation and irregular villous shape with trophoblastic pseudoinclusions and syncytiotrophoblastic knuckles.

**8. Correct choice: B.**

Often an incidental microscopic finding, exaggerated placental site (EPS) is a benign change that is simply an exaggeration of a physiologic process. An EPS may occur in association with normal pregnancy, an abortion, or a hydatidiform mole. An EPS is composed of implantation site intermediate trophoblastic cells that extensively infiltrate the endomyometrium and are p63 immunoreactive. Despite the extensive infiltration by intermediate trophoblastic cells, the overall architecture of the implantation site is not disturbed. The smooth muscle cells of the myometrium are separated by cords, nests, and individual implantation site intermediate trophoblastic cells that diffusely infiltrate the myometrium without producing necrosis. EPS is a benign trophoblastic lesion that involutes following curettage and is not associated with increased risk of persistent gestational trophoblastic disease. Morphologically, EPS overlaps with placental site trophoblastic tumor (PSTT), also of intermediate trophoblastic origin. Mitotic activity and Ki-67 labeling index are close to 0 in EPS, whereas PSTT has mitoses and Ki-67 labeling index higher than 10%.

**9. Correct choice: D.**

Placental site nodule (PSN) is a well-circumscribed hyalinized lesion composed of chorionic-type intermediate trophoblastic cells that are normally located in chorion laeve (fetal membrane). Typically, it is incidentally found in an endometrial biopsy, endocervical curettage, or cervical biopsy from a woman in the reproductive age group. PSNs are benign. The chorionic-type intermediate trophoblastic cells within the PSN are arranged singly, in nests and cords. They are embedded in abundant eosinophilic fibrillar extracellular matrix protein, which is a prominent feature. Epithelioid trophoblastic tumors (ETTs) are larger and display substantial necrosis and focal calcification. PSN is much less cellular than ETT. In addition, the trophoblastic cells in PSN in contrast to an ETT are bland and mitotic activity is low or absent. The Ki-67 index in ETTs is significantly higher (>12%) versus in PSN (<8%). These so-called atypical PSN may represent a tumor transformation from a classical PSN to an ETT. Intermediate trophoblastic tumor (placental site trophoblastic tumor [PSTT] or ETT) can emerge from a preexisting atypical PSN. Atypical PSNs usually contain more abundant lesional tissues in specimens and appear more cellular than PSNs.

**10. Correct choice: E.**

Approximately 50% of gestational choriocarcinomas follow a molar pregnancy (almost always complete hydatidiform mole), 25% ectopic pregnancy, and 25% normal pregnancy. The more abnormal the pregnancy, the more likely that it will be followed by choriocarcinoma. This aggressive cancer is highly responsive to chemotherapy regimens, with a nearly 100% survival. It consists of a mixture of extremely pleomorphic cytotrophoblastic and syncytiotrophoblastic cells. It is richly vascularized and often leads to hemorrhage. Chorionic villi are not a component of choriocarcinoma. Choriocarcinoma disseminates hematogenously, and the lungs are most frequently involved, with other common sites including the brain, liver, and gastrointestinal tract. Syncytiotrophoblast and intermediate trophoblast are hormonally active and will show immunolabeling to β-human chorionic gonadotropin (β-hCG) or human placental lactogen (hPL). One of the most unusual features of this neoplasm is its relationship with blood group type; women with group A married to men with the same group have the highest risk.

**11. Correct choice: E.**

Placental site trophoblastic tumor (PSTT) is a rare tumor that originates from the intermediate trophoblastic cells of the implantation site. It occurs usually in parous women, sometimes long after the last known pregnancy. Its usual location is in the fundus, where it infiltrates the endometrium and myometrium up to the serosa. PSTT is composed of intermediate trophoblastic cells that display a marked propensity to invade vessel walls and is associated with fibrin deposition in the vessel wall (as shown in the image). In choriocarcinoma, there is a combination of mononucleated trophoblastic and syncytiotrophoblastic cells, accounting for a biphasic pattern. An epithelioid trophoblastic tumor is also of intermediate trophoblastic origin, but it resembles a squamous cell carcinoma. An exaggerated implantation site overlaps morphologically with PSTT, from which it is difficult to differentiate in curettage specimens. A placental site nodule is usually an incidental finding in an endometrial biopsy or curettage samples.

**12. Correct choice: B.**

Epithelioid trophoblastic tumor (ETT) is a rare trophoblastic tumor composed of chorionic-type intermediate trophoblast. ETT arises in the uterine corpus, lower uterine segment, or endocervix and grows in a nodular expansile manner. Histologically, ETT resembles a carcinoma, and it is uniquely able to replace and reepithelialize endocervical and/or endometrial surface epithelium, furthering its potential mimicry. The tumor cells have distinct cell borders and abundant eosinophilic or vacuolated cytoplasm. A prominent feature is multifocal necrosis with accumulation of a fibrinoid, eosinophilic material similar to that found in placental site nodule (PSN). The tumor behaves in a benign fashion in two-thirds of patients but recurs and metastasizes in the remaining third. A simple step-by-step algorithm in the immunohistochemical analysis of trophoblastic tumors is shown in Figure 1.

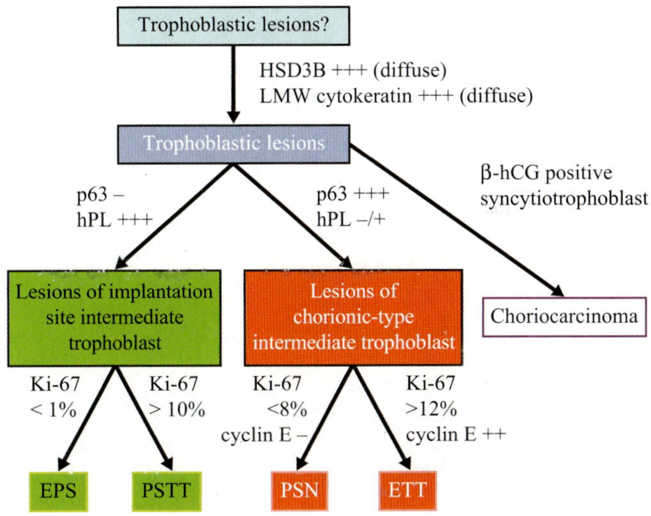


**Fig. 1**

# 50 Placenta

1. A long umbilical cord is associated with increased fetal morbidity and mortality. A diagnosis of long umbilical cord is made when the length exceeds

   A. 40 cm.
   B. 50 cm.
   C. 60 cm.
   D. 70 cm.
   E. 80 cm.

2. Figure 1 shows an abnormality of cord insertion that may lead to

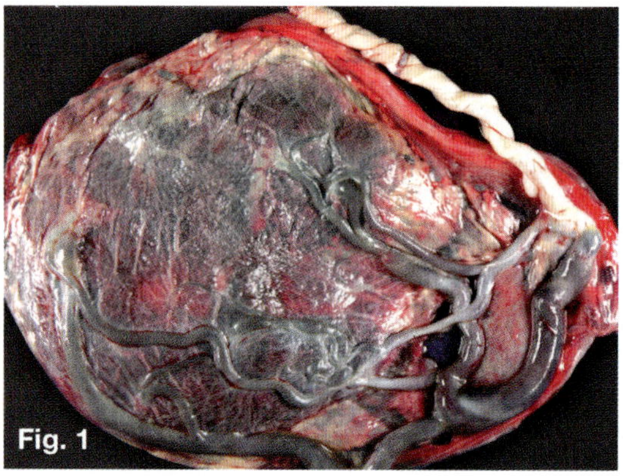

Fig. 1

   A. cord torsion.
   B. oligohydramnios.
   C. placenta previa.
   D. premature rupture of membranes.
   E. vasa previa.

3. What does the finding in the umbilical cord shown in Figure 1 most likely correspond to?

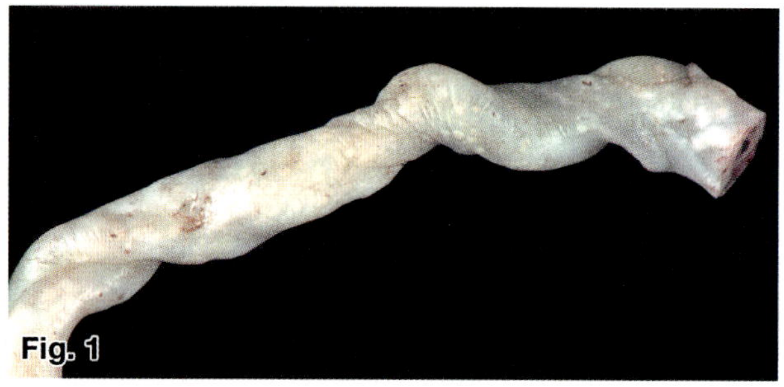

Fig. 1

   A. Acute chorioamnionitis
   B. *Candida* infection
   C. Prolonged cord compression
   D. Prolonged meconium exposure
   E. Retention of an intrauterine fetal demise

4. The umbilical cord of a placenta from a preterm delivery is narrow and wrinkled. A 10-cm segment adjacent to the placental disk is flattened. Which of the following conditions is most likely associated with these changes?

   A. Abruptio placentae
   B. Ectopic implantation
   C. Infection
   D. Maternal history of cocaine use
   E. Oligohydramnios

5. Figure 1 demonstrates a significant gross finding, which is associated with which of the following conditions?

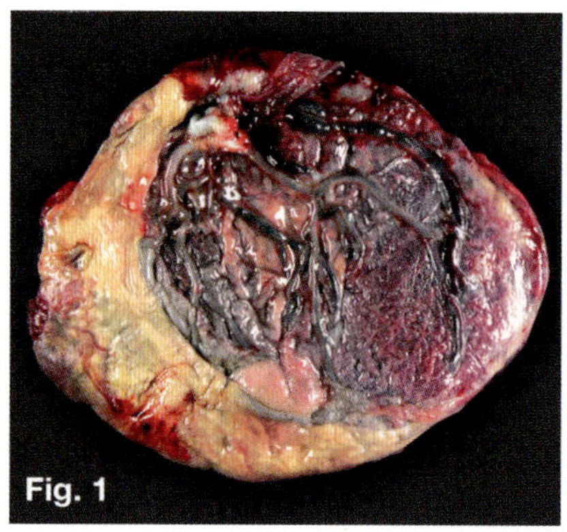

Fig. 1

   A. Chronic abruption
   B. Infection
   C. Prolonged cord compression
   D. Prolonged meconium exposure
   E. Vasa previa

---

All figures in this chapter are from Longacre TA, Greenson JK, Hornick JL, Reuter VE, eds. *Mills and Sternberg's Diagnostic Surgical Pathology*. 7th ed. Wolters Kluwer; 2022 except for those noted at the end of this book.

6. A 35-year-old pregnant woman presents with fever, uterine tenderness, and leukocytosis. She delivers a male baby at 30 weeks gestation. Histologic examination of the placenta and amniotic sac reveals the changes shown in Figure 1. Which of the following is the most likely infectious agent of this condition?

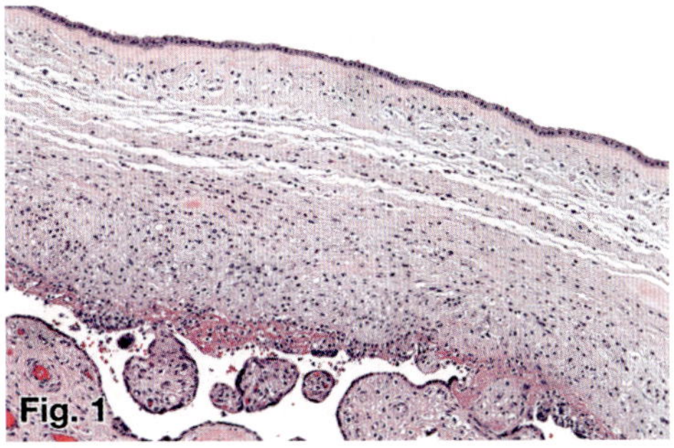


A. *Bacteroides fragilis*
B. *Chlamydia trachomatis*
C. *Escherichia coli*
D. *Fusobacterium*
E. Group B streptococci

7. Microscopic examination of a term placenta reveals a diffuse neutrophilic infiltration of villi and intervillous spaces, with scattered microabscesses, as shown in Figure 1. This histologic presentation is usually caused by

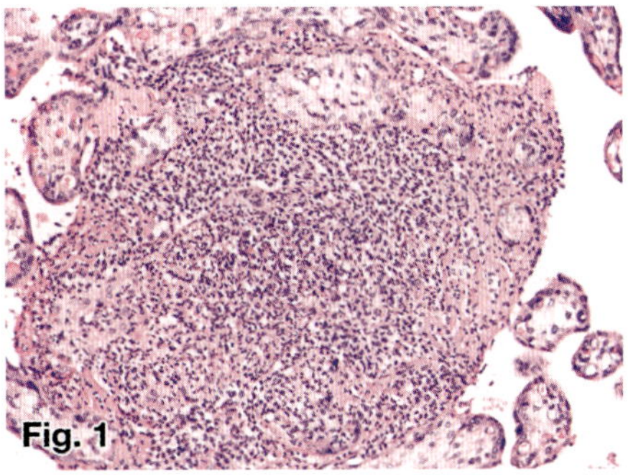


A. cytomegalovirus.
B. group B streptococci.
C. *Listeria monocytogenes.*
D. syphilis.
E. *Toxoplasma.*

8. Figure 1 depicts a case of villitis of unknown etiology (VUE). What is the cause in most cases?

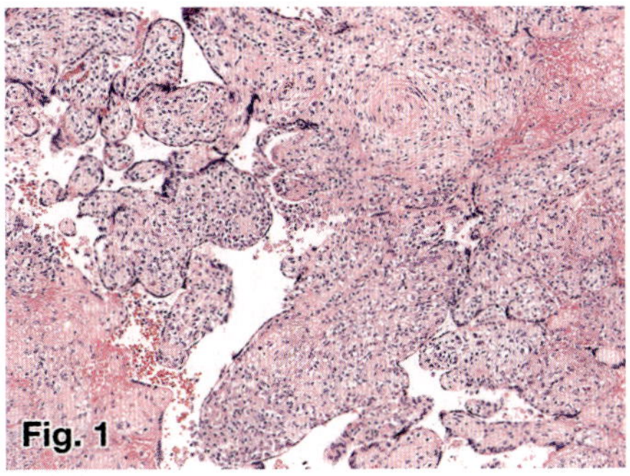


A. Ascending infection
B. Chronic hypoxia
C. Hematogenous infection
D. Immunologic reaction
E. Malformative process

9. Which of the following infectious agents is most likely responsible for the microscopic changes seen in Figure 1 of placenta from a preterm delivery?

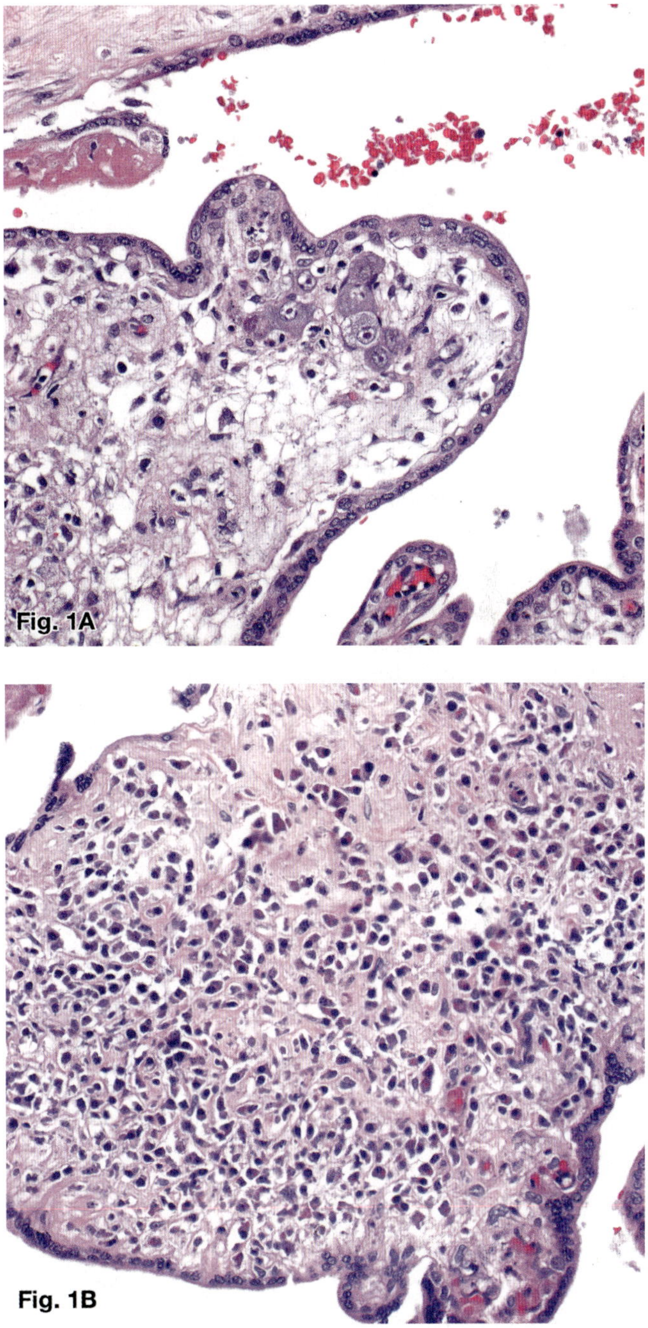


A. Cytomegalovirus
B. Group B streptococci
C. *Listeria monocytogenes*
D. Syphilis
E. *Toxoplasma*

10. Additional workup for which of the following infectious agents should be sought when the histologic features shown in Figure 1 are encountered in a placenta from a preterm delivery?

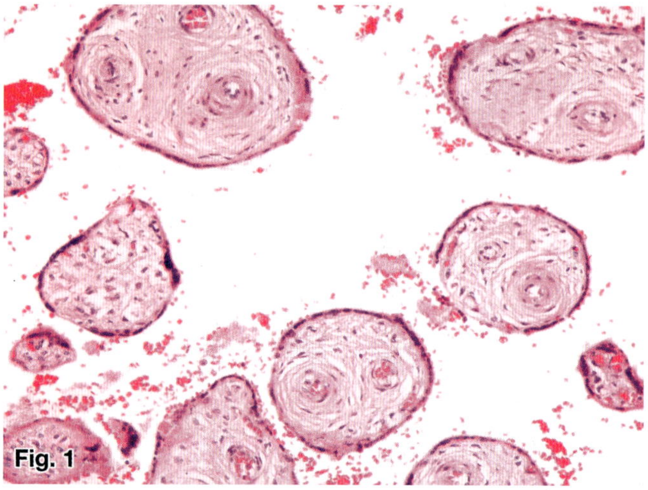

Fig. 1

A. Cytomegalovirus
B. Group B streptococci
C. *Listeria monocytogenes*
D. Syphilis
E. *Toxoplasma*

11. Which of the following is a possible cause of fetal vascular malperfusion?

A. Thin umbilical cord in diameter
B. Umbilical cord compression
C. Umbilical cord hypercoiling
D. Velamentous cord insertion
E. All of the above

12. Which of the following maternal disorders may show changes related to maternal vascular malperfusion in the placenta?

A. Antiphospholipid syndrome
B. Diabetes
C. Drug use (particularly vasoconstrictive drugs like cocaine)
D. Preeclampsia
E. All of the above

13. Which of the following conditions results in the abnormalities of villous maturation illustrated in Figure 1 of a 30-week preterm gestation?

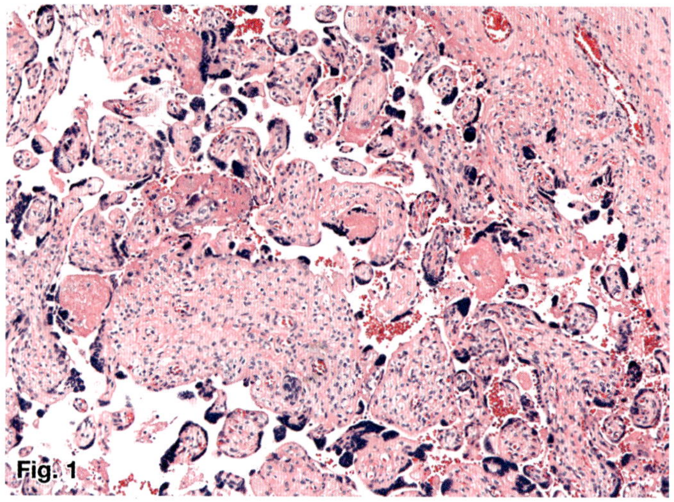

Fig. 1

A. Chorangiosis
B. Generalized villous dysmaturity
C. Meconium exposure
D. Placental malperfusion
E. Villitis of unknown etiology

14. A placenta is submitted for gross and histologic evaluation in a case of clinically diagnosed abruptio placentae. Which of the following microscopic findings is most compatible with this diagnosis?

A. Intravillous and intervillous hemorrhage
B. Meconium-laden macrophages in amniotic membrane
C. Myocytes and hemorrhage in the maternal plate
D. Neutrophil-rich infiltration of membranes
E. Thrombi in fetal blood vessels

15. Figure 1 depicts chorionic villi with a change that may be produced by chronic fetal-placental hypoxia. In the diffuse and multifocal form shown by the arrows in Figure 2, it may be associated with infant anomalies (including cardiac, renal, intestinal). Which of the following is it?

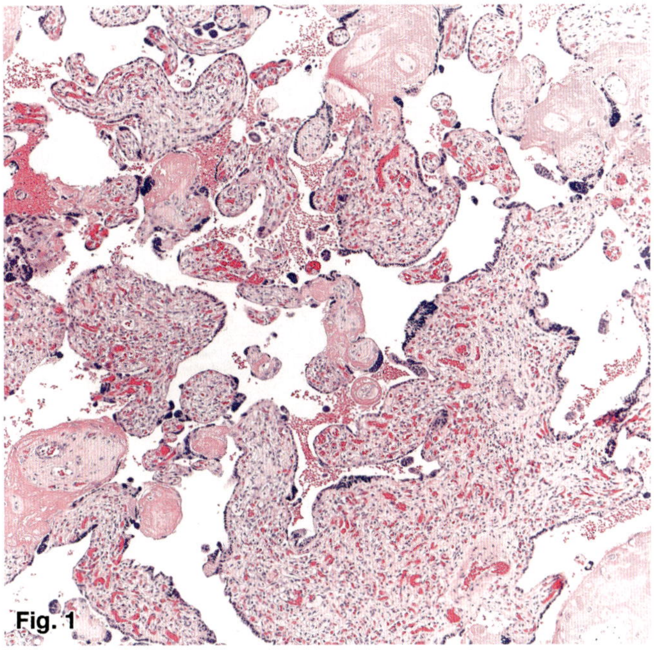
Fig. 1

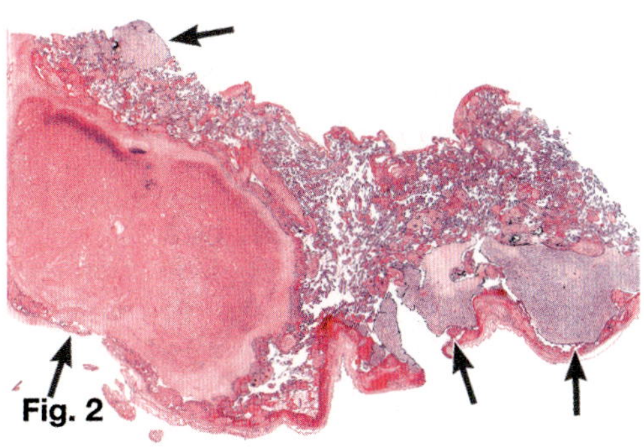
Fig. 2

A. Chorangiomatosis
B. Chorioamnionitis
C. Intravillous hemorrhage
D. Villitis of unknown origin
E. Villous dysmaturity

16. Which of the following types of multiple pregnancies is associated with the highest risk of twin-to-twin transfusion syndrome?

A. Dichorionic diamniotic with fused placental disks
B. Dichorionic diamniotic with separate placental disks
C. Monochorionic diamniotic
D. Monochorionic monoamniotic

17. Figure 1 demonstrates the terminal villi in a 38-week gestational age placenta with delayed villous maturation. This histologic finding can be seen in which of the following conditions?

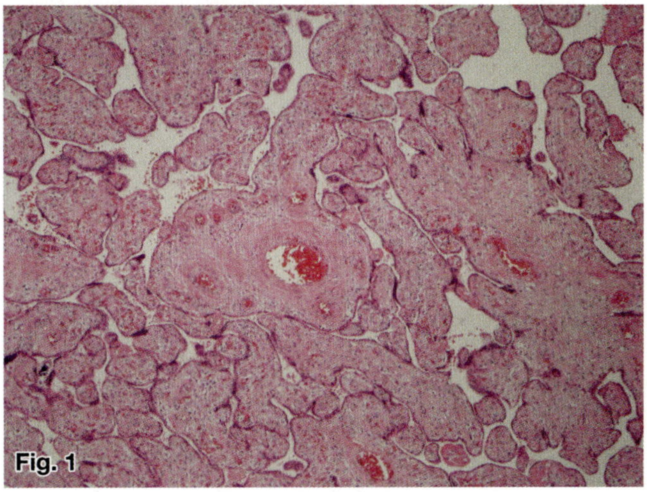
Fig. 1

A. Beckwith-Wiedemann syndrome
B. Gastroschisis
C. Gestational diabetes
D. Opioid maintenance therapy
E. All of the above

18. A tan-green discoloration of a placenta and its membranes is noticed on gross examination. Histologically, numerous meconium-laden macrophages are found in the superficial plate, extraplacental amniotic membrane, and Wharton jelly of the umbilical cord, as shown by the arrows in Figure 1. There is focal necrosis of umbilical arteries as depicted in Figure 2. These changes are compatible with an antenatal meconium exposure of at least

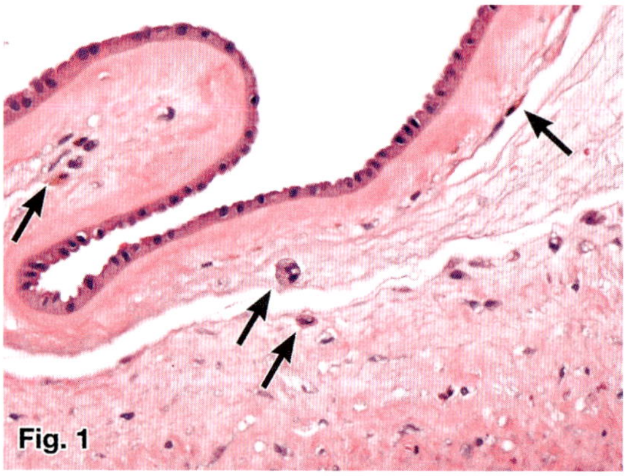
Fig. 1

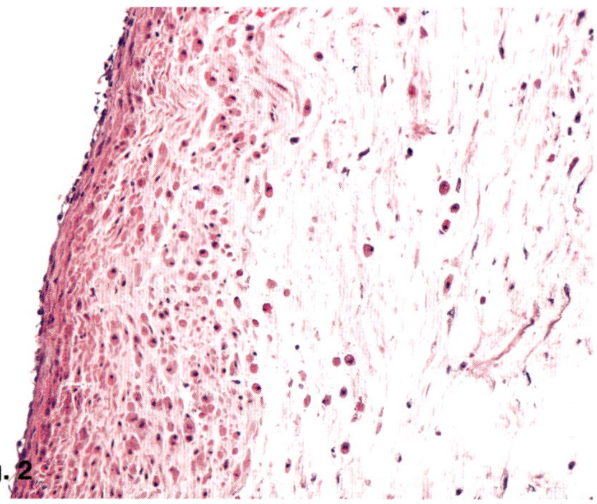
Fig. 2

A. few minutes.
B. 1 hour.
C. 3 hours.
D. 12 hours.
E. 24 to 48 hours.

19. A 30-year-old woman has a spontaneous abortion at 30 weeks gestation. On histologic examination of the placenta, the maternal floor contains an extensive perivillous deposition of eosinophilic fibrinoid material with numerous intermediate cells. A histopathologic diagnosis of maternal floor infarction is made. This condition is associated with an increased risk of

A. abruptio placentae.
B. ectopic pregnancies.
C. fetal hydrops.
D. postmaturity.
E. recurrent reproductive failure.

20. Figure 1 demonstrates the histologic findings of the terminal villi of a boggy, pale, and large-for-gestational-age placenta. Which of the following conditions can be associated with these placental findings?

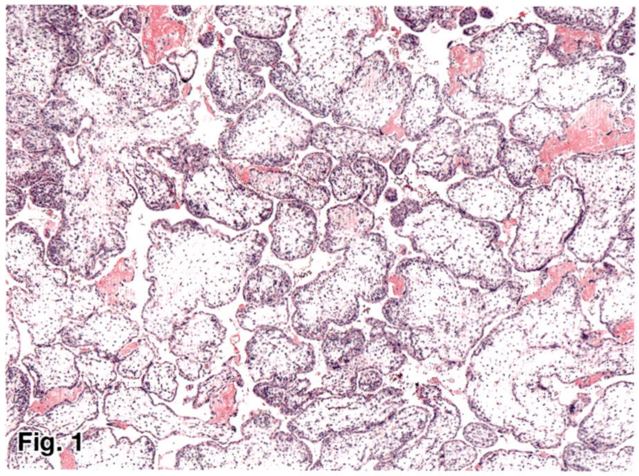
Fig. 1

A. Fetal anemia
B. Fetal cardiovascular defects
C. Fetal hemoglobinopathies
D. Fetal metabolic disorders
E. All of the above

21. Which of the following infectious agents is most likely responsible for the microscopic changes seen in Figure 1 in a large-for-gestational-age placenta?

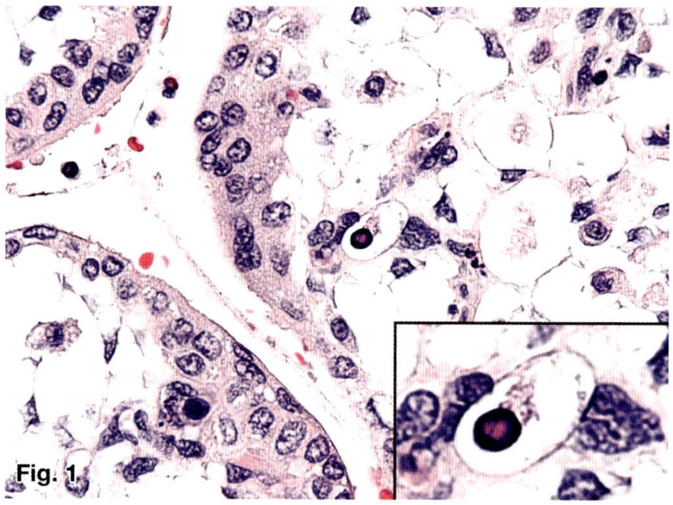
Fig. 1

A. Adenovirus
B. Cytomegalovirus
C. Parvovirus
D. Syphilis
E. *Toxoplasma*

22. Figure 1 demonstrates the histologic findings in a hysterectomy specimen performed for postpartum hemorrhage, following difficult extraction of placenta requiring manual removal after delivery. What is the new terminology used for this disorder?

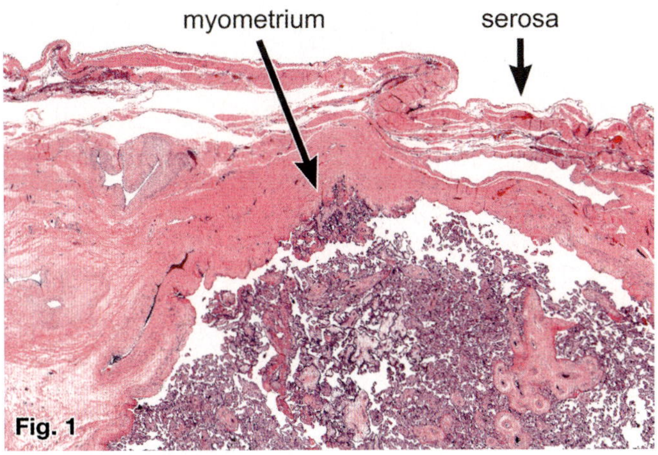


A. Invasive placenta accreta spectrum (PAS) Grade 2
B. Invasive PAS Grade 3A
C. Noninvasive PAS Grade 1
D. Placenta accreta
E. Placenta increta

# ANSWERS AND EXPLANATIONS

**1. Correct choice: D.**

The length of the umbilical cord should be documented in pathology reports. The mean length is 50 to 60 cm. A long cord measures more than 70 cm and is more prone to knots, entanglement, torsion, prolapse, and compression, which may result in reduced blood flow and place additional workload on the fetal heart that may be involved with increased morbidity and mortality. Conversely, a short cord is defined as measuring less than 32 cm. It is associated with conditions of restricted fetal movements.

**2. Correct choice: E.**

Normally, the cord is located centrally or near the center of the placental disk. Marginal insertion refers to a cord that inserts within less than 2 cm from the disk margin. The image shows a velamentous insertion, which is the most clinically significant abnormality of cord insertion. A velamentous cord inserts into the fetal membranes, so the vessels traveling through the membranes are susceptible to compression, thrombosis, and rupture. Velamentous insertion can cause vasa previa, in which the umbilical vessels within the membrane present before the fetus during delivery and may undergo rupture, leading to catastrophic fetal hemorrhage. It is important to measure and sample any membranous vessels (even if not associated with velamentous insertion) to check for thrombosis, inflammation, or necrosis.

**3. Correct choice: B.**

Cord color is an important part of the gross examination of the placenta. The color of the umbilical cord is normally white tan; this feature can be altered by infection, meconium, or fetal demise. *Candida* infections, white spots may be noted on the surface of the umbilical cord that correspond to peripherally located microabscesses, as depicted in the image. In severe acute chorioamnionitis, the umbilical cord may appear green or yellow. With prolonged meconium exposure, the cord may be green brown and feel slippery or slimy. Retention of an intrauterine fetal demise of more than 6 hours results in a brown/red discoloration of the umbilical cord.

**4. Correct choice: E.**

Oligohydramnios indicates an abnormally reduced volume of amniotic fluid. The reduced available space leads to fetal deformities as well as to umbilical cord compression. In these cases, meconium discharge is usually associated.

**5. Correct choice: A.**

The fetal membranes (chorion and amnion) normally insert onto the edge of the placental disk. When the membranes insert further in from the edge, leaving a rim of fibrin or thrombus between the chorionic membranes and the underlying placental tissue, it is termed circummarginate or circumvallate. These two types of insertion are distinguished by the presence of a palpable ridge of folded membranes in the case of circumvallate membranes versus a smooth edge in the case of circummarginate membranes. Circumvallate membranes are associated with more significant and chronic marginal bleeding and the clinical syndrome of chronic abruption. The resulting lifting up of the membranes/chorionic plate by the hemorrhage results in the ridge seen grossly. Remote hematomas and hemosiderin can be seen microscopically.

**6. Correct choice: E.**

The image shows an example of chorioamnionitis, which results from infectious organisms traveling through the birth canal to the amniotic cavity. Both mother and fetus respond to the infection. Maternal neutrophils migrate from the decidua to the chorion and later into the amniotic membrane. Fetal neutrophils migrate from chorionic vessels to the amnion and from the umbilical cord vessels as well (funisitis). Staging and grading of chorioamnionitis is based on assessment of both maternal and fetal responses. In term pregnancy, chorioamnionitis usually follows rupture of membranes. In preterm pregnancies, chorioamnionitis predisposes to premature rupture of membranes and various fetal complications. Group B streptococci are the most frequent etiologic agents of severe fetal/neonatal sepsis. Clinical criteria for a diagnosis of chorioamnionitis include maternal fever during labor, leukocytosis, uterine tenderness, and maternal or fetal tachycardia. Assessment of the severity of the inflammatory response is clinically useful because the degree of fetal inflammatory response seems to correlate with the risk for adverse neurologic outcomes.

**7. Correct choice: C.**

Acute villitis and intervillositis are characterized by neutrophilic infiltration of villi and intervillous spaces and result from hematogenous spread of maternal infection to the placenta and fetus. Acute villitis with mild intervillositis is usually caused by group B streptococci or gram-negative organisms. Acute villitis with severe intervillositis and microabscesses is typically due to *Listeria monocytogenes* infection, as shown in the image, although it can be seen with *Campylobacter*, coccidioidomycosis, psittacosis, tularemia, and brucellosis. Gram and silver stains should be performed in case of villitis and intervillositis in order to identify the infectious agent.

**8. Correct choice: D.**

Chronic villitis is defined by lymphohistiocytic, giant cell, or lymphoplasmacytic infiltration of the villi. This change is found in approximately 5% to 15% of all placentas. In most cases, no specific infectious agent can be identified. However, in about 1% of cases, chronic villitis is caused by the diverse group of microorganisms referred to as TORCH: *Toxoplasma gondii*, rubella virus, cytomegalovirus (CMV), herpes simplex virus (HSV), and other organisms including *Treponema pallidum*, varicella-zoster virus, Epstein-Barr virus, and human immunodeficiency virus (HIV). Thus, the pathologist's role is to investigate possible infectious etiologies by special stains or molecular tests when indicated. Noninfectious cases of villitis of unknown etiology (VUE) are thought to result from a maternal immunologic reaction against placental antigens, which would explain why it tends to recur in subsequent pregnancies. VUE is more frequently associated with small-for-gestational-age newborns and intrauterine growth retardation.

**9. Correct choice: A.**

TORCH infections are the classic infectious causes of chronic villitis. The term "TORCH" refers to congenital infections caused by *Toxoplasma gondii*, rubella virus, cytomegalovirus (CMV), herpes simplex virus, and other organisms such as *Treponema pallidum* (syphilis), varicella-zoster virus, and Epstein-Barr virus. CMV and syphilis are the most common TORCH infections in the United States. CMV-associated villitis classically demonstrates a plasma cell component, as illustrated in Figure 2, which is often accompanied by hemosiderin. Rarely, intranuclear inclusions can be identified in the villous stromal cells, as shown in Figure 1. There is an immunohistochemical stain for CMV; however, studies have shown that this may not be adequately sensitive compared to CMV DNA polymerase chain reaction (PCR) from paraffin-embedded tissue.

**10. Correct choice: D.**

TORCH infections are the classic infectious causes of chronic villitis. The term "TORCH" refers to congenital infections caused by *Toxoplasma gondii*, rubella virus, cytomegalovirus (CMV), herpes simplex virus, and other organisms such as *Treponema pallidum* (syphilis), varicella-zoster virus, and Epstein-Barr virus. Congenital syphilis placentas are often large (heavy) and pale with a histiocyte-rich infiltrate, prominent stem villous vasculitis often with an "onion skin" appearance, as illustrated in the image, and necrotizing umbilical periphlebitis with chronic inflammation.

**11. Correct choice: E.**

Most cases of fetal vascular malperfusion are associated with umbilical cord abnormalities, resulting in cord compression and stasis rather than true hereditary thrombophilias, as once thought. These cord abnormalities include velamentous insertion, entanglement, thin umbilical cord in diameter (<0.8 cm at term), kinking, obstruction from the presenting part, and hypercoiling.

**12. Correct choice: E.**

The term "maternal vascular malperfusion" is an umbrella term replacing "uteroplacental underperfusion" and has been used to refer generically to maternal disorders with a component of vascular disease, which result in placental pathology of ischemia. Such disorders include preeclampsia, eclampsia, chronic hypertension, pregnancy-induced hypertension, lupus, antiphospholipid syndrome, diabetes, maternal thrombophilias, and drug use (particularly vasoconstrictive drugs like cocaine).

**13. Correct choice: D.**

This condition refers to chronic placental ischemia resulting from maternal vascular disorders such as preeclampsia, eclampsia, chronic hypertension, systemic lupus erythematosus, antiphospholipid syndrome, diabetes, thrombophilias, and illicit drug use (especially cocaine). Microscopically, the placenta shows a feature known as accelerated villous maturation, characterized by paucity of intermediate-sized villi, increased syncytial knots, and avillous knots. Presence of syncytial knots in preterm placentas is diagnostic of accelerated villous maturation. Malperfused placentas tend to have infarcts of the usual type.

**14. Correct choice: A.**

Placental abruption is a potentially catastrophic clinical syndrome that is caused by premature separation of the placenta from the uterine wall prior to delivery of the fetus. Predisposing factors to acute and subacute abruption include the causes of maternal vascular malperfusion, maternal abdominal trauma, tobacco smoking, and uterine distention (such as multiple gestations). Placental abruption can be an acute, subacute, or chronic phenomenon, and all have different gross and histopathologic findings. The most typical histopathologic correlates of abruptio placentae include intravillous and intervillous hemorrhage. Intravillous hemorrhage, imparting a characteristic "bag of blood" appearance, is the most specific change, although not always present. The finding of hemorrhage and myocytes between basal decidual cells is suggestive of placenta accreta.

**15. Correct choice: A.**

Normally, each chorionic villus contains no more than five capillary lumina. Chorangiosis refers to an abnormal increase in the number of capillaries within villi. The original diagnostic criteria required finding at least 10 fields with 10 villi, with 10 capillaries per villus. Chorangioma is a mass lesion, an angioma, occurring within a villus. Chorangiomatosis is a chorangioma associated with stromal proliferation. Chorangiomatosis can be multifocal. These conditions are thought to derive from protracted fetal-placental hypoxia, which is consistent with the high incidence of chorangiosis and chorangiomas in pregnant mothers living at high altitudes. Fetal nucleated red blood cells are also a consequence of fetal-placental hypoxia. There is an association of the diffuse multifocal chorangiomatosis, shown in the image, with fetal/infant anomalies (including cardiac, renal, and intestinal).

**16. Correct choice: C.**

Twin-to-twin transfusion syndrome (TTTS) complicates about 15% of monochorionic twin pregnancies and results in unequal blood flow between fetuses. The donor twin is small and anemic, while the recipient twin is large and congested. The syndrome is due to the fact that the fetal vascular trees within a monochorionic placenta are interconnected and lead to development of anastomoses. Arterioarterial and venovenous anastomoses do not have appreciable hemodynamic effects and seem to counteract the potentially unequal flow caused by deep artery-to-vein anastomoses, which are always present in monochorionic placentas and result in TTTS if sufficiently extensive and not counteracted by the superficial shunts. TTTS is uncommon in monochorionic monoamniotic placentas, because the vascular bed is more evenly distributed. Dichorionic diamniotic twins do not share vascular channels in vascular anastomoses and thus are at the lowest risk for TTTS.

**17. Correct choice: E.**

Delayed villous maturation is a phenomenon in which the terminal villi appear less mature for the gestational age, with increased large distal villi containing prominent stromal cells and sometimes edema; the placentas are often large for gestational age. This constellation of findings is most commonly seen in association with stillbirth, chromosomal anomalies, gastroschisis, or gestational diabetes and may be a feature of placentas exposed to opioid maintenance therapy. This finding has also been associated with fetal death and thought to be a primary placental maturational arrest. Similar changes are noted in placentas from infants with

Beckwith-Wiedemann syndrome, which is characterized by fetal overgrowth in multiple organs.

**18. Correct choice: E.**

Passage of meconium in utero at the time of delivery is a frequent, probably physiologic, event. It may occur as a response to acute hypoxic events or chronic hypoxia. By itself, meconium is toxic to the fetus, as it contains vasoconstrictive substances that cause tissue hypoperfusion. Furthermore, aspiration of meconium can cause inflammatory pneumonitis, surfactant inactivation, and airway obstruction. This is the basis of meconium aspiration syndrome, a potentially severe condition that occurs in approximately 5% of meconium-exposed newborns. Pathologic changes correlate with the time of antenatal exposure to meconium:

a. 1 hour: meconium appreciable grossly (green-discolored membranes and chorionic plate); meconium-laden macrophages in amnion
b. 2 to 3 hours: meconium-laden macrophages within fetal-placental chorionic plate
c. 6 to 12 hours: meconium-laden macrophages in extraplacental membranes and umbilical cord; amnion necrosis
d. 24 to 48 hours: necrosis of umbilical vessels, with occasional umbilical ulcerations

**19. Correct choice: E.**

Maternal floor infarction is characterized histologically by massive perivillous fibrin deposition and hyperplasia of intermediate cells. Studies show that 50% of women with this complication have suffered from previous abortions or stillbirths. Association with maternal antiphospholipid antibody syndrome has been described. Maternal serum major basic protein is typically elevated.

**20. Correct choice: E.**

Placental hydrops is a common end point of many disorders rather than a distinct disorder in itself. Grossly, the placenta is boggy, somewhat pale, and large for gestational age (usually >95 percentile) by weight. Microscopically, there is diffuse villous edema with accumulation of fluid in the villous stroma, villous enlargement, and an increase in the proportion of villous stroma to capillaries. The etiology of placental hydrops parallels the differential diagnosis for fetal hydrops and includes both immune and nonimmune causes. Generally, the more common causes include fetal anemia, cytogenetic abnormalities, hypoproteinemia, or cardiac failure due to anomalies or other forms of failure. Immune hydrops results from fetal hemolysis from maternally derived circulating antibodies. Nonimmune hydrops includes a diverse array of conditions, including fetal cardiovascular defects, fetal hemoglobinopathies, parvovirus infection, fetomaternal hemorrhage, twin-twin transfusion, fetal infections, chromosomal disorders, metabolic disorders (eg, inborn errors of metabolism), fetal hematologic malignancies, and fetal tumors.

**21. Correct choice: C.**

Awareness of parvovirus B-19 infection is important because this is not always clinically suspected. Many (50%) pregnant women infected with the virus are asymptomatic, but the virus can still be transmitted to the fetus. In symptomatic infections, the symptoms may include erythema infectiosum, fever, arthralgia, and headache. Parvovirus infects the fetal red blood cell precursors and results in hemolysis and anemia. In cases of placental and/or fetal hydrops of unknown cause, it is worthwhile to scan the villous capillaries for virally infected cells. Parvovirus-infected red cell precursors are enlarged, and the nuclear chromatin is pushed to the edges and surrounds a glassy pink-purple inclusion of viral particles, as illustrated in the image. An immunohistochemical stain for parvovirus is available and can confirm the diagnosis.

**22. Correct choice: B.**

Placenta accreta spectrum (PAS) disorder refers to a placenta that is abnormally adherent to the uterine wall; it is the result of deficient decidua at the site of implantation and is a common cause of postpartum bleeding. The older terminology includes accreta, increta, and percreta. Placenta accreta is defined as implantation of the placenta directly on the myometrium without adequate intervening decidua. The terms "placenta increta and percreta" are used to describe more severe forms of creta in which the chorionic villi invade deeply into the myometrium and through the myometrium to the serosa surface of the uterus, respectively. PAS is the preferred term for all cretas, which are differentiated as either "invasive" (as in the older term increta or percreta) or noninvasive (as in the older term accrete). The image demonstrates placenta increta with villi adjacent to very thin myometrium, with no intervening decidua. The following table delineates the new International Federation of Gynecology and Obstetrics (FIGO) system, which proposes subcategories of PAS as grades based on the depth of invasion and involvement of extrauterine structures (see Table 1).

**TABLE 1 PAS Disorder FIGO System Grading Schema**

| Grade | Diagnostic Criteria |
|---|---|
| PAS Grade 1 | Noninvasive; lack of decidua; smooth myometrial interface without thinning |
| PAS Grade 2 | Superficial invasion; irregular placental-myometrial interface with maintenance of the outer layer of myometrium |
| PAS Grade 3A | Deep invasion; invasion of the placenta to the outer 25% of the myometrium |
| PAS Grade 3B | Deep invasion through the uterine serosa |
| PAS Grade 3C | Deep invasion with placental adherence to extrauterine tissues (eg, bladder) |

FIGO, International Federation of Gynecology and Obstetrics; PAS, placental accreta spectrum.

# 51 Vulva and Vagina

1. Which of the following is the most common type of vulvar cyst in the adult?

   A. Bartholin duct
   B. Epidermoid
   C. Hymenal
   D. Pilonidal
   E. Skene duct/paraurethral

2. The lesion known as *condyloma latum* is caused by

   A. *Calymmatobacterium granulomatis.*
   B. *Chlamydia trachomatis.*
   C. *Haemophilus ducreyi.*
   D. human papillomavirus.
   E. *Treponema pallidum.*

3. A 39-year-old female presents with a large 14-cm, slow-growing, polypoid mass in the pelvic soft tissue. Histologically, there is no nuclear atypia, tumor cell necrosis, or mitotic figures as shown in Figure 1. Blood vessels of various caliber are typically widely dilated. The lesion lacks marginal circumscription. Which of the following is the most likely diagnosis?

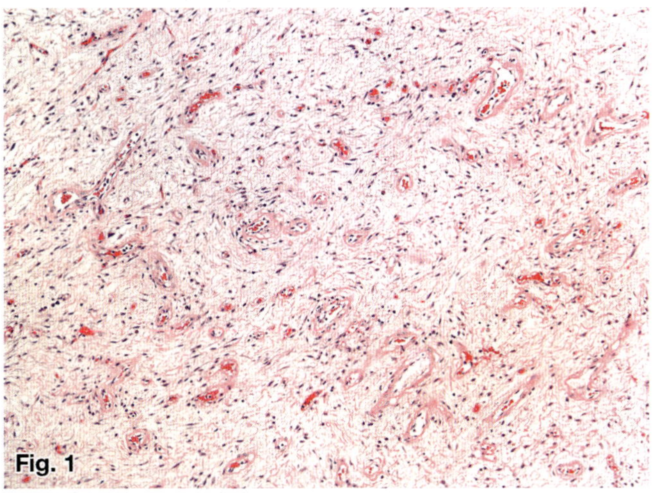

Fig. 1

   A. Angiomyofibroblastoma
   B. Cellular angiofibroma
   C. Deep (aggressive) angiomyxoma
   D. Superficial angiomyxoma
   E. Superficial myofibroblastoma

4. A biopsy of a dry, itchy plaque on the vulva of a 55-year-old woman shows the histologic changes seen in Figure 1. Which of the following is the most likely diagnosis?

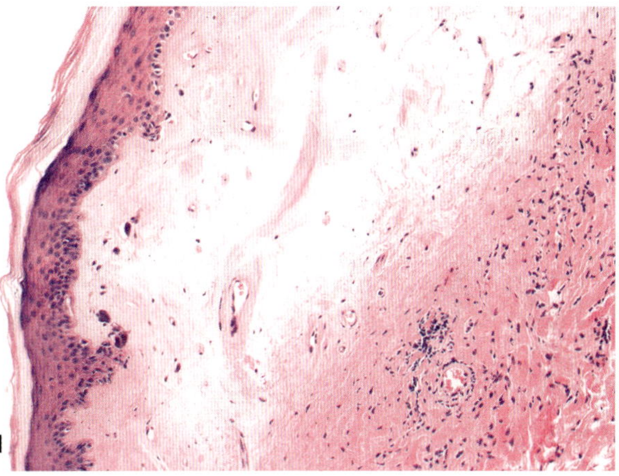

Fig. 1

   A. Atrophic squamous epithelium
   B. High-grade squamous intraepithelial lesion
   C. Lichen sclerosus
   D. Lichen simplex chronicus
   E. Low-grade squamous intraepithelial lesion

All figures in this chapter are from Longacre TA, Greenson JK, Hornick JL, Reuter VE, eds. *Mills and Sternberg's Diagnostic Surgical Pathology.* 7th ed. Wolters Kluwer; 2022 except for those noted at the end of this book.

5. Figure 1 represents a vulvar biopsy of a lesion from a 74-year-old woman. Which of the following is incorrect?

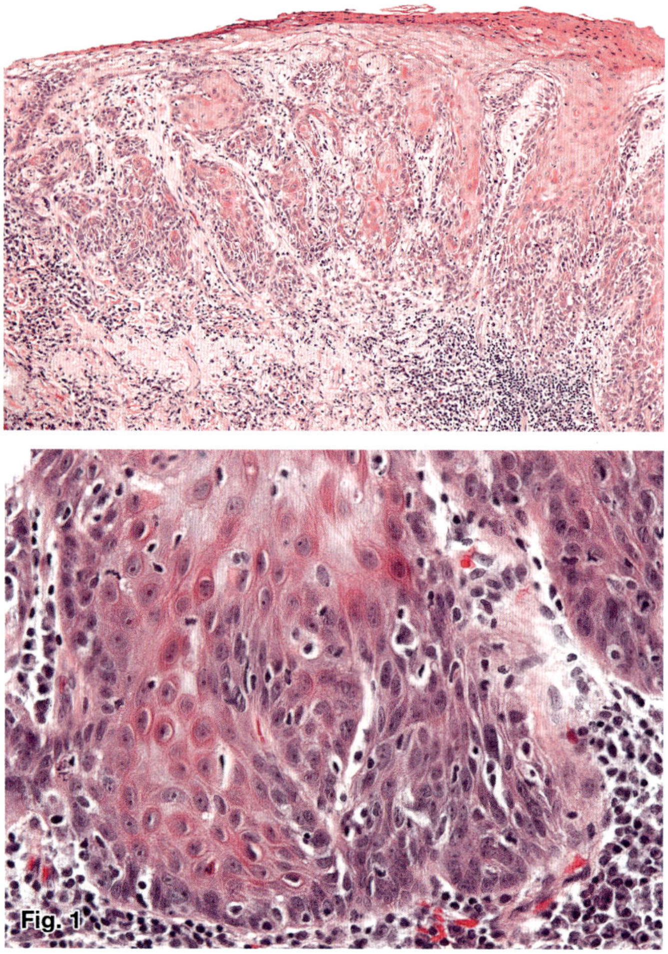

Fig. 1

A. Aberrant p53 expression by immunohistochemistry is present.
B. Extension into skin appendages is uncommon.
C. It is associated with high-risk human papillomavirus (HPV) infection.
D. Lichen sclerosus is commonly observed.
E. Treatment is complete excision with follow-up for recurrence/progression to invasive cancer.

6. Which of the following key factors does not determine the prognosis for vulvar invasive squamous cell carcinoma?

A. Age of patient
B. Distant metastasis
C. Extension into surrounding structures
D. Status of the groin and pelvic lymph nodes
E. Tumor size

7. A postmenopausal white woman has a slow-growing lesion primary to the vulva, clinically thought to represent chronic dermatitis. A biopsy of the lesion shows the findings in Figure 1. CK7 immunohistochemical stain highlights the lesional cells in Figure 2. The lesional cells will be negative for which immunohistochemical stain?

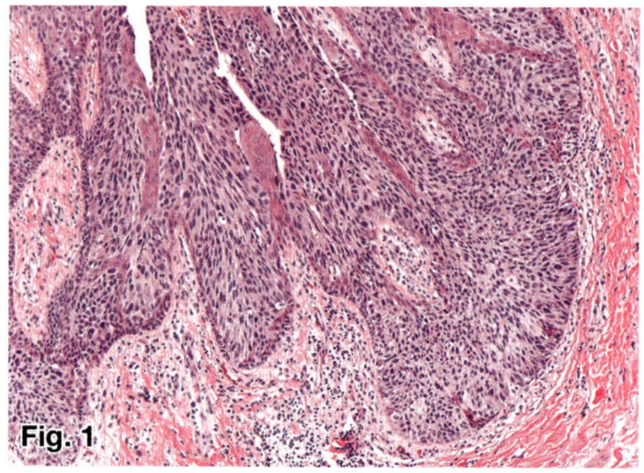

Fig. 1

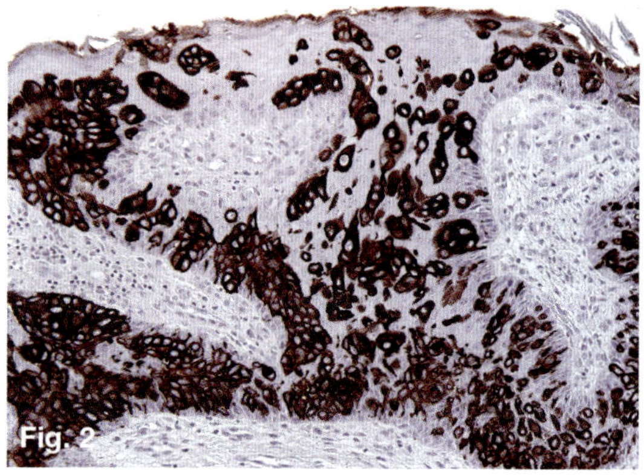

Fig. 2

A. Carcinoembryonic antigen (CEA)
B. CK20
C. Cytokeratin
D. Epithelial membrane antigen (EMA)
E. Gross cystic disease fluid protein 15 (GCDFP-15)

8. A 35-year-old White woman undergoes excision of a small, well-circumscribed, ulcerated nodule located on the labia majora. The histologic features of the lesion are shown in Figure 1. Which of the following is false with regard to this entity?

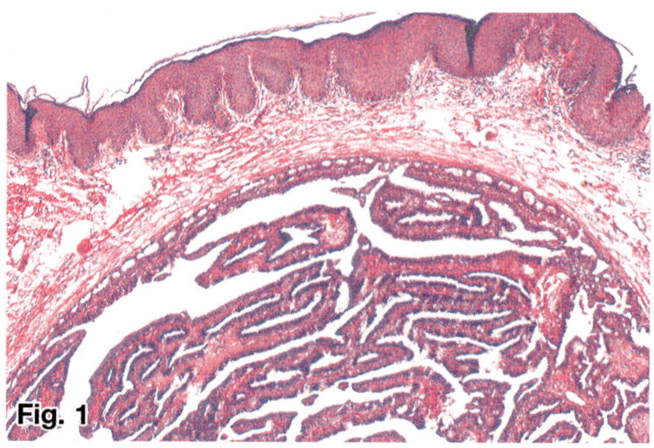

Fig. 1

A. Likely derives from anogenital mammary-like glands
B. Majority occur on the labia majora or labia minora
C. Most commonly seen in prepubertal women
D. Often resembles intraductal papilloma or nipple adenoma of the breast

9. Which of the following is false with regard to vaginal adenosis?

   A. It commonly occurs in the upper one-third of the vagina.
   B. It rarely progresses to adenocarcinoma.
   C. It results from in utero exposure to diethylstilbestrol (DES).
   D. There are no identifiable lesions on clinical examination.
   E. With age, it is replaced by squamous metaplasia.

10. Which of the following is the most frequent site of malakoplakia when it occurs in the female genital tract?

   A. Cervix
   B. Endometrium
   C. Perineum
   D. Vagina
   E. Vulva

11. Which of the following is a common pathogen causing vaginitis?

   A. *Candida albicans*
   B. *Candida glabrata*
   C. *Mycoplasma*
   D. *Neisseria gonorrhoeae*
   E. *Ureaplasma urealyticum*

12. An incidental soft pedunculated vaginal polyp measuring 2 cm is found along the lateral wall of the lower one-third of the vagina in a 41-year-old female during her annual gynecologic exam. The histologic features are demonstrated in Figure 1. What is the diagnosis?

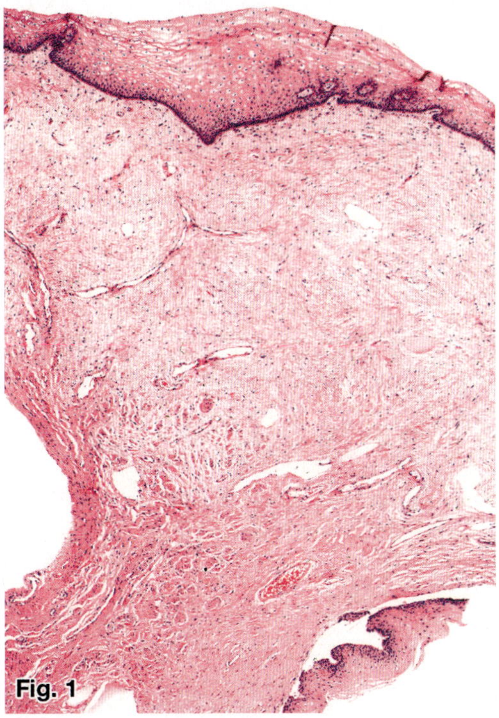

Fig. 1

   A. Embryonal rhabdomyosarcoma
   B. Fibroepithelial stromal polyp
   C. Granulation tissue
   D. Tubulosquamous polyp
   E. Vaginal mixed tumor

13. A vaginal polypoid mass is excised from a 43-year-old woman. Histologically, it is composed of large strap cells with cross-striations in a fascicular arrangement as shown in Figure 1. No cambium layer is present underneath the epithelial layer. Which of the following is the most likely diagnosis?

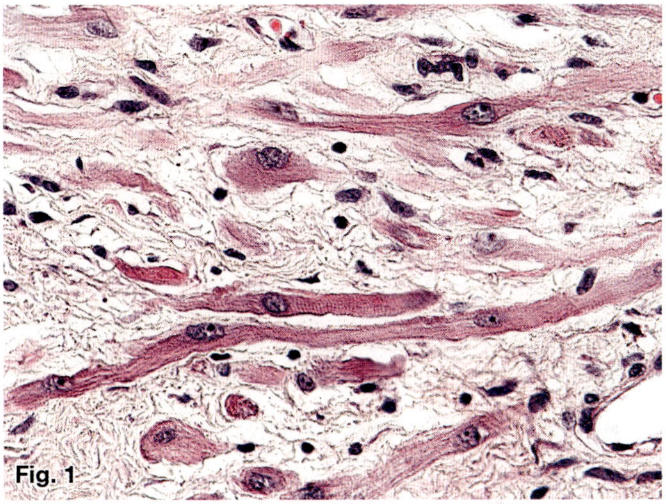

Fig. 1

   A. Aggressive angiomyxoma
   B. Embryonal rhabdomyosarcoma
   C. Fibroepithelial stromal polyp
   D. Rhabdomyoma
   E. Vaginal mixed tumor

14. Which is the most common vaginal mesenchymal neoplasm?

   A. Angiomyofibroblastoma
   B. Angiomyolipoma
   C. Leiomyoma
   D. Neurofibroma
   E. Rhabdomyoma

15. Which of the following is not associated with in utero diethylstilbestrol (DES) exposure?

   A. Cervical clear cell carcinoma
   B. Cervical microglandular hyperplasia
   C. Congenital abnormalities of the vagina
   D. Vaginal adenosis
   E. Vaginal clear cell carcinoma

16. Figure 1 shows the histologic features of a vaginal tumor that occurs in children and adolescents. Which of the following is a known risk factor for the development of this tumor?

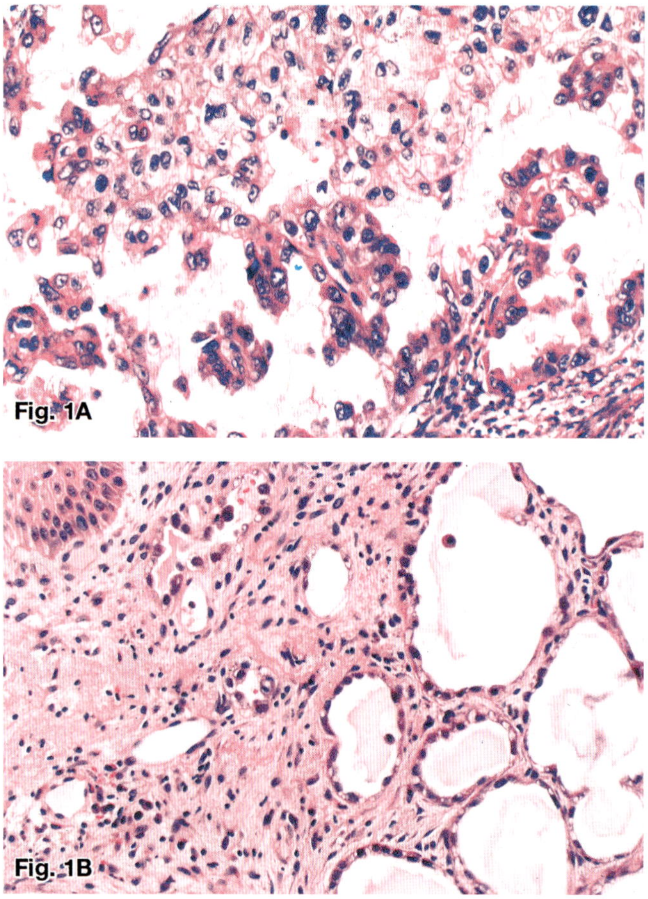

Fig. 1A

Fig. 1B

A. Bacterial vaginosis
B. High-risk human papillomavirus (HPV) infection
C. Postnatal exposure to estrogens
D. Prenatal exposure to diethylstilbestrol (DES)
E. Vaginal endometriosis

17. A 2-year-old girl presented with a polypoid vaginal tumor, with histologic features shown in Figure 1. She has no in utero exposure to diethylstilbestrol (DES). What is the most likely diagnosis?

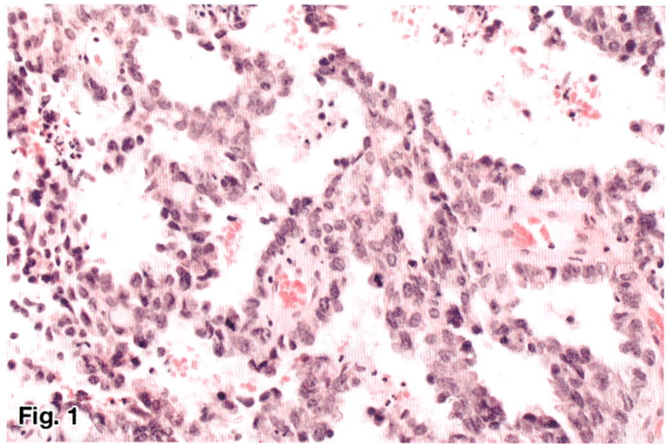

Fig. 1

A. Arias-Stella reaction
B. Clear cell carcinoma
C. Embryonal rhabdomyosarcoma
D. Microglandular hyperplasia
E. Yolk sac tumor

18. A 4-year-old girl was found to have a soft polypoid tumor protruding out of the vagina. On clinical examination, it was noted to arise from the anterior vaginal wall. Figure 1 shows the histologic features of the tumor, which included a cambium layer. What is the most likely diagnosis?

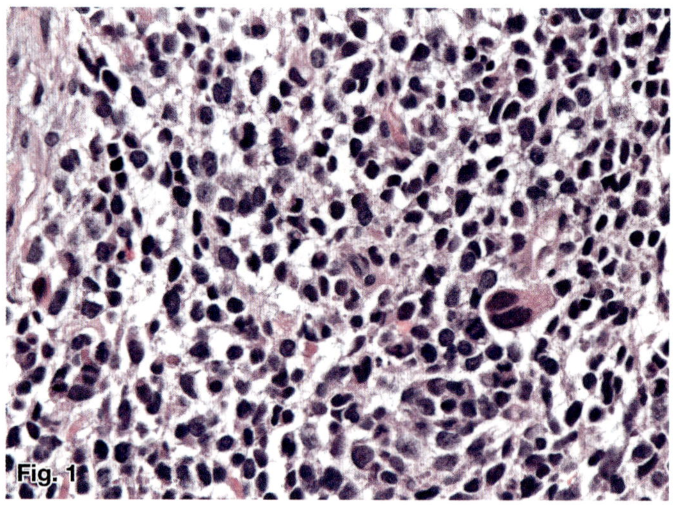

Fig. 1

A. Clear cell carcinoma
B. Embryonal rhabdomyosarcoma
C. Rhabdomyoma
D. Yolk sac tumor

# ANSWERS AND EXPLANATIONS

**1. Correct choice: B.**

Epidermoid cysts are the most common vulvar cysts. They are usually located in the anterior half of the labia majora. Hymenal cysts are the most common type in newborns. Vulvar cysts other than epidermoid are listed in the following table:

| Type | Origin | Lining |
|---|---|---|
| Bartholin duct cyst | Bartholin duct | Transitional |
| Pilonidal cyst | Hair follicle | Squamous |
| Hymenal cyst | Hymen | Squamous |
| Skene duct cyst | Skene duct | Transitional |
| Cyst of canal of Nuck | Processus vaginalis | Mesothelium |
| Mucinous cyst | Minor vestibular glands | Mucus secreting |
| Gartner duct cyst | Mesonephric/Wolffian | Non-mucus-secreting cuboidal |
| Fox-Fordyce disease | Apocrine glands | Hair follicle wall |
| Endometriotic cyst | Endometriotic foci | Endometrium |

**2. Correct choice: E.**

*Condyloma latum* is a manifestation of secondary syphilis and develops 3 to 6 weeks following primary infection (also known as the chancre). It consists of gray-white soft papules or plaques and is highly contagious. Histologically, the lesions are composed of plasma cell infiltration and obliterative endarteritis, with conspicuous overlying pseudoepitheliomatous hyperplasia, which must not be confused with squamous cell carcinoma when florid. Tertiary syphilis is rarely encountered in the vulva. *Calymmatobacterium granulomatis* (recently renamed *Klebsiella granulomatis*) causes *granuloma inguinale*, which is rare in the United States and is mostly confined to southern states. Serotypes L1 to L3 of *Chlamydia trachomatis* cause *lymphogranuloma venereum*, and serotypes D to K cause sexually transmitted diseases. *Haemophilus ducreyi* is the etiologic agent of the rare *chancroid.*

**3. Correct choice: C.**

Deep (aggressive) angiomyxoma occurs in the vulva, vagina, perineum, inguinal area, or pelvic soft tissues of women in their third and fourth decade of life and presents as a large, slow-growing, polypoid mass or swelling. Most are greater than 10 cm in size. Histologic features include a hypocellular proliferation of stellate and spindle-shaped small bland mesenchymal cells embedded in a loose myxoid stroma with a few collagen fibers. Small- or medium-sized veins and arteries within the tumor often are grouped together and may show medial hypertrophy. Blood vessels of various calibers are typically widely dilated with extravasation of red blood cells. Light microscopic features of angiomyofibroblastoma that distinguish it from deep angiomyxoma include marginal circumscription, higher cellularity, larger numbers of blood vessels lacking hyalinization or hypertrophy, often plump stromal cells with perivascular accentuation, a paucity of stromal mucin, and only rare extravasated erythrocytes. Cellular angiofibroma is a benign spindle cell tumor of the vulva that measures 1.2 to 2.5 cm in size. Microscopically, the tumor consists of a monotonous spindle cell proliferation, often admixed with small foci of mature fat and coarse collagen fibers. Superficial angiomyxoma is a rare, small cutaneous lesion that exhibits a multilobulated growth pattern and has a significant potential for local but nondestructive recurrence. These lesions are centered in the dermis and superficial subcutaneous tissue and feature abundant myxoid stroma with bland fibroblasts; scattered inflammatory cells; and thin-walled, capillary-sized vessels. Superficial myofibroblastoma occurs more commonly in the cervix but can present in the vulva and vagina. This tumor occurs in a wide age range (23-80 years) and measures 1 to 6.5 cm. The tumor is well circumscribed and typically exhibits a variety of architectural patterns. The constituent cells are bland, ovoid to spindle-shaped, often with wavy nuclei set in a finely collagenous stroma. Stromal edema or myxoid change and/or hyalinized areas with thick, dense collagen bundles may be seen.

**4. Correct choice: C.**

Lichen sclerosus is a condition that usually affects postmenopausal women, involving the vulva and occasionally extending to adjacent regions. Initially, the lesions are dry, scaly, and itchy, which evolve into parchment-like plaques. The microscopic features include (a) epithelial thinning with loss of rete pegs, and hyperkeratosis; (b) basal cell vacuolation; (c) atrophic, edematous dermis; and (d) loss of skin adnexa. Lichen sclerosus is often found in a close spatial relationship with differentiated vulvar intraepithelial neoplasia (VIN) and vulvar human papillomavirus (HPV)-independent squamous cell carcinoma.

**5. Correct choice: C.**

Human papillomavirus (HPV)-independent differentiated vulvar neoplasia lacks typical morphologic features of HPV infection and is characterized by prominent cytologic atypia in the basal layer, with or without expansion of nuclear atypia into the parabasal layers with abrupt, abnormal keratinocyte maturation. p53 is often strongly expressed in the basal and suprabasal epithelium. In contrast to HPV-associated high-grade squamous intraepithelial lesion (HSIL), extension into skin appendages is very uncommon. It typically occurs in postmenopausal women, often with a history of lichen sclerosus. Differentiated vulvar intraepithelial neoplasia (VIN) carries a high risk of progression to invasive squamous cell carcinoma (SCC), so treatment is complete excision with close follow-up.

**6. Correct choice: A.**

The key factors that determine prognosis for vulvar invasive squamous cell carcinoma (SCC) are tumor size, extension into surrounding structures, status of the groin and pelvic lymph nodes, and distant metastasis. Human papillomavirus (HPV) status is a significant prognostic marker in vulvar SCC. Within the HPV-negative vulvar SCCs, about 74% are associated with abnormal p53 expression/TP53 mutation, which is associated with a poorer prognosis than SCCs demonstrating a wild-type pattern of expression of p53. Age is not a key prognostic factor.

**7. Correct choice: B.**

The H&E (hematoxylin and eosin) image is of vulvar extramammary Paget disease, which is a slowly growing neoplasm of long duration that sometimes is mistaken clinically for a chronic, intractable dermatitis. Most cases occur in postmenopausal white women, commonly in the seventh decade of life. Microscopically, Paget disease consists of large, pale cells, predominantly in the basal layer of the epidermis. Single cells, nests, and well-formed glands are present and sometimes extend into the upper layers of the epithelium. Immunohistochemically, Paget cells are reactive for carcinoembryonic antigen (CEA), cytokeratin, epithelial membrane antigen (EMA), gross cystic disease fluid protein, which is also found in normal eccrine and apocrine cells, and CK7. CK20 reactivity with gross cystic disease fluid protein 15 (GCDFP-15) negativity may be a clue to an associated internal gastrointestinal or urothelial adenocarcinoma. Human epidermal growth factor receptor 2 (HER2) overexpression may occur in vulvar Paget disease.

**8. Correct choice: C.**

Hidradenoma papilliferum (papillary hidradenoma) is virtually nonexistent in prepubertal women. Eighty percent are on the labia majora or labia minora, often in or near the interlabial sulcus. Hidradenoma papilliferum often resembles intraductal papilloma or nipple adenoma of the breast. It likely derives from anogenital mammary-like glands, which often are found in or around the hidradenoma.

**9. Correct choice: D.**

Vaginal adenosis appears as red nodules on clinical examination and manifests with excessive mucus discharge in postpubertal age. It develops in almost all women who had in utero diethylstilbestrol (DES) exposure. It consists of Müllerian-type epithelium within the vaginal mucosa, which may be of the endocervical (mucus-producing) type or tubal/endometrium (clear cell) type. Vaginal adenosis seldom progresses to adenocarcinoma and is gradually replaced by squamous metaplasia. Microglandular hyperplasia develops in foci of vaginal adenosis, especially after oral contraceptive use.

**10. Correct choice: D.**

The vagina is the most frequent site of malakoplakia when it occurs in the female genital tract. *Escherichia coli* is often cultured from the urine or the specific lesion of genital malakoplakia.

**11. Correct choice: A.**

*Candida* (usually *Candida albicans*) is a common pathogen causing vaginitis. It is mostly observed in women during the childbearing years and manifests as mucosal erythema or a thick, white exudate. Histologically, there is mild acanthosis and spongiosis, with congestion and edema of the lamina propria. The organism resides on the epithelial surface and does not penetrate the mucosa and can be highlighted by periodic acid-Schiff (PAS) special stains. Necrotic debris, neutrophils, and yeast form a surface exudate. About 10% of fungal vaginitis is caused by *Candida glabrata*. *Mycoplasma* spp. and *Ureaplasma urealyticum* normally inhabit the vagina, but, rarely, each may be the predominant isolate in cases of vaginitis. *Neisseria gonorrhoeae* rarely causes vaginitis in adults but may infect children who have less resistance to vaginal squamous epithelium.

**12. Correct choice: B.**

Benign vaginal fibroepithelial (stromal) polyps are generally found in adults. They are polypoid or pedunculated, less than 4 cm in size, and found along the lateral walls of the lower one-third of the vagina. The underlying fibrovascular stroma is loose or dense and contains abundant blood vessels. Approximately one-half of the cases have atypical stromal cells with large nuclei and abundant cytoplasm, designated as fibroepithelial stromal polyp. Unlike embryonal rhabdomyosarcoma, which usually occurs in young children, it lacks rapid growth, invasion of adjacent tissues, hypercellularity, a cambium layer, and cells with cytoplasmic cross-striations. Tubulosquamous polyps typically occur in the upper vagina in postmenopausal females, are generally small, and composed of a well-circumscribed proliferation of tubules and bland squamous nests with central necrosis or keratinization set within a cellular fibrous stroma. The tubules may be positive for prostatic markers as these polyps are thought to be derived from paraurethral Skene glands. Vaginal mixed tumor is situated most often just above the hymenal ring in adults. Microscopically, it is composed of small spindle cells that surround nests of mature squamous cells and glands lined by mucinous epithelium. Granulation tissue, commonly found in the vaginal vault after hysterectomy, often occurs within a few weeks or months after surgery, and is frequently biopsied because it simulates carcinoma clinically and is of concern in women who have had a prior hysterectomy for neoplasia.

**13. Correct choice: D.**

It is important to distinguish benign rhabdomyoma, which usually occurs in adult patients, from botryoid rhabdomyosarcoma, which affects children under the age of 5 years. Rhabdomyoma is composed of very large strap cells with evident cross-striations. Cross-striations are difficult to identify in rhabdomyosarcoma of the embryonal type (botryoid). The latter exhibits a characteristic accumulation of neoplastic cells underneath the epithelium, known as the cambium layer. Vaginal mixed tumor is composed of basophilic cells arranged in cords, glandular structures, and squamous nests. Fibroepithelial stromal polyp is a pedunculated polyp composed of a dense fibrovascular core covered by intact epithelium, with scattered atypical stromal cells with large nuclei and abundant cytoplasm in the stroma.

**14. Correct choice: C.**

Leiomyoma is the most common vaginal mesenchymal neoplasm. Leiomyomata with epithelioid features are very uncommon in the vagina.

**15. Correct choice: B.**

The association of vaginal and cervical clear cell carcinoma with in utero exposure to diethylstilbestrol (DES) is well known. Congenital abnormalities of the vagina that result from in utero exposure to DES include mucosal membrane abnormalities, corolla-like mucosal elevation, fibrous band, apical narrowing, forniceal obliteration, transverse or longitudinal vaginal septa, and vaginal adenosis. There is no association between DES exposure and cervical microglandular hyperplasia, which consists of small, uniform, crowded glands containing mucin without prominent intervening stroma, nuclear pleomorphism, or prominent nucleoli.

**16. Correct choice: D.**

Clear cell carcinoma of the vagina develops in children and adolescents with a history of prenatal exposure to diethylstilbestrol (DES), a medication previously used for the treatment of threatened abortion. Morphologically, the tumor resembles analogous uterine or ovarian neoplasms arising in older women. It is composed of cells with clear glycogen-filled cytoplasm, which acquire the characteristic hobnail appearance when lining papillary structures, and predominantly show tubulocystic growth pattern. In utero DES exposure leads most commonly to vaginal adenosis or anatomic abnormalities such as mucosal membranes, apical narrowing, vaginal septa, among others.

**17. Correct choice: E.**

Yolk sac tumor of the vagina occurs in girls 3 years of age or younger. Grossly, the neoplasm is sessile or polypoid, with areas of ulceration. Vaginal yolk sac tumor is microscopically identical to pure yolk sac tumors of the ovary and testis. Clear cell carcinoma develops in children and adolescents with a history of prenatal exposure to diethylstilbestrol (DES). Morphologically, the tumor resembles analogous uterine or ovarian neoplasms arising in older women and is composed of cells with clear glycogen-filled cytoplasm, which acquire the characteristic hobnail appearance when lining papillary structures, and predominantly show tubulocystic growth pattern. Embryonal rhabdomyosarcoma is found in infants or children up to 6 years of age. It is composed of small, round, or spindle-shaped cells with scanty cytoplasm embedded in a myxoid stroma. A characteristic subepithelial condensation of malignant cells (cambium layer) and rhabdomyoblasts are observed. Vaginal microglandular hyperplasia develops in foci of vaginal adenosis, especially after oral contraceptive use, and consists of small, uniform, crowded glands containing mucin without prominent intervening stroma, nuclear pleomorphism, or prominent nucleoli. Arias-Stella reaction is a hormone-related reactive phenomenon of the endometrium characterized by hypertrophy and vacuolization of glandular epithelial cells showing marked enlargement, nuclear pleomorphism, and hyperchromasia.

**18. Correct choice: B.**

Embryonal rhabdomyosarcoma is found in infants or children up to 6 years of age. The neoplasm often arises from the anterior vaginal wall and presents as soft, botryoid nodules that fill and often protrude out of the vagina. It is composed of small, round, or spindle-shaped cells with scanty cytoplasm embedded in a myxoid stroma. A characteristic subepithelial condensation of malignant cells (cambium layer) and rhabdomyoblasts are observed. Yolk sac tumor of the vagina occurs in girls 3 years of age or younger. Grossly, the neoplasm is sessile or polypoid, with areas of ulceration. Vaginal yolk sac tumor is microscopically identical to pure yolk sac tumors of the ovary and testis. Clear cell carcinoma develops in children and adolescents with a history of prenatal exposure to diethylstilbestrol (DES). Morphologically, the tumor resembles analogous uterine or ovarian neoplasms arising in older women and is composed of cells with clear glycogen-filled cytoplasm, which acquire the characteristic hobnail appearance when lining papillary structures, and predominantly show tubulocystic growth pattern. Rhabdomyoma is a benign tumor seen in adults, composed of very large strap cells with evident cross-striations.

# 52 Cervix

1. Which of the following two pathogens cause characteristic histologic findings upon cervical infection?

   A. *Bacterial vaginosis*
   B. Herpes simplex virus (HSV)
   C. *Neisseria gonorrhoeae*
   D. *Trichomonas vaginalis*

2. Which of the following is not a change associated with high-grade squamous intraepithelial lesions (HSILs) during colposcopic examination after application of 3% to 5% acetic acid to the cervix?

   A. Acetowhite changes
   B. Atypical vessels
   C. Mosaicism
   D. Punctation
   E. Sloughing

3. A cervical biopsy demonstrates the changes shown in Figure 1. There are no atypical mitotic figures. These changes should be reported as

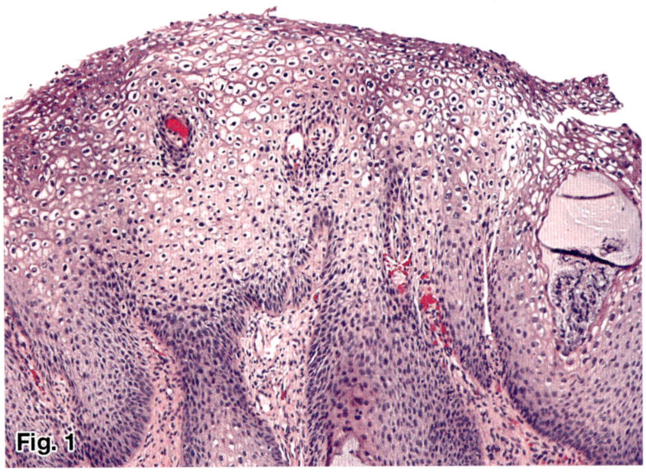


   A. condyloma.
   B. high-grade squamous intraepithelial lesion (HSIL).
   C. low-grade squamous intraepithelial lesion (LSIL).
   D. reactive changes, negative for dysplasia.

4. The nuclear changes in the cervical epithelium shown in Figure 1 are best described as

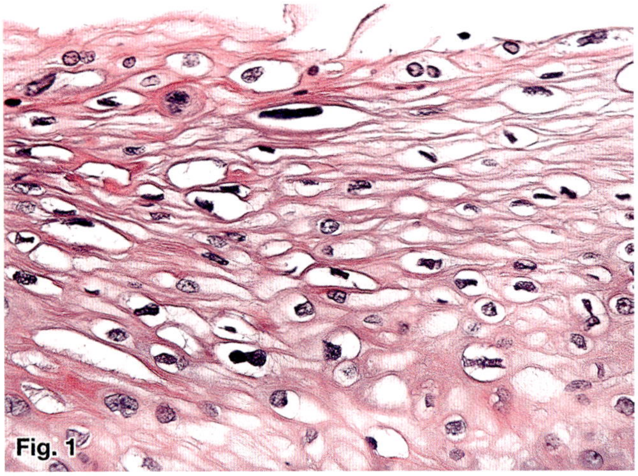


   A. degenerative.
   B. glycogenation.
   C. inflammatory halos.
   D. koilocytosis.
   E. smudgy.

5. A cervical biopsy reveals the changes shown in Figure 1. Which of the following is the best diagnosis?

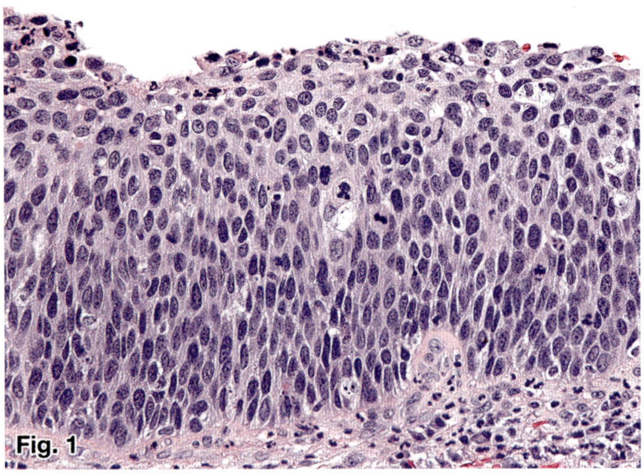


   A. Atrophy
   B. High-grade squamous intraepithelial lesion (HSIL)
   C. Immature squamous metaplasia
   D. Low-grade squamous intraepithelial lesion (LSIL)
   E. Transitional metaplasia

All figures in this chapter are from Longacre TA, Greenson JK, Hornick JL, Reuter VE, eds. *Mills and Sternberg's Diagnostic Surgical Pathology*. 7th ed. Wolters Kluwer; 2022 except for those noted at the end of this book.

6. According to the recommendations of the Lower Anogenital Squamous Terminology (LAST) project, the molecular marker most useful in the diagnostic evaluation of cervical squamous dysplasia is

   A. immunohistochemistry for cyclin E.
   B. immunohistochemistry for Ki-67.
   C. immunohistochemistry for p16.
   D. immunohistochemistry for ProEx C.
   E. in situ hybridization for HPV16 (human papillomavirus 16) and 18.

7. According to the Lower Anogenital Squamous Terminology (LAST) project recommendations, p16 immunohistochemistry (IHC) should not be performed in which of the following situations?

   A. In the differential diagnosis between high-grade squamous intraepithelial lesion (HSIL) and a dysplasia-mimicking lesion (ie, immature squamous metaplasia, atrophy, reactive changes, tangential sectioning)
   B. When a precancer lesion is not found in a biopsy from a patient with prior cytologic diagnosis of HSIL, atypical squamous cells-HSIL (ASC-H), atypical glandular cells-not otherwise specified (AGC-NOS), or atypical squamous cells of undetermined significance (ASC-US) with positive HPV type 16 (HPV16+)
   C. When morphology is unequivocally negative or diagnostic of LSIL (CIN1) or HSIL (CIN3)
   D. When the lesion shows features of CIN2
   E. When there is lack of consensus among pathologists in the diagnosis of HSIL

8. Which of the following may mimic superficially invasive squamous cell carcinoma of the cervix?

   A. Decidualization of the cervical stroma in pregnant women
   B. Displacement of benign or dysplastic squamous epithelium into lymphatic-vascular channels
   C. High-grade squamous intraepithelial lesion (HSIL) with extension into underlying endocervical glands
   D. Prior biopsy site
   E. All of the above

9. By definition, which of the following criteria must be met for the diagnosis of superficially invasive squamous cell carcinoma on a resection specimen?

   A. No endometrial involvement
   B. No grossly visible lesion
   C. No invasion
   D. No lymph node metastasis
   E. No vaginal involvement

10. Figure 1 shows a metaplastic change that may mimic endocervical adenocarcinoma in situ. What is the diagnosis?

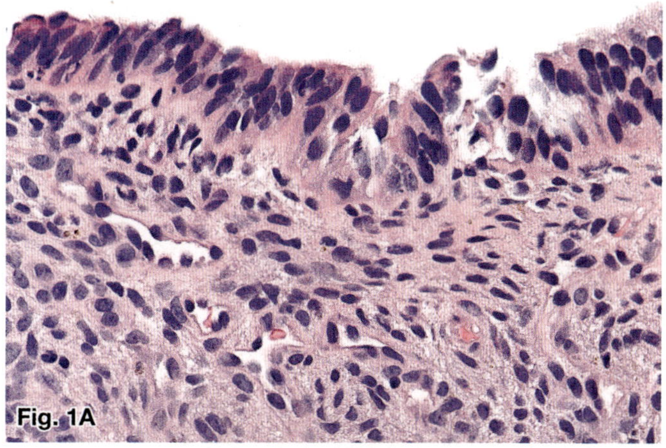

Fig. 1A

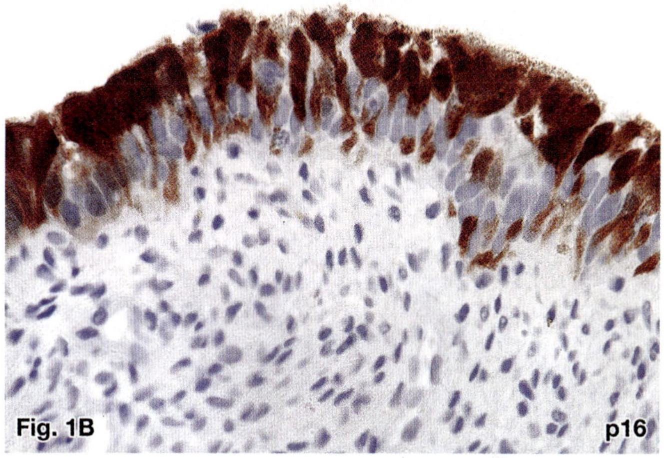

Fig. 1B p16

   A. Atypical oxyphilic metaplasia
   B. Endometriosis
   C. Endosalpingiosis
   D. Misplaced Skene glands
   E. Tuboendometrioid metaplasia

11. Figure 1 shows a glandular hyperplastic lesion of the endocervix that is known to be associated with oral contraceptive use, which can become florid and clinically present as an endocervical polyp or cervical erosion. Which of the following is it?

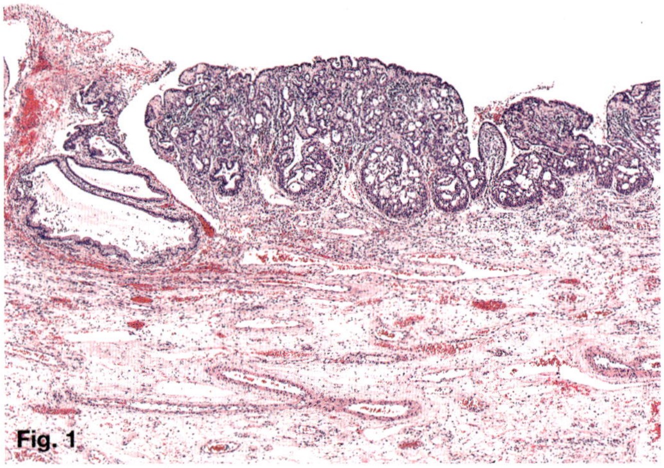

Fig. 1

A. Adenoid basal hyperplasia
B. Diffuse laminar endocervical glandular hyperplasia
C. Lobular endocervical glandular hyperplasia
D. Microglandular hyperplasia
E. Nabothian cyst

12. The endocervical reactive change demonstrated in Figure 1 is due to

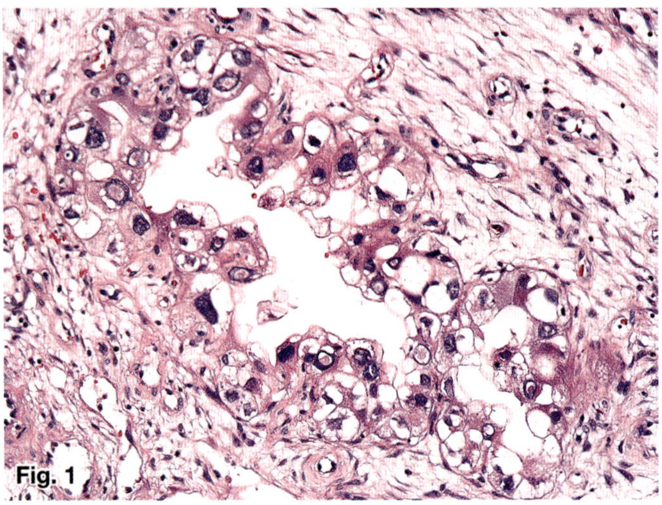

Fig. 1

A. Arias-Stella reaction.
B. clear cell carcinoma.
C. gastric-type endocervical adenocarcinoma.
D. papillary endocervicitis.
E. radiation.

13. The endocervical reactive change demonstrated in Figure 1 is due to

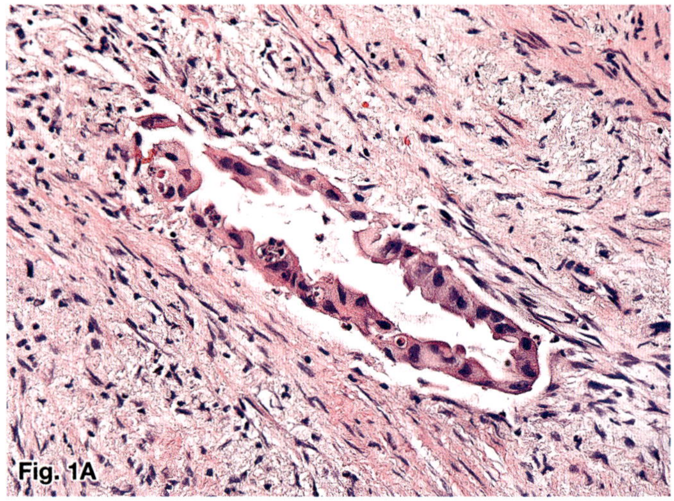

Fig. 1A

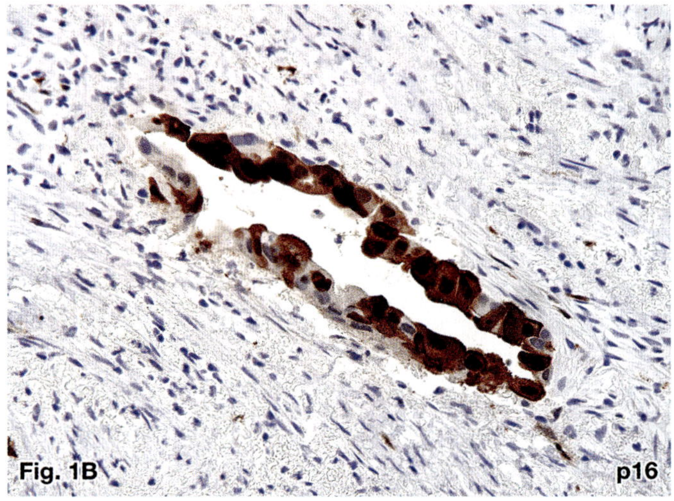


Fig. 1B

A. Arias-Stella reaction.
B. clear cell carcinoma.
C. gastric-type endocervical adenocarcinoma.
D. papillary endocervicitis.
E. radiation.

14. Figures 1 and 2 show a lesion detected in a cervical biopsy from a 40-year-old woman. Which of the following is true about this lesion?

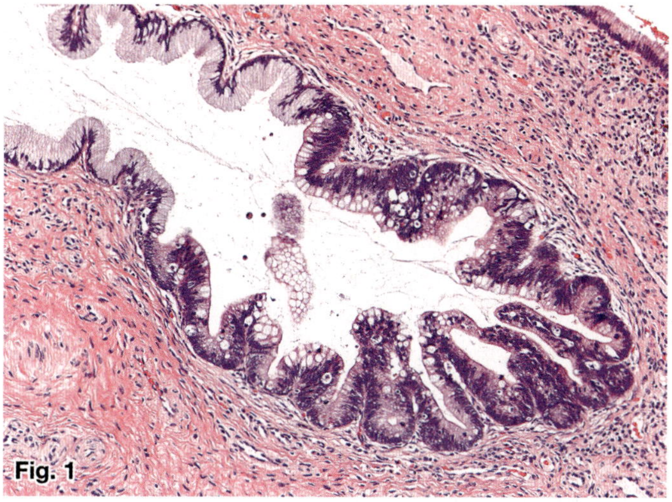
Fig. 1

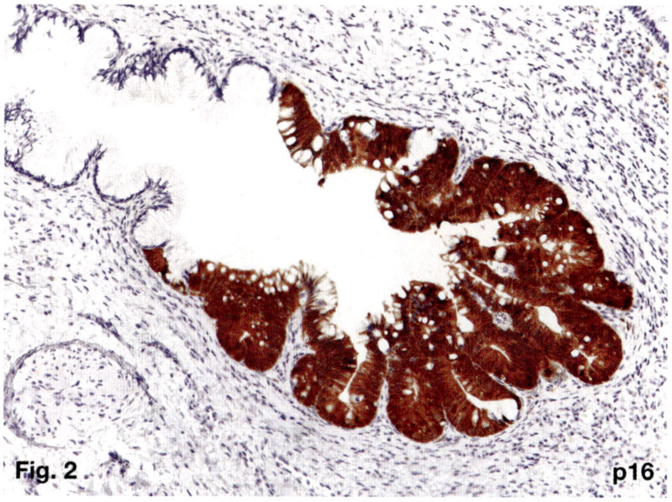

Fig. 2

A. Arises from reserve cells at the squamocolumnar junction
B. Associated with human papillomavirus (HPV) in the majority of cases
C. Often associated with squamous intraepithelial lesion
D. Usually seen next to invasive adenocarcinoma
E. All of the above

15. Figure 1 shows a lesion that was identified in the cervical biopsy of a 38-year-old female who had a prior atypical squamous cells cannot exclude high-grade squamous intraepithelial lesion (ASC-H), high-risk human papillomavirus (HPV)-positive Pap screening cytology. What is the most likely diagnosis?

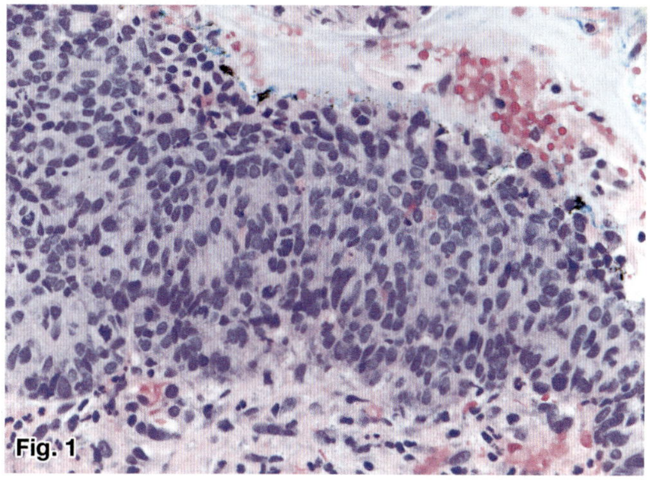
Fig. 1

A. High-grade squamous intraepithelial lesion
B. Immature squamous metaplasia
C. Microglandular hyperplasia
D. Stratified mucin-producing intraepithelial lesion
E. Transitional metaplasia

16. An endocervical adenocarcinoma displaying diffuse, strong immunoreactivity for p16, but is negative for estrogen receptor (ER) and vimentin, is most likely of

A. endocervical origin.
B. endometrial origin.

17. Which of the following cervical adenocarcinoma is associated with the worst prognosis?

A. Clear cell carcinoma
B. Gastric-type adenocarcinoma
C. Mesonephric adenocarcinoma
D. Usual-type adenocarcinoma
E. Villoglandular adenocarcinoma

18. Which of the following statements is false regarding the tumor seen in Figure 1, an incidental finding in a 60-year-old female who underwent excision for high-grade squamous intraepithelial lesion (HSIL) with high-risk human papillomavirus type 16 (HPV16) positive abnormal Pap smear?

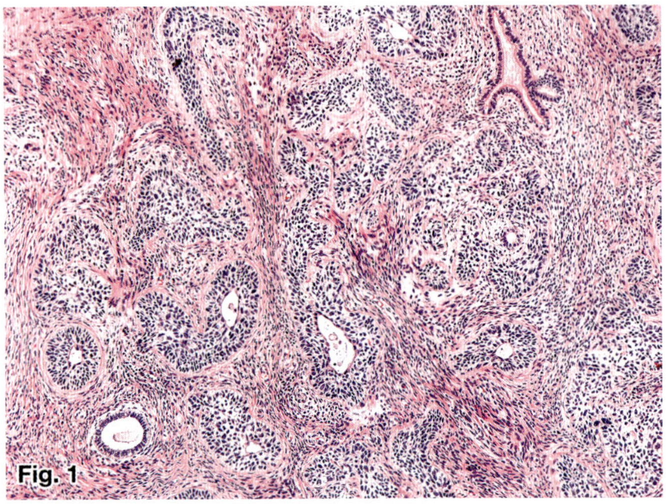


A. Can have basaloid, squamous, and glandular differentiation and is composed of cytologically bland mitotically inactive cells
B. Has a poor prognosis
C. Invasion not usually associated with desmoplastic stromal reaction
D. May be superficial
E. May extend deeply into the cervical stroma

19. A 50-year-old female presented with a polypoid cervical mass and underwent hysterectomy. The histologic features of the tumor are shown in Figure 1. The tumor cells are positive for p16, synaptophysin, and chromogranin and negative for p63 and desmin. Ki-67 proliferation index is markedly increased (>90%). What is the most likely diagnosis?

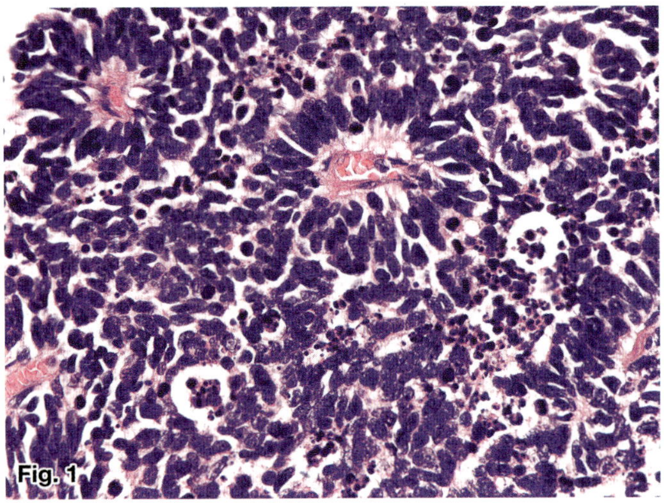


A. Endocervical adenocarcinoma, human papillomavirus (HPV)-associated
B. Large-cell neuroendocrine carcinoma
C. Poorly differentiated squamous cell carcinoma, HPV-associated
D. Rhabdomyosarcoma
E. Small-cell neuroendocrine carcinoma

20. A 15-year-old teenager presents with a cervical polypoid mass that is protruding from the introitus. The histologic features of the lesion are shown in Figure 1. Foci of benign cartilage are noted. The atypical cells show positive nuclear staining with myogenin and MyoD1. Which of the following germline mutations is associated with this tumor?

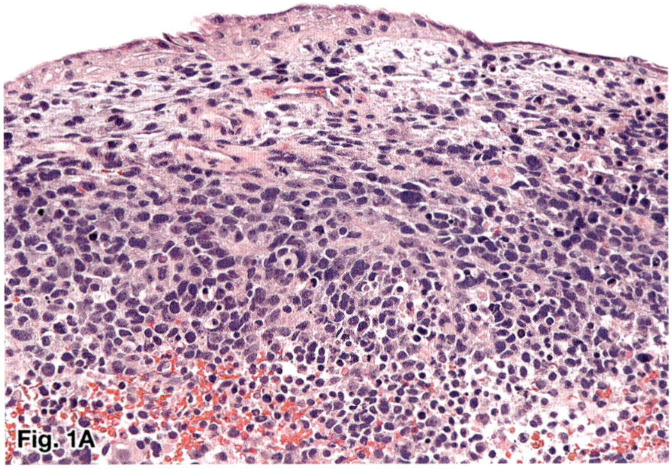


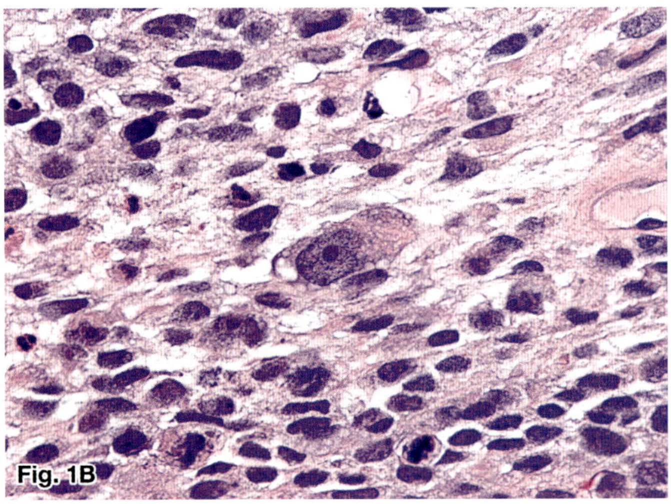


A. *APC*
B. *DICER1*
C. *MSH2*
D. *STK11*
E. *TP53*

# ANSWERS AND EXPLANATIONS

**1. Correct choice: B.**

Herpes simplex virus (HSV) and *Chlamydia trachomatis* cause characteristic histologic findings, whereas *Trichomonas vaginalis* and *Neisseria gonorrhoeae* do not. HSV is associated with mucosal ulceration. Mucosal cells infected with HSV can be identified at the edge of the ulcer and exhibit the characteristic nuclear changes of multinucleation, margination of chromatin, and nuclear molding. In cases where characteristic nuclear inclusions are not identified, immunohistochemical stain for HSV can be helpful. In contrast to HSV, infections with chlamydia, trichomonas, and gonorrhea are rarely associated with ulceration. Chlamydia infections are characterized by follicular cervicitis with well-formed germinal centers and a marked plasmacytic infiltrate.

**2. Correct choice: A.**

Precursor lesions can only be visualized by colposcopic examination after application of 3% to 5% acetic acid to the cervix. Low-grade squamous intraepithelial lesions (LSILs) often appear white, leading to the designation of an acetowhite lesion, whereas high-grade squamous intraepithelial lesions (HSILs) tend to demonstrate changes such as punctation, mosaicism, and atypical vessels.

**3. Correct choice: C.**

The image depicts a low-grade squamous intraepithelial lesion (LSIL). There is acanthosis and mild parabasal atypia without atypical mitotic figures. By definition, cytologic atypia is limited to the lower third of the epithelium. Koilocytic changes, which are cytopathic effects due to human papillomavirus (HPV) infection, are present in the upper two-thirds. Exophytic LSIL (condyloma acuminatum) is characterized by exophytic growth and papillomatosis, associated with low-risk HPV types 6 and 11 and occurs more frequently in the vulva. Reactive, inflammatory changes and glycogenation can be associated with binucleation and cytoplasmic halos. With reactive change, the halo is round, uniform, and less distinct, and the nuclei are minimally enlarged and normochromic.

**4. Correct choice: D.**

The image demonstrates the nuclear changes due to human papillomavirus (HPV) cytopathic effect. Affected cells, named koilocytes, contain enlarged, wrinkled, raisin-like nuclei surrounded by a punched-out halo and cytoplasmic thickening. The halos are irregular in shape, and the nuclei are variably located within the halo. Binucleated and trinucleated cells are commonly seen. The question is aimed at emphasizing the two cytologic changes that may be confused with koilocytosis. Reactive changes, including inflammatory halos, are associated with round, uniform, ill-defined halos, whereas the nuclei are minimally enlarged and normochromic. Glycogenation produces uniform cytoplasmic clearing, and nuclei are not atypical. The nuclei are centrally located within the halo in both glycogenation and reactive changes.

**5. Correct choice: B.**

A diagnosis of high-grade squamous intraepithelial lesion (HSIL) implies that dysplastic changes are present in the lower and upper epithelial cell layers. The list of choices reflects the range of lesions to be considered in the differential diagnosis of HSIL. The distinction of low-grade squamous intraepithelial lesion (LSIL) from HSIL is based on the nuclear-to-cytoplasmic (N:C) ratios of the dysplastic cells and extent of mucosal involvement. In LSIL, cytologic atypia is limited to the lower third of the epithelium by definition. Atrophy can be difficult to distinguish from thin HSIL because both can have cells with high N:C ratios and hyperchromatic nuclei. However, with atrophy, the nuclei should be relatively uniform with even chromatin and smooth nuclear contours. Mitotic activity should be absent. Immature squamous metaplasia represents a proliferation of reserve, basal-type cells that replace and undermine endocervical columnar mucosa. The cells are not crowded or disorganized, and although there is loss of maturation to the surface and the cells have high N:C ratios, the nuclei are uniform, bland, and round to oval in shape. Prominent nucleoli may be present and are a sign of reactive changes. Mitotic activity may be present, but no abnormal mitotic figures should be identified. Transitional metaplasia is associated with atrophy. The hyperplastic mucosa consists of basal and parabasal cells that morphologically resemble urothelium with vertically oriented, oval nuclei that often have longitudinal nuclear grooves. Along the surface, the nuclei may have a horizontal orientation and streaming appearance, similar to umbrella cells.

**6. Correct choice: C.**

Positive immunoreactivity for p16 has been shown to indicate the presence of high-risk human papillomavirus (HPV) integrated into the host genome, which supports a diagnosis of squamous intraepithelial lesion (SIL). The Lower Anogenital Squamous Terminology (LAST) Project defines positive p16 stain as a continuous strong nuclear or nucleocytoplasmic stain of the basal layer involving at least one-third of the epithelial thickness. Cytoplasmic staining only or focal staining should be considered negative.

**7. Correct choice: C.**

The answer choices A through D summarize the specific situations in which p16 immunohistochemistry (IHC) is recommended in the evaluation of squamous dysplastic lesions in cervical biopsies by the Lower Anogenital Squamous Terminology (LAST) project. The LAST project recommends that p16 IHC should *not* be used routinely, particularly if the morphology of the lesion is unequivocal, whether negative or diagnostic of low-grade squamous intraepithelial lesion (LSIL, CIN1) or high-grade squamous intraepithelial lesion (HSIL, CIN3).

**8. Correct choice: E.**

Superficial invasion is usually associated with stromal desmoplastic response, blurring of the epithelial-stromal interface, and loss of nuclear polarity at the infiltrating border. All of the choices listed are mimickers of superficially invasive squamous cell carcinoma. A diagnosis of high-grade squamous intraepithelial lesion (HSIL) is supported by retention of nuclear polarity, no confluent growth, and a smooth interface between epithelium and submucosa. Prior biopsy sites can produce mimics of invasion such as displaced epithelium into the submucosa or irregular epithelial-stromal interface. Artifactual displacement of benign or dysplastic squamous epithelium into lymphatic-vascular channels can easily mimic lymphatic-vascular invasion.

**9. Correct choice: B.**

By definition, superficially invasive squamous cell carcinomas are not grossly visible, but may be visible by colposcopy after application of 3% to 5% acetic acid to the cervix. Before defining a lesion as superficially invasive, it is essential that the invasive component is completely excised. More advanced invasive carcinomas can be exophytic, endophytic, or ulcerative. With hysterectomy specimens, care should be taken to determine macroscopic tumor size, depth of invasion, and, if present, involvement of vaginal, endometrial, and parametrial tissue.

**10. Correct choice: E.**

Pathologists should be familiar with many different types of benign endocervical changes that could potentially be mistaken for malignancy. Tuboendometrioid metaplasia refers to endocervical glands displaying tubal differentiation with terminal bars and cilia. Atypical oxyphilic metaplasia occurs in superficial endocervical glands lined by large cuboidal-polygonal cells with abundant eosinophilic cytoplasm and variable nuclear atypia, which can mimic radiation change. Endometriosis in the cervix is morphologically identical to endometriosis in other locations. Endosalpingiosis is common in pelvic and lower abdominal peritoneum, pelvic, and paraaortic lymph nodes. Misplaced Skene glands are paraurethral Skene glands, which are the female equivalent of prostatic glands. Ectopic Skene glands can be found in the ectocervix, where it consists of tubular structures around squamous epithelium.

**11. Correct choice: D.**

Microglandular hyperplasia is a frequent condition that is often discovered incidentally in women using oral contraceptives but is also found in women of postmenopausal age. It is benign, but it may be misdiagnosed as carcinoma when some atypia or mitotic activity (both features usually absent or minimal) is present. It consists of clusters of small glandular structures lined by cuboidal or flat epithelial cells. Atypical features, such as signet-ring cells, pseudoinfiltrative pattern of growth, myxoid stroma, hobnail cells, and mild-to-moderate nuclear atypia, can lead to consideration of malignancy.

**12. Correct choice: A.**

Arias-Stella reaction commonly involves the endometrium as a result of pregnancy or hormonal therapy. Sometimes, it involves endocervical glands, where it can be misinterpreted as a malignancy process such as clear cell carcinoma and gastric-type endocervical adenocarcinoma. Morphologic changes suggesting Arias-Stella reaction include vacuolated clear or oxyphilic cytoplasm, intraglandular tufting, hobnail cells, and intranuclear inclusions. Estrogen receptor (ER) immunohistochemical stain is helpful in this important differential, with positive staining in Arias-Stella reaction and negative expression in clear cell carcinoma and gastric-type endocervical adenocarcinoma. Papillary endocervicitis is due to chronic inflammation resulting in a papillary appearance. When florid, it may mimic endocervical adenocarcinoma, but the lesion shows minimal nuclear atypia and no mitotic activity. Radiation change can produce long-lasting nuclear atypia (>10 years) and is characterized by marked nuclear enlargement, bizarre nuclear shapes, multinucleated cells, hyperchromasia, and prominent nucleoli. Low nucleocytoplasmic ratio and lack of nuclear crowding favor radiation change.

**13. Correct choice: E.**

Radiation change can lead to significant nuclear atypia that persists for more than a decade after treatment. Radiation therapy can lead to marked nuclear enlargement with multinucleated or bizarre forms, hyperchromasia, and prominent eosinophilic nucleoli. The cells lack nuclear crowding and have low nuclear-to-cytoplasmic (N:C) ratios with abundant eosinophilic cytoplasm that may be bubbly or vacuolated. The nuclei often appear smudged or degenerated, and mitotic activity is uncommon. Stromal cells may also exhibit radiation atypia with similar nuclear changes, as well as fibrosis, hyalinization, edema, chronic inflammation, and calcifications. Vessels may appear ectatic with intimal thickening. Arias-Stella reaction can be misinterpreted as a malignancy process such as clear cell carcinoma and gastric-type endocervical adenocarcinoma. Morphologic changes suggesting Arias-Stella reaction include vacuolated clear or oxyphilic cytoplasm, intraglandular tufting, hobnail cells, and intranuclear inclusions. Papillary endocervicitis is due to chronic inflammation resulting in a papillary appearance. When florid, it may mimic endocervical adenocarcinoma, but the lesion shows minimal nuclear atypia and no mitotic activity.

**14. Correct choice: E.**

The picture shows the sudden transition from normal endocervical epithelium (Figure 1) to endocervical adenocarcinoma in situ (AIS) (Figure 2), the latter showing crowded, stratified nuclei and mucin depletion. Mitotic figures at the luminal aspect ("floating mitoses") are common. This is a recognized precursor of invasive cervical adenocarcinoma. AIS usually occurs at or close to the transformation zone and arises from reserve cells. High-risk human papillomavirus (HPV) is present in nearly 90% of cases. In approximately 30% to 60% of AIS, there is coexistent squamous intraepithelial lesion (SIL).

**15. Correct choice: D.**

Stratified mucin-producing intraepithelial lesion resembles high-grade squamous intraepithelial lesion (HSIL) but is distinguished by the presence of cells with cytoplasmic mucin in the form of discrete vacuoles or cytoplasmic clearing dispersed throughout the lower to middle epithelial layers, which can be highlighted by mucicarmine stain. Microglandular hyperplasia is benign and consists of clusters of small glandular structures lined by cuboidal or flat epithelial cells. Transitional metaplasia shows hyperplastic mucosa consisting of basal and parabasal cells that morphologically resemble urothelium with vertically oriented, oval nuclei that often have longitudinal nuclear grooves. Immature squamous metaplasia represents a proliferation of reserve, basal-type cells that replace and undermine endocervical columnar mucosa. The cells are not crowded or disorganized, and although there is loss of maturation to the surface and the cells have high nuclear-to-cytoplasmic (N:C) ratios, the nuclei are uniform, bland, and round to oval in shape. Prominent nucleoli may be present and are a sign of reactive changes. Mitotic activity may be present, but no abnormal mitotic figures should be identified.

**16. Correct choice: A.**

Endocervical adenocarcinoma typically shows diffuse and strong nuclear or nucleocytoplasmic immunoreactivity for p16, but it is negative for estrogen receptor (ER) and vimentin. On the other hand, endometrial adenocarcinoma is negative or only patchy positive for p16 and positive for ER and vimentin (basolateral membrane pattern). These findings apply to human papillomavirus (HPV)-associated endocervical adenocarcinomas (the majority) and to low-grade endometrial endometrioid adenocarcinomas. High-grade endometrial carcinomas and serous or clear cell carcinomas may have diffuse p16 reactivity even if they are not associated with HPV. Conversely, HPV-independent endocervical adenocarcinomas (minimal deviation adenocarcinoma and mesonephric adenocarcinoma) are negative for p16. In such cases, the site of origin can be determined only by correlating gross, clinical, and radiologic data.

**17. Correct choice: B.**

Gastric-type adenocarcinomas of the cervix are generally associated with a worse prognosis than usual cervical adenocarcinoma. Although, overall, cervical adenocarcinomas behave similarly to cervical squamous cell carcinomas, it is now recognized that certain variants (ie, invasive stratified mucin-producing and gastric-type) are associated with a worse prognosis.

**18. Correct choice: B.**

The prognosis is excellent when adenoid basal carcinoma occurs in pure form, and because of this, it has been suggested that this tumor type be renamed adenoid basal epithelioma. Pure adenoid basal carcinoma is cytologically bland without appreciable mitotic activity, lacks destructive stromal invasion, and is not associated with other variants of invasive carcinoma. The tumor is usually superficial but can extend deeply into the cervical stroma. Complete excision with negative margins is required to exclude the presence of a more aggressive variant of invasive carcinoma.

**19. Correct choice: E.**

It is important to distinguish small-cell neuroendocrine carcinoma (SCNEC) from non–neuroendocrine carcinomas and to exclude metastasis because their management differs significantly. They behave aggressively and are associated with a poor prognosis, even when detected early. A subset is associated with ectopic hormone production. Human papillomavirus 18 (HPV18) is reported as the predominant HPV subtype in SCNEC, while HPV16 is reported as the predominant HPV subtype in large-cell neuroendocrine carcinomas (LCNEC). Neuroendocrine carcinomas often grow as solid sheets with extensive areas of necrosis and abundant mitotic and apoptotic activity but can also exhibit insular or trabecular architecture and rosette formation. The tumor cells in the small-cell type have nuclei with smudgy or stippled chromatin, scant cytoplasm, and nuclear molding; crush artifact is common. In contrast, the tumor cells in the large-cell type have larger nuclei with more abundant cytoplasm and prominent nucleoli. A diagnosis of SCNEC can be made on the basis of characteristic morphologic features, but a diagnosis of LCNEC requires confirmation of neuroendocrine differentiation by expression of at least one neuroendocrine marker.

**20. Correct choice: B.**

Embryonal rhabdomyosarcoma (sarcoma botryoides) can occur as a cervical primary and/or a polypoid mass protruding from the introitus and is associated with *DICER1* germline mutations. When it occurs in the cervix, the patients are older (mean age 12.4-18 years) compared to when it presents in the vagina (<5 years of age). The characteristic histologic finding is the presence of a cambium layer with increased stromal cellularity beneath the surface epithelium and around benign glandular elements. Elongated cells or globular cells with abundant eosinophilic cytoplasm (rhabdomyoblasts) may be seen, but cross-striations are not identifiable in all cases and are not required for the diagnosis. Positive nuclear staining with the skeletal muscle markers myogenin and MyoD1 can assist in the diagnosis. Rare cases of cervical embryonal rhabdomyosarcoma have been associated with ovarian Sertoli-Leydig cell tumor and pleuropulmonary blastoma and are thought to be due to an underlying *DICER1* mutation. There is no association of cervical embryonal rhabdomyosarcoma with the other mutations listed.

# 53 Uterine Corpus: Epithelial

1. Which of the following is false with respect to endometrial sampling through dilatation and curettage versus endometrial biopsy?

   A. Allows for the removal of focal lesions
   B. Carries a risk of perforation and postprocedural adhesions
   C. Is the preferred first-line approach
   D. Represents a complete sampling of the endometrial cavity
   E. Requires the use of anesthesia

2. What phase of the normal cycling endometrium is depicted in Figure 1?

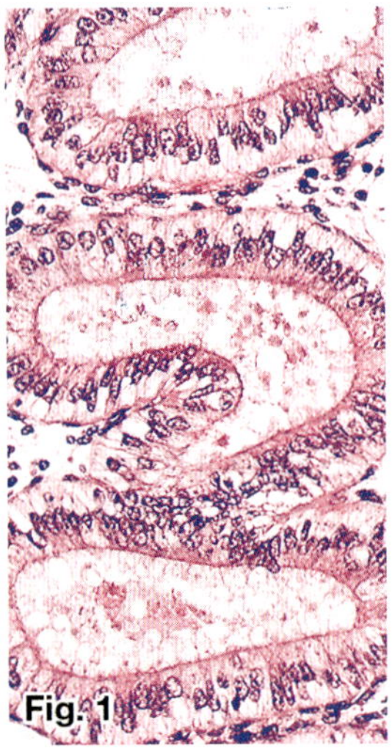

Fig. 1

   A. Early secretory
   B. Late secretory
   C. Menstrual
   D. Mid secretory
   E. Proliferative

3. What phase of the normal cycling endometrium is depicted in Figure 1?

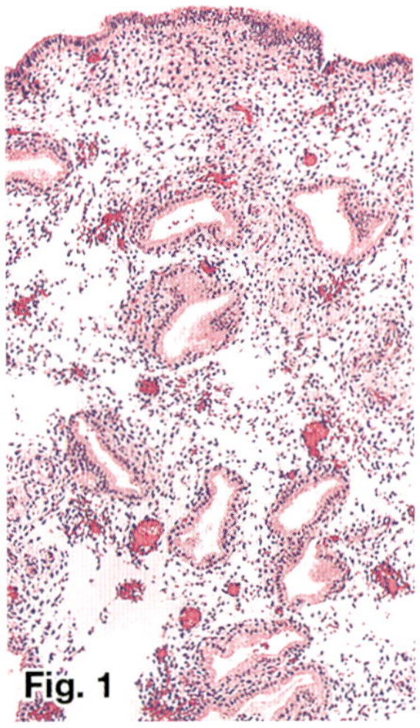

Fig. 1

   A. Early secretory
   B. Late secretory
   C. Menstrual
   D. Mid secretory
   E. Proliferative

4. An endometrial biopsy reveals endometrial glands lined by cells with pleomorphic large nuclei and abundant clear cytoplasm, as shown in Figure 1. Mitotic figures are not seen. This histologic appearance is not associated with which of the following conditions?

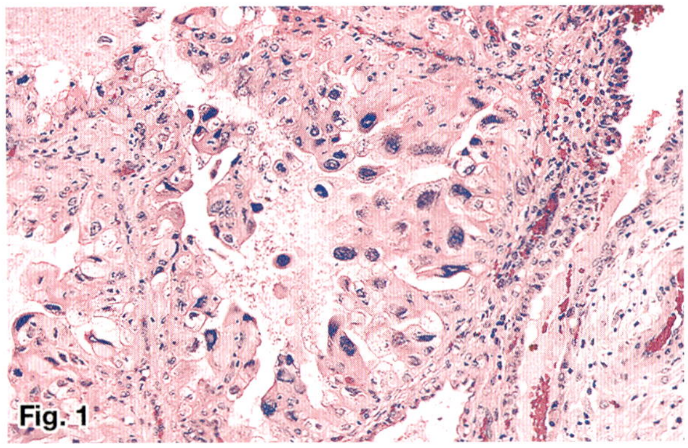

Fig. 1

   A. Ectopic pregnancy
   B. Exogenous hormonal administration
   C. Gestational trophoblastic disease
   D. Intrauterine pregnancy
   E. Postmenopause

All figures in this chapter are from Longacre TA, Greenson JK, Hornick JL, Reuter VE, eds. *Mills and Sternberg's Diagnostic Surgical Pathology.* 7th ed. Wolters Kluwer; 2022 except for those noted at the end of this book.

5. Which of the following features is not helpful in differentiating Arias-Stella reaction from clear cell carcinoma?

    A. Background of decidual changes
    B. Clinical scenario
    C. Expression of Napsin-A
    D. Lack of mitotic activity

6. A 48-year-old woman undergoes an endometrial biopsy for evaluation of abnormal uterine bleeding. The main histologic findings are illustrated in Figure 1. There are mitoses in the glandular epithelium, but no cytologic atypia. Foci of ciliated cell metaplasia are seen. Which of the following is the most likely diagnosis?

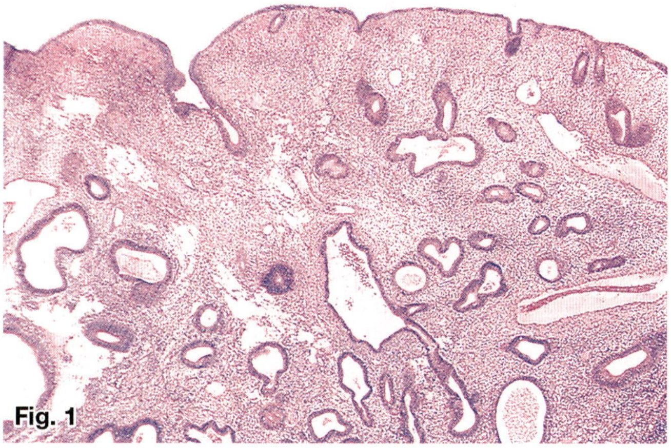

Fig. 1

    A. Complex hyperplasia without atypia
    B. Disordered proliferative endometrium
    C. Endometrial atrophy with ciliated cell metaplasia
    D. Inactive (weakly proliferative) endometrium
    E. Simple hyperplasia without atypia

7. Which of the following findings in the endometrial biopsy depicted in Figure 1 is false?

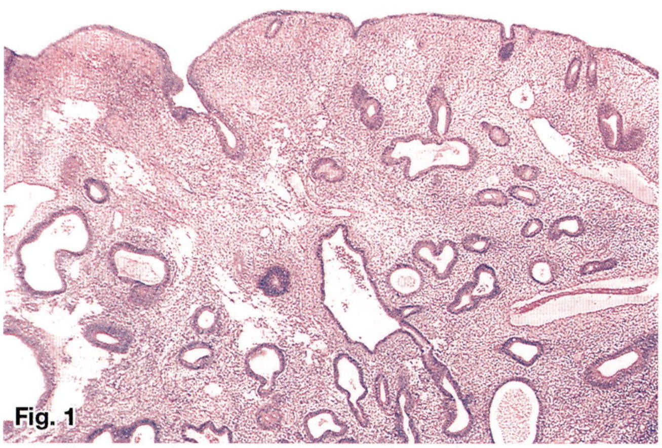

Fig. 1

    A. Can be seen in the context of exogenous hormone administration
    B. Is common in perimenopause
    C. Is consistent with cystic endometrial atrophy with ciliated cell metaplasia
    D. Results from dyssynchronous gland development
    E. May represent a harbinger of incipient endometrial hyperplasia

8. Which of the following is false concerning the entity in the endometrial curettage specimen shown in Figure 1?

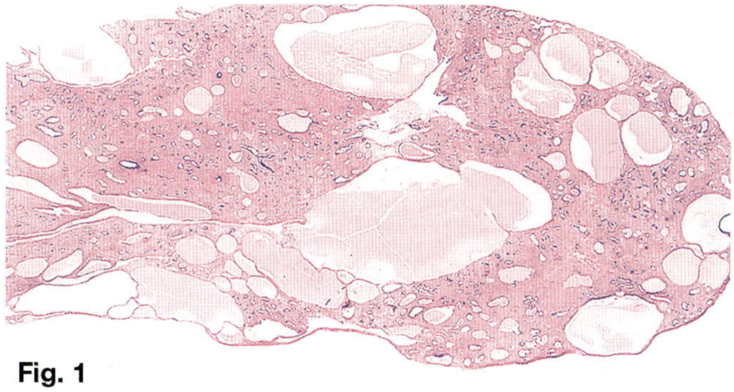

Fig. 1

    A. Focal gland crowding is diagnostic of hyperplasia in this context.
    B. Patients with tamoxifen exposure often develop an associated endometrial carcinoma.
    C. The entity can be the cause of significant abnormal uterine bleeding.
    D. The entity is a common site for uterine serous carcinoma in postmenopausal women.
    E. Thick-walled blood vessels are a key feature of the entity.

9. An endometrial biopsy from a 30-year-old patient with an intrauterine device is evaluated for assessment of possible chronic endometritis. This diagnosis would be confirmed by finding

    A. granulomas.
    B. lymphocytic infiltration.
    C. neutrophilic infiltration.
    D. plasmacytic infiltration.
    E. viral inclusions.

10. Which of the following endometrial changes represent the most typical effects of treatment with synthetic progesterone receptor antagonists such as mifepristone?

    A. Atrophic non-coiled glands in a spindle cell pre-decidualized stroma
    B. Decidualization of endometrial stroma and marked secretory changes
    C. Glandular and stromal proliferation
    D. Polyps with staghorn vessels and myxoid stroma
    E. Shift in gland-to-stroma ratio with prevalence of stroma

11. Which of the following statements about endometrial hyperplasia is false?

    A. Current practice is to divide it into simple or complex hyperplasia, with or without cytologic atypia.
    B. It is a nonobligate precursor to endometrioid carcinoma.
    C. It is defined as architecturally crowded proliferative endometrium.
    D. It is most often related to prolonged exposure to unopposed estrogen.
    E. It may occur in premenopausal, perimenopausal, and postmenopausal women.

12. Which of the following is false regarding the endometrial glandular abnormality depicted in Figure 1?

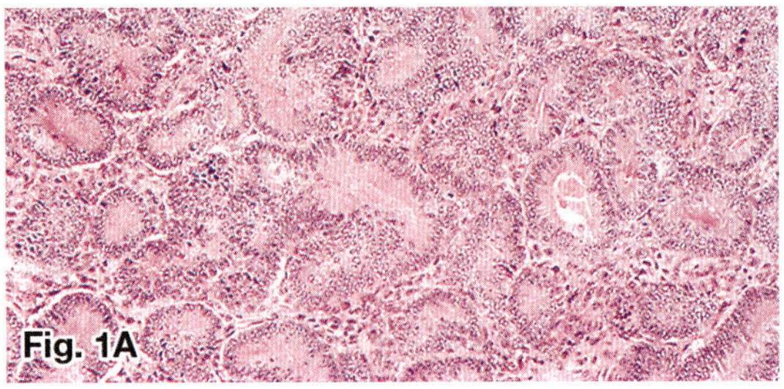


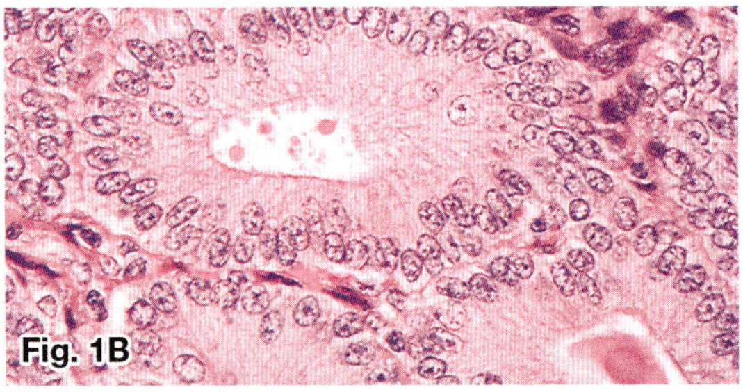


A. It carries a significantly higher risk of both concurrent carcinoma and progression to carcinoma.
B. It has very high interobserver reproducibility among pathologists.
C. It is associated with molecular alterations, including *PTEN* mutations and concomitant loss of PTEN (phosphatase and tensin) protein expression.
D. The diagnosis is a critical flag for clinicians and triggers further interventions.
E. The diagnosis requires either cytologic atypia exceeding what is expected in proliferative endometria or a cytologically distinct population of glands not attributable to metaplasia.

13. Which of the following is not a molecular signature identified by The Cancer Genome Atlas (TCGA)?

A. *BRCA* mutations
B. High copy number abnormalities
C. Hypermutation/mismatch repair deficiency/microsatellite instability
D. Low copy number abnormalities
E. Ultra-mutation/polymerase ε (*POLE*) mutations

14. The International Federation of Gynecology and Obstetrics (FIGO) grading system of the endometrial neoplasm shown in Figure 1 is based on

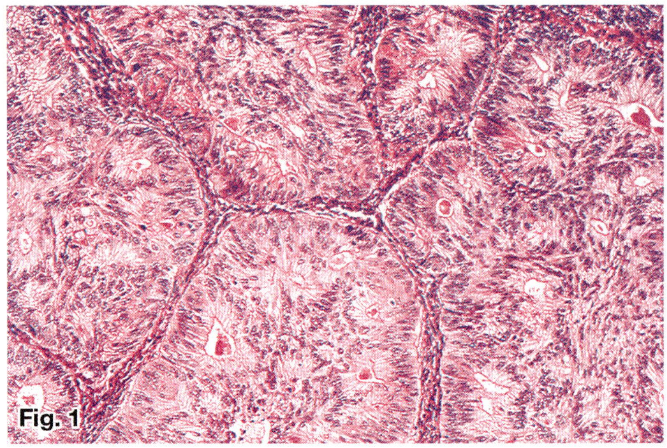


A. architectural features.
B. architectural features and nuclear atypia.
C. hormone receptor status.
D. mitotic rate.
E. nuclear atypia.

15. Figure 1 shows a type of endometrial carcinoma that does not develop in association with hyperestrinism and is characterized by extremely aggressive behavior. What is the most likely oncogenic mutation in this tumor?

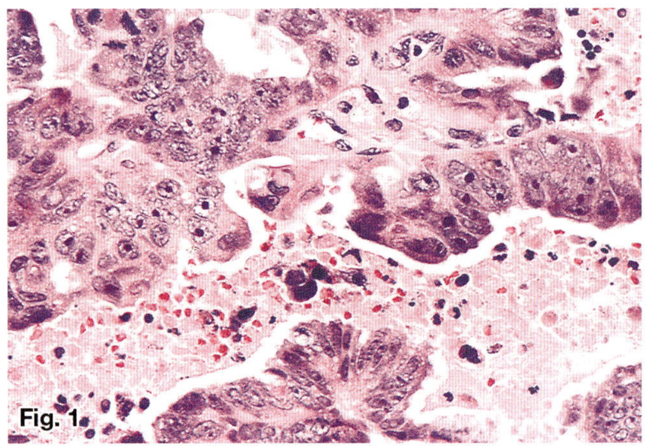


A. *ARID1A*
B. *MLH1*
C. *PIK3CA*
D. *PTEN*
E. *TP53*

16. Figure 1 demonstrates the invasive front of an endometrioid carcinoma. Which of the following is false regarding this pattern?

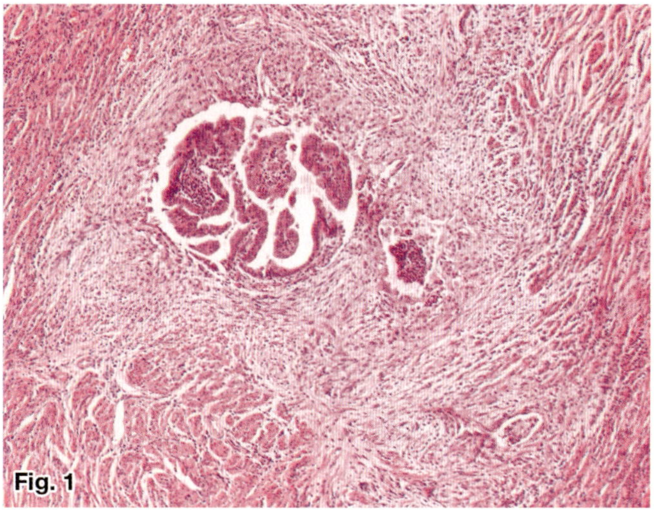

Fig. 1

A. It is adenomyosis involved with carcinoma.
B. It is associated with an increased risk of lymphovascular invasion and nodal metastases.
C. It is characterized by the microcytic, elongated, and fragmented (MELF) pattern of invasion.
D. It may be mistaken for lymphovascular involvement.
E. It shows a unique myxoinflammatory stromal response.

17. Figure 1 shows a high-grade aggressive uterine carcinoma found on the surface of an endometrial polyp in a postmenopausal woman. Which of the following is not an expected immunoprofile of this tumor?

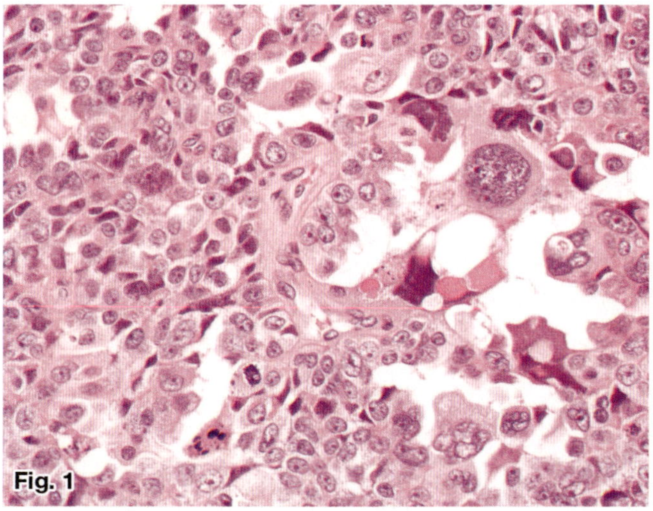

Fig. 1

A. Cytoplasmic expression of p53
B. Null (absent) expression of PTEN (phosphatase and tensin)
C. Null (absent) expression of p53
D. Overexpression of p53
E. Strong and diffuse p16

18. Figure 1 depicts the findings in an irregular exophytic mass in the uterine cavity of a nulliparous woman with a significant smoking history. What is the best diagnosis?

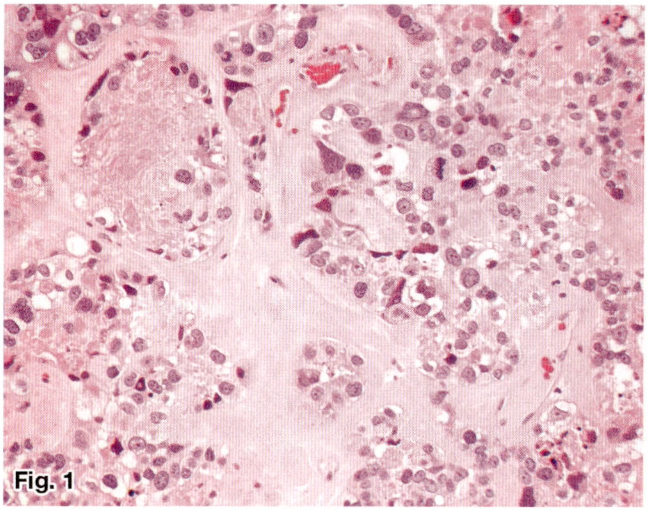

Fig. 1

A. Arias-Stella reaction
B. Clear cell carcinoma
C. Endocervical adenocarcinoma, gastric-type, human papillomavirus (HPV)-independent
D. Endometrioid carcinoma, secretory variant
E. Serous carcinoma

19. A hysterectomy specimen from a 70-year-old woman reveals a large polypoid mass consisting of an epithelial glandular component admixed with a sarcoma-like component, as shown in Figure 1. The latter includes cellular anaplastic elements resembling the normal endometrial stroma and neoplastic cells with cross-striations and myoglobin immunoreactivity. Which of the following is true about this cancer?

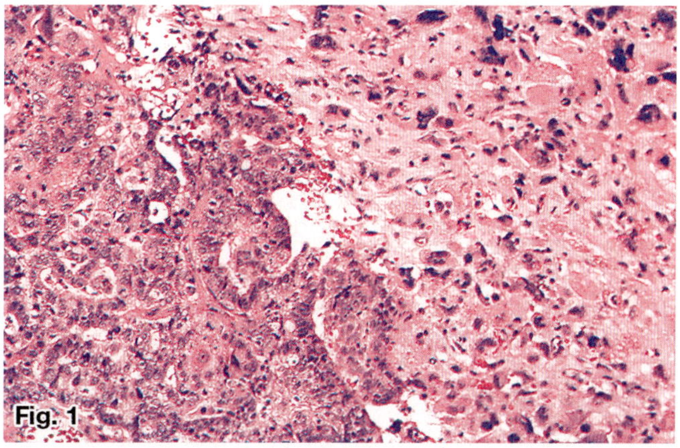

Fig. 1

A. It usually occurs in women of reproductive age.
B. The cancer has a better prognosis than endometrial adenocarcinoma.
C. The carcinomatous component has the highest metastatic potential.
D. The histology is reminiscent of phyllodes tumors.
E. The neoplastic components often include skin and thyroid tissue.

20. A 55-year-old female presents with an exophytic uterine mass that involves the lower uterine segment. Regional necrosis is seen on gross examination. Figure 1 shows the histology features of the tumor. Epithelial membrane antigen (EMA) immunoreactivity is seen in all components of the tumor. SMARCA4/BRG1 immunostaining shows loss of expression. What is the best diagnosis?

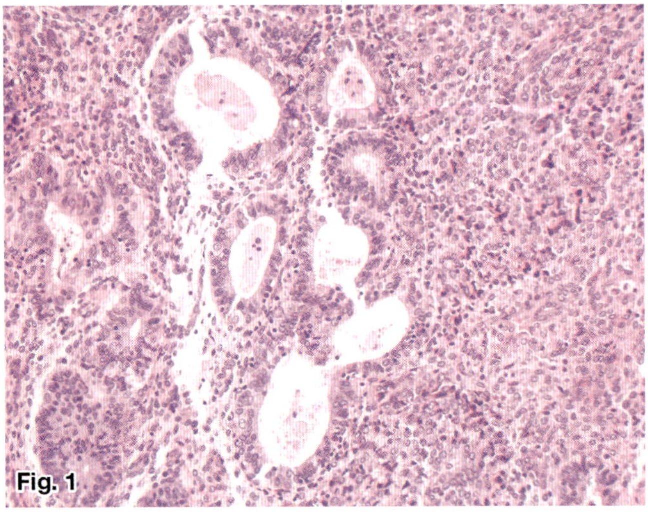
Fig. 1

A. Adenosarcoma
B. Carcinosarcoma
C. Dedifferentiated endometrial carcinoma
D. Endometrial adenocarcinoma, the International Federation of Gynecology and Obstetrics (FIGO) grade 3
E. Undifferentiated endometrial carcinoma

21. Figure 1 demonstrates a section of a uterine mass found in a 40-year-old female. She later developed lung metastases. Molecular analysis identified a *KRAS* mutation. What is the most likely diagnosis?

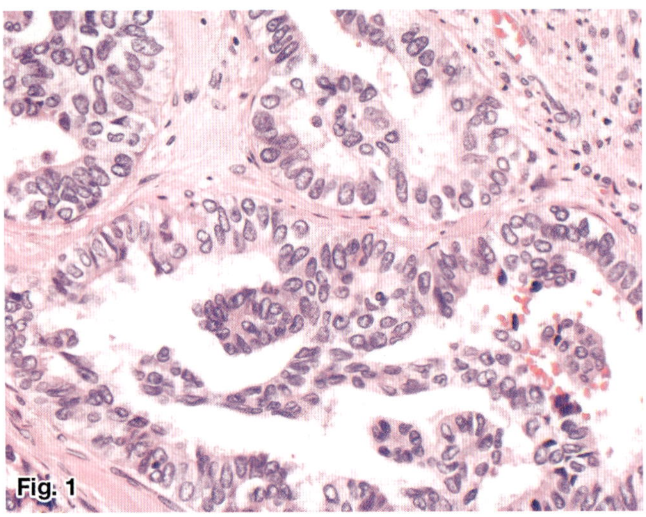
Fig. 1

A. Adenomyosis involved by low-grade endometrioid carcinoma
B. Clear cell carcinoma
C. Endometrial carcinoma, the International Federation of Gynecology and Obstetrics (FIGO) grade 1
D. Mesonephric-like carcinoma
E. Serous carcinoma

22. The tumor in Question 21 will show which of the following immunoprofile?

A. ER+, PR+, p53 aberrant, PTEN (phosphatase and tensin) intact, p16 positive
B. ER+, PR+, p53 wild type, PTEN loss, p16 patchy
C. ER−, PR−, p53 wild type, PTEN intact, p16 patchy
D. ER−, PR−, p53 wild type, PTEN intact, p16 positive
E. ER−, PR−, p53 wild type, TTF-1 positive, p16 patchy

23. A 34-year-old G0 female is found to have endometrioid carcinoma of both the uterus and ovary. Which of the following features favors an endometrial primary with metastasis to the ovary, rather than synchronous primaries?

A. Absence of lymphovascular invasion
B. Deep myometrial invasion
C. Endometriosis associated with the ovarian tumor
D. Intermediate-grade histology
E. Low-grade histology

# ANSWERS AND EXPLANATIONS

**1. Correct choice: C.**

Endometrial samplings are obtained either through endometrial biopsy (EMB) or through dilatation and curettage (D&C). EMB is typically the preferred first-line approach because it can be performed in the office with minimal patient discomfort and expense. However, EMB may be insufficient for the diagnosis and removal of focal lesions, such as polyps. D&C represents a complete sampling of the endometrial cavity. Unlike EMB, D&C allows for the removal of focal lesions, such as polyps and submucosal leiomyomas. Because this procedure requires anesthesia and carries some risk of both perforation and post-curettage adhesions, which can lead to secondary amenorrhea (Asherman syndrome), it is less commonly enlisted than EMB.

**2. Correct choice: A.**

Early secretory endometrium is seen on postovulatory days 2 to 5 and manifests microscopically with coiled glands, with at least half of the cells bearing large cytoplasmic vacuoles. The background stroma lacks predecidual change, and mitotic figures should be sparse.

**3. Correct choice: B.**

Late secretory phase endometrium is characterized by coiled glands without any vacuoles or mitotic activity embedded in edematous stroma. Predeciduation begins around postovulatory day 10 and appears first as thickening of the spiral arteries with adjacent stromal cuffing. Over the ensuing days, these predecidual changes extend beyond the periarterial regions and become confluent.

**4. Correct choice: E.**

Arias-Stella reaction is an exaggerated hypersecretory response of the endometrium to human chorionic gonadotropin (hCG) stimulation, which may be observed in normal or ectopic pregnancy, gestational trophoblastic disease, exogenous administration of hormones, and even in foci of endometriosis. Because of its striking nuclear pleomorphism, it may be mistaken for adenocarcinoma. In the Arias-Stella reaction, the nuclei contain smudged chromatin (vs coarse chromatin in adenocarcinoma) and mitoses are rare.

**5. Correct choice: C.**

Arias-Stella reaction is characterized by hypersecretory glands lined by large cells bearing abundant eosinophilic to clear cytoplasm with enlarged, pleomorphic nuclei bearing smudgy, hyperchromatic chromatin. Mitotic figures should be rare if present at all. Because clear cytoplasm is often pronounced, Arias-Stella reaction may mimic clear cell carcinoma. Caution should be exercised in such cases because Arias-Stella reaction commonly expresses Napsin-A and is, therefore, of no value in resolving this differential. Instead, pathologists should rely on the lack of mitotic activity, clinical scenario, and the background milieu of decidual changes to differentiate Arias-Stella reaction from clear cell carcinoma.

**6. Correct choice: B.**

Disordered proliferative endometrium is found most commonly in association with anovulatory cycles in women of perimenarchal and perimenopausal age. Patients usually present with dysfunctional uterine bleeding. This is due to desynchronization of glandular maturation. The gland-to-stroma ratio is approximately 1, but glands vary in size and shape. Some glands are markedly dilated, whereas others show budding. Although it is considered a normal finding in the perimenopausal period, in truly postmenopausal patients, this pattern may represent a harbinger of incipient hyperplasia.

**7. Correct choice: C.**

Disordered proliferative endometrium consists of irregularly shaped glands lined by bland columnar cells with readily appreciable mitotic activity. The glands range from small caliber and rounded to cystically dilated. These glands are embedded in abundant proliferative-type, mitotic active stroma, and the glands-to-stroma ratio remains low ($\leq 1$). The presence of mitoses and proliferative-type glands allows for its differentiation from cystic atrophy. Disordered proliferative glands demonstrate dyssynchrony rather than uniform development. Metaplasia, particularly tubal metaplasia, is common. It can be seen in the context of exogenous hormone administration and is commonly encountered with anovulatory cycles, particularly in the years surrounding menopause. Although it is considered a normal finding in the perimenopausal period, in truly postmenopausal patients, this pattern may represent a harbinger of incipient hyperplasia.

**8. Correct choice: A.**

Endometrial polyps are typically pedunculated growths composed of fibrous stroma containing variably dilated glands, which range from atrophic to weakly proliferative. Thick-walled blood vessels are requisite for the diagnosis. Focal crowding can be seen and does not necessarily warrant a diagnosis of hyperplasia in this context. Endometrial polyps may be entirely asymptomatic but can also cause bleeding, which is significant in some cases. Although polyps are not independently associated with an increased risk of cancer, they represent a common site for serous carcinoma in postmenopausal women. In addition, patients with tamoxifen exposure seem particularly prone to polyp-associated endometrial carcinomas.

**9. Correct choice: D.**

Chronic endometritis is most often associated with intrauterine device (IUD) use, retained products of conception, and pelvic inflammatory disease (of which Chlamydia and gonococcus are the most frequent etiologic agents). Although lymphocytes and lymphoid follicles are found in the normal endometrium, plasma cells are abnormal and represent the essential criterion for a diagnosis of chronic endometritis. Glandular disarray usually accompanies chronic endometritis and makes dating of the endometrium not feasible. Cytomegalovirus is the most common cause of viral endometritis.

**10. Correct choice: E.**

Compounds like mifepristone (progesterone receptor inhibitor) are used as an "emergency contraceptive" and for treatment of endometriosis and leiomyomas. These compounds produce a range of endometrial changes, the most frequent of which include cystically dilated glands lined by atrophic/inactive epithelium, shift of gland-to-stroma ratio with predominance of stroma, appearance of thick-walled vessels lying just below the surface epithelium, and ciliary metaplasia. The changes described in C and D are associated with administration of tamoxifen, which acts as an estrogen receptor antagonist in the breast and agonist in the endometrium. The changes mentioned in A and B are seen with administration of progestins, alone or in combination with estrogens.

**11. Correct choice: A.**

Hyperplasia is defined as architecturally crowded proliferative endometrium, where the glands may be crowded secondary to enlargement or to budding, and when budding is prominent, it can generate complex structures with branching and infoldings. The intervening endometrial stroma is decreased in tandem with this increase in epithelium. Hyperplasia is further classified as nonatypical and atypical. This binary approach represents an evolution from the four-tier system originally endorsed by the 1994 World Health Organization (WHO) Classification, which categorized hyperplasia into simple hyperplasia without atypia, simple hyperplasia with atypia, complex hyperplasia without atypia, and complex hyperplasia with atypia. Although some pathologists and gynecologists remain most comfortable with this terminology, it is outmoded and should be avoided in favor of the two-tier classification system of nonatypical versus atypical hyperplasia.

**12. Correct choice: E.**

A diagnosis of atypical hyperplasia requires either cytologic atypia in excess of what is expected in proliferative endometrium or a cytologically distinct population of glands that is not attributable to metaplasia. This latter criterion was introduced through the integration of the endometrial intraepithelial neoplasia (EIN) system for classifying endometrial precancerous lesions, which accounts for the fact that some morphologically banal proliferations can progress to carcinoma at rates similar to those with frank cytologic atypia. The 2014 and 2020 editions of the World Health Organization (WHO) incorporated the EIN system and collapsed the terms "atypical hyperplasia" and "EIN" such that these are now essentially synonymous. Neither the EIN system nor the hyperplasia classification systems that preceded it have perfect interobserver reproducibility. Nonetheless, it is clear that a binary system is more diagnostically reproducible and more clinically useful and that the presence of clonally distinct subpopulations is prognostically important even in the absence of overt atypia.

**13. Correct choice: A.**

In 2013, The Cancer Genome Atlas (TCGA) revealed that on detailed genetic analysis, endometrial cancer is classified into four molecular groups, defined by the following molecular signatures: (1) ultra-mutation/polymerase ε (*POLE*) mutations, (2) hypermutation/mismatch repair deficiency/microsatellite instability, (3) low copy number abnormalities, and (4) high copy number abnormalities. The *POLE*-mutated group bears a strikingly good prognosis, whereas cancers with high copy number abnormalities show the worst outcomes. Mismatch repair-deficient and copy number-low tumors track closely together and fall in between these extremes. Although *BRCA* mutations are classically associated with ovarian and breast cancers, recent evidence suggests that women with *BRCA* mutations may also have a slightly increased risk of developing uterine serous carcinoma.

**14. Correct choice: B.**

The figure shows a grade I endometrioid adenocarcinoma. Endometrioid carcinoma is the most frequent morphologic type of endometrial cancer. The International Federation of Gynecology and Obstetrics (FIGO) grading system is based on assessment of architectural features (ie, solid vs glandular growth) and nuclear atypia. Degree of architectural differentiation is divided into: grade 1 is equal to 5% or less of a nonsquamous or nonmorular solid growth pattern; grade 2 is equal to 6% to 50% of a nonsquamous or nonmorular solid growth pattern; and grade 3 50% or more of a nonsquamous or nonmorular solid growth pattern. Cytologic features to be used in formulating final grade include notable diffuse nuclear atypia, inappropriate for the architectural grade, which raises the grade of a grade 1 or grade 2 tumor by one level. Because endometrioid adenocarcinoma often contains villous and papillary projections, this feature does not by itself warrant the diagnosis of serous carcinoma, which is a very aggressive subtype characterized by extreme cellular pleomorphism. Estrogen/progesterone receptors are present in the majority of endometrioid carcinomas. These are the recognized variants of endometrioid carcinoma: usual (including glandular and villoglandular); secretory, with squamous differentiation; and ciliated. It should be emphasized that the FIGO grading system does not apply to special variants of uterine cancer such as serous carcinoma and clear cell carcinoma.

**15. Correct choice: E.**

Uterine serous carcinoma is a highly aggressive tumor that resembles ovarian serous carcinoma. It has a predilection for women older than 60 years. In contrast to the endometrioid type, it is not associated with clinical or morphologic evidence of hyperestrinism (anovulatory cycles or endometrial hyperplasia). The tumor arises on a background of atrophy and is frequently found on the surface of endometrial polyps. It is very important to differentiate this type from an endometrioid carcinoma with a prominent villous/papillary component. Underlying *TP53* mutation is the oncogenic driver in this tumor, which can be demonstrated by aberrant p53 expression using immunohistochemistry. All of the other mutations listed are found in endometrioid carcinomas.

**16. Correct choice: A.**

Microcystic elongated and fragmented (MELF) invasion is a pattern of invasion in endometrial carcinoma, characterized by singly dispersed, cytologically bland glands with attenuated lining cells, demonstrating moderate-to-abundant cytoplasm and a squamoid-to-histiocytoid appearance. The surrounding stroma shows a unique myxoinflammatory response. The MELF pattern may be mistaken for lymphovascular involvement because of the attenuated glandular lining and frequent presence of intraluminal malignant cell clusters. MELF is also associated with an increased risk of true lymphovascular invasion and nodal metastases.

**17. Correct choice: B.**

p53 is commonly enlisted in the diagnosis of uterine serous carcinoma as abnormal expression is a fairly reliable surrogate for the *TP53* mutations that underlie these tumors. Two-thirds of cases will show strong, diffuse overexpression because of mutations that result in an abnormal, degradation-resistant protein. One-quarter show complete absence of expression (null pattern) either because of completely absent p53 protein production or because of the generation of a truncated protein that fails to react with the immunohistochemical antibody. Approximately 5% of total cases show aberrant cytoplasmic staining with variable, low-intensity nuclear expression; this pattern has been associated with *TP53* mutations, disrupting the nuclear localization domain, and should be interpreted as abnormal. Serous carcinomas typically demonstrate strong diffuse p16 expression. Loss of PTEN (phosphatase and tensin) expression is a common feature of the low copy number group of endometrioid carcinomas because of the frequency of *PTEN* mutations.

**18. Correct choice: B.**

Clear cell carcinoma, like serous carcinoma, affects old women without a history of conditions leading to hyperestrinism and typically arises in a background of atrophic endometrium. The neoplastic cells are organized in papillary, tubulocystic, and solid arrangements with variable amounts of associated eosinophilic hyaline stroma (as seen in the image). Scattered mitoses are often appreciated. It is morphologically indistinguishable from its ovarian counterpart and the cervicovaginal clear cell carcinoma arising in women with a history of in utero exposure to diethylstilbestrol (DES).

**19. Correct choice: C.**

Carcinosarcomas (malignant mixed Müllerian tumors) are highly aggressive neoplasms that consist of two histologic high-grade malignant components: epithelial and mesenchymal. The epithelial portion of carcinosarcoma may be serous, endometrioid, clear cell, undifferentiated, or mixed, whereas the mesenchymal component can be either homologous (smooth muscle or endometrial stromal) or heterologous (rhabdomyomatous, cartilaginous, osteoid, and lipomatous differentiation). The great majority of cases arise in women of postmenopausal age. The carcinomatous component is the one that usually metastasizes. The prognosis of carcinosarcoma is generally worse than the most aggressive of endometrial carcinomas. Genetic studies have demonstrated that both cellular elements of carcinosarcoma originate from the same precursor; it is therefore considered to be a poorly differentiated carcinoma with metaplastic components.

**20. Correct choice: C.**

Dedifferentiated endometrial carcinomas are defined by the immediate juxtaposition of endometrioid carcinomas showing well-formed glands with regions of confluent undifferentiated growth, creating an abrupt transition. The undifferentiated portion is composed of loosely cohesive, fairly monotonous intermediate-sized cells, which fail to form glands or other structures. The accurate distinction of these cases from conventional endometrioid tumors is important, as many behave worse than stage-matched the International Federation of Gynecology and Obstetrics (FIGO) grade 3 endometrioid cancers. Immunostaining is important for confirming the epithelial nature of undifferentiated carcinomas, which will simultaneously rule out the diagnosis of carcinosarcoma and adenosarcoma. Although dedifferentiated carcinomas typically fail to express most cytokeratins, they should have at least focal staining for epithelial membrane antigen (EMA) and CK18. A subset of dedifferentiated and undifferentiated carcinomas also demonstrate abnormal expression of proteins in the switch/sucrose nonfermenting (SWI/SNF) complex pathway, including BRG1/SMARCA4 loss, which occurs in approximately one-third of cases and has been associated with rhabdoid morphology. Undifferentiated endometrial carcinomas are morphologically equivalent to the high-grade areas of dedifferentiated endometrial carcinomas but lack the gland-forming endometrioid component.

**21. Correct choice: D.**

Mesonephric-like carcinoma of the endometrium is a rare and recently described malignancy that carries a poor prognosis. These tumors arise across a wide age spectrum, with reported ages ranging from early 30s to over 80 years of age. They follow an aggressive clinical course, with a predilection for lung metastases. Mesonephric-like carcinomas show a variety of architectural configurations, including tubular, ductal, papillary, retiform, and solid growth patterns, with glomeruloid structures often present. The solid areas may assume a somewhat spindled appearance. The constituent cells are relatively monotonous and bear vesicular oval-to-angulated nuclei, often with optical nuclear clearing reminiscent of papillary thyroid carcinoma nuclei. Glandular spaces often bear brightly eosinophilic intraluminal material. They often demonstrate deep myometrial invasion, typically without an associated desmoplastic response. While their bland appearance and frequent gland formation most often result in misdiagnosis as endometrioid carcinoma, they can also show loss of polarity suggestive of serous carcinoma and hobnail cells suggestive of clear cell carcinoma.

**22. Correct choice: E.**

Immunohistochemistry is extremely useful in distinguishing mesonephric-like carcinoma from other endometrial malignancies. Mesonephric-like carcinoma is typically negative for estrogen receptor (ER) and progesterone receptor (PR) and strongly positive for the mesonephric markers TTF-1 and GATA-3, although some tumors will only express one of the two. Many cases also show luminal CD10 expression. p53 is typically wild type, p16 is patchy, and PTEN expression is preserved. Choice A is most commonly seen in serous carcinoma. Choice B is seen in low-grade endometrioid carcinoma. Choice C is an immunoprofile found in clear cell carcinoma. Choice D is associated with human papillomavirus (HPV)-associated usual-type endocervical adenocarcinoma.

**23. Correct choice: B.**

Ovarian endometrioid carcinomas occur in tandem with endometrial endometrioid carcinomas in as many as 20% of cases, and the majority of these tumors represent dual primaries. Most synchronous primaries are due to somatic causes and tied to an estrogenic field effect, which is evidenced by the high body mass index, frequent nulliparity, and young age of many women with synchronous ovarian and endometrial endometrioid primaries. Features supporting independent primaries include low- to intermediate-grade histology, the absence of lymphovascular invasion, and endometriosis associated with the ovarian tumor. The presence of high-grade histology, deep myometrial invasion, lymphovascular involvement, and bilateral ovarian involvement is more indicative of an endometrial primary with metastatic spread to the ovary.

# 54 Uterine Corpus: Mesenchymal Tumors

1. Which of the following features favors microscopic adenomyosis over low-grade endometrial stromal sarcoma?

   A. Infiltration of myometrium in tongues
   B. Presence of a mass lesion
   C. Presence of muscular hypertrophy
   D. Presence of solid extrauterine masses greater than 3 cm
   E. Sparse or absent endometrial glands throughout

2. Figure 1 shows the microscopic appearance of a well-demarcated myometrial tumor with bulging and trabeculated cut surfaces. In the differential diagnosis with an endometrial stromal tumor, which of the following favors leiomyoma?

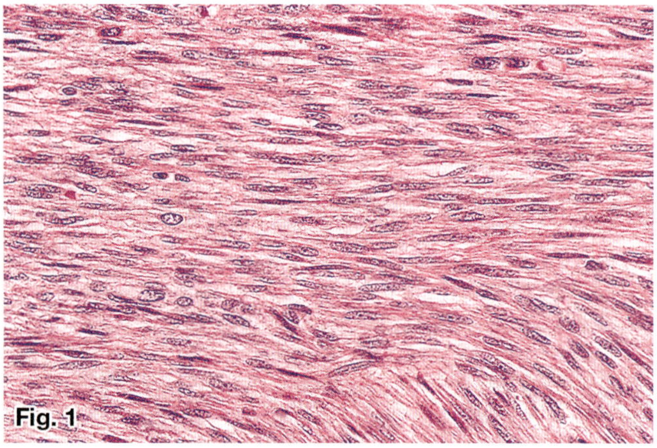

Fig. 1

   A. Negative immunostain for CD10
   B. Positive immunostain for h-caldesmon
   C. Presence of numerous mast cells
   D. Thick-walled blood vessels
   E. All of the above

3. Which of the following features cannot be used to distinguish a leiomyoma from leiomyosarcoma?

   A. Location of mitotic figures
   B. Morphology of mitotic figures
   C. Nuclear atypia
   D. Surrounding tissue infiltration
   E. Type of tissue necrosis

4. A myometrial tumor expressing smooth muscle actin, desmin, and h-caldesmon displays multiple foci of tissue necrosis, as shown in Figure 1. More than 10 mitotic figures per high-power field are found, and significant cellular atypia is appreciated. Which of the following is the most likely diagnosis?

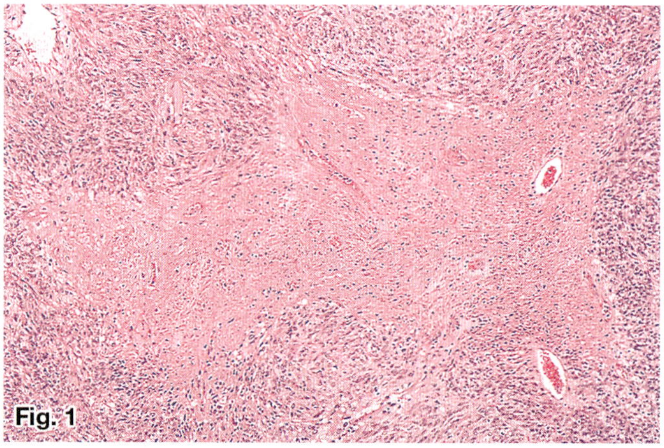

Fig. 1

   A. Atypical leiomyoma
   B. Cellular leiomyoma
   C. Endometrial stromal sarcoma, high grade
   D. Leiomyosarcoma
   E. Mitotically active leiomyoma

---

All figures in this chapter are from Longacre TA, Greenson JK, Hornick JL, Reuter VE, eds. *Mills and Sternberg's Diagnostic Surgical Pathology.* 7th ed. Wolters Kluwer; 2022 except for those noted at the end of this book.

5. A 26-year-old female with cutaneous benign smooth muscle tumors presents with abnormal uterine bleeding and is found to have a fibroid uterus. The histologic features of the uterine lesions are shown in Figure 1, which demonstrate desmin immunopositivity. Which of the following is false regarding the syndrome for which she should be evaluated for?

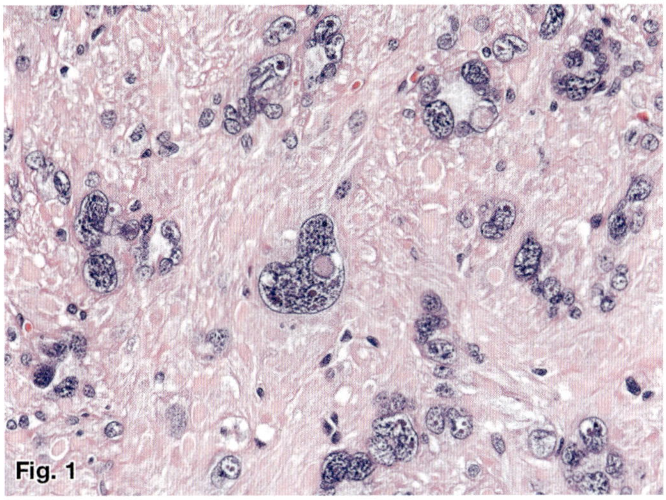

Fig. 1

A. Fumarate hydratase (FH) immunohistochemistry shows loss of expression.
B. It is a rare autosomal dominant disorder due to germline mutation in the *FH* gene.
C. Multiple uterine leiomyomas in conjunction with multiple cutaneous leiomyomas may occur.
D. Subset of affected patients develops type II renal cell papillary carcinoma.
E. Women most often develop symptomatic uterine leiomyomas in postmenopausal age.

6. Which of the following is true regarding the type of tissue necrosis in a uterine smooth muscle tumor of a 50-year-old woman in Figure 1?

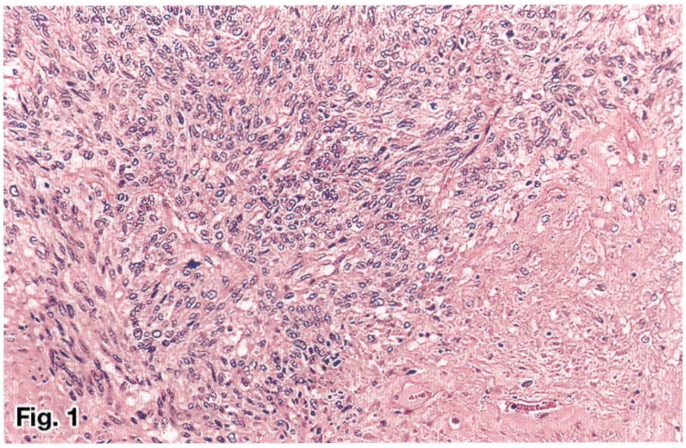

Fig. 1

A. It features an abrupt transition between necrotic cells and preserved cells.
B. It should be distinguished from infarct necrosis.
C. Tumors with this pattern of tissue necrosis behave aggressively.
D. Tumors with this pattern of tissue necrosis favor a diagnosis of leiomyosarcoma.
E. All of the above are correct.

7. A myxoid smooth muscle neoplasm is found in the uterus of a 55-year-old woman. Myometrial infiltration is seen, along with the histologic features shown in Figure 1. The tumor cells show immunolabeling with desmin, with negative expression for ALK-1 immunostain. What is the diagnosis?

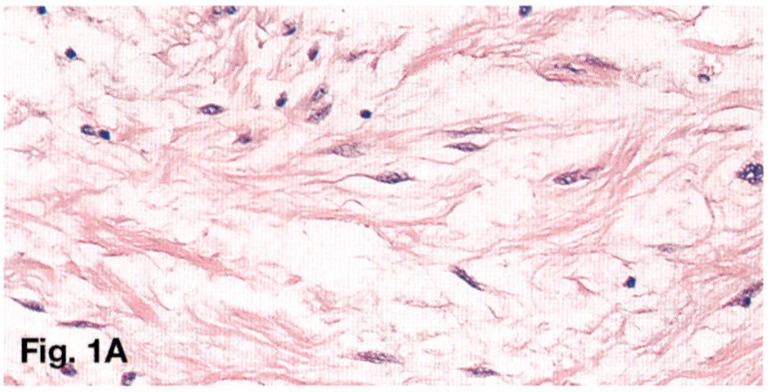

Fig. 1A

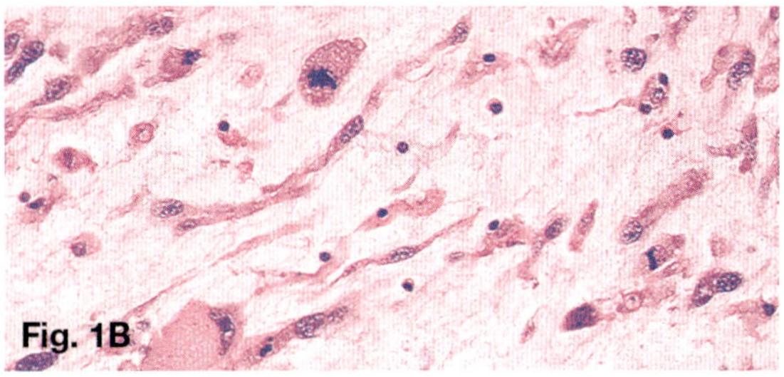

Fig. 1B

A. Degenerating leiomyoma with myxoid and hydropic change
B. Dissecting or cotyledonoid leiomyoma
C. Inflammatory myofibroblastic tumor (IMT)
D. Myxoid leiomyoma
E. Myxoid leiomyosarcoma

8. A 43-year-old G5P4 woman with a recent pregnancy was found to have an infiltrating uterine mass, with histologic features shown in Figure 1. Based on the clinical history and histomorphology of the tumor, which of the following must be considered in the differential diagnosis?

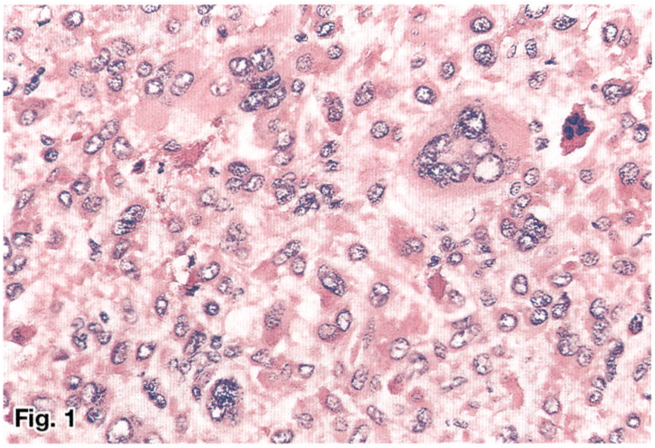

Fig. 1

A. Epithelioid leiomyosarcoma
B. Epithelioid trophoblastic tumor
C. Perivascular epithelioid cell tumor (PEComa)
D. Placental site trophoblastic tumor
E. All of the above

9. A 35-year-old woman is incidentally found to have multiple small peritoneal nodules (ranging from 1 to 1.5 cm) at the time of her cesarean section following an uneventful pregnancy. The surgeon is worried about metastatic disease and removes as many of the nodules as possible. Figure 1 shows the histologic features of the well-sampled nodules. A potentially malignant process must be considered when these lesions occur in which of the following clinicopathologic contexts?

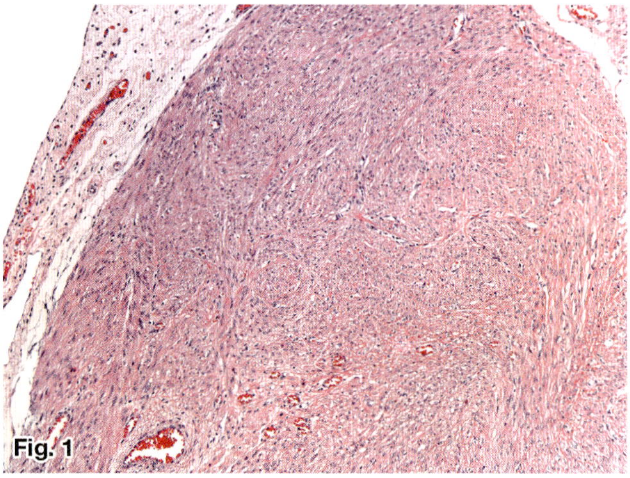
Fig. 1

A. Absence of concomitant uterine leiomyomas
B. Absence of exogenous hormone treatment
C. Absence of recent pregnancy
D. Negative estrogen receptor (ER) and progesterone receptor (PR) expression by immunohistochemistry
E. Any of the above

10. A 35-year-old woman, with a history of uterine fibroids status post remote myomectomy, is incidentally found to have two small pelvic nodules (ranging from 3 to 4 cm) at the time of her appendectomy for appendicitis. Intraoperatively, the nodules are noted to be distributed near the region of the round ligament. Microscopic examination reveals mitotically inactive, cytologically bland, nonnecrotic smooth muscle tumors that show strong immunopositivity for desmin, h-caldesmon, and estrogen receptor (ER). What is the best diagnosis?

A. Benign metastasizing leiomyoma
B. Disseminated peritoneal leiomyomatosis (DPL)
C. Intravascular (intravenous) leiomyomatosis
D. Leiomyosarcoma
E. Parasitic leiomyoma

11. A tumor within the myometrium shows the histologic features and pattern of infiltration shown in Figure 1. Immunohistochemically, it is diffusely positive for CD10 and negative for h-caldesmon. The mitotic count is 5 per 10 high-power field (HPF). What is the diagnosis?

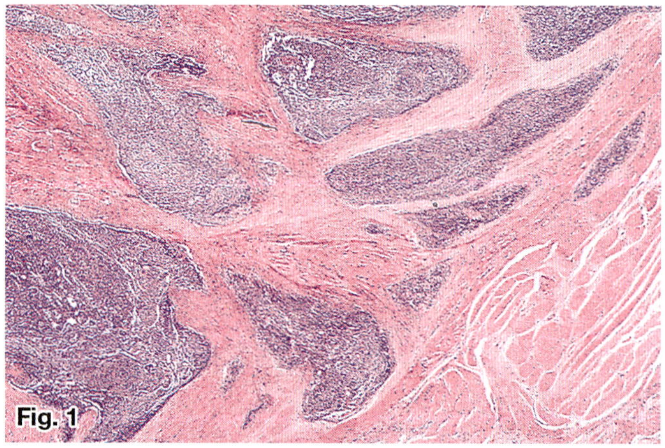
Fig. 1

A. Cellular leiomyoma
B. Endometrial stromal nodule
C. Endometrial stromal sarcoma, high grade
D. Endometrial stromal sarcoma, low grade
E. Leiomyosarcoma

12. The diagnosis of low-grade endometrial stromal sarcoma can almost always be made reliably on an endometrial biopsy. Is this true or false?

A. True
B. False

13. A 48-year-old woman is found to have a myometrial mass. A hysterectomy is performed, and the tumor demonstrates the histologic features shown in Figure 1. Tumor cell necrosis is not identified. Immunohistochemical workup shows expression for cyclin D1, with no immunopositivity for desmin, estrogen receptor (ER), progesterone receptor (PR), or CD10. What is the most likely diagnosis?

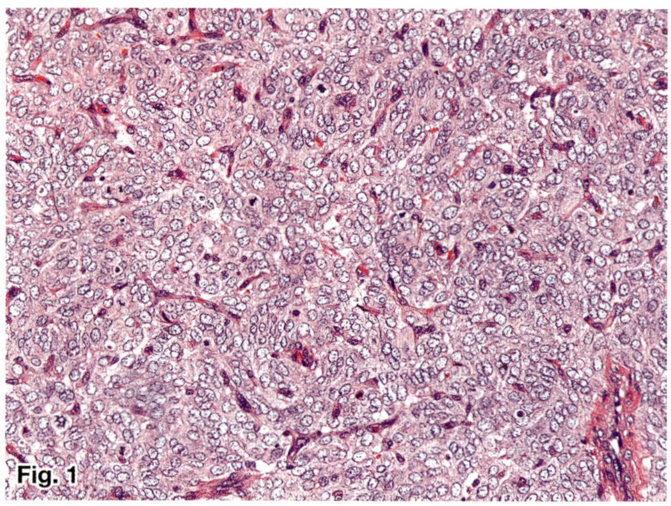
Fig. 1

A. Epithelioid leiomyosarcoma
B. High-grade endometrial stromal sarcoma (HGESS)
C. Low-grade endometrial stromal sarcoma
D. Perivascular epithelioid cell tumor (PEComa)
E. Undifferentiated uterine sarcoma

14. A 48-year-old woman is found to have a myometrial mass. A hysterectomy is performed, and grossly, the tumor is myxoid in appearance. The tumor demonstrates the histologic features shown in Figure 1. Additional workup demonstrates the tumor cells express CD10, B-cell corepressor (BCOR), estrogen receptor (ER), and progesterone receptor (PR), with limited smooth muscle actin (SMA) and desmin expression. What is the diagnosis?

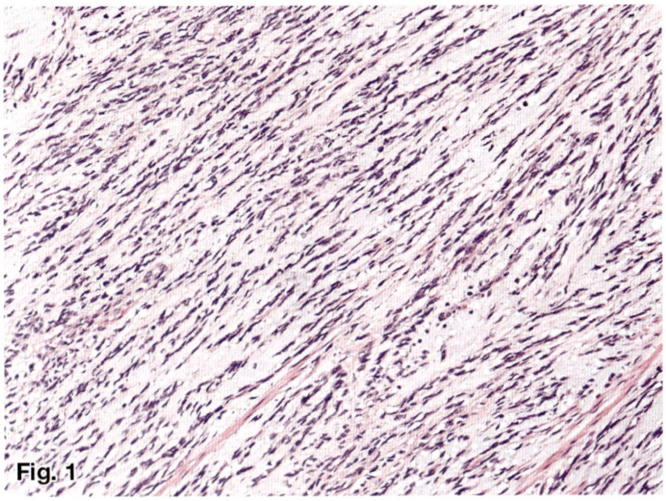
Fig. 1

A. High-grade endometrial stromal sarcoma (HGESS)
B. Inflammatory myofibroblastic tumor (IMT)
C. Myxoid leiomyosarcoma
D. *NTRK*-rearranged uterine sarcoma
E. Undifferentiated uterine sarcoma

15. A 31-year-old woman presents with post–coital bleeding, and imaging reveals a 7-cm cervical mass. A hysterectomy is performed, and the tumor is found to have the histologic features shown in Figure 1. Immunohistochemically, the tumor cells express cyclin D1, CD34, and S100, with no expression of desmin, estrogen receptor (ER), progesterone receptor (PR), or B-cell corepressor (BCOR). What is the most likely diagnosis?

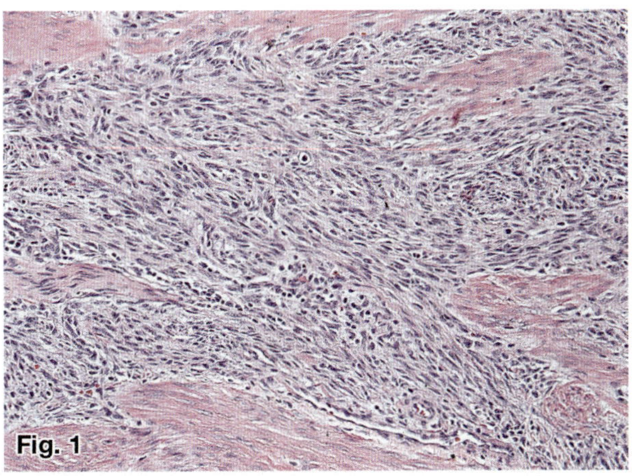
Fig. 1

A. *COL1A1-PDGFB*–rearranged uterine sarcoma
B. High-grade endometrial stromal sarcoma with *ZC3H7B-BCOR* fusion
C. Inflammatory myofibroblastic tumor
D. Myxoid leiomyosarcoma
E. *NTRK*-rearranged uterine sarcoma

16. A 51-year-old woman with abnormal uterine bleeding is found to have a myometrial mass. The tumor shows the histologic features shown in Figure 1. Immunohistochemical workup fails to demonstrate prominent expression of lineage markers, including cyclin D1, CD10, desmin, smooth muscle actin (SMA), erythroblast transformation-specific transcription factor (ERG), epithelial membrane antigen (EMA), and estrogen receptor (ER). What is the most likely diagnosis?

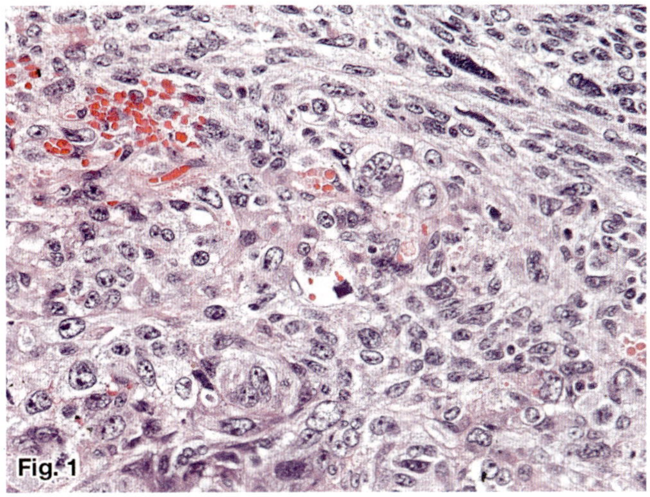
Fig. 1

A. Angiosarcoma
B. Leiomyosarcoma
C. Osteosarcoma
D. Rhabdomyosarcoma
E. Undifferentiated uterine sarcoma (UUS)

17. Figure 1 shows the histologic features of a myometrial tumor found in a 45-year-old woman. The epithelioid cells in this tumor are arranged in cords and trabeculae and have scanty to eosinophilic or clear cytoplasm, indistinct cell margins, and round nuclei. The tumor cells are immunopositive for inhibin, SF1, calretinin, WT-1, keratin, epithelial membrane antigen (EMA), smooth muscle actin (SMA), and desmin. Which genetic mutation is not associated with this neoplasm?

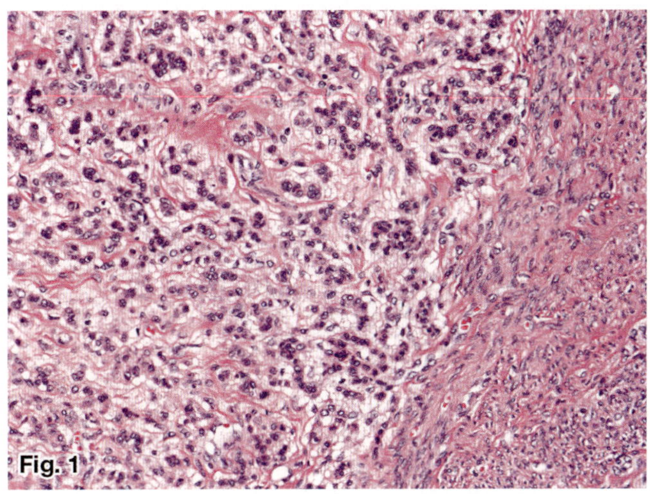
Fig. 1

A. *DICER1*
B. *ESR1*
C. *GREB1*
D. *NCOA2*
E. *NCOA3*

18. A 33-year-old woman who presents with abnormal uterine bleeding is found to have a cervical polyp. Histologic features of the cervical polyp are shown in Figure 1. Which of the following is true with regard to the diagnosis?

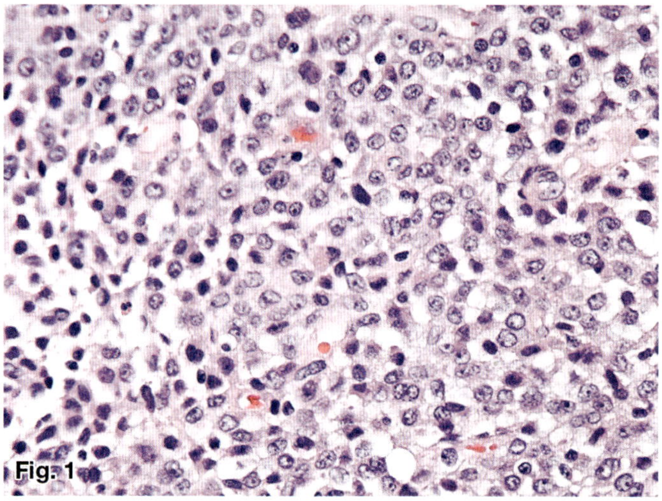

Fig. 1

A. Cellular condensation beneath epithelial surfaces (cambium layer) is present.
B. Differential diagnosis includes uterine adenosarcoma.
C. Expression of smooth muscle actin (SMA) and h-caldesmon is usually negative.
D. When syndromic, it is related to mutations in *DICER1* gene.
E. All of the above are correct.

19. Figure 1 demonstrates a uterine mass composed of nests of large polygonal cells with granular eosinophilic cytoplasm, vesicular nuclei, and distinct nucleoli. The tumor cells fail to show smooth muscle actin (SMA), desmin, h-caldesmon, or melanocytic immunopositivity. Which of the following is true regarding this uterine tumor?

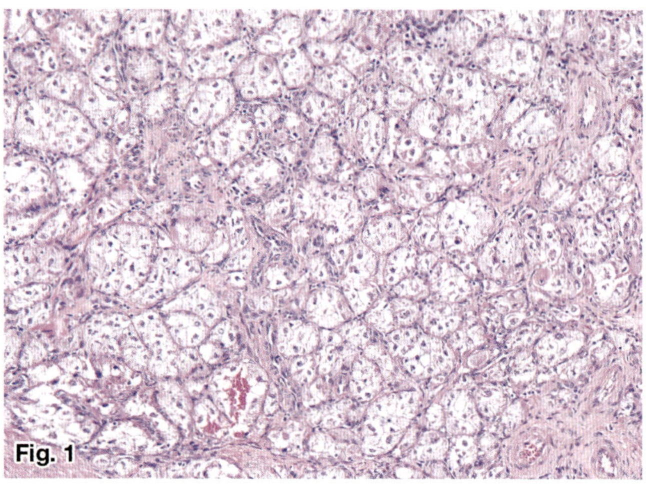

Fig. 1

A. It is characterized by *ASPSCR1/TFE3* gene fusion.
B. It has an indolent clinical course.
C. Recurrences and/or metastases may respond to selective MET inhibitor therapy.
D. Tumor cells show strong TFE3 nuclear expression.
E. All of the above are correct.

20. A 34-year-old woman is found to have a uterine mass at the time of cesarean section following an uneventful pregnancy. The mass has the histologic features shown in Figure 1. The tumor shows immunopositivity for desmin, CD10, h-caldesmon, and ALK. What is the diagnosis?

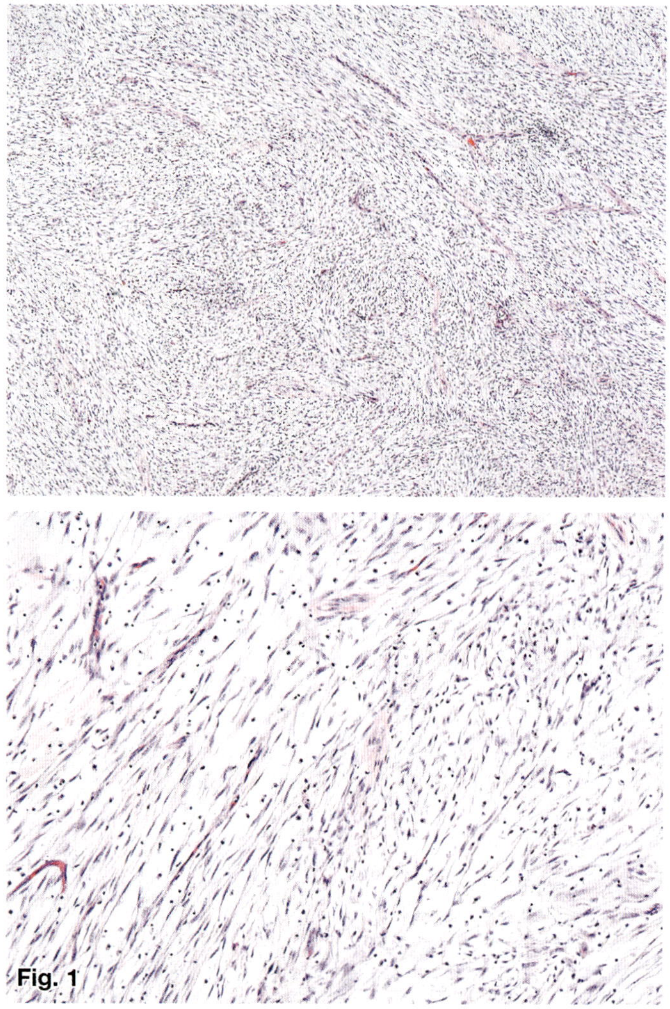

Fig. 1

A. High-grade endometrial stromal sarcoma
B. Inflammatory myofibroblastic tumor (IMT)
C. Low-grade endometrial stromal sarcoma
D. Myxoid leiomyosarcoma
E. *NTRK*-rearranged uterine sarcoma

21. Figure 1 demonstrates the histologic features of a myometrial mass that shows immunolabeling with desmin, cathepsin k, melan-A, and HMB45. Which of the following is not a prognostic variable for this tumor?

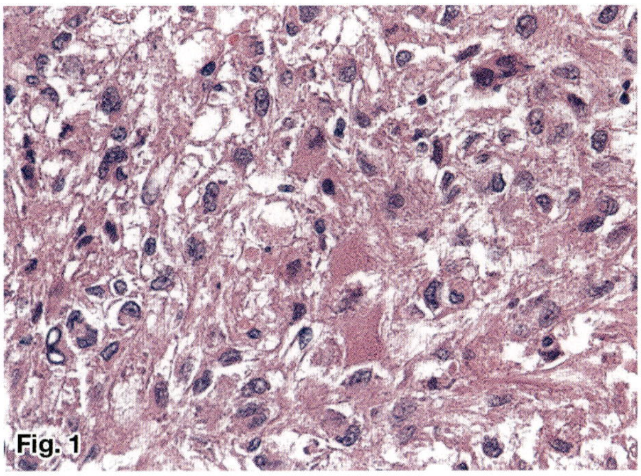

A. High-grade atypia
B. Mitotic index greater than 1 mitotic figure per 50 HPF (high-power field)
C. Myometrial infiltration
D. Necrosis
E. Tumor size greater than or equal to 5 cm

22. A 40-year-old G0 woman is found to have a lower uterine polypoid mass. Figure 1 demonstrates the characteristic histologic features of this lesion from low and high power. There is no significant cytologic atypia or mitotic activity identified. What is the diagnosis?

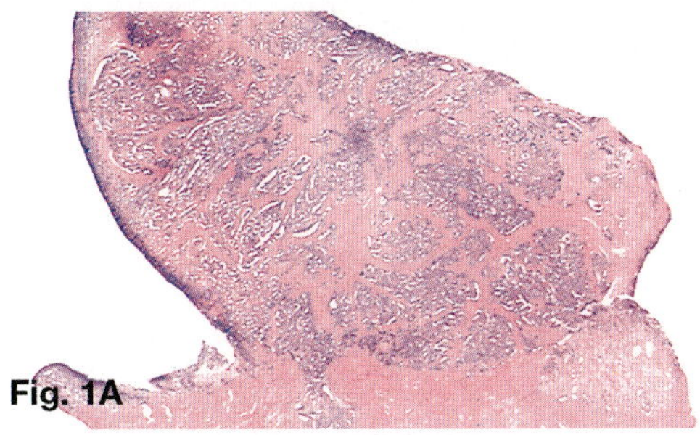

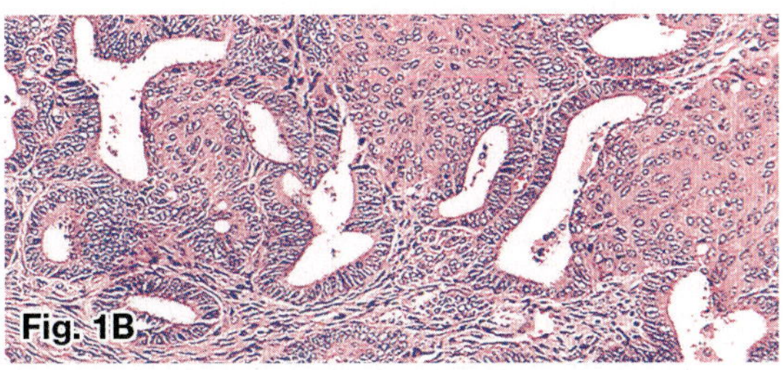

A. Atypical polypoid adenomyoma (APA)
B. Endometrial polyp
C. Myoinvasive low-grade endometrioid adenocarcinoma with squamous morular metaplasia
D. Polypoid adenomyoma
E. Polypoid atypical endometrial hyperplasia

23. A 55-year-old woman undergoes excision of a recurrent endometrial polyp. Figure 1 demonstrates the histologic features of the most recent specimen. What is the diagnosis?

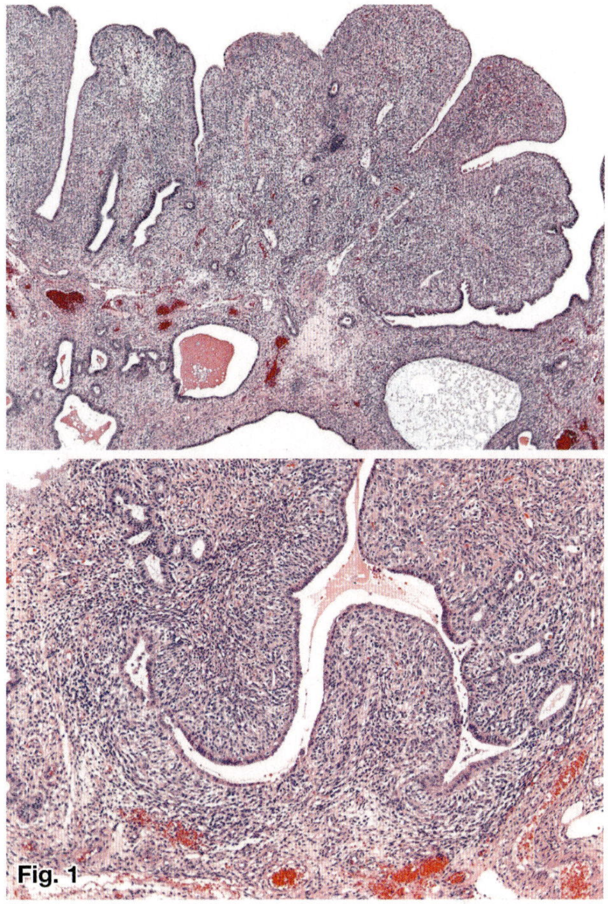

A. Adenosarcoma
B. Atypical polypoid adenomyoma
C. Embryonal rhabdomyosarcoma
D. Endometrial polyp
E. *NTRK*-rearranged uterine sarcoma

# ANSWERS AND EXPLANATIONS

**1. Correct choice: C.**

Adenomyosis is endometrial tissue (glands and stroma) that is ectopic in the uterus and often located deep in the myometrium. The glands in adenomyosis may be sparse or absent, which may pose concern for low-grade stromal sarcoma. This scenario (gland-poor adenomyosis) typically occurs in postmenopausal women. The islands of gland-poor adenomyosis are often circumscribed by hypertrophic myometrium, but there is no associated mass lesion. Diffuse adenomyosis may raise the question of low-grade stromal sarcoma with glands. Adenomyosis does not infiltrate the myometrium in tongues, as does stromal sarcoma, and the muscular hypertrophy characteristic of adenomyosis is largely absent in stromal sarcoma. It is also very rare for endometrial stromal sarcoma to contain small, regular glands diffusely spread throughout the lesion.

**2. Correct choice: E.**

The image shows the classic cellular morphology of a leiomyoma, an extremely common tumor usually found in women of reproductive age. There are several variants: (a) cellular, with increased cellular density; (b) epithelioid, composed of round epithelioid-like cells; (c) atypical (symplastic), containing scattered cells with atypical nuclei; (d) lipoleiomyoma, consisting of an admixture of classic leiomyoma and mature fat; and (e) myxoid, with spindle cells in a myxoid background. Benign metastasizing leiomyoma is an ordinary leiomyoma that has spread to the lungs, pelvis, or lymph nodes, usually following procedures such as dilatation and curettage (D&C), myomectomy, and hysterectomy. Intravascular leiomyomatosis refers to leiomyomatous tissue growing into the uterine and pelvic veins (it may grow into the inferior vena cava and extend to the right atrium). The differential diagnosis between cellular leiomyoma and endometrial stromal tumors relies on the features listed in the answer choices.

**3. Correct choice: D.**

The margins of most leiomyomas are microscopically circumscribed, but a few benign tumors demonstrate apparent infiltration. Consequently, infiltration is not a criterion of malignancy for smooth muscle tumors. Conversely, most leiomyosarcomas infiltrate; therefore, evaluation of histologic features of apparently infiltrating smooth muscle tumors must be performed carefully. Submucous leiomyomas may display extensive necrosis, often with acute inflammatory cells, particularly if they protrude into the endometrial cavity. Not infrequently, there will be increased mitotic activity in the tumor cells near the areas of necrosis. The coagulative tumor cell necrosis that is typical of leiomyosarcoma is usually not associated with acute inflammation, and ghost outlines of cells are prominent; such cells are inconspicuous or absent in infarct necrosis. In addition, the mitotic figures seen in conjunction with inflammatory necrosis are small and normal, whereas they may be large and abnormal in leiomyosarcomas.

**4. Correct choice: D.**

Leiomyosarcoma is the most common sarcoma of the uterus. Three features distinguish leiomyosarcoma from leiomyoma: coagulative tumor cell necrosis, diffuse moderate-to-severe atypia, and increased mitotic activity. True coagulative tumor cell necrosis is characterized by a sharp border between the necrotic area and surrounding viable tumor (as shown in the image). Leiomyosarcomas may occur in women of both premenopausal and postmenopausal age, with a peak incidence between 40 and 60 years. They frequently metastasize to the lungs, bone, and brain. A mitotically active leiomyoma has a mitotic index but is not associated with a good prognosis similar to usual leiomyomas.

**5. Correct choice: E.**

The presence of multiple leiomyomas in the uterus in conjunction with multiple cutaneous leiomyomas may occur in the setting of hereditary leiomyomatosis and renal cell carcinoma (HLRCC) syndrome, which is associated with germline mutations in the *FH* gene. Fumarate hydratase (FH)-deficient uterine leiomyomas typically exhibit increased cellularity, multinucleation, nuclear atypia, large orangeophilic nucleoli surrounded by a perinuclear halo, and hemangiopericytomatous (staghorn) blood vessels. A particularly distinctive feature is the presence of eosinophilic cytoplasmic inclusions. Immunohistochemistry for FH can be helpful in detecting FH deficiency, which typically manifests as complete loss of staining. HLRCC is a rare autosomal dominant disorder due to germline mutation in the *FH* gene, a gene that encodes an enzyme involved in the mitochondrial tricarboxylic acid cycle. A subset of affected patients develops aggressive type II renal cell papillary carcinoma. Because almost all women with HLRCC develop symptomatic uterine leiomyomas resulting in surgery at a young age, early detection of these patients is important in order to implement surveillance for renal cell carcinoma.

**6. Correct choice: E.**

Coagulative tumor cell necrosis features an abrupt transition between necrotic cells and preserved cells. The nuclei of the necrotic cells often retain their basophilia, and inflammatory cells are unusual. A cuff of viable cells may be seen around blood vessels. This pattern of necrosis is common in clinically malignant smooth muscle tumors and should never be ignored. In contrast, hyalinizing necrosis exhibits a zone of usually eosinophilic collagen interposed between the dead cells and the preserved cells, a pattern reminiscent of a region of infarction being organized by granulation tissue. Dead nuclei in areas of hyalinizing necrosis are uniform, with often faint chromatin, compared with the nuclear hyperchromasia and pleomorphism still visible in tumor cell necrosis. Tumors containing areas of unequivocal coagulative tumor cell necrosis behave aggressively, often enough to be considered leiomyosarcoma or tumors of uncertain malignant potential, regardless of other morphologic features.

**7. Correct choice: E.**

Myxoid leiomyosarcoma demonstrates smooth muscle cells widely separated by myxoid material. The characteristic low cellularity partly accounts for the presence of only a few mitotic figures per 10 HPF (high-power field). There is myometrial infiltration in most cases, and some invade blood vessels. In myxoid leiomyosarcomas, not only is the stroma myxoid, but the cells are enlarged with hyperchromatic nuclei; pleomorphism is usually obvious. Myxoid leiomyosarcoma should be distinguished from inflammatory myofibroblastic tumor (IMT), which may express smooth muscle markers. The latter tumor often expresses anaplastic lymphoma kinase-1 (ALK-1); patients with uterine tumors that harbor *ALK* gene rearrangements may benefit from targeted therapy. Many leiomyomas exhibiting gross degeneration on microscopic evaluation feature islands of collagenated smooth muscle set in a sea of edematous connective tissue, which may appear myxoid. Large-caliber vessels are characteristically suspended in these myxoid areas, which is termed *perinodular hydropic degeneration.* Dissecting leiomyoma demonstrates an irregular interface with the surrounding myometrium, characterized by wormlike or nodular protrusions. This permeative growth pattern may extend into the parametrial tissue and broad ligament, creating a "cotyledonoid" appearance. Myxoid leiomyoma is uncommon, with small and uniform cells, absent or at most mild atypia, and low mitotic index (<2 mitotic figures per 10 HPF [high-power field]). Areas of ordinary leiomyoma should be present focally in these lesions. Importantly, the margins of a myxoid leiomyoma are circumscribed, and there is no tumor cell necrosis.

**8. Correct choice: E.**

Epithelioid leiomyosarcomas exhibit predominant (>50%) epithelioid differentiation in addition to the usual features of malignancy seen in conventional leiomyosarcoma, that is, moderate-to-severe cytologic atypia, and/or tumor cell necrosis or elevated mitotic index (≥5 mitotic figures per 10 high-power field [HPF]). These tumors are characterized by round or polygonal cells with eosinophilic, but occasionally clear cytoplasm, which may exhibit rhabdoid or sex cord–like elements. The cells are typically arranged in nests, cords, large nodules, or diffuse sheets. Epithelioid leiomyosarcoma should be distinguished from placental site trophoblastic tumor and epithelioid trophoblastic tumor. A history of a recent pregnancy and/or elevated serum human chorionic gonadotropin (β-hCG) levels may suggest the diagnosis of placental site trophoblastic tumor; the presence of tumor cells interposed between preexisting smooth muscle bundles is also a useful distinguishing feature. Confirmation of the diagnosis can usually be made with immunohistochemistry for keratin and human platelet lysate (hPL). Although premenopausal and perimenopausal women can develop leiomyosarcoma, placental site trophoblastic tumor should be considered in this age group before a diagnosis of leiomyosarcoma (particularly epithelioid variants) is made. Uterine perivascular epithelioid cell tumor (PEComa), which can have a nested growth pattern composed of epithelioid cells, should also be excluded.

**9. Correct choice: E.**

Disseminated peritoneal leiomyomatosis (DPL) is a rare, benign, hormonally induced proliferation characterized by multiple peritoneal nodules composed of an admixture of fibroblasts and bland smooth muscle cells. The nodules are usually small (<2 cm), and they stud the surface of the peritoneum, mimicking metastatic disease. Expression of estrogen receptor (ER) and progesterone receptor (PR) is almost always present. It almost always occurs in young women subject to an altered hormonal milieu, usually pregnancy. Consequently, it is most often discovered incidentally at the time of cesarean section. Postpartum spontaneous regression is the rule, but all nodules that are surgically removed should be adequately sampled to exclude a potentially malignant smooth muscle neoplasm. Occasionally, the peritoneal nodules may contain benign endometrial glands, mimicking endometriosis. Women who present with suspected DPL in the absence of (a) uterine leiomyomas, (b) exogenous or increased endogenous estrogen exposure, or (c) hormone receptor expression on immunohistochemical studies should be regarded as harboring potentially malignant tumors and followed closely.

**10. Correct choice: A.**

Women with mitotically inactive, cytologically bland, nonnecrotic uterine smooth muscle tumors may develop similarly benign extrauterine smooth muscle deposits (often in the lungs but also in the pelvis and lymph nodes) in the absence of a primary smooth muscle malignancy in the gastrointestinal tract, retroperitoneum, or other nonuterine areas; this has been termed *benign metastasizing leiomyoma.* These tumors usually demonstrate high estrogen receptor (ER) and progesterone receptor (PR) expression levels. The pulmonary nodules usually progress slowly, sometimes to the point of producing pulmonary insufficiency, but they may respond to hormonal treatment and are often treated by excision. Benign metastasizing leiomyoma usually presents as one or more pulmonary nodules. When it occurs within the pelvis and abdomen, there are usually only one or two nodules, the nodules are larger than those in disseminated peritoneal leiomyomatosis (DPL), and they tend to be distributed near the region of the round ligament or iliac veins. Although both lesions are associated with intrauterine leiomyomas, the extrauterine lesions in benign metastasizing leiomyoma often present years after the previous resection of the uterine leiomyoma, whereas in DPL, the uterine leiomyomas are concomitant. On rare occasions, leiomyomas have been reported to detach from their initial subserosa location and attach themselves to some other pelvic site through the mediation of a combination of infarction and inflammatory adhesions, earning the term *parasitic leiomyoma.* The definition of intravascular leiomyomatosis requires the presence of benign smooth muscle within the vascular lumina or within the chambers of the heart. By definition, leiomyosarcoma will have a combination of malignant histologic features, including mitotic activity, cytologic atypia, and coagulative tumor cell necrosis.

**11. Correct choice: D.**

Low-grade endometrial stromal sarcoma, by definition, is composed of cells resembling those of the normal proliferative-phase endometrium and has infiltrative margins and/or intravascular intrusion. The cells are almost always CD10 positive, with weaker variable expression of smooth muscle markers. The pattern of myometrial infiltration is often distinctive and consists of irregularly shaped tongues or islands of tumor cells randomly placed between bundles of smooth muscle cells. An arborizing vascular pattern is characteristic of this neoplasm. Endometrial stromal nodule is a well-circumscribed, noninfiltrative, typically spherical mass of endometrial stromal cells without an intravascular component. High-grade endometrial stromal sarcoma exhibits more cellularity, and the cytologic atypia and mitotic index are beyond that seen in the usual low-grade endometrial stromal sarcoma.

**12. Correct choice: B.**

Endometrial stromal nodule is a well-circumscribed, noninfiltrative, typically spherical mass of endometrial stromal cells without an intravascular component. The cells are identical to those found in proliferative endometrium or in low-grade endometrial stromal sarcoma. The distinction between a stromal nodule and low-grade endometrial stromal sarcoma depends on the absence of myometrial infiltration or vascular invasion; these nodules cannot be reliably distinguished from low-grade stromal sarcoma in endometrial samplings and myomectomy specimens unless fragments with vascular or myometrial invasion are unequivocally present. Hysterectomy may be required to make this distinction when the entire uterus and margin of the lesion are available for microscopic examination.

**13. Correct choice: B.**

High-grade endometrial stromal sarcoma (HGESS) is a cellular neoplasm with infiltrating margins, usually with extensive myometrial infiltration. The tumor often demonstrates greater than 10 mitotic figures per 10 HPF (high-power field) and tumor cell necrosis. The image shows the high-grade round cell component, but frequently, a low-grade spindle cell component with fibromyxoid features is identified as well. The high-grade round cell component will show immunopositivity for cyclin D1, with no expression of CD10, estrogen receptor (ER), or progesterone receptor (PR). The low-grade spindle cell component is positive for CD10, ER, and PR and variably positive for cyclin D1. This particular subtype of HGESS harbors *YWHAE-NUTM2* gene fusion. Extrauterine extension of HGESS is common at diagnosis, metastasis is possible, and behavior is intermediate between that of low-grade endometrial stromal sarcoma and undifferentiated uterine sarcoma.

**14. Correct choice: A.**

High-grade endometrial stromal sarcoma (HGESS) with *ZC3H7B-BCOR* fusion is a subtype of HGESS that is uniformly cellular neoplasm with infiltrating margins, similar in appearance to that of low-grade endometrial stromal sarcoma; however, the cells are uniformly more atypical than those in usual low-grade endometrial stromal sarcoma. This tumor will often exhibit greater than 10 mitotic figures per 10 high-power fields as well as tumor cell necrosis. The spindled cells are variably associated with a myxoid matrix and collagen plaques and are positive for CD10, B-cell corepressor (BCOR), estrogen receptor (ER), and progesterone receptor (PR) with limited smooth muscle actin (SMA) and desmin. They may be positive for cyclin D1 as well. As with HGESS with *YWHAE-NUTM2* gene fusions, extrauterine extension is common at diagnosis in this subtype as well. The tumors can also metastasize, and their behavior is intermediate between that of low-grade endometrial stromal sarcoma and undifferentiated uterine sarcoma.

**15. Correct choice: E.**

*NTRK*-rearranged uterine sarcoma occurs in the uterine cervix and, rarely, in the corpus, in young patients (mean age is 31 years). The size of these tumors ranges from 3 to 12 cm. The tumors are composed of spindle-shaped cells with ovoid nuclei, inconspicuous nucleoli, and scant cytoplasm. Atypia is mild to moderate, although scattered markedly atypical symplastic-like cells may be present in some cases. Mitotic index is variable and ranges from 1 to 50 mitotic figures per 10 high-power fields. Tumor cell necrosis and staghorn vessels may be present. Immunohistochemically, these tumors express CD34, S100, pan-TRK, and cyclin D1. *COL1A1-PDGFB*–rearranged uterine sarcoma is a cervical sarcoma that exhibits a more cellular herringbone architectural pattern and more uniform cells. This tumor harbors a *COL1A1-PDGFB* rearrangement and expresses CD34 and cyclin D1, but not S100 or pan-TRK.

**16. Correct choice: E.**

Undifferentiated uterine sarcoma (UUS) exhibits no morphologic evidence of endometrial stromal or smooth muscle differentiation. Most undifferentiated uterine sarcomas are composed of enlarged, pleomorphic cells with numerous mitotic figures. However, some may exhibit a more uniform appearance. UUS behaves in a highly aggressive manner. UUS are characterized by complex karyotypic abnormalities but lack a unifying tumor-specific alteration. Pure sarcomas containing cells differentiating along recognizable mesenchymal lines are named in a way that reflects their differentiation, that is, leiomyosarcoma, osteosarcoma, rhabdomyosarcoma, and angiosarcoma.

**17. Correct choice: A.**

The neoplastic cells of uterine tumor resembling ovarian sex cord tumor (UTROSCT) that give the tumor its name are typically arranged in cords, hollow tubules, trabeculae, and/or sheets resembling epithelial cells, and they most often have scanty cytoplasm, indistinct cell margins, and round nuclei. In some tumors, however, the constituent cells may have abundant eosinophilic or clear cytoplasm. The cells composing the sex cord–like areas are often positive for inhibin, SF1, calretinin, and WT1; they may also express keratin, epithelial membrane antigen (EMA), smooth muscle actin (SMA), desmin, and/or h-caldesmon. Despite the striking similarity to a sex cord-stromal tumor in the ovary, UTROSCT does not harbor *FOLX2* or *DICER1* mutations, which are characteristic of ovarian adult-type granulosa cell tumors and Sertoli-Leydig cell tumors, respectively. UTROSCT appears to harbor recurrent fusions involving *NCOA2/3* (either *ESR1-NCOA3*, *ESR1-NCOA2*, or *GREB1-NCOA2*), and these fusions may stratify patients at risk for recurrence. Specifically, *GREB1*-rearranged tumors, which tend to be larger, more mitotically active, and occur in older women, may behave more aggressively than *ESR1*-rearranged UTROSCT. In general, UTROSCT is associated with significantly lower rates of extrauterine spread and recurrence when compared to low-grade endometrial stromal sarcoma.

**18. Correct choice: E.**

Adult patients with uterine embryonal rhabdomyosarcoma range in age from 20 to 89 years. Uterine rhabdomyosarcoma can present as a cervical polyp or uterine mass. Cellular condensation beneath epithelial surfaces (cambium layer) and occasional elongated or globular cells with eosinophilic cytoplasm are also present. The tumor cells express desmin, muscle-specific actin, myogenin, and MyoD1, as well as PAX7. Desmin expression may be minimal or absent in tumors that occur in patients older than 40 years. Expression of smooth muscle actin (SMA) and h-caldesmon is usually negative. Embryonal rhabdomyosarcoma has been associated with ovarian Sertoli-Leydig cell tumors and/or pleuropulmonary blastoma, and this has been related to mutations in *DICER1* (DICER syndrome). Adult uterine embryonal rhabdomyosarcoma has a worse prognosis than the pediatric cervical-vaginal form. The chief differential diagnosis is uterine adenosarcoma, which typically also exhibits periglandular stromal condensation and may contain areas of cartilaginous differentiation. However, adenosarcoma, even when exhibiting sarcomatous overgrowth, should maintain at least some foci of phyllodes growth pattern with intraluminal polypoid projections.

**19. Correct choice: E.**

Alveolar soft-part sarcoma may rarely occur in the uterine corpus and cervix. It is composed of a distinctive epithelioid cell population organized in an alveolar growth pattern. The neoplastic cells exhibit strong TFE3 nuclear expression but typically lack smooth muscle actin (SMA), desmin, h-caldesmon, and melanocytic (melan-A, HMB45) expression. Alveolar soft-part sarcoma is characterized by an *ASPCR1/TFE3* gene fusion that leads to MET (mesenchymal epithelial transition) transcriptional upregulation. Unlike their soft tissue counterpart, most uterine alveolar soft-part sarcomas appear to have an indolent clinical course. Recurrences and/or metastases may respond to selective MET inhibitor therapy.

**20. Correct choice: B.**

Inflammatory myofibroblastic tumor (IMT) involving the uterus has a strong association with pregnancy, but the mean age of presentation is 40 years. The tumor exhibits two main morphologic patterns: the more characteristic pattern is myxoid (also described as myxoid/vascular or hypocellular), which is characterized by the presence of plump spindle cells with open chromatin set in a prominent myxoid and edematous matrix, imparting a fasciitis or tissue culture–like appearance. A less common pattern is fascicular (also described as compact spindle cell), where the spindled cells form intersecting bundles and have eosinophilic cytoplasm, resembling smooth muscle. In contrast to smooth muscle, the nuclei exhibit a more open chromatin pattern with fusiform or tapered (as opposed to blunt-ended) nuclei and a variably prominent inflammatory component. Uterine IMT expresses anaplastic lymphoma kinase (ALK) protein on immunohistochemistry in up to 80% of cases. As in other sites, uterine IMT harbors rearrangement of the *ALK* gene located at 2p23.13. Those that occur during pregnancy appear to harbor specific fusion partners involved in placentation, and limited data suggest these tumors may have a benign clinical course. The presence of *ALK* gene rearrangements provides potential targeted therapy for clinically aggressive tumors with tyrosine kinase inhibitors (crizotinib or ceritinib).

**21. Correct choice: C.**

Perivascular epithelioid cell tumors (PEComas) belong to a family of HMB45–positive epithelioid cell proliferations with clear to lightly eosinophilic cytoplasm that tends to develop around blood vessels. In addition to PEComas, this family includes angiomyolipomas, lymphangioleiomyomas, and clear cell tumors of the lungs. The constituent cells of uterine PEComas often coexpress muscle markers, including desmin, smooth muscle actin (SMA), and h-caldesmon, as well as cathepsin k, microphthalmia transcription factor, melan-A, and, rarely (and focally), S100 protein. Prognostic variables include tumor size greater than or equal to 5 cm, mitotic index greater than 1 mitotic figure per 50 HPF (high-power field), high-grade atypia, necrosis, and lymphovascular invasion. About 15% of uterine PEComas are associated with tuberous sclerosis complex and/or lymphangioleiomyomatosis; these are associated with mutations in *TSC1* and *TSC2*. A subset of PEComa carry gene rearrangements involving *TFE3*; these tumors tend to be composed of epithelioid cells with clear cytoplasm arranged in an alveolar architecture, round nuclei; they label strongly for TFE3 and HMB45 with minimal expression of muscle markers. These tumors may respond to mTOR-targeted therapy.

**22. Correct choice: A.**

Atypical polypoid adenomyoma (APA) features a biphasic proliferation of irregularly dispersed, architecturally complex, and cytologically atypical endometrial glands within a mitotically active myofibromatous stroma, often forming a polyp in the lower uterine segment. Polypoid adenomyoma and atypical polypoid adenomyoma differ in the complexity of the architecture of the glandular component, which is complex in APA and simple in polypoid adenomyoma. Polypoid atypical endometrial hyperplasia lacks the characteristic myofibromatous stroma, as does endometrial polyp; instead, both show endometrial glands separated by endometrial stroma. The major differential diagnostic problem presented by APA is the exclusion of well-differentiated endometrial carcinoma with myoinvasion. In this case, discrete septa of myometrial smooth muscle surround carcinomatous glands, often with an associated stromal inflammatory response.

**23. Correct choice: A.**

Adenosarcoma is an uncommon, predominantly low-grade malignant biphasic tumor that is composed of sarcomatous stroma and benign epithelial elements. When it occurs in the uterine corpus, adenosarcoma often presents as a polys or polypoid lesion, which may protrude through the cervical os or appear to arise from the cervix or lower uterine segment with uterine enlargement. Often, there is a history of recurrent polyps, which may represent early or subtle forms of adenosarcoma. Histologically, broad papillary fronds that resemble phyllodes tumor of the breast and cystically enlarged glands are present with areas of abundant, cellular stroma, which can compress the glands. Angiosarcomas fall into three groups, depending on the atypicality of the stroma and the presence of stromal overgrowth: group 1: low-grade adenosarcoma, with nondescript stromal component and mitotic count of 2 to 4 per 10 HPF (high-power field); group 2: high-grade adenosarcoma with histologically malignant stroma, most often with rhabdomyosarcomatous differentiation, but chondroid, smooth muscle, and undifferentiated sarcoma may also be seen; and group 3: adenosarcoma with stromal overgrowth, defined as containing pure stroma, comprising more than 25% of the tumor volume. It contains high-grade sarcomatous stroma, often with heterologous differentiation (typically rhabdomyosarcoma), and it is associated with a poor prognosis.

# 55 Ovarian Epithelial-Stromal Tumors

1. Which of the following statements about ovarian tumors is correct?

   A. Majority of ovarian tumors in older women are malignant.
   B. Minority of ovarian tumors in patients less than 45 years of age are malignant.
   C. One of the most important clinical features is the patient's age.
   D. Primitive germ cell tumors are rarely seen in women more than 50 years of age.
   E. All of the above are correct.

2. Which of the following findings often accompany primary ovarian cancers?

   A. Adenofibromatous background
   B. Endometriosis
   C. Endometriotic cysts
   D. Teratoma
   E. All of the above

3. Which of the following germline mutations are not associated with hereditary epithelial ovarian cancers?

   A. *BRCA1*
   B. *BRCA2*
   C. *DICER1*
   D. *MSH2*
   E. *MSH6*

4. Ovarian serous tumors are composed of an epithelium that microscopically and ultrastructurally resembles which of the following?

   A. Endocervical epithelium
   B. Endometrial epithelium
   C. Intestinal epithelium
   D. Transitional epithelium
   E. Tubal epithelium

5. The lining of a cystic ovarian tumor from a 40-year-old woman displays complex polypoid projections into the lumen. The areas shown in Figure 1 comprise most of the cyst lining. Tumor cells appear similar to tubal epithelial cells. No stromal invasion is found after thorough sampling. What is the most likely diagnosis?

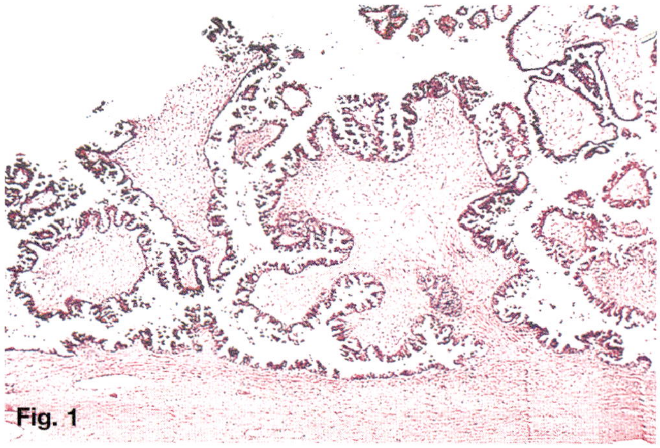


**Figure 1** Republished with permission of Springer, from Scully RE. Histological classification of ovarian tumours. In: World Health Organization, ed. *Histological Typing of Ovarian Tumours: International Histological Classification of Tumours*. Springer; 1999. doi .org/10.1007/978-3-642-58564-7_2. Copyright © 1999 Springer-Verlag, Berlin, Heidelberg; permission conveyed through Copyright Clearance Center, Inc.

   A. Low-grade serous carcinoma
   B. Serous borderline tumor
   C. Serous cystadenofibroma
   D. Serous cystadenoma
   E. Serous cystadenoma with focal epithelial proliferation

All figures in this chapter are from Longacre TA, Greenson JK, Hornick JL, Reuter VE, eds. *Mills and Sternberg's Diagnostic Surgical Pathology*. 7th ed. Wolters Kluwer; 2022 except for those noted at the end of this book.

6. The lining of a cystic ovarian tumor from a 45-year-old woman demonstrates epithelium similar to that of the fallopian tube, with only a minor focus of complex polypoid projections into the lumen comprising less than 10% of the cyst lining, such as that shown in Figure 1. Thorough sampling fails to identify stromal invasion. What is the most likely diagnosis?

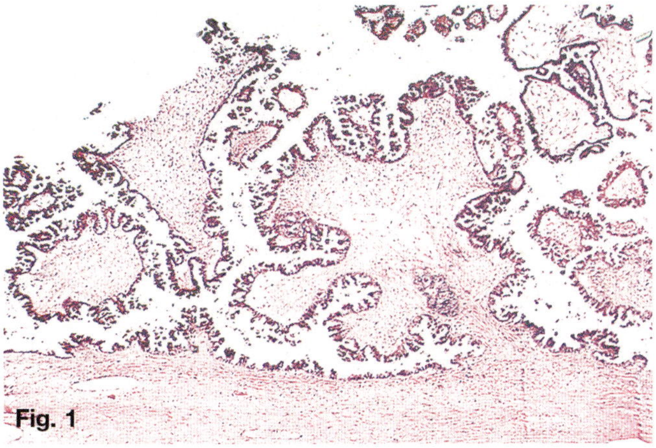


**Figure 1** Republished with permission of Springer, from Scully RE. Histological classification of ovarian tumours. In: World Health Organization, ed. *Histological Typing of Ovarian Tumours: International Histological Classification of Tumours.* Springer; 1999. doi.org/10.1007/978-3-642-58564-7_2. Copyright © 1999 Springer-Verlag, Berlin, Heidelberg; permission conveyed through Copyright Clearance Center, Inc.

A. Low-grade serous carcinoma
B. Serous borderline tumor
C. Serous cystadenofibroma
D. Serous cystadenoma
E. Serous cystadenoma with focal epithelial proliferation

7. A 43-year-old woman is found to have bilateral ovarian masses that show the histologic features depicted in Figure 1. After thorough sampling, there is no evidence of invasive disease noted. Which of the following is true of this distinct pattern of serous borderline tumor (SBT) when compared to typical SBTs?

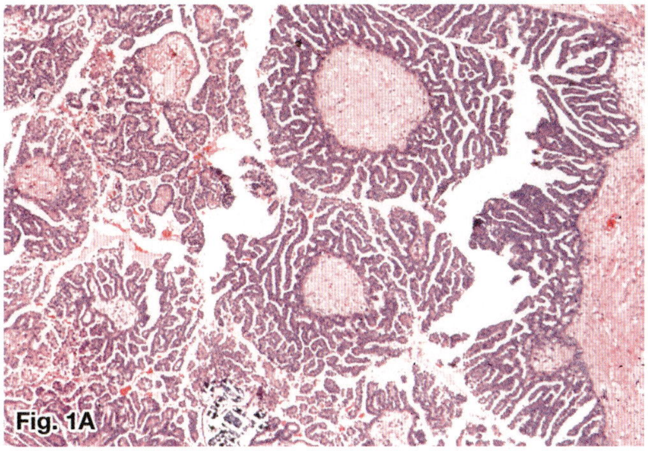


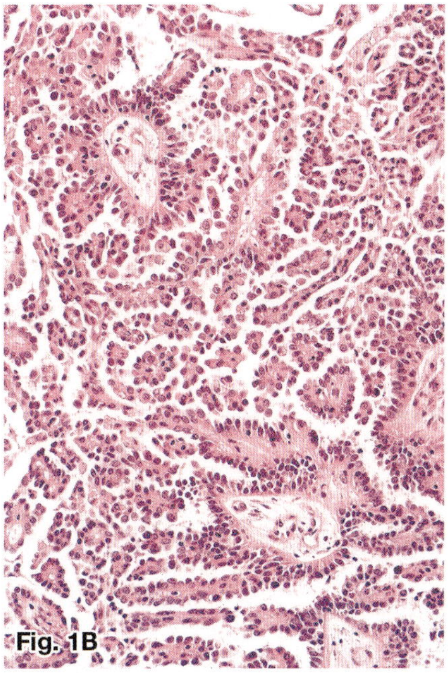


A. They include SBTs with micropapillary and/or cribriform pattern.
B. They have a higher frequency of bilaterality.
C. They have a higher frequency of implants, which tend to be invasive.
D. They have a higher frequency of surface involvement.
E. All of the above are correct.

8. A 40-year-old woman is found to have an ovarian serous borderline tumor. During her surgical staging, multiple peritoneal implants are biopsied. The histomorphologic feature of one of these biopsies is shown in Figure 1. What is the correct diagnosis of this implant?

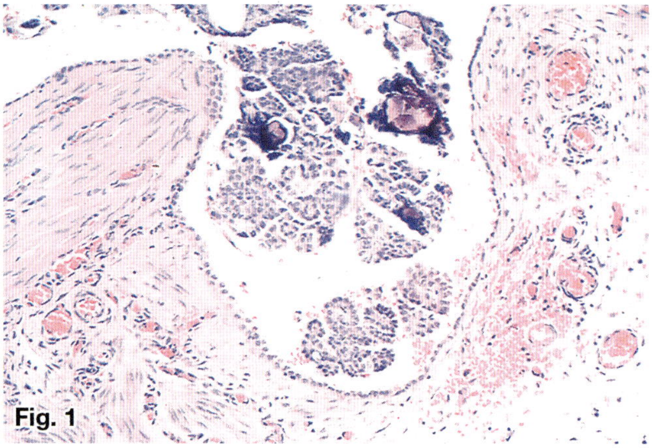
Fig. 1

A. Endosalpingiosis
B. Invasive implant
C. Low-grade serous carcinoma
D. Noninvasive implant, desmoplastic subtype
E. Noninvasive implant, epithelial subtype

9. A 40-year-old woman is found to have an ovarian serous borderline tumor. During her surgical staging, multiple peritoneal implants are biopsied. The histomorphologic feature of one of these biopsies is shown in Figure 1. What is the correct diagnosis of this implant?

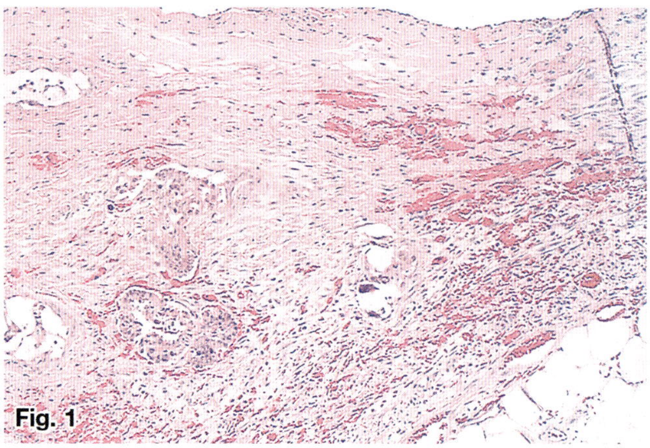
Fig. 1

A. Endosalpingiosis
B. Invasive implant
C. Low-grade serous carcinoma
D. Noninvasive implant, desmoplastic subtype
E. Noninvasive implant, epithelial subtype

10. A 40-year-old woman is found to have an ovarian serous borderline tumor. During her surgical staging, her omentum was resected and demonstrated foci of microscopic disease after thorough sampling. The histomorphologic feature of one of these areas is shown in Figure 1. What is the correct designation of her omental disease?

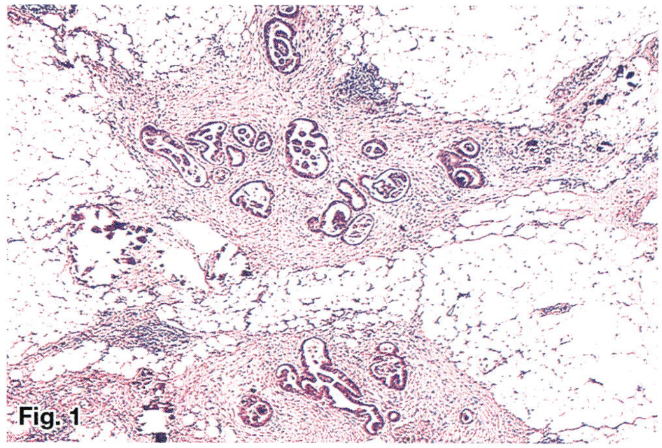
Fig. 1

A. Endosalpingiosis
B. Involvement by serous borderline tumor
C. Low-grade serous carcinoma
D. Noninvasive implant, desmoplastic subtype
E. Noninvasive implant, epithelial subtype

11. Which of the following factors is not associated with the transformation of a serous borderline tumor to low-grade serous carcinoma?

A. Micropapillary serous borderline tumor
B. Presence of desmoplastic noninvasive implant
C. Presence of invasive implant
D. Presence of microinvasion
E. Serous borderline tumor with cribriform pattern

12. The ovarian neoplasm shown in Figure 1 was diagnosed as a high-grade serous carcinoma. Which of the following is the primary feature used to differentiate this neoplasm from low-grade serous carcinoma?

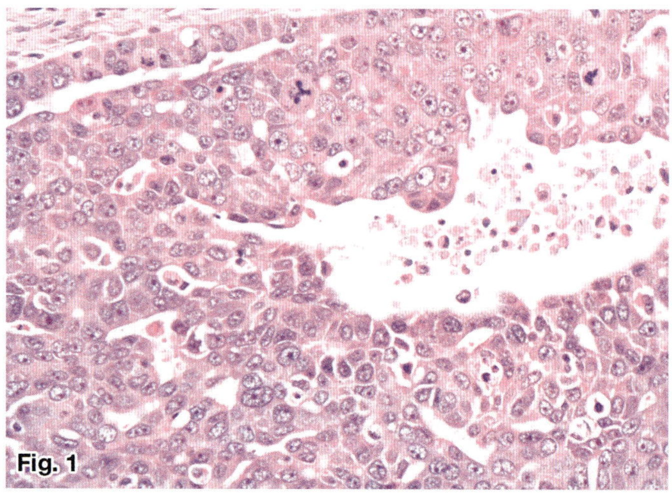
Fig. 1

A. Architecture
B. Infiltration pattern
C. Mitotic index
D. Nuclear size
E. Tumor size

13. Which of the following molecular alterations is not associated with high-grade serous carcinoma?

A. Aneuploidy
B. Chromosomal instability
C. Complex karyotypes
D. *PTEN* mutations
E. *TP53* mutations

14. A 43-year-old female is found to have a serous borderline tumor in her left ovary. Staging surgery revealed the findings shown in Figure 1. Which of the following alterations is not part of the molecular profile of this tumor?

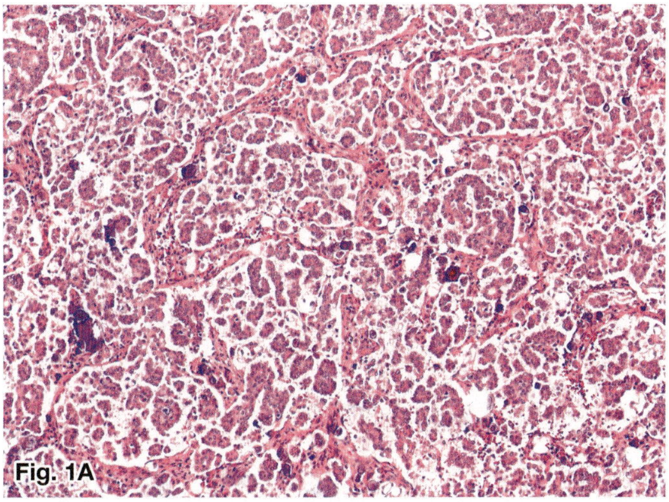

Fig. 1A

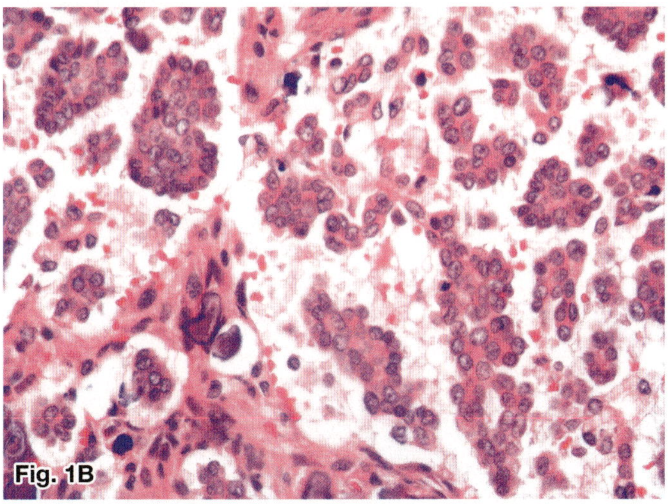

Fig. 1B

A. *BRAF* mutations
B. Chromosomal stability
C. Diploidy
D. *KRAS* mutations
E. *TP53* mutations

15. Which of the following is not a criterion for the diagnosis of psammocarcinoma?

A. Invasion of the ovarian stroma/intraperitoneal tissue or its lymphovascular spaces
B. Mild-to-moderate nuclear atypia
C. Presence of psammoma bodies in at least 75% of papillae or nests
D. Significant nuclear size variation
E. Small epithelial nests, no greater than 15 cells in their largest linear dimension

16. When assigning primary site of origin in a case of high-grade serous carcinoma, which of the following features of distribution of disease fulfill the criterion for its designation as an ovarian primary?

A. Carcinoma being confined to the ovarian surface and the only site of intraperitoneal disease
B. Carcinoma of invasive type in the ovary
C. No overgrowth of both fallopian tubes by carcinoma
D. No situ or invasive disease involving the mucosa of both fallopian tubes
E. All of the above

17. Ovarian mucinous tumors are composed of an epithelium that microscopically and ultrastructurally resembles which of the following?

A. Endocervical epithelium
B. Endometrial epithelium
C. Ovarian surface epithelium
D. Transitional epithelium
E. Tubal epithelium

18. A 52-year-old woman undergoes excision of a large multilocular ovarian cyst containing thick mucinous fluid. Microscopically, the wall consists of nonciliated columnar cells arranged mostly in a single layer and papillary projections, with some foci of increased cytologic atypia and stratification, as shown in Figure 1. Stromal invasion is absent. These features are most consistent with which of the following?

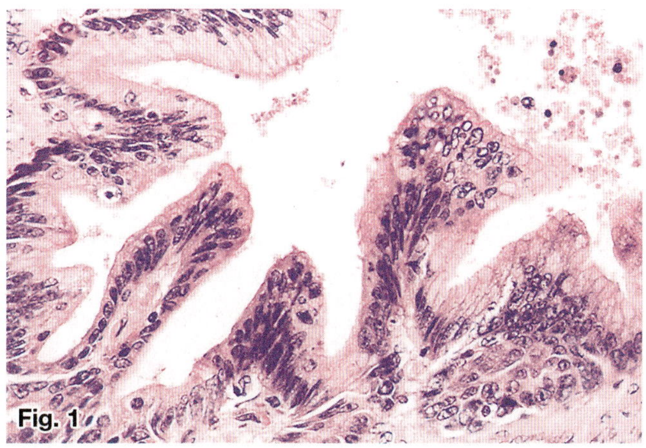

Fig. 1

A. Mucinous borderline tumor
B. Mucinous carcinoma
C. Mucinous cystadenoma
D. Seromucinous borderline tumor
E. Serous cystadenoma

19. A 50-year-old woman undergoes excision of a large multilocular ovarian cyst containing thick mucinous fluid. Microscopically, the wall consists of nonciliated columnar cells arranged mostly in a single layer and papillary projections, with foci of severely atypical lining cells, as shown in Figure 1. Stromal invasion is absent. These features are most consistent with which of the following?

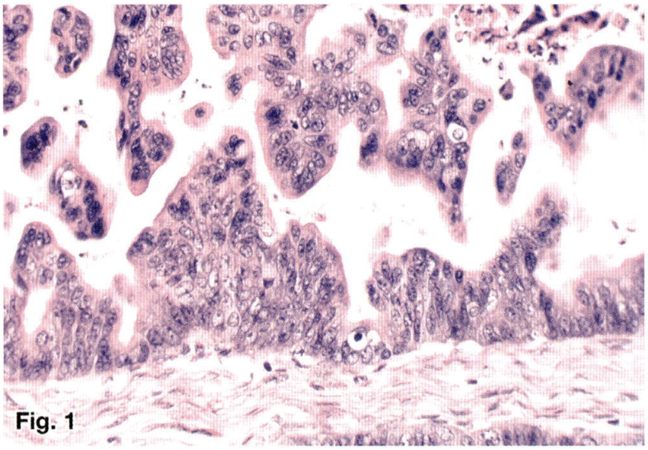

Fig. 1

A. Mucinous borderline tumor
B. Mucinous borderline tumor with intraepithelial carcinoma
C. Mucinous carcinoma
D. Mucinous cystadenoma
E. Seromucinous borderline tumor

20. A 48-year-old woman is found to have a 20-cm multiloculated mucinous cystic tumor. Microscopic examination reveals foci shown in Figure 1. Which of the following is true regarding this tumor?

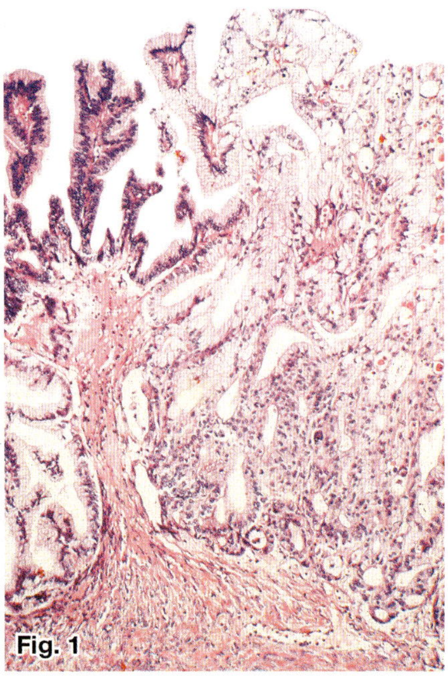

Fig. 1

A. Characterized by a confluent growth of back-to-back glands lined by malignant epithelium
B. Greatest linear dimension of greater than 5 mm
C. Have a low risk of recurrence
D. Is most likely a stage I tumor
E. All of the above

21. A 40-year-old female is found to have a large unilateral multiloculated mucinous borderline tumor of the ovary. Figure 1 shows the histologic features of one of the solid nodules that was found in the wall during macroscopic examination. What is the correct diagnosis?

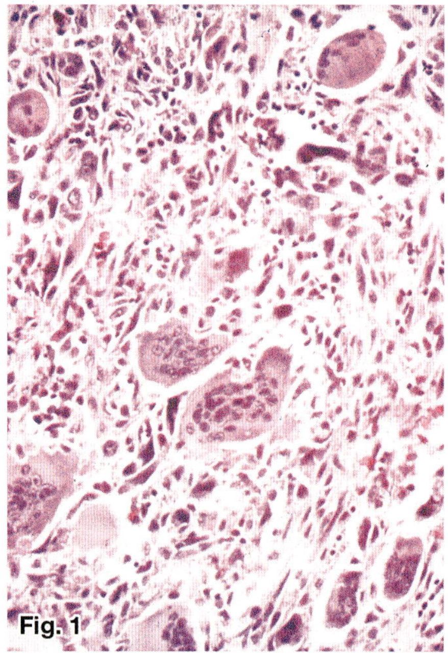

Fig. 1

A. Anaplastic carcinoma nodule
B. Focus of invasive mucinous carcinoma
C. Mucin granuloma
D. Sarcoma-like mural nodule
E. Sarcomatous nodule

22. A 40-year-old female is found to have a large unilateral multiloculated mucinous borderline tumor of the ovary. Figure 1 shows the histologic features of one of the solid nodules that was found in the wall during macroscopic examination. The features are concerning for which of the following?

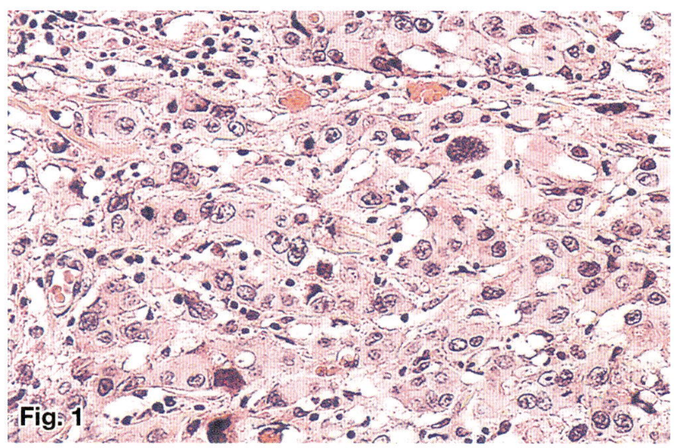

Fig. 1

A. Anaplastic carcinoma nodule
B. Focus of invasive mucinous carcinoma
C. Mucin granuloma
D. Sarcoma-like mural nodule
E. Sarcomatous nodule

23. Which of the following is true regarding seromucinous carcinomas?

A. Considered to be endometrioid carcinomas
B. Considered to be high-grade serous carcinomas
C. Considered to be low-grade serous carcinomas
D. Considered to be mucinous carcinomas
E. Considered to be seromucinous carcinomas

24. Figure 1 shows the histologic features of bilateral unilocular ovarian tumors found in a 38-year-old female with a history of pelvic endometriosis. What is the most likely diagnosis?

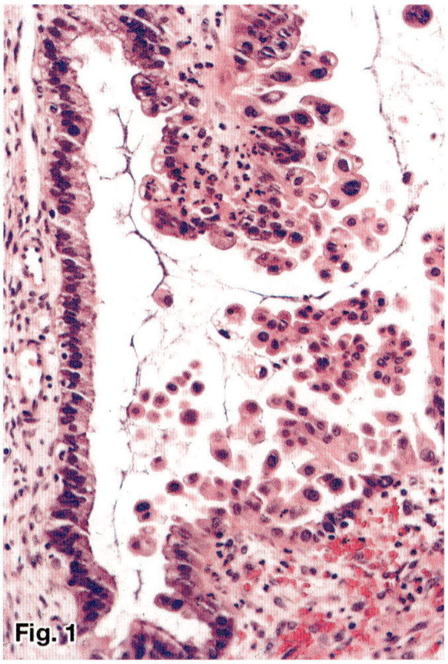
Fig. 1

A. Atypical endometriosis
B. Clear cell borderline tumor
C. Mucinous borderline tumor
D. Seromucinous borderline tumor
E. Serous borderline tumor

25. Which of the following tumors is not associated with endometriosis?

A. Clear cell carcinoma
B. Endometrioid carcinoma
C. High-grade serous carcinoma
D. Mesonephric-like carcinoma
E. Seromucinous borderline tumor

26. A 37-year-old woman with pelvic endometriosis is found to have the ovarian lesion shown in Figure 1. What is the best classification of this lesion?

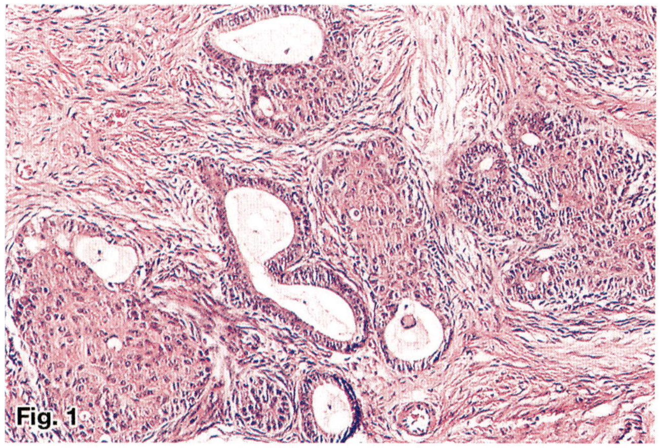
Fig. 1

A. Endometrioid adenoacanthofibroma
B. Endometrioid adenofibroma
C. Endometrioid borderline tumor
D. Endometrioid carcinoma
E. Endometrioid hyperplasia

27. A 52-year-old woman with abnormal uterine bleeding is found to have a uterine endometrioid adenocarcinoma. During her surgical staging, she is found to have a unilateral ovarian mass, which demonstrates the histologic features shown in Figure 1. What is the most likely diagnosis?

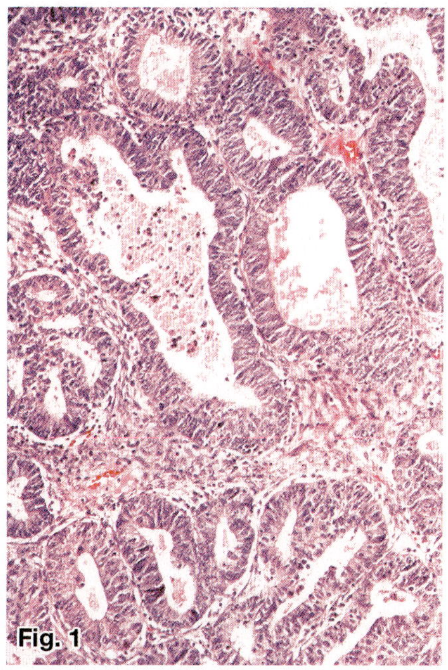
Fig. 1

A. Adult granulosa cell tumor
B. Atypical endometriosis
C. Endometrioid borderline tumor
D. Endometrioid carcinoma
E. Sertoli cell tumor

28. Which of the following histologic features and components may be encountered in ovarian endometrioid carcinomas?

A. Corded and hyalinized variant
B. Mucin secretion
C. Secretory pattern
D. Yolk sac tumor
E. All of the above

29. A 48-year-old woman is found to have uterine endometrioid adenocarcinoma during her workup for abnormal uterine bleeding. During her surgical staging, she is found to have a unilateral ovarian mass as well. Which of the following macroscopic and histologic features support independent primary tumors in this case?

A. Both tumors are confined to the organ.
B. Both tumors are low grade.
C. There is no deep myometrial invasion and/or lymphovascular invasion.
D. There is no ovarian surface involvement.
E. All of the above are correct.

30. The ovarian tumor whose typical morphology is shown in Figure 1 is most frequently associated with ovarian/pelvic endometriosis and increased risk of thrombosis. Which one is it?

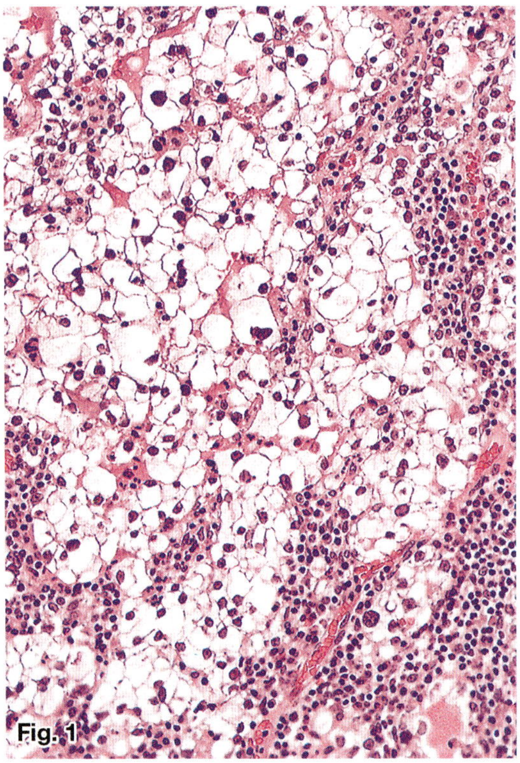

Fig. 1

A. Clear cell carcinoma
B. Dysgerminoma
C. Endometrioid carcinoma
D. High-grade serous carcinoma
E. Mucinous carcinoma

31. A solid ovarian tumor histologically shows nests of transitional-like epithelium separated by fibroblastic stroma, as shown in Figure 1. Scattered small microcystic spaces are present that contain dense eosinophilic material or mucin. The cells have clearly outlined borders and frequent nuclear grooving. The patient is a 40-year-old woman with signs of hyperestrinism. What is the most likely diagnosis?

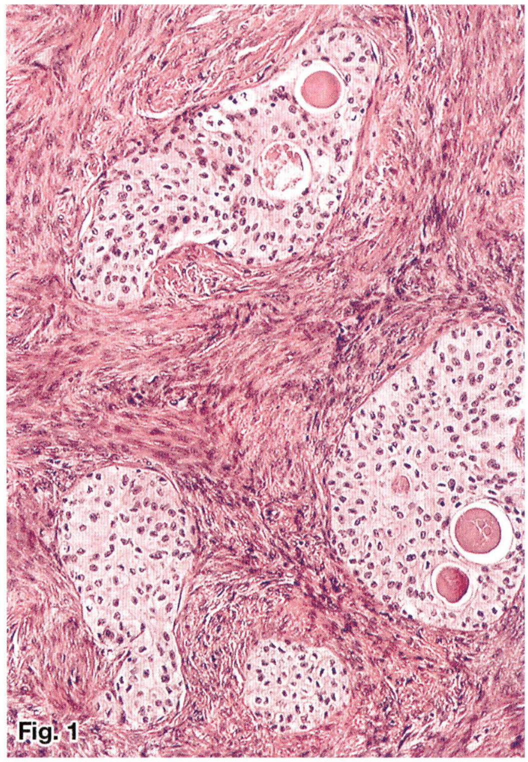

Fig. 1

A. Borderline Brenner tumor
B. Brenner tumor
C. Malignant Brenner tumor
D. Metastatic urothelial carcinoma
E. Squamous cell carcinoma

# ANSWERS AND EXPLANATIONS

**1. Correct choice: E.**

There is an important correlation between age and certain types of ovarian tumors, which may help in the differential diagnosis. Most ovarian tumors affecting women younger than 45 are benign. The percentage of malignant tumors increases with age. The peak incidence of ovarian germ cell tumors occurs around 20 years of age.

**2. Correct choice: E.**

Certain gross and microscopic ovarian findings that often accompany primary cancers may provide helpful diagnostic clues and also evidence that they are primary rather than metastatic. Among these are endometriotic cysts and endometriosis, which are associated especially with clear cell carcinomas, endometrioid carcinomas, and seromucinous borderline tumors. Squamous cell carcinomas and other primary tumors (eg, malignant melanoma, struma ovarii, and carcinoids) can arise within dermoid cysts or may have only microscopic evidence of teratoma. Similarly, some carcinomas, particularly those of endometrioid and clear cell type, arise within an adenofibroma.

**3. Correct choice: C.**

More than 15% of epithelial ovarian cancers are hereditary. Two autosomal dominant cancer susceptibility syndromes account for a large majority of these cases: hereditary breast and ovarian cancer syndrome, secondary to germline *BRCA1* and/or *BRCA2* mutations, with a number of other less common mutations also associated with the syndrome, and Lynch syndrome, or hereditary nonpolyposis colorectal cancer (HNPCC) syndrome, secondary to mutations in DNA-mismatch repair (MMR) enzymes, with *MLH1*, *MSH2*, *MSH6*, and *PMS2* being the most commonly mutated genes in this syndrome. Hereditary breast and ovarian cancer syndrome accounts for 90% of hereditary ovarian cancer, almost all of which are high-stage high-grade serous carcinomas. Ovarian carcinoma is less common than either colorectal or endometrial carcinoma in patients with Lynch syndrome, and only 10% of patients with the syndrome will develop an ovarian carcinoma. The type of carcinomas associated with Lynch syndrome appears to be endometrioid and clear cell carcinomas that predominate.

**4. Correct choice: E.**

The cysts, as well as the polypoid excrescences of benign serous tumors (which may be exophytic or endophytic or both), are typically lined by epithelium similar to that of the fallopian tube, including focal or diffuse ciliation. Tumors lined entirely by nonciliated cuboidal or columnar epithelium that resembles ovarian surface epithelium are also generally included in the serous category, despite their indifferent appearance. The epithelial cells of benign serous tumors may secrete mucin but, when present, are confined to the lumina of cysts and the apical cytoplasm of the lining cells.

**5. Correct choice: B.**

The image depicts the typical intricate branching pattern of the epithelium lining the cyst of a serous borderline tumor. The fact that tumor cells resemble tubal epithelium places this tumor in the serous category. Borderline tumors are designated as such when the epithelial proliferation comprises greater than 10% of the cyst lining. Borderline tumors are separated from malignant serous tumors by their lack of stromal invasion.

**6. Correct choice: E.**

The image depicts tumor cells that resemble tubal epithelium, which places this tumor in the serous category. The typical intricate branching pattern of the epithelium shown is consistent with borderline neoplasia (nuclear stratification and atypia). An otherwise typical benign cystic serous tumor that contains very minor foci (<10% of the cyst lining after thorough sampling) of borderline neoplasia is retained in the benign category and is referred to as serous cystadenoma with focal epithelial proliferation. Borderline tumors are designated as such when the epithelial proliferation comprises greater than 10% of the cyst lining, after thorough sampling to exclude the presence of stromal invasion.

**7. Correct choice: E.**

Five to 10% of serous borderline tumors (SBTs) have a micropapillary and/or a cribriform, which is associated with a higher frequency of bilaterality, surface involvement, and implants when compared to typical SBTs lacking these patterns. The implants associated with SBTs with micropapillary features are more frequently invasive than in typical SBTs. The micropapillary pattern is characterized by a nonhierarchical pattern of branching. It has been suggested that the micropapillae should be 5 times as long as wide. The neoplastic cells forming the micropapillary and cribriform patterns are round and nonciliated and have scanty cytoplasm, mild-to-moderate nuclear atypia, and often a small nucleolus. The cells are more monomorphic than those in typical SBTs. These tumors, however, should be thoroughly sampled to exclude foci of invasion.

**8. Correct choice: E.**

Peritoneal implants of serous borderline tumors may be grossly visible as small nodules or plaques but are often microscopic. The implants have been subclassified as noninvasive and invasive, with the former subdivided into epithelial and desmoplastic subtypes. In epithelial noninvasive implants, papillary proliferations of atypical serous cells with a minor or absent stromal component are present on the surface of the peritoneum in smoothly contoured peritoneal invaginations or in invaginations between lobules of omental fat. The cytologic atypia of these implants usually approximates that in the primary ovarian tumor. In both forms of noninvasive implants, psammoma bodies may be present and are occasionally conspicuous. In some cases, the peritoneal foci are composed of benign-appearing serous cells, which are not considered neoplastic, but possibly preneoplastic, and have been designated endosalpingiosis.

**9. Correct choice: D.**

Peritoneal implants of serous borderline tumors (SBTs) may be grossly visible as small nodules or plaques but are often microscopic. The implants have been subclassified as noninvasive and invasive, with the former subdivided into epithelial and desmoplastic subtypes. Desmoplastic noninvasive implants are characterized by a predominance of reactive stroma and are layered onto the peritoneal surfaces, including those lining invaginations between omental fat lobules. Within these implants, small glands and papillae lined by atypical serous cells, as well as single cells and psammoma bodies, are entrapped in granulation and scar tissue, which is often infiltrated by acute and chronic inflammatory cells. The glands and papillae may lie in clear spaces, possibly caused by secretory activity of the neoplastic cells. Necrosis, fibrin deposition, and hemorrhage are occasionally seen and may play a role in inducing the desmoplasia. In both forms of noninvasive implants, psammoma bodies may be present and are occasionally conspicuous.

**10. Correct choice: C.**

Invasive implants of serous borderline tumor (SBTs) are foci of extraovarian disease and are best considered foci of low-grade serous carcinoma (LGSC). They are diagnosed as such; thus, the term *invasive implant* is now synonymous with LGSC. This designation is based on the prognosis of patients with invasive implants being much inferior to that of patients whose SBTs have noninvasive implants. Invasive implants/LGSC are much less common than noninvasive implants. Invasive implants are characterized by an irregular infiltration and destruction of underlying tissue, identical to LGSC. It is important to note that assessment of implants as noninvasive versus invasive is only relevant in the context of SBT and is not applicable for high-grade serous carcinoma. In cases of high-stage SBTs, the presence of invasive implants is the most significant prognostic indicator.

**11. Correct choice: B.**

Serous borderline tumors (SBTs) associated with clinically progressive disease have frequently transformed to a low-grade serous carcinoma (LGSC), and this finding is a strong adverse factor. This complication may occur more commonly with micropapillary SBTs and those with cribriform pattern. Transformation correlated positively with the presence of microinvasion and/or invasive implants.

**12. Correct choice: D.**

It has become apparent that high-grade serous carcinomas (HGSC) and low-grade serous carcinomas (LGSC) are entirely different neoplasms. The distinction is based on variability in nuclear size, which is greater than 3-fold in HGSC. Mitotic index can be used as an alternative parameter if assessing nuclear size is problematic. HGSC shows greater than 12 mitotic figures per 10 HPFs (high-power fields). By immunohistochemistry (IHC), serous carcinomas express CK7, WT1, and estrogen receptor (ER). The following is a list of key features of HGSC and LGSC:

- HGSC: More frequent; originates from the tubal or ovarian surface epithelia, not from LGSC; spreads early on; has p53 gene mutations resulting in high or absent immunoreactivity for p53 protein; has complex karyotypes and marked intratumoral genetic heterogeneity; the cytology is high grade throughout the tumor.
- LGSC: Much less common than HGSC; most develop from serous borderline tumors (SBTs); psammoma bodies are frequent; cytology is low grade throughout the tumor.

**13. Correct choice: D.**

High-grade serous carcinomas (HGSCs) almost all have *TP53* mutations, resulting in either high-level expression of p53 protein or complete loss of p53 immunoreactivity ("all or nothing" staining pattern) indicative of abnormal p53. HGSCs are chromosomally unstable, with complex karyotypes, aneuploidy, and considerable intratumoral genetic heterogeneity. *PTEN* mutations are characteristic of endometrioid carcinomas, which can be harnessed by loss of PTEN (phosphatase and tensin) expression by immunohistochemistry.

**14. Correct choice: E.**

The molecular profile, in addition to the histomorphologic features, differ between low-grade (LGSC) and high-grade serous carcinoma (HGSC). LGSCs differ from HGSCs in being diploid or near-diploid, with relatively few mutations. *BRAF* and *KRAS* mutations are common in both serous borderline tumors (SBTs) and LGSCs, but not in HGSCs. HGSCs have TP53 mutations, in addition to being chromosomally unstable, with complex karyotypes and aneuploidy.

**15. Correct choice: D.**

A rare variant of low-grade serous carcinoma (LGSC) with an apparently favorable prognosis is the psammocarcinoma. This tumor, which is often primary in the peritoneum, appears to behave clinically more like a serous borderline tumor (SBT) than a serous carcinoma, but it differs in its microscopic features from the former by infiltrating the ovarian stroma or other peritoneal organs. Four criteria have been recommended for the diagnosis of psammocarcinoma: (a) invasion of the ovarian stroma or its lymphovascular spaces (or, in extraovarian areas of involvement, invasion of any intraperitoneal tissue or its lymphovascular spaces), (b) no more than mild-to-moderate nuclear atypia, (c) epithelial nests no greater than 15 cells in their largest linear dimension, and (d) the presence of psammoma bodies in at least 75% of papillae or nests. Significant nuclear size variation is a criterion for the diagnosis of high-grade serous carcinoma.

**16. Correct choice: E.**

The distinction between primary ovarian, tubal, and peritoneal high-grade serous carcinoma (HGSC) based on "dominant tumor mass" does not accurately indicate the primary site and underestimates the number of tumors originating in the fallopian tube. The propensity of secondary ovarian involvement by carcinoma to result in tumor masses larger than the primary tumor is well known (eg, ovarian metastases from carcinomas of the vermiform appendix, stomach, endocervix, and colon). Because there are no morphologic or molecular markers that can distinguish between HGSCs originating in the ovary, fallopian tube, or peritoneum, it may not be possible to determine the primary site in some cases of advanced-stage HGSC. The convention is that an HGSC is considered an ovarian primary tumor only if the fallopian tubes are normal, that is, there is no in situ or invasive disease involving the mucosa of the fallopian tubes, and there is no overgrowth of fallopian tube by carcinoma, a common finding in advanced-stage HGSC. The treatment is the same for all three primary sites so that accurate, determination of primary site is not necessary for clinical management, and it is acceptable to acknowledge that primary site cannot be determined with certainty in a given case. If the carcinoma is confined to the ovarian surface and is the only or almost only intraperitoneal tumor, it is considered to be of ovarian origin; if the ovarian tumor is invasive, it is considered primary.

**17. Correct choice: A.**

This group constitutes approximately 15% of all ovarian tumors. Benign mucinous tumors of the ovary are lined by a single layer of nonciliated mucus-producing cells similar in appearance to endocervical or intestinal epithelium. They develop in middle-aged or older women, rarely in those of younger age. Most tumors are large multilocular cysts filled with mucinous fluid. Of all ovarian mucinous tumors, approximately 75% are benign, 10% are borderline, and 15% are carcinomas. Grossly, they appear as multilocular cysts, whereas serous tumors are usually unilocular.

**18. Correct choice: A.**

In mucinous borderline tumors (MBTs), the epithelium shows cytologic atypia and architectural disorganization, but no stromal invasion. Areas of nodularity or increased thickness in the cyst wall should be carefully evaluated for stromal invasion. MBTs may be classified further into those with epithelium of the endocervical or intestinal type. Most MBTs are of the intestinal type. In mucinous carcinoma, on the other hand, there is unequivocal expansile or stromal invasion. The absence of ciliated columnar epithelium removes the consideration of serous and seromucinous tumors.

**19. Correct choice: B.**

In mucinous borderline tumors (MBTs), the lining cells are often stratified, generally to two or three layers, and exhibit nuclear atypia that is usually only mild or moderate. The presence of severely atypical lining cells warrants a diagnosis of MBT with intraepithelial carcinoma. In such cases, the carcinomatous cells usually (but not invariably) exhibit marked cellular stratification or stroma-free papillae or a cribriform pattern or combinations thereof. MBTs with intraepithelial carcinoma warrant more extensive sampling than usual to rule out foci of invasion. These tumors are almost invariably stage I and associated with a favorable prognosis, although rare tumors have recurred, especially if stage IC.

**20. Correct choice: E.**

The image shows a mucinous carcinoma with expansile invasion associated with a small focus of borderline tumor in the top left corner. Expansile invasion in mucinous carcinomas is characterized by a confluent growth of back-to-back or almost back-to-back glands or cysts lined by malignant epithelium, with a greatest linear dimension of greater than 5 mm. In some cases, the expansile pattern is intracystic. Mucinous carcinomas with expansile invasion are almost invariably stage I and recur in only about 5% of cases, a recurrence risk similar to that of intestinal mucinous borderline tumors (IMBTs) with intraepithelial carcinoma and/or microinvasive carcinoma.

**21. Correct choice: D.**

Mural nodules are occasionally found in mucinous tumors (benign, borderline, or malignant), which display a morphology entirely different from the main tumor. There are three types: (1) sarcoma-like mural nodules (shown in the picture), composed of pleomorphic mitotically active cells admixed with osteoclast-like or epulis-type giant cells. The osteoclastic cells stain for CD68. They are almost always multiple and well circumscribed. They appear to be reactive and have no influence on the prognosis of the underlying tumor. (2) Anaplastic carcinoma nodules, which consist of a poorly differentiated invasive epithelial neoplasm, composed of sheets of large, polygonal epithelial cells with high-grade nuclei and often abundant eosinophilic cytoplasm. They may be single or multiple and are usually poorly circumscribed. They are associated with poor prognosis. (3) Sarcomatous nodules, which may have features of fibrosarcoma, rhabdomyosarcoma, undifferentiated sarcoma, or giant cell sarcoma. They are associated with poor prognosis. Mucinous borderline tumors often contain small, circumscribed pools of extravasated mucin in the stroma, sometimes associated with a histiocytic and foreign body giant cell reaction, called mucin granuloma. Infiltrative invasion of mucinous carcinoma is diagnosed when there is irregular penetration of the stroma by often-misshapen glands, clusters, cords, or nests of cells, typically evoking a stromal response.

**22. Correct choice: A.**

Mural nodules are occasionally found in mucinous tumors (benign, borderline, or malignant), which display a morphology entirely different from the main tumor. There are three types: (1) sarcoma-like mural nodules (shown in the picture), composed of pleomorphic mitotically active cells admixed with osteoclast-like or epulis-type giant cells. The osteoclastic cells stain for CD68. They are almost always multiple and well circumscribed. They appear to be reactive and have no influence on the prognosis of the underlying tumor. (2) Anaplastic carcinoma nodules, which consist of a poorly differentiated invasive epithelial neoplasm, composed of sheets of large, polygonal epithelial cells with high-grade nuclei and often abundant eosinophilic cytoplasm. They may be single or multiple and are usually poorly circumscribed. They are associated with poor prognosis. (3) Sarcomatous nodules, which may have features of fibrosarcoma, rhabdomyosarcoma, undifferentiated sarcoma, or giant cell sarcoma. They are associated with poor prognosis. Mucinous borderline tumors often contain small, circumscribed pools of extravasated mucin in the stroma, sometimes associated with a histiocytic and foreign body giant cell reaction, called mucin granuloma. Infiltrative invasion of mucinous carcinoma is diagnosed when there is irregular penetration of the stroma by often-misshapen glands, clusters, cords, or nests of cells, typically evoking a stromal response.

**23. Correct choice: A.**

Seromucinous tumors, also known as endocervical-like or Müllerian-type mucinous tumors in the past, are now recognized as a separate category, distinct from the mucinous tumors with respect to clinical and pathologic features. The borderline category is the best characterized subtype. In the fifth edition of the World Health Organization (WHO) Classification of Female Genital Tract Tumours, the category of seromucinous carcinoma was eliminated; only a handful of such tumors have been reported, and based on the morphologic, immunohistochemical (IHC), and molecular findings, they are now considered to be endometrioid carcinomas.

**24. Correct choice: D.**

Seromucinous borderline tumor occurs in patients who are in the early reproductive age group (mean ages 35-39 years) and are associated with pelvic endometriosis in 30% to 50% of the cases, with some tumors arising within endometriotic cysts. They are synchronously or metachronously bilateral in 20% to 40% of cases. They tend to be smaller than their mucinous counterparts, being typically 8 to 10 cm in diameter, and are usually unilocular or contain three or fewer locules. Most tumors have grossly visible intracystic papillae like those in serous borderline tumors, which may be edematous, with the epithelial lining composed of columnar mucin-containing cells, as well as polygonal cells with abundant eosinophilic cytoplasm, which are usually located at the tips of papillae. The nuclei exhibit mild to focally severe atypia. A prominent acute inflammatory cell infiltrate in the stroma, within the neoplastic epithelium, and in the cyst lumina is found in most cases.

**25. Correct choice: C.**

Clear cell carcinoma, endometrioid carcinoma, mesonephric-like carcinoma, and seromucinous borderline tumors can all arise out of endometriosis and endometriotic cysts. There is no association of endometriosis with high-grade serous carcinoma.

**26. Correct choice: A.**

Endometrioid tumors are characterized by tubular glands variably resembling those of proliferative, secretory, hyperplastic, or adenocarcinomatous endometrium. An intimate association with endometriosis may be seen. Endometrioid adenofibromas with focal squamous differentiation are called endometrioid adenoacanthofibromas, which may have a reactive fibroblastic stromal proliferation that should not be interpreted as a desmoplastic response to invasion. In endometrioid borderline tumors, the glandular epithelium is severely atypical or has an appearance of low-grade carcinoma but is neither confluent nor does it irregularly infiltrate the stroma. Typical endometrioid adenocarcinomas are characterized by the presence of distinctive tubular glands lined by stratified, mucin-free epithelium.

**27. Correct choice: D.**

Endometrioid carcinoma represents up to 10% of ovarian tumors. Its histologic features are very similar to endometrial endometrioid adenocarcinoma: glandular structures with tall pseudostratified epithelial cells and centrally placed nuclei. Most of these tumors are probably derived from endometriosis or from benign or borderline adenofibromas, which themselves may be derived from endometriosis. Hyperestrogenic states appear to have a role in the malignant transformation of endometriosis. Up to one-third of ovarian endometrioid carcinomas are accompanied by endometrioid adenocarcinoma of the uterine corpus. In endometrioid borderline tumors, the glandular epithelium is severely atypical or has an appearance of low-grade carcinoma but is neither confluent nor does it irregularly infiltrate the stroma. Tubular glands of endometrioid carcinomas may mimic the tubules of Sertoli cell tumor or Call-Exner bodies of adult granulosa cell tumors.

**28. Correct choice: E.**

Basal vacuolization similar to that seen in the 16-day secretory endometrium is occasionally observed in ovarian endometrioid carcinomas (secretory carcinomas), as it is in a small percentage of uterine endometrioid adenocarcinomas. Abundant mucin secretion may be encountered in endometrioid carcinomas, but typically, the mucin is secreted from the surfaces of the cells or accumulates only in the uppermost portion of their cytoplasm. Rare, otherwise typical endometrioid adenocarcinomas contained a component of yolk sac tumor. Rare variants of endometrioid carcinoma encountered in the uterus may also be seen in the ovary, such as the corded and hyalinized variant, composed of cords of epithelial cells, spindled cells, and hyalinized stroma.

**29. Correct choice: E.**

Various approaches have been used to assess whether concurrent endometrioid carcinomas of the ovary and endometrium are independent primary tumors or the result of metastasis from one organ to the other, but genetic studies have conclusively demonstrated a clonal relationship between the ovarian and endometrial tumors in a large majority of cases. These molecular studies notwithstanding, the prognosis when the tumor is low grade and confined to the ovary and uterus, with no ovarian surface involvement or deep myometrial invasion/lymphovascular invasion is similar to that of carcinoma restricted to one or the other organ, that is, the behavior is equivalent to that of independent primary tumors.

**30. Correct choice: A.**

Clear cell carcinoma accounts for 5% to 10% of ovarian cancers and is the neoplasm found in association with endometriotic foci more often than any other ovarian tumor, including endometrioid carcinoma. Also, clear cell carcinoma gives rise to paraendocrine hypercalcemia more frequently than any other ovarian neoplasm, excluding small cell carcinoma of the hypercalcemic type. Thromboembolic complications are another significant association. Histologically, clear cell carcinoma is composed of clear cells lining tubules, papillae, or cystic spaces. Neoplastic cells have clear cytoplasm in most cases, but a hobnail appearance is frequent, which may be mistaken for high-grade serous carcinoma. Frequently, clear cell carcinoma contains a diffuse lymphoplasmacytic infiltrate that may mimic dysgerminoma.

**31. Correct choice: B.**

The typical benign Brenner tumor is composed of rounded to elongated, sharply demarcated, small nests of epithelial cells lying within an abundant fibromatous. The nests may be solid or have a central lumen that contains dense eosinophilic material or mucin. Most of the neoplastic cells are polygonal to ovoid and have pale cytoplasm and oval nuclei, some of which may have a central longitudinal groove. Borderline Brenner tumors are usually characterized by cysts into which the protrude papillae are lined by proliferating cells that are mainly of transitional cell type. The lining cells resemble those of papillary urothelial carcinoma of the urinary tract. No invasion of the stroma is evident, and a benign Brenner component is also definitionally present. Malignant Brenner tumors also contain a component of benign Brenner tumor as well as nests of urothelial cell carcinoma or, occasionally, squamous cell carcinoma (which is usually focal) that irregularly infiltrate the stromal component of the tumor. Borderline and malignant Brenner tumors are distinguished from metastatic urothelial carcinoma by the finding of benign Brenner nests or glands lined by mucinous epithelium in the former tumors. Squamous cell carcinomas of the ovary are rare and usually arise in dermoid cysts, less often from endometriosis, and rarely in Brenner tumors or mucinous borderline tumor of Müllerian/endocervical type.

# 56 Sex Cord-Stromal, Steroid Cell, and Germ Cell Tumors of the Ovary

1. A 30-year-old woman presents with abnormal uterine bleeding and abdominal pain. Imaging reveals a large 13-cm unilocular ovarian mass that seems to be mostly solid. Gross examination of the tumor following oophorectomy demonstrates solid lobulated yellow tissue. Figure 1 shows the histologic features of the tumor cells, which are immunopositive for inhibin and show loss of reticulin network around groups of neoplastic cells on reticulin special stain. Which of the following is the diagnosis?

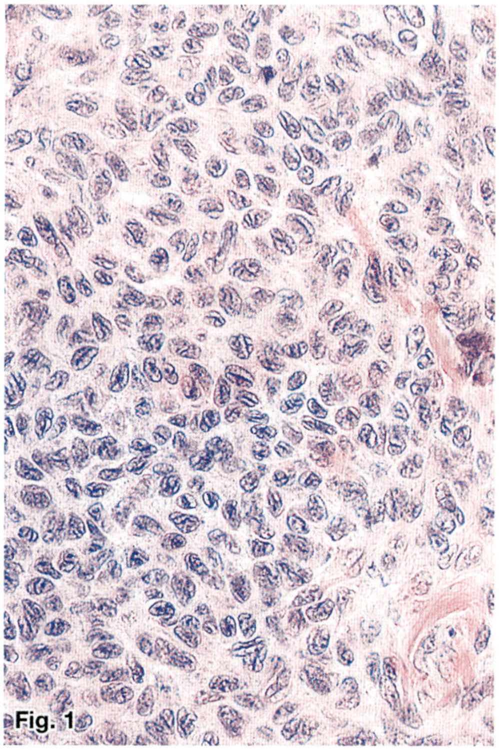

Fig. 1

A. Adult-type granulosa cell tumor
B. Fibroma
C. Juvenile-type granulosa cell tumor
D. Sertoli-Leydig cell tumor
E. Thecoma

2. Which of the following immunostains is positive in most cases of sex cord-stromal tumors?

A. Calretinin
B. Inhibin
C. Melan-A
D. Steroidogenic factor 1 (SF-1)
E. All of the above

3. An 8-year-old girl presents with precocious puberty, and a pelvic ultrasound reveals a right ovarian mass. The histologic appearance of the tumor is shown in Figure 1. What is the diagnosis?

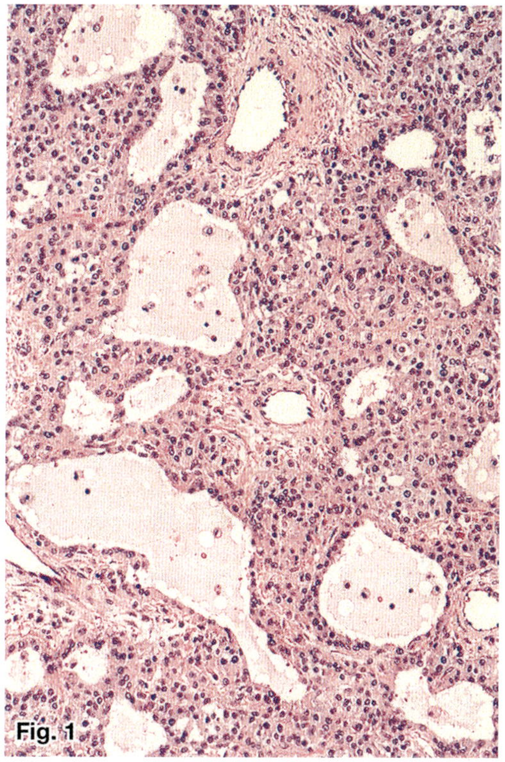

Fig. 1

A. Adult-type granulosa cell tumor
B. Clear cell carcinoma
C. Juvenile-type granulosa cell tumor
D. Sertoli-Leydig cell tumor
E. Thecoma

4. A syndrome characterized by a large (>10 cm) ovarian tumor, ascites, and right pleural effusion is typically associated with what?

A. Fibroma
B. Granulosa cell tumor
C. Leydig cell tumor
D. Sclerosing stromal tumor
E. Thecoma

All figures in this chapter are from Longacre TA, Greenson JK, Hornick JL, Reuter VE, eds. *Mills and Sternberg's Diagnostic Surgical Pathology*. 7th ed. Wolters Kluwer; 2022 except for those noted at the end of this book.

5. A 48-year-old woman presenting with abdominal pain is found to have a 6-cm unilateral solid ovarian mass. Histologic features of the tumor are shown in Figure 1, which are noted to displace follicles. Immunohistochemical workup reveals the tumor cells expressing steroidogenic factor (SF-1), calretinin, variably inhibin, smooth muscle actin (SMA), estrogen receptor (ER), and progesterone receptor (PR), with no expression of CD10. Reticulin special stain demonstrates pericellular accentuation of the reticulin fibrils. What is the most likely diagnosis?

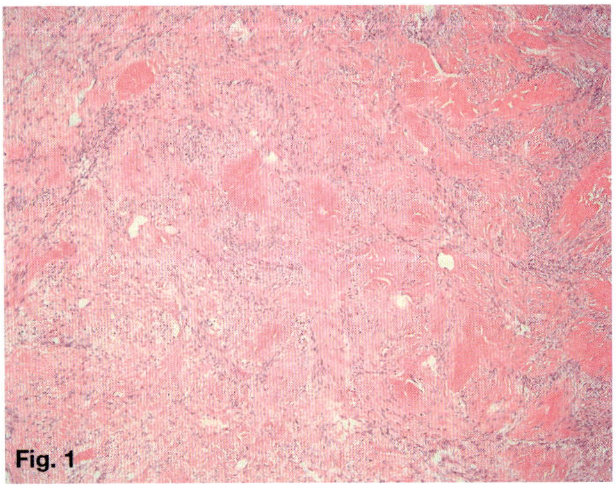
Fig. 1

A. Adult granulosa cell tumor
B. Fibroma
C. Fibromatosis
D. Leiomyoma
E. Ovarian endometrial stromal sarcoma

6. An ovarian tumor is found to have the histologic features shown in Figure 1, with diffuse minimal cytologic atypia and up to 10 mitoses per 10 HPF (high-power field). The neoplastic cells are immunopositive for steroidogenic factor 1 (SF-1), calretinin, inhibin, WT-1, estrogen receptor (ER), and progesterone receptor (PR), with no expression of smooth muscle actin (SMA) or desmin. These tumors are almost always benign, but cases have been known to rarely recur. What is the most likely diagnosis?

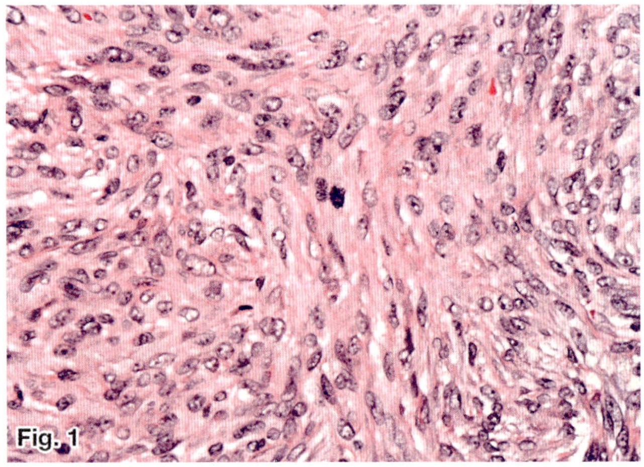
Fig. 1

A. Cellular fibroma
B. Fibrosarcoma
C. Gastrointestinal stromal tumor
D. Leiomyosarcoma
E. Mitotically active cellular fibroma

7. Figure 1 shows an ovarian neoplasm from a postmenopausal woman presenting with abnormal uterine bleeding. Which of the following immunohistochemical or special stains is most useful in differentiating this neoplasm from adult granulosa cell tumor?

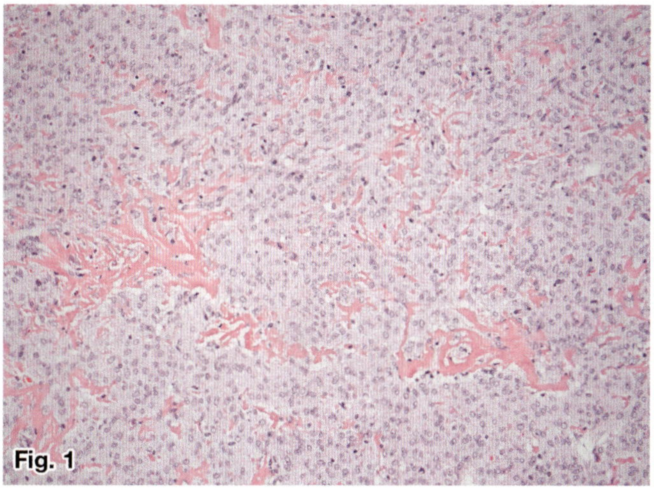
Fig. 1

A. FOXL2
B. Inhibin
C. Masson trichrome stain
D. Reticulin stain
E. Steroidogenic factor 1 (SF-1)

8. A 33-year-old female is found to have bowel obstruction and bilateral irregular ovarian lesions, upon presenting with abdominal pain and ascites. Figure 1 shows the gross findings of the ovary, with Figure 2 demonstrating the histologic features, with brisk mitotic activity noted. The spindled cells are immunopositive for desmin and estrogen receptor (ER), with no expression of inhibin or calretinin. The luteinized cells are diffusely positive for inhibin and calretinin. Gross examination reveals the bowel obstruction to be a result of omental septal involvement that produces a distinctive lobulated pattern. What is the most likely diagnosis?

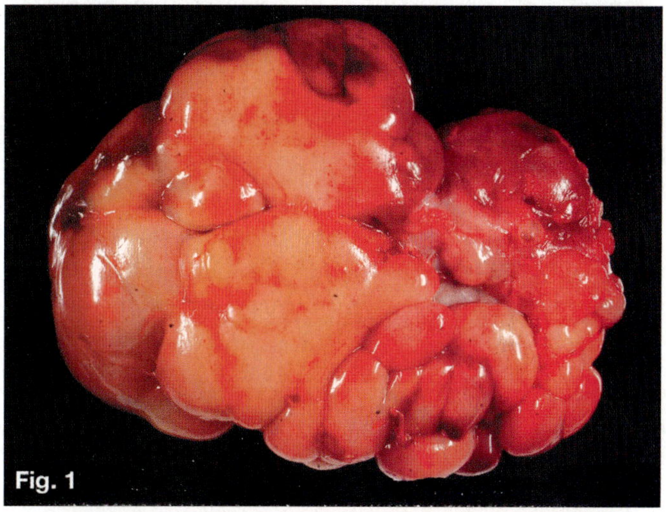
Fig. 1

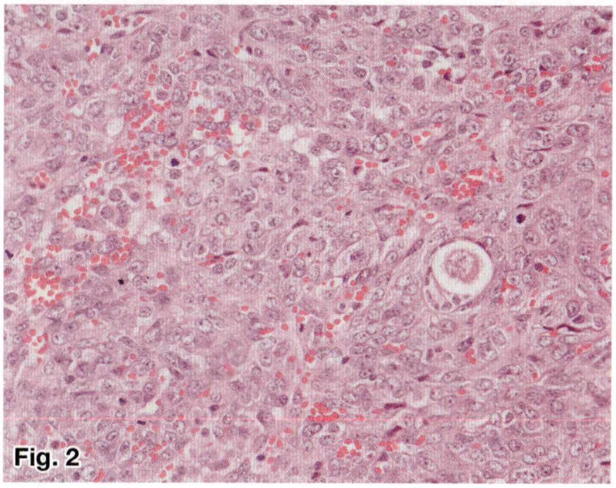
Fig. 2

A. Cellular fibroma
B. Fibromatosis
C. Luteinized thecoma associated with sclerosing peritonitis
D. Massive edema of the ovary
E. Sclerosing stromal tumor

9. A 24-year-old female presents with nonspecific abdominal pain. Imaging workup reveals a unilateral solid and cystic ovarian mass, measuring 6.5 cm. Gross examination of the oophorectomy specimen shows a predominantly solid ovarian mass with occasional cysts, with a white to yellow cut surface. Microscopic examination demonstrates ill-defined cellular pseudolobules containing distinctive network of thin-walled, often ectatic blood vessels, sometimes with a staghorn-like morphology, within and in between the nodules that are separated by connective tissue, as shown in Figure 1. Figure 2 highlights the two cell types that are intermingled within the nodules: spindle cells producing collagen and round to oval cells with small, dark nuclei, consistent with lutein cells. Immunohistochemical workup shows the tumor is positive for calretinin, estrogen receptor (ER), progesterone receptor (PR), and FOXL2, with weak inhibin expression. What is the most likely diagnosis?

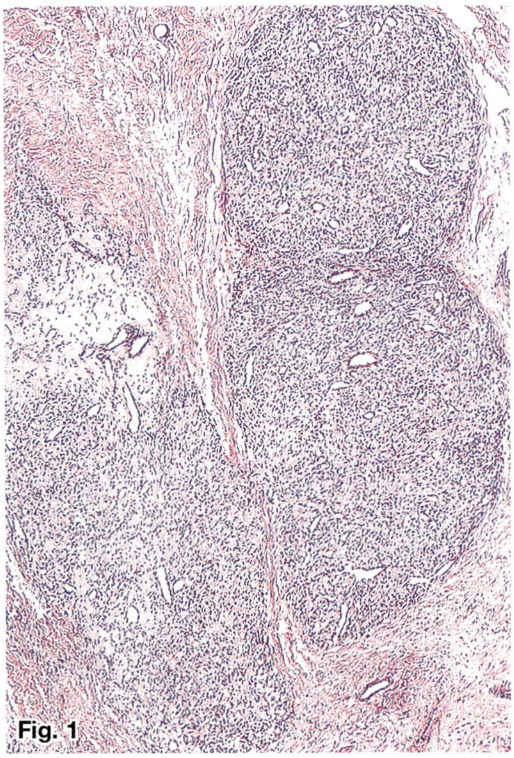
Fig. 1

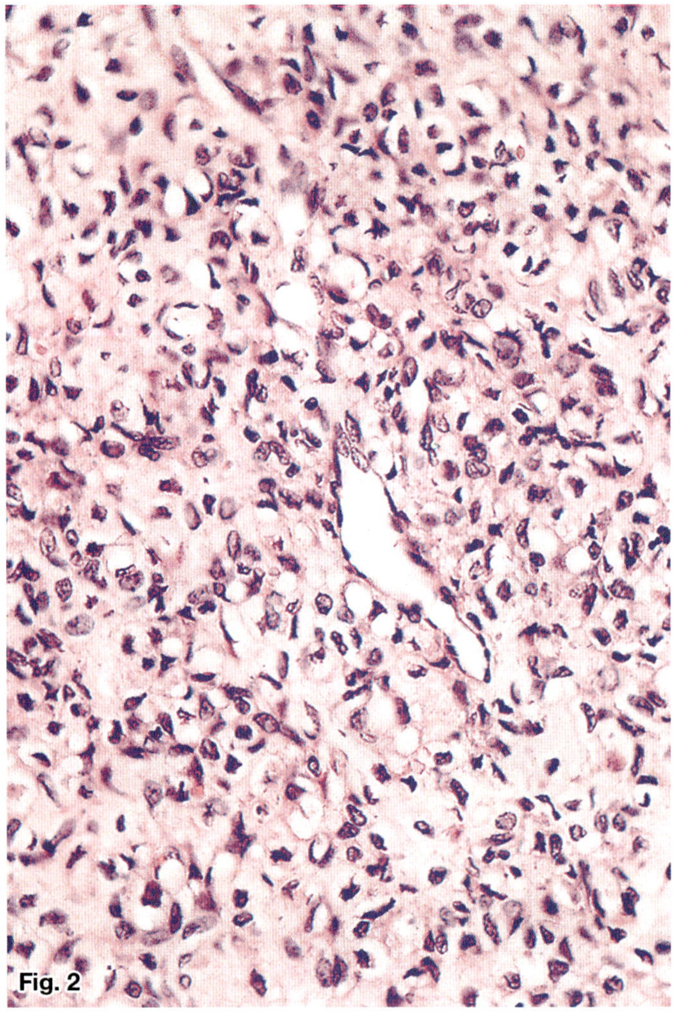
Fig. 2

A. Adult granulosa cell tumor
B. Krukenberg tumor
C. Luteinized thecoma associated with sclerosing peritonitis
D. Sclerosing stromal tumor
E. Signet-ring stromal tumor

10. A 25-year-old woman with menstrual irregularities undergoes resection of a unilateral 8-cm ovarian tumor, which has solid yellow cut surface on gross examination. The histologic appearance of the tumor is shown in Figure 1. Mitotic activity is low. Immunoreactivity for inhibin, calretinin, and steroidogenic factor 1 (SF-1) is seen throughout the tumor. These features are most consistent with the diagnosis of what?

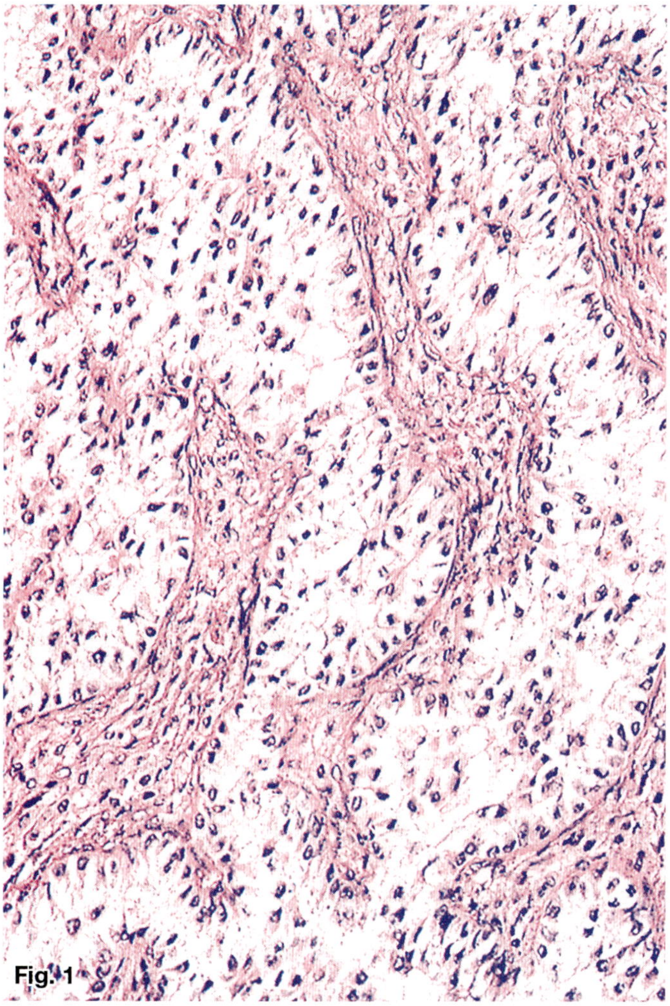

Fig. 1

A. Leydig cell tumor
B. Sclerosing stromal tumor
C. Sertoli cell tumor
D. Sertoli-Leydig cell tumor
E. Sex cord tumor with annular tubules (SCTATs)

11. The ovarian tumor shown in Figure 1 is most frequently associated with the production of which of the following?

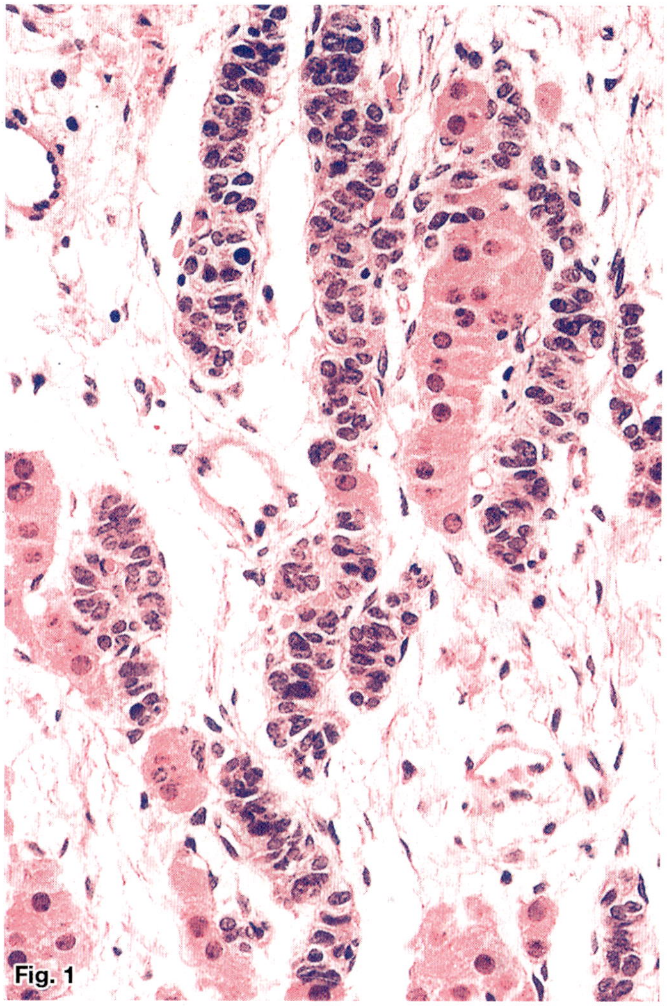

Fig. 1

A. α-Fetoprotein (AFP)
B. Androgens
C. Estrogens
D. Human chorionic gonadotropin (hCG)
E. Placental alkaline phosphatase (PLAP)

12. A 15-year-old adolescent girl is found to have an ovarian mass by imaging during the working up for generalized abdominal pain. She undergoes oophorectomy, and the gross examination reveals large edematous "vesicle-like" structures that protrude from the opened cystic mass. Histologic examination demonstrates a tumor with slit-like spaces and polyps within the cysts. The polyps have edematous stroma and budding papillae with a complex branching pattern and contain edematous to hyalinized cores, as shown in Figure 1. Which of the following is true regarding this entity?

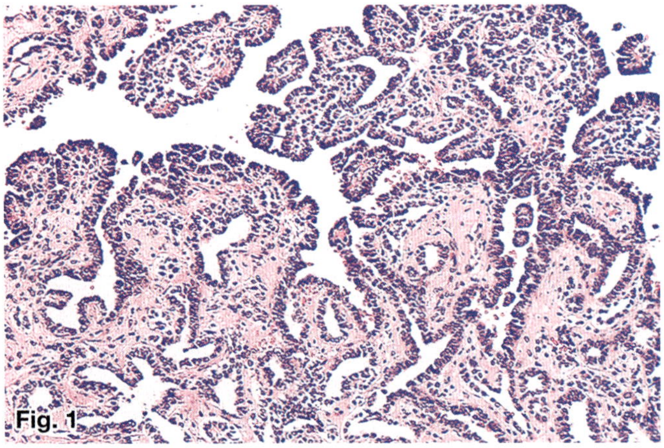


A. Histologic features simulate serous borderline tumors.
B. Pattern simulates those of the rete testis.
C. This is found in younger patients with other Sertoli-Leydig tumor cell subtypes.
D. This pattern is only present in intermediate- or poorly differentiated Sertoli-Leydig cell tumor.
E. All of the above are correct.

13. A 48-year-old woman with oral melanin pigmentation and abnormal uterine bleeding undergoes appendectomy for acute appendicitis. Intraoperatively, she is noted to have bilateral enlargement of her ovaries, with multifocal tumors noted with calcified areas. She undergoes bilateral oophorectomy, and microscopic examination reveals the tumor morphology depicted in Figure 1. Which of the following is true regarding the tumor in this particular patient?

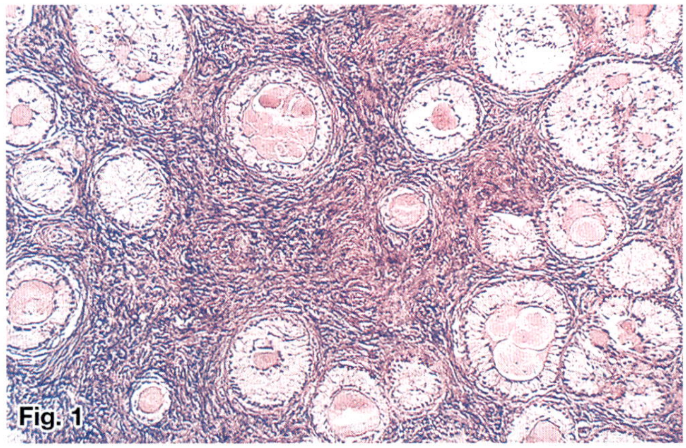


A. She most likely has *STK11* germline mutation.
B. The tumors in this patient may contain foci of typical germ cell tumors or solid tubular Sertoli cell tumor.
C. The tumors in this patient may show prominent cysts with cystic degeneration.
D. The tumors in this patient show cytologic atypia and increased mitotic activity.
E. The tumors pursue a malignant clinical course in 25% of patients.

14. Figure 1 demonstrates the most significant histopathologic findings in a unilateral 4-cm tumor located in the ovarian hilus of a 55-year-old female with clinical signs of virilization. Fibrinoid degeneration of large blood vessel walls is noted on microscopic examination. Which of the following is the most likely diagnosis?

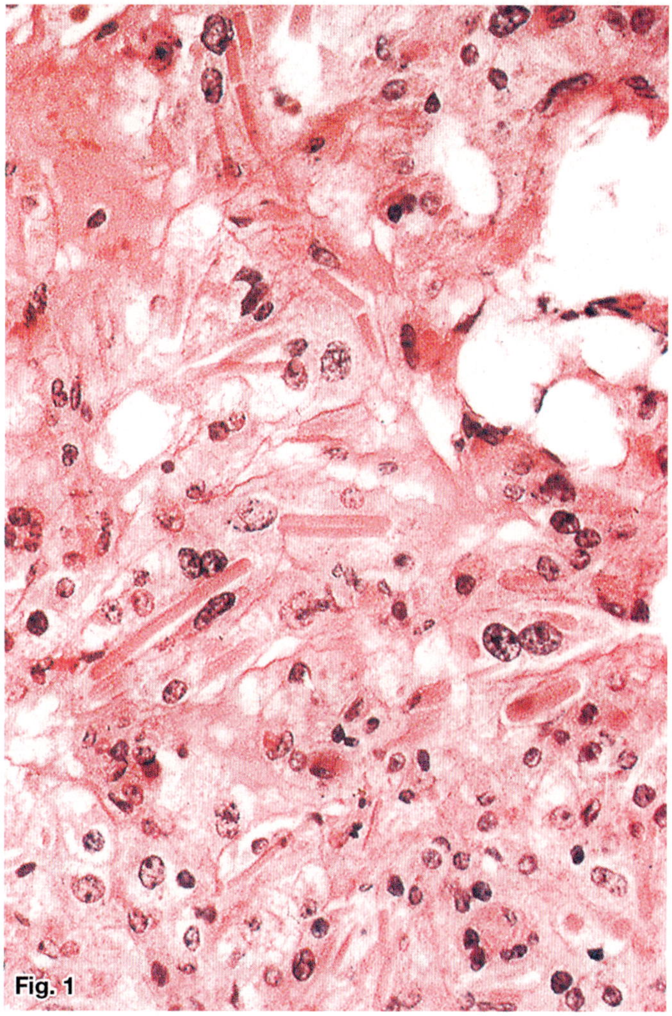

Fig. 1

A. Leydig cell tumor
B. Luteinized thecoma
C. Sertoli cell tumor
D. Steroid cell tumor, not otherwise specified (NOS)
E. Stromal luteoma

15. A 25-year-old woman is found to have a unilateral ovarian mass during a workup for persistent abdominal pain. Figure 1 demonstrates the histologic features seen in the majority of her tumor. In addition, scattered isolated foci of gland-like structures that are immunoreactive for α-fetoprotein (AFP) and keratin are also identified. This immunohistochemical pattern is evidence of differentiation toward which of the following?

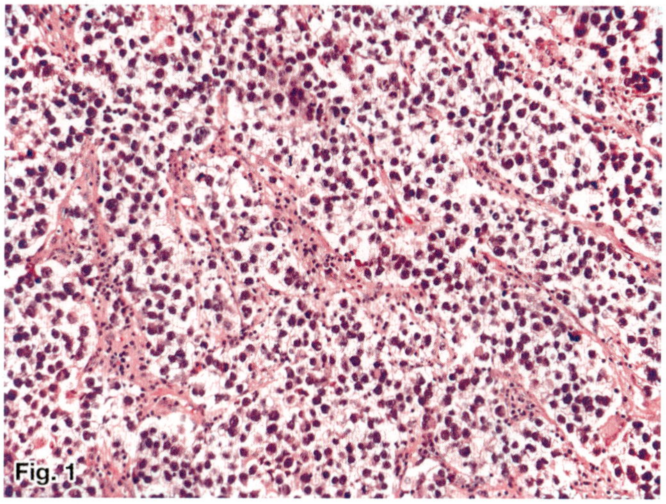

Fig. 1

A. Choriocarcinoma
B. Early carcinomatous differentiation
C. Embryonal carcinoma
D. Yolk sac tumor
E. None of the above

16. Which of the following is correct regarding ovarian dysgerminomas?

A. *C-kit* mutations appear to be associated with advanced stage at presentation.
B. Rarely, the tumors may have paraneoplastic hypercalcemia.
C. Rarely, the tumors produce human chorionic gonadotropin (hCG).
D. The tumor has a high sensitivity to chemotherapy and radiation therapy.
E. All of the above are correct.

17. An ovarian neoplasm composed of interlacing cords of cuboidal cells, pseudopapillary formations around a central vessel, as shown in Figure 1, and intra- and extracellular periodic acid-Schiff (PAS)-positive droplets will exhibit immunoreactivity for which of the following?

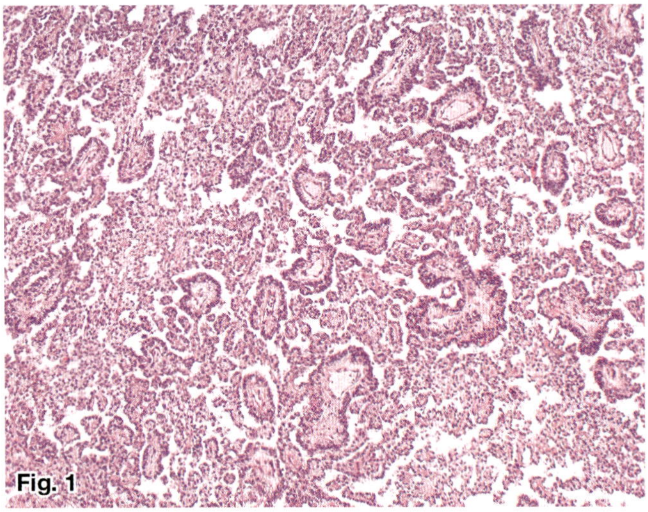

Fig. 1

A. α-Fetoprotein (AFP)
B. Human chorionic gonadotropin (hCG)
C. Human placental lactogen (hPL)
D. Placental alkaline phosphatase (PLAP)
E. Synaptophysin

18. Microscopic examination of multifocal peritoneal nodules in a 12-year-old girl shows the findings shown in Figure 1 with positive immunoreactivity with antibodies to glial fibrillary acidic protein (GFAP). Which of the following accounts for this condition?

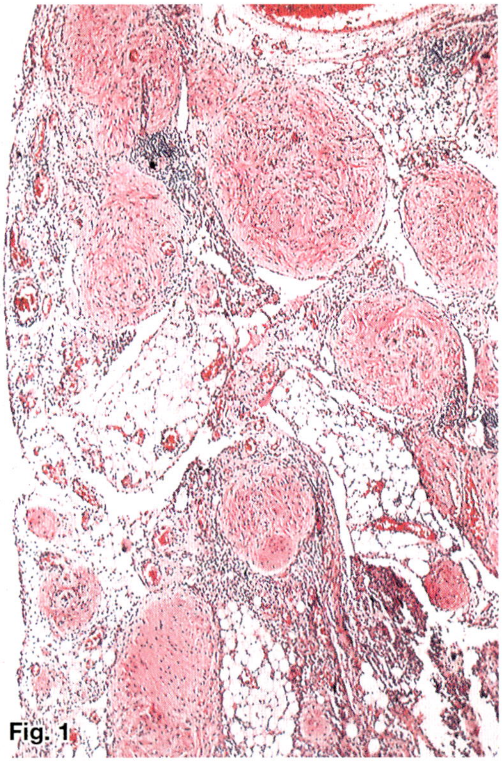

Fig. 1

A. Carcinoid tumor of the ovary
B. Development from autochthonous neural tissue
C. Ectopic neural tissue
D. Metastasis of glioblastoma multiforme
E. Ovarian teratoma

19. Which of the following is true regarding the tumor shown in Figure 1?

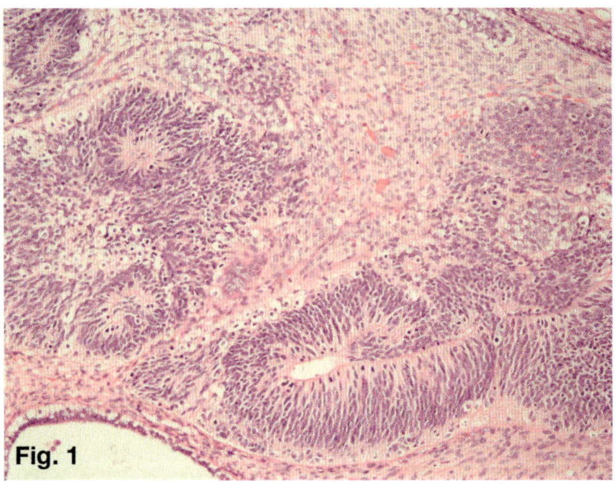

Fig. 1

A. Grade 1 tumors have rare foci of tissue, occupying less than one 40 times field in any slide.
B. Grade 2 tumors have moderate quantities of tissue, occupying two to three 40 times fields in any slide.
C. Grade 3 tumors contain large quantities of tissue, occupying four or more 40 times fields in any slide.
D. It is positive for SALL-4.
E. All of the above are correct.

20. A 55-year-old woman presents with complaints of skin flushing on her face and neck, as well as chronic diarrhea. She is found to have a large 10-cm unilateral ovarian mass. She undergoes oophorectomy and finds relief in her systemic symptoms soon thereafter. Figure 1 demonstrates the histologic features of her ovarian tumor. Immunohistochemical workup reveals CDX-2 expression in the tumor cells. What is the most likely diagnosis?

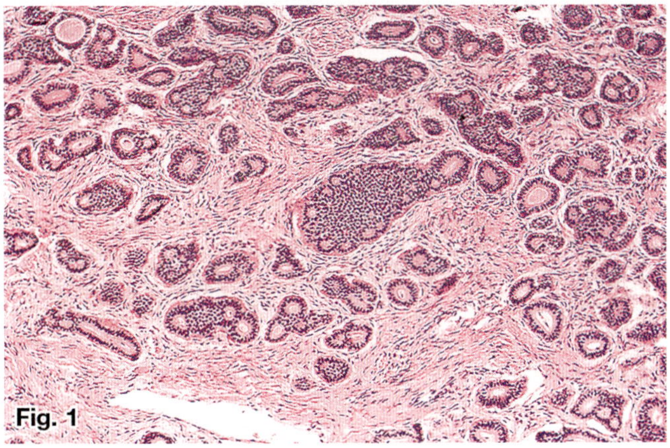


A. Adult granulosa cell tumor
B. Brenner tumor
C. Gastrointestinal carcinoid tumor
D. Ovarian carcinoid tumor
E. Sertoli-Leydig cell tumor

21. Which of the following is true regarding the ovarian tumor shown in Figure 1, which was discovered in a 35-year-old woman with nonspecific abdominal pain?

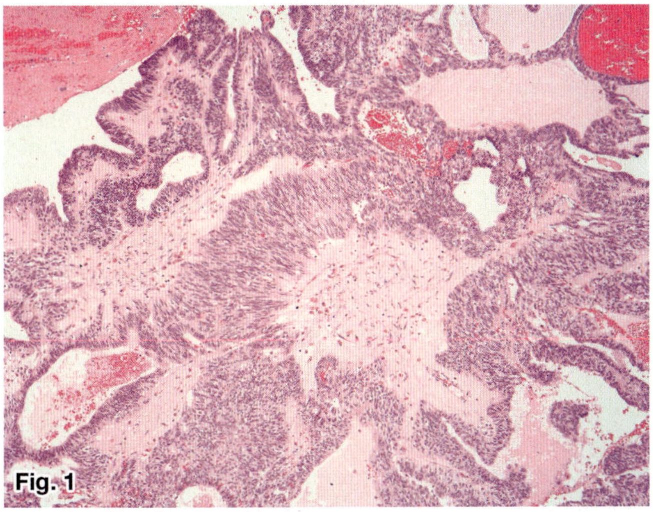


A. The tumor has a favorable prognosis even with extraovarian spread.
B. The tumor is immunoreactive for glial fibrillary acidic protein (GFAP).
C. The tumor is not usually associated with a background teratoma.
D. The tumor may express estrogen receptor (ER) and progesterone receptor (PR).
E. All of the above are correct.

22. An ovarian tumor that occurs predominantly in patients with gonadal dysgenesis is shown in Figure 1. What is the most likely diagnosis?

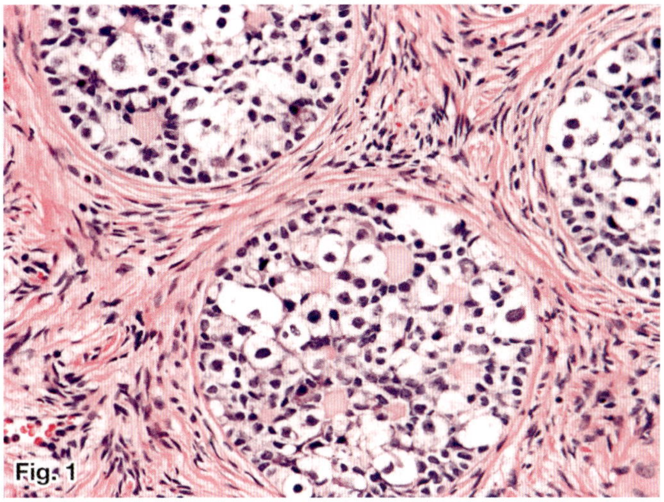


A. Gonadoblastoma
B. Immature teratoma
C. Sertoli-Leydig cell tumor
D. Sex cord tumor with annular tubules (SCTAT)
E. Steroid cell tumor

# ANSWERS AND EXPLANATIONS

**1. Correct choice: A.**

Granulosa cell tumors (GCTs) are divided into two types, juvenile (JGCT) and adult (AGCT). AGCT may have diffuse (the most common, shown in the picture), microfollicular, or macrofollicular patterns. The most typical architectural feature of AGCT, but found in a minority of cases, is the small follicle known as Call-Exner body. The grooved nucleus of tumor cells is the most typical cytologic feature. Approximately 75% of granulosa cell tumors secrete estrogens, thus giving rise to isosexual pseudoprecocity in prepubertal girls, and endometrial hyperplasia and/or uterine endometrioid adenocarcinoma. Almost all cases of AGCT harbor *FOXL2* mutations, which are absent in other sex cord tumors. Survival at 10 years is 90%. AGCT may recur decades after removal. The differential diagnosis is with cellular fibromas (no or weak positivity for inhibin) and thecoma (rich pericellular reticulin network).

**2. Correct choice: E.**

All sex cord-stromal tumors express inhibin. Inhibin expression is variable in fibromas and absent in fibrosarcoma, carcinomas (eg, small cell carcinoma of hypercalcemic type), and carcinoid. Up to 20% of adult granulosa cell tumor (AGCT) are inhibin negative. Calretinin is more sensitive but less specific for sex cord and steroid cell tumors. Epithelial membrane antigen (EMA) or CK7 should be used in the differential diagnosis of carcinomas. SF-1 (steroidogenic factor 1) is the most sensitive marker of sex cord-stromal tumors, being more frequently positive than inhibin and calretinin. Immunoreactivity for FOXL2 is also detected in AGCT but is also positive in other sex cord-stromal tumors. Other markers in AGCT and other sex cord-stromal tumors include melan-A, CD99, WT1, CD56, CD10, and CKAE1/AE3.

**3. Correct choice: C.**

In contrast to adult granulosa cell tumor (AGCT), juvenile granulosa cell tumor (JGCT) displays irregularly sized and shaped follicles, nuclei lack their characteristic grooves, and there are no Call-Exner bodies. Mitotic activity and nuclear atypia are more pronounced in JGCT compared to AGCT, with the neoplastic cells of JGCT showing nuclear immaturity. JGCT represents 5% of ovarian tumors in childhood/adolescence. Immunostains for inhibin and calretinin are usually not necessary; however, germ cell tumors (ie, yolk sac tumor) or melanoma need to be ruled out.

**4. Correct choice: A.**

The syndrome of large (>10 cm) ovarian fibroma, right pleural effusion, and ascites is known as Meigs syndrome. Meigs syndrome resolves once the ovarian neoplasm is excised. Ovarian fibromas are also part of basal cell nevus (Gorlin) syndrome and are almost always bilateral, multinodular, and calcified. Ovarian fibroma is the most frequent of sex cord-stromal tumors and develops most commonly in women of reproductive age without producing endocrine abnormalities. It is a benign tumor composed of well-differentiated fibroblasts arranged in densely packed fascicles with a storiform pattern. In contrast, thecoma produces estrogens and develops in women of postmenopausal age. Thecomas show a characteristic yellow cut surface owing to their rich steroid content. Histologically, thecomas consist of spindle-shaped cells with vacuolated cytoplasm that stains with oil red O special stain.

**5. Correct choice: B.**

Fibromas represent approximately 4% of all ovarian neoplasms and occur at an average age of 48 years. The main presenting symptom is abdominal pain, reported in approximately 40% of patients. Fibromas average 6 cm in diameter, with typically a uniform solid, firm, white appearance, but they may be soft and edematous. The classic appearance is that of spindle cells resembling fibroblasts associated with collagen and hyaline plaques, sometimes arranged in a storiform pattern. These tumors are more often positive for calretinin and steroidogenic factor (SF-1) than inhibin and are typically CD10 negative. They are also positive for estrogen receptor (ER) and progesterone receptor (PR) and can be positive for smooth muscle actin (SMA). The cellularity of endometrial stromal tumors equates with that of cellular fibromas and may show fibroblastic or fibromatous differentiation. Primary ovarian endometrioid stromal tumors are frequently associated with endometriosis. Endometrial stromal tumors are typically CD10 positive, in contrast to fibromas. Fibromatosis of the ovary may resemble a fibroma, but it envelops follicles and their derivatives in contrast to fibroma, which typically displaces them, and it is often bilateral. Fibromas can be distinguished from the uncommon smooth muscle of the ovary based on standard criteria used at other sites. Of note, when using immunohistochemistry, it is important to be aware that fibromas can be positive for SMA. Furthermore, fibromas and smooth muscle tumors share expression of ER, PR, WT1, and CD56.

**6. Correct choice: E.**

Cellular fibromas are densely cellular with closely packed nuclei and often associated with an increased mitotic rate, with an average of less than or equal to 3 mitoses per 10 HPFs (high-power fields; but higher than that of a typical fibroma). A higher mitotic index is still compatible with a diagnosis of mitotically active cellular fibroma, provided there is no appreciable cytologic atypia. Cellular and/or mitotically active fibromas are almost always benign, unless they are adherent to surrounding tissues or ruptured, but even in the absence of these features, they may rarely recur. Fibrosarcomas are typically large and fleshy and exhibit moderate to marked nuclear atypia and brisk mitotic activity. The absence of smooth muscle differentiation, supported by a lack of expression for smooth muscle actin (SMA) and desmin immunostains, lends no support for leiomyoma or leiomyosarcoma. Gastrointestinal stromal tumors (GISTs) may secondarily involve the ovary and grow in fascicles of fairly uniform spindle-shaped cells, but these tumors typically lack the storiform growth of some fibromas. GISTs are typically positive for c-kit and DOG1 and, frequently, CD34. Although some fibromas may be locally positive for CD34, they are negative for c-kit and DOG1.

**7. Correct choice: D.**

Thecomas are benign tumors consisting of large cells with ill-defined borders and pale cytoplasm, arranged in patternless sheets or nodules, with intermixed hyaline collagenous plaques or bands. The tumor secretes estrogens and most commonly affects postmenopausal women who present with abnormal uterine bleeding due to hyperestrinism. The main differential diagnosis is with adult granulosa cell tumor, which may contain significant thecomatous components. Immunohistochemistry is not useful because of the extensive overlap in immunoprofiles between the two neoplasms. Reticulin stain will demonstrate abundant, pericellular reticulin in thecomas, but not in adult granulosa cell tumor. Nuclear expression of FOXL2 is often seen in thecomas, even if they lack the gene mutation (which is present only in adult granulosa cell tumor).

**8. Correct choice: C.**

Luteinized thecoma associated with sclerosing peritonitis should be distinguished from various nonneoplastic lesions, including massive edema or fibromatosis, and neoplastic conditions, such as edematous/cellular fibroma or sclerosing stromal tumor. Fibromatosis and massive edema share with luteinized thecoma with sclerosing peritonitis frequent bilateral ovarian involvement as well as entrapment of follicles, but they lack the cellularity, microcystic change, as well as the brisk mitotic activity seen in the latter. Edematous/cellular fibroma and sclerosing stromal tumor are typically unilateral and lack other features, including the brisk mitotic activity usually seen in the luteinized thecomas.

**9. Correct choice: D.**

The heterogeneous gross and microscopic appearance of sclerosing stromal tumor contrasts with the relative homogeneity of fibromas and thecomas. Although fibromas may be edematous and vascular, edema is generally diffuse rather than focal, and pseudolobules and lutein cells are absent or rare. Hyaline plaques, a conspicuous feature of many fibromas and thecomas, are rare in sclerosing stromal tumors, whereas lutein cells typically appear degenerate, in contrast to their typical robust appearance in other stromal tumors. The vacuolated cells of a sclerosing stromal tumor may have eccentric, compressed nuclei and simulate signet-ring cells of a Krukenberg tumor; however, there are many clinical, gross, and microscopic features that help in this uncommon differential diagnosis. While sclerosing stromal tumor can show FOXL2 immunopositivity, they do not harbor a *FOXL2* mutation that is characteristic of adult granulosa cell tumor. Signet-ring stromal tumor lacks the characteristic pseudolobulation, lipid-rich cells, and prominent vascularity of a sclerosing stromal tumor.

**10. Correct choice: C.**

Sertoli cell tumor is a rare benign neoplasm with a peak age at presentation of 30 years. It may produce estrogens, especially in the lipid-rich variant (as in the image), manifesting with menstrual abnormalities or sexual precocity. The morphology is characterized by tightly packed hollow or solid tubules. Solid tubules are lined by cells with eosinophilic or pale cytoplasm. The prognosis is excellent in the vast majority of patients; the tumors are usually confined to the ovary at the time of diagnosis, but approximately 10% are associated with an adverse outcome. These tumors often harbor *DICER1* mutations. Sertoli-Leydig cell tumors are distinguished from Sertoli cell tumors by the finding of more than rare Leydig cells within the tumor. While histologic overlap exists with sclerosing stromal tumor when a lipid-rich variant is encountered, Sertoli cell tumors lack the characteristic pseudolobulation and prominent vascularity of a sclerosing stromal tumor.

**11. Correct choice: B.**

Sertoli-Leydig cell tumor (SLCT) is a rare neoplasm that affects young women and manifests in up to 50% of cases with signs of virilization, oligo-/amenorrhea, and loss of secondary sex characteristics. Occasionally, there are estrogenic manifestations. Cases without endocrine abnormalities present with nonspecific signs of an ovarian mass. Histologically, the tumor recapitulates various stages of testicular development and is classified into five subtypes (well differentiated, intermediate differentiated, poorly differentiated, retiform, and with heterologous elements). The one shown in the image is of intermediate differentiation and consists of cords of immature Sertoli cells intermixed with clusters of Leydig cells (larger, with eosinophilic cytoplasm). Patients with well- or intermediate-differentiated tumors have an excellent to good prognosis, whereas poorly differentiated tumors or those with heterologous mesenchymal elements (mostly rhabdomyosarcoma) are often associated with adverse outcomes. About 5% of SLCTs recur or metastasize. SLCTs may be part of the gynecologic manifestations associated with DICER1 syndrome occurring at a young age. Rarely, SLCTs tumors have been associated with elevated serum α-fetoprotein (AFP) levels but are generally lower than that seen with yolk sac tumors.

**12. Correct choice: E.**

Retiform patterns simulating those of the rete testis are found in approximately 10% of Sertoli-Leydig cell tumor (SLCT), but only approximately 10% of these tumors are purely retiform, and these patterns are only present in intermediate- or poorly differentiated tumors. Retiform SLCTs are seen typically in patients who are younger (average age 15 years) than patients with other subtypes of SLCTs and often differ grossly. The growth patterns include slit-like spaces, cysts sometimes containing polyps with edematous stroma, papillae containing edematous to hyalinized cores, or cellular papillae that bud and simulate those of serous neoplasms. The papillae may be simple or have a complex branching pattern with a lining of stratified atypical cells; glomeruloid structures are often present. The stroma varies from hyalinized (most common among sex cord-stromal tumors) to edematous to densely cellular; the first two types in association with the retiform areas being quite distinctive, and the third suggests carcinosarcoma. Somatic *DICER* hotspot mutations are commonly seen in intermediate- and poorly differentiated SLCTs, but not in their well-differentiated counterpart. There is no association between *DICER1* mutation status and the presence of heterologous or retiform differentiation in these tumors and/or different overall morphologic features.

**13. Correct choice: A.**

One-third of sex cord tumor with annular tubules (SCTATs) are associated with Peutz-Jeghers syndrome (PJS; gastrointestinal polyposis, oral and cutaneous melanin pigmentation, and, rarely, cervical gastric type adenocarcinoma) and are almost always benign. Patients with the PJS often display *STK11* germline mutations. In patients with PJS, the tumor has almost always been an incidental finding at operation or autopsy, whereas in patients without the syndrome, it is detected clinically and pursues a malignant course in approximately one-fourth of patients. Estrogenic manifestations are present in approximately 40% of patients, with or without PJS. The appearance differs depending on whether the patient has PJS. In patients with the syndrome, the tumors are typically bilateral, multifocal, calcified, and up to 3 cm in diameter. Tumors from patients without PJS are almost always unilateral and usually larger, solid, and yellow and are rarely calcified. Cysts are occasionally present and rarely predominate, with focal cystic degeneration seen in tumors not associated with the PJS. Cytologic atypia and mitotic activity are only increased in SCTAT unassociated with the PJS. In large tumors unassociated with PJS, foci of typical germ cell tumor or solid tubular Sertoli cell tumor or both may be present.

**14. Correct choice: A.**

Steroid cell tumors are rare ovarian neoplasms composed of cells resembling lutein, Leydig, or adrenocortical cells. When a steroid cell tumor contains crystals of Reinke (as in the image), it is, by definition, a Leydig cell tumor (LCT). LCT usually originates in the ovarian hilus and manifests with hirsutism or virilization in postmenopausal women. Stromal luteoma is another form of steroid cell tumor composed of luteinized cells and manifesting with hyperestrinism in 60% of cases, with virilization in 10%. When a steroid cell tumor lacks features characteristic of stromal luteoma or LCT, it is diagnosed as a steroid cell tumor, not otherwise specified (NOS). Currently, steroid cell tumors NOS constitute the majority of tumors in this category. They are often hormonally active, 50% androgenic, and 10% estrogenic.

**15. Correct choice: D.**

Ovarian dysgerminoma is analogous to testicular seminoma. The histology is, therefore, identical, characterized by an admixture of placental alkaline phosphatase (PLAP)-positive large cells with clear cytoplasm and prominent nucleoli, admixed with nonneoplastic lymphocytes. Often, dysgerminomas are admixed with yolk sac or choriocarcinomatous foci. Yolk sac components are positive for keratin and α-fetoprotein (AFP), and choriocarcinoma is immunoreactive for human chorionic gonadotropin (hCG). Positivity for keratin may be strongly enhanced in early carcinomatous differentiation (also referred to as anaplastic dysgerminoma). Ovarian dysgerminomas are often large tumors with a convoluted, cerebroid surface.

**16. Correct choice: E.**

Rare patients with dysgerminomas that produce human chorionic gonadotropin (hCG) may experience hormonal manifestations, typically estrogenic (isosexual precocity, menstrual irregularities) but occasionally androgenic, clinically mimicking an ectopic or intrauterine pregnancy or a hydatidiform mole. Rare patients may have paraneoplastic hypercalcemia secondary to tumoral synthesis of parathyroid hormone–related protein (PTHrP) or 1,25-dihydroxyvitamin D, which typically resolves after tumor resection. The presence of *c-kit* mutations appears to be associated with advanced stage at presentation. Because of the sensitivity of dysgerminomas to chemotherapy and radiation therapy, the 5-year survival rate for patients with higher stage or recurrent disease is currently greater than 80%.

**17. Correct choice: A.**

Ovarian yolk sac tumor develops usually in children/adolescents, as do all germ cell tumors of the ovary. The histologic appearance is comparable to testicular yolk sac tumor. Schiller-Duval bodies are pseudopapillary structures consisting of a central small vessel surrounded by a double layer of cuboidal cells, which contain intracytoplasmic and extracellular periodic acid-Schiff (PAS)-positive globules (shown in image). Cells with yolk sac differentiation express both α-fetoprotein (AFP) and keratin. This immunohistochemistry pattern is useful in identifying yolk sac elements in mixed germ cell tumors, the most common of which is dysgerminoma plus yolk sac tumor. Serum AFP level is almost always elevated preoperatively and can also be used to monitor recurrences and response to therapy.

**18. Correct choice: E.**

Ovarian teratoma is a neoplasm of germ cell origin consisting of tissues originating from the ectoderm, mesoderm, and endoderm. Typically, teratomas develop in children or adolescents. Mature teratomas consist of well-differentiated elements, whereas immature teratomas include atypical components with a propensity for metastatic spread. Tissue of neuroectodermal origin is the most frequent immature component and consists of sheets, rosettes, and tubules of poorly differentiated cells resembling a primitive neuroectodermal tumor. Other times, the neuroectodermal component consists of glial fibrillary acidic protein (GFAP)-positive glial tissue. Peritoneal spread is the most common path of dissemination. Gliomatosis peritonei refers to the presence of peritoneal implants of otherwise mature glial tissue spreading from a teratoma. Its presence does not affect prognosis. Dermoid cyst is the most common form of mature teratoma and consists of a cyst lined by keratinizing squamous epithelium and skin appendages. A monodermal teratoma is composed exclusively of a single tissue of endodermal or ectodermal origin, of which struma ovarii is the most common form.

**19. Correct choice: E.**

Immature teratoma is composed of immature, embryonic-type tissue that varies from small foci to large areas and is primarily of neuroectodermal elements. These elements consist of neuroepithelial rosettes and tubules or cellular mitotically active glia. The diagnosis of immature teratoma relies on histologic examination, but immature tissues including immature neuroectoderm are SALL-4 positive. Immature teratomas have been traditionally graded from 1 to 3 based on the amount of immature, almost always neural, tissue. Grade 1 tumors have rare foci of embryonal neural tissue occupying less than one low-power (40 times) field in any slide; grade 2 tumors contain moderate quantities of embryonal neural tissue, occupying greater than one but less than four low-power fields in any slide; and grade 3 tumors contain large quantities of embryonal neural tissue, occupying four or more low-power fields in any slide.

**20. Correct choice: D.**

Approximately one-third of ovarian insular carcinoids are accompanied by carcinoid syndrome, which disappears after the removal of the tumor. Patients with carcinoid syndrome are usually greater than 50 years and have tumors greater than 7 cm. Evidence favoring or establishing the diagnosis of metastasis includes definite or probable carcinoid in the gastrointestinal tract or elsewhere, extraovarian metastases, bilaterality, intraovarian multinodular growth, and persistence of the carcinoid syndrome or increased 5-hydroxyindoleacetic acid levels in the urine after removal of the ovarian tumor. Insular carcinoids may express CDX-2 expression, creating a pitfall to assigning the site of origin. In contrast to the acini of carcinoids, the Call-Exner bodies of adult granulosa cell tumors have irregular outlines and contain watery or hyaline material and often shrunken nuclei. Moreover, these cells typically have pale, grooved, haphazardly oriented nuclei instead of round, finely, and coarsely stippled nuclei of carcinoid tumors. The sex cords in Sertoli-Leydig cell tumors of intermediate differentiation are shorter, less uniform, and more sparsely distributed than the elongated ribbons of trabecular carcinoid. In contrast to carcinoid tumors, the cells of Brenner tumors have a distinct transitional appearance with grooved nuclei, and the most inner epithelial layer is often composed of mucinous cells.

**21. Correct choice: E.**

Ependymomas are usually not associated with a background teratoma and have a favorable prognosis even with extraovarian spread. These tumors are encountered most often during the second to fourth decades. The initial symptoms are usually nonspecific, but occasionally, there are hormonal manifestations as a result of secondary stromal luteinization. Ependymomas may be estrogen receptor (ER) and progesterone receptor (PR) positive, and in approximately 50% of cases, they express glial fibrillary acidic protein (GFAP).

**22. Correct choice: A.**

Gonadoblastoma, a rare tumor, is the most common ovarian neoplasm seen almost exclusively in patients with an underlying gonadal disorder, especially in association with gonadal dysgenesis. It may very rarely occur, however, in otherwise normal females as well. Histologically, discrete well-circumscribed oval nests with sex cord cells (which expresses steroidogenic factor 1 [SF-1]) at the periphery and germ cells punctuating their more central regions are seen, as well as acini containing basement membrane–like material. The germ cells are similar to those of dysgerminoma and seminoma in most tumors, usually exhibit mitotic activity, and are immunopositive for OCT3/4 and SALL-4. Gonadoblastoma can be confused with pure dysgerminoma (especially if dissecting variant) and sex cord tumor with annular tubules (SCTATs). Dysgerminoma or seminoma in a patient with maldeveloped gonads, and a Y chromosome should raise the question of its origin in a gonadoblastoma. SCTAT resembles gonadoblastoma in its growth pattern, basement membrane material, and calcification, but it lacks a germ cell component.

# 57 Miscellaneous Primary Tumors, Secondary Tumors, and Nonneoplastic Lesions of the Ovary

1. Which is the most common malignant mesenchymal tumor of the ovary?

   A. Endometrial stromal sarcoma
   B. Fibrosarcoma
   C. Leiomyosarcoma
   D. Osteosarcoma
   E. Rhabdomyosarcoma

2. A 65-year-old woman is found to have large bilateral ovarian masses during laparoscopy for imaging findings that were concerning for peritoneal carcinomatosis. The ovarian masses are found to be fleshy and gray to pink in color on gross examination. Figure 1 demonstrates the histologic features of her tumor masses. Diffuse infiltration of the adjacent fallopian tube and broad ligament are also noted. What is the most likely diagnosis?

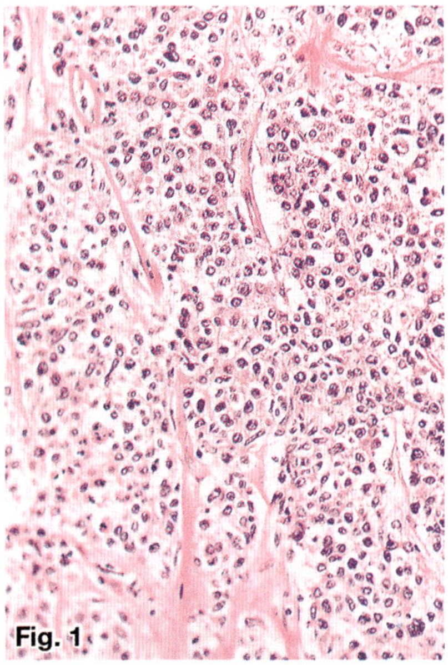

Fig. 1

   A. Dysgerminoma
   B. Extramedullary myeloid tumors
   C. Lymphoma
   D. Small cell carcinoma of the hypercalcemic type
   E. Undifferentiated carcinoma

3. A 22-year-old woman is found to be hypercalcemic. Clinical workup identified a large unilateral predominantly solid ovarian mass, with the histologic features shown in Figures 1 and 2. The tumor cells show immunopositivity to WT-1 (antibodies directed against the *N*-terminus only), cytokeratin, epithelial membrane antigen (EMA), calretinin, CD10, and p53, with loss of SMARCA4/BRG1 expression. This neoplasm is known to have a very poor prognosis. The tumor in this patient will have histopathologic features resembling which of the following?

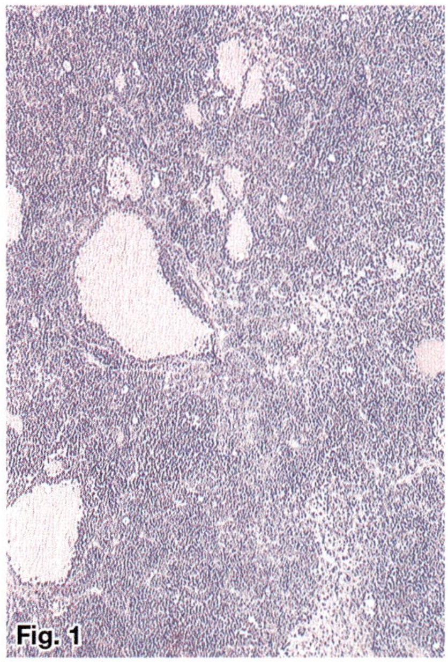

Fig. 1

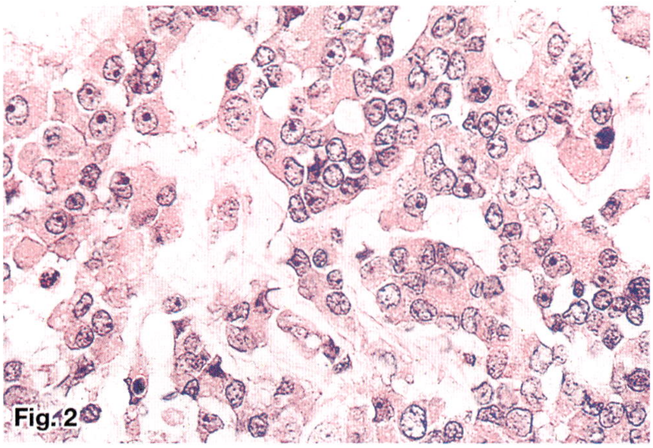

Fig. 2

   A. Brenner tumor
   B. Dysgerminoma
   C. Embryonal carcinoma
   D. Gonadoblastoma
   E. Small cell carcinoma, hypercalcemic type

All figures in this chapter are from Longacre TA, Greenson JK, Hornick JL, Reuter VE, eds. *Mills and Sternberg's Diagnostic Surgical Pathology*. 7th ed. Wolters Kluwer; 2022 except for those noted at the end of this book.

4. Which of the following macroscopic or microscopic features favors a primary ovarian neoplasm over metastasis?

   A. Expansile growth pattern
   B. Microscopic surface mucin
   C. Multinodular invasive growth
   D. Prominent vascular invasion
   E. Single-cell invasion

5. The ovaries of a 50-year-old patient show a multinodular appearance. Histologically, the lesions are composed of scattered single cells within a spindle cell stroma, as shown in Figure 1. Statistically, which of the following is the most likely origin of this tumor?

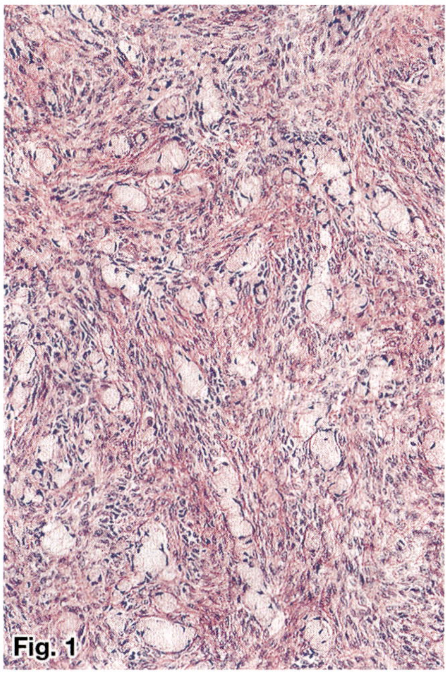

Fig. 1

   A. Appendix
   B. Breast
   C. Colon
   D. Ovary
   E. Stomach

6. Figure 1 shows a mucinous neoplasm identified in the ovary of a 50-year-old woman. Which of the following should the pathologist perform in order to be able to correctly diagnose this tumor?

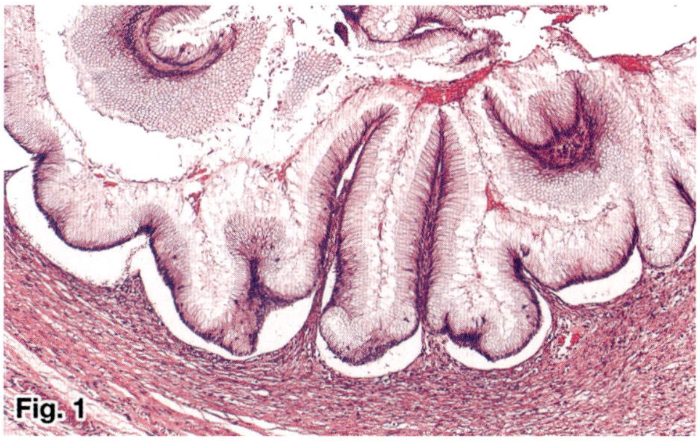

Fig. 1

   A. Advise surgeon at time of frozen section to perform an appendectomy.
   B. Carefully examine the ovary for a teratomatous component.
   C. Carefully examine the ovary for mucin granulomas.
   D. Carefully examine the ovary for pseudomyxoma ovarii.
   E. All of the above are correct.

7. A unilateral 10-cm ovarian mass is found to have the histologic features shown in Figure 1. Which of the following is in the differential diagnosis for this tumor?

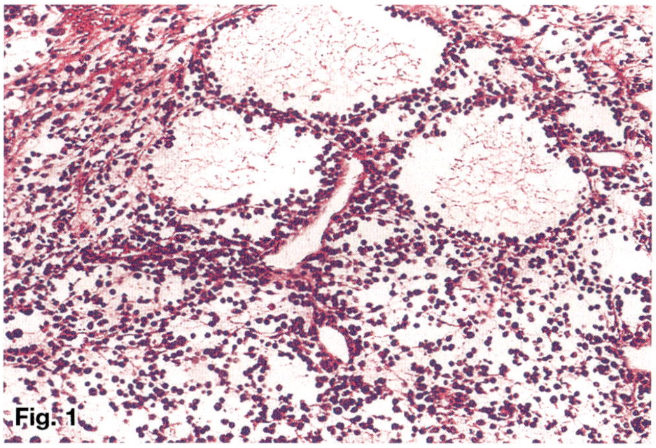

Fig. 1

   A. Juvenile granulosa cell tumor
   B. Metastatic melanoma
   C. Pregnancy luteoma
   D. Small cell carcinoma of the hypercalcemic type
   E. All of the above

8. Figure 1 demonstrates the histologic features of bilateral ovarian tumors found in a 45-year-old woman with endometriosis. Which of the following immunohistochemical stains will be the most helpful in confirming the diagnosis?

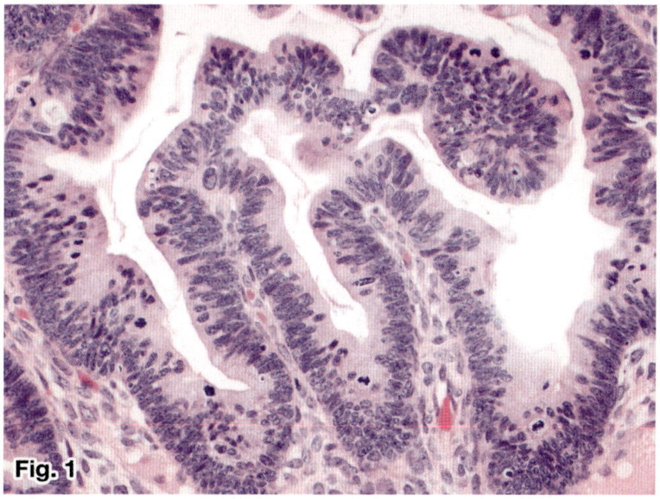

Fig. 1

   A. CK7
   B. CK20
   C. PAX-8
   D. p16
   E. SATB2

9. The majority of ovarian infections in the United States are secondary to what?

   A. Acute appendicitis
   B. Malakoplakia
   C. Pelvic inflammatory disease (PID)
   D. Pelvic tuberculosis
   E. Use of an intrauterine device (IUD)

10. Which of the following is correct regarding ovarian epithelial inclusion glands?

    A. Most are incidental microscopic findings.
    B. Most are lined by a single layer of columnar epithelium that may be ciliated.
    C. The glands arise from cortical invaginations of the surface epithelium.
    D. They measure up to 1 cm.
    E. All of the above.

11. Which of the following features is typically absent in ovaries associated with polycystic ovarian disease (Stein-Leventhal syndrome)?

    A. Corpora lutea and corpora albicantia
    B. Cystic follicles
    C. Follicle cysts
    D. Luteinization of theca interna
    E. Stromal hyperplasia/hyperthecosis

12. Examine these five gross images: Figure 1 to Figure 5. Match each of the diagnoses below with its corresponding image.

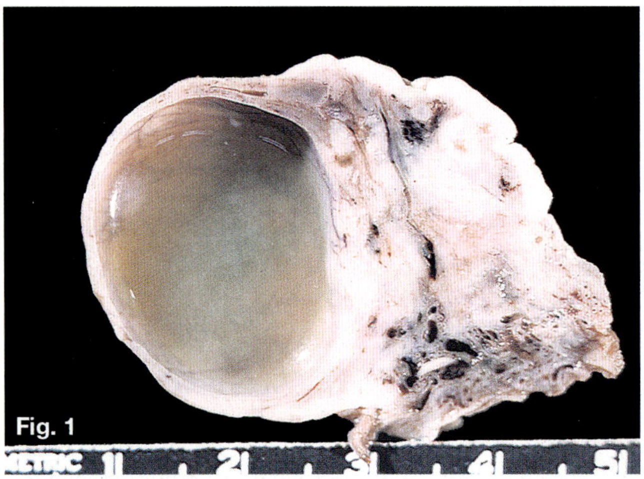

Fig. 1

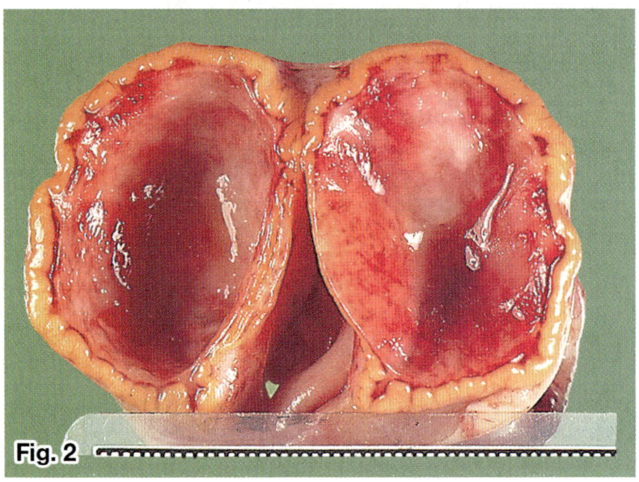

Fig. 2

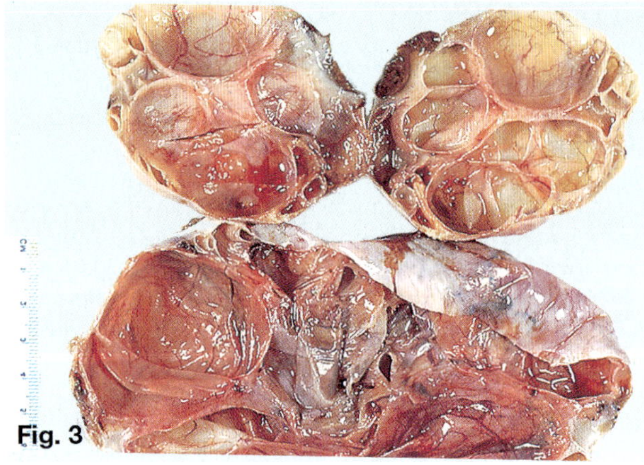

Fig. 3

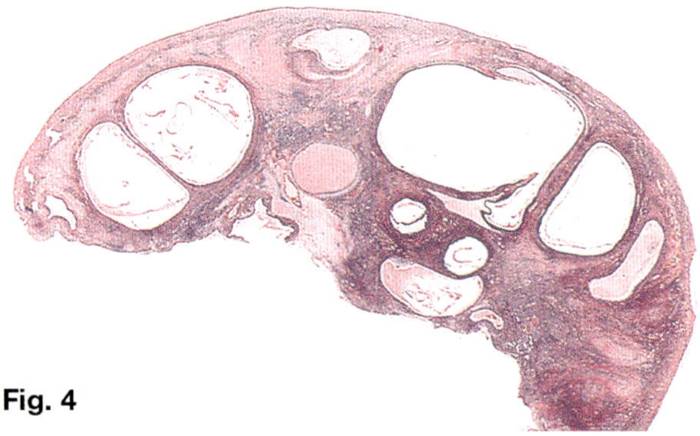

Fig. 4

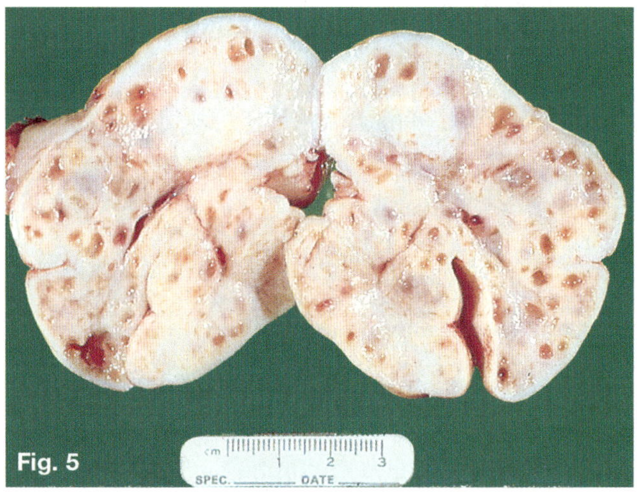

Fig. 5

    A. Corpus luteum
    B. Fibromatosis
    C. Follicle cyst
    D. Hyperreactio luteinalis
    E. Polycystic ovary syndrome

13. Which of the following is the pathologic substrate of an ovarian condition known as hyperreactio luteinalis?

    A. Bilateral luteinized follicle cysts
    B. Decidual reaction of ovarian stroma
    C. Massive ovarian edema
    D. Stromal hyperplasia and hyperthecosis
    E. Unilateral luteoma

# ANSWERS AND EXPLANATIONS

**1. Correct choice: B.**

Fibrosarcoma is the most frequent of ovarian sarcomas. Leiomyosarcoma and endometrioid stromal sarcoma account for the majority of the remainder, while all other types are very rare. Morphologically, ovarian sarcomas have morphologic features that are indistinguishable from analogous tumors occurring in other locations. Fibrosarcomas lie at the malignant end of a spectrum of stromal neoplasms, including fibroma, cellular fibroma, and mitotically active cellular fibroma. Ovarian fibrosarcomas usually present as large, fleshy tumors with significant nuclear atypia and high mitotic rate. Fibrosarcomas are negative for inhibin and CD10.

**2. Correct choice: C.**

Lymphoma in the ovary may be confused with several primary ovarian tumors. In such cases, it is helpful that diffuse infiltration of the adjacent fallopian tube and broad ligament is much more common in lymphomas than in most of the tumors in the differential diagnosis. Lymphomas may be indistinguishable on gross examination from dysgerminomas; however, they are bilateral in 50% of cases, in contrast to up to 10% of dysgerminomas. Although these tumors may resemble each other superficially on microscopic examination, the difference in their nuclei and immunohistochemical profile are helpful. The single-file arrangement of lymphoma and leukemic cells may simulate metastatic carcinoma, particularly one of breast origin. Diffuse lymphoma can resemble undifferentiated carcinoma, or small cell carcinoma of the hypercalcemic type on low magnification, but differences in immunoprofile will help identify tumors as lymphomas. Extramedullary myeloid tumors can be distinguished with immunopositivity for myeloperoxidase or chloroacetate esterase staining. The cells extramedullary myeloid tumors have more finely dispersed nuclear chromatin and may have more abundant cytoplasm, which may be deeply eosinophilic, compared to lymphoma cells with nuclei of the same size. Identification of eosinophilic myelocytes with confirmatory immunostaining may be crucial in making the diagnosis.

**3. Correct choice: E.**

Small cell carcinoma of hypercalcemic type is a rare tumor that has the usual features of small cell carcinomas, including evidence of neuroendocrine differentiation. The presence of scattered follicle-like microcysts may mimic the Call-Exner bodies of granulosa cell tumors. Hypercalcemia strongly favors a diagnosis of small cell carcinoma, and evidence of estrogen excess strongly favors a diagnosis of giant cell tumor (GCT). In addition, extraovarian spread is much more common for small cell carcinomas than GCTs. Immunohistochemical staining for inhibin supports a diagnosis of GCT. Dysgerminoma, which occurs in an age group similar to that of the small cell carcinoma and may be grossly identical to it, is also sometimes associated with hypercalcemia. Rare small cell carcinomas have cells with clear cytoplasm and fibrous stroma that may impart a very superficial resemblance to a dysgerminoma on low-power examination; however, the difference in immunoprofiles is most helpful. Small cell carcinomas can also be confused with lymphomas and the pulmonary form of small cell carcinoma. A variety of features of these three neoplasms, particularly their cytologic features, should distinguish them, and if necessary, immunohistochemical stains facilitate their distinction.

**4. Correct choice: A.**

Gross and microscopic patterns that favor metastases include bilateral involvement, multiple nodules, hilar location, prominent vascular invasion, single-cell infiltration, surface mucin, and signet-ring cells. Features favoring primary tumors include expansile growth, a complex papillary architecture, and large size (>10 cm). The following are the most common sources of ovarian metastases:

- Stomach: This organ is the most frequent source of Krukenberg tumors.
- Uterus-fallopian tubes: Ovarian involvement is around 40% at autopsy and 15% at surgery.
- Breast: One-third of patients develop ovarian metastases (particularly lobular carcinoma) during the course of the disease.
- Large bowel: 2% to 10% of patients develop ovarian metastases.

**5. Correct choice: E.**

The designation of Krukenberg tumor applies to the occurrence of bilateral nodular masses in the ovaries secondary to the metastatic spread of a signet-ring cell carcinoma. Neoplastic cells may be arranged in nests, glands, or tubules or distributed as single cells within a cellular stroma. Gastric carcinomas are the most common source, but Krukenberg tumors have been described in association with other intra-abdominal signet-ring cell cancers, including appendix, colon, and so on. The breast is the commonest primary site outside the gastrointestinal tract. Primary Krukenberg tumors are exceedingly rare.

**6. Correct choice: E.**

Although distinguishing metastatic low-grade appendiceal mucinous neoplasms (LAMNs) from primary ovarian mucinous cystadenomas and cystadenomas of borderline malignancy may be difficult, the former tumors are bilateral much more often, and they usually have a jellylike consistency on gross examination. Pseudomyxoma ovarii is frequently present, a finding that is much less common in primary ovarian mucinous tumors. Conversely, histiocytic aggregates ("mucin granulomas") are generally not seen in appendiceal metastases but are common in primary mucinous tumors. The difference in immunoprofiles using the panel of markers consisting of CK7, CK20, CDX2, and MUC2 has shown to be helpful. Rare cases of pseudomyxoma peritonei are associated with primary ovarian mucinous tumors arising in a background of teratoma. The morphology and immunoprofile is similar to LAMNs metastatic to the ovaries. Teratoma-associated mucinous neoplasms are typically unilateral, however, and accurate diagnosis of such cases requires a careful search for teratomatous components in the ovary and rigorous pathologic evaluation of the appendix.

**7. Correct choice: E.**

The image shows an example of metastatic melanoma to the ovary. Both ovaries are involved in approximately one-third of the cases. Tumors average 10 cm in size. Only a minority are black or brown in color. A confusing feature is the presence of follicle-like spaces in approximately 40% of tumors, which can lead to confusion with juvenile granulosa cell tumor or small cell carcinoma of the hypercalcemic type. Metastatic melanomas may closely resemble lipid-poor steroid cell tumors or even pregnancy luteomas, the latter of which, like melanomas, are often bilateral. Immunohistochemical staining is almost always helpful in confirming or excluding the diagnosis of malignant melanoma; S100, HMB45, and MART-1 will be positive in most melanomas.

**8. Correct choice: D.**

Cervical adenocarcinomas metastasize to the ovaries approximately 5 times as frequently as cervical squamous cell carcinomas. The risk of ovarian spread increases with the involvement of the outer third of the cervical wall, the parametrium, and/or lymph nodes. Most of the reported cases in this category have been adenocarcinomas of the usual type and have a picture that can mimic endometrioid carcinoma. The typical somewhat amphophilic cytoplasm and "floating mitoses" of usual endocervical adenocarcinoma are helpful, as is the absence of squamous metaplasia that is seen in many endometrioid carcinomas but is relatively rare in endocervical adenocarcinomas. Positivity for p16 suggests metastatic endocervical adenocarcinoma, confirming the underlying human papillomavirus (HPV)-driven process.

**9. Correct choice: C.**

Most cases of ovarian infection are due to the ascending spread of pelvic inflammatory disease (PID). With resolution of the infection, the only sequelae may be tubo-ovarian fibrous adhesions; occasionally, a healed abscess is converted into a tubo-ovarian cyst, which may mimic an ovarian cystic neoplasm at operation. Actinomycotic ovarian infections are rare and usually due to the use of intrauterine devices (IUDs). A unilateral or bilateral ovarian abscess without tubal involvement is much rarer than a tubo-ovarian abscess. The former is the result of direct or lymphatic spread from a nongynecologic pelvic inflammatory process (diverticulitis, appendicitis, inflammatory bowel disease, postoperative pelvic infection) or, uncommonly, of a blood-borne infection.

**10. Correct choice: E.**

Epithelial inclusion glands arise from cortical invaginations of the surface epithelium that have lost their connection with the surface. They can be seen in all age groups. These inclusions can measure up to 1 cm in diameter, and they may be visible grossly, but most are incidental microscopic findings in the form of multiple glands or cysts scattered either singly or in clusters throughout the superficial cortex; less commonly, they are found in the deeper cortical or medullary stroma. They may be accompanied by surface fibrous adhesions. The inclusion cysts are typically lined by a single layer of columnar epithelium that may be ciliated, but, less often, the lining is a single layer of endometrioid or, rarely, mucinous epithelium.

**11. Correct choice: A.**

Polycystic ovary syndrome (PCOS) is a condition that affects 10% to 20% of the female population. Key pathophysiologic elements are excessive ovarian production of androgens and insulin resistance. Such hormonal imbalances manifest with recurrent anovulatory cycles, oligo-/amenorrhea, infertility, hirsutism, acne, and obesity. The ovaries develop numerous follicle cysts, prominent luteinization of the theca interna, and stromal hyperplasia with variable hyperthecosis. Corpora lutea and corpora albicantia are absent. Unopposed hyperestrinism leads to endometrial hyperplasia.

**12. Correct choices: A 2; B 5; C 1; D 3; E 4.**

The images demonstrate the gross appearance of common ovarian cysts:

A. Corpus luteum cysts (Figure 2) are also common in women of reproductive age. They are unilocular and contain thick blood-tinged fluid. The wall is yellow and convoluted and consists of luteinized granulosa theca cells intermixed with theca cells and surrounded by a thick rim of fibrous tissue. They are usually asymptomatic.
B. Fibromatosis (Figure 5) manifests in young women (average 25 years of age) with menstrual irregularities and abdominal pain. This process is usually unilateral and consists of diffuse proliferation of fibrous tissue, resulting in enlarged ovaries (6-14 cm in diameter) with firm, white, solid cut surfaces containing scattered cystic follicles.
C. Follicle cysts (Figure 1) are very common in all ages and result from abnormal enlargement of a follicle due to abnormal gonadotropin stimulation. By definition, they are greater than 2 cm in diameter (if <2 cm, they are called cystic follicles). Grossly, follicle cysts are unilocular and thin walled and contain clear fluid. The wall is lined by an inner layer of granulosa cells and an outer layer of theca interna cells. Usually asymptomatic, they may rupture or present as a palpable mass.
D. Hyperreactio luteinalis (Figure 3) results in bilateral development of numerous luteinized follicle cysts so that both ovaries are transformed into large multicystic sacs. Microscopically, the cyst wall shows marked luteinization of the theca interna and granulosa cell layers.
E. Polycystic ovary syndrome (Figure 4) leads to numerous follicle cysts with prominent luteinization of the theca interna and stromal hyperplasia. Corpora lutea and corpora albicantia are absent.

**13. Correct choice: A.**

Hyperreactio luteinalis is a condition that usually occurs in association with disorders leading to high levels of human chorionic gonadotropin (hCG), such as gestational trophoblastic disease, multiple pregnancies, or fetal hydrops. It is characterized by bilateral multiple luteinized follicle cysts. It manifests with pain and/or a pelvic mass and may complicate with torsion or cyst rupture. Both ovarian decidual reaction and pregnancy luteoma develop during pregnancy, and both of them are probably related to abnormal endocrine influences. Massive ovarian edema is usually seen in young women and manifests with pelvic pain, a palpable mass, and menstrual irregularities. Stromal hyperplasia and hyperthecosis are common in perimenopausal women, but usually asymptomatic; in younger women, it may cause hypertension, virilization, glucose intolerance, and obesity.

# 58 Fallopian Tube and Broad Ligament

1. Which of the following are possible etiologies of granulomatous salpingitis?

   A. Crohn disease
   B. Foreign body
   C. Fungal infection
   D. Tuberculosis
   E. All of the above

2. A postmenopausal woman with a history of sterility undergoes hysterectomy with bilateral salpingo-oophorectomy for endometrial hyperplasia. Gross examination of the fallopian tubes reveals bilateral nodular enlargement of the isthmic segment. Microscopically, the enlarged segments consist of gland-like spaces of varying size and shape surrounded by a rim of thick smooth muscle as shown in Figure 1. Which of the following is the most likely diagnosis?

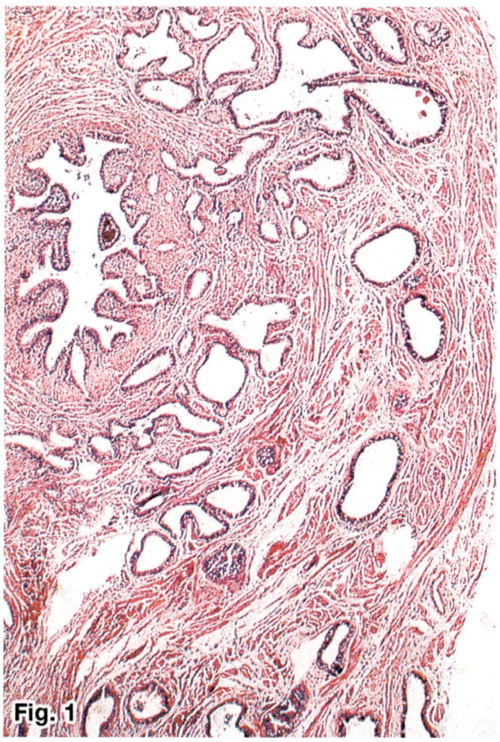


   A. Endometriosis
   B. Endosalpingiosis
   C. Salpingitis isthmica nodosa
   D. Tubal adenocarcinoma
   E. Usual-type tubal hyperplasia

3. Figure 1 shows the incidental finding in the salpingectomy specimen of a 48-year-old woman with a history of Peutz-Jeghers syndrome. Diagnostic consideration must be given to which of the following?

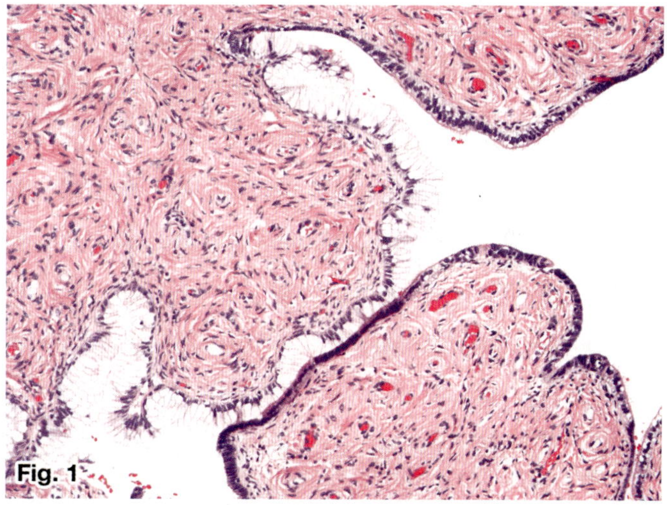


   A. Mucinous metaplasia
   B. Well-differentiated mucinous tumor from the appendix
   C. Well-differentiated mucinous tumor from the cervix
   D. Well-differentiated mucinous tumor from the ovary
   E. All of the above

All figures in this chapter are from Longacre TA, Greenson JK, Hornick JL, Reuter VE, eds. *Mills and Sternberg's Diagnostic Surgical Pathology*. 7th ed. Wolters Kluwer; 2022 except for those noted at the end of this book.

4. A 50-year-old female undergoes salpingectomy. Gross examination reveals a 1.8-cm well-circumscribed, firm, yellow mural nodule that projects from the tubal serosa. The histologic features of the lesion are shown in Figure 1. Cells range from flattened to cuboidal with abundant eosinophilic cytoplasm containing inconspicuous vacuoles. The lesional cells express WT-1, CK5/6, D2-40, and calretinin. What is the most likely diagnosis?

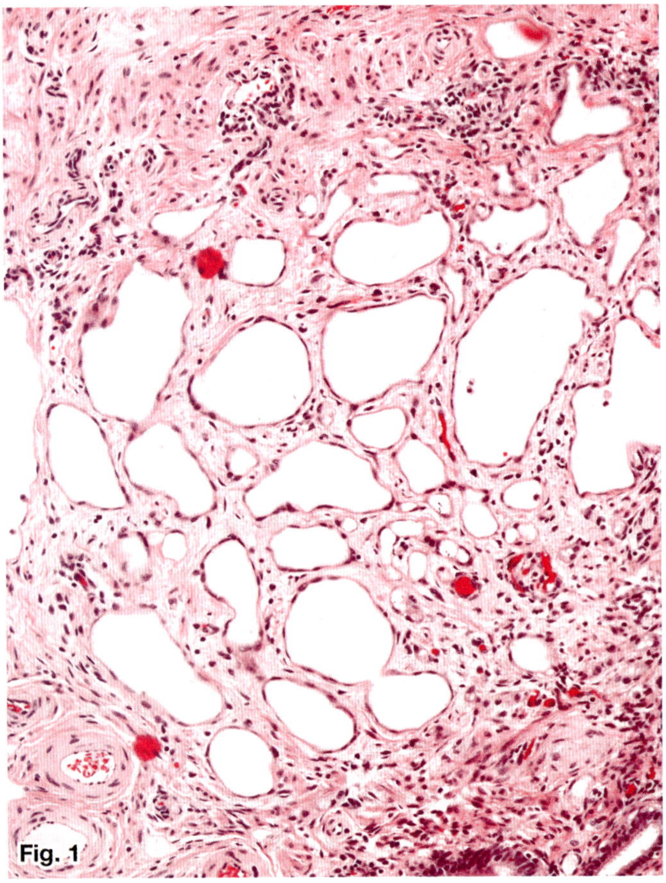
Fig. 1

A. Adenomatoid tumor
B. Hemangioma
C. Leiomyoma
D. Lymphangioma
E. Well-differentiated adenocarcinoma

5. Fallopian tube carcinoma is encountered with increased frequency in patients with which deleterious germline mutation?

A. *BRCA1*
B. *BRCA2*
C. *RAD51C*
D. *RAD51D*
E. All of the above

6. What is the most frequent morphologic type of fallopian tube adenocarcinoma?

A. Clear cell
B. Endometrioid
C. Mucinous
D. Serous
E. Undifferentiated

7. Carriers of *BRCA1* and *BRCA2* mutations have markedly increased risk of developing tubal carcinoma. Genetic counseling and risk-reducing bilateral salpingo-oophorectomy (RRSO) are recommended for women at increased risk of tubo-ovarian cancers. According to recommended protocols concerning pathologic examination of RRSO specimens, the segment of the fallopian tube that should be extensively sampled and examined is which of the following?

A. Ampulla
B. Broad ligament
C. Fimbriae
D. Intramural
E. Isthmus

8. What is the suggested Ki-67 proliferation index cutoff for the diagnosis of serous tubal intraepithelial carcinoma (STIC)?

A. 5%
B. 10%
C. 40%
D. 50%
E. 80%

9. A 75-year-old woman undergoes hysterectomy with bilateral salpingo-oophorectomy for uterine prolapse. One of the fallopian tube fimbriae harbors an incidental lesion with the histologic features shown in Figure 1. A p53 immunostain performed shows the expression pattern shown in Figure 2. Ki-67 proliferation index is shown in Figure 3. What is the most likely diagnosis?

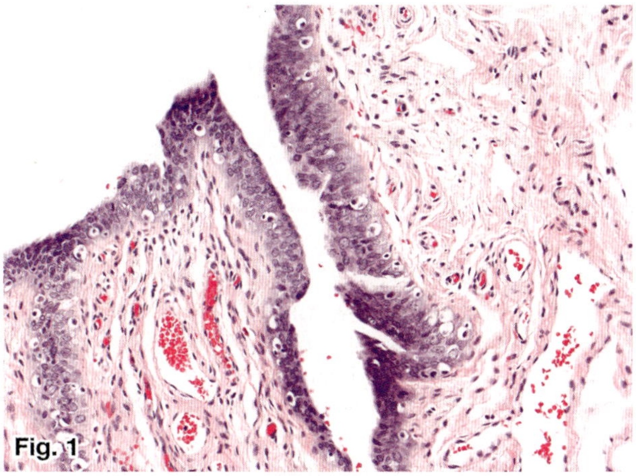
Fig. 1

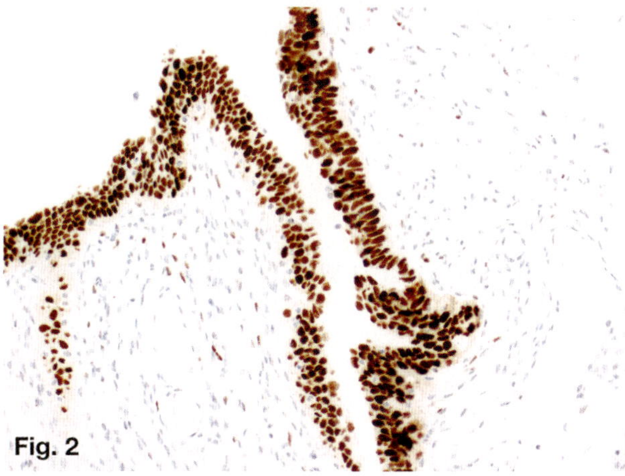
Fig. 2

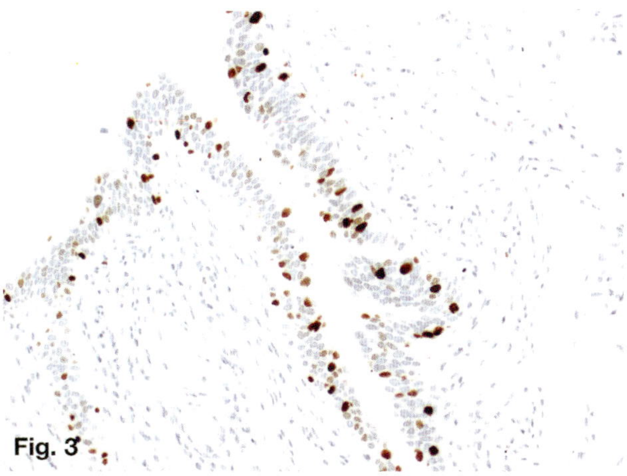
Fig. 3

A. High-grade serous carcinoma
B. Reactive tubal epithelium
C. Serous tubal intraepithelial carcinoma (STIC)
D. Serous tubal intraepithelial lesion (STIL)
E. Usual-type tubal hyperplasia

10. A 75-year-old woman undergoes hysterectomy with bilateral salpingo-oophorectomy for uterine prolapse. One of the fallopian tube fimbriae harbors an incidental lesion with the histologic features shown in Figure 1. A p53 immunostain performed shows the expression pattern shown in Figure 2. Ki-67 proliferation index is 5%. What is the most likely diagnosis?

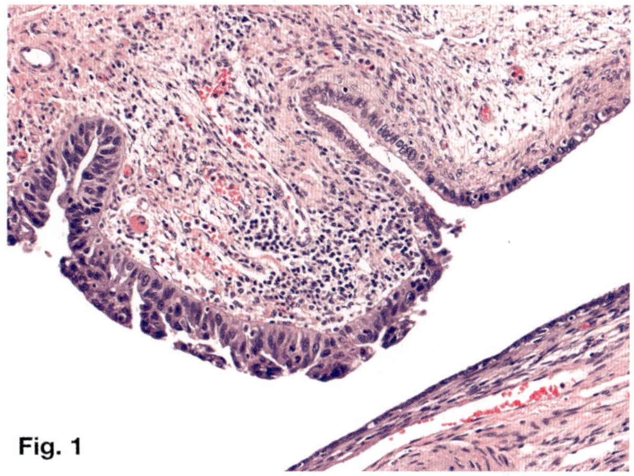
Fig. 1

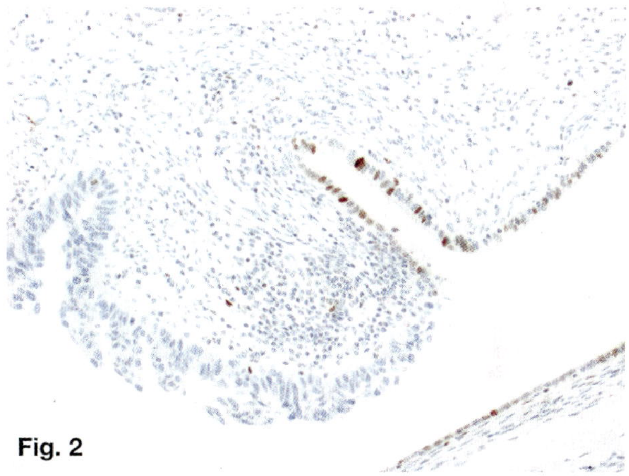
Fig. 2

A. High-grade serous carcinoma
B. Reactive tubal epithelium
C. Serous tubal intraepithelial carcinoma (STIC)
D. Serous tubal intraepithelial lesion (STIL)
E. Usual-type tubal hyperplasia

11. A 60-year-old woman with endometriosis undergoes hysterectomy with bilateral salpingo-oophorectomy for atypical endometrial hyperplasia. Noninvasive International Federation of Gynecology and Obstetrics (FIGO) grade 1 endometrioid adenocarcinoma is found in her uterus. An incidental lesion is seen in her fallopian tube, the histologic features of which are shown in Figure 1. Tubal endometriosis is noted. Which of the following features favor synchronous primary tumors of the fallopian tube and endometrium?

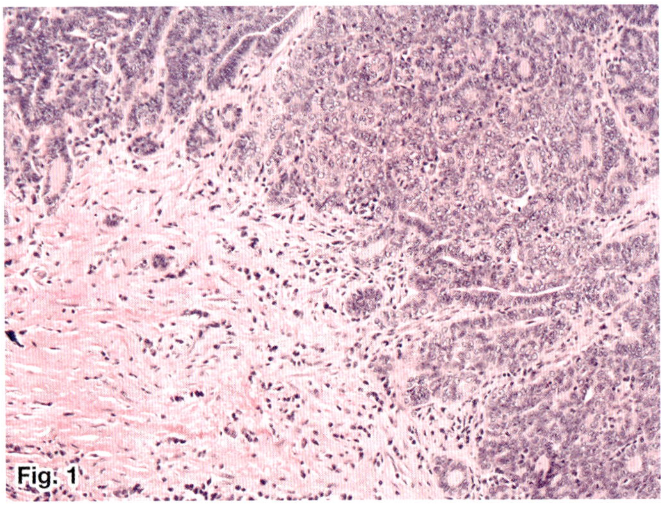
Fig. 1

A. Absence of tubal endometriosis
B. Lack of continuity among the tumors
C. Lymphovascular invasion in the uterine tumor
D. Morphologic similarity between the tumors
E. Outer half myometrial invasion in the uterine tumor

12. A unilateral tumor found in a 47-year-old woman localized to the broad ligament appears as a well-circumscribed, solid, bosselated mass with yellow-white cut surfaces. Its histologic appearance is shown in Figure 1. The lesional cells are immunopositive for pan-cytokeratin, Cam5.2, CK7, SF-1, GATA-3, and PAX-8. Which of the following is the most likely diagnosis?

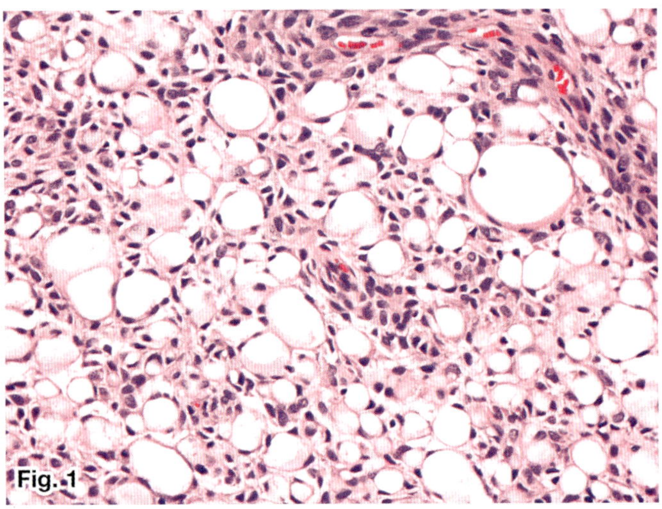
Fig. 1

A. Adenomatoid tumor
B. Endometrioid adenocarcinoma
C. Ependymoma
D. Female adnexal tumor of Wolffian origin (FATWO)
E. Sertoli cell tumor

13. A unilateral tumor found in a 47-year-old woman localized to the broad ligament appears as a well-circumscribed and lobulated mass with gray-tan, solid to cystic cut surfaces. Hemorrhage and necrosis are present. The histologic features are shown in Figure 1. The lesional cells are immunopositive for glial fibrillary acidic protein (GFAP), CD99, WT-1, S100, CAM5.2, and estrogen receptor (ER). Which of the following is the most likely diagnosis?

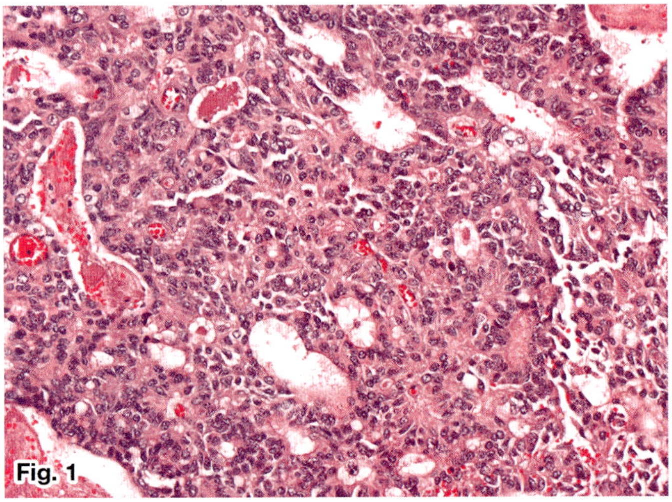
Fig. 1

A. Adenomatoid tumor
B. Endometrioid adenocarcinoma
C. Ependymoma
D. Female adnexal tumor of Wolffian origin (FATWO)
E. Sertoli cell tumor

# ANSWERS AND EXPLANATIONS

**1. Correct choice: E.**

The most common etiology of granulomatous salpingitis is *Mycobacterium tuberculosis* or *Mycobacterium bovis*. Genital tuberculosis is rarely due to primary infection of the genitalia and is more frequently secondary to hematogenous spread from other sites of disease, particularly primary pulmonary infection. The fallopian tube is the most common female genital tract organ affected by tuberculosis; approximately 90% of women with genital tuberculosis have tubal involvement. Fungi that may cause granulomatous salpingitis or tubo-ovarian abscesses include *Blastomyces dermatitidis*, *Coccidioides immitis*, *Candida glabrata*, and *Aspergillus*. Crohn disease of the lower gastrointestinal tract may secondarily involve the fallopian tube to produce a granulomatous salpingitis, tubo-ovarian abscess, or tubo-intestinal fistula. Granulomatous salpingitis may arise secondary to irritants, including surgical talc, suture material, lubricant, or mineral oil. Pulse granulomas can also occur in the fallopian tube.

**2. Correct choice: C.**

Salpingitis isthmica nodosa consists of diverticula of tubal epithelium involving the myosalpinx of the isthmus. It is usually associated with chronic salpingitis. It typically affects young women and may cause infertility and ectopic tubal pregnancy. Variably sized and shaped glands lined by a single layer of bland tubal epithelium are present within an often thickened, hyperplastic myosalpinx. Glands may be cystically dilated. In contrast to adenocarcinoma, the glands in salpingitis nodosa isthmica are regularly distributed and lack atypia. Endosalpingiosis refers to ectopic tubal epithelium found on the serosal surface of the fallopian tube, a process analogous to endometriosis. In tubal hyperplasia, the epithelium shows nuclear crowding and stratification, loss of polarity, tufting, and usually mild cytologic atypia.

**3. Correct choice: E.**

The tubal epithelium can undergo mucinous metaplasia characterized by endocervical-like cells. It may be associated with Peutz-Jeghers syndrome and mucinous tumors of the female genital (ovary, cervix) and gastrointestinal tracts (appendix). However, approximately 50% of cases of mucinous metaplasia of the fallopian tube occur incidentally in the absence of gynecologic or appendiceal neoplasia and are often accompanied by chronic inflammation and/or other metaplastic changes.

**4. Correct choice: A.**

Adenomatoid tumor is the most frequent benign tumor of the fallopian tube. It is usually asymptomatic and found incidentally. This tumor is of mesothelial origin, and the tumor cells express cytokeratin, vimentin, calretinin, D2-40, and WT-1, with no expression of endothelial markers, such as CD34 or ERG (ETS [E26 transformation-specific]-related gene). The differential diagnosis includes other benign lesions, such as lymphangioma and leiomyoma. Cytokeratin expression and the absence of endothelial markers distinguish adenomatoid tumors from vascular neoplasms. While adenomatoid tumors may mimic leiomyoma macroscopically and contain smooth muscle, the presence of characteristic gland-like spaces is lacking in smooth muscle neoplasms. Adenomatoid tumors may also be confused with cancers, including malignant mesothelioma and adenocarcinoma, especially of signet-ring cell type. However, gross tumor circumscription, bland cytologic features, and lack of mitotic activity facilitate the diagnosis of adenomatoid tumor.

**5. Correct choice: E.**

Fallopian tube carcinoma is now encountered with increased frequency in patients with deleterious germline mutations in *BRCA1*, *BRCA2*, and, less commonly, *BRIP1*, *RAD51C*, and *RAD51D* genes. Carriers of these mutations also have higher risk of developing breast, ovarian, and peritoneal carcinomas. The frequency of hereditary tubal carcinoma is currently unknown. However, germline mutations have been detected in 15% to 43% of patients with tubal carcinoma. The lifetime risk of developing tubal carcinoma is 0.6 in *BRCA* mutation carriers and 0.2 in the general population. Genetic counseling and risk-reducing salpingo-oophorectomy (RRSO) after completion of childbearing or by age 35 to 40 years have thus been recommended for women with *BRCA* germline mutations since the benefit diminishes with age. RRSO between 45 and 50 years of age may be considered in women with *BRIP1*, *RAD51C*, and *RAD51D* mutations.

**6. Correct choice: D.**

Over half of tubal carcinomas are serous carcinomas. Endometrioid carcinoma accounts for the second most common subtype type. Other histologic types are rare.

**7. Correct choice: C.**

Carriers of mutations of the *BRCA1* and *BRCA2* genes have higher risk of breast, ovarian, peritoneal, and tubal carcinomas. Germline mutations have been detected in up to 43% of patients with tubal carcinoma. The lifetime risk for tubal cancer is 0.2% in the general population and 6% in *BRCA1/2* mutation carriers. A risk-reducing bilateral salpingo-oophorectomy (RRSO) following completion of childbearing has been shown to reduce such risk to 0.04%. The so-called SEE-FIM protocol (protocol for Sectioning and Extensively Examining the FIMbriated end of the fallopian tube) consists of the following steps: (a) immediate fixation of the specimen in formalin to prevent loss of epithelium, (b) transection of the fimbriated end, (c) sectioning the fimbriated end at 2-mm intervals, and (d) transverse sectioning of the remaining segments of the fallopian tube and ovary at 2-mm intervals. Invasive or intraepithelial carcinoma is found in 2% to 10% of RRSO specimens from *BRCA1/2* mutation carriers by using this examination of the SEE-FIM protocol.

**8. Correct choice: B.**

The proliferation index, as measured by Ki-67, is typically high in serous tubal intraepithelial carcinoma (STIC), but it may be variable. A Ki-67 cutoff level of 10% in the lesional epithelium has been suggested. Reported mean Ki-67 proliferation indices of STIC range from 36% to 72%.

**9. Correct choice: C.**

Histologically, serous tubal intraepithelial carcinoma (STIC) is characterized by markedly atypical, nonciliated tubal epithelium without invasion of the underlying lamina propria. Cytologic abnormalities include nuclear enlargement and pleomorphism, high nuclear-to-cytoplasmic ratio, hyperchromasia or uneven chromatin pattern, prominent nucleoli, and nuclear stratification as shown in the image. Mitotic figures are usually present, and apoptotic bodies may be seen. It often occurs in the distal or fimbriated end of the fallopian tube and may originate at or near the tuboperitoneal junction. Any lesions that are unequivocal or suspicious for STIC histologically may be diagnosed as such in the setting of aberrant p53 (overexpression or null phenotype) and high Ki-67 proliferation index.

**10. Correct choice: D.**

An algorithmic approach to tubal epithelial lesions has been proposed to improve the diagnostic reproducibility of serous tubal intraepithelial carcinoma (STIC). Serous tubal intraepithelial lesion (STIL) may be considered in the setting of unequivocal or suspicious STIC morphology with abnormal p53 and low Ki-67 proliferation index. STIL is not currently diagnosed in the clinical and pathologic settings.

**11. Correct choice: B.**

Features that favor synchronous primary tumors of the fallopian tube and endometrium include the lack of continuity among neoplasms, morphologic distinction between tumors, and the presence of tubal endometriosis. Features favoring fallopian tube metastasis of a uterine primary include outer half myometrial invasion, lymphovascular invasion, and morphologic, immunophenotypic, and molecular similarities between the tumors.

**12. Correct choice: D.**

Female adnexal tumor of Wolffian origin (FATWO) is usually localized in the broad ligament, occurs at a mean age of 47 years, and may manifest with abdominal pain and swelling. Microscopically, it consists of cells arranged in solid sheets or in a characteristic sievelike pattern. The cells are typically bland, cuboidal to columnar to flattened, and occasionally spindled or fusiform with scant eosinophilic cytoplasm. Nuclei are usually small, round to oval, and pale. Mitotic figures are few, if present. Occasional tumors may demonstrate foci of markedly atypical cells with increased mitotic activity. Focally prominent fibrous or hyalinized stroma may be present. Most cases are benign, but malignant forms occur.

**13. Correct choice: C.**

Extra-axial ependymomas have been reported in the broad ligament and uterosacral ligament. They have been reported in patients aged 13 to 48 years and range in size from 1 to 14 cm. Grossly, tumors are well circumscribed and lobulated with gray-tan, solid to cystic cut surfaces. Hemorrhage and necrosis may be present. Compared to their central nervous system counterparts, extra-axial ependymomas tend to exhibit greater variation in architectural patterns, including perivascular pseudorosettes and, occasionally, true ependymal rosettes, along with papillary, pseudopapillary, tubuloglandular, cystic, solid, trabecular, cribriform, and myxopapillary areas. They diffusely express glial fibrillary acidic protein (GFAP), with preferential expression CK18, 34βE12, CAM5.2, CK7, estrogen receptor (ER), and progesterone receptor (PR), and, less frequently, demonstrate CD99 and S100 protein positivity. WT-1 expression is found in 50% of tumors. Extraneural ependymomas are indolent tumors that may recur after many years but rarely cause death.

# 59 Peritoneum

1. Scattered white miliary-like nodules are found in the visceral peritoneum during an exploratory laparotomy in a patient who underwent a previous abdominal surgery. On microscopic examination, the nodules consist of granulomas with periodic acid-Schiff (PAS)-positive birefringent granules within histiocytes and giant cells. These granules display a Maltese cross pattern under polarized light. What is this material?

   A. Barium
   B. Cellulose
   C. Paraffin
   D. Starch
   E. Talc

2. Which of the following may cause florid granulomatous peritonitis?

   A. Keratin exfoliated from endometrioid carcinoma with squamous differentiation
   B. Leakage of amniotic fluid
   C. Ruptured diverticulitis
   D. Spillage of bile
   E. All of the above

3. A 14-year-old adolescent presents with bowel obstruction. Intraoperative findings include an abdominal cocoon. Histologic features of the lesion are shown in Figure 1. Which of the following are possible causes of the secondary form of this rare, potentially fatal disorder?

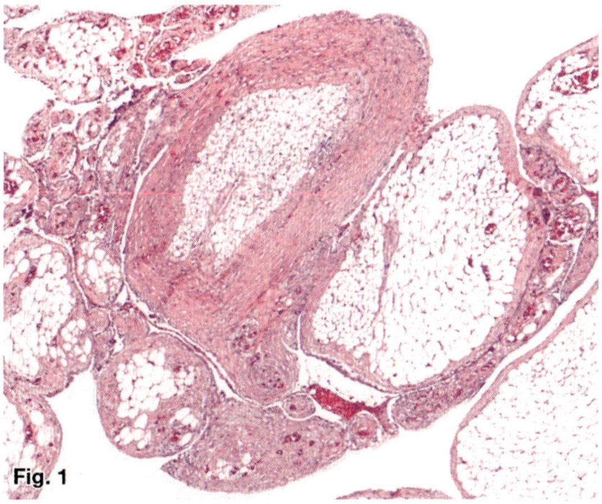

Fig. 1

   A. Lupus erythematosus
   B. Ovarian fibrothecomatous tumors
   C. Practolol therapy
   D. Sarcoidosis
   E. All of the above

4. The major differential diagnosis of mesothelial hyperplasia is peritoneal mesothelioma. The presence of which of the following favors the malignant process?

   A. Grossly visible nodules
   B. Necrosis
   C. Severe nuclear pleomorphism
   D. Tissue invasion
   E. All of the above

5. A 40-year-old woman with a history of pelvic inflammatory disease presents with lower abdominal pain. Pelvic ultrasound reveals a multicystic lesion, which is surgically excised. The gross appearance of the surgical specimen is shown in Figure 1. Pathologic examination reveals a multiloculated cystic mass consisting of thin-walled cysts lined by flattened mesothelial cells. What is the most likely of the pathogenesis of this lesion?

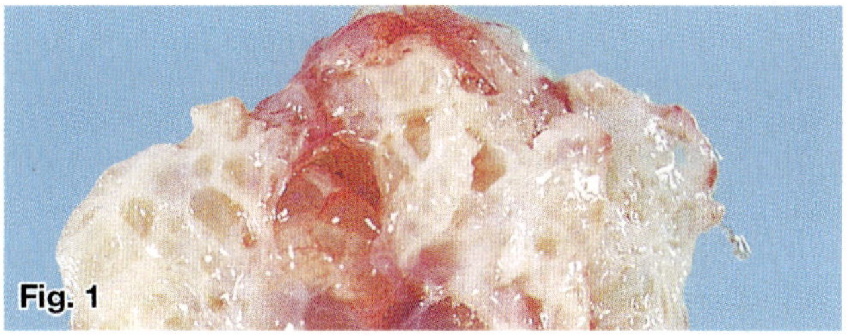

Fig. 1

   A. Asbestos related
   B. Iatrogenic
   C. Inflammatory
   D. Malformative
   E. Neoplastic

All figures in this chapter are from Longacre TA, Greenson JK, Hornick JL, Reuter VE, eds. *Mills and Sternberg's Diagnostic Surgical Pathology*. 7th ed. Wolters Kluwer; 2022 except for those noted at the end of this book.

6. During an exploratory laparotomy on a 40-year-old woman, multiple gray-white nodules are incidentally discovered within the pelvic peritoneum. The histologic appearance of these nodules is shown in Figure 1. Which of the following is the most likely diagnosis?

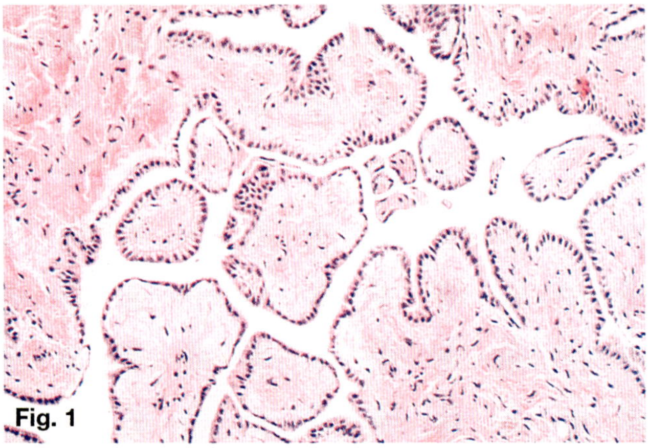
Fig. 1

A. Adenomatoid tumor
B. Gliomatosis peritonei
C. Müllerian metaplasia
D. Solitary fibrous tumor
E. Well-differentiated papillary mesothelial tumor

7. Which of the following is true about peritoneal malignant mesothelioma?

A. Accounts for 50% of all malignant mesotheliomas
B. 1:1 male-to-female ratio
C. Nonepithelioid being the most frequent histologic type
D. Results from malignant transformation of mesothelial hyperplasia
E. Unrelated to asbestos exposure in males

8. Which of the following is not considered a favorable prognostic factor for peritoneal malignant mesothelioma?

A. Age greater than 60 years
B. Lack of deep tissue invasion
C. Low mitotic count
D. Low nuclear grade
E. Minimal residual disease after cytoreduction

9. Figure 1 demonstrates that the histologic features of a localized lesion in the peritoneal cavity have been slowly growing per serial imaging studies. There is no appreciable marked cytologic pleomorphism or increased mitotic rate. Immunohistochemical workup reveals expression of CD34, vimentin, and STAT6 in the tumor cells, with no expression of cytokeratin, CD117, or desmin. What is the most likely diagnosis?

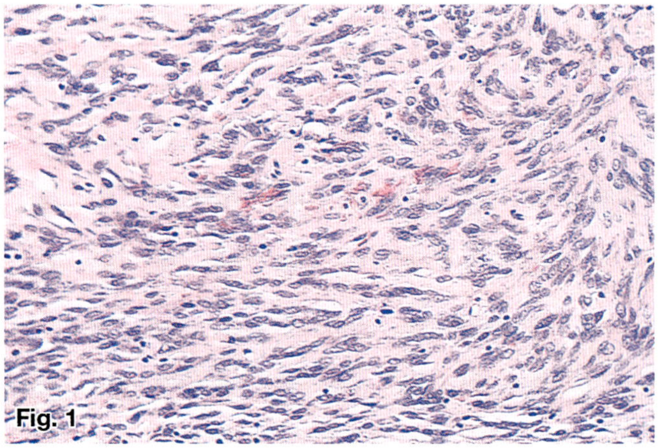
Fig. 1

A. Desmoplastic mesothelioma
B. Gastrointestinal stromal tumor
C. Leiomyosarcoma
D. Mesenteric desmoid fibromatosis
E. Solitary fibrous tumor

10. A 24-year-old man presents with ascites. Imaging studies reveal a multinodular tumor in the pelvic cavity, which is resected. Histologic examination reveals the neoplasm shown in Figure 1. Neoplastic cells show cytoplasmic immunoreactivity for low-molecular-weight keratin, synaptophysin, vimentin, and desmin and nuclear expression of WT1 protein. Reverse polymerase chain reaction (rPCR) on paraffin-embedded tissue shows the presence of t(11;22) involving the Ewing sarcoma (*EWS*) and Wilms tumor (*WT1*) genes. Which of the following is the most likely diagnosis?

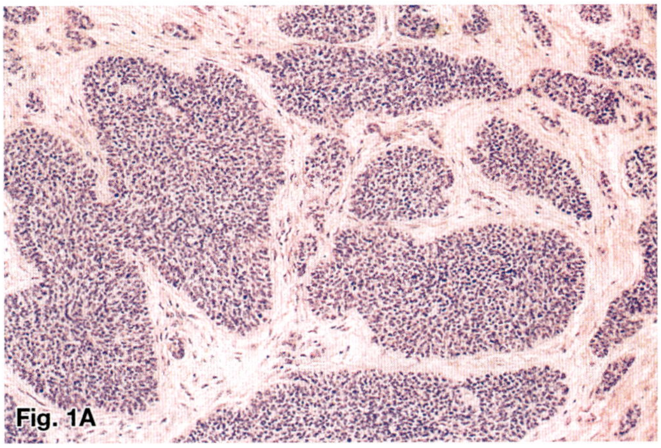
Fig. 1A

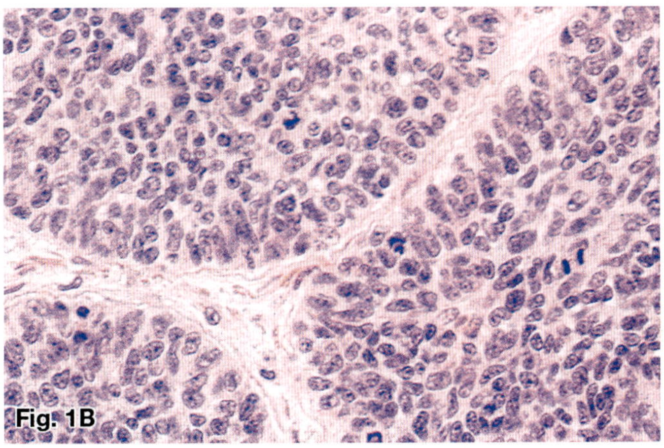
Fig. 1B

A. Ewing sarcoma
B. Intra-abdominal desmoplastic small round cell tumor
C. Lymphoma
D. Neuroblastoma
E. Wilms tumor

11. Figure 1 demonstrates the histologic features of an abdominal lesion in a 19-year-old male who presented with fever and weight loss. The spindle cells show cytoplasmic immunopositivity for anaplastic lymphoma kinase-1 (ALK-1). Which of the following is true regarding this tumor?

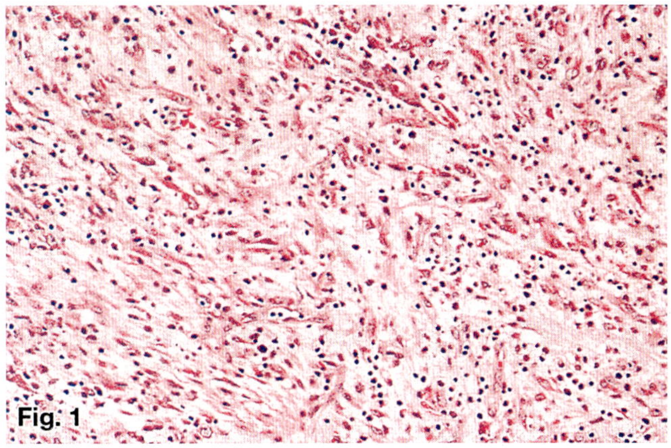
Fig. 1

A. Abdominopelvic tumors have a higher recurrence rate than those in other anatomic sites.
B. *ALK*-negative tumors are more likely to be associated with metastases.
C. Chromosomal translocations involving the *ALK* gene are seen in 50% of the cases.
D. It is regarded as tumor of intermediate biologic behavior, given the tendency for local recurrence.
E. All of the above are correct.

12. A patient with ascites undergoes paracentesis, which yields mucinous fluid with fragments of neoplastic glandular epithelium. Which of the following is the most common source of this condition?

A. Adenocarcinoma of the colon
B. Goblet cell carcinoma of the appendix
C. Mucinous carcinoma of the ovary
D. Mucinous tumor of the appendix
E. Signet-ring cell carcinoma of the gastrointestinal tract

13. Figure 1 demonstrates the histologic appearance of a red-brown peritoneal lesion, described as "powder burn" in the surgeon's operative report, that was removed from a woman with cyclic abdominal pains. At the time of surgery, which hormonal status is the patient most likely to be in?

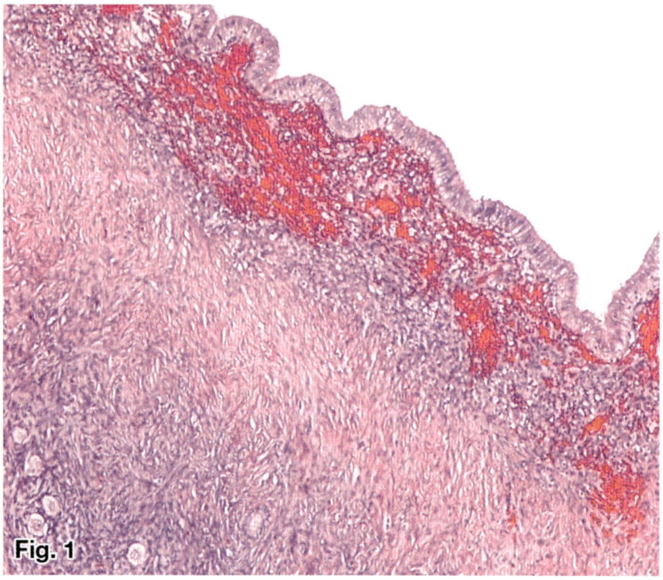

Fig. 1

A. Estrogen replacement therapy
B. Postmenopause
C. Pregnancy
D. Proliferative phase of menstrual cycle
E. Secretory phase of menstrual cycle

14. A 48-year-old female with a history of ovarian endometrioid carcinoma is found to have a colonic stricture. Resection of her bowel identified the following histologic finding shown in Figure 1. What is the most likely diagnosis?

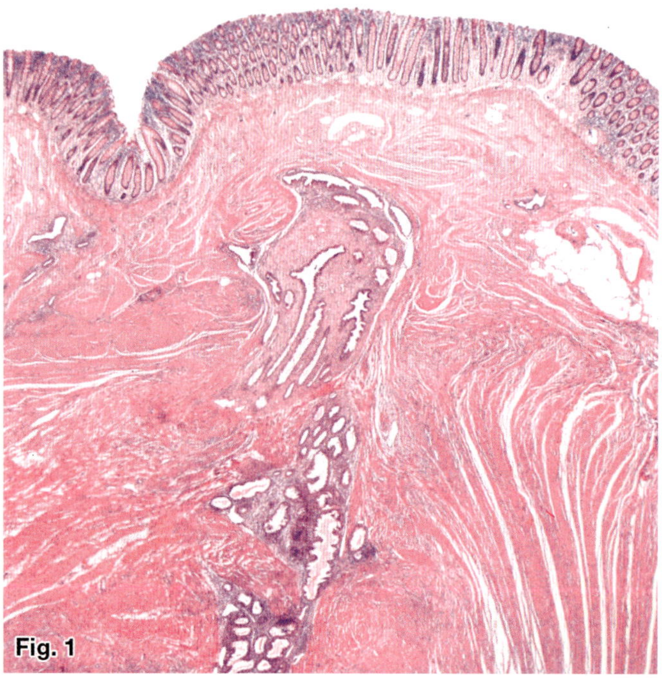

Fig. 1

A. Colonic adenocarcinoma
B. Endometriosis
C. Metastatic adenosarcoma
D. Metastatic endometrioid carcinoma
E. Metastatic low-grade endometrial stromal sarcoma

15. Which of the following is the most frequent primary peritoneal carcinoma?

A. Endometrioid carcinoma
B. High-grade serous carcinoma
C. Mucinous carcinoma
D. Squamous cell carcinoma
E. Transitional cell carcinoma

16. Figure 1 shows an incidental finding in the para-aortic lymph node in a female patient undergoing a staging surgery for ovarian high-grade serous carcinoma. Which of the following histologic features favor a benign diagnosis?

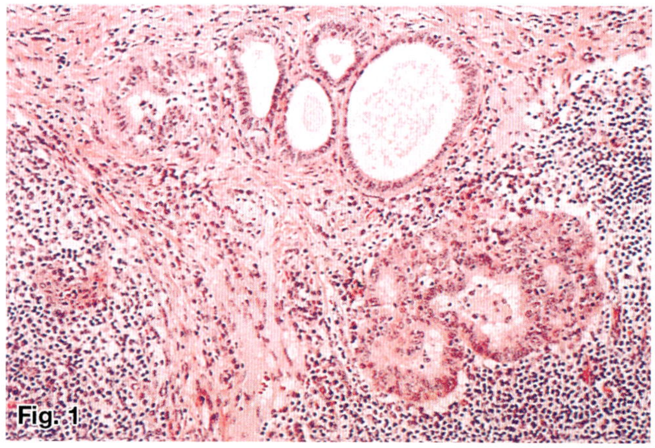

Fig. 1

A. Absence of a desmoplastic stromal reaction
B. Capsular or interfollicular location of the glands
C. Lack of significant cellular atypia and mitotic activity
D. Lining cells of multiple types, including ciliated forms
E. All of the above

17. Figure 1 shows an incidental finding in the pelvic lymph node in a recently pregnant female patient undergoing a staging surgery for cervical squamous cell carcinoma. Which of the following histologic features favor a benign entity?

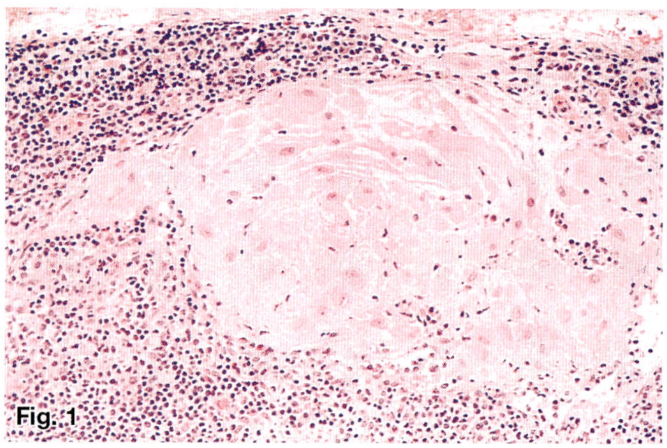

Fig. 1

A. Absence of cytokeratin immunoreactivity
B. Increased mitotic activity
C. Presence of diffuse cytologic atypia
D. Presence of keratinization
E. Presence of stromal desmoplasia

# ANSWERS AND EXPLANATIONS

**1. Correct choice: D.**

A Maltese cross pattern is characteristic of starch (specifically cornstarch), which is used for surgical gloves and has replaced talc. Cellulose from disposable gowns is another potential peritoneal contaminant. All of the named materials may induce a granulomatous reaction, mimicking infection or Crohn disease.

**2. Correct choice: E.**

Escaped bowel contents, including vegetable matter, food-derived starch, can produce a peritoneal foreign body reaction. Sebaceous material and keratin from ruptured dermoid cysts typically evoke an intense granulomatous, lipogranulomatous, and fibrosing peritoneal inflammatory reaction that may mimic a neoplasm at operation. The use of an endoscopic retrieval bag in the laparoscopic removal of dermoid cysts can reduce the risk of intraoperative spillage and subsequent granulomatous peritonitis. Granulomatous inflammation can occur to keratin exfoliated from uterine and ovarian endometrioid carcinomas with squamous differentiation. Leakage of amniotic fluid antenatally or its spillage at cesarean section can result in contamination of the peritoneal cavity by vernix caseosa (lanugo hair, squamous cells, keratin) and meconium (bile and pancreatic and intestinal secretions), resulting in a granulomatous peritonitis. Chronic bile peritonitis may be associated with granulomatous inflammation and fibrosis; cholesterol crystals and bile pigment may be identifiable within giant cells. Granulomatous peritonitis has also been described secondary to Crohn disease, sarcoidosis, and Whipple disease. Spillage of bile or gallstones during laparoscopic cholecystectomy may also be a source of peritoneal granulomatous inflammation.

**3. Correct choice: E.**

Sclerosing peritonitis is a rare, potentially fatal disorder characterized by a fibrous peritoneal thickening. Pearly white thickening of the peritoneum is seen, as either discrete plaques or continuous sheets involving the hepatic, splenic, and diaphragmatic peritoneum. More recent reports have described a similar lesion that encases the small bowel ("abdominal cocoon"), causing bowel obstruction. It occurs in an idiopathic form, typically affecting adolescent girls, or it may be secondary to practolol therapy, chronic ambulatory peritoneal dialysis, sarcoidosis, the use of a peritoneovenous or ventriculoperitoneal shunts, lupus erythematosus, or ovarian fibrothecomatous tumors or tumor-like lesions. In the last situation, the peritoneal lesions may be misinterpreted intraoperatively or even on microscopic examination as metastatic tumor.

**4. Correct choice: E.**

The major differential diagnosis of mesothelial hyperplasia is that of peritoneal malignant mesothelioma. The presence of grossly visible nodules, necrosis, conspicuous large cytoplasmic vacuoles, severe nuclear pleomorphism, and invasion favors malignant mesothelioma over mesothelial hyperplasia. Some of these features, however, such as severe nuclear atypia, are often not present, or they may only be present focally within malignant mesothelioma. Loss of BAP1 immunoreactivity, particularly in combination with homozygous deletion of 9p21 and p16 by fluorescent in situ hybridization, is highly characteristic of malignant mesothelioma, whereas these alterations have not been observed in reactive mesothelial proliferations.

**5. Correct choice: C.**

Peritoneal inclusion cysts develop almost exclusively in women of reproductive age. Single cysts are usually incidental findings at laparotomy. Multilocular peritoneal cysts may reach considerable size (up to 20 cm) and present with abdominopelvic pain or palpable mass. This condition is called *multilocular peritoneal inclusion cysts* (MPICs). MPICs are usually attached to pelvic organs and clinically may mimic cystic ovarian tumors. The lining consists of flattened mesothelial cells, which may form papillary protrusions. The great majority of patients with MPICs have a history of prior abdominal surgery, pelvic inflammatory disease (PID), and endometriosis, which is consistent with the hypothesis that MPICs result from chronic inflammation of the peritoneum. Asbestos does not cause MPICs. On the other hand, hormonal changes may play a pathogenetic role. The main differential diagnosis is with lymphangiomas, which occur in children and are usually not located in the pelvis. Their contents may be chylous, and histologic examination often reveals mural lymphoid aggregates and smooth muscle, which are rare findings in MPICs.

**6. Correct choice: E.**

Well-differentiated papillary mesothelial tumor (formerly known as well-differentiated papillary mesothelioma) is an uncommon BENIGN lesion of the peritoneal mesothelium that usually represents an incidental finding at surgery or autopsy and occurs most commonly in women of reproductive age. It may be solitary or multiple, measuring less than 2 cm. It appears as a vascularized nodule composed of fibrous papillary structures lined by a single layer of cuboidal cells resembling choroid plexus. Adenomatoid tumor is much more common in the genital tract. Gliomatosis peritonei is due to peritoneal dissemination of glial tissue from an ovarian teratoma. Solitary fibrous tumor has been reported in the peritoneum. Müllerian metaplasia occurs in women and leads to foci of endometrium, tubal epithelium, or reactive decidua in the pelvic peritoneum.

**7. Correct choice: B.**

Peritoneal malignant mesothelioma (PMM) represents 10% to 20% of all malignant mesotheliomas, of which pleural-based origin is the most common. It has equal prevalence in males and females (M:F is 1:1). A definite relationship with asbestos exposure is proven in males with PMM, but not in females. Mesothelial hyperplasia is usually an incidental finding, which may generate some difficulties in the differential diagnosis with PMM, but it is not a premalignant precursor. PMM presents in middle-aged or older patients with abdominal discomfort, ascites, digestive problems, and weight loss. Cytologic diagnosis can be made in the ascitic fluid, but exploratory laparotomy with biopsy is usually necessary. Grossly, the tumor appears as diffuse plaque-like multinodular thickening of the peritoneal lining, only rarely being localized. Most tumors are epithelioid type.

**8. Correct choice: A.**

Favorable prognostic factors for peritoneal mesothelioma include an age less than 60 years, low nuclear grade, low mitotic count, minimal residual disease after cytoreduction, and lack of deep invasion. Rare tumors that are localized may also have a better prognosis. Decreased overall survival has been associated with tumors that exhibit solid architecture, sarcomatoid growth, and depth of invasion.

**9. Correct choice: E.**

Localized fibrous tumors of the type that involve the pleura are extremely rare in the peritoneal cavity. Their clinical and pathologic features, including a patternless proliferation of spindled to ovoid cells and variably collagenous stroma with staghorn vessels, strong immunoreactivity for STAT6, vimentin, and CD34 and negativity for cytokeratin, as well as their usually indolent behavior are similar to those encountered in the pleura and elsewhere and facilitate their distinction from desmoplastic mesotheliomas. Rare tumors with focal hypercellularity, marked nuclear pleomorphism, and a high mitotic rate have not been found to have an adverse outcome.

Mesenteric desmoid fibromatosis contains longer fascicles and more collagenous stroma and expresses nuclear β-catenin. Gastrointestinal stromal tumors show a hypercellular, syncytial appearance with limited intervening stroma, with CD117 and DOG-1 immunoreactivity.

**10. Correct choice: B.**

Intra-abdominal desmoplastic small round cell tumor (DSRCT) is a small cell tumor of young adults, with an M:F ratio of 4:1, that arises from serosal membranes, more frequently in the pelvic and abdominal peritoneum. The mean age at presentation is 22 years. DSRCT has a unique chromosomal translocation t(11;22) that results in the fusion of the Ewing sarcoma (*EWS*) gene with the Wilms tumor (*WT1*) gene. The EWS-WT1 gene fusion transcript is detectable by reverse polymerase chain reaction (rPCR) on paraffin-embedded tissue. Its immunohistochemical phenotype is highly characteristic: positivity for epithelial markers (low-molecular-weight cytokeratins, EMA [epithelial membrane antigen]), neuroendocrine markers (NSE [neuron-specific enolase], synaptophysin), and muscle markers (desmin), as well as vimentin. Nuclear immunoreactivity for the C-terminal region of WT1 is present in most cases, which distinguishes DSRCT from Ewing sarcoma and primitive neuroectodermal tumor. DSRCT is highly malignant and has a dismal prognosis.

**11. Correct choice: E.**

Inflammatory myofibroblastic tumor (IMT) was once referred to as plasma cell granuloma, owing to the presence of mature plasma cells and small lymphocytes percolating through the myofibroblastic spindle cells. The abdominal lesions are typically encountered in patients younger than 20 years of age who present with a mass, fever, growth failure or weight loss, hypochromic anemia, thrombocytosis, and polyclonal hypergammaglobulinemia. The spindle cells show cytoplasmic immunopositivity for anaplastic lymphoma kinase-1 (ALK-1), with associated chromosomal translocations, in approximately 50% of cases. IMTs may be associated with an uneventful postoperative course but are regarded as tumors of intermediate biologic behavior, given the tendency for local recurrence and very rare cases that have behaved in a malignant manner. It has also been reported that abdominopelvic tumors have a higher recurrence rate than those arising in other anatomic sites and that ALK-negative tumors are more likely to be associated with metastases.

**12. Correct choice: D.**

Pseudomyxoma peritonei consists of the accumulation of mucinous fluid and microscopic fragments of neoplastic glandular epithelium within the peritoneal cavity. Floating neoplastic fragments seed the peritoneal cavity, producing macroscopically identifiable nodules. The patient will develop intestinal obstruction, infective peritonitis, and other complications resulting from the invasion of pelvic organs. Mucinous appendiceal tumors, most commonly a mucinous cystadenoma, represent the most common cause, although ovarian cystadenoma and mucinous carcinoma may occasionally be the source. Coexisting appendiceal and ovarian mucinous tumors are seen in some of these cases, which raise the question as to which of the two neoplasms is the primary tumor.

**13. Correct choice: D.**

In addition to changes related to the duration of disease, the histology of endometriotic foci varies in response to endogenous or exogenous hormonal influences. The example shown here is characterized by endometrial glands with a proliferative appearance. During pregnancy, stromal cells are decidualized, whereas the glandular epithelium is flat. Menopause leads to glandular atrophy. Estrogen replacement therapy may cause a variety of hyperplastic changes similar to those in the uterus. Atypical hyperplasia in endometriosis has the same potential for malignant transformation. Most cases of endometriosis-related carcinomas are clear cell carcinoma and endometrioid carcinoma. The ovary is by far the most common site of endometriosis-related cancer, followed by the rectovaginal pouch.

**14. Correct choice: B.**

Endometriosis that involves the hollow viscera is typically associated with striking proliferation of the indigenous smooth muscle, creating a stricture. The muscularis propria is thickened by hyperplastic smooth muscle that surrounds the foci of endometriosis and can mimic invasion of a local tumor. The absence of glandular atypical hyperplasia precludes the diagnosis of endometrioid carcinoma in this case. Rare examples of recurrent or metastatic low-grade endometrial stromal sarcomas with benign-appearing or atypical endometrial glands may be confused with endometriosis. Differential features from endometriosis include foci of typical endometrial stromal sarcoma devoid of glands, at least mild atypia of the stromal cells, sex cord–like elements, and prominent vascular invasion. Polypoid endometriosis can sometimes be confused with adenosarcoma; in contrast to the latter, however, its stroma lacks atypia and typically does not form periglandular cuffs or intraglandular papillae.

**15. Correct choice: B.**

Most primary peritoneal serous neoplasms are high-grade serous carcinomas (HGSCs) that extensively involve the peritoneum. They are about one-tenth as common as their tubo-ovarian counterparts. Germline *BRCA* mutations occur in peritoneal HGSCs with the same frequency as they do in their tubo-ovarian counterparts. For *BRCA1* mutation carriers, the risk of developing HGSC is approximately 4% at 20 years post-prophylactic salpingo-oophorectomy. It has been suggested that some tumors interpreted as HGSC in patients with BRCA may actually represent spread of an unrecognized serous carcinoma of the tubal fimbria. It is also prudent that a diagnosis of peritoneal serous carcinoma be made only after the exclusion of an endometrial serous carcinoma, which can be microscopic. It has been recommended that HGSC with associated serous tubal intraepithelial carcinoma (STIC) be assigned as primary fallopian tube origin. As such, only rare cases are likely of true primary peritoneal origin, and this diagnosis requires confirmation of benign findings in completely embedded fallopian tubes, ovaries, and endometrium.

**16. Correct choice: E.**

The image captures both typical and atypical endosalpingiotic glands in the subcapsular region of a lymph node. Four glands (top) in the capsule of the node are lined by a single layer of benign, ciliated columnar cells. In several other glands, the lining cells are atypical, and they form cribriform arrangements. As Müllerian glandular inclusions are most common in the para-aortic nodes, which receive drainage from the ovaries, and because of their association with ovarian serous borderline tumors (SBTs), it has been suggested that in some cases, the "inclusions" are metastatic SBTs that have undergone maturation. In most cases, the distinction between glandular inclusions and metastatic adenocarcinoma is not difficult unless a primary ovarian serous tumor of low malignant potential is present, in which case the distinction may be difficult or impossible. Features favoring a benign diagnosis include a capsular or interfollicular location of the glands; lining cells of multiple types, including ciliated forms; a lack of significant cellular atypia and mitotic activity; periglandular basement membranes; and an absence of a desmoplastic stromal reaction.

**17. Correct choice: A.**

Ectopic decidua has been described as a rare, incidental microscopic finding in para-aortic and pelvic lymph nodes that have usually been removed as part of a radical hysterectomy for carcinoma of the cervix in pregnant patients. The decidual nests typically occupy the subcapsular sinus and superficial cortex, although more central parts of the lymph node may also be involved. The cells appear benign, but they may contain occasional bizarre, hyperchromatic nuclei, thus mimicking metastatic squamous cell carcinoma. The absence of mitotic activity, keratinization, stromal desmoplasia, and cytokeratin reactivity should facilitate the diagnosis. Metastatic squamous cell carcinoma may, however, be present in the same node.

# INDEX

Note: Locators followed by letter 't' refer to tables.

# FIGURE CREDITS

The figures in the following questions are new for *Mills & Sternberg's Diagnostic Surgical Pathology Review*, Third Edition, and appear in print for the first time:

Question 32.7

Question 32.10

Question 34.1

Question 35.5

Question 35.7

Question 36.14

Question 36.18